THE VETERINARY

ICU Book

Edited by

Wayne E. Wingfield, MS, DVM
Diplomate, American College of Veterinary Emergency and Critical Care
Diplomate, American College of Veterinary Surgeons
Professor and Chief, Emergency and Critical Care Medicine
Department of Clinical Sciences
College of Veterinary Medicine and Biomedical Sciences
Colorado State University
Ft. Collins, Colorado

Marc R. Raffe, DVM, MS
Diplomate, American College of Veterinary Emergency and Critical Care
Diplomate, American College of Veterinary Anesthesia
Professor and Head, Critical Care Unit
Department of Veterinary Clinical Medicine
College of Veterinary Medicine
University of Illinois
Urbana, Illinois

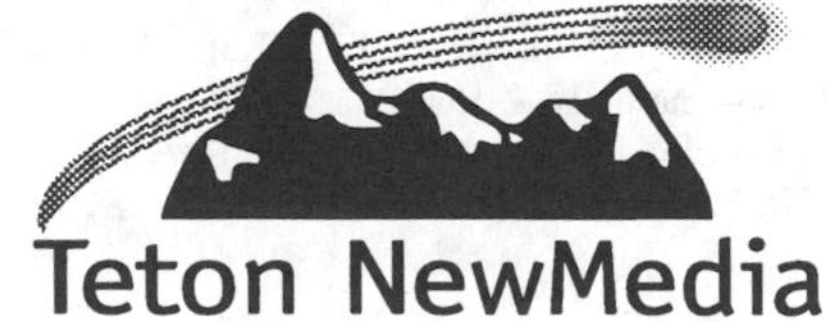
Teton NewMedia
Jackson Hole, Wyoming

Executive Editor: Carroll C. Cann
Developmental Editor: Susan L. Hunsberger
Editor: Cynthia J. Roantree
Design and Production: Anita B. Sykes
Composition: Achorn Graphics, Worcester, MA
Printer: Ink On Paper, Alpine, WY

Teton NewMedia
PO Box 4833
4125 South Highway 89
Suite 1
Jackson, WY 83001

1-888-770-3165
www.tetonnm.com
www.veterinarywire.com

PRINTED IN THE UNITED STATES OF AMERICA

ISBN 1-893441-13-X

Print number 5 4 3 2 1

Library of Congress Cataloging-in-Publication Data

The veterinary ICU book / edited by Wayne E. Wingfield, Marc R. Raffe.
p. ; cm.
Includes bibliographical references and index.
ISBN 1-893441-13-X (alk. paper)
1. Veterinary critical care. I. Wingfield, Wayne E. II. Raffe, Marc R.
[DNLM: 1. Intensive Care—methods. 2. Veterinary Medicine—methods. 3. Animal Diseases—therapy. 4. Critical Illness—therapy. 5. Hospitals, Animal. 6. Wounds and Injuries—veterinary. SF 778 V586 2001]
SF778.V58 2001
636.089′6028—dc21

2001027037

"When GOD has laid His hands upon the patient, take yours off!"
Ken Mattox, MD

Dedication

To our entrusting animal owners for their love of their animals and faith in our veterinary medicine practitioners.

To my parents, Opal and Bud, thank you for this lifetime of happiness in doing what I do best. To my kids, Shawna and Yvonne, you brighten my life daily. To my wife Suzanne, you make my heart beat with joy. To our dogs, Sage and Loretta, you initiate our smiles. To my CCU nurses, thank you for your caring. And to my colleagues, who make each of us better every day. Your eyes show me the way.

WEW

To my parents, Milly and Phil who pointed the way. To my wife, Mayda, who showed me the way. To my children, Jennifer and Daniel, who taught me the way. To all the talented technicians, students, interns, and residents who teach me every day.

MRR

Acknowledgment

We wish to thank Dr. John L. Mara of Hill's Pet Nutrition for his unwavering support of emergency and critical care medicine for veterinarians and veterinary technicians. Without Dr. Mara's support it is unlikely our specialty would have grown so rapidly and thus offered our patients such significant improvements in quality of care. Dr. Mara is our beacon of support. We are forever indebted to him as a leader, colleague, friend, and fearless parasailor! Thank you, Dr. Mara!

Preface

In 1985, a group of dedicated visionary veterinarians began the process of developing emergency and critical medicine into a recognized specialty discipline. Through their efforts, the American College of Veterinary Emergency and Critical Care was formed and selected its charter diplomates in 1990. This event was a milestone in the recognition of emergency and critical care medicine as a formal discipline. The unique information and skills needed to practice emergency and critical care medicine have rapidly expanded over the past decade. Originally, this discipline emphasized the care of severely injured animals and postoperative complications. It has now evolved into an integrated veterinary health care discipline that focuses on illnesses and injuries requiring specialized therapies. Practitioners of this discipline are generally personnel with advanced educational experiences. They apply their skills and knowledge to the most seriously injured and ill patients while struggling with ethical dilemmas associated with the limits of current medical knowledge. These unique qualities, in conjunction with an emphasis on technological innovation, often foster the mistaken impression that critical care medicine is somehow different in principle and practice from more traditional branches of veterinary medicine. In reality, the management of the critically ill veterinary patient requires the same basic skills common to all veterinary medicine: astute observation, careful differentiation diagnosis, and analytical therapeutic decision-making.

The Veterinary ICU Book is dedicated to these fundamental skills. Expert contributors representing core clinical disciplines have written a concise, clinically specific resource for the specialists, residents in training, veterinary practitioners and technicians, and students. The strength of this book is that it's interdisciplinary approach clearly defines the physiologic and clinical principles that are fundamental to the management of the critically ill veterinary patient.

The contributing authors and editors wish to acknowledge the help of our friends and colleagues in the completion of this book. Specifically, we would like to thank Paul L. Marino, MD. He grabbed our interest and ignited our enthusiasm for this specialty with his milestone text entitled *The ICU Book*. The tireless efforts of Carroll Cann, Susan Hunsberger, Cindy Roantree, and John Spahr of Teton NewMedia were indispensable and extraordinary. And most importantly, we acknowledge our patients. We develop an unwavering bond and trust with these animals and promise to them we will provide each with our best critical care skills.

Our clients expect more from veterinarians than ever before. Critical care medicine over the past 10 years has matured to meet this need. The coming decade will see even more advancement in the skills we are capable of mustering. We are a part of the most exciting specialty in veterinary medicine. Jump on board and enjoy the ride!

Wayne E. Wingfield, MS, DVM
Marc R. Raffe, DVM, MS

Contributor List

Rodney S. Bagley, DVM, DACVIM
Associate Professor
Department of Veterinary Clinical Sciences
College of Veterinary Medicine
Washington State University
Pullman, Washington

June A. Boon, MS
Cardiology Services Coordinator
Department of Clinical Sciences
College of Veterinary Medicine and Biomedical Sciences
Colorado State University
Ft. Collins, Colorado

Dawn Merton Boothe, DVM, Ph.D, DACVIM
Texas A&M University
College Station, Texas

R. A. Bowen, DVM, Ph.D
Associate Professor
Department of Physiology
Colorado State University
Ft. Collins, Colorado

Janice McIntosh Bright, BSN, MS, DVM
Associate Professor of Cardiology
College of Veterinary Medicine and Biomedical Sciences
Colorado State University
Ft. Collins, Colorado

David R. Brown, Ph.D
Professor
Department of Veterinary PathoBiology
College of Veterinary Medicine
University of Minnesota
St. Paul, Minnesota

Terry W. Campbell, MS, DVM, Ph.D
Associate Professor
Department of Clinical Sciences
College of Veterinary Medicine and Biomedical Sciences
Colorado State University
Ft. Collins, Colorado

Anthony P. Carr, Dr. med. Vet., DACVIM
Associate Professor
Small Animal Clinical Sciences
Western College of Veterinary Medicine
University of Saskatchewan
Saskatoon, Canada

Leslie Carter, RVT, VTS
Head Nurse
Intensive Care unit
Section of Critical Care
School of Veterinary Medicine
University of Pennsylvania
Philadelphia, Pennsylvania

Gregory Conger, M.Ed.
Veterinary Teaching Hospital
Colorado State University
Ft. Collins, Colorado

Harold Davis, BA, RVT, VTS
Supervisor, Emergency Nursing Service
Veterinary Medical Teaching Hospital
School of Veterinary Medicine
University of California
Davis, California

Curtis W. Dewey, DVM, MS, DACVIM
Long Island Veterinary Specialists
Plainview, New York

Nishi Dhupa, DVM
Department head
Specialty Medical Services
Angel Memorial Animal Hospital
Boston, Massachusetts

Kenneth J. Drobatz, DVM, DACVIM, DACVECC
Associate Professor
Section of Critical Care
Department of Clinical Studies
School of Veterinary Medicine
University of Pennsylvania
Philadelphia, Pennsylvania

Dana Durrance, MA
Veterinary Teaching Hospital
Colorado State University
Ft. Collins, Colorado

Leah S. Faudskar, DVM, DACVECC
Affiliated Emergency Veterinary Service
Golden Valley, Minnesota

Martin J. Fettman, DVM, MS, Ph.D
Martin L. Morris Chair in Clinical Nutrition
Department of Pathology
College of Veterinary Medicine and Biomedical Sciences
Colorado State University
Ft. Collins, Colorado

Patrick R. Gavin, DVM, Ph.D, DACVR
Professor
Department of Veterinary Clinical Sciences
College of Veterinary Medicine
Washington State University
Pullman, Washington

Juliet R. Gionfriddo, DVM, MS, DACVOphth
Veterinary Teaching Hospital
College of Veterinary Medicine and Biomedical Sciences
Colorado State University
Ft. Collins, Colorado

Deborah S. Greco, DVM, Ph.D, DACVIM
Professor
Small Animal Medicine
Department of Clinical Sciences
Colorado State University
Ft. Collins, Colorado

Maura T. Green, LAHT, Veterinary Specialist II
Manager, Blood Donor Program
Small Animal Medicine
Colorado State University
Ft. Collins, Colorado

Timothy Hackett, DVM, MS, DACVECC
Assistant Professor
Department of Clinical Sciences
Colorado State University
Ft. Collins, Colorado

Kevin A. Hahn, DVM, Ph.D, DACVIM
Gulf Coast Veterinary Diagnostic Imaging and Oncology
Houston, Texas

Joseph Harari, MS, DVM, DACVS
Visiting Associate Professor
Veterinary Clinical Medicine
College of Veterinary Medicine
University of Illinois
Urbana, Illinois

Ashley Harvey, MS
Veterinary Teaching Hospital
Colorado State University
Ft. Collins, Colorado

Peter W. Hellyer, DVM, MS, DACVA
Associate Professor of Anesthesiology
Department of Clinical Sciences
College of Veterinary Medicine and Biomedical Sciences
Colorado State University
Ft. Collins, Colorado

Michael S. Henson, DVM
Department of Small Animal Clinical Sciences
College of Veterinary Medicine
University of Minnesota
St. Paul, Minnesota

Dez Hughes, DVSc, MRCVS, ACVECC
Senior Lecturer
London Department of Small Animal Medicine
Royal Veterinary College
North Mymms
Hatfield
Herefordshire

Leslie G. King, MVB
Diplomate ACVECC, ACVIM
Associate Professor
Section of Critical Care
School of Veterinary Medicine
University of Pennsylvania
Philadelphia, Pennsylvania

Charlotte A. Lacroix, DVM, JD
Priority Veterinary Consultants
Yardley, Pennsylvania

Michael S. Laguchik, DVM, MS
Diplomate ACVECC
Lieutenant Colonel
United States Army Veterinary Corps
Ft. Leavenworth, Kansas

Lorna Lanman, DVM
President
American Academy on Veterinary Disaster Medicine
Sun City West, Arizona

Jody P. Lulich, DVM, PhD
Associate Professor
Department of Small Animal Clinical Sciences
College of Veterinary Medicine
University of Minnesota
St. Paul, Minnesota

Douglass K. Macintire, DVM, MS
Diplomate, ACVIM and ACVECC
Professor of Acute Medicine and Critical Care
Department of Veterinary Clinical Sciences
College of Veterinary Medicine
Auburn University
Auburn, Alabama

Catriona M. MacPhail, DVM
Surgical Fellow, Soft tissue and Oncology
Department of Clinical Sciences
School of Veterinary Medicine
Colorado State University
Ft. Collins, Colorado

Paul L. Marino, MD, PhD
Physician in Chief
St. Clare's Hospital and Health Center
New York, New York

Julie M. Martin, DVM
Resident in Cardiology
College of Veterinary Medicine and Biomedical Sciences
Colorado State University
Ft. Collins, Colorado

Michael E. Matz, DVM
Diplomate ACVIM
Staff Internist
Southwest Veterinary Specialty Center
Tucson, Arizona

Elisa M. Mazzaferro, DVM, MS
Resident
Emergency and Critical Care Medicine
Veterinary Teaching Hospital
Colorado State University
Ft. Collins, Colorado

Sheila McCullough, DVM, MS
Clinical Assistant Professor
Small Animal Medicine and Emergency/Critical Care
Department of Veterinary Clinical medicine
University of Illinois
Urbana, Illinois

Brendan C. McKiernan, DVM, Dip. ACVIM
Denver Veterinary Specialists
Wheat Ridge, Colorado

Carrie Miller, DVM
Denver Veterinary Specialists
Wheat Ridge, Colorado

Charles W. Miller, MS, PhD
Professor and Interim Department Head
Department of Biomedical Sciences
College of Veterinary Medicine
Colorado State University
Ft. Collins, Colorado

Eric Monnet, DVM, PhD
Dipl ACVS, ECVS
Department of Clinical Sciences
College of Veterinary Medicine and Biomedical Sciences
Colorado State University
Ft. Collins, Colorado

Deidre Noling
Research Assistant
Priority Veterinary Consultants
Yardley, Pennsylvania

Robert T. O'Brien, DVM, Dipl. ACVR
Clinical Associate Professor
Chief of Staff Small Animal Services
School of Veterinary Medicine
University of Wisconsin—Madison
Madison, Wisconsin

Gregory K. Olgilvie, DVM, Dipl. ACVIM
Professor
Animal Cancer Center
Department of Clinical Services
College of Veterinary Medicine and Biomedical Sciences
Colorado State University
Ft. Collins, Colorado

E. Christopher Orton, DVM, PhD, Dipl. ACVS
Professor
Department of Clinical Sciences
Colorado State University
Ft. Collins, Colorado

Carl A. Osborne, DVM, PhD
Professor
Department of Small Animal Clinical Sciences
College of Veterinary Medicine
University of Minnesota
St. Paul, Minnesota

Elizabeth O'Toole, DVM, DVSc
Fellow in Emergency Critical Care Medicine
College of Veterinary Medicine
University of Illinois
Urbana, Illinois

Cynthia M. Otto, DVM, PhD, Dipl ACVECC
Assistant Professor, Critical Care
Department of Clinical Studies
School of Veterinary Medicine
University of Pennsylvania
Philadelphia, Pennsylvania

Sheldon Padgett, DVM, MS, DACVS
Metropolitan Veterinary Hospital
Akron, Ohio

Joane Parent, DVM, MvetSc, ACVIM
Professor
Department of Veterinary Clinical Studies
Ontario Veterinary College
University of Guelph
Guelph, Ontario, Canada

Michael M. Pavletic, DVM, Dipl. ACVS
Head
Department of Surgery
Angel Memorial Animal Hospital
Boston, Massachusetts

Davis J. Polzin, DVM, PhD
Professor
Department of Small Animal Clinical Sciences
College of Veterinary Medicine
University of Minnesota
St. Paul, Minnesota

Roberto Poma, DVM, DVSc
Staff Veterinarian
Veterinary Teaching Hospital
Ontario Veterinary College
University of Guelph
Guelph, Ontario, Canada

Cynthia C. Powell, DVM, MS, Dipl ACVO
College of Veterinary Medicine and Biomedical Sciences
Veterinary Teaching Hospital
Colorado State University
Ft. Collins, Colorado

Jeffrey Proulx, DVM, Dipl. ACVECC
Director of Veterinary Services
Society for Prevention of Cruelty to Animals
San Francisco, California

Marc R. Raffe, DVM, MS
Dipl. ACVECC, ACVA
Professor
Emergency and Critical Care
College of Veterinary Medicine
University of Illinois
Urbana, Illinois

Kenneth M. Rassnick, DVM, DACVIM
Comparative Cancer Program
Department of Clinical Sciences
College of Veterinary Medicine
Cornell University
Ithaca, New York

Adam J. Reiss, DVM
Denver Veterinarian Specialists
Wheat Ridge, Colorado

Bernard E. Rollin, PhD
University Distinguished Professor
Department of Philosophy
Colorado State University
Ft. Collins, Colorado

Sheri J. Ross, DVM
Resident
Clinical Nutrition and Internal Medicine
Department of Small Animal Clinical Services
College of Veterinary Medicine
University of Minnesota
St. Paul, Minnesota

Rene Scalf, CVT, VTS (ECC)
Veterinary Teaching Hospital
College of Veterinary Medicine and Biomedical Sciences
Colorado State University
Ft. Collins, Colorado

Stephanie A. Smith, DVM
Dipl. ACVIM
Department of Small Animal Clinical Sciences
College of Veterinary Medicine
University of Minnesota
St. Paul, Minnesota

Andrew J. Staatz, DVM
Resident, Small Animal Surgery
Department of Clinical Sciences
College of Veterinary Medicine and Biomedical Sciences
Colorado State University
Ft. Collins, Colorado

Sara Sugarman
Veterinary Teaching Hospital
Colorado State University
Ft. Collins, Colorado

DeWayne Townsend IV, DVM
Department of Veterinary Pathobiology
College of Veterinary Medicine
University of Minnesota
St. Paul, Minnesota

Russell Tucker, DVM, DACVR
Associate Professor
Department of Clinical Sciences
College of Veterinary Medicine
Washington State University
Pullman, Washington

Julia K. Veir, DVM
Resident, Small Animal Medicine
Department of Clinical Sciences
Colorado State University
Ft. Collins, Colorado

Lori S. Waddell, DVM
Diplomate ACVEEC
Intensive Care Unit
Section of Critical Care
School of Veterinary Medicine
University of Pennsylvania
Philadelphia, Pennsylvania

J. Michael Walters, DVM
Staff Veterinarian
Park Cities Animal Hospital
Dallas, Texas

Ronald S. Walton, DVM, DACVIM, ACVECC
Chief of Experimental Surgery
US Army Institute of Surgical Research
Fort Sam Houston, Texas

Craig B. Webb, DVM, PhD
Resident, Small Animal Medicine
Department of Clinical Sciences
Colorado State University
Ft. Collins, Colorado

Donald S. Westfall, DVM
Department of Clinical Sciences
College of Veterinary Medicine and Biomedical Sciences
Colorado State University
Ft. Collins, Colorado

Suzanne G. Barker Wingfield, RVT, VTS
Veterinary Teaching Hospital
College of Veterinary Medicine and Biomedical Sciences
Colorado State University
Ft. Collins, Colorado

Wayne E. Wingfield, DVM
Diplomate ACVS, ACVECC
Emergency and Critical Medicine
Department of Clinical Sciences
College of Veterinary Medicine and Biomedical Sciences
Colorado State University
Ft. Collins, Colorado

Robert H. Wrigley, DVR, MRCVS
Dipl ACVR, ECVDI
Professor
Department of Radiological Health Sciences
Veterinary Teaching Hospital
Colorado State University
Ft. Collins, Colorado

Contents

Section I: Physiology Review

Section II: Standard Practices in Patient Care

Section III: Monitoring the Critically Ill Animal

Section IV: Cardiovascular Disorders

Section V: Respiratory Failure

Section VIII: Endocrine Disorders

Section IX: Neurologic Disorders

Section X: Trauma

Section XI: Toxicology and Environmental

SECTION I
Physiology Review

1
Applied Cardiovascular Physiology

C. W. Miller

"I began to think whether there might not be a motion, as it were, in a circle."
William Harvey

In 1628, William Harvey's observations of the characteristics of blood flow in arteries and veins led him to describe the flow of blood as a "circulatory" pattern, rather than a "tidal" pattern similar to the back and forth motion of air flow in and out of the airways. The "circulatory" pattern of flow permits the delivery of oxygen and other essential elements to virtually every cell in the body while removing carbon dioxide and other metabolic waste products from tissues. If circulation ceases or declines below critical levels, metabolic processes are disrupted and irreversible damage to tissues results.

One of the hallmarks of animals with serious illness is the direct link between the cardiac performance and patient performance. If the heart fails, the patient fails! Therefore, it is of paramount importance one understands the forces that influence cardiac output of the heart also influence patient outcome. This chapter reviews these important forces of cardiac function, blood flow, and their regulation.

DESIGN OF THE CARDIOVASCULAR SYSTEM

The cardiovascular system consists of a right pump that provides circulation to the pulmonary circuit and a left pump that supplies the systemic circuit. Both systems operate simultaneously in a series arrangement and as such their outputs, over more than a few heartbeats, is normally equal. The output per minute from either the right or left ventricles is called the cardiac output (CO). The stroke volume (SV), the volume of blood ejected per beat by either ventricle multiplied by the heart rate (HR) equals the CO.

$$CO = SV \times HR$$

The right ventricle, which is relatively thin walled, pumps blood into the lower pressure, lower resistance pulmonary circuit, while the thicker walled left ventricle ejects blood into the higher pressure, higher resistance, systemic circuit. CO is equal to the venous return (VR) or the volume of blood returning to the heart from the veins in the thoracic cavity.

$$CO = VR$$

Vascular beds, in contrast to the relationship between the systemic and pulmonary circuits, are generally arranged in parallel with each other, thus permitting diversion of blood from one vascular bed to another during periods of vasodilation and vasoconstriction. Normally, the arterial blood pressure is maintained relatively constant. The perfusion pressure or the difference in pressure between the inflow to, and the outflow from, an organ provides the driving force to move blood from the heart to the tissues. The arterial blood pressure is determined by the product of the CO and the resistance (R) to flow.

$$BP = CO \times R$$

PERFORMANCE OF THE HEART

Preload, Contractility, and Afterload

The ability of the myocardium to generate an appropriate SV to meet the demands of the tissues is critical to normal tissues function. The SV, an indicator of adequacy of cardiac function, can be routinely estimated in most animals noninvasively using echocardiographic techniques.[1] The principal physical factors affecting the SV or performance of the heart are preload, afterload, and contractility. Changes in preload and contractility directly affect SV, whereas afterload inversely affects SV. The pressure-volume curve for the left ventricle shown in Figure 1-1 is a convenient graphic method to illustrate the effect of changes in preload, afterload, and contractility on cardiac function.

The pressure-volume curve in Figure 1-1 depicts the filling phase from A-B, the isovolumic contraction phase from B-C, the ejection phase of systole from C-D, and the isovolumic relaxation phase from D-A. The letters indicate points at which valves open or close. The volume of blood in the ventricle at "B" is referred to as the end-diastolic volume (EDV), whereas the volume of blood in the ventricle at the end of the ejection period is called the end-systolic volume (ESV).

$$SV = EDV\text{-}ESV$$

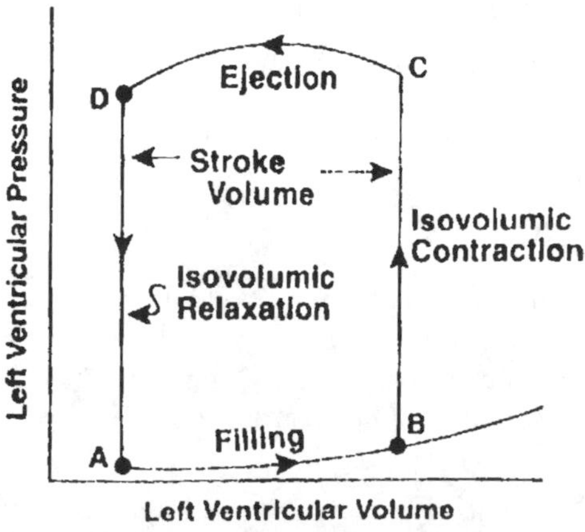

Figure 1-1
Pressure-volume curve for a ventricle. The letters A, B, C, and D refer respectively to the opening of the atrioventricular valve, closure of atrioventricular valve, opening of semilunar valve, and closure of semilunar valve.

Preload

The "all-or-none" law of the heart[2] implies that cardiac muscle either contracts maximally for those conditions or it does not contract at all. These inherent conditions of the heart are now termed "contractility" or relative degree of activation. The cardiac muscle also possesses inherent characteristics that allow its output to be adjusted to venous return. In 1884, William Howell and later in 1895, Otto Frank, showed that within limits, increases in diastolic volume and pressure affected the magnitude of the "all-or-none response." In 1918, Ernest Starling, using earlier data from Frank and others,[3] formally stated the fact that "within limits, the greater the stretch on the myocardial muscles prior to contraction, the greater is the force of contraction." This phenomenon is known as the Frank-Starling law of the heart. Figure 1-2 shows the relationship between end-diastolic pressure and SV depicting the Frank-Starling law. This fundamental principle of cardiac physiology explains the beat-to-beat adjustments that occur in balancing the output of the right and left ventricles as occurs during normal respiration. Changes in muscle fiber length appear to affect the number of active force-generating sites on the myocardial cell as well as the sensitivity to Ca^{++}.[4] The preload-dependent regulation of cardiac performance is referred to as heterometric autoregulation.

Figure 1-3 shows the impact of changes in preload on cardiac performance using the pressure-volume curves. Preload may change, for example, as a result of blood loss or gain, alterations in venous tone, peripheral resistance and body position, fluid changes due to kidney dysfunction, atrial contraction, skeletal muscle contraction, and changes in intrapleural and pericardial pressures. Certain cardiac arrhythmias may also affect preload when filling time is substantially increased or decreased. Preload can be determined by recording the volume of the ventricle at end-diastole using echocardiographic or radiographic methods. The ventricular end-diastolic pressure, although useful if the com-

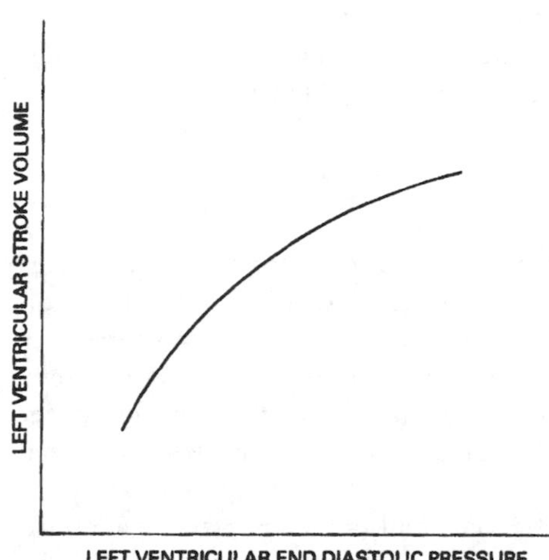

Figure 1-2
Illustration of the Frank-Starling law of the heart depicting the direct relationship between end-diastolic pressure (preload) and stroke volume.

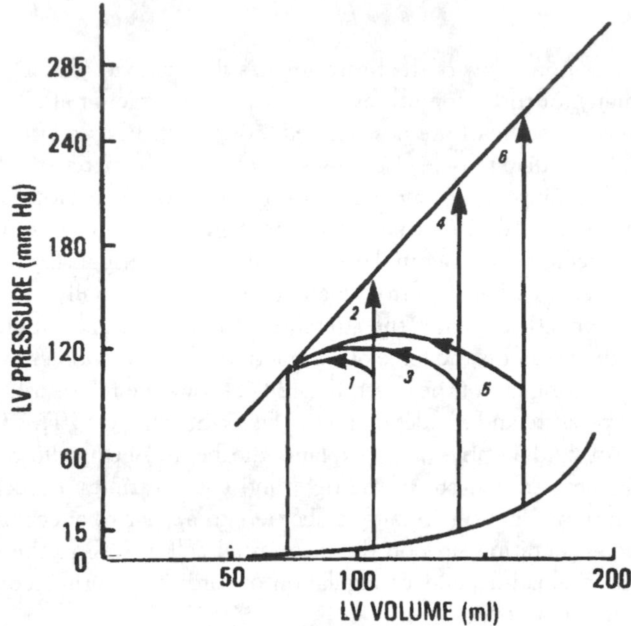

Figure 1-3
Pressure-volume curves showing the impact of progressively increasing end-diastolic volume on left ventricular pressure. Heartbeat numbers 1, 2, and 3 indicate the role increasing end-diastolic volume has on increasing stroke volume. Isometric contractions, 2, 4, and 6 show the impact increasing fiber length has on peak isometric pressure development.

pliance of the heart is known, provides a poor indicator of preload if compliance of the heart is unknown because the end-diastolic pressure would be elevated for a given filling volume if the heart is less compliant. The pulmonary capillary wedge pressure or the pressure recorded by "wedging" a catheter into the pulmonary arterioles provides an approximate estimate of the left atrial blood pressure and as such provides an estimate of the preload for the left ventricle.

Afterload

Afterload has a negative impact on SV of the heart. Afterload is the pressure in either the aorta or pulmonary artery that must be overcome during systole before the blood can be ejected into the vessel from the respective ventricle. If a weight representing the afterload is attached to a muscle as it begins to shorten, the force developed by the contracting muscle must be greater than that of the weight before shortening will occur. The degree of shortening in the intact heart is defined by the end-systolic pressure volume relationship represented by the sloped line in Figure 1-4. Afterload is the sum of all the loads against which the myocardium must develop tension during systole to shorten. The Laplace law incorporates factors that contribute to the afterload and is as follows:

$$\text{Wall stress } (\sigma) = (P \times r)/h$$

where ventricular pressure = P, chamber radius = r, and wall thickness = h. The relationship shows that as the ventricular pressure or chamber size increases, the wall stress or afterload increases. A thinner ventricular wall will also increase the wall stress. The greater the afterload, less shortening of the muscle produces lower stroke volume. The amount of blood in the ventricle at the end of diastole (preload) also affects the wall tension and afterload. The extent of shortening also will affect the diastolic characteristics of the heart and thus the preload. Figure 1-4 shows that as the afterload increases, the ESV is elevated contributing to a smaller SV. The systolic blood pressure of the ventricle provides a reasonable indicator for the afterload. Heartbeat numbers 1, 2, and 3 represent progressively increasing afterloads. The isometric contraction depicted by the vertical arrow shows that the afterload is elevated sufficiently so that no shortening occurs and thus no ejection of blood can occur.

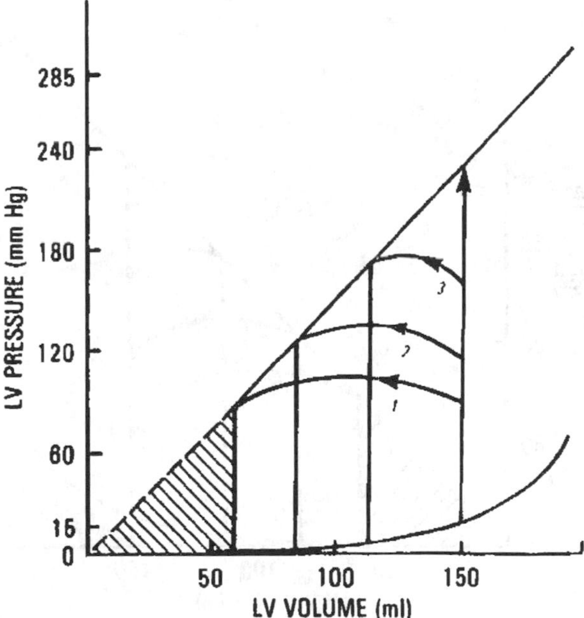

Figure 1-4
Pressure-volume curves for the left ventricle showing the effect of progressively increasing afterload (1 → 2 → 3) on the stroke volume. The end-systolic volume progressively increases as the afterload increases. Likewise, if the afterload diminishes as the arterial blood pressure or the heart size decreases, the stroke volume would increase as the end-systolic volume declines.

Contractility

The ability of the heart to develop tension independently of changes in preload or afterload is referred to as the "contractility" or inotropic state of the heart. Contractility is reflected in the speed and degree of shortening of the myocardium at a given load (preload/afterload). Activation of the sympathetic nervous system and the resultant increase in release of norepinephrine augments the contractility of the myocardium as more calcium is available for binding with contractile components of the muscle. Changes in contractility reflect a qualitative change in the force generated by the activated sites irrespective of a change in number of active sites. The biochemical events associated with changes in contractility remain the subject of active investigation. Decreases in sympathetic nervous system activation diminishes contractility.[5,6] A change in cardiac performance as a result of altered contractility is known as "homeometric autoregulation." Contractility in the intact heart can be estimated from the ejection fraction (EF = SV/EDV) and the change in ventricular pressure/time during the isovolumetric contraction time (dP/dt). Figure 1-5 shows the effect of alterations in contractility on performance of the heart.

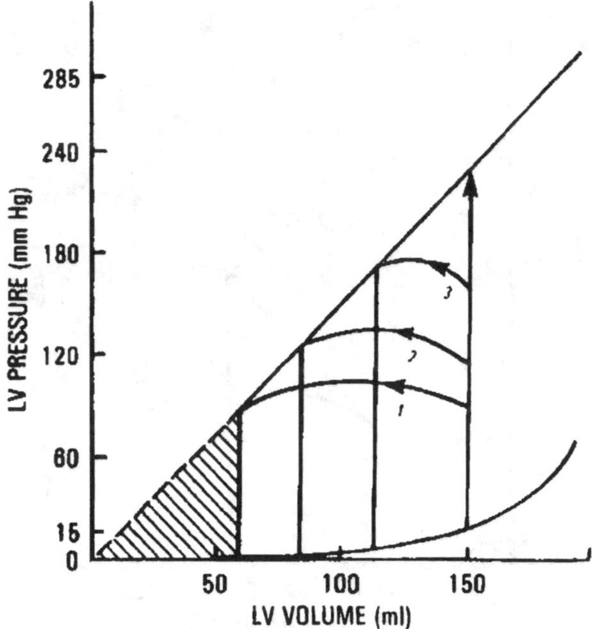

Figure 1-5
Pressure-volume curve for the left ventricle depicting the effect of changes in contractility on the extent of shortening of the myocardium (heartbeat numbers 1, 3, and 5) as well as on the peak pressure generated by the left ventricle during isometric contractions (heartbeat numbers 2, 4, and 6). Heartbeat numbers 1 and 2 depict normal contractility.

The greater the contractility, the lower the ESV and the greater the SV. The lower the contractility, the higher the ESV and the lower the SV. In many circumstances preload, afterload, and contractility may be changing simultaneously, producing an outcome that is a combination of the interactions. For example, an increase in preload (due to cardiac rhythm changes that allow longer filling times) in combination with diminished sympathetic nervous system activation might produce an unaltered SV.

MECHANICS OF BLOOD FLOW

The cardiovascular system is comprised of a network of conduits designed to transport blood to the trillions of cells in the body. A summary of important characteristics of the major vessel types of the circulation is shown in Table 1-1.

The changes in average blood velocity, blood pressure, total cross-sectional area, and percentage blood volume are shown in Figure 1-6. Summary highlights include the following: The blood pressure declines from the large artery (aorta or pulmonary artery) to the veins returning blood to the heart; blood velocity declines to a minimum in the exchange vessels (capillaries) where diffusion and bulk flow occur across the thin capillary wall and then returns to moderate levels in the veins; the total cross-sectional area of the vessel types is large (in the order of many square meters for larger animals) in the capillary region; blood volume is highest in venules and veins (60%–70% of the total blood volume); the resistance (R) (not shown in Fig. 1-6) to blood flow (Q) is greatest at the level of the arterioles where vascular tone is highest.

The design of the cardiovascular system allows a limited amount of circulating blood volume to control the chemical make-up of the internal environment. The rate of flow of these substances in blood is determined by certain physical factors that have been carefully characterized using simple model systems.[7] Although the assumptions governing flow of water in rigid tubes pumped by simple (steady flow) pumps do not strictly apply to the complexities of flow in the cardiovascular system, the analogy is extremely useful. Figure 1-7 depicts the physical factors affecting flow in vessels.

Table 1-1. Summary Characteristics of the Major Vessel Types

Vessel Type	Vessel Characteristics
Aorta	High pressure, high velocity, distensible walls, low resistance, pulsatile flow
Smaller arteries	Distributing vessels
Arterioles	Site of majority of resistance to flow; vasodilation or vasoconstriction affects local flow.
Capillaries	Thin walled exchange vessels, large total cross-sectional area, extremely low blood velocity, site of diffusion
Venules and veins	Low pressure, intermittent blood flow, low blood velocity, 60%–70% of blood volume stored in veins, venous valves.

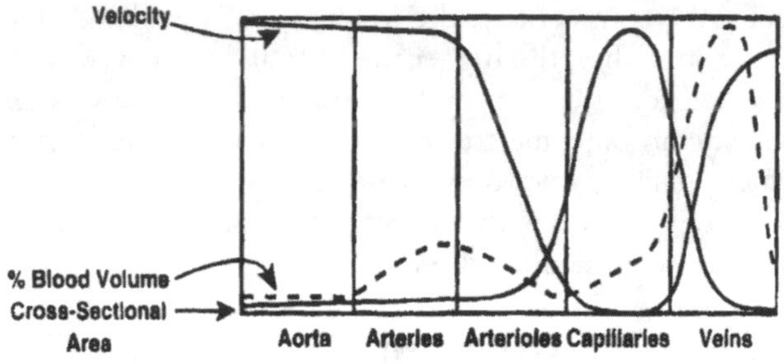

Figure 1-6
The changes in average blood velocity, blood pressure, total cross-sectional area, and percentage blood volume.

The Poiseuille equation or "law" was established in a flow model by the French physician J. Poiseuille. The equation states the relationship between Q = blood flow, ΔP as perfusion pressure, r is the radius of the tube, L the length of the tube, and η is blood viscosity. A simplified version of the equation is $Q = \Delta P/R$, where R = resistance to blood flow ($R = 8\,\eta L/\pi r^4$). Because the viscosity changes are fairly minimal in most situations, it should be apparent that the major factors that affect blood flow to an organ are changing pressure gradient across the vascular bed or changing vascular resistance. The latter variable plays the predominate role in altering blood flow primarily due to the huge impact of radius (r^4) on blood flow and the fact that the arterial blood pressure normally is fairly constant.

Continuity Equation

One of the confusing issues related to blood flow is the apparent contradiction between the Poiseuille law and the continuity equation ($Q = V \times A$). As flow occurs along the cardiovascular system and encounters the small high resistant arterioles, one would predict that the flow rate would decrease in that area.

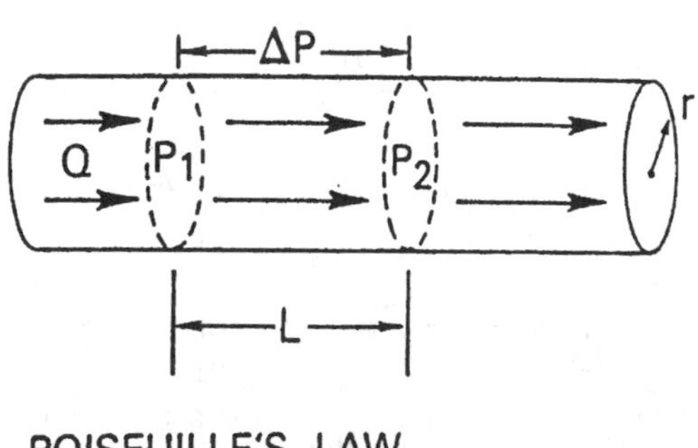

Figure 1-7
Model of vessel showing the factors that affect blood flow (Q). In this figure, ΔP is the perfusion pressure, r is the radius of the tube, L the length of the tube, and η is blood viscosity.

Because $Q = V \times A$, where V = blood velocity and A = total cross-sectional area, one can predict that since the flow rate must be the same in each composite vessel segment, the velocity will decrease as the total cross-sectional area increases. This basic equation also explains why the blood velocity decreases with the huge total cross-sectional area comprising the capillaries. It also provides the basic rationale for the blood velocity increasing in the venous segments as the total cross-sectional area declines compared to the capillaries.

Bernoulli Equation

The energy required to transport blood at a given velocity and the blood pressure exerted on the vessel wall are connected by the Bernoulli principle. The total energy associated with blood flow in a vessel is the sum of the potential energy (pressure exerted on the vessel wall) and the kinetic energy due to the velocity of blood (kinetic energy = $\frac{1}{2}\rho V^2$ where ρ = density and V = velocity). The total energy (E) at a given point in the vessel is a constant and is provided by the following equation:

$$E = P + \rho gh + \frac{1}{2}\rho V^2$$

In this equation, ρgh represents the pressure resulting from the hydrostatic pressure of a column of blood. As the blood velocity increases, the distending pressure exerted on the vessel wall declines. This principle is applied in clinical situations such as a valvular narrowing where the lateral or distending pressure is diminished proportionally to the severity of the narrowing and as the kinetic energy increases. The Bernoulli equation can be simplified to the following:

$$\Delta P = 4(V_1 - V_2)$$

where ΔP = the pressure gradient, V_1 = the blood velocity proximal to the obstruction, and V_2 = blood velocity distal to the obstruction. This equation is used to predict the pressure gradient across a narrowed vessel or heart valve. Narrowing in arteries may cause such elevated velocities that the lateral pressure is diminished producing a vessel that will collapse in the presence of enhanced vascular tone.

Laminar and Turbulent Flow

For the most part, flow in arteries and veins is streamlined or laminar indicating that cellular elements do not move among the other laminae. Figure 1-8 depicts the nature of flow in streamlined (laminar) flow. A stream of dye injected into a vessel containing laminar flow will be located precisely in that lamina at locations below the injection site if the flow remains laminar. Fluid flow that behaves in a nonlaminar way exhibits movement of fluid elements among laminae. Turbulent flow produces a type of flow in which the velocity of elements are chaotic with variable degrees of interchange among laminae. At one point a red blood cell might be in one lamina and the next instant it is in another. The presence of turbulence can be estimated using Reynold's number (Re #):

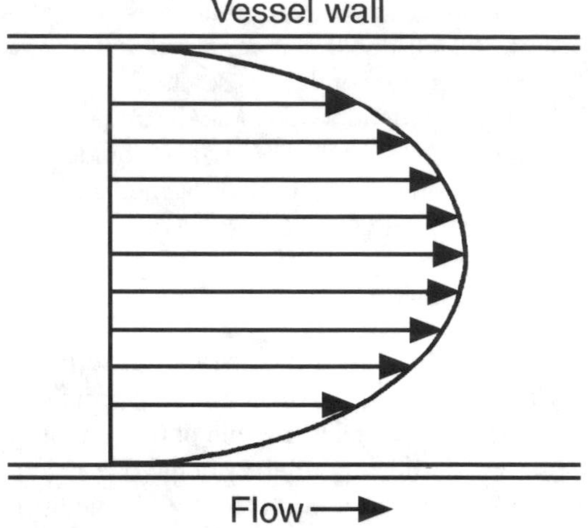

Figure 1-8
Schematic of "streamlines" in laminar flow. The blood velocity in streamline or laminar flow is highest in the vessel center and lowest at the vessel wall.

$$\text{Re \#} = (D \times V \times \rho)/\eta$$

The Re # is a nondimensional number that is the ratio between the kinetic energy and the viscous component. The higher the kinetic energy, the greater the possibility for turbulence and the lower the viscosity, the higher the potential for turbulence. Values greater than 2000 indicate the possibility for turbulence. The relationship between blood velocity and perfusion (pressure gradient) pressure are different for laminar and turbulent flow (Fig. 1-9). In laminar flow, flow is directly proportional to pressure, whereas in turbulent flow, flow is proportional to the square root of pressure. In other words, more pressure energy is required in turbulent flow to achieve a comparable flow to laminar flow.

INTERRELATIONSHIPS BETWEEN CARDIAC OUTPUT AND VENOUS RETURN

Because the heart is connected to a "circulatory system" comprised of an arterial system that is separated from a more compliant venous system by resistance ves-

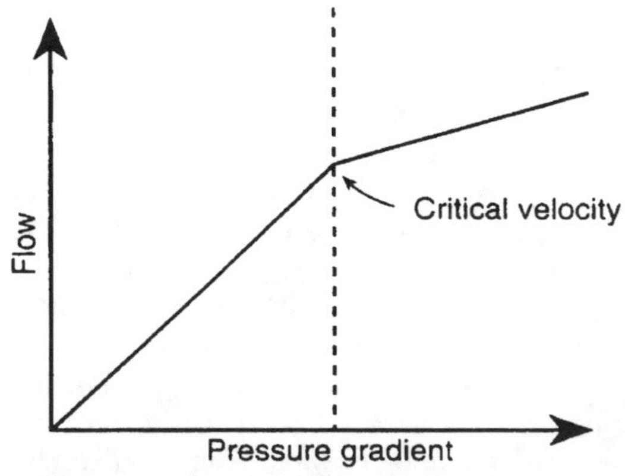

Figure 1-9
Relationship between pressure gradient and flow in a tube. At a critical velocity when flow becomes turbulent, the pressure gradient required to produce a comparable flow in laminar flow must increase.

sels, the CO and the venous return at equilibrium must be equal. CO is controlled by heart rate, myocardial contractility, preload, and afterload. The first two factors are cardiac factors, whereas the latter two are coupling factors because they constitute a functional coupling between the heart and the vasculature.[8,9] The preload and afterload are determined by cardiac factors and by characteristics unique to the vasculature. A simple model (Fig. 1-10) shows the effect of changing CO on the central venous pressure (CVP) and arterial blood pressure. When the pump is stopped and CO/VR are zero, the pressure in the entire circulatory system is approximately 7 mm Hg. The pressure in the vascular system when the CO is zero is termed the mean circulatory pressure (MCP) or simply the static pressure. This pressure is a function of the average compliance of the circulatory system as well as the blood volume. The mean circulatory pressure increases when blood volume increases and it decreases as the blood volume declines. It is from this value that the arterial blood pressure increases with CO and the venous pressure decreases. In the example, when the CO increases to 4 L/min, the CVP decreases to 3 mm Hg and the arterial pressure increases to 103 mm Hg.

The ratio of venous compliance to arterial compliance is approximately 24:1 meaning that for every 25 mm Hg pressure difference between the arterial and venous compartments, 24 mm Hg of pressure is added to the MCP of the arterial side and 1 mm Hg pressure is subtracted from the MCP for the venous side. In our example in Figure 1-10, assuming a peripheral resistance of 25 peripheral resistance units (PRU) and a CO of 4 L/min, the pressure gradient is 100 mm Hg and thus the pressure on the arterial side would be 96 mm Hg plus 7 mm Hg, or 103 mm Hg, and that for the venous would be 7 mm Hg minus 4 mm Hg or 3 mm Hg. In other words, once the "heart" begins to pump, blood will be transferred to the arterial system and will be removed from the venous system until the pressure in the arterial system rises and the venous pressure falls to a

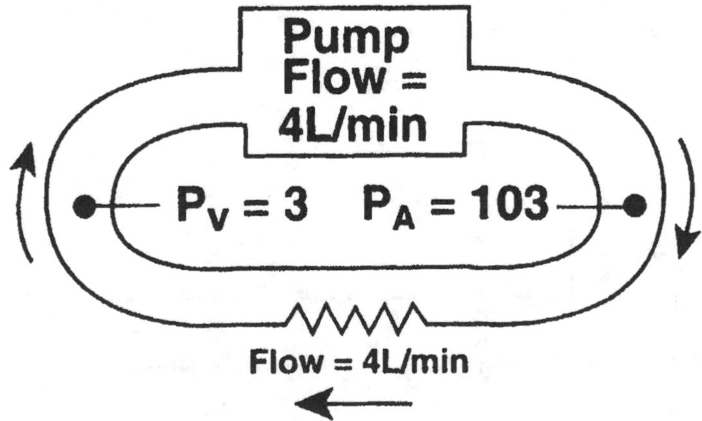

Figure 1-10
Schematic of a flow model demonstrating the effect of flow rate on venous blood pressure and arterial blood pressure.

new equilibrium at which the VR = CO. Similar analogies apply to a falling CO with the arterial pressure dropping and the venous pressure rising. These interactions can be analyzed using a combination of cardiac function curves that are an extension of the Frank-Starling law and vascular function curves that depict the inverse relationship between CO or VR and venous pressure (preload). Figure 1-11 shows cardiac function and vascular function curves plotted as a function of the venous pressure. The cardiac function curve shows that factors that augment the preload increase CO. A shift to the left indicates higher contractility and a shift in the curve to the right indicates lower contractility. The vascular function curve shows that the CO is inversely related to the venous pressure. Factors such as venous capacitance, blood volume, and vascular resistance affect the vascular function curves. The curve shifts to the right with lower vascular resistance, increased venous tone (decreases venous compliance), and higher blood volumes. The opposite will shift the vascular curve to the left. Figure 1-12 shows the effects of alterations in both cardiac function and vascular function. At the normal equilibrium point "A" when CO = VR, the venous pressure is approximately 3 mm Hg. If the blood volume is expanded or venous tone increases, the CO increases to point "B" even though the myocardial contractility remains unchanged. If the venous tone decreases or blood volume is depleted but cardiac contractility remains unchanged, the CO (VR) declines to "C." If the cardiac contractility decreases but the vascular function remains

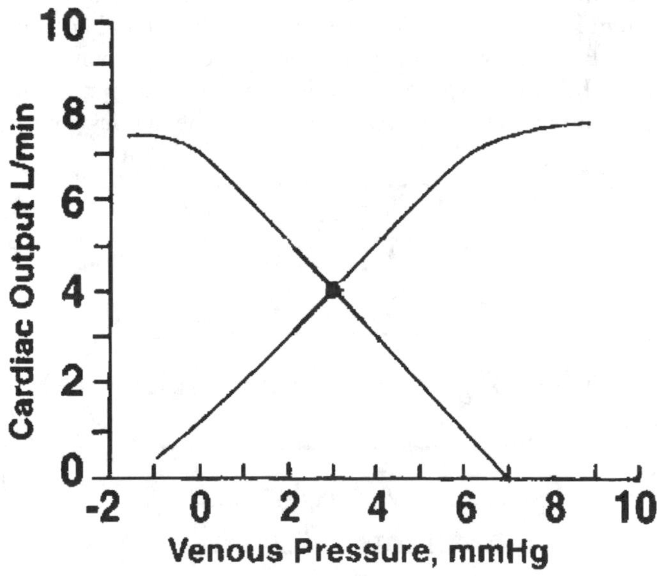

Figure 1-11
Cardiac function (Frank-Starling curve) and vascular function curve depicting that at equilibrium, the cardiac output and the venous return are equal.

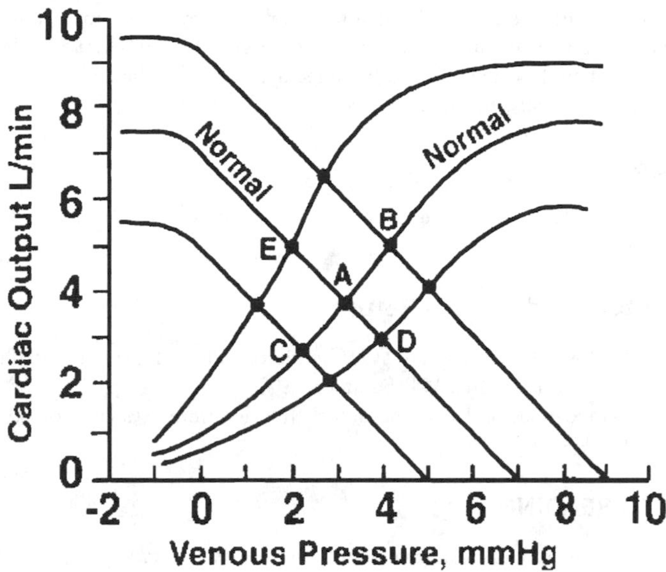

Figure 1-12
Effects of alterations in both cardiac function and vascular function. See text for explanation.

unchanged, the CO drops to "D." If the contractility increases but vascular function remains unchanged, the CO rises to "E." Other points where the vascular function and cardiac function curves intersect represent other points of equilibrium where the VR = CO. Thus, the vascular function (VR) and cardiac function (CO) interact to determine the specific CVP at a given time. Clinically though it is nearly impossible to generate cardiac function or vascular function curves, measurements of CVP can shed light on the cardiac or vascular status. If a patient presents with abnormally elevated CVP, the CO is either depressed or the blood volume is elevated (or both). If the CVP is depressed, the CO is either significantly increased or the blood volume is low (or both).

REFERENCES

Cardiac Performance

1. Boon, JA: Manual of Veterinary Echocardiography. Baltimore, Williams & Wilkins, 1998, 478.
2. Schlant RC, Sonnenblick EH, Katz AM: Normal physiology of the cardiovascular system. *In* Alexander RW, Schlant RC, Fuster V, ed.: Hurst's The Heart, 9th ed. New York, McGraw Hill, 1998, 81.
3. Wiggers CJ: Some factors controlling the shape of the pressure curve in the right ventricle. *Am J Physiol* 33:382, 1914.
4. Allen DG, Kentish JG: The cellular basis of the length-tension relation in cardiac muscle. *J Mol Cell Cardiol* 17:821, 1985.

5. Lakatta EG: Starling's law of the heart is explained by an intimate interaction of muscle length and myofilament calcium interaction. *J Am Coll Cardiol* 10:1157, 1987.
6. Babu A, Sonnenblick EH, Gulati J: Molecular basis for the influences of muscle length on myocardial performance. *Science* 240:74, 1988.

Blood Flow

7. Lee RT, Kamm RD: Vascular mechanics for the cardiologist. *J Am Coll Cardiol* 23: 1289, 1994.

Cardiac Output and Venous Return

8. Guyton AC, Jones CE, Coleman TG: Circulatory Physiology: Cardiac Output and Its Regulation. Philadelphia, WB Saunders, 1973.
9. Levy MN: The cardiac and vascular factors that determine systemic blood flow. *Circ Res* 44:739, 1979.

SUGGESTED READING

Hicks GH: Cardiopulmonary Anatomy and Physiology. Philadelphia, WB Saunders, 2000.

2
Respiratory Gas Transport

Marc R. Raffe

Uptake, transport, and delivery of O_2 to tissues is essential in maintaining physiologic integrity and cell viability. Concurrent removal of metabolic by-products including CO_2 from tissues is equally critical to maintain homeostasis. Because these processes have a common purpose, they are frequently linked together and referred to as respiratory gas transport.

The purpose of this chapter is to review the processes involved in oxygen (O_2) transport from the ambient environment to the living cell and carbon dioxide (CO_2) transport from the cell to the ambient environment. A common thread in this relationship is hemoglobin (Hb) and its role in supporting both processes.

O_2 TRANSPORT

The process of transporting O_2 from the external environment to the cell is elegantly simple in concept but complex in practice. The transport process may be divided into four phases: (1) pulmonary gas exchange, (2) O_2 interaction with Hb, (3) O_2 delivery to tissues, and (4) extraction of O_2 at the tissues. Each step is critical to ensure that a steady O_2 source is supplied to cells for metabolism.

Pulmonary Gas Exchange

The respiratory system is comprised of several anatomic regions that blend together to facilitate gas transport to the alveolus. Gas transport and distribution begins at the nares and ends with gas delivery to the pulmonary alveolus. Upper conducting elements of the respiratory system include the nares, maxilla, frontal sinuses, nasopharnyx, larynx, trachea, bronchi, bronchioles, and alveoli. The bronchioles and alveoli are incorporated into the lung structure. Sequential branching of the conducting airways from the trachea to the alveoli occurs in mammalian lungs and contributes to the compact space in which millions of alveolar units reside. The sequential branching is referred to as airway generations. Depending on species, there are between 22 and 26 airway generations between the trachea and alveolus.

Pulmonary gas exchange is the process that encompasses bulk movement of gas from the ambient environment to the terminal respiratory units of the lung. This process requires metabolic energy to perform. Under normal conditions, lung expansion occurs in concert with chest wall and diaphragm motion.

Tension generated by the diaphragm and respiratory muscles produces mechanical expansion of the thoracic cavity; this act produces concurrent pulmonary tissue expansion and generates a subatmospheric pressure gradient. Gas enters the respiratory passages, pharynx, and upper airways and produces a reduction in the transrespiratory pressure gradient to a static level at the end of inspiration. Expiration is generally a passive event that is initiated by relaxation of the respiratory muscles and diaphragm. Muscle relaxation permits elastic tissue elements in the lung to retract, thus facilitating alveolar emptying into the conducting pathways and, ultimately, the ambient atmosphere.

Movement of O_2 from the external environment to the blood requires the process outlined above. Transport of O_2 into the conducting pathways of the pulmonary tree occurs during each breath. Once O_2 enters the conducting pathways, movement to the alveolus occurs by a combination of bulk transfer and diffusion. Bulk transfer occurs in the first six airway generations; diffusion occurs in the remaining pathways to the alveolus. Diffusion is effective because O_2 partial pressures in the conducting pathways are greater than those in the alveolus, thus facilitating gas transfer to the alveolar level. This relationship is dynamic and constantly changes as gas diffusion occurs back and forth between the alveolus and the pulmonary circulation.

Once in the alveolus, oxygen diffusion occurs across the capillary-alveolar membrane. The rate of diffusion is governed by transmembrane partial pressures and gas solubility in tissue. Solubility is related to molecular weight; O_2 (mw = 32) has a slightly higher solubility coefficient than CO_2 (mw = 44). The magnitude of partial pressure gradient influences speed of diffusion. O_2 has a high partial pressure gradient (~100 mm Hg in the alveolus, ~38 mm Hg in venous blood). Thus, the difference in partial pressure gradient between venous and arterial blood facilitates rapid diffusion across the alveolar membrane.

The above discussion assumes ideal balance between alveolar gas exchange (V) and pulmonary blood flow (Q) past the alveolus. This does occur in a significant portion of healthy lung; it has long been recognized that physical forces affect the optimal balance in certain lung zones. Any V/Q imbalance affects gas exchange across the capillary-alveolar interface. Either increased V/Q (dead space) or decreased V/Q (shunt) will affect pulmonary O_2 uptake before affecting CO_2 exchange. Increasing respiratory rate in the normal patient will not significantly increase O_2 levels because O_2 partial pressure is unchanged. Supporting ventilation during anesthesia or during pulmonary disease will improve O_2 distribution and uptake in the lung. Disturbances in V/Q are generally amenable to increased inspired O_2 levels. Increased O_2 level will increase the diffusion gradient favoring O_2 uptake in the blood.

O_2 Interaction with Hb

Oxygen is predominantly carried on the Hb molecule once it enters the vascular network. Hb has remarkable characteristics in that it has the ability to carry four O_2 molecules per Hb molecule. O_2 that chemically complexes on the Hb molecule does not exert a partial gas pressure. A small percent of O_2 remains

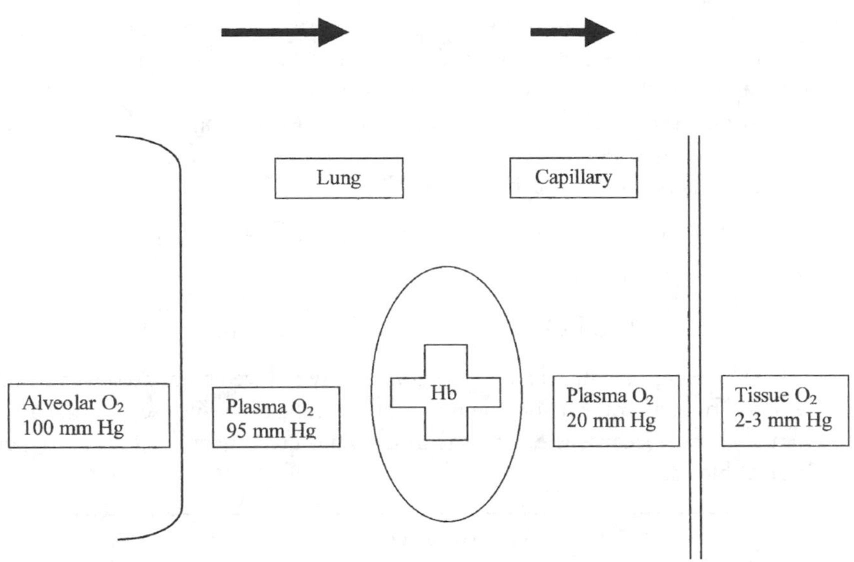

Figure 2-1
Schematic indicates O_2 transport from the alveolus to tissue beds. Note that the direction of O_2 diffusion is governed by the O_2 partial pressure in the local capillary-tissue environment. Plasma O_2 plays a key role in determining directional "flow."

in physical solution in the plasma compartment. This plasma soluble O_2 provides directional movement to or away from Hb in the diffusion process (Figure 2-1).

Each gram of Hb carries approximately 1.30 mL O_2 (there is a slight species difference in this value). A dog (cat) generally has between 12 and 15 g Hb/dL blood. An animal that has 15 g Hb/dL would have a Hb capacity of 1.34 (mL O_2/g Hb) × 15 g Hb/dL = 20.0 mL O_2/dL blood. This is the total amount of O_2 complexed with Hb. It is assumed that under normal conditions, O_2 interacts with all available sites (>97% O_2 saturation [SaO_2]) on the Hb molecule. As noted above, there is a small amount of O_2 in physical solution; the amount of O_2 in plasma (solution) is about 0.3 mL/dL/100 mm Hg O_2 partial pressure. The total amount of O_2 content (CaO_2) per blood deciliter (100 mL) is the sum of the O_2 complexed on the Hb molecule and O_2 in physical solution. This may be mathematically described as follows:

$$CaO_2 = (1.34 \times Hb \times SaO_2) + (0.003 \times PaO_2)$$

In this example, a normal patient breathing room air would have a total O_2-carrying capacity (O_2 content) of 20.0 + 0.3 = 20.3 mL O_2/dL.

Several issues can markedly affect O_2-carrying capacity. The first issue is Hb saturation. Any disease process affecting cardiovascular or respiratory function has the potential to reduce O_2 uptake at the lung. Under these conditions, the O_2 partial pressure is lower than expected producing incomplete Hb saturation. This is the reason that SaO_2 must be factored into calculating O_2 content.

The second issue is Hb concentration. If Hb concentration is reduced, marked change in CaO_2 will occur, even if blood O_2 tension (partial pressure) is unchanged. Because the quantity of O_2 carried in physical solution is small and will be constant irrespective of Hb level, it is safe to assume that total O_2-carrying capacity is directly proportional to Hb concentration. The following example underscores this point. A patient has an Hb level of 6 g/dL.

$$\text{Hb bound } O_2 - 6 \text{ g} \times 1.34 \text{ mL}/O_2/\text{g Hb} = 7.80 \text{ mL } O_2$$

$$O_2 \text{ in plasma}/100 \text{ mm Hg} = 0.3 \text{ mL } O_2$$

$$\text{Total } O_2 \text{ carried} = 8.10 \text{ mL } O_2/\text{dL}$$

Note that the total carrying capacity is significantly reduced compared to normal Hb levels. This patient will not demonstrate significant response to increased inspired O_2 levels because the defect is in the absolute O_2-carrying capacity per deciliter of blood.

Learning Points

Hemoglobin levels have a larger impact on oxygen carrying capacity than PaO_2.

Moderate hypoxemia plays a relatively minor role in arterial oxygenation if the oxygen saturation remains relatively normal.

Factors in Hb O_2-Carrying Capacity

As each molecule is attached, the stereochemistry of Hb is altered. Thus, as O_2 molecules three and four are attached, their binding is such that they may be freely unbound at appropriate points in the circulation based on local tissue O_2 tension. As O_2 is detached, the Hb molecule will subsequently release additional O_2 molecules in a more energy-efficient manner. Analysis of the physiologic properties of Hb led to construction of the oxyhemoglobin dissociation curve (Fig. 2-2).

Note that the curve is "sigmoid" in configuration. If one plots normal venous O_2 tension (PvO_2 = 40 mm Hg) and arterial O_2 tension (PaO_2 = 100 mm Hg), one notes that O_2 uptake and release occurs in the 75% to 100% Hb saturation range. This is the most energy efficient portion of the curve with large "reserve" capacity still available.

P_{50} is an analysis that is used to help understand real-time Hb physiology. Hb has the ability to change its affinity for O_2; this produces "shifts" in the Hb curve. P_{50} is the value at which Hb is 50% saturated. Normal P_{50} value is 27 to 35 mm Hg, depending on conditions. Factors that may influence P_{50} are listed in Table 2-1.

Increased P_{50} values indicate decreased O_2 affinity, meaning that O_2 is less likely to attach to the Hb molecule but is more likely to be released in low O_2 pressure environments. Decreased P_{50} value indicates increased O_2 affinity for Hb, meaning that Hb is less likely to donate O_2 at tissue sites that have low O_2

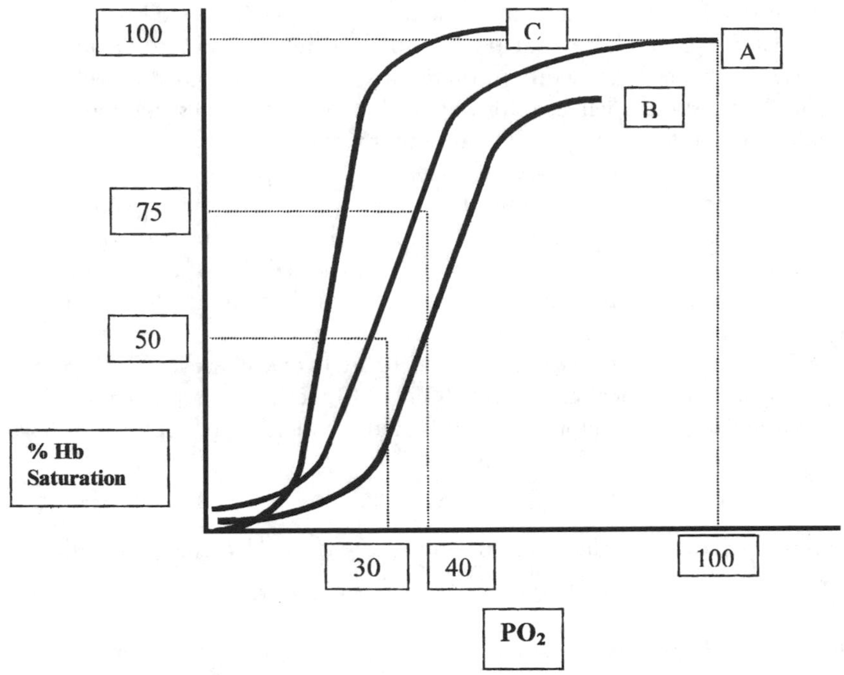

Figure 2-2
Oxyhemoglobin dissociation curves. Curve A represents the normal physiologic relationship between Hb and O_2. Curve B represents decreased oxyhemglobin affinity. Curve C represents increased oxyhemoglobin affinity.

partial pressure. Plot out O_2 tensions versus percent saturation with normal and shifted Hb curves to convince yourself of this principle.

Tissue O_2 Delivery

Once O_2 is attached to the Hb molecule, it must be transported to organ systems and tissues in a time- and energy-efficient manner. Tissue blood flow

Table 2-1. Factors That Influence the P_{50} Value of Hb

Decreased O_2 affinity (increased P_{50} value)	Increased O_2 affinity (decreased P_{50} value)
Acidemia	Alkalemia
Hyperthermia	Hypothermia
Hypercarbia (CO_2)	Hypocarbia
Increased 2,3-DPG activity	Decreased 2,3-DPG activity

DPG, 2,3-diphosphoglycerate.

(perfusion) is dictated by a complex series of events. As noted above in the first equation, blood O_2 content (CaO_2) must be high enough to facilitate O_2 transfer at tissue beds. In addition, there must be adequate blood flow (cardiac output) to constantly deliver oxygenated blood to tissues. Distribution of cardiac output must occur according to the metabolic needs of various tissue beds. This is determined by a coordinated action of neurogenic and humoral control mechanisms. Global control is under the autonomic nervous system which modulates local vascular tone to match blood flow to tissue metabolic demands. Moment-to-moment regulation is provided by local neurohumoral control mechanisms (nitric oxide and adenosine) that provide fine control of blood flow velocity through capillary beds.

It is not possible to measure cellular O_2 delivery. However, we can infer this by quantifying global O_2 delivery. Global O_2 delivery is a product of blood O_2 content and cardiac output (flow). It is mathematically represented as follows:

$$DO_2 = Q \times CaO_2$$

where Q is cardiac output in L/min and CaO_2 is calculated as previously discussed.

Tissue O_2 Uptake

Tissue O_2 uptake is the product of cardiac output and the difference in O_2 content between arterial and venous blood. The mathematical expression is as follows:

$$\dot{V}O_2 = Q \times (CaO_2 - CvO_2)$$

Because Hb characteristics ($1.3 \times Hb = CO_2$) are similar in arterial and venous blood, the equation can be modified as follows:

$$\dot{V}O_2 = Q \times 13.4 \times Hb \times (SaO_2 - SvO_2)$$

In this last equation, Hb content is multiplied by 10 to correct unit differences.

O_2 Extraction Ratio

The O_2 extraction ratio (OER) is the ratio of O_2 uptake to O_2 delivery ($\dot{V}O_2/DO_2$). It represents the fraction of O_2 delivered to tissues by the microcirculation that diffuses into the tissues. The ratio can be multiplied by 100 to express OER as a percentage. The normal OER in humans is 0.2 to 0.3 indicating that approximately 20% to 30% of O_2 delivered is extracted into the tissue spaces and is used in metabolism. This is adjustable based on a variety of factors including disease, stress, exercise, and metabolism. All these physiologic states will increase OER. The ability of the body to adjust for OER is critical in certain disease states as described below.

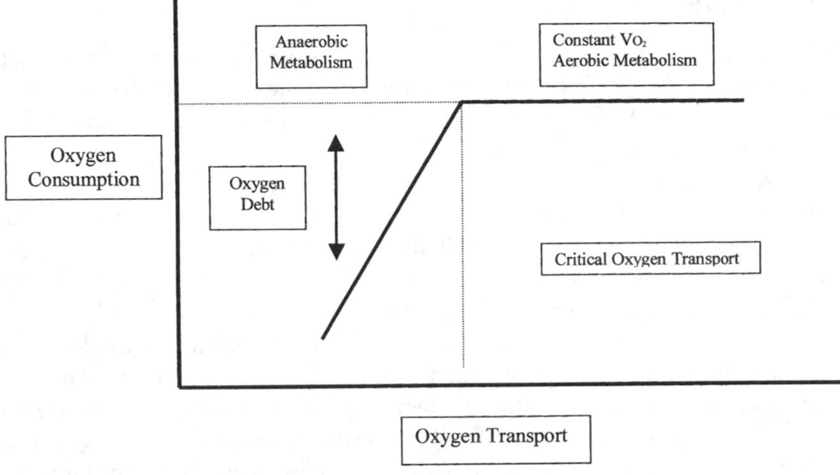

Figure 2-3
Graphic representation of the relationship between O_2 transport (DO_2) and O_2 consumption ($\dot{V}O_2$). The relationship of O_2 transport and consumption ($\dot{V}O_2/DO_2$) is referred to as the O_2 extraction ratio (OER).

Control of O_2 Uptake

Aerobic metabolism requires a steady stream of O_2 ($\dot{V}O_2$) to maintain normal biochemical processes. As a rule of thumb, an O_2 consumption value of 5 mL/kg/min is used to calculate O_2 demand by the patient under normal metabolic conditions. This requirement occurs irrespective of the ability to supply adequate O_2 levels (DO_2) at any moment in time. O_2 demand may change with many factors including metabolic rate, body temperature, age, disease, and organ failure or dysfunction. Because of moment-to-moment changes in O_2 delivery, the OER changes during normal daily activity. This is not apparent in healthy patients because the OER is never high enough to tax O_2 reserves available on the Hb molecule. Abnormal conditions in which Hb is low, perfusion is poor, or metabolic demands increase during fixed O_2 delivery may create a serious disturbance in O_2 availability by increasing the percent of O_2 extraction. Under these conditions, a state of critical O_2 delivery may be reached. Critical O_2 delivery is defined as the point where $\dot{V}O_2$ is limited by the DO_2. The point at which critical O_2 delivery is reached is referred to as supply-dependent $\dot{V}O_2$ (Fig. 2-3). Conceptually it represents the condition where tissue O_2 uptake is limited by the O_2 supplied, not by the metabolic demand. This scenario is not uncommon in critically ill patients for reasons described above. The reasons for this conversion are not fully understood, but appear to be related to an inherent $\dot{V}O_2/DO_2$ imbalance related to the underlying disorder.

CO_2 TRANSPORT

Carbon dioxide is the major end-product of oxidative metabolism. The body is exquisitely sensitive to CO_2; it is the dominant substance on which respiratory control is monitored. The ventilatory control systems are designed to regulate CO_2 and facilitate its clearance in the lung.

Based on partial gas pressures, CO_2 diffuses from intracellular sites to plasma compartment. When CO_2 comes in contact with plasma water, it forms carbonic acid, a potentially damaging product if allowed to accumulate. To minimize potential damage, CO_2 is buffered in the vascular compartment until it can be "off loaded" at the lung for excretion. The transport of CO_2 can occur using one of three mechanisms: (1) A small percentage of CO_2 is maintained in physical solution due to its plasma (water) solubility. This small amount is important because it facilitates the direction of diffusion much as plasma soluble O_2 does in arterial blood. The absolute amount of soluble CO_2 is small compared to other transport mechanisms. (2) CO_2 may continue to diffuse in plasma and gain entry into red blood cells. Approximately 20% of CO_2 combines with Hb forming carbaminohemoglobin. This CO_2 molecule is exchanged for O_2 during pulmonary gas exchange (arterialization). As O_2 is attached, this physiologically enhances CO_2-Hb dissociation; this phenomenon is called the Bohr effect. (3) The majority of CO_2 is transported following chemical interconversion. Erythrocyte cytoplasm (and renal tubular cells) possesses an enzyme system called carbonic anhydrase (CA). This enzyme facilitates CO_2 hydration and chemical interconversion into carbonic acid. The hydrogen ion from carbonic acid dissociates and interacts with available binding sites on the Hb molecule. The residual molecule from this process is bicarbonate ion; it is exchanged into plasma for chloride ion (chloride shift). In this way, CO_2 is dismantled for transport and is rebuilt at the lung. By complexing acid elements, tissue damage is minimized. The events may be summarized in the mass action reaction:

$$CO_2 + H_2O \rightleftarrows H_2CO_3 \rightleftarrows H^+ + HCO_3$$

In this reaction, CA expedites step 1; step 2 occurs spontaneously.

The Role of Hb in CO_2 Transport

Hemoglobin is a major buffer system in the blood. As noted above, it is integral in neutralizing hydrogen ion for transport from cells to the lung. Hb has a six-fold higher buffering capacity than plasma protein. This is mainly due to the massive Hb pool that is available in normal blood. The pK of Hb (7.0) is closer to normal body pH (7.4). This further enhances the contribution of Hb to total blood buffering capacity. It also makes Hb the primary buffer system for CO_2 transport.

Hemoglobin has a greater buffering capacity in its deoxygenated (desaturated) state. This characteristic is referred to as the Haldane effect. This effect is physiologically favorable because it increases Hb affinity for CO_2 and shortens the time that free CO_2 can interconvert to hydrogen ion instead of being directly complexed or dismantled for transport on the Hb molecule.

Once desaturated blood reaches the lung, it reassembles CO_2 by reversing the mass action reaction or releases it from the Hb molecule. CO_2 is released from the blood and diffuses into the alveolus and upward through the respiratory tract to be environmentally excreted. The Hb molecule changes stereochemical configuration as CO_2 and hydrogen ion are released. This characteristic is referred to as the Bohr effect. The release speed of CO_2 can be estimated by the arterial-venous difference in pCO_2. This can be formalized by a modification of the Fick equation. The Fick equation describes the relationship between content difference for a specific gas (in this case CO_2) in arterial and venous blood and perfusion (cardiac output). For CO_2, it may be defined as follows:

$$\dot{V}CO_2 = Q \times (CvCO_2 - CaCO_2)$$

where Q = perfusion (cardiac output), $CvCO_2$ = venous content of CO_2, and $CaCO_2$ = arterial content of CO_2.

This concept is essential to daily acid–base regulation. As noted in the acid–base section, CO_2 is the acid partner with bicarbonate. The ability to buffer CO_2 for transport and excretion at the pulmonary level is critical to maintain overall acid–base balance in the body. This is an important role that Hb plays in overall homeostasis. On a daily basis, over 10,000 mEq acid per day is excreted by this route.

SUMMARY

Transport of respiratory gases is crucial to maintaining cellular and systemic homeostasis. A number of steps are required in the process; disturbance at any level may produce harmful consequences to the patient. It is important to understand the sequence of steps associated with gas transport so that accurate problem identification and therapeutic intervention may be performed before significant deleterious consequences develop.

SUGGESTED READINGS

Comroe JH: Physiology of Respiration, 2nd ed. Chicago, Yearbook Medical Publishers, 1974.

Bryan-Brown CW, Guitterez G: Pulmonary gas exchange, transport and delivery. *In* Shoemaker W, Ayres S, Grenvik A, Holbrook P, eds.: Textbook of Critical Care, 3d ed. Philadelphia, WB Saunders, 1995, 776.

Marino PL: The ICU Book, 2nd ed. Baltimore, Williams & Wilkins, 1999, 19.

Szaflarski NL: Pulmonary and tissue gas exchange. *In* Parsons PE, Wiener-Kronish JP, eds.: Critical Care Secrets. Philadelphia, Hanley and Belfus, 1992, 7.

3
Oxidant Injury

Paul L. Marino

The management of critically ill organisms is dominated by the notion that promoting the supply of oxygen (O_2) to the vital organs is necessary to sustain life. As a result, O_2 is provided in a liberal and unregulated fashion, whereas the tendency for O_2 to degrade and decompose organic (carbon-based) matter is usually overlooked. In fact, in contrast to the notion that O_2 protects cells from injury in the critically ill, the accumulated evidence over the past 15 years suggests that O_2 may be responsible for the cell injury that accompanies critical illness. The possibility for O_2 to act as a toxic rather than life-sustaining force has monumental implications for the way we manage the critically ill. This chapter summarizes the mechanisms by which O_2 can promote tissue injury and presents some of the endogenous mechanisms used by aerobic organisms to protect themselves from O_2-induced tissue injury.

THE OXIDATION REACTION

An oxidation reaction is a chemical reaction between O_2 and another chemical species. Because O_2 removes electrons from other atoms and molecules, oxidation is also described as the loss of electrons by an atom or molecule. The chemical species that removes the electrons is referred to as an "oxidizing agent" or oxidant. The companion process (*i.e.*, the gain of electrons by an atom or molecule) is called a "reduction" reaction, and the chemical species that donates the electrons is referred to as a "reducing agent." Because oxidation of one atom or molecule must be accompanied by reduction of another atom or molecule, the overall reaction is often referred to as a "redox" reaction.

When an organic molecule (*i.e.*, a molecule with a carbon skeleton) reacts with O_2, electrons are removed from carbon atoms in the molecule. This disrupts one or more covalent bonds, and as each of these covalent bonds ruptures, energy is released in the form of heat and light (and sometimes sound). The organic molecule then breaks into smaller fragments.[1] When oxidation is complete, the parent molecule is broken down into the smallest molecules capable of independent existence. Because organic matter is composed mainly of carbon and hydrogen, the final end-products of oxidation are simple combinations of O_2 with carbon and hydrogen, that is, carbon dioxide (CO_2) and water (H_2O).

METABOLISM OF O_2

Oxygen itself is a weak oxidizing agent, but some of its metabolites are potent oxidants capable of producing lethal cell injury. This tendency for a weakly oxidizing parent molecule (O_2) to form metabolites that are powerful oxidants is explained by the atomic structure of the O_2 molecule, which is described below.

The O_2 Molecule

Oxygen in its natural state is a diatomic molecule, as shown by the familiar O_2 symbol at the top of Figure 3-1. The orbital diagram to the right of the O_2

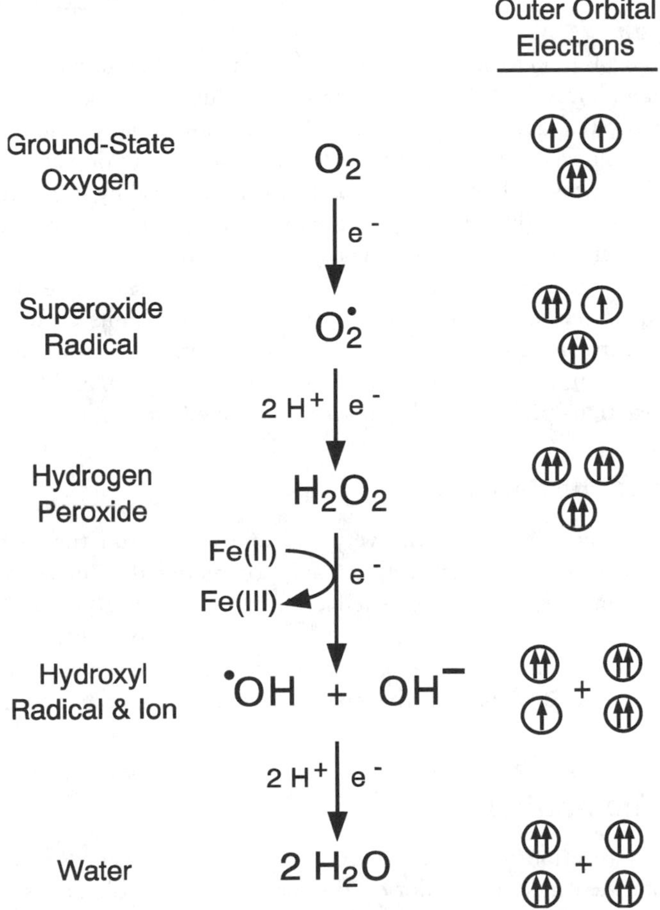

Figure 3-1
The metabolism of molecular oxygen to water. Orbital diagrams on the right side of the figure show the electron configuration (indicated by the arrows) in the outer orbitals (small circles) of each reactant. Highest orbitals in each diagram are furthest from the nucleus. Single electron reductions indicated by e^-. See text for explanation.

symbol shows how the outer electrons of the O_2 molecule are arranged. The circles in the diagram represent orbitals, which are energy fields that can be occupied by electrons. The arrows in the diagram represent electrons that are spinning in the direction indicated by the arrows. Note that one of the O_2 orbitals contains two electrons with opposing spins, whereas the other two orbitals each contain a single electron spinning in the same direction. The orbital with the paired electrons is obeying one of the basic rules of the quantum atom: an electron orbital can be occupied by two electrons, but only if they have opposing spins. The two outermost orbitals with single electrons are thus only half-full, and their electrons are "unpaired." An atom or molecule that has one or more unpaired electrons in its outer orbitals is called a free radical.[2] (The term "free" indicates that the atom or molecule is capable of independent existence; *i.e.*, it is free-living).

Free radicals tend to be highly reactive by virtue of their unpaired electrons. However, not all free radicals are highly reactive. This is the case with O_2, which is not a highly reactive molecule despite having two unpaired electrons. The reason for the sluggish reactivity of O_2 is the directional spin of its two unpaired electrons. As mentioned above, no two electrons can occupy the same orbital if they have the same directional spin (the exclusion principle, proposed by the Austrian physicist Wolfgang Pauli). Thus, an electron pair cannot be added to O_2 because one orbital would have two electrons with the same directional spin, which is a quantum impossibility. This "spin restriction" limits O_2 to reduction reactions that involve single electron additions. This means that more than one reduction reaction is needed to reduce molecular O_2 to H_2O, and this series of reduction reactions produces highly reactive intermediates.

The Metabolic Pathway

Oxygen is metabolized at the very end of the electron transport chain, where the electrons and protons that have completed the transport process are left to accumulate. The complete reduction of molecular O_2 to H_2O requires the addition of four electrons and four protons, as shown in the reaction sequence in Figure 3-1. Each metabolite in this sequence is accompanied by an orbital diagram to demonstrate the changes occurring at each point in the pathway.

Superoxide Radical

The first reaction adds one electron to O_2 and produces the superoxide radical. Note the superscripted dot on the superoxide symbol. This signifies an

$$O_2 + e^- \rightarrow O_2^{\bullet}$$

unpaired electron, and it is the conventional symbol for a free radical. The superoxide radical has one unpaired electron, and thus is less of a free radical than O_2. Superoxide is neither a highly reactive radical nor a potent oxidant.[3] Nevertheless, it has been implicated in conditions associated with widespread tissue damage, such as the "reperfusion injury" that follows a period of tissue ischemia.[2] The toxicity of superoxide may be due to the large daily production of this molecular species, which is estimated at 1 billion molecules per cell, or 1.75 kg (4 lb) for a 70-kg adult human.[4]

Hydrogen Peroxide

The addition of one electron to the superoxide radical creates hydrogen peroxide (H_2O_2), which, although not a free radical, is a strong oxidizing agent.[5]

$$O_2^{\bullet} + e^- + 2H^+ \rightarrow H_2O_2$$

Hydrogen peroxide is very mobile and crosses cell membranes easily. It is a powerful cytotoxin and is well known for its ability to damage endothelial cells. Although it is not a free radical, it may have to generate a free radical (*i.e.*, hydroxyl radical) to express its toxicity.

Hydrogen peroxide is loosely held together by a weak O_2-O_2 bond (this bond is represented by the lower orbital in the orbital diagram for H_2O_2). This bond ruptures easily, producing two hydroxyl radicals ($^{\bullet}OH$), each with one unpaired electron. An electron is donated to one of the hydroxyl radicals, creating one hydroxyl ion (OH^-) and one hydroxyl radical ($^{\bullet}OH$). The electron is donated by iron in its reduced form, Fe(II), which serves as a catalyst for the reaction. Iron is involved in many free radical reactions and is considered an powerful pro-oxidant. The role of transition metals in free radical reactions will be discussed again later in the chapter.

Hydroxyl Radical

The iron-catalyzed dissociation of H_2O_2 proceeds as follows:

$$H_2O_2 + Fe(II) \rightarrow OH^- + {}^{\bullet}OH + Fe(III)$$

(Note that Roman numerals are used instead of plus signs to designate the oxidation state of iron, as recommended by the International Union of Chemistry.) The hydroxyl radical is the king of free radicals. It is one of the most reactive molecules known in biochemistry; that is, it often reacts with another chemical species within five molecular diameters from its point of origin.[2] Because of this high degree of reactivity, the hydroxyl radical is considered the single most potent oxidizing agent in all of biochemistry.

Hypochlorous Acid

The metabolism of oxygen in neutrophils has an additional pathway (not shown in Fig. 3-1) that uses a myeloperoxidase enzyme to "chlorinate" H_2O_2, producing hypochlorous acid (hypochlorite).

$$H_2O_2 + 2\ Cl^- \rightarrow 2\ HOCl$$

When neutrophils are activated, the conversion of O_2 to superoxide increases 20-fold. This is called the "respiratory burst" (which is an unfortunate term, because the increased O_2 consumption has nothing to do with energy metabolism). When the increased metabolic traffic reaches H_2O_2, about 40% is diverted to hypochlorite production, and the remainder forms hydroxyl radicals.[6] Hypochlorite is the active ingredient in household bleach. It is a powerful germicidal agent and requires only milliseconds to produce lethal damage in bacteria.[7]

Water

The final reduction reaction in the metabolism of O_2 involves the addition of one electron to the hydroxyl radical. This reaction produces two molecules of H_2O, as shown below.

$$OH^- + {}^{\bullet}OH + e^- + 2H^+ \rightarrow 2\ H_2O$$

Summary

In summary, the metabolism of one molecule of O_2 requires four chemical reactions, each involving the addition of a single electron. This process requires four reducing equivalents (electrons and protons), and it produces three potentially toxic chemical intermediates (*i.e.*, superoxide radical, H_2O_2, and the hydroxyl radical). Under normal conditions, about 98% of O_2 metabolism is completed, and less than 2% of the intermediary metabolites escape into the cytoplasm.[3] This is a tribute to cytochrome oxidase, which carries on the reactions in a deep recess that effectively blocks any molecular escape.

Once the O_2 metabolites escape the confines of cytochrome oxidase, their mobility and toxicity differ. The superoxide radical and H_2O_2 are mobile but nontoxic, whereas the hydroxyl radical is toxic but not very mobile (remember the hydroxyl radical reacts within five molecular diameters of its origin, and this hinders its mobility). Thus, the more mobile, nontoxic oxidants (*i.e.*, $O_2^{\bullet}$ and H_2O_2) can move readily and reach distant sites, and once they reach their destination, they can then generate hydroxyl radicals to produce the tissue injury.[3] According to this scheme, the superoxide radical and H_2O_2 serve as transport vehicles for oxidant injury, and the hydroxyl radical is the actual "hit man" for the tissue injury caused by O_2 metabolites.

FREE RADICAL REACTIONS

The damaging effects of oxidation are largely the result of free radical reactions. This section describes the two basic types of free radical reactions, that is, those involving a free radical and a nonradical, and those involving two free radicals.

Radical and Nonradical

When a free radical reacts with a nonradical, the nonradical loses an electron and is transformed into a free radical. Therefore, the union of a radical and a nonradical begets another radical. Because free radicals are often highly reactive in nature, this type of radical-regenerating reaction tends to become repetitive, creating a series of self-sustaining reactions known collectively as a chain reaction.[3] The tendency to produce chain reactions is one of the most characteristic features of free radical reactions (a burning flame is one example of a chain reaction involving free radicals). A chain reaction that is capable of producing widespread organ damage is described next.

Lipid Peroxidation

Oxidative decomposition of polyunsaturated fatty acids (PUFAs) in foods produces what is known as "rancidity" in decaying food.[8] This same process of "lipid peroxidation" is also responsible for oxidative damage of membrane lipids. The lipophilic interior of the cell membranes is rich in PUFAs, and the low melting point of these fatty acids may be responsible for the "fluidity" of cell membranes. Oxidation increases the melting point of membrane fatty acids and reduces membrane fluidity. The membranes eventually lose their selective permeability and become "leaky," predisposing cells to osmotic disruption.[8]

The peroxidation of membrane lipids proceeds as shown in Figure 3-2. The reaction sequence is initiated by a strong oxidant like the hydroxyl radical, which

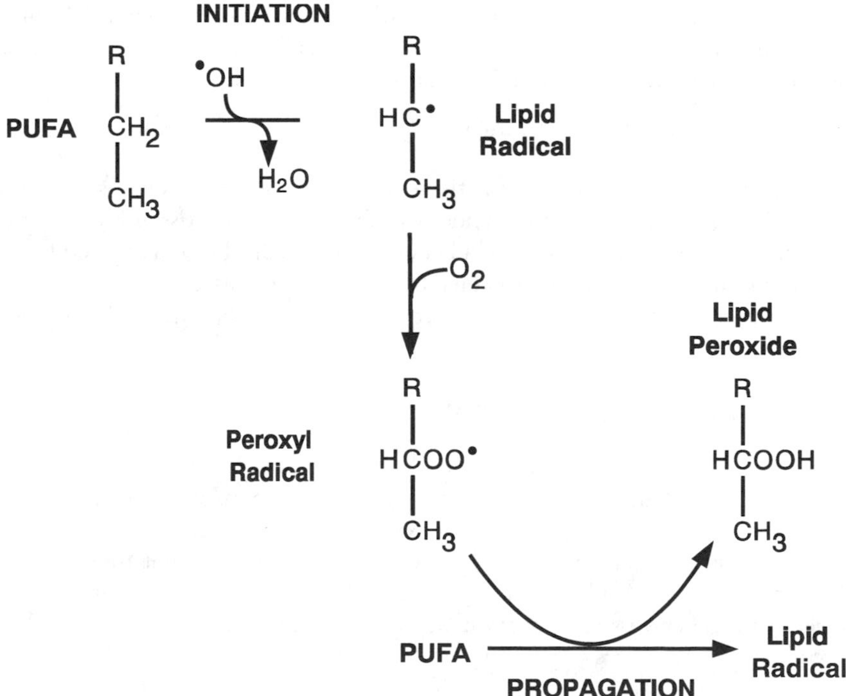

Figure 3-2
The reaction sequence for the peroxidation of polyunsaturated fatty acids (PUFAs) in cell membranes. See text for explanation.

removes an entire hydrogen atom (proton and electron) from one of the carbon atoms in a PUFA. This creates a carbon-centered radical ($C^\bullet$), which is then transformed into an O_2-centered "peroxy radical" ($COO^\bullet$) that can remove a hydrogen atom from an adjacent fatty acid and initiate a new series of reactions. The final "propagation reaction" creates a self-sustaining chain reaction that will continue until the substrate (*i.e.*, fatty acid) is exhausted or until something interferes with the reaction. (The latter mechanism is the basis for the antioxidant action of vitamin E, which is described later.)

Radical and Radical

Two radicals can react by sharing electrons to form a covalent bond. This eliminates the existence of free radicals but it does not eliminate the risk for toxicity. In the example below, the product of a radical-radical reaction is much more destructive than both radicals combined.

Nitric Oxide Transformation

Nitric oxide is a free radical that has been placed in a category of its own because of its beneficial actions as a vasodilator, neurotransmitter, and bactericidal agent.[9] However, despite its favorable reputation, nitric oxide can become a problem in the presence of superoxide. The reaction of superoxide ($O_2^\bullet$) with nitric oxide ($NO^\bullet$) generates a powerful oxidant called peroxinitrite, which is 2000 times more potent than H_2O_2 as an oxidizing agent.[10]

$$NO^{\bullet\bullet} + O_2^\bullet \rightarrow ONOOO^- \text{ (peroxynitrite)}$$

Peroxinitrite can either cause direct tissue damage, or it can decompose to form hydroxyl radicals and nitrogen dioxide, which then produce tissue injury. This transformation of nitric oxide from a beneficial free radical into a source of oxidant injury demonstrates how O_2 metabolites ($O_2^\bullet$ in this case) can promote oxidant injury indirectly, by changing the character of the chemical environment.

ANTIOXIDANT PROTECTION

Any chemical species that can reduce or delay the oxidation of a substrate is called an antioxidant.[2] Most aerobic organisms have a host of endogenous antioxidants that protect the organism from oxidant injury. Evidence for endogenous antioxidant protection is provided by the simple observation that the moment of death (when antiodxidant production ceases) is marked by an accelerated rate of decay in the carcass. This section will present the chemical substances that play a major role in this protection (Table 3-1).

Enzyme Antioxidants

Three enzymes function as antioxidants, and each is shown in Figure 3-3.

Table 3-1. Endogenous and Exogenous Antioxidants

Antioxidant	Action(s)	Comment
Selenium	A cofactor for glutathione peroxidase	Although an essential nutrient, is not routinely provided in feeding formulas. Can be given IV as sodium selenite. RDA in humans is 55–70 µg/d.
Glutathione	A reducing agent by virtue of an SH group on its cysteine residue	A major intracellular antioxidant. Synthesized de novo in cells and does not readily cross cell membranes.
N-Acetylcysteine	A commercially available mucolytic agent that acts as a glutathione analog	Crosses cell membranes. Has proven effective as an exogenous source of glutathione in cases of acetaminophen poisoning.
Vitamin E	Blocks propagation of lipid peroxidation in cell membranes.	The major antioxidant for oxidant injury in lipid-laden structures.
Vitamin C	A reducing agent normally. Can act as a pro-oxidant by maintaining iron as Fe(II).	A major extracellular antioxidant. Use in the critically ill may be limited by its ability to act as a pro-oxidant.
1. Ceruloplasmin 2. Transferrin 3. Albumin 4. Uric acid	Major antioxidants in plasma. Most act by binding free iron and copper. Albumin is a potent scavenger of hypochlorite.	Ceruloplasmin accounts for a majority of the antioxidant activity in plasma.

Superoxide Dismutase

Superoxide dismutase (SOD) is an enzyme that facilitates the "dismutation" of superoxide radicals to form H_2O_2. Because SOD promotes the formation of an oxidant (*i.e.*, H_2O_2), its role as an antioxidant has been questioned. In fact, when SOD promotes the formation of H_2O_2, but the catalase and peroxidase enzymes (described below) are unable to reduce the H_2O_2 to H_2O, then SOD will serve as a "pro-oxidant" rather than an antioxidant.[11] Thus, exogenously administered SOD is not advised unless the stores of the other enzyme antioxidants are adequate.

Catalase

Catalase is an iron-containing heme protein that reduces H_2O_2 to H_2O. It is present in most cells but is lowest in cardiac cells and neurons. Inhibition of the catalase enzyme does not enhance the toxicity of H_2O_2 for endothelial cells,[12] so the role of this enzyme as an antioxidant is unclear.

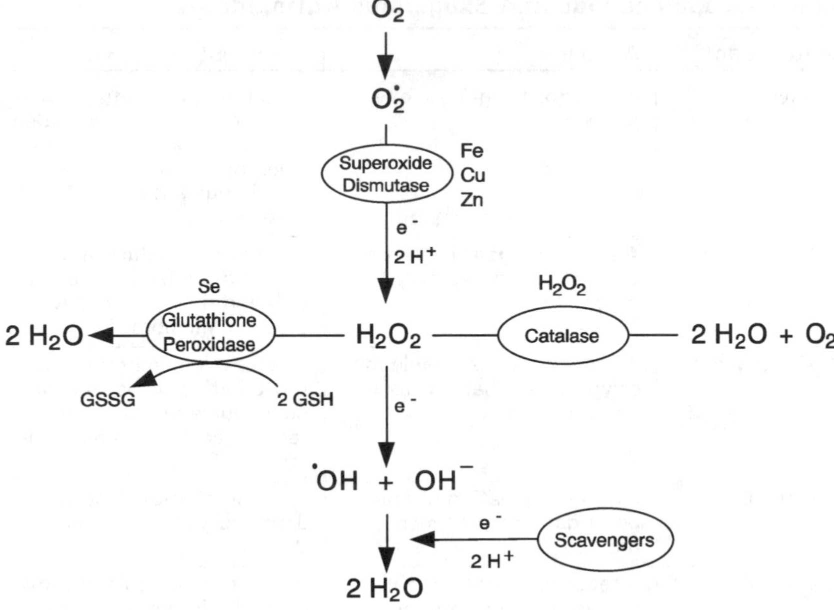

Figure 3-3
The actions of three antioxidant enzymes and a free radical scavenger. Reaction sequence depicts oxygen metabolism, as shown in Figure 3-1. Cofactors for superoxide dismutase are iron (Fe), zinc (Zn), and copper (Cu), but are never present as a triad on the same enzyme. Cofactor for glutathione peroxidase is selenium (Se). GSH, reduced glutathione, GSSG, oxidized glutathione as a dipeptide.

Glutathione Peroxidase

The peroxidase enzyme reduces H_2O_2 to H_2O by removing electrons from glutathione in its reduced form and then donating the electrons to H_2O_2. The peroxidase reaction can be written as follows:

$$H_2O_2 + 2\ GSH \rightarrow 2\ H_2O + GSSG$$

where GSSG and GSH are oxidized and reduced glutathione, respectively.

Selenium

The activity of the glutathione peroxidase enzyme is dependent on the trace element selenium. Selenium is an essential nutrient with a recommended dietary allowance (RDA) of 70 μg/d for men and 55 μg/d for women.[13] The absence of dietary selenium produces measurable differences in glutathione peroxidase activity after just 1 week,[14] so the routine administration of selenium seems justified. However, selenium, has no clear-cut deficiency syndrome, and this creates little impetus to provide selenium as a nutritional supplement on a routine basis.

[Ed note: Selenium deficiency is commonly recognized in sheep and cattle as "white muscle disease," a serious, often fatal disease of striated muscle.]

Selenium status can be monitored with whole blood selenium levels. The normal range (in humans) is 0.5 to 2.5 mg/L. Selenium can be provided intravenously as sodium selenite.[15] The highest daily dose that is considered safe (in humans) is 200 μg/d, given in divided doses: that is, 50 μg IV q 6 h.

Nonenzyme Antioxidants

In addition to the enzyme antioxidants just presented, there are a host of nonenzyme substances that serve as endogenous antioxidants. These are listed in Table 3-1.

Glutathione

One of the major antioxidants in the human body is glutathione, a tripeptide (glycine-cysteine-glutamine) found in molar concentrations (0.5–10 mM/L) in most cells.[16,17] Glutathione acts as a reducing agent by virtue of the sulfhydryl group in its cysteine residue. It is normally in the reduced state (GSH), and the normal ratio of reduced to oxidized forms is 10:1. The major antioxidant action of glutathione is to reduce H_2O_2 directly to H_2O. This diverts H_2O_2 from producing the highly toxic hydroxyl radicals. Glutathione is found in all organs but is particularly prevalent in the lung, liver, endothelium, and intestinal mucosa. It is primarily an intracellular antioxidant, and plasma levels of glutathione are three orders of magnitude lower than intracellular levels.

Glutathione does not cross cell membranes directly. It is synthesized in every cell of the body and largely remains sequestered within cells. Glutathione administered exogenously thus has little effect on intracellular levels,[18] and this limits the therapeutic value of this agent.

N-*Acetylcysteine*

N-Acetylcysteine (NAC) is a glutathione analogue that is used as a mucolytic agent (Mucomyst). The benefit of NAC is its ability to readily cross cell membranes (unlike glutathione), which makes NAC a potentially valuable treatment for glutathione-deficient states. In fact, NAC has proven effective in treating acetaminophen toxicity, which is the result of an overwhelmed glutathione detoxification pathway.

It is also possible that NAC will prove valuable as an antioxidant for therapeutic use in a variety of other conditions. It has been shown to protect the myocardium from ischemic injury and has been successful in reducing the incidence of reperfusion injury during cardiac catheterization.[19] It has also been used with some success in treating critically ill patients with acute respiratory distress syndrome and inflammatory shock syndromes.[20,21]

Vitamin E

Vitamin E (α-tocopherol) is a lipid-soluble vitamin that antagonizes the peroxidative injury of membrane lipids.[22] In fact, vitamin E is the only antioxi-

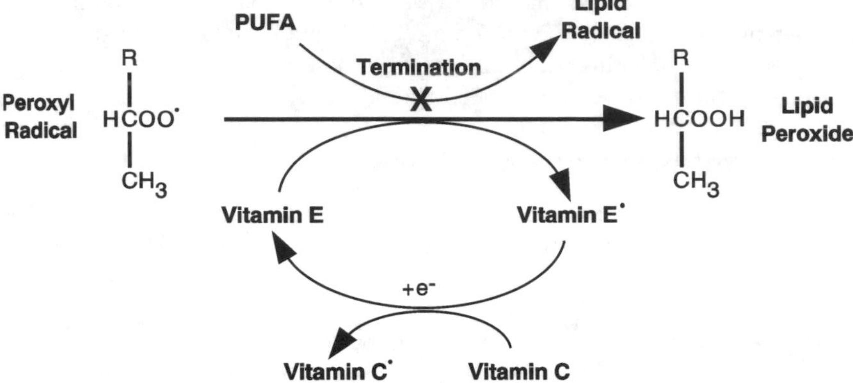

Figure 3-4
The "chain-breaking" action of vitamin E that terminates lipid peroxidation in cell membranes. Free radicals indicated by superscripted dots, as before. See text for explanation.

dant capable of halting the propagation of lipid peroxidation. The mechanism for this action is shown in Figure 3-4. Vitamin E is present in the lipophilic interior of cell membranes, which is rich in oxidizable PUFAs. When a propagating wave of lipid peroxidation reaches vitamin E, it transforms the vitamin E into a free radical that is poorly reactive. This reaction thus spares the adjacent PUFAs from oxidation and halts the propagation of the peroxidation reactions. In this capacity, vitamin E acts as a "chain-breaking" antioxidant. When the vitamin E radical is formed, it must be transformed back to vitamin E, and this reaction uses vitamin C as the electron donor. Therefore, vitamin C deficiency can hinder the ability of vitamin E to act as an antioxidant.

Vitamin C

Vitamin C (ascorbic acid) is a reducing agent that can donate electrons to free radicals and fill their electron orbitals. It is a water-soluble antioxidant and operates primarily in the extracellular space. Vitamin C is found in abundance in the lung, where it may play a protective role in inactivating pollutants that enter the airways. This would be a valuable function in ventilator-dependent subjects, whose airways are constantly bombarded with O_2-rich gas mixtures.

The problem with vitamin C is its tendency to promote (rather than retard) the formation of oxidants in the presence of iron and copper.[23–25] Vitamin C reduces iron to the Fe(II) state, and this normally aids in the absorption of iron from the intestinal tract. However, Fe(II) can promote the production of hydroxyl radicals, as described earlier. Thus, vitamin C can function as a pro-oxidant by maintaining iron in its reduced or Fe(II) state. The reactions involved are shown below

$$\text{Ascorbate} + \text{Fe(III)} \rightarrow \text{Fe(II)} + \text{Dehydroascorbate}$$

$$\text{Fe(II)} + H_2O_2 \rightarrow {}^{\bullet}OH + OH^- + \text{Fe(III)}$$

Several conditions that are common in the critically ill can promote an increase in free iron. Among these are inflammation, blood transfusions, and reductions in iron-binding proteins. The prevalence of these conditions raises serious concerns about the use of vitamin C as an exogenous antioxidant in the ICU.

Plasma Antioxidants

The plasma components with antioxidant activity are listed at the very bottom of Table 3-1. Most of the antioxidant activity in plasma can be traced to two proteins that make up only 4% of total plasma protein pool: ceruloplasmin (the copper transport or storage protein) and transferrin.[24] Transferrin binds iron in the Fe(III) state, and ceruloplasmin oxidizes iron from the Fe(II) to Fe(III) state. Therefore, ceruloplasmin helps transferrin to bind iron, and both proteins then act to limit free iron in plasma. For this reason, iron sequestration has been proposed as the major antioxidant activity in plasma.[25] This is consistent with the ability of Fe(II) to promote free radical production, as shown in Figure 3-1.

OXIDANT STRESS

The risk of oxidation-induced tissue injury is determined by the balance between the activities of oxidant and antioxidant compounds. When oxidant activity exceeds the neutralizing capacity of the antioxidants, the excess or unopposed oxidant activity can promote tissue injury. This condition of unopposed biologic oxidation is known as oxidant stress.[26]

Clinical Disease

Oxidant stress has been implicated in the pathogenesis of more than 100 clinical diseases,[27] and the ones most likely to be encountered in the ICU are listed in Table 3-2. Unopposed biologic oxidation (*i.e.*, oxidant stress) has been documented in each of these clinical conditions in humans,[27–32] and there is no reason to believe that the situation is any different in animals.

Inflammation

Most of the clinical conditions in Table 3-2 are accompanied by inflammation, and the conditions with multiorgan involvement are often associated with a progressive, systemic inflammatory response. As a result, inflammation has been proposed as a principal offender in pathologic forms of oxidant injury. The release of free radicals from activated neutrophils and macrophages creates an oxidant-intense environment, and the ability of host cells to withstand this "oxidative assault" may be the important factor in determining the clinical course of inflammatory conditions. In the desirable world, leukocyte-derived oxidants would annihilate all invading microbes but would spare the host cells. In the undesirable world, the inflammatory oxidants would destroy both the invader and the host. This proposed scheme is intuitively appealing and emphasizes the value of antioxidant therapy in inflammatory illnesses.

Table 3-2. Clinical Conditions Accompanied by Oxidant Stress*

Target Organ	Clinical Conditions	Comments
Lung	1. ARDS 2. Asthma 3. Acid aspiration 4. Pulmonary O_2 toxicity	The lung is vulnerable to oxidant injury from two directions: the airways and the pulmonary capillaries.
Heart	1. Acute myocardial infarction 2. Reperfusion injury 3. Cardiomyopathy	Oxidant injury may play a role in the "stunned myocardium" associated with reperfusion injury.
Nervous system	1. Stroke 2. Traumatic brain injury 3. Postresuscitation injury 4. Spinal cord injury	Because the nervous system is rich in lipids, it is vulnerable to lipid peroxidation.
Gastrointestinal tract	1. Peptic ulcer disease 2. Stress ulceration 3. Intestinal ischemia	The gut is susceptible to reperfusion injury, possibly due to an abundance of xanthine oxidase, which generates superoxide radicals during periods of ischemia.
Kidneys	Acute renal failure due to: 1. Aminoglycosides 2. Ischemia 3. Myoglobinuria	Iron and hydrogen peroxide may have important roles in oxidant injury of the kidneys.
Multiple organs	1. Multiorgan failure 2. Multisystem trauma 3. Septic shock 4. Thermal injury	The systemic inflammatory response plays a major role in the oxidant injury in these conditions.

* Includes only conditions likely to be seen in the CCU.
ARDS, acute respiratory distress syndrome.

Metabolic Support

The tendency for aerobic metabolism to generate toxins is a concern that deserves more attention because it has significant implications for the appropriate method of providing metabolic support in critically ill patients. When metabolically generated oxidants are overwhelming the body's antioxidant defenses, the common practice of supporting metabolism by promoting the availability of O_2 and nutrients will only serve to generate more toxic metabolites. The proper maneuver here is to support the antioxidant defenses. This approach adds another dimension to the concept of metabolic support by considering the output side of metabolism and the value of eliminating the cell injury induced by metabolically generated toxins. Remember that metabolism is an engine (*i.e.*, an energy converter), and like all engines, it has an exhaust that contains noxious by-products of combustion. The exhaust from an automobile engine adds pollutants to the atmosphere; the exhaust from a metabolic engine adds pollutants to the "biosphere."

REFERENCES

Oxidants

1. Chance B, Sies H, Boveris A: Hydroperoxide metabolism in mammalian organs. *Physiol Rev* 59:527, 1979.
2. Halliwell, B, Gutteridge JM: Free Radicals in Biology and Medicine, 2nd ed. Clarendon, England: Oxford University Press, 1989, 2.
3. Liochev SI, Fridovich I: The role of $O_2^{\bullet}$ in the production of $HO^{\bullet}$ in vitro and in vivo. *Free Radic Biol Med* 16:29, 1994.
4. Frei B: Reactive oxygen species and antioxidant vitamins: mechanisms of action. *Am J Med* 97(suppl 3A): 5S, 1994.
5. Thompson AM: The oxidizing capacity of the earth's atmosphere: probable past and future changes. *Science* 256:1157, 1992.
6. Anderson BO, Brown JM, Harken A: Mechanisms of neutrophil-mediated tissue injury. *J Surg Res* 51:170, 1991.
7. Bernovsky C: Nucleotide chloramines and neutrophil-mediated cytotoxicity. *FASEB J* 5:295, 1991.
8. Halliwell B, Gutteridge JM: Free radicals in biology and medicine, 2nd ed. Clarendon, England: Oxford University Press, 1989, 188.
9. Anggard E: Nitric oxide: mediator, murderer, and medicine. *Lancet* 343:1199, 1994.
10. Freeman B: Free radical chemistry of nitric oxide. Looking at the dark side. *Chest* 105(suppl):79S, 1994.

Antioxidants

11. Michiels C, Raes M, Toussant O, Remacle J: Importance of Se-glutathione, peroxidase, catalase, and CU/ZN-SOD for cell survival against oxidative stress. *Free Radic Biol Med* 17:235, 1994.
12. Suttorp N, Toepfer W, Roka L: Antioxidant defense mechanisms of endothelial cells: glutathione redox cycle versus catalase. *Am J Physiol* 251:C671, 1986.
13. National Research Council Subcommittee on the Tenth Edition of the RDAs: RDAs, 10th ed. Washington, DC: National Academic Press, 1989, 220.
14. Sando K, Hoki M, Nezu R, *et al.*: Platelet glutathione peroxidase activity in long term total parenteral nutrition with and without selenium supplementation. *JPEN J Parenter Enteral Nutr* 16:54, 1992.
15. World Health Organization: Selenium. Environmental Health Criteria 58. Geneva, Switzerland, 1987.
16. Meister A: On the antioxidant effects of ascorbic acid and glutathione. *Biochem Pharmacol* 44:1905, 1992.
17. Cantin AM, Begin R: Glutathione and inflammatory disorders of the lung. *Lung* 169:123, 1991.
18. Robinson M, Ahn MS, Rounds JD, *et al.*: Parenteral glutathione monoester enhances tissue antioxidant stores. *JPEN J Parenter Enteral Nutr* 16:413, 1992.
19. Ferrari R, Ceconi C, Curello S, *et al.*: Oxygen free radicals and myocardial damage: protective role of thiol containing agents. *Am J Med* 91(suppl 3C):95S, 1991.
20. Henderson A, Hayes P: Acetylcysteine as a cytoprotective antioxidant in patients with severe sepsis: potential new use for an old drug. *Ann Pharmacother* 28:1086, 1994.

21. Suter PM, Domenighetti G, Schaller MD, *et al.*: *N*-Acetylcysteine enhances recovery from acute lung injury in man: a randomized, double-blind placebo-controlled clinical study. *Chest* 105:190, 1994.
22. Meydani M: Vitamin E. *Lancet* 345:170, 1995.
23. Herbert V, Shaw S, Jayatilleke E: Vitamin C supplements are harmful to lethal for over 10% of Americans with high iron stores. *FASEB J* 8:A678, 1994.
24. Halliwell B, Gutteridge JMC: Role of free radicals and catalytic metal ions in human disease. *Methods Enzymol* 186:1, 1990.
25. Herbert V, Shaw S, Jayatilleke E, Stopler-Kasdan T: Most free-radical injury is iron-related: it is promoted by iron, hemin, haloferritin and vitamin C, and inhibited by desferrioxamine and apoferritin. *Stem Cells* 12:289, 1994.

Oxidant Stress

26. Smith CV: Correlations and apparent contradictions in assessment of oxidant stress in vivo. *Free Radic Biol Med* 10:217, 1991.
27. Gutteridge JMC: Free radicals in disease processes: a compilation of cause and consequence. *Free Radic Res Commun* 19:41, 1993.
28. Weitz ZW, Birnbaum AI, Sobotka PA, *et al.*: High breath pentane concentrations during acute myocardial infarction. *Lancet* 337:933, 1991.
29. Cross CE, van der Vilet A, O'Neill CA, Eiserich JP: Reactive oxygen species and the lung. *Lancet* 344:930, 1994.
30. Grace PA: Ischemia-reperfusion injury. *Br J Surg* 81:637, 1994.
31. Deitch EA: Multiple organ failure. *Ann Surg* 216:117, 1992.
32. Natanson C, Hoffman WD, Suffredini AF, *et al.*: Selected treatment strategies for septic shock based on proposed mechanisms of pathogenesis. *Ann Intern Med* 120: 771, 1994.

SUGGESTED READINGS

Center SA: Chronic liver disease: current concepts of disease mechanisms. *J Small Anim Pract* 40:106, 1999.

Davies KJA, Ursini F, eds.: The Oxygen Paradox. Padova, Italy: CLEUP University Press, 1995.

Freeman LM, Brown DJ, Rush JE: Assessment of degree of oxidative stress and antioxidant concentration in dogs with idiopathic dilated cardiomyopathy. *J Am Vet Med Assoc* 215:644, 1999.

Grisham MB: Reactive Metabolites of Oxygen and Nitrogen in Biology and Medicine. Austin, TX: RG Landes, 1992.

Halliwell B, Gutteridge JM: Free Radicals in Biology and Medicine, 2nd ed. Clarendon, England: Oxford University Press, 1989.

Impellizeri JA, Lau RE, Azzara FA: Fourteen week clinical evaluation of an oral antioxidant as a treatment for osteoarthritis secondary to canine hip dysplasia. *Vet Q* 20(suppl 1): S 107, 1998.

Lantz GC, Badylak SF, Hiles MC, *et al.*: Treatment of reperfusion injury in dogs with experimentally induced gastric dilatation-volvulus *Am J Vet Res* 53:1594, 1992.

Meydani SN, Hayek M, Wu D, *et al.*: Vitamin E and immune response in aged dogs. *In* Reinhart GA, Carey DP, eds.: Recent Advances in Canine and Feline Nutrition, vol II. Wilmington, OH: Orange Frazier Press, 1998, p 295.

Moslen MT, Smith CV: Free Radical Mechanisms of Tissue Injury. Boca Raton, FL: CRC Press, 1992.

Sies H, ed.: Oxidative Stress II: Oxidants and Antioxidants. New York: Academic Press, 1991.

Xiaobing F, Huimin T, Zhiyong S, *et al.*: Multiple organ injuries after abdominal high energy wounding in animals and the protective effect of antioxidants. *Chin Med Sci J* 7:86, 1992.

Yagi K, ed.: Active Oxygens, Lipid Peroxides, and Antioxidants. Boca Raton, FL: CRC Press, 1993.

4
The Gastrointestinal Barrier

R. A. Bowen

The gastrointestinal (GI) mucosa forms a barrier between the body and a lumenal environment, which not only contains nutrients, but also is laden with potentially hostile microorganisms and toxins. The challenge is to allow efficient transport of nutrients across the epithelium while rigorously excluding passage of harmful molecules and organisms. The exclusionary properties of the gastric and intestinal mucosa are referred to as the "gastrointestinal barrier."

It is clear that a number of primary GI diseases lead to disruption of the mucosal barrier, allowing escalation to systemic disease. It is equally clear that many systemic disease processes result in damage to the GI barrier, thereby adding further insult to an already compromised system. Understanding the nature of the barrier can assist in predicting such events and aid in prophylactic or active therapies.

THE NORMAL GI MUCOSA

Sheets of epithelial cells that form the defining structure of the mucosa line the alimentary canal. With few exceptions, epithelial cells in the stomach and intestines are circumferentially tied to one another by tight junctions, which seal the paracellular spaces and thereby establish the basic barrier. Throughout the digestive tube, maintenance of an intact epithelium is thus critical to the integrity of the barrier. In general, toxins and microorganisms that are able to breach the single layer of epithelial cells have unimpeded access to the systemic circulation.

Epithelial Cell Dynamics

The GI epithelium is populated by a variety of functionally mature cells derived from proliferation of stem cells. Many of these cells, including mucous cells in the stomach and absorptive cells in the small intestine, show rapid turnover rates, and maintenance of epithelial integrity thus requires a precise balance between cell proliferation and cell death.

In the epithelium of the stomach, stem cells in the middle of the gastric glands proliferate to repopulate mucous neck and surface cells, which are replaced every 2 to 4 days. The same stem cells probably are also the source of parietal, chief (pepsinogen-secreting) and G (gastrin-secreting) cells that populate the lower reaches of the glands.

Epithelial cell dynamics of the small intestine have been well studied. Fixed stem cells located within each crypt proliferate continually to supply cells that then differentiate into absorptive enterocytes, mucous-secreting goblet cells, enteroendocrine cells, and Paneth cells. Except for Paneth cells, which remain in the crypts, the other cells differentiate into their mature forms as they migrate up from the crypts to replace cells extruded from the tips of the villi. This migration takes about 3 to 6 days. A similar system exists in the colon, with stem cells located toward that base of the crypts providing a zone of proliferating cells that migrate up to replace extruded neck and surface cells.

Many local and systemic factors influence the processes of epithelial cell proliferation, differentiation, and death. Several of the enteric hormones, including gastrin, have been demonstrated to enhance rates of proliferation. Different forms of injury to the epithelium can lead to either enhanced or suppressed rates of cell proliferation. For example, it has been demonstrated that resection of a portion of the canine small intestine is followed by epithelial cell hyperplasia and increased villous length in animals fed orally. Animals fed parenterally failed to show the same compensatory hyperplasia, indicating that, among other factors, local nutrients play an important role in cell dynamics.

Mucosal Permeability

There are two routes for transport across the epithelium of the GI tract: through the plasma membranes and cytosol of the epithelial cells (transcellular) and across tight junctions between epithelial cells (paracellular). Both routes, for instance, transport some molecules, such as water. Tight junctions seem to be essentially impermeable to ions and most organic molecules, which are transported by the transcellular route via a large array of membrane transporters.

Within the intestine, there is a proximal-to-distal gradient in osmotic permeability, with a decrease in effective pore size from duodenum to colon. This means that the duodenum is much more "leaky" to water than the ileum and that the ileum is more leaky than the colon. These regional differences in permeability are due almost entirely to differences in conductivity across the paracellular path.

NATURE OF THE MUCOSAL BARRIER

The GI barrier can be conceived as having intrinsic and extrinsic properties. The intrinsic barrier is composed of the epithelial cells themselves, along with their associated tight junctions. Tight junctions used to be viewed as passive structures akin to welds, but recent studies indicate that these structures are quite dynamic, and their permeability may be regulated by a number of factors that affect the epithelial cells. As might be anticipated, there is diversity among different types of epithelial cells in specific barrier functions. For example, the apical plasma membranes of gastric parietal and chief cells have atypically low permeability to protons, which probably aids in preventing damaging back diffusion of acid into the cells. Additionally, a large number of hormones, cytokines, and even nutrients have been demonstrated in experimental models to modulate epithelial cell integrity and thus barrier function.

Extrinsic barrier functions are secretions and other influences that are not physically part of the epithelium. These attributes likely have the greatest potential for therapeutic manipulation.

Mucus and Bicarbonate

The entire GI epithelium is coated with mucus, which is synthesized by cells that form part of the epithelium. Mucus serves an important role in mitigating shear stresses on the epithelium and contributes to barrier function in several ways. The abundant carbohydrates on mucin molecules bind to bacteria, which aids in preventing epithelial colonization and, by causing aggregation, accelerates clearance. Diffusion of hydrophilic molecules is considerably lower in mucus than in aqueous solution, which is thought to retard diffusion of a variety of damaging chemicals, including gastric acid, to the epithelial surface.

In addition to being coated with a mucous layer, gastric and duodenal epithelial cells secrete bicarbonate ion on their apical faces. This serves to maintain a neutral pH along the epithelial plasma membrane, even though highly acidic conditions exist in the lumen.

Finally, most of the GI tract is bathed in secretory immunoglobulin A (IgA). This class of antibody is secreted from subepithelial plasma cells and transcytosed across the epithelium into the lumen. Lumenal IgA provides an antigenic barrier by binding bacteria and other antigens. Importantly, this barrier function is specific for particular antigens and requires previous exposure for development of the response.

Hormones and Cytokines

Normal proliferation of gastric and intestinal epithelial cells, as well as proliferation in response to injury such as ulceration, is known to be affected by a large number of endocrine and paracrine factors.

Prostaglandins, particularly prostaglandin E_2 and prostacyclin have long been known to have "cytoprotective" effects on the GI epithelium. A common clinical correlate in many mammals is that use of aspirin and other nonsteroidal anti-inflammatory drugs (NSAIDs), which inhibit prostaglandin synthesis, are commonly associated with gastric erosions and ulcers. Dogs and cats are particularly sensitive to this side effect. Prostaglandins are synthesized within the mucosa from arachidonic acid, through the action of cyclooxygenases. Their cytoprotective effect appears to result from a complex ability to stimulate mucosal mucous and bicarbonate secretion, to increase mucosal blood flow and, particularly in the stomach, to limit back diffusion of acid into the epithelium. Considerable effort is underway to develop NSAIDs that fail to inhibit mucosal prostaglandin synthesis.

Two peptides that have received attention for their potential role in barrier maintenance are epidermal growth factor (EGF) and transforming growth factor-α (TGF-α). EGF is secreted in saliva and from duodenal glands, and TGF-α is produced by gastric epithelial cells. Both peptides bind to a common receptor and stimulate epithelial cell proliferation. In the stomach, they also enhance mucous secretion and inhibit acid production. Other cytokines such as fibroblast growth factor and hepatocyte growth factor enhance healing of GI ulcers in experimental models.

Trefoil proteins are a family of small peptides that are secreted abundantly by goblet cells in the gastric and intestinal mucosa and coat the apical face of the epithelial cells. Their distinctive molecular structure appears to render them resistant to proteolytic destruction. A number of studies have demonstrated that trefoil peptides play an important role in mucosal integrity and repair of lesions, and in limiting epithelial cell proliferation. They have been shown to protect the epithelium from a broad range of toxic chemicals and drugs. Trefoil peptides also appear to be a central player in the restitution phase of epithelial damage repair, where epithelial cells flatten and migrate from the wound edge to cover denuded areas. Mice with targeted deletions in trefoil genes showed exaggerated responses to mild chemical injury and delayed mucosal healing.

Another molecule that plays a crucial role in mucosal integrity and barrier function is nitric oxide (NO). Paradoxically, NO also contributes to mucosal injury in a number of digestive diseases. This molecule is synthesized from arginine through the action of one of three isoforms of nitric oxide synthease (NOS). Much of the clinical research in this area has focused on understanding the effects of applying NO donors such as glyceryltrinitrate or NOS inhibitors. In several models, NO donors significantly reduced the severity of mucosal injury induced by toxic chemicals (*e.g.*, ethanol) or associated with ischemia and reperfusion. Similarly, healing of gastric ulcers in rats has been accelerated by application of NO donors. Another intriguing observation is that coadministration of NO donors and NSAIDs results in anti-inflammatory properties comparable to NSAIDs alone, but with less damage to the GI mucosa. NOS inhibitors are under investigation for treatment of situations in which NO is overproduced and contributes to mucosal injury.

Antibiotic Peptides

An important part of barrier function is to prevent transit of bacteria from the lumen through the epithelium. Paneth cells are epithelial granulocytes located in small intestinal crypts of many mammals. They synthesize and secrete several antimicrobial peptides, chief among them isoforms of α-defensins known also as cryptdins ("crypt defensin"). These peptides have antimicrobial activity against of number of potential pathogens, including several genera of bacteria, some yeasts, and *Giardia* trophozoites. Their mechanism of action is likely similar to neutrophilic α-defensins, which permeabilize target cell membranes.

DISRUPTION OF BARRIER FUNCTION

Ischemia and Reperfusion Injury

Varying degrees of damage to the GI barrier due to ischemia and reperfusion injury is a common and serious condition in many critical care patients. Ischemia occurs when blood flow is insufficient to deliver an amount of oxygen and nutrients necessary for maintenance of cell integrity. Reperfusion injury occurs when blood flow is restored to ischemic tissue.

Gastrointestinal ischemia results from two fundamental types of disorders. Nonocclusive ischemia results from systemic conditions such as circulatory shock, sepsis, or cardiac insufficiency. Occlusive ischemia refers to conditions that directly block the vascular system of the GI tract, such as strangulation, volvulus, or embolism. In both cases, the epithelial barrier can be compromised, most likely due to direct effects of tissue hypoxia.

Reperfusion injury to the GI wall, especially the mucosa, is thought to be due primarily to generation of reactive oxygen species, including superoxide, hydrogen peroxide, and hydroxyl radicals (see Chapter 3). These oxidants are generated within the mucosa and also in the numerous local leukocytes activated during the course of ischemia.

Oxygen-derived free radicals generated during reperfusion initiate a series of events that causes mucosal damage and disruption of the barrier. They directly damage cell membranes by forming lipid peroxides, which also leads to production of a number of inflammatory mediators derived from phospholipids (*e.g.*, platelet-activating factor and leukotrienes). These proinflammatory agents function as chemoattractants for neutrophils, which migrate into the mucosa, release their own reactive oxygen metabolites, and cause further damage to the intrinsic epithelial barrier. An initially minor effect from ischemia is thus amplified into significant damage to barrier function. Additionally, the inflammatory mediators generated in the GI tract can harm distant tissues.

The observed effects of ischemia-reperfusion injury range from increased vascular permeability and consequent subepithelial edema, to massive loss of epithelial cells and villi. Even relatively mild damage to the epithelium disrupts barrier function and can lead to translocation of bacteria and toxins from the lumen into the systemic circulation. A number of treatments are being developed and tested to prevent this cascade of damage, including application of antioxidants such as superoxide dismutase and use of drugs such as platelet-activating factor antagonists to block the effect of inflammatory mediators.

Neutrophils and Mucosal Injury

Diverse insults to the intestinal mucosa, including infectious processes, ischemia, and damaging chemicals, promote infiltration of neutrophils. This common end-point results because many types of injuries lead to local production of neutrophil chemoattractants such as leukotrienes, interleukins, and activated complement components. In response to chemoattractants, neutrophils migrate out of capillaries, infiltrate the subepithelial mucosa, and often transmigrate through the gastric or intestinal epithelium. In crossing the epithelium, neutrophils must break junctional complexes between epithelial cells. This "impalement" through tight junctions necessarily causes transient increases in permeability. When the insult is minor, the junctions reseal quickly, but transmigration of large numbers of neutrophils induces significant damage to barrier function. In addition to physically disrupting epithelial connections, infiltrating neutrophils themselves release reactive oxygen species and proteases that accentuate the damage to the epithelium and microvasculature. Blocking or suppressing the infiltration of neutrophils with such treatments as antibodies to integrins and other cell adhesion molecules may aid in protecting the mucosal barrier, but would likely have to be administered early in the course of disease.

Effects of Stress

Stress comes in a myriad of forms and is an integral part of all illness and trauma. The response to stress involves modulation of literally dozens of hormones and cytokines, as well as significant effects on neurotransmission. However, the foremost effect of stress is to decrease mucosal blood flow and thereby compromise the integrity of the mucosal barrier. Among other things, reduced mucosal blood flow suppresses production of mucus and bicarbonate and limits the ability to remove back-diffusing protons. As a consequence, significant stress is almost always associated with mucosal erosions, particularly in the stomach. A majority of these lesions are subclinical, but GI hemorrhage and sepsis are not infrequent consequences.

Restitution and Healing After Injury

The critical first task following disruption of the GI epithelium is to cover the denuded area and re-establish the intrinsic barrier. A process called restitution accomplishes this rapid restoration of epithelium; epithelial cells adjacent to the defect flatten and migrate over the exposed basement membrane. In the small intestine, this process is aided by a rapid contraction and shortening of the affected villi, which reduces the area of basement membrane that must be covered.

Restitution provides a rapid mechanism for covering a defect in the barrier and does not involve proliferation of epithelial cells. It results in an area that, while protected, is not physiologically functional. Healing requires that the epithelial cells on the margins of the defect proliferate, differentiate, and migrate into the damaged area to restore the normal cellular architecture and function.

Restitution has been shown to be stimulated by a number of mostly paracrine regulators. Local prostaglandins and trefoil proteins are clearly involved in this process, and suppression of their production significantly delays restitution. Another group of molecules involved in restitution includes the polyamines such as spermine, spermidine, and putrescine. These molecules are present in many diets and also synthesized by the GI mucosa. Enteral administration of polyamines has been shown in experimental models to accelerate restitution and healing of mucosal lesions.

SUGGESTED READINGS

Blikslager AT, Roberts MC: Mechanisms of intestinal mucosal repair. *J Am Vet Med Assoc* 211:1437, 1997.

Dieckgraefe BK, Stenson WF, Alpers DH: Gastrointestinal epithelial response to injury. *Curr Opin Gastroenterol* 12:109, 1996.

Filep J, Herman F, Braquet P, Mozes T: Increased levels of platelet-activating factor in blood following intestinal ischemia in the dog. *Biochem Biophys Res Commun* 158: 353, 1989.

Gayle JM, Blikslager AT, Jones SL: Role of neutrophils in intestinal mucosal injury. *J Am Vet Med Assoc* 217:498, 2000.

Kubes P, Hunter J, Granger ND: Ischemia/reperfusion-induced feline intestinal dysfunction: importance of granulocyte recruitment. *Gastroenterology* 103:807, 1992.

Lichtenberger LM: The hydrophobic barrier properties of gastrointestinal mucus. *Ann Review Physiol* 57:565, 1995.

Mashimo H, Wu D, Podolsky DK, Fishman M: Impaired defense of intestinal mucosa in mice lacking intestinal trefoil factor. *Science* 274:262, 1996.

Moore RM: Clinical relevance of intestinal reprefusion injury in horses. *J Am Vet Med Assoc* 211:1362, 1997.

Murphy MS: Growth factors and the gastrointestinal tract. *Nutrition* 14:771, 1998.

Muscara MN, Wallace JL: Nitric oxide V. Therapeutic potential of nitric oxide donors and inhibitors. *Am J Physiol* 276:G1313, 1999.

Thompson JS: The intestinal response to critical illness. *Am J Gastroenterol* 90:190, 1995.

Wallace JL, Miller MJ: Nitric oxide in mucosal defense: a little goes a long way. *Gastroenterology* 119:515, 2000.

5
Receptor Physiology

DeWayne Townsend, IV and David R. Brown

INTRODUCTION

All cells in living organisms can potentially communicate with each other in distance and time. They synthesize and release a wide array of chemically diverse signaling molecules, such as neurotransmitters, growth factors, cytokines, and hormones. These molecules reach a concentration in the extracellular fluid surrounding target cells that is sufficient to trigger cellular responses. Receptors allow cells to recognize specific extracellular signaling molecules, which we will henceforth refer to as *endogenous ligands*. Information encoded in the ligand-receptor recognition event is subsequently conveyed to the interior of the cell where it is transduced and amplified, resulting in altered cellular function.

Many drugs used in critical care medicine are, in essence, chemical analogs of endogenous ligands that have accepted therapeutic utility. Drugs acting as agonists stimulate receptors and produce biologic responses of varying magnitudes. Nearly all known endogenous ligands act as agonists. Minor modifications in a ligand or drug molecule can diminish its ability to produce a maximal activation; in other words, drug agonism exists on a continuum. Drugs interacting with a common receptor that produce submaximal activation are termed partial *agonists*, and drugs capable of occupying a receptor but incapable of producing a biologic response are termed *antagonists*. Drugs acting as competitive antagonists have great clinical importance as reversal agents (such as naloxone does in reversing the respiratory depressant action of morphine at opioid receptors) or in interrupting the actions of endogenous agonists (such as vecuronium does to acetylcholine neurotransmission at nicotinic cholinergic receptors).

This chapter is intended to update the clinician in some recent advances and evolving concepts that are occurring in the field of receptor biology, particularly in the context of the critically ill patient. The drug-receptor concept and its theoretical underpinnings were formulated beginning in the late 19th century and continue to undergo revisions as new information is obtained. Receptors are now defined functionally by strict pharmacologic criteria, that is, by relative potencies of agonists, selective antagonism, and stereoselectivity. Under this definition, it is important to note that many important drug targets are not receptors in the pharmacologic sense. Some examples of commonly used drugs or drug classes that do not act through receptors to produce their effects are listed in Table 5-1. Properly functioning receptors and their associated signal transduction pathways are critical for homeostasis and health. They may be inappropri-

Table 5-1. Representative Drugs That Do Not Act Through Receptors

Drug or Drug Class	Drug Target
Antibiotics	Wide variety of bacterial enzymes and transport molecules
Captopril, enalapril	Angiotensin-converting enzyme
Cardiac antiarrhythmic drugs	Voltage-gated cardiac ion channels
Cardiac glycosides	Sodium-potassium ATPase
Fluoxetine (Prozac)	Serotonin transport protein
Furosemide, thiazides, and related diuretics	Renal ion transport proteins
Local anesthetics	Voltage-gated sodium channel
Methylxanthines, such as theophylline	Phosphodiesterase enzymes
Neostigmine; edrophonium	Acetylcholinesterase
Nonsteroidal anti-inflammatory drugs	Cyclooxygenase enzymes
Omeprazole	Hydrogen-potassium ATPase
Plasma volume expanders	Blood

ately activated or unresponsive in the critically ill patient. Not only do receptors play a key role in the pathophysiologic underpinnings of several diseases, they offer us the ability to modify a wide variety of disease processes.

CLASSES OF RECEPTORS

G-Protein–Coupled Receptors (GPCR)

Receptors that are coupled to intracellular guanine nucleotide-binding proteins, the so-called G-protein–coupled receptors (GPCRs) constitute a large superfamily of glycoproteins that consists of some 1000 to 2000 members. Although individual GPCRs specifically recognize a particular molecule or small group of chemically related molecules, as a whole this superfamily of receptors is activated by a wide variety of substances ranging from large proteins (thrombin) to small soluble chemicals (epinephrine) and even subatomic particles (photons).[1,2] Nevertheless, GPCRs have several structural characteristics in common. Perhaps the most striking characteristic is their seven transmembrane domains, which anchor the receptor protein in a cell plasma membrane (Fig. 5-1). These transmembrane domains are clustered together within the membrane, and in many receptors, these domains form a hydrophilic pocket that is in contact with the extracellular fluid. The amino (N)-terminus of GPCRs is located extracellularly, as are three smaller extracellular loops. Amino acids within these extracellular regions and hydrophilic pocket often form a binding region for a receptor's particular endogenous ligand.[3]

Similar to the extracellular face of GPCRs, the intracellular surface of GPCR contains a long carboxy (C)-terminus and three intracellular loops. These

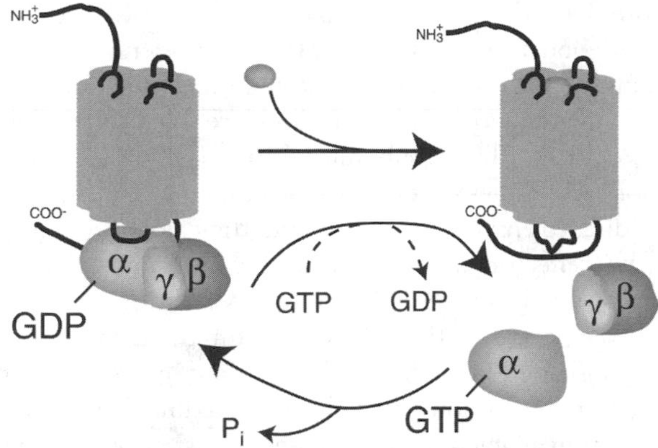

Figure 5-1
Model of G-protein–coupled receptor activation. Agonist is depicted by oval and intracellular G-protein subunits are shown. See text for details.

loops are generally quite short, but in some GPCRs the third intracellular loop can be quite long. The intracellular regions of GPCR interact with a heterotrimeric molecule, consisting of α, β, and γ subunits. The α subunit is a guanine nucleotide-binding protein (G-protein). In addition to binding guanosine triphosphate (GTP), it has the ability to enzymatically convert GTP to guanosine diphosphate (GDP); that is, it has GTPase activity.[4] There are approximately 20 distinct α subunits, divided into three major classes (G_s, G_i, and $G_{q/11}$). In addition, there are about 5 β subunits and 11 γ subunits. It is the α subunit that determines the specificity of the interaction between the G-protein and the receptor itself.[5] The properties of the intracellular domains of a particular GPCR determine which type(s) of G-protein will interact with the receptor and therefore what downstream effector pathways will be affected.[3]

Binding of an endogenous ligand or an agonist drug to the extracellular binding domain of a GCPR will change the conformation of the receptor. This conformational change is conveyed across the cell membrane and induces the G protein α subunit to exchange a molecule of GDP, already bound to the subunit, for GTP. GTP binding to the α subunit results in the dissociation of the G protein into two separate proteins: an α subunit and a β/γ subunit. Both of these proteins then carry out a wide variety of preprogrammed responses through a wide diversity of effector systems (*i.e.*, enzymes in biochemical pathways, ion channels, etc.) that modulate cellular function. Stimulated receptors are able to activate multiple G-proteins, which greatly amplifies the small signal produced by the agonist-receptor interaction.[6] The heterotrimeric G-proteins are activated for only a short period of time, however. The intrinsic GTPase activity of the α subunit eventually hydrolyzes GTP to GDP. When this subunit enters the GDP bound form, it reassociates with the β/γ subunits. The reassembled G-protein is then ready to interact with another GPCR.

The G-protein–coupled receptors are linked to a variety of intracellular second messenger pathways, chiefly through the α subunit. The G_s class of α subunit (G_s) stimulates the enzyme adenylate cyclase, which catalyzes the production of the second messenger molecule cyclic adenosine monophosphate (cAMP); this same enzyme is inhibited by α subunits of the G_i class. Cyclic AMP mediates many cellular functions, most of which are the result of the activation of protein kinase A (PKA). The α subunits of the $G_{q/11}$ class mediate the release of another major second messenger molecule, calcium. Calcium affects cellular processes by binding to enzymes directly or via the calcium-binding protein calmodulin. Together, effector pathways linked to cAMP and calcium underlie the effects mediated by a large number of GPCRs. In addition to the α subunit, the β/γ subunits also appear to activate a significant number of effector systems, including cell membrane ion channels.[6] Within any given tissue, the ability of the agonist-receptor interaction to produce a maximal effect depends on the number of receptors available to recognize an agonist as well as the levels of G-proteins and downstream second messenger molecules that are linked to receptor stimulation.[7]

Ion Channel Receptors

To function properly, all cells in the body must maintain an electrical potential ("voltage") across their plasma membranes. In excitable cells, such as neurons and muscle cells, the membrane potential can undergo transient depolarization, which, if it attains a sufficient magnitude, is propagated along the length of the cell. These "action potentials" can affect major cellular functions, such as the release of neurotransmitters or muscle contraction. Action potentials are produced after the excitable cell membrane reaches a threshold for depolarization; such depolarizations are often mediated by ligand-gated ion channels. Agonist binding to these receptors is associated with the production of an ionic current across the cell membrane, leading to a change in membrane potential. The ability to recognize a particular endogenous ligand or drug molecule makes these ion channels distinct from many other types of ion channels, and this is one characteristic that defines them as receptors. Some of these receptors allow cations to enter the cell, resulting in membrane depolarization, which in turn may lead to the production of an action potential. An example of this type of receptor is the nicotinic cholinergic receptor present in skeletal muscle and autonomic ganglia. These receptors conduct cations across cell membranes after binding to two acetylcholine molecules; the resulting action potentials evoke muscle contraction and transmitter release from ganglia, respectively. Glutamate receptors in the central nervous system also conduct cations; these receptors are blocked by certain sedatives and dissociative anesthetics such as barbiturates or ketamine. Another class of ion channel receptors is permeable to anions; currents mediated by them tend to stabilize the membrane potential, inhibiting cellular activation. An example of this type of ion channel receptor is the A subtype of the γ-aminobutyric acid ($GABA_A$) receptor. After GABA binds to it, the receptor permits the influx of chloride ions, causing neuronal inhibition. Benzodiazepines and barbiturates, respectively, modulate the frequency at which the chloride channel opens and the duration of time the channel remains open

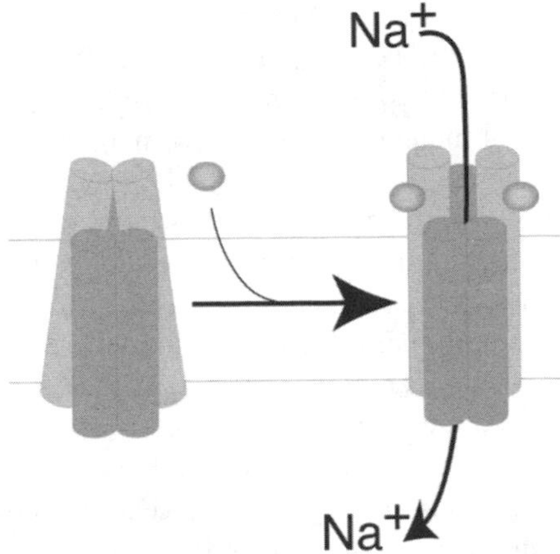

Figure 5-2
Model for ion channel receptor showing activation of a sodium conductance after drug (oval) binding. See text for details.

in response to GABA. As is the case with many drugs that interact with ion channel receptors, barbiturates and benzodiazapines bind to $GABA_A$ receptors at sites distinct from the binding site for the endogenous ligand, GABA.

Both classes of receptor proteins are composed of five subunits, with a pore in the center that allows ions to selectively pass through when agonist is bound (Fig. 5-2). The endogenous ligands for these receptors are generally small molecules, which, after their release into the extracellular fluid, are quickly removed by enzymes or transport proteins. Ion channel receptors are unique in that their activation has an immediate and direct effect on cellular function. The cellular consequences of ion channel receptor stimulation, that is, the flux of millions of ions across the cell membrane in a short period of time, occur within milliseconds of agonist binding, whereas agonist effects mediated by GPCRs are detected in seconds to minutes.

Enzyme-Linked Receptors

Although GPCRs are often linked through G-proteins to enzyme-catalyzed biochemical cascades that serve to amplify the agonist-receptor binding event, other families of receptor proteins contain an intrinsic enzymatic activity within their amino acid sequence. These receptors are often divided into two groups: the receptor tyrosine kinases (RTKs) and the guanylyl cyclases (GCs). The GCs can be further classified as soluble and membrane-bound forms; the soluble GC will be discussed later.[8] Unlike GPCRs, these two classes of receptor proteins pass through the cell membrane only once. Like GPCRs, they have an extracellular N-terminus that is involved in the binding of their respective endogenous ligands. Moreover, their C-termini are located on the intracellular side of the cell membrane; some amino acids in the C-terminus form a catalytic domain and others can associate with several intracellular proteins involved in signal transduction.[9] The ligands for these receptors are generally water-soluble peptides (such as atrial natriuretic peptide, an endogenous GC ligand) or proteins (such as insulin, an endogenous ligand for the insulin RTK), but in some instances they bind integral membrane proteins in neighboring cells.[8,10]

Activation of membrane-bound GCs or RTKs requires that two identical receptor molecules combine to form a receptor homodimer. Some dimers are created by two receptors binding to a single molecule of the endogenous ligand (as is the case with receptors for platelet-derived growth factor); others are formed by changes in receptor conformation that favor receptor dimer (the epidermal growth factor receptor serves as an example of this mechanism); or they may be biosynthesized as dimers (such as is the case with the insulin receptor). Dimerization allows the catalytic domains of the two receptor monomers to interact and form a functional enzyme (Fig. 5-3). The enzymatic activity of the receptor GCs result in the formation of cyclic guanosine monophosphate (cGMP), which functions as a second messenger within the cell. Like cAMP, cGMP alters cellular function by the activation of a protein kinase G pathway. The RTKs also activate a cascade of intracellular protein kinases by catalyzing the addition of a phosphate group on tyrosine residues of key intracellular proteins, but these receptors do not produce a second messenger. The RTK cascades rely on protein-to-protein interactions to activate downstream effectors. Proteins phosphorylated in these cascades are important in both cell proliferation and differentiation. It should be mentioned that receptor tyrosine phosphatases also exist. Activation of these receptors catalyzes the removal of phosphate groups from tyrosine residues in proteins. These receptors, which include the common lymphocyte antigen CD45, have structural features similar to cell adhesion molecules, and their potentially important roles in health and disease are now under intense investigation.[11]

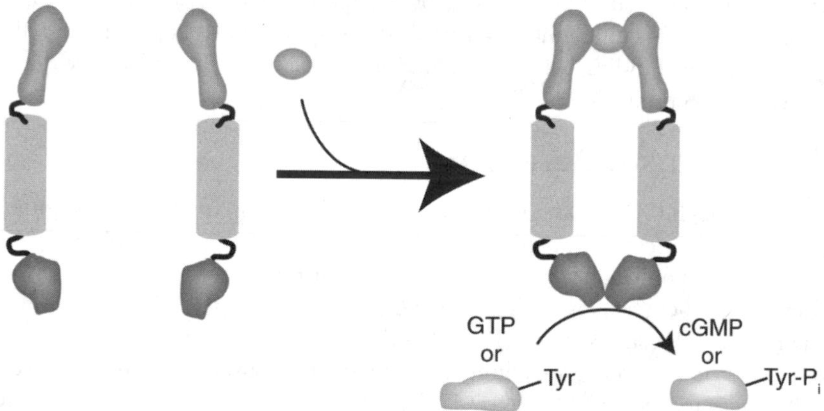

Figure 5-3
Model of enzyme-linked receptor with one transmembrane domain. Agonist (right oval) binding induces receptor homodimerization and intracellular catalytic activity. The model is pertinent to both guanylyl cyclase rceptors and receptor tyrosine (tyr) kinases.

The gaseous transmitter substance, nitric oxide (NO), has an important role in vasodilation, neurotransmission, and immune function, and, when produced in high concentrations, it can act as a free radical in host defense processes.[12] The nonpolar NO freely diffuses across cell membranes to reach its intracellular receptor, the soluble GC present in the cell cytoplasm. This receptor consists of two subunits that combine around a heme group. On activation by NO, the soluble GC produces cGMP, which activates cellular processes similar to those activated by the membrane-bound guanylyl cyclase.[8]

Nuclear Factor Receptors

Another major superfamily of receptors in mammalian cells includes the nuclear factor receptors. These receptors, which recognize steroid hormones, vitamin A and its derivatives, thyroid hormones, or a group of lipid-soluble molecules called peroxisome-proliferator activators, are located in the cell cytoplasm or nucleus, rather than on cell membranes. Accordingly, the endogenous ligands and drugs that interact with these receptors are very hydrophobic, a property that allows them to freely cross the cell membrane and gain access to the receptors within the cell.

The most understood class of receptors, the steroid hormone receptors, possess at least two separate domains that allow them to bind hormone and specific DNA sequences in genes called *responsive elements* that regulate gene transcription (Fig. 5-4). Like the enzyme-linked receptors discussed above, steroid receptors dimerize when bound to agonist ligands, which allows them to translocate from the cytoplasm to the nucleus where the hormone-receptor complex can bind to DNA.[13] Once the activated receptor binds to its response element; the hormone-receptor-DNA complex can interact with a variety of other nuclear proteins, which act to stabilize RNA polymerase II in the promoter region of the gene. This effect leads to an increase in the transcription of genes that contain response elements within their promoter.[14]

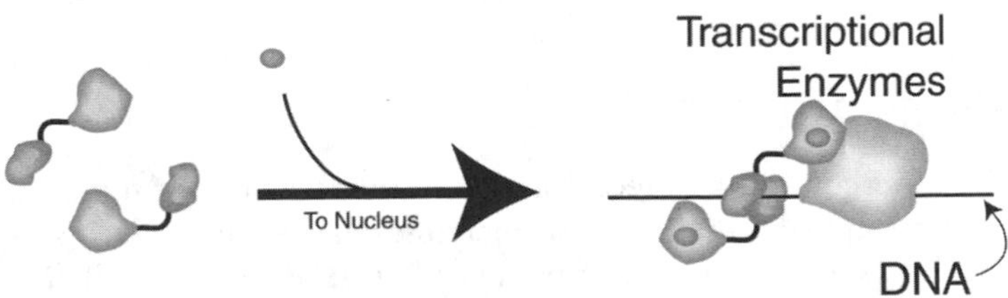

Figure 5-4
Model of nuclear factor receptor. Receptor monomers unbound to hormone exist in cytoplasm. Binding of hormone (oval) induces receptor homodimerization and translocation of the hormone-receptor complex to the nucleus, where it binds to specific responsive elements on DNA to enhance gene transcription. Additional details can be found in the text.

Considering the period of time that must elapse for alterations in gene transcription to influence the production of messenger RNA, the translation of RNA to proteins, and the often extensive post-translational processing of proteins before the proteins are functional, it is not surprising that cellular responses to the stimulation of nuclear factor receptors occur on a time scale of minutes to hours and thus are slow relative to the other families of receptors described above.

Receptor Regulation and Disease

The excessive stimulation of receptors by endogenous ligands or through continuous drug administration in the course of some diseases may result in receptor down-regulation, whereas lack of stimulation often increases receptor numbers. In critical care medicine, continuous exposure of adrenergic receptors by norepinephrine and epinephrine is not uncommon. This leads to clinically significant alterations in cardiovascular responses to drugs that target these receptors, such as "tolerance," that is, decreased drug sensitivity with continued drug administration, which is particularly apparent after the administration of drugs acting as full agonists. In addition, chronic diseases such as congestive heart failure are associated with high levels of circulating catecholamines, which can result in adrenergic receptor dysfunction.[15]

The mechanisms underlying ligand-mediated receptor regulation are best described for GPCRs, but they are a current topic of research for other receptor families as well.[16,17] As mentioned above, the activation of GPCRs results in the breakdown of a multi-subunit G-protein. One of the proteins activated by the β/γ-subunit is the G-protein–coupled receptor kinase (GRK). As its name implies, this protein phosphorylates GPCRs that are in the active conformation. Receptor phosphorylation prevents the receptor from activating any more G-proteins; in addition to this receptor-transducer uncoupling, the phosphorylated receptor attains an affinity for a class of proteins called *arrestins*. The arrestins bind to both phosphorylated receptors and cytoskeletal components and appear to be involved in the endocytosis of GPCRs, making them unavailable for binding with extracellular ligands.[2,16] Internalization is also a common form of down-regulation for RTKs.[17] The internalization of receptors occurs relatively rapidly, often taking place only minutes after agonist stimulation. Table 5-2 lists drugs whose actions are mediated by receptors.

RECEPTORS AND DISEASE

Given the important role that receptors play in the regulation of normal physiology, it is not surprising that receptor function changes in various physiologic and pathophysiologic states. This is particularly true for the critically ill patient where altered receptor function may dictate which therapeutic options will be most effective. This final section will focus on some of the general roles members of each receptor superfamily play in various disease processes.

Subtle mutations in receptor sequences or their associated signal transduction pathways occurring as the result of genetic mutations can result in profound changes in receptor function, leading to disease or altered responses to drugs in

Table 5-2. Representative Drugs Whose Actions Are Mediated by Receptors

Drug	Receptor Type (Receptor Family)
Albuterol	β_2-adrenergic receptor (GPCR)
Atropine	Muscarinic cholinergic receptors (GPCR)
Cimetidine, famotidine, ranitidine	H_2-histamine receptor (GPCR)
Dobutamine	α_1-Adrenergic receptor (GPCR)
Propranolol	β_1-adrenergic receptors (GPCR)
Neuromuscular blockers (atracurium, vecuronium)	Nicotinic cholinergic receptor (ion channel receptor)
Barbiturates, ketamine	NMDA-type glutamate receptor (ion channel receptor)
Insulin	Insulin receptor (receptor tyrosine kinase)
Tumor necrosis factor (TNF)	TNF receptor (receptor tyrosine kinase)
Dexamethasone	Glucocorticoid receptor (nuclear receptor)
Levothyroxine	Thyroid receptor (nuclear receptor)

individual patients.[18] For example, mutations in the V_2-vasopressin receptor are now known to be responsible for some of the manifestations of nephrogenic diabetes insipidus.[19] The fields of pharmacogenetics and pharmacogenomics are offering genetic explanations for idiosyncratic drug effects in humans and clues for the discovery of new drugs capable of treating specific patient subpopulations, and this knowledge base will eventually extend to veterinary medicine as well.[20,21] Table 5-3 contains a brief list of several receptor-mediated disease conditions.

The GPCRs are often involved in the pathophysiology and treatment of

Table 5-3. Some Diseases Linked to Receptor Dysfunction

Disease	Receptor (Receptor Family)
Anaphylaxis	H_1-histamine receptor; leukotriene receptors (GPCR)
Congestive heart failure	Adrenergic receptors (GPCR)
Hyperthyroidism	Thyroid-stimulating hormone receptor (GPCR)
Stress-related gastrointestinal ulceration	H_2-histamine receptor (GPCR)
Diabetes insipidus	Vasopressin receptor (GPCR)
Myasthenia gravis	Nicotinic cholinergic receptor (ion channel receptor)
Status epilepticus	$GABA_A$ receptor (ion channel receptor)
Diabetes mellitus, type 2	Insulin receptor (RTK)

several diseases commonly encountered in critical care medicine. The minute-to-minute regulation of the cardiovascular and respiratory systems relies heavily on adrenergic receptors, all of which are GPCRs. These same receptors are also used to stabilize the critically ill patient. G-protein–coupled receptors also play a significant role in the pathophysiology of several endocrine disorders, such as those involving the parathyroid hormone and calcitonin receptors, which control body calcium homeostasis.[22] Inflammation and allergy are mediated by several different GPCRs, including the H_1-histamine receptor and several different leukotriene receptors. The H_2-histamine receptors, on the other hand, may mediate aspects of stress-related gastrointestinal ulceration, and H_2-histamine receptor blockers are effective in mitigating this condition.

Ion channel receptors are common in the peripheral and central nervous systems. Some of these receptors may be involved in the pathogenesis of epilepsy. Indeed, inappropriate activation of excitatory ion channel receptors can result in uncontrolled neuronal stimulation, leading to generalized seizures. Strychnine, for example, blocks the inhibitory ion channel receptor for glycine and produces convulsions. In myasthenia gravis, on the other hand, skeletal muscle weakness is attributable to decreased cholinergic transmission at nicotinic cholinergic receptors in the neuromuscular junction because these receptors are under autoimmune attack.[23]

Insulin receptor dysfunction in non-insulin–dependent (type 2) diabetes mellitus is the best described example of an enzyme-linked receptor leading to a disease state. In this form of diabetes, cells expressing the insulin receptor become unresponsive to the presence of insulin, due in part to the uncoupling of the receptor from its intracellular signal transduction pathway.[17] Several other members of the RTK receptor family are proto-oncogenes, and mutations in these proteins can lead to uncontrolled cell proliferation and neoplasia.

The down-regulation of nuclear factor receptors after long-term administration of their cognate ligands, such as occurs with glucocorticoid receptors in secondary adrenocortical insufficiency, is a frequent cause of disease. However, the involvement of nuclear factor receptors in chronic disease conditions, such as asthma, atherosclerosis, cancer, obesity, and osteoporosis is under increasing scrutiny. Their involvement in these and other disease states will certainly expand in coming years.

SUMMARY

Receptors are critical elements in the physiologic regulation of homeostatic balance and in the actions of drugs. New receptors and their endogenous ligands continue to be discovered and characterized, which will lead to the design and development of new drugs. Furthermore, abnormalities in receptors and their associated signal transduction pathways have been elucidated that are clearly associated with acute and chronic diseases. Because there is considerable "cross-talk" between members of the same and different receptor superfamilies, changes in the function of a particular receptor may have an impact on other receptor systems. Because the actions of agonists on members of different receptor superfamilies have different temporal characteristics, interventions to treat diseases where receptors are involved should take into account both short- and long-term regulatory mechanisms associated with these diverse receptor systems and their effectors.

REFERENCES

1. Bockaert J, Pin JP: Molecular tinkering of G protein-coupled receptors: an evolutionary success. *EMBO J* 18:1723, 1999.
2. Morris AJ, Malbon CC: Physiological regulation of G protein-linked signaling. *Physiol Rev* 79:1373, 1999.
3. Gether U. Uncovering molecular mechanisms involved in activation of G protein-coupled receptors. *Endocr Rev* 21:90, 2000.
4. Forse RA: Biology of heterotrimeric G-protein signaling. *Crit Care Med* 28:N53, 2000.
5. Bourne HR: How receptors talk to trimeric G proteins. *Curr Opin Cell Biol* 9:134, 1997.
6. Gudermann T, Kalkbrenner F, Schultz G: Diversity and selectivity of receptor-G protein interaction. *Annu Rev Pharmacol Toxicol* 36:429, 1996.
7. Kenakin T: Pharamacologic Analysis of Drug-Receptor Interactions, 3rd ed. Philadelphia: Lippincott-Raven, 289.
8. Garbers DL: The guanylyl cyclase receptors [editorial]. *Methods* 19:477, 1999.
9. McInnes C, Sykes BD: Growth factor receptors: structure, mechanism, and drug discovery. *Biopolymers* 43:339, 1997.
10. Acuto O, Cantrell D: T cell activation and the cytoskeleton. *Annu Rev Immunol* 18:165, 2000.
11. Hunter T: The phosphorylation of proteins on tyrosine: its role in cell growth and disease. *Philos Trans R Soc London B Biol Sci* 353:583, 1998.
12. Colasanti M, Suzuki H: The dual personality of NO. *Trends Pharmacol Sci* 21:249, 2000.
13. Egea PF, Klaholz BP, Moras D: Ligand-protein interactions in nuclear receptors of hormones. *FEBS Lett* 476:62, 2000.
14. Whitfield GK, Jurutka PW, Haussler CA, Haussler MR: Steroid hormone receptors: evolution, ligands, and molecular basis of biologic function. *J Cell Biochem* Suppl 32–33:110, 1999.
15. Post SR, Hammond HK, Insel PA: Beta-adrenergic receptors and receptor signaling in heart failure. *Annu Rev Pharmacol Toxicol* 39:343, 1999.
16. Grady EF, Bohm SK, Bunnett NW: Turning off the signal: mechanisms that attenuate signaling by G protein-coupled receptors. *Am J Physiol* 273:G586, 1997.
17. Gustafson TA, Moodie SA, Lavan BE: The insulin receptor and metabolic signaling. *Rev Physiol Biochem Pharmacol* 137:71, 1999.
18. Shenker A: G protein-coupled receptor structure and function: the impact of disease-causing mutations. *Baillieres Clin Endocrinol Metab* 9:427, 1995.
19. Birnbaumer M: Vasopressin receptor mutations and nephrogenic diabetes insipidus. *Arch Med Res* 30:465, 1999.
20. Roses AD: Pharmacogenetics and the practice of medicine. *Nature* 405:857, 2000.
21. Emilien G, Ponchon M, Caldas C, *et al.*: Impact of genomics on drug discovery and clinical medicine. *QJM* 93:391, 2000.
22. Brown EM, Segre GV, Goldring SR: Serpentine receptors for parathyroid hormone, calcitonin and extracellular calcium ions. *Baillieres Clin Endocrinol Metab* 10:123, 1996.
23. Lindstrom JM: Acetylcholine receptors and myasthenia. *Muscle Nerve* 23:453, 2000.

SECTION II
Standard Practices in Patient Care

6
Emergency Vascular Access and Intravenous Catheterization

Suzanne G. Barker Wingfield

INTRODUCTION

Emergency access to the venous system is vitally important to all veterinary practitioners. This access most commonly requires catheterization of peripheral veins to facilitate treatment of patients in shock or cardiopulmonary arrest. Oftentimes, venous access is challenging and difficult because of poor perfusion, the size of the patient, exotic veterinary species, edematous patients, obesity, or the lack of technical skills of the veterinarian or technician. Therefore, alternative methods to access the circulatory system must be employed. The purpose of this chapter is to provide a discussion of the techniques and alternative access routes to the venous circulation for purposes of emergency fluid and drug administration. Additionally, this chapter will discuss the use of intravenous catheterization for total and peripheral parenteral nutrition.

SITES FOR EMERGENCY VENOUS ACCESS

Peripheral veins continue to be the primary sites for emergency placement of catheters. These sites include the jugular, cephalic, medial saphenous, and lateral saphenous veins. When these veins are unavailable, the most logical site depends on the need for emergency access. If the animal is in cardiopulmonary arrest, intratracheal administration of drugs is commonly employed. If the animal is an exotic species, in severe shock, or numerous attempts at peripheral veins have failed, the intraosseous route is preferred. In seizure patients, the per rectum or intranasal route is preferred.

PERIPHERAL INTRAVENOUS CATHETERIZATION

Intravenous use of catheters involves the selection of a catheter, proper vein selection, preparation of the venipuncture site, insertion, bandaging, maintenance of the catheter, and an awareness of potential complications.

Selection of a Catheter

Three types of catheters are commonly used in veterinary medicine: the winged-tip or butterfly, the through-the-needle catheter, and the over-the-needle catheter. The butterfly catheter is adequate for one-time administration of drugs or fluids but is unsatisfactory for long-term fluid therapy. Through-the-needle catheters are safe for longer-term fluid administration, including that of hypertonic solutions, and for monitoring central venous pressure measurements when inserted into the jugular vein. Over-the-needle catheters are most useful for short-term fluid administration (12–24 hours). These catheters are more difficult to secure and are more likely to cause phlebitis and vessel irritation because of their rigid texture.

Most commonly, a large-gauge catheter (14, 16, or 18) is selected for rapid administration of fluids. In most cases, these large catheters are inserted into the largest vein available.

Selection of a Vein

Choose a vein that is the least stressful for the patient and least likely to become contaminated. When selecting this vein, consider the following questions:

1. Is the patient in shock and therefore in need of rapid volume replacement?
2. Is the patient demonstrating seizure activity and in need of anticonvulsive medication?
3. Is the patient in respiratory distress and intolerant to excessive handling required for the placement of the catheter?
4. Does the patient have a bleeding disorder, thrombi-forming disease (*e.g.*, hyperadrenocorticism and immune-medicated hemolytic anemia)?
5. Does the animal have diarrhea, vomiting, polyuria, or a vaginal discharge?
6. Is the animal able to move or paralyzed?
7. Will central venous pressure be monitored?
8. Does the animal have a fracture?

Table 6-1 will help you to determine the best catheter insertion site for the patient.

Maintenance of the Catheter and Insertion Site

Strict aseptic technique must be practiced in the intravenous insertion and maintenance of a catheter. The protective bandage covering the catheter should be marked with the date of catheter insertion and the type of catheter inserted. Catheters and administration sets must be examined every 8 hours and changed when soiled. Close observation for heat, swelling, swollen toes, or pain at the site of catheter insertion should alert you to potential complications. Tubing

Table 6-1. Selecting an Appropriate Venous Access in Dogs and Cats

Clinical Problem	Recommended Venous Access Site
Cardiopulmonary arrest	Peripheral vein, jugular vein, intratracheal, intraosseous
Bleeding disorder	Peripheral vein
Dehydration	Peripheral vein, jugular vein, intraosseous
Renal failure	Jugular vein
Respiratory distress	Peripheral vein
Seizures	Per rectum, intranasal, peripheral vein
Shock	Peripheral vein, jugular vein, intraosseous

should be kept off the cage floor to avoid contamination, and all fluids and administration sets should be maintained as sterile solutions and equipment. All open containers of fluids should be discarded and administration sets and tubing changed every 24 hours.

The need for an intravenously placed catheter should be assessed daily. When no longer required, prompt removal is advocated. The longer a catheter remains in a vein, the more likely it is that complications will develop. At present, intravenously placed catheters are usually changed every 72 hours. If continued intravenous therapy is required, a new catheter is inserted. Matthews et al. have questioned the need for changing the catheter. Their study indicates that an intravenously placed catheter can remain in place for >24 hours if a polyetherurethane and not a Teflon catheter is used. They also stress the importance of continuous catheter care and monitoring for complications. Interestingly, Matthews et al. also calculated that establishing and maintaining a peripherally inserted catheter and delivery set at the Ontario Veterinary College is $79.90 for 6 days. Changing the catheter every 48 to 72 hours, changing the fluid and delivery system change every 24 hours, and the use of sterile gloves would cost approximately $200.00. In fact, greater complications result when the catheter is routinely changed in human patients. Thus, one should support maintaining catheter change times based on clinical findings instead of defined time limits.

Complications

Catheter complications arise from 2 sources: 1) the animal and its environment and 2) the personnel working with the catheter. Strict attention to cleanliness of the patient and cage minimizes complications. Occasionally, physical restraint devices (*i.e.*, Elizabethan collar) are required to prevent mutilation of the catheter. Cleanliness of hospital personnel must include strict hand-washing policy between handling of patients and the use of examination gloves, if not sterile surgical gloves, when handling the catheter for blood sampling, drug administration, or inspection of the catheter insertion site.

Venous Cutdown Procedures

The decision to perform a venous cutdown procedure for venous access is unusual in these days of highly skilled veterinary technicians. Occasionally, an animal may be so hypovolemic or hypotensive that a cutdown may be required. Two types of cutdown procedures are generally employed in small animals. The first is a full cutdown procedure and the more common is a minicutdown. With both techniques, sterile conditions are mandatory. Occasionally, a solution of lidocaine warmed to the body temperature of the animal is injected subcutaneously for local analgesia. Following skin incision a strand of sterile suture material is passed around the vein proximal to the intended puncture site. A second strand of suture is passed distal to the intended puncture site. Total occlusion of the vessel with these sutures is not required. Retraction on these sutures occludes venous flow, and a small incision or the catheter needle is then placed into the vessel lumen. The catheter is advanced into the vein, and the two sutures are then secured around the catheter to stabilize and provide hemostasis. The subcutaneous tissue and skin incisions are closed in a routine fashion. The minicutdown procedure requires a smaller skin incision than the full cutdown. Usually, the vein can be easily viewed, and the needle and catheter can then be placed and advanced into the lumen.

Use of a venous cutdown procedure is contraindicated if the patient has a coagulopathy, systemic infection, thrombocytopenia, or is immune compromised. Hemorrhage and infection are the main complications seen with cutdown procedures. Providing pressure over the wound and covering the wound with clean, sterile bandages minimizes these complications.

INTRATRACHEAL VENOUS ACCESS

The intratracheal route for the administration of drugs is reserved for severe emergencies such as cardiopulmonary resuscitation (CPR). Rationale for this route is more direct access to the coronary arteries via the pulmonary veins, left atrium, and left ventricle. Most drugs used during CPR need to get to the coronary arteries to have any effect and, therefore, rapid access through the left ventricle is advantageous.

The drug is delivered via a tube inserted through the endotracheal tube and a large breath given to drive the drug as deeply into the airways as possible. Administration of the drug is commonly followed by either a flush of saline or sterile water followed by another breath. Importantly, the dosage of drugs administered intratracheally is three (3) times the dosage given intravenously. Also, the presence of pulmonary edema, hemorrhage, or pneumonia contraindicates this venous access route because of the patient's impaired absorptive capacity. Table 6-2 lists the drugs that can be administered by the intratracheal route. Sodium bicarbonate should never be given intratracheally because it will inactivate pulmonary surfactant.

Table 6-2. Drugs That Can Be Effectively Administered Via an Intraosseous Catheter

Aminophylline	Dexamethasone	Epinephrine
Atropine	Diazepam	Insulin
Calcium gluconate	Digitalis	Morphine
Naloxone	Diphenhydramine	Thiopental
Cefoxitin	Dobutamine	Dextrose
Whole blood	Plasma	Colloids and crystalloids

INTRAOSSEOUS VENOUS ACCESS

There is a resurgence of interest in the intraosseous route for administration of drugs and fluids. This is an excellent route for the emergency administration of drugs, fluids, whole blood and plasma transfusions, and dextrose.

The most common site for intraosseous insertion of a catheter is the trochanteric fossa of the femur. Alternative sites include the greater tubercle of the humerus, wing of the ilium, the distal femur just proximal to the patella and, rarely, the tibial tuberosity. In birds, the ulna is usually selected in order to avoid bones connecting with the air sacs. Additionally, local anesthesia is usually avoided in birds. The hair is clipped from the insertion site, the skin is surgically prepared, and an anesthetic such as lidocaine, bupivacaine, or carbocaine is locally applied to the skin, muscle, and periosteum. A large-bore catheter is selected (Table 6-3). This catheter can be a simple hypodermic needle for neonates but is more commonly a catheter with an indwelling trocar. For animals <4 months of age, spinal needles work well. For others, a bone marrow needle or a commercial catheter for intraosseous administration is used.

Transfusions and any drugs that can be given intravenously can be administered by the intraosseous route. It is possible to deliver fluids at shock volumes via the intraosseous route when pressure is applied to the fluid container. Rapid administration of fluids or drugs is often painful to the animal. Therefore, fluids are usually warmed before rapid intraosseous administration to avert pain.

Table 6-3. Selecting an Intraosseous Catheter for Dogs and Cats

Animal	Suggested Catheter	Size of Catheter
Adult dogs and cats	Bone marrow needle	16 to 20 gauge
Dogs and cats <4 months of age	Spinal needle	18 to 22 gauge
Neonates	Hypodermic needle	18 to 25 gauge
Any of the above	Commercial intraosseous catheter	12 to 15 gauge

Currently, the intraosseous route is used only for emergency patients and is usually exchanged for a peripheral venous catheter within 12 to 24 hours. Complications are few, and the technique is invaluable in small, neonatal, or exotic species.

INTRARECTAL ADMINISTRATION OF DRUGS IN EMERGENCIES

Seizures are common in small animals, and diazepam is the drug of choice for treating status epilepticus. Most commonly, diazepam is administered intravenously, but there are occasions when this route of administration may not be possible. Oral administration of diazepam to a convulsing animal is not practical and absorption is unpredictable. Absorption after intramuscular administration of diazepam is characterized as variable and erratic, depending on the site of injection, and may induce necrosis at the injection site. An alternative route is per rectum. Studies in humans indicate that diazepam is absorbed systemically when administered via the rectum and induces anticonvulsive effects in patients with status epilepticus and clusters of seizures. Results of a clinical trial in children indicate that rectal administration of diazepam is effective for treatment of seizures at home.

In dogs, per rectum administration of diazepam for management of cluster seizures was evaluated over a 16-month period. In this clinical study, rectal administration of diazepam at a dosage of 0.5 mg/kg was an effective method of home treatment. Because diazepam is rapidly metabolized by the liver in dogs, it is subject to high hepatic clearance, consistent with a first-pass effect. Most of the gastrointestinal tract, including the proximal portion of the rectum, is drained by the portal vein, whereas the distal rectum (hemorrhoidal veins) is drained into the caudal vena cava via the internal iliac vein. A drug administered orally is absorbed from the portal vein and must pass through the liver before it can have a systemic effect, whereas drainage from the distal portion of the rectum bypasses the liver. Studies in dogs have confirmed that diazepam is absorbed after rectal administration, and the pharmacologic effects are probably caused by the active metabolites, not the parent drug.

When administering diazepam per rectum, care must be taken to avoid injecting the drug into the feces. With most dogs, a 3-ml syringe (with the needle removed) is lubricated with K-Y jelly, introduced through the anus, directed toward the mucosa, and the drug is expelled into the rectum. If the animal is receiving chronic administration of phenobarbital, the total benzodiazepine concentration will be reduced after intravenous or per rectum administration. This is likely because of increased hepatic clearance of diazepam and its metabolites oxazepam and nordiazepam. Despite this finding, administration of diazepam rectally at 2 mg/kg may be a clinically useful alternative to intravenous administration for the emergency treatment of seizures when intravenous therapy is not possible in dogs with a history of chronic phenobarbital therapy.

INTRANASAL ADMINISTRATION OF DIAZEPAM

Intranasal administration of anticonvulsants has been used successfully to treat status epilepticus in humans. Following intranasal administration of midazolam, triazolam, and flurazepam in dogs, maximum plasma concentrations are achieved within 15 minutes. Diazepam administered at a dosage of 0.5 mg/kg via the intranasal route results in systemic availability of diazepam and its metabolites of 80.1%. This bioavailability is slightly higher than that reported following rectal administration. Additionally, the time to peak concentration was three times as fast with intranasally versus per rectum administered diazepam. This rapid response time may be an indication of a direct pathway from the nasal cavity to the brain. Rapid clearance of the drug from the nasal arterial circulation into the brain and fat has been proposed as the mechanism to explain these rapid effects.

DELIVERY OF NUTRITIONAL SUPPORT

Enteral delivery of nutritional support is the preferred method when the gastrointestinal tract is functional. This is because it preserves the integrity of the gastrointestinal mucosal barrier and function, helps maintain the animal's appetite, and is less expensive. When enteral delivery of nutritional support is not possible, parenteral delivery should be considered.

Two methods of parenterally delivered nutritional support are used in animals: total parenteral nutrition and peripheral parenteral nutrition. Total parenteral nutrition (TPN) is recommended when the gastrointestinal (gastrointestinal) tract is not functional or in patients in which it is undesirable to use the gastrointestinal tract (*e.g.*, those with malassimilation or prolonged ileus and after some gastrointestinal surgeries). Because of the high osmolality of infused TPN solutions (>800 mOsm/L), it is recommended they be administered via a central vein in order to prevent thrombosis of a peripheral vein.

Solutions used for peripheral parenteral nutritional (PPN) are lower in osmolality and therefore can be administered via a peripheral vein (cephalic or lateral saphenous). Patients that are good candidates for PPN include those in which a short term (<7 days) of nutritional support is needed. Other patients that benefit from PPN are those in which the jugular vein cannot be catheterized (*e.g.*, those with bleeding disorders), animals needing adjunctive nutrition because their enteral feeding does not completely meet their needs, and animals needing short-term nutritional support before anesthesia for placement of a gastrostomy or enterotomy tube (see Nutrition in Critical Care).

Intravenously placed catheters for delivery of parenteral nutrition should be reserved solely for this purpose. Additional catheters placed in other veins can be used for blood sampling and fluid and drug administration. Catheters for parenteral nutrition must be placed by sterile technique (*i.e.*, clip, surgical scrub, sterile gloves). Usually, Betadine ointment is applied over the catheter insertion site, and the catheter is wrapped with sterile gauze. Meticulous cleanliness of the animal and minimal handling of the catheter is advised. Daily examination of the catheter site is required. If the bandage is soiled or wet, it must be changed. All TPN and PPN solutions should be changed every 24 hours. This also applies to the tubing and extension sets. If possible, the use of a 1.2-micron filter, placed in-line, is advocated. This reduces the occurrence of thromboembolism with lipid solutions. Polyurethane or silicon catheters are the least thrombogenic.

Complications of Parenteral Nutrition

Mechanical complications involving catheters used for parenteral nutrition include occlusion, accidental removal, or line disconnection. If a break in aseptic integrity is suspected, remove and replace the catheter. The development of venous thromboembolism is the most severe potential complication of parenteral nutrition in humans and animals. This manifests as redness, swelling, and pain at the catheter site. The initiating factors that result in thromboembolism include damage to the vessel wall and endothelium during insertion of the catheter and movement of the catheter within the vein. Fibrin, white blood cells, red blood cells and platelets adhere to the catheter within the first few hours of insertion. Endothelial damage leads to venoconstriction, which increases endothelial irritation and decreases dilution of the infusion solution. Local release of inflammatory and vasoactive mediators escalates the inflammatory response and causes platelet aggregation, and then both can result in thrombosis. Occasionally, signs of acute respiratory distress will manifest indicating the presence of pulmonary thromboembolism.

The location of the catheter tip also influences the formation of thromboemboli. When the catheter tip is positioned near a joint, movement of the tip may increase endothelial damage. The longer a catheter remains in place, the more likely it is that thrombi will form. In human patients, the development of thromboembolism is diminished when the catheter is changed every 24 hours and the administration of the solution is limited to 12 hours. Changing the catheter every 24 hours is impractical and prohibitively expensive, but administering the infusion over 12 hours is reasonable. The obvious disadvantage is the necessity of infusing larger volumes during this shortened interval.

Solutions with an osmolality >600 mOsm/L are more likely to cause thromboembolism than those with an osmolality of <600 mOsm/L, although the osmolality rate (osmolality of solution x infusion rate) may be more important than osmolality alone. Use of lipids reduces the osmolality, and these solutions appear to have a protective effect on the venous endothelial wall.

Addition of a low dose of heparin (0.5 to 1 U/ml) to the infusion solution minimizes fibrin clots around the catheter tip. Adding a low dose of hydrocortisone (5 mg/L) to the solution decreases venous inflammation. Application of transdermal glycerol trinitrate over the anticipated site of the catheter tip induces venodilation and stimulates prostacyclin synthesis. Finally, topical administration of a nonsteroidal anti-inflammatory ointment over the catheter site may also reduce the development of thromboembolism.

CONCLUSIONS

Use of catheters for access to the venous system is safe, relatively inexpensive, easy to maintain, and frequently lifesaving to the patient. These techniques require rigorous attention to detail regarding proper catheter and site selection to fit the clinical needs of the patient. Meticulous cleanliness and frequent monitoring of both the patient and catheter site and bandage cannot be overemphasized. Complications occasionally develop but should not deter their use.

SUGGESTED READINGS

Burrows CF: Inadequate skin preparation as a cause of intravenous catheter-related infection in the dog. *J Am Vet Med Assoc* 180:747, 1982.

Chandler ML, Guilford WG, Payne-James J: Use of peripheral parenteral nutritional support in dogs and cats. *J Am Vet Med Assoc* 216:669, 2000.

Collins E, Lawson L, Lau MT, *et al.*: Care of central venous catheters for total parenteral nutrition. *Nutr Clin Pract* 11:109, 1996.

Crowe DT: Performing life-saving cardiovascular surgery. *Vet Med* 84:77, 1989.

Dunn DL, Lenihan SF: The case for the saline flush. *Am J Nurs* 87:798, 1987.

Eyer S, Brummitt C, Crossley K, *et al.*: Catheter-related sepsis: prospective, randomized study of three methods of long-term catheter maintenance. *Crit Care Med* 18:1073, 1990.

Fulton RB, Hauptman JG: *In vitro* and *in vivo* rates of fluid flow through catheters in peripheral veins of dogs. *J Am Vet Med Assoc* 198:1622, 1991.

Hoffman KK, Weber DJ, Samsa GP, *et al.*: Transparent polyurethane film as an intravenous catheter dressing: a meta-analysis of the infection risks. *J Am Vet Med Assoc* 267:2072, 1992.

Linares J, Sitges-Serra A, Garau J *et al.*: Pathogenesis of catheter sepsis: a prospective study with quantitative and semi-quantitative cultures of catheter hub and segments. *J Clin Microbiol* 21:357, 1985.

Loo S, van Heerden PV, Gollege CL, *et al.*: Infection in central lines: antiseptic-impregnated vs standard non-impregnated catheters. *Anaesth Intensive Care* 25:637, 1997.

Maki DG, Band JD: A comparative study of polyantibiotic and iodophor ointments in prevention of vascular catheter-related infection. *Am J Med* 70:739, 1981.

Maki DG, Stolz SS, Wheeler S, *et al.*: A prospective, randomized trial of gauze and two polyurethane dressings for site care of pulmonary artery catheters: implications for catheter management. *Crit Care Med* 22:1729, 1994.

Martin GJ, Rand JS: Evaluation of a polyurethane jugular catheter in cats placed using a modified Seldinger technique. *Aust Vet J* 77:250, 1999.

Matthews KA, Brooks MJ, Valliant AE: A prospective study of intravenous catheter contamination. *J Vet Emerg Crit Care* 6:33, 1996.

Norwood S, Ruby A, Civetta J, *et al.*: Catheter-related infections and associated septicemia. *Chest* 99:968, 1991.

Otto CM, Kaufman GM, Crowe DT: Intraosseous infusion of fluids and therapeutics. *Compend Contin Educ Pract Vet* 11:421, 1989.

Papich MG, Alcorn J: Absorption of diazepam after its rectal administration in dogs. *Am J Vet Res* 56:1629, 1995.

Payne-James JJ, Khawaja HT: First choice for total parenteral nutrition: the peripheral route. *J Parenter Enteral Nutr* 17:468, 1993.

Peterson FY, Kirchhoff KT: Analysis of the research about heparinized versus non-heparinized intravascular lines. *Heart Lung* 20:631, 1991.

Platt SR, Randell SC, Scott KC, *et al.*: Comparison of plasma benzodiazepine concentrations following intranasal and intravenous administration of diazepam in dogs. *Am J Vet Res* 61:651, 2000.

Poundstone M: Intraosseous infusion of fluids in small animals. *Vet Tech* 13:407, 1992.

Powell LL: Emergency venous access. *In* Wingfield WE, ed.: Veterinary Emergency Medicine Secrets. Philadelphia: Hanley and Belfus, 2001, 446.

Rottman SJ, Larmon B, Manix T: Rapid volume infusion in prehospital care. *Prehospital Disaster Med* 5:225, 1990.

Sacchetti A: Large-bore infusion catheters (Seldinger technique for vascular access). *In* Roberts JR, Hedges JR, eds.: Clinical Procedures in Emergency Medicine. Philadelphia: WB Saunders, 1985, 289.

Tillson DM, Brewer WG, Lenz SD: Cannulated bone screws for chronic intraosseous access. [Abstract 79]. *Vet Surg* 28: 404, 1999.

Treston-Aurand J, Olmsted RN, Allen-Bridson K, *et al.*: Impact of dressing materials on central venous catheter infection rates. *J Intravenous Nurs* 20:201, 1997.

Wagner SO, Sams RA, Podell M: Chronic phenobarbital therapy reduces plasma benzodiazepam concentrations after intravenous and rectal administration of diazepam in the dog. *J Vet Pharmacol Ther* 21:335, 1998.

7
Pain Management

Peter W. Hellyer

PAIN IN THE VETERINARY ICU—AN OVERVIEW

It is the obligation of all veterinarians to minimize pain and suffering in patients under their care.[1] This obligation is even greater for those veterinary personnel who strive to care for the critically injured and sick animal.

Critically ill patients frequently suffer from pain and distress associated with trauma or disease. The well-intentioned medical and surgical interventions designed to prolong or save lives often induce additional tissue trauma and pain. Many of these same patients are too debilitated or compromised to display behaviors indicative of pain that would prompt the ICU staff to administer analgesic therapy. Consequently, many of these patients divert energy to coping with pain instead of getting the rest and sleep required for a full recovery. In other words, the process of recovery is prolonged and the metabolic cost to the animal is increased. The potential benefits of aggressive diagnostic, surgical, and lifesupport procedures must be weighed against the pain and distress that the animal will likely experience. Withholding analgesics, or simply neglecting the issue of patient pain and comfort, subjects animals in the ICU to unacceptable suffering.[1] There is no question that many people would be unwilling to put their own pets through painful procedures if there was no hope of alleviating their pain. In fact, fear of unrelieved pain and suffering prevents some clients from pursuing additional diagnostic or therapeutic procedures, opting for euthanasia instead.

Appropriate analgesic therapy is designed to help the animal cope with pain, induce rest and sleep, reduce stress, and promote a more rapid recovery.[2] In cases where recovery is unlikely, analgesic therapy is a key component to ensuring comfort at the end of life.

CAUSES OF PAIN

A reasonable clinical rule of thumb is that the greater the tissue trauma the more severe the pain.[3-6] Patients with neuropathic pain, pain arising from an injured or cut nerve, may be an exception to this rule. Severe neuropathic pain may be present even though the amount of tissue trauma appears minor.[7] Patients with multiple traumas, including superficial and deep musculoskeletal injuries, long bone and pelvic fractures, superficial abrasions, and degloving injuries are obvious patients that would be expected to be in severe pain.[8] Patients with extensive cellulitis or burn injuries are in severe pain. Postoperative patients are generally expected to be in pain for at least the first 24 to 72 hours, if not longer. Any surgical procedure can induce pain; however, fore or hind limb amputation, hemipelvectomy, thoracotomy, and laparotomy usually induce severe pain in dogs and cats.[8] A laparotomy should be considered more painful than an ovariohysterectomy, primarily because the amount of tissue trauma is greater due to the length of the incision, the amount of time spent exploring the abdomen, and the degree of abdominal wall retraction required for a thorough exploration of the abdomen.

Some relatively healthy patients may require intensive care after surgery simply to manage postoperative pain effectively. For example, patients undergoing radical mastectomy, total ear canal ablation, laminectomy, cranial cruciate ligament repair, or arthrotomy often experience severe pain that can best be managed with round-the-clock analgesic therapy and monitoring. Patients with pancreatitis and peritonitis may have severe abdominal pain in addition to nausea, vomiting, and diarrhea. Less obvious sources of pain include multiple intravenous (IV) catheterizations, intramuscular (IM) or subcutaneous (SQ) injections, multiple venipunctures to obtain blood samples, changing of bandages, urinary catheterization, chest tube irritation, distended bladders in animals unable or unwilling to urinate in their cage, and any other invasive diagnostic or therapeutic procedure.

IDENTIFYING PAIN IN ICU PATIENTS

Clinical Signs of Pain in the Dog and Cat

The clinical signs of pain may range from subtle to obvious, depending on the degree and type of pain, intensity of pain, and the individual patient's response to pain.[8–12] Dogs tend to demonstrate pain behaviors more readily than cats; however, some dogs show few outward signs of pain despite severe injuries. Exaggerated, violent behaviors, such as thrashing, lunging, paddling, or climbing the cage walls (cats) tend to be observed most commonly during recovery from anesthesia following painful surgical procedures. Head pressing or head banging may be observed with severe abdominal pain. Less obvious signs of pain include restlessness (constantly getting up and down), shifting positions, reluctance to move or lie down and sleep, favoring a part of the body, or excessively licking or mutilating an area. Any dog or cat that is falling asleep standing up or propped against the cage wall should be considered to be in severe pain until proven otherwise. Vocalizing (including grunting, whining, crying, and howling) may be indicative of pain; however, it is not a sensitive or specific indicator of pain. Nevertheless, many dogs do stop vocalizing following administration of an analgesic drug. Dogs are much more likely to vocalize than cats. Dilated pupils, staring off into the distance (star gazing), grimacing, having ears flattened against the head, shivering or shaking, or appearing obtunded are more subtle signs of pain. Excessive salivation may indicate nausea or pain. Change in demeanor may be an extremely important clinical sign of pain that is particularly difficult to recognize in a clinical setting.[13]

Changes in Monitored Physiologic Parameters

In general, heart rate, arterial blood pressure, and respiratory rate increase as a result of sympathetic stimulation in response to noxious/painful stimuli. Less commonly, noxious/painful events will induce a vagal response characterized by decreases in heart rate and arterial blood pressure, and possibly loss of consciousness. Monitoring of physiologic parameters may be useful in assessing acute pain and the effect of analgesic drugs; however, two important clinical rules should be considered. First, physiologic parameters may be within the normal range despite the patient experiencing pain and distress.[9] Second, changes in physiologic parameters may occur as a result of underlying metabolic derangements that have nothing to do with pain. For example, a dog with sinus tachycardia after surgery may be in pain, but may also be hypovolemic, hypotensive, or hypoxemic, or have some other type of acid–base or metabolic abnormality. A careful examination of the patient is required to determine the cause of the tachycardia.

Factors Confounding the Identification of Pain

The standard for determining whether or not pain is adequately controlled in a person is to ask that person. Because that option is not available in veterinary medicine, behavioral observations play a key role in determining whether an animal is in pain and how well that animal is coping with the pain. Unfortunately, some behaviors indicative of pain are similar if not identical to some behaviors indicative of anxiety. Furthermore, some behaviors such as vocalization can be induced by opioid analgesics or may be unrelated to pain. Because some animals (especially cats) mask their signs of pain so well, relying solely on observed behaviors to determine if an animal is in pain will result in some animals receiving inadequate or no treatment at all. A dog may not demonstrate pain behaviors when interacting with a caregiver, but may appear restless and uncomfortable when observed undisturbed in its cage as has been demonstrated in dogs recovering from ovariohysterectomy.[10,14] A consideration of the animal's demeanor, amount of tissue trauma incurred, underlying disease process, overall physical status, and the likelihood that the animal has the ability to demonstrate pain behaviors must be considered when deciding if the behaviors observed are indicative of pain. If unsure, observing for any behavioral changes after a trial dose of an opioid analgesic is usually a safe method to determine if the behavior is related to pain.

Rationale for Treating Pain

The benefits of adequate analgesic therapy on morbidity and mortality have been most clearly demonstrated in critically ill people. Studies are lacking in veterinary medicine; however, it is reasonable to assume that similar principles apply. Critically ill people are the least able to cope with the metabolic and energy demands imposed by severe, untreated pain. Providing critically ill people effective analgesia improves their ability to rest, improves immune function, improves mobility, decreases the stress response with its concomitant catabolic abnormalities, decreases pneumonia and deep venous thrombosis, decreases ICU stays, and has been shown to improve survival in neonatal infants following cardiac surgery.[15,16]

Healthy animals, like people, recover from surgery or trauma more quickly if their pain is controlled and they are given the opportunity to rest. Uncontrolled pain in this population of patients may not result in increased mortality, but may initiate a cascade of neural changes that leads to exaggerated pain states (wind-up) or chronic pain.[4] Requiring our patients to endure severe pain needlessly is inhumane and unethical, especially considering the ready availability of effective analgesic drugs.

Therapeutic Approach

Analgesic drugs should be administered on a regular basis before the patient displays signs of pain or anxiety.[2] It bears repeating that if there is any doubt as to whether the patient may be in pain, analgesic drugs should be administered.[17] If an IV catheter is in place, a constant rate infusion (CRI) of the analgesic drug provides the most stable and predictable levels of analgesia. Alternatively, intermittent IV administration of drugs is usually preferable to SQ or IM injections. If an IV catheter is not in place, SQ injections are much less painful and are better tolerated that repeated IM injections. The onset time following SQ injections is generally within 20 to 30 minutes as compared to 10 to 15 minutes for IM injections. Anxiety often intensifies the pain experience and prevents patients from getting the rest they need. If anxiety cannot be alleviated through environmental changes and good nursing care, it should be treated pharmacologically as described below.

When Should Analgesic Therapy Be Withheld?

Analgesic therapy is usually withheld in critically ill patients during initial patient assessment and stabilization. Particular attention should be paid to neurologic, cardiovascular, and respiratory function during the initial work-up. Opioid analgesics are frequently the first-line analgesic drugs administered to critically ill or traumatized patients. Opioids are likely to induce sedation in animals in pain; therefore, the potential for neurologic injury should be determined before administering the first dose of an opioid. Follow-up evaluations of neurologic function will need to be timed so that the animal can be assessed as the sedative effects of the opioid are waning. On occasion, analgesic drugs must be administered prior to a complete assessment in painful, difficult to handle cases.

Opioid analgesics should be avoided in patients with head trauma, particularly those with an abnormal neurologic examination. Opioid-induced respiratory depression can lead to increases in $PaCO_2$ and decreases in PaO_2, resulting in an increase in cerebral blood flow and intracranial pressure.[18] Global or regional brain ischemia or brainstem herniation may result from excessive increases in intracranial pressure. In addition, opioid-induced sedation will make it difficult if not impossible to determine if neurologic function is deteriorating. On the other hand, some animals with head trauma also have multiple other traumas necessitating the use of opioids for analgesia and sedation. Administering low doses of opioids to effect and supplementing oxygen to the patient will help prevent opioid-induced respiratory depression.

Analgesic drugs should be withheld from hypothermic, obtunded patients that are not regaining consciousness as typically occurs in critically ill patients recovering from anesthesia. Under these circumstances, opioids may further obtund the patient and contribute to further loss of body temperature and prolonged recoveries. Once the patient has begun to warm and regain consciousness, opioid analgesics may be administered. In contrast, hypothermic patients that recover from anesthesia rapidly and are likely to be in pain may be given reduced dosages of opioids until they regain a normal body temperature.

OPIOID ANALGESICS

Mechanism of Action

Opioids are the safest, most effective, and most commonly administered analgesic and sedative drugs used to treat acute pain in dogs and cats in the ICU and in the immediate postoperative period.[17,19] Opioid analgesics mimic the effect of endogenous opiate peptides (endorphins, enkephalins, dynorphin) and bind to specific μ-, δ-, and κ-opioid receptors. These receptors are located principally in the central nervous system (CNS) with large concentrations in the dorsal horn of the spinal cord and multiple supraspinal sites, including the cerebral cortex.[20] Stimulation of these receptors decreases the transmission of nociceptive impulses and decreases the perception of pain.[20] Opioid receptors have been identified in peripheral tissues and in joints; however, these receptors play a secondary role in the management of pain in the ICU.[21] Opioids are typically classified as μ-receptor agonists, agonist-antagonists, partial agonists, or antagonists. Of the opioids, the μ-receptor agonists (*e.g.*, morphine, oxymorphone, hydromorphone, and fentanyl) are the most effective and commonly used opioids in the veterinary ICU.[19,22] Due to their limited efficacy to treat severe pain, opioid agonist-antagonists (*e.g.*, butorphanol) and partial agonists (*e.g.*, buprenorphine) play a secondary role in pain management of the critically ill patient.[2,17,19]

Side Effects

The side effects of opioids include sedation, dysphoria or excitement, respiratory depression, bradycardia, histamine release (morphine, meperidine), vomiting, and constipation.[2,19,23,24] Sedation, with the possibility of sleeping, may be viewed as a beneficial or detrimental effect of the opioids depending on the circumstance. Simply relieving pain, thereby allowing the animal to relax, may induce sleep. If the amount of sedation is excessive, decreasing the dose or discontinuing the opioid may be all that is needed. At the other end of the behavioral spectrum, opioids may induce excitement or dysphoria. Excitement rarely, if ever, occurs in critically ill or traumatized patients. Excitement is most likely to occur when opioids are administered to excitable, healthy dogs or cats that are not experiencing pain as may occur in some anesthetic protocols. Excitement can be reversed by antagonizing the opioid with naloxone or by concurrently administering a tranquilizer (*e.g.*, acepromazine). Opioids can induce dysphoria, a term loosely used to refer to behavior that appears agitated or disoriented, and frequently includes some form of vocalization. Frequently, pain-induced behaviors are misdiagnosed as dysphoria, simply because it is known that the animal received an opioid. Administering an additional dose of an opioid is usually a safe way to differentiate pain and dysphoria. If the animal relaxes, it is likely that the clinical signs are due to pain. If the animal does not improve or becomes more agitated, dysphoria is the likely diagnosis and naloxone can be used to reverse the opioid or acepromazine can be administered to sedate the animal.

Respiratory depression is the side effect that causes the most concern, particularly in the critically ill patient. Opioids alter respiratory center sensitivity to carbon dioxide, with the potential of causing hypoventilation and respiratory acidosis. In the animal breathing room air, clinically significant hypoventilation will lead to hypoxemia. In general, dogs and cats are relatively resistant to the respiratory depressant effects of the opioids. Clinically significant respiratory depression from opioids is most likely to occur in the presence of other centrally depressant drugs given during general anesthesia. Nevertheless, care must be taken when administering opioids to animals that are obtunded (particularly those with head trauma or organic brain disease), excessively sedated (as may occur upon recovery from anesthesia), or have pre-existing respiratory disease. Administering reduced dosages of μ-receptor agonists to effect is a safe method of providing analgesia while minimizing the respiratory depressant effect of the drug. Alternatively, administering an opioid agonist-antagonist (*e.g.*, butorphanol) decreases the potential for respiratory compromise because there is "ceiling effect" to the respiratory depression induced by this class of drugs.[19,24] For example, brachycephalic dogs with severe upper airway obstruction tolerate butorphanol much better than low doses of morphine or oxymorphone.

Bradycardia may occur as a result of an increase in vagal tone, a decrease in sympathetic tone as pain perception is decreased, or the animal falling asleep. The reduction in heart rate usually does not require treatment, provided the pulse is strong and regular. In contrast, combining an opioid with an α_2-agonist such as xylazine or medetomidine frequently results in bradycardia that must be treated. If needed, bradycardia can be treated with atropine or glycopyrrolate.

Vomiting can occur with any opioid; however, vomiting is observed most frequently with the first dose of morphine in an ambulatory patient. Subsequent doses of morphine are unlikely to cause vomiting. The incidence of vomiting with oxymorphone and fentanyl appears to be less than that observed with morphine. Occasionally, opioids will continue to cause nausea and vomiting in susceptible individuals. Switching to an opioid agonist-antagonist sometimes alleviates the problem. Alternatively, administering an antiemetic or a subanesthetic dose of propofol (Propoflo, Abbott Labs, 0.5–1 mg/kg, slowly IV) can break the cycle of vomiting. Opioids frequently induce constipation; however, this is more of a problem with the chronic administration of opioids. Morphine causes constriction of the sphincter of Oddi, which can lead to biliary stasis and abdominal pain.[24] An alternative opioid (*e.g.*, fentanyl [Fentanyl Citrate Injection, Abbott Labs], oxymorphone [Numorphan, Dupont Merck Pharma]) may be used in animals with hepatobiliary disease.

Histamine release is most likely to occur with the IV administration of morphine or meperidine. Morphine is frequently used in ICU settings with little problem. Administering morphine as a slow IV bolus (over 60 seconds) or as a continuous IV infusion decreases the likelihood that clinically significant histamine release will occur.

Tolerance develops to the analgesic, sedative, and adverse side effects of the opioids, with the possible exception of constipation. For the treatment of acute pain, the requirements for opioid analgesics usually decrease over a matter of days as tissue healing occurs as the animal recovers. In cases of severe and on-going injuries, or in some forms of chronic pain, tolerance develops and increased doses of opioids are required to maintain the same level of pain relief. How quickly tolerance develops is open to debate; however, it is likely that it can occur in some individuals in less than a day. Increasing the opioid dose incrementally until the patient appears comfortable is a safe way to avoid excessive side effects while still providing adequate analgesia. High doses of continuous opioids may induce a form of dependence that has been termed "therapeutic dependence." Therapeutic dependence simply means that the opioid is required for the patient to cope with the pain and to maintain a given level of comfort, much as a diabetic may be dependent on insulin to maintain glucose homeostasis. The longer the animal is maintained on opioids, and the higher the doses used, the more important it is to wean the animal off the opioid when recovery has progressed to the point that analgesic therapy may be discontinued.

Species Considerations: Dog Versus Cat

Opioids can be used successfully to treat pain in both dogs and cats. Opioids tend to have greater sedative effects in dogs than cats; however, opioids will often sedate painful, ill, and geriatric cats satisfactorily. In cats, opioid doses are generally one quarter to one half the dose administered to dogs to avoid excitatory side effects. Opioids typically cause mydriasis in cats, whereas they cause miosis in dogs. Aside from the differences in the potential for excitement, the advantages and disadvantages of opioids are the same in dogs and cats.

Regulatory Issues

It is not possible to aggressively treat pain and provide state-of-the-art critical care to dogs and cats without using scheduled (controlled) drugs. In other words, there is no excuse for not using these drugs, particularly in a specialty or referral clinic. The μ-opioid agonists (*e.g.*, morphine, oxymorphone, fentanyl), butorphanol, diazepam, and ketamine are all scheduled drugs. Maintaining accurate records of these drugs is essential; however, it is not an exceptionally difficult task. Noting the drug administered, dose, route, and time in the patient record should just be part of maintaining good patient records. In addition, maintaining a running inventory of scheduled drugs used becomes second nature and ensures that the entire content of a bottle is accounted for. Unfortunately, our societal fears of drug addiction have spilled over into veterinary medicine. Although veterinary patients may develop a therapeutic dependence on opioid analgesics while they are in pain, addiction is not a problem in our patients. Even among people given large doses of opioids, actual addiction is quite rare.

SPECIFIC OPIOIDS

Morphine

Morphine is the prototypical μ-opioid agonist, which is assigned an analgesic potency index of one. Morphine is an exceptionally useful opioid for the ICU setting, primarily because it provides equivalent analgesia to other μ agonists and is very inexpensive; therefore, effective analgesic levels can be obtained without significantly adding to the costs of the ICU stay. Because of its relatively long duration of action, morphine may be administered IV, SQ, or IM on a fixed dose schedule (Table 7-1). Fluctuations in plasma concentrations of morphine, and analgesic effect, are avoided if morphine is administered as a CRI. IV boluses of morphine should be given slowly (over approximately 60 seconds) to avoid histamine release with accompanying vasodilation, hypotension, or bronchoconstriction. Morphine should be used cautiously in patients with mast cell tumors or a history of asthma. Vomiting is more likely with morphine than with some of the other opioids; however, repeated episodes of vomiting are uncommon after the first dose of morphine. Importantly, morphine may be administered orally for continued analgesic therapy when the patient is discharged from the hospital.[25–27] The bioavailability of oral morphine is approximately 15% to 17% for sustained-release and nonsustained-release morphine in dogs.[26]

Table 7-1. Opioid Analgesia in Dogs and Cats

Drug	Dog Dose/Route/Frequency	Cat Dose/Route/Frequency
Morphine	0.25–0.5 mg/kg, IV q 1–2 h 0.1–0.5 mg/kg/h CRI 0.5–1 mg/kg, SQ, IM q 3–4 h 1–5 mg/kg, PO, q 4–6 h SR 1–5 mg/kg, PO, q 8–12 h	0.1–0.25 mg/kg, IV q 1–2 h 0.05–0.25 mg/kg/h CRI 0.25–0.5 mg/kg, SQ, IM q 3–4 h 0.5–2 mg/kg, PO q 4–6 h 0.5–2 mg/kg, PO q 8–12 h
Oxymorphone	0.025–0.05 mg/kg, IV q 1–2 h 0.05–0.1 mg/kg, SQ, IM q 3–4 h	0.01–0.025 mg/kg, IV q 1–2 h 0.025–0.05 mg/kg, SQ, IM q 3–4 h
Fentanyl	0.001–0.002 mg/kg, IV bolus 0.001–0.006 mg/kg/h, CRI up to 0.01 mg/kg/hr, CRI (severe pain)	0.001–0.002 mg/kg, IV bolus 0.001–0.004 mg/kg/h, CRI
Butorphanol	0.1–0.2 mg/kg, IV q 1 h 0.2–0.5 mg/kg, SQ, IM q 1–2 h	0.1–0.2 mg/kg, IV q 1–2 h 0.2 to 0.4 mg/kg, SQ, IM q 2–4 h

CRI, constant rate infusion; SR, sustained-release oral formulation.

Morphine is metabolized by the liver with one of the metabolites, morphine-6-glucoronide, having pharmacologic activity.[24] Considering the confounding factors of low oral bioavailability and the potential for accumulation of an active metabolite, it is recommended that the veterinarian work closely with the client to adjust the patient's dose of morphine as indicated by response to drug therapy.

Oxymorphone and Hydromorphone

Oxymorphone has similar properties to morphine with the exception that oxymorphone is more potent than morphine (potency ~10–15), it does not cause histamine release, and it is less likely to cause vomiting (see Table 7-1). Oxymorphone may sedate cats a little more than morphine; however, this finding is inconsistent. The primary disadvantage of oxymorphone is cost, so much so that it often becomes prohibitively expensive to provide effective analgesia over a 1- to 2-day hospital stay.

Hydromorphone is also a μ-opioid agonist that is approximately five times more potent than morphine. It is reportedly used at a dose of 0.05 to 0.4 mg/kg, IV, SQ, or IM in both dogs and cats.[19,22] The actions and side effects of hydromorphone are similar to those of oxymorphone. Hydromorphone is used as an alternative to oxymorphone because it is less expensive.

Fentanyl

Fentanyl is an effective and relatively inexpensive opioid making it an extremely useful analgesic for the ICU setting. Fentanyl is a μ-opioid agonist that is approximately 100 times more potent than morphine (see Table 7-1). The terminal elimination phase of fentanyl in dogs anesthetized with enflurane was 199 ± 17 minutes; however, a single IV bolus of fentanyl has a clinical duration of action of approximately 15 minutes, due largely to extensive redistribution.[28] Fentanyl should be administered as a loading dose followed by a CRI. Failure to start with a loading dose will result in a period of at least 4 to 5 hours before therapeutic plasma concentrations of fentanyl are reached. Patients that were administered large doses of fentanyl in the intraoperative period may already have relatively high plasma concentrations of fentanyl and may not need a loading dose of fentanyl when recovering from anesthesia. Fentanyl infusion rates may be incrementally increased if the patient requires additional analgesia, or decreased if the patient is too obtunded or it is time to wean the patient off the infusion. When increasing the rate of fentanyl administration for patients in pain, it is recommended that an additional bolus of fentanyl be administered to hasten the onset of higher fentanyl plasma concentrations. Fentanyl boluses of 1 to 2 μg/kg IV are well tolerated with little clinical evidence of respiratory depression. Fentanyl is also available as a transdermal patch (Duragesic, Janssen Pharmaceutica) that delivers a constant rate of fentanyl over approximately 72 hours. Attaining effective plasma concentrations of fentanyl from the transdermal patch is quite variable in dogs and cats and may take from 12 to 24 hours, with some animals never reaching effective plasma concentrations.[29,30] Due to this inconsistency, fentanyl transdermal patches should never be the sole source of analgesia for the animal that is critically ill, traumatized, or in pain. Weaning a patient off fentanyl CRI on to a fentanyl patch appears to work well with some patients. Fentanyl may cause some dogs to become more vocal (primarily whining), which needs to be differentiated from a behavior suggesting uncontrolled pain. If an additional bolus of fentanyl does not stop the vocalization, a low dose of acepromazine will usually correct the problem (assuming that acepromazine is an acceptable drug for that patient).

Butorphanol

Butorphanol is an opioid agonist-antagonist that has limited utility in the ICU setting (see Table 7-1). Butorphanol has traditionally been used to treat mild to moderate pain in dogs and cats or to partially antagonize the effects of μ-agonists such as morphine.[32] The effect of butorphanol on μ- and κ-opioid receptors probably varies with species and dose. Some evidence suggests that there may be additive, rather than antagonistic, effects between butorphanol and oxymorphone administered to cats.[33] The potential for interaction between butorphanol and other opioids requires further investigations; therefore, it is not recommended at this time that the two classes of drugs be routinely combined. Butorphanol may be preferentially selected over a μ-opioid agonist in patients with marked respiratory disease, such as brachycephalic dogs with upper airway obstruction. Clinically, it appears that these patients tolerate the respiratory depressant effects of butorphanol better than μ-opioid agonists. Butorphanol may also be preferentially selected for patients that have excessive nausea or vomiting with the μ-agonists, as may occur in some dogs with pancreatitis.

NONOPIOID ANALGESICS

Ketamine

Ketamine may play a unique role as an adjunct analgesic to treat or prevent the development of hyperalgesia in the ICU patient in severe pain.[34–39] Ketamine blocks the actions of the excitatory neurotransmitter glutamate at the *N*-methyl-D-aspartate (NMDA) receptor in the CNS. Glutamate and the NMDA receptor have been implicated in the phenomenon of wind-up, with its resultant states of exaggerated pain and hyperalgesia, which is purported to occur in the nociceptive pathways in the dorsal horn of the spinal cord.[38,39] Glutamate is an important neurotransmitter in the development of memory and may be involved in creating a memory for pain. In addition, the NMDA receptor has been implicated in the development of morphine tolerance.[40] The intraoperative administration of low-dose ketamine to people decreased the requirements for postoperative analgesics, well beyond the expected duration of effect of ketamine.[35–37] Ketamine has been administered to terminally ill people who were opioid tolerant and in severe pain.[34] Ketamine improved patient comfort and markedly decreased opioid requirements. In veterinary medicine, ketamine has been used extensively for the

Table 7-2. Sedation/Anesthesia in the ICU Dog and Cat

Drug	Dose	Frequency
Acepromazine	0.01–0.02 mg/kg, IV 0.02–0.05 mg/kg, SQ, IM	q 2–4 h q 4–6 h (as needed)
Diazepam	0.1–0.5 mg/kg, IV	q 1–2 h
Midazolam	0.1–0.5 mg/kg, IV, SQ, IM	q 1–2 h
Medetomidine	0.001–0.002 mg/kg, IV, IM	q 1–2 h
Xylazine	0.1–0.2 mg/kg, IV, SQ, IM	q 1–2 h
Propofol	0.5–4 mg/kg, slow IV administration to induce unconsciousness 0.5–1 mg/kg, IV as needed to maintain unconsciousness 0.05–0.4 mg/kg/min CRI	

CRI, constant rate infusion.

induction and maintenance of anesthesia in a wide variety of species. Ketamine to treat pain requires doses that are generally considered to be subanesthetic (Table 7-2). The doses of ketamine used for analgesia have been extrapolated from the human literature and appear to work well in dogs and cats based on clinical experience. To date, no controlled dose-response studies have been performed to determine the ideal dose of ketamine in the treatment of pain. Clearly, excessively high doses of ketamine may cause marked behavioral abnormalities or even induce anesthesia. The optimal duration of administration of a ketamine CRI also has not been established. Ketamine may be administered during the intraoperative period or for 24 hours after a surgical or traumatic event. Because of the potential for ketamine to interact with the opioid receptor and prevent the development of opioid tolerance, ketamine is typically administered in conjunction with an opioid analgesic. The safety of a CRI of subanesthetic doses of ketamine in patients with elevated intracranial pressure (*e.g.*, head trauma, intracranial tumor), heart disease, or glaucoma has not been established; therefore, ketamine should not be used in these patients.

α_2-Agonists

The α_2-agonists (*e.g.*, xylazine, medetomidine [Domitor, Pfizer Animal Health]) have not typically been used in the ICU patient because of the marked cardiopulmonary effects of these drugs.[41,42] In particular, clinically significant decreases in heart rate, myocardial contractility, and cardiac output limit their usefulness in compromised dogs and cats. Decreases in heart rate can be treated with anticholinergics; however, returning heart rate to normal values does not necessarily improve cardiac output. Medetomidine-induced decreases in cardiac output do not appear to be dose dependent; in that cardiac output was decreased similarly over a dose range of 1 to 20 μg/kg IV in dogs.[41] Nevertheless, combinations of α_2-agonists and opioids can induce additive or synergistic analgesic and sedative effects. In animals in severe pain, addition of low doses of either xylazine or medetomidine can markedly improve patient comfort (see Table 7-2). The IV administration of a low dose of xylazine or medetomidine appears to exert an effect for less than an hour. The goal of α_2-agonist therapy in the ICU should be to "buy some time" in the patient in severe pain for other analgesic interventions to improve patient comfort.

Nonsteroidal Anti-inflammatory Drugs (NSAIDs)

The NSAIDs are clearly effective analgesic adjuncts, particularly in the presence of tissue inflammation.[43–46] NSAIDs may exert some analgesic effects within the CNS; however, they are classically thought of as inhibitors of prostaglandin synthesis.[24,44,47] Prostaglandins are synthesized by the actions of cyclooxygenase enzyme on arachidonic acid, located within cell membranes. Prostaglandins serve as key mediators in the inflammatory cascade, sensitize nociceptors in the periphery, and may exert a role in the CNS transmission of nociceptive impulses. Prostaglandins also have important homeostatic functions such as maintenance of gastric mucosal lining, platelet function, and maintenance of renal blood flow during periods of hypovolemia. At least two different isoforms of cyclooxygenase (prostaglandin endoperoxide synthase) exist, COX-1 and COX-2. COX-1 purportedly synthesizes basal levels of prostaglandins responsible for homeostatic functions, whereas COX-2 is the inducible form synthesized by macrophages and inflammatory cells involved in the response to tissue injury.[47] The characterization of NSAIDs relative to COX-1 versus COX-2 inhibitory effects is dependent on the methodology used and is therefore confusing and somewhat contradictory.[48] In addition, clinical studies assessing the safety of NSAIDs in critically ill dogs and cats are lacking. At this time, preferential COX-2 inhibitors are not available in the United States in injectable form, further limiting their usefulness in the ICU patient. Ketoprofen (Ketofen, Fort Dodge Laboratories) is not a selective COX-2 inhibitor, but it has been used in healthy patients that are treated in the ICU for severe postoperative pain (see Table 7-3). Oral NSAIDs may be useful drugs when sending an animal home

Table 7-3. Nonopioid Analgesics

Drug	Dose/Route	Species
Ketamine	Loading dose: 0.25–0.5 mg/kg, IV CRI: 2–10 μg/kg/min, IV	Dog/cat
IV Lidocaine	Loading dose: 0.25–2 mg/kg, IV CRI: 15–30 μg/kg/min, IV	Dog
Intrapleural/Intraperitoneal		
Bupivacaine	1.5–2 mg/kg, q 3–6 h	Dog/cat
Epidural bupivacaine (with preservative-free morphine at 0.1 mg/kg)	0.1–0.5 mg/kg 0.1–0.2 mg/kg	Dog Cat
Ketoprofen	1–2 mg/kg, IV, SQ, IM q 24 h	Dog/cat

CRI, constant rate infusion.

after its stay in the ICU, provided there are no contraindications. Unfortunately, there is minimal dosing information for most NSAIDs in cats. NSAIDs should not be used in patients that are hypovolemic or hypotensive, or have renal disease, gastrointestinal ulceration or diarrhea, or a coagulopathy.[45,49,50]

Local Anesthetics

Local anesthetics (*e.g.*, lidocaine, bupivacaine) block the generation and transmission of nociceptive impulses and have the unique ability to completely block the sensation of pain. Because local anesthetics need to be infiltrated into tissues or injected close to sensory nerves, the use of local and regional blocks is primarily used in the perioperative period to decrease pain after surgery. The uses of these techniques as adjuncts to general anesthesia in small animal practice have gained acceptance recently and several exceptional reviews are available.[51–53] Local and regional anesthetic techniques are excellent methods to improve recovery and prevent central sensitization of nociceptive pathways after painful surgical procedures. The routine use of these techniques in the ICU patient is somewhat limited because repeated infiltration of local anesthetics is technically difficult and may be painful in the conscious patient. Nevertheless, some of these techniques are effective and provide excellent analgesia without sedation.

Intrapleural administration of local anesthetics may be used to decrease thoracic and cranial abdominal pain. The duration of action of bupivacaine (4-6 hours) is longer than that of lidocaine (1–2 hours) making it the preferred drug for this technique (see Table 7-3). Bupivacaine may be administered through the chest tube every 3 to 6 hours for post-thoracotomy pain. Rapid intrapleural administration of bupivacaine can be painful. The addition of sodium bicarbonate to bupivacaine (1 part sodium bicarbonate to 9 parts bupivacaine) and diluting the bupivacaine with physiologic saline (0.9% NaCl) help to decrease pain on injection. Injecting bupivacaine through the chest tube slowly and ensuring that the bupivacaine is close to body temperature before injection (warm syringe in hand or pocket) also help to decrease injection pain. Administration of intrapleural bupivacaine for cranial abdominal pain is somewhat more difficult but may be accomplished using a butterfly catheter or an over-the-needle catheter in a sedated patient. Alternatively, diluted bupivacaine may be injected into the peritoneal space at the level of the umbilicus.[53] With both intrapleural and intraperitoneal injections, it is often helpful to gently place the patient in different positions (dorsal and ventral recumbency) to increase the distribution of the bupivacaine.

Epidural administration of local anesthetics and opioids is an excellent means to decrease abdominal and hindlimb pain (see Table 7-1).[54–56] Depending on the drugs and doses selected, epidural techniques may also help to treat thoracic and forelimb pain. The primary advantage of epidurally administered drugs is the attainment of excellent analgesia with reduced side effects as compared to treating pain with systemically administered analgesics. Epidural administration of analgesics typically occurs one time in an anesthetized or heavily sedated patient. Repeated epidural injections or continuous infusion of epidural drugs may be accomplished through an epidural catheter.[57] Regardless of the technique selected, strict adherence to aseptic technique is essential to prevent infections in the epidural space. A detailed description of these techniques is beyond the scope of this chapter and the reader is referred to recent excellent reviews.[56,57] The two most common complications that occur with the administration of epidural analgesics are temporary hindlimb paresis and urine retention. Accordingly, a urinary catheter should be placed in all patients receiving epidural drugs. Following a single epidural injection, these effects resolve within 24 hours with the vast majority of cases.

Intravenous infusions of lidocaine administered in low doses (sub-antiarrhythmic) may induce mild sedation and augment opioid-induced analgesia in dogs (see Table 7-3). Lidocaine infusions are generally reserved for dogs in severe pain that appear resistant to relatively high doses of opioid analgesics. The evidence to support the use of lidocaine in this manner is mostly empirical, and the selection of lidocaine versus some other adjunct analgesic, such as ketamine CRI, is based on the clinician's judgment. Lidocaine infusions are quite safe because it is administered well below the toxic dose and may be most useful in dogs that are compromised and require some additional sedation.

ANXIETY

The clinical signs of anxiety are often indistinguishable from some of the signs attributable to pain. Typically, dogs may react with clinical signs such as incessant barking or whining, shaking, pacing, reluctance to rest, panting, having a wide-eyed appearance, and often difficulty in handling. Cats are usually difficult to restrain and may be fearful. Anxiety and pain interact in such a way as to exacerbate each other. Anxiety can sometimes be effectively treated simply by treating the patient's pain with an analgesic, by changing the environment (*e.g.*, moving to a larger or quieter cage), or by providing attention from a caregiver. Sometimes taking a dog outside to urinate will relieve discomfort and ease anxiety. Dogs and cats that still appear anxious should be administered acepromazine, a benzodiazepine, or an α_2-agonist depending on their health status.

ICU SEDATION/ANESTHESIA

Acepromazine

Acepromazine is an effective tranquilizer in dogs, particularly when it is combined with an opioid.[58] Acepromazine can be used in cats; however, it is a less predictable drug in cats and the degree of sedation is generally less than in dogs. Acepromazine has a relatively long duration of action that may last from 3 to 4 hours to over 24 hours in compromised patients. Acepromazine induces dose-dependent vasodilation, which will result in hypotension in hypovolemic or compromised patients. There is no antagonist for acepromazine and the adverse effects are dose dependent; therefore, the lowest doses possible should be used (Table 7-3). Acepromazine is also purported to lower the seizure threshold and should not be used in patients with pre-existing seizure history or neurologic disorders. Acepromazine interferes with platelet function and should not be administered to patients that are hemorrhaging or that have bleeding disorders. In general, acepromazine is only used in ICU patients if it is absolutely necessary and no good alternatives exist.

Benzodiazepines

Diazepam and midazolam (Versed, Roche) may be used as an alternative to acepromazine for sedation. Midazolam is similar to diazepam, with the exception that midazolam is more potent than diazepam, has a shorter duration of action, and is water soluble.[59] Benzodiazepines are poor sedatives in young healthy animals, but they are effective in compromised dogs and cats, especially when combined with an opioid. Thus, benzodiazepines are reserved for anxious animals that require some sedation and are unlikely to tolerate the adverse side effects of acepromazine (see Table 7-2). Although it is rarely necessary in animals, both diazepam and midazolam can be reversed with flumazenil (0.1 mg, IV total dose), a specific benzodiazepine antagonist.

Propofol

Occasionally ICU patients require deep sedation to the point of unconsciousness (anesthesia) to facilitate a diagnostic or therapeutic intervention. Propofol is widely used for this purpose in both dogs and cats. The rapid onset, short duration of action, rapid recovery, and limited residual effects of propofol are useful attributes in the ICU setting.[60] Propofol may be administered repeatedly as small IV boluses or by CRI (see Table 7-2). Repeated dosing does not prolong the effect of propofol in dogs, although propofol infusions longer than 1 hour or propofol anesthesia repeated daily might result in longer recoveries in cats. Despite its usefulness, propofol does have its limitations that could have adverse consequences in high-risk patients. Propofol causes marked vasodilation in dogs and cats leading to hypotension. Administering propofol slowly to effect, while diluting it with IV fluids, helps to decrease the incidence of hypotension. Propofol should not be administered to hypovolemic or dehydrated patients. Administering an opioid or benzodiazepine premedication before propofol also helps to reduce the dose of propofol and decrease the incidence of hypotension. Propofol is a profound respiratory depressant that will cause hypoventilation and may induce apnea and hypoxemia. Decreasing the rate of injection and dose of propofol will help to minimize the severity of hypoventilation. All critical animals should be preoxygenated using a loose-fitting facemask and high oxygen flow rate prior to induction with propofol to prevent hypoxemia. The trachea should be intubated and the patient maintained on oxygen throughout the procedure. If the patient cannot be intubated for any reason, it should be maintained on oxygen delivered through the facemask until complete recovery. Propofol is an excellent medium for bacterial and fungal growth; therefore, aseptic technique must be used when handling the drug and opened bottles should be discarded. Propofol may interfere with immune function, which may be particularly problematic in immunocompromised patients requiring multiple sedations/

anesthesias.[61,62] Propofol has no residual analgesia beyond the duration of unconsciousness; therefore, patients should be administered analgesics if invasive procedures are performed.

REFERENCES

1. McMillan FD: Comfort as the primary goal in veterinary medicine. *J Am Vet Assoc* 212:1370, 1998.
2. Hellyer PW, Gaynor JS: How I treat: acute postsurgical pain in dogs and cats. *Compend Contin Educ* 20:140, 1998.
3. Carr DB, Goudas LC: Pain: acute pain. *Lancet* 353:2051, 1999.
4. Besson JM: Pain: the neurobiology of pain. *Lancet* 353:1610, 1999.
5. Cervero F, Laird JMA: Pain: visceral pain. *Lancet* 353:2145, 1999.
6. Chapman CR, Gavrin J: Pain: suffering: the contributions of persistent pain. *Lancet* 353:2233, 1999.
7. Woolf CJ, Mannion RJ: Pain: neuropathic pain: aetiology, symptoms, mechanisms, and management. *Lancet* 353:1959, 1999.
8. Carroll GL: Small Animal Pain Management. Lakewood, CO: AAHA Press, 1998.
9. Hansen BD, Hardie EM, Carroll GS: Physiological measurements after ovariohysterectomy in dogs: what's normal? *Appl Anim Behav Sci* 51:101, 1997.
10. Hardie EM, Hansen BD, Carroll GS: Behavior after ovariohysterectomy in the dog: what's normal? *Appl Animal Behav Sci* 51:111, 1997.
11. Cambridge AJ, Tobias KM, Nowberry RC, *et al.*: Subjective and objective measurements of postoperative pain in cats. *J Am Vet Med Assoc* 217:685, 2000.
12. Smith JD, Allen SW, Quandt JE, *et al.*: Indicators of postoperative pain in cats and correlation with clinical criteria. *Am J Vet Res* 57:1674, 1996.
13. Firth AM, Haldane SL: Development of a scale to evaluate postoperative pain in dogs. *J Am Vet Med Assoc* 214:651, 1999.
14. Hansen B: Through a glass darkly: using behavior to assess pain. *Semin Vet Med Surg (Small Anim)* 12:61, 1997.
15. Whipple JK, Lewis KS, Quebbeman EJ, *et al.*: Analysis of pain management in critically ill patients. *Pharmacotherapy* 15:592, 1995.
16. Anand KJ, Hickey PR: Halothane-morphine compared with high-dose sufentanil for anesthesia and postoperative analgesia in neonatal cardiac surgery. *N Engl J Med* 326:1, 1992.
17. Mathews KA: Pain assessment and general approach to management. *Vet Clin North Am Small Anim Pract* 30:729, 2000.
18. Cornick JL: Anesthetic management of patients with neurologic abnormalities. *Comp Contin Educ* 14:163, 1992.
19. Pascoe PJ: Opioid analgesics. *Vet Clin North Am Small Anim Pract* 30:757, 2000.
20. Yaksh TL: Pharmacology and mechanisms of opioid analgesic activity. *Acta Anaesthesiol Scand* 41:94, 1997.
21. Stein C: Peripheral mechanisms of opioid analgesia. *Anesth Analg* 76:182, 1993.
22. Pettifer G, Dyson D: Hydromorphone: a cost-effective alternative to the use of oxymorphone. *Can Vet J* 41:135, 2000.
23. Thurmon JC: Preanesthetics and anesthetic adjuncts. *In* Thurmon JC, Tranquilli WJ, Benson GJ, eds.: *Lumb & Jones' Veterinary Anesthesia*, 3rd ed. Baltimore: Williams & Wilkins, 1996, p. 183.
24. Papich MG: Pharmacologic considerations for opiate analgesis and nonsteroidal anti-inflammatory drugs. *Vet Clin North Am Small Anim Pract* 30:815, 2000.

25. Barnhart MD, Hubbell JA, Muir WW, *et al.*: Pharmacokinetics, pharmacodynamics, and analgesic effects of morphine after rectal, intramuscular, and intravenous administration in dogs. *Am J Vet Res* 61:24, 2000.
26. Dohoo SE, Tasker RAR: Pharmacokinetics of oral morphine sulfate in dogs: a comparison of sustained release and conventional formulations. *Can J Vet Res* 61:251, 1997.
27. Dohoo S: Steady-state pharmacokinetics of oral sustained-release morphine sulphate in dogs. *J Vet Pharmacol Therap* 20:129, 1997.
28. Murphy MR, Olson WA, Hug CC Jr: Pharmacokinetics of ^{3}H-fentanyl in the dog anesthetized with enflurane. *Anesthesiology* 50:13, 1979.
29. Egger CM, Duke T, Archer J, *et al.*: Comparison of plasma fentanyl concentrations by using three transdermal fentanyl patch sizes in dogs. *Vet Surg* 27:159, 1998.
30. Scherk-Nixon M: A study of the use of a transdermal fentanyl patch in cats. *J Am Anim Hosp Assoc* 32:19, 1996.
31. Twycross RG: Opioids. *In* Wall PD, Melzack R, eds.: Textbook of Pain, 4th ed. Edinburgh: Churchill Livinstone, 1999, p 1187.
32. Carroll GL, Howie LB, Slater MR, *et al.*: Evaluation of analgesia provided by postoperative administration of butorphanol to cats undergoing onychectomy. *J Am Vet Med Assoc* 213:246, 1998.
33. Briggs SL, Sneed K, Sawyer DC: Antinociceptive effects of oxymorphone-butorphanol-acepromazine combination in cats. *Vet Surg* 27:466, 1998.
34. Bell RF: Low-dose subcutaneous ketamine infusion and morphine tolerance. *Int Assoc Study Pain* 83:101, 1999.
35. Fu ES, Miguel R, Scharf JE: Preemptive ketamine decreases postoperative narcotic requirements in patients undergoing abdominal surgery. *Anesth Analg* 84:1086, 1997.
36. Menigaux C, Fletcher D, Dupont X, *et al.*: The benefits of intraoperative small-dose ketamine on postoperative pain after anterior cruciate ligament repair. *Anesth Analg* 90:129, 2000.
37. Stubhaug A, Breivik H, Eide PK, *et al.*: Mapping of punctuate hyperalgesia around a surgical incision demonstrates that ketamine is a powerful suppressor of central sensitization to pain following surgery. *Acta Anaesthesiol Scand* 41:1124, 1997.
38. Dickenson AH: NMDA receptor antagonists: interactions with opioids. *Acta Anaesthesiol Scand* 41:112, 1997.
39. Dickenson AH: Plasticity: implications for opioid and other pharmacological interventions in specific pain states. *Behav Brain Sci* 20:392, 1997.
40. Mao J, Price DD, Mayer DJ: Mechanisms of hyperalgesia and morphine tolerance: a current view of their possible interactions. *Pain* 62:259, 1995.
41. Pypendop BH, Verstegen JP: Hemodynamic effects of medetomidine in the dog: a dose titration study. *Vet Surg* 27:612, 1998.
42. Cullen LK: Medetomidine sedation in dogs and cats: a review of its pharmacology, antagonism and dose. *Br Vet J* 152:519, 1996.
43. Lascelles BDX, Crippa PJ, Jones A, *et al.*: Efficacy and kinetics of carprofen, administered preoperatively or postoperatively, for the prevention of pain in dogs undergoing ovariohysterectomy. *Vet Surg* 27:568, 1998.
44. Yaksh TL, Dirig DM, Malmberg AB: Mechanism of action of nonsteroidal anti-inflammatory drugs. *Cancer Inv* 16:509, 1998.
45. Mathews KA: Nonsteroidal anti-inflammatory analgesics: indications and contraindications for pain management in dogs and cats. *Vet Clin North Am Small Anim Pract* 30:783, 2000.

46. Slingsby LS, Waterman-Pearson AE: Comparison of pethidine, buprenorphine and ketoprofen for postoperative analgesia after ovariohysterectomy in the cat. *Vet Rec* 143:185, 1998.
47. Jones CJ, Budsberg SC: Physiological characteristics and clinical importance of the cyclooxygenase isoforms in dogs and cats. *J Am Vet Med Assoc* 217:721, 2000.
48. Livingston A: Mechanism of action of nonsteroidal anti-inflammatory drugs. *Vet Clin North Am Small Anim Pract* 30:773, 2000.
49. Forsyth SF, Guilford WG, Haslett SJ, *et al.*: Endoscopy of the gastroduodenal mucosa after carprofen, meloxicam and ketoprofen administration in dogs. *J Small Anim Pract* 39:421, 1998.
50. Ko JCH, Miyabiyashi T, Mandsager RE, *et al.*: Renal effects of carprofen administered to healthy dogs anesthetized with propofol and isoflurane. *J Am Vet Med Assoc* 217:346, 2000.
51. Quandt JE, Rawlings CE: Reducing postoperative pain for dogs: Local anesthetic and analgesic techniques. *Comp Cont Educ* 18:101, 1996.
52. Pascoe P: Local and regional anesthesia and analgesia. *Semin Vet Med Surg Small Anim Pract* 12:94, 1997.
53. Lemke KA, Dawson SD: Local and regional anesthesia. *Vet Clin North Am Small Anim Pract* 30:839, 2000.
54. Popilskis S, Kohn D, Sanchez JA, *et al.*: Epidural vs. intramuscular oxymorphone analgesia after thoracotomy in dogs. *Vet Surg* 20:462, 1991.
55. Hendrix PK, Raffe MR, Robinson EP, *et al.*: Epidural administration of bupivacaine, morphine, or their combination for postoperative analgesia in dogs. *J Am Vet Med Assoc* 209: 598, 1996.
56. Torske KE, Dyson DH: Epidural analgesia and anesthesia. *Vet Clin North Am Small Anim Pract* 30:859, 2000.
57. Swalander DB, Crowe DT, Hittenmiller DH, *et al.*: Complications associated with the use of indwelling epidural catheters in dogs: 82 cases (1996–1999). *J Am Vet Med Assoc* 216:368, 2000.
58. Jacobson JD, McGrath CJ, Smith EP: Cardiorespiratory effects of four opioid-tranquilizer combinations in dogs. *Vet Surg* 23:299, 1994.
59. Jones DJ, Stehling LC, Zauder HL: Cardiovascular response to diazepam and midazolam maleate in dogs. *Anesthesiology* 51:430, 1979.
60. Quandt JE, Robinson EP, Rivers WJ, *et al.*: Cardiorespiratory and anesthetic effects of propofol and thiopental in dogs. *Am J Vet Res* 59:1137, 1998.
61. Heldmann E, Brown DC, Shofer F: The association of propofol usage with postoperative wound infection rate in clean wounds: a retrospective study. *Vet Surg* 28:256, 1999.
62. Kelbel I, Koch T, Weber A, *et al.*: Alterations of bacterial clearance induced by propofol. *Acta Anaesthesiol Scand* 43:71, 1999.

8
Oximetry and Capnography

Marc R. Raffe

Noninvasive methods for monitoring oxygen (O_2) and carbon dioxide (CO_2) have been available for over a decade. The development of these technologies significantly changed clinical practice habits in critical care medicine. The ability to continuously monitor O_2 and CO_2 without serial blood sample collection and laboratory analysis dramatically improved patient care and decreased the amount of blood lost for laboratory evaluation. These technologies are becoming increasingly popular in veterinary medicine and have been recognized as providing valuable information in both the anesthesia and critical care areas. Despite their routine use, a survey in human medicine indicates that over 90% of clinicians and support staff do not understand how these technologies operate. The goal of this presentation is to provide background in how these technologies work and their value to the critically ill patient.

BACKGROUND

Spectrophotometry is an optical detection method that uses light reflection properties of molecules to measure the concentration of a chemical species in a gaseous or liquid medium. All molecules and atoms share the property of absorbing or reflecting light of specific wavelengths. Absorption and reflection are unique to that molecular structure and occur in specific portions of the light spectrum.

Both O_2 and hemoglobin (Hb) reflect light in the infrared and red spectrums. The technique of measuring the amount of (Hb) that has O_2 attached versus nonoxygenated hemoglobin is called oximetry. Similarly, the technique for measuring the amount of CO_2 in exhaled gas is called capnography.

OXIMETRY

Hemoglobin changes its stereochemical configuration when it interacts with or releases O_2 from its chemical structure. This change in molecular configuration affects light absorption and reflection. The patterns associated with oxygenated hemoglobin (HbO_2, oxyhemoglobin) are distinct from deoxygenated hemoglobin (Hb, reduced or deoxyhemoglobin). This difference in light absorption and reflectance is one reason that arterialized blood (oxyhemoglobin) has a more intense red color than venous blood (reduced Hb). HbO_2 reflects more readily in the red spectrum of light. At 660 nm, maximum light absorption occurs for

HbO_2 compared to Hb. The opposite occurs at 940 nm; reduced Hb has maximum reflectance. This relationship is useful to understand because it is the basis of all oximetric measurement techniques.

Oximetry uses the reflectance relationship of HbO_2 and reduced Hb to determine the degree of Hb saturation; that is, the quantity of Hb that has O_2 attached. The absolute concentration of HbO_2 and Hb are measured and inserted in a mathematical expression to determine the percent oxyhemoglobin saturation (SaO_2). The formula used for this calculation is:

$$SaO_2 = (HbO_2/HbO_2 + Hb) \times 100$$

CLINICAL OXIMETRY MEASUREMENT

Currently, there are two main methods for evaluation of oximetry in veterinary medicine, namely, pulse oximetry and co-oximetry.

Pulse Oximetry

The application of pulse oximetry has increased over the last 10 years in veterinary medicine. Any patient at risk of developing hypoxemia or requiring circulatory monitoring may benefit from pulse oximetry monitoring. The value of pulse oximetry is in early detection of changes in microcirculatory blood flow and hypoxemia associated with capillary blood flow disturbances. Therefore, it is indicated when noninvasive, continuous monitoring of arterial Hb saturation and development of hypoxemic episodes is warranted.

The term pulse oximetry represents a fusion of two physiologic principles. Oximetry, the measurement of HbO_2, is quantitated using the principles described above. Pulsatile capillary blood flow is simultaneously evaluated using the principle of plethysmography. Pulsatile flow monitored by plethysmography is used as a "signal" to confirm that a correct site for oximetry measurement is identified. The way in which this is accomplished is that the probe views only pulsatile or "arterial" blood flow in determining the Hb saturation. Nonpulsatile components are not evaluated (Fig. 8-1). The plethysmographic signal is counted and reported as either heart or pulse rate on the digital display.

Following signal detection and measurement at the tissue level, data are reported to the base device, which interprets and displays the information. The information is reported as heart or pulse rate and HbO_2 saturation at the tissue bed (SaO_2 or SpO_2). These parameters are digitally displayed. More sophisticated units also permit visualization of the "pulse" signal on a screen display to aid in evaluating the signal strength and characteristics. Most units also have a light-emitting diode (LED) "bar" display or numerical indicator that will assist in determining correct probe placement and indicate the signal strength. Built-in alarms will alert the operator to incorrect probe placement, loss of signal quality, low and high heart rate limits, and low saturation levels. At clinically acceptable levels of arterial oxygenation ($>$70% Hb saturation), the Hb saturation reported by pulse oximetry is very close (within 3%) to laboratory-based oximetry measurements.

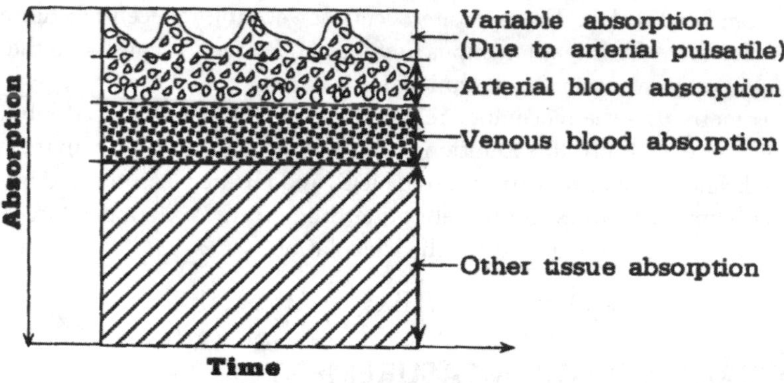

Figure 8-1
Components of a pulse oximeter waveform. Note the variable absorption component of the waveform; this is the key component that the pulse oximeter detects and integrates during signal processing.

Probe placement technique and detection sites are critical to ensure accurate results. Several probe types are commercially available. The most common probe design is a transflectance probe. In this probe style, the two infrared wavelengths (660, 940 nm) are emitted from a phototransmitter diode through a thin tissue bed. A photodetector on the opposite side of the tissue bed detects reflected light at both band widths and sends the information to the base module. A second probe style is a reflectance probe. In this design, both the phototransmitter and photodetector are on the same side of the tissue bed. Light emitted from the phototransmitter reflects off hard tissue such as bone or cartilage and is measured by the photodetector. A variation of this approach can be used in soft tissue by modifying the intensity of the light source and photodetector sensitivity.

Reported measurement sites in companion animals include tongue, lip, nasal septum, toe web, axilla, inguinal area, ventral surface of the tail base, and rectum. The most consistent detection sites are the tongue, lip, and tail base. This poses a limitation in awake animals necessitating use of the tail base for continuous measurement or intermittent measurement techniques.

A number of factors have been reported to influence pulse oximeter accuracy. Motion at the detection site is the most common artifact. Accurate and consistent results are difficult to obtain in patients that move during measurement. Dyshemoglobinemias represented by carboxyhemoglobin and methemoglobin artificially elevate oximetry readings. Hypotension and vasoconstriction affect the pleythysmographic reading of pulsatile blood flow resulting in inaccurate saturation measurement. Dark skin pigmentation can reduce readings by dampening the light source and detection capability. Severe anemias (<3 g/dL) may result in underestimation of Hb saturation. Several clinical studies have shown the superiority of pulse oximetry over periodic blood gas analysis in detecting hypoxemic episodes in critically ill patients. However, these studies also show that despite the improved detection ability, no difference in morbidity or mortality occurred. This may reflect the impact of operator decision-making rather than technology limitation.

Co-Oximetry

In vitro oximetry is performed using a co-oximeter instrument. The principle of co-oximetry is similar to pulse oximetry. The difference in methodologies is that the co-oximeter is a laboratory-based instrument that requires an anaerobically collected blood sample. An additional distinction is that co-oximetry does not monitor pulsatile flow due to the in vitro analytical methodology.

Four separate red spectrum wavelengths are simultaneously emitted and passed through a chamber containing the anaerobic blood sample. A photodetector on the opposite side of the measurement chamber quantitates the light transmission. This measurement is reported for four hemoglobin species: HbO_2, reduced Hb, carboxyhemoglobin, and methemoglobin. A total Hb value is also reported. Each Hb species is reported as a percent of total Hb. The sum of all Hb species is approximately 100%; slight differences in individual measurement may make the sum of all species slightly less (*i.e.*, 99.7%).

Co-oximetry is generally performed in conjunction with a blood gas analysis to determine Hb saturation. New devices have simplified the methodology and have excellent accuracy on small amounts of blood (50 μL).

CO_2 DETECTION AND CAPNOGRAPHY

Detection and measurement of CO_2 in pulmonary gas is an important part of evaluating ventilatory efficiency in healthy and critically ill patients. Several technologies have evolved that support these functions.

Colorometric CO_2 Detection

A disposable device that colorometrically detects CO_2 is available. The device is composed of a plastic housing with molded fittings to interface with an endotracheal tube and breathing circuit. The center part of the plastic housing contains a filter paper disk that is impregnated with a color-sensitive pH indicator. Exhaled respiratory gas is hydrated by a liquid film on the paper; the resulting pH is detected and displayed as a color in the disk section. The zone surrounding the disk contains a "ring" that has different color-coded areas that represented different CO_2 concentrations. The color ranges from purple (0%) to yellow (>2%). The color shades are not entirely accurate for predicting end-tidal CO_2 levels; the major use for this device has been to confirm endotracheal tube placement into the proximal airway.

The system is easy and accurate in all but low perfusion and respiratory states. The detector is not accurate in patients with cardiopulmonary arrest because CO_2 levels are essentially zero until spontaneous circulation is reestablished. Patients with excessive gastrointestinal gas (carbonated beverages) may also demonstrate a false-positive result. Despite these shortcomings, the device is easy to use and accurate under most conditions.

Infrared Capnometry

Infrared light analysis of respiratory gases provides a quantitative method for detection and measurement. This principle is applied to measurement of CO_2 in respiratory gases. The key factor is to identify a light wavelength that provides maximal measurement ability without interference from other respiratory gases.

For CO_2 measurement, a wavelength of 4.28 μm provides analysis without interference from other gas agents such as nitrous oxide. An LED generates a steady light beam that passes through a measuring chamber. A photodetector on the opposite side of the chamber measures transmitted light intensity. The detected light intensity is inversely proportional to the concentration of CO_2 in the analyzed gas sample. The light intensity measured at the photodetector is analyzed and quantitated for display to the user.

The are two principal designs for CO_2 detection and measurement. A mainstream analyzer uses an optical chamber that is attached to the patient's face or breathing circuit. An LED and photodetector unit surround the optical chamber for measurement. This design has the advantage of maintaining a "closed" breathing system to the patient without loss of gas volume. The main disadvantage is moisture condensation in the optical chamber that can affect accurate measurement. A sidestream analyzer has a sampling port and a small-bore tubing connection that is incorporated into the breathing circuit or attached to a facemask. Exhaled gas is continuously sampled by active withdrawal through the sampling port. A small suction pump housed in the analyzer base unit performs this function. After withdrawal of gas, it passes through a moisture trap/desiccation chamber to remove condensation. Following moisture removal, it is introduced into the measurement chamber, analyzed, and purged to the atmosphere. Measurements are integrated and displayed on the front panel of the analyzer.

Two types of CO_2 monitors are available. A capnogram displays only a digital value that corresponds to the end-tidal CO_2 concentration (described below). A capnograph displays the digital information and also has a waveform display in the monitor unit. This ability to visualize and interpret the CO_2 waveform provides additional useful information to the clinician.

Capnogram

The signal detected by the infrared detector has a rapid response time and can be plotted during different phases of an individual breath on a moment-to-moment basis. The graphical plot of the changes in CO_2 concentrations versus time is called a capnogram. Capnogram waveforms can be useful in diagnosis and management of acute changes in respiratory function. An individual breath waveform is comprised of five component areas (Fig. 8-2). A zero baseline represents exhaled gas that has been in the anatomic dead space of the large conducting pathways, oropharynx, and nasopharnyx. This part of the waveform tracing is the A-B region. The rapid upstroke representing gas from the intermediate airways containing both fresh and exhaled gases is the B-C region. The flat plateau area representing mixed alveolar gas is the C-D region. The distinct endpoint of the plateau that represents true end-tidal gas is the D point. The rapid

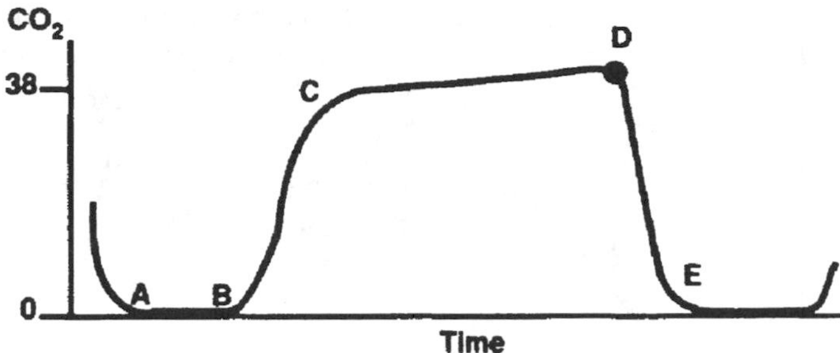

Figure 8-2
Components of a normal capnograph waveform. Segment A-B represents the zero baseline. Segment B-C represents the rapid, sharp rise associated with gas from the intermediate airways. Segment C-D represents the flat alveolar plateau associated with alveolar gas detection. Point D is the $ETCO_2$ concentration found in the alveolus. Segment D-E represents inspiration of fresh gas devoid of CO_2.

downstroke of the curve associated with inspiration is the D-E region. This waveform component is devoid of CO_2.

Under conditions of normal lung health and physiology, the graphical point on the plateau just prior to downward inflection represents the mixed alveolar CO_2 level. This value is referred to as end-tidal CO_2 ($ETCO_2$, P_{ETCO2}). $ETCO_2$ values approximate blood CO_2 levels; however, the gradient is species dependent.

Capnogram Waveforms

When pulmonary gas exchange is impaired, less CO_2 is eliminated with each breath due to the reduced zones of diffusion attendant with most forms of pulmonary disease. In these cases, the $PaCO_2 - ETCO_2$ gradient increases due to a decreased $ETCO_2$. The conditions that may contribute to this response are listed in Table 8-1.

Capnogram waveform changes in fall into one of two categories: change in individual waveform characteristics and change in waveform across time (trend monitoring). Changes may be noted in any phase of the capnogram waveform. In most cases, the point of change involves the plateau (C-D) end-tidal (D), and expiratory (D-E) waveform phases. Several characteristic patterns have been noted (Figs. 8-3, 8-4, 8-5, and 8-6).

Table 8-1. Factors in $PaCO_2 - ETCO_2$ Gradient Increase

Increased Anatomic Dead Space	Increased Physiologic Dead Space
Open ventilator circuit	Obstructive lung disease
Shallow breathing	Low cardiac output
	Pulmonary thromboembolism
	Excessive lung inflation

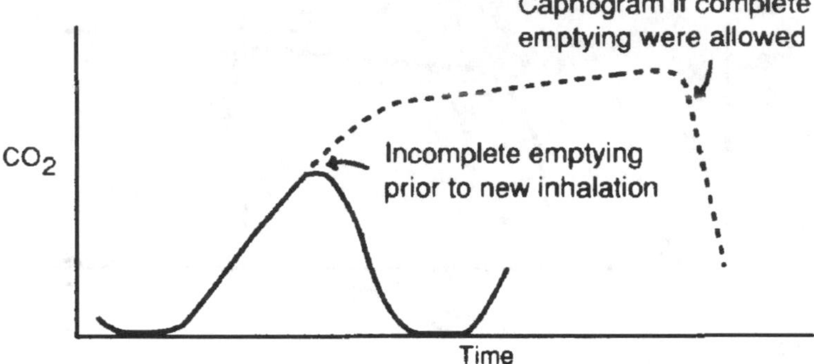

Figure 8-3
Change in alveolar waveform indicating incomplete alveolar emptying. Incomplete emptying may be associated with asthma, upper airway obstruction, partial endotracheal tube obstruction, or chronic obstructive pulmonary disease (COPD). This is one example of a waveform change indicating a clinical problem. (Good VS: Continuous End Tidal Carbon Dioxide Monitoring. *In* McHale DJ, Carlson KK: AACN Procedure Manual for Critical Care, 4th ed. Philadelphia: WB Saunders, 2001.)

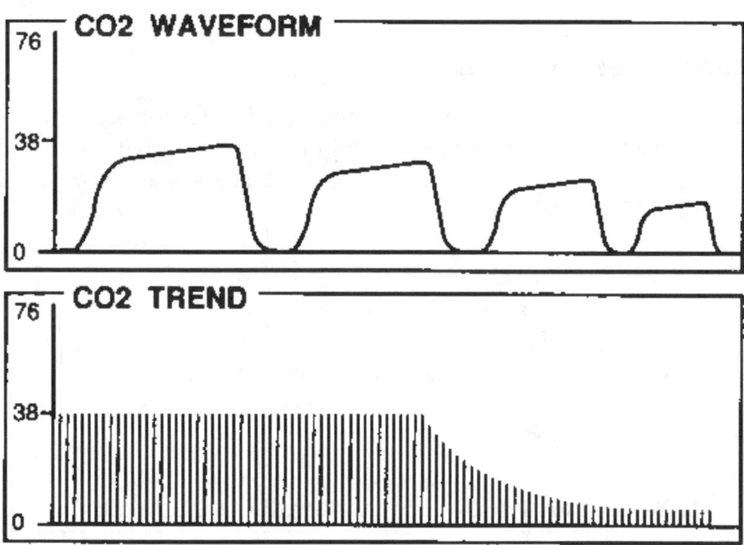

Figure 8-4
Exponential fall in $ETCO_2$ indicating pulmonary embolism, severe pulmonary hypoperfusion, or cardiopulmonary arrest. (Good VS: Continuous End Tidal Carbon Dioxide Monitoring. *In* McHale DJ, Carlson KK: AACN Procedure Manual for Critical Care, 4th ed. Philadelphia: WB Saunders, 2001.)

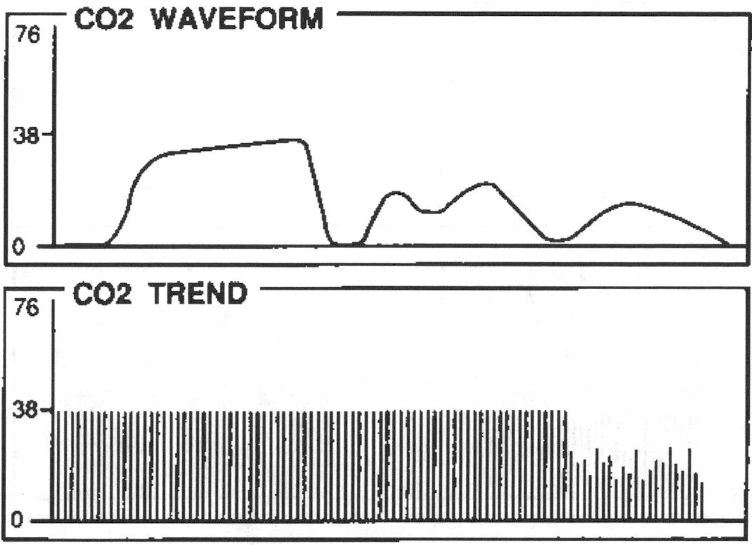

Figure 8-5
Sudden fall in $ETCO_2$ indicating mechanical airway leak. Possible reasons include breathing circuit leak or disconnection, accidental extubation, partial airway obstruction, and ventilator leak. (Good VS: Continuous End Tidal Carbon Dioxide Monitoring. *In* McHale DJ, Carlson KK: AACN Procedure Manual for Critical Care, 4th ed. Philadelphia: WB Saunders, 2001.)

Waveforms with a normal appearance but a higher scalar plateau represent elevated $ETCO_2$ partial pressure reflecting hypercapnia. A gradual rise in $ETCO_2$ reflects increased metabolism, hyperthermia, sepsis, hypoventilation, neuromuscular weakness, and reduced alveolar gas exchange. A stable, sustained rise in $ETCO_2$ reflects sedative or anesthetic drugs, metabolic alkalosis, or hypoventilation. A gradual rise in both baseline and $ETCO_2$ reflects rebreathing of CO_2 gas.

A decreased $ETCO_2$ with a stable plateau phase reflects hyperventilation, hypothermia, and metabolic acidosis. A sudden fall in $ETCO_2$ to low values reflects airway leak, partial airway obstruction, disconnection from a breathing circuit, or mechanical ventilator malfunction. A sudden fall in $ETCO_2$ to zero indicates a dislodged airway, complete airway obstruction, breathing circuit disconnection, mechanical ventilator malfunction, or esophageal intubation. It may also be associated with cardiopulmonary arrest, pulmonary thromboembolism, or severe pulmonary hypoperfusion. A sustained low $ETCO_2$ without alveolar plateau indicates partial airway obstruction, bronchospasm, small airway mucous plugs, or incorrect ventilator settings.

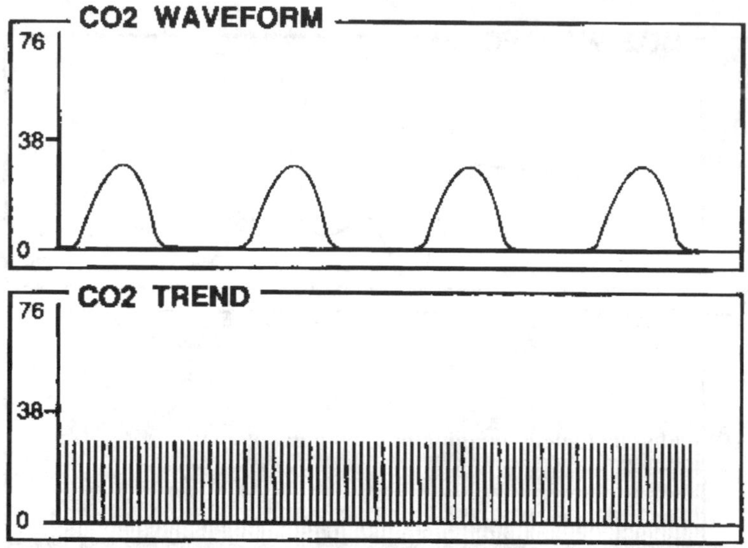

Figure 8-6
Sustained fall in $ETCO_2$ indicating incomplete alveolar emptying, endotracheal tube leak, bronchospasm, mucous plugging of the airway, or improper gas sampling technique. (Good VS: Continuous End Tidal Carbon Dioxide Monitoring. *In* McHale DJ, Carlson KK: AACN Procedure Manual for Critical Care, 4th ed. Philadelphia: WB Saunders, 2001.)

Comparison of $PaCO_2$ and $ETCO_2$ Values

In small animal species, a difference of 5 mm Hg or less is reported to be normal between arterial blood gas and $ETCO_2$ values ($PaCO_2$ − $ETCO_2$). $ETCO_2$ values will be lower than arterial values due to intrapulmonary dead space ventilation.

Almost all cardiac or respiratory diseases produce an increase in the $PaCO_2$ − $ETCO_2$ gradient. In these cases, arterial blood gas analysis remains the definitive method for evaluating CO_2 dynamics. Once the $PaCO_2$ − $ETCO_2$ gradient is established, continued monitoring using $ETCO_2$ may be more practical.

Additional Information from $ETCO_2$ Measurement

Trends in $ETCO_2$ can be used to monitor cardiac output. Studies have shown that $ETCO_2$ measurement correlates well with cardiac output measurements during volume resuscitation and during cardiopulmonary resuscitation. $ETCO_2$ has also proven useful in early detection of pulmonary thromboembolism, atelectasis, low cardiac output, pneumonia, and pulmonary edema. It is also useful in monitoring ventilator management by reporting ventilator-related mishaps and monitoring controlled hyperventilation. $ETCO_2$ is also useful for monitoring patients during discontinuation of ventilatory support ("weaning").

SUGGESTED READINGS

Boggs RL, Wooldridge-King M: AACN Procedure Manual for Critical Care, 3rd ed. Philadelphia: WB Saunders, 1993, 206.

Haskins SC: Monitoring the anesthetized patient. *In* Thurmon JC, Tranquilli WJ, Benson GJ, edd.: Veterinary Anesthesia, 3rd ed. Baltimore: Williams & Wilkins, 1996, p 413.

Marini JJ, Wheeler AP: Critical Care Medicine: The Essentials, 2nd ed. Baltimore: Williams & Wilkins, 1997, 75.

Marino PL: The ICU Book, 2nd edition. Baltimore: Williams & Wilkins, 1998, 339.

Parbrook GD, Davis PD, Parbrook EO: Basic Physics and Measurement in Anaesthesia, 3rd ed. Oxford, England: Butterworths, Heinneman, 1992, 232.

9
Principles of Mechanical Ventilation

Marc R. Raffe

INTRODUCTION

Mechanical ventilation has become a key support modality in emergent and critically ill patients. Principles and practice in this area have changed markedly in the past decade due to increased understanding of disease pathophysiology and improvements in ventilator technology. Increased demand for ventilatory support is based on better understanding of how to recognize need and institute therapy, increased availability of technology and support staff to implement therapy, and increased consumer awareness and demand for this level of support.

The classic mechanical ventilator has changed into a sophisticated support device that can be used to implement support strategies that were unheard of a decade ago. Improved technology and increased "choice" of support techniques has raised the level of practice. However, application of newer support techniques must be based on individual patient need to avoid undue risk and complications associated with mechanical ventilation. This chapter introduces current principles and practices of mechanical ventilation in clinical veterinary patients.

INDICATIONS FOR MECHANICAL VENTILATION

There are a number of clinical indications for mechanical ventilation. When surveying reasons for mechanical ventilation, there are four core profiles in which mechanical ventilation is indicated (Table 9-1).

Table 9-1. Indications for Mechanical Ventilation

- Inadequate ventilation to maintain blood pH level
  - Decreased ability to remove CO_2
    - Primary pulmonary disease
    - Chest wall/diaphragm injury
  - CNS injury
    - Apnea
- Inadequate tissue oxygenation
  - Pulmonary disease that impairs O_2 uptake
- Increased work of breathing
  - Increased O_2 consumption
  - Respiratory muscle fatigue
- Cardiovascular support
  - Congestive heart failure
  - Circulatory shock

PRINCIPLES AND THEORY OF MECHANICAL VENTILATION

Each breath is divided into inspiration and expiration. Inspiration is an active process in which respiratory muscle contraction produces pulmonary expansion secondary to changes in intrathoracic volume and pressure. Expiration is a passive process in which respiratory muscle relaxation permits shortening of elastic fibers in lung tissue producing volume reduction and gas expulsion.

Mechanical ventilators are classified as positive or negative pressure. Their design is based on their method for achieving pulmonary inflation. Ventilators are classified as "positive pressure" if they require application of positive airway pressure to inflate lungs. This principle of breath delivery requires an artificial airway to deliver adequate breath volume. Ventilator designs are based on the pulmonary compliance relationship. All ventilator designs control either applied airway pressure or delivered gas volume per breath. Ventilators that control airway pressure are pressure cycled; ventilators that control delivered breath volume are flow (volume) cycled. Breaths delivered in a pressure cycled mode are called "pressure-targeted" breaths. Breaths delivered in a flow-cycled mode are called "volume-targeted" breaths. Flow-cycled ventilators have become the standard ventilator design because they deliver a reliable breath volume independent of physiologic changes in lung tissue or chest wall. New ventilator designs have the ability to operate in either pressure- or flow-cycled ventilation. These designs increase operator ability to modify individual elements of a breath to reduce hazardous side effects associated with positive pressure ventilation.

A second factor is whether each breath is delivered using controlled or assisted mode. Controlled ventilation delivers each breath at a set time interval irrespective of the patient's needs. In this mode, the ventilator replaces both breathing function and central respiratory control. Assisted ventilation senses patient's need to breathe and provides a preprogrammed breath in response to patient efforts. Controlled ventilation is preferred when central nervous system (CNS) depression (anesthesia) is anticipated. Assisted ventilation is preferred when central regulation is intact.

A third key factor in providing optimal ventilatory support is delivering individual breaths that are patient appropriate. Each breath is a composite of inspiratory and expiratory components as described in the Cournand relationship (Fig. 9-1). Inspiration begins when the ventilator initiates breath support and stops when pulmonary inflation produces an inflation volume appropriate for the patient. Factors in optimizing inspiration include duration of the delivered breath, speed at which the breath is delivered, pattern of delivery, and whether a brief breath "hold" is needed. Expiration begins when pulmonary inflation is complete. Factors in optimizing expiration include duration of breath release, speed of breath release, and whether the stop point for breath release is at or above ambient pressure.

Over time, guidelines for ventilator settings have been developed in both human and veterinary medicine (Table 9-2). The guidelines are valuable for initial set up and support of the patients. These guidelines are empirical because each patient has unique pulmonary physiology. "Fine tuning" of support parame-

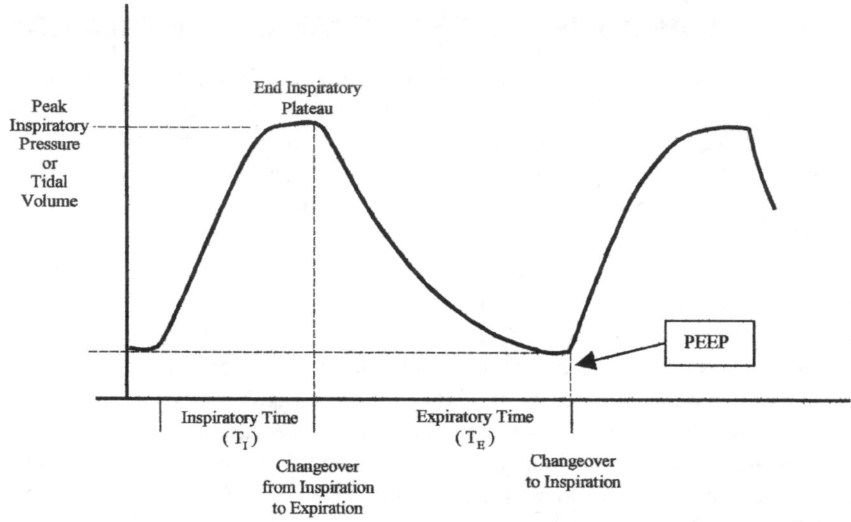

Figure 9-1
Graph of a ventilator-delivered breath. Breath components are identified. The plot also indicates PEEP reflected as an elevated interbreath baseline.

ters requires dynamic, real-time information regarding patient response to the mechanically delivered breath. These factors are based on airway monitoring, arterial blood gases, and cardiovascular measurements. The goal is to optimize pulmonary gas exchange and to confirm that the breath is delivered in a "physiologically compatible" manner.

It is important to understand that ventilatory support produces global physiologic effects on the cardiovascular, renal, hepatic, and gastrointestinal systems. Cardiovascular effects include changes in cardiac output, blood pressure, venous return (preload), and systemic vascular tone (afterload). Increased sympathetic activity in the kidney is noted by redistribution of intrarenal blood flow, and increased circulating levels of antidiuretic hormone, renin-angiotensin-

Table 9-2. Initial Ventilator Settings for Dogs and Cats

Parameter	Dog	Cat
Ventilator rate (breaths/min)	16–20	20
Tidal volume (ml/kg)	8–15	8–10
Minute volume (ml/kg/min)	150–250	160–200
Peak inspiratory pressure (cm H_2O)	15–18	12
Inspiratory time (sec)	1.5–2.0	1.0–1.5
Inspiratory period (% breath cycle)	33	33
End-inspiratory pause (% breath cycle)	10–15	10

aldosterone, and atrial natriuretic peptide. Elevated hepatic vascular resistance and bile retention have been reported during ventilatory support. Increased incidence of gastrointestinal hemorrhage has also been associated with positive pressure ventilation.

MODES OF VENTILATORY SUPPORT

Mechanical ventilation requires an artificial airway to interface the patient to the ventilator. There is a hesitancy to undertake mechanical ventilation due to the concern for placement and maintenance of an artificial airway. Although this is not a trivial issue, it should also not be a determinant for whether therapy is indicated. Several key points should be remembered during the decision-making process:

1. The indication for intubation and mechanical ventilation is *thinking* of it.
2. Endotracheal tubes are not a *disease*, ventilators are not an addiction
3. Intubation is not an act of weakness, it is an act of kindness.

Conventional Mechanical Ventilation

Conventional mechanical ventilation (CMV) remains the foundation of ventilatory support. CMV is delivered as either a pressure-cycled or flow-cycled breath. Individual breath components must be programmed and monitored to ensure that the support fits the patient's demands. The procedure will be outlined below.

Initially, four parameters are "patient adjusted" during ventilator setup. The first variable is programming assist/control or controlled ventilation. In general, assist-control mode is selected to permit patient participation in breath initiation. A "baseline" ventilator rate is included (control programming) to ensure that a minimum breath rate is delivered. The second variable is tidal volume. Tidal volume is set at 8 to 15 mL/kg/breath. As previously noted, this may be modified based on individual characteristics. The third variable is respiratory rate. This will vary depending on ventilator technology. Generally, a rate of 16 to 20 breaths/min is initially selected. Finally, the delivered oxygen (O_2) concentration is selected. Most ventilators have an O_2 mixer whose purpose is to provide a known concentration of O_2 delivery to the patient. The mixer may deliver O_2 concentrations that vary from 21% (room air) to 100%. The goal is to achieve adequate arterial O_2 level (>80 mm Hg) with the minimum O_2 concentration required. This strategy is used because it has been recognized that administering high O_2 concentrations for long time periods produce acute lung injury (ALI) associated with O_2 toxicity.

After the global settings are complete, individual breath configuration is programmed. Each breath is divided into inspiratory and expiratory components. Inspiratory flow rate determines the speed of breath delivery to the patient. The easiest way to adjust this is to breathe with the ventilator. If the breath seems comfortable, then the flow rate is appropriate for the patient. Inspiratory time determines the time over which the breath is delivered. Inspiratory time should be adjusted to deliver the breath in 1.5 to 2.5 seconds. Inspiratory time is not a specific adjustment on some ventilators; it is derived from the respiratory rate and the percentage of each breath that comprises the inspiratory period. Inspiratory pause (end-inspiratory pressure [EIP]) may also be provided during the later stage of inspiration. This is a short time (10%–15% of the total breath) in which the lung is "held" at full inspiration. The value of EIP is to facilitate uniform gas distribution in lower airway and alveolar units. This phase of the breath cycle should be monitored to ensure that gas trapping associated with ventilator settings (auto-positive end-expiratory pressure [PEEP]) does not occur.

A critical setting is change over from inspiratory to expiratory phase. One of two key parameters determines changeover point. Pressure-targeted ventilation is when the ventilator is programmed to stop gas flow and volume delivery at a predetermined airway pressure. If pressure-targeted mode is elected, key parameters in ventilator setup include speed of breath delivery (inspiratory time), flow rate associated with breath delivery (inspiratory flow rate), and maximum airway pressure (peak inspiratory pressure [PIP]) at which the inspiratory cycle is stopped (Figs. 9-2 and 9-3). Advantages of pressure-targeted ventilation include reduced risk for dangerous peak airway pressure and pulmonary tissue injury (baro-

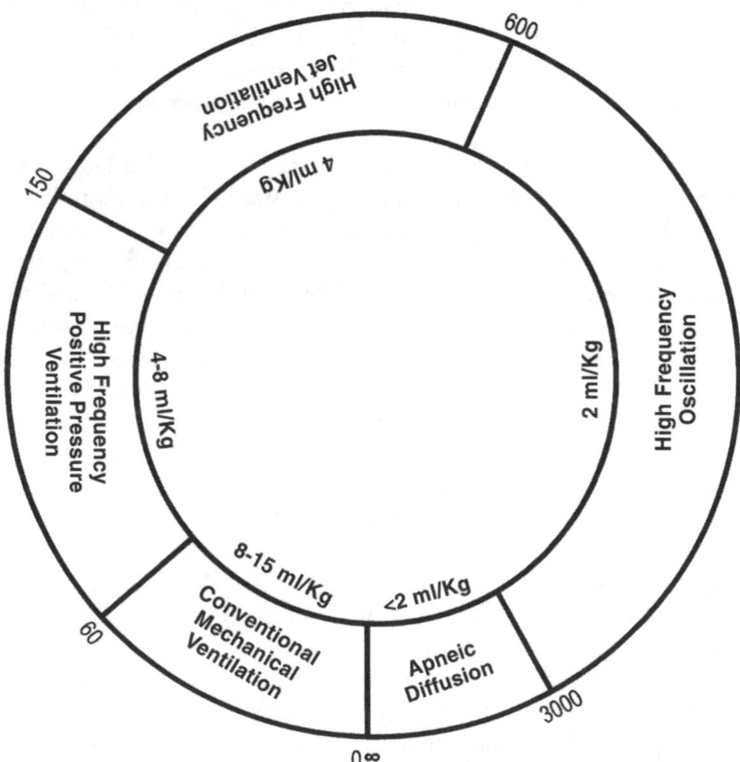

Figure 9-2
Comparison of ventilatory rates and tidal volume with different ventilator principles.

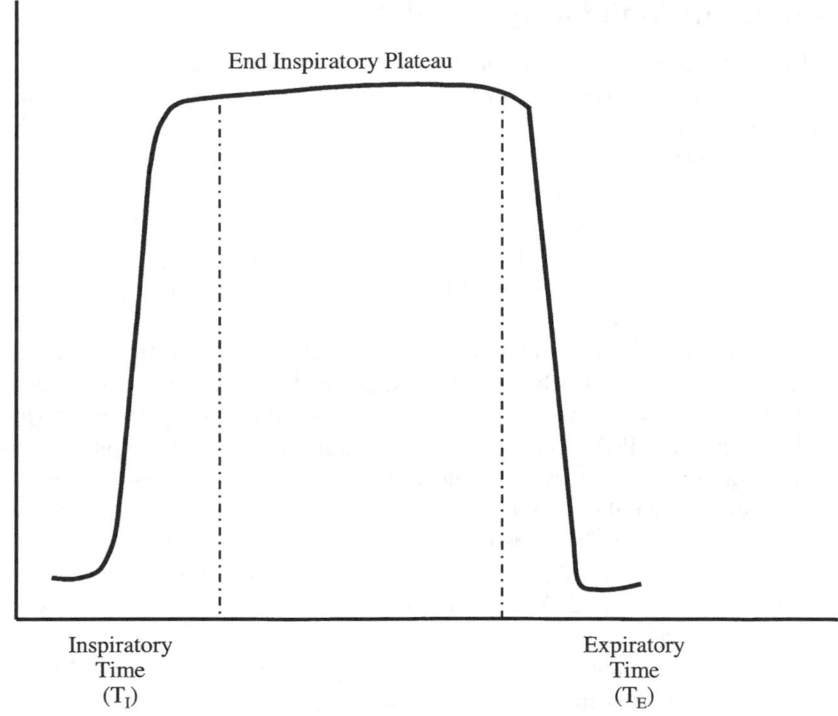

Figure 9-3
Graph of an inverse ratio breath. Note that the inspiratory period is short compared to a standard breath with an extended plateau period.

trauma). The major disadvantage of pressure-targeted ventilation is that tidal volume depends on mechanical properties of the lung. In general, pulmonary compliance is reduced in disease states affecting lung tissue (pneumonia, acute respiratory distress syndrome [ARDS]) or pleural space (pneumothorax, hemothorax). In these cases, tidal volume varies with dynamic changes that occur during mechanical support.

Volume-targeted ventilation delivers a constant tidal volume during each breath. In this mode, a calculated tidal volume or minute volume (tidal volume multiplied by rate) is delivered to meet patient needs. The advantage of volume-targeted ventilation is that a constant tidal volume is delivered during each breath. The disadvantage is that overinflation may produce parenchymal injury (volutrauma) in diseased lung tissue. Regional damage can occur even if overall airway pressure and tidal volume are within acceptable parameters. Regional damage is associated with reduced regional compliance that produces excessive pulmonary pressure and volutrauma.

Currently, most ventilator practitioners use pressure-targeted ventilation as a basis for CMV support. Volume-targeted ventilation is reserved for specific situations where fixed volume delivery is preferred.

Intermittent Mandatory Ventilation

Intermittent mandatory ventilation (IMV) is a support mode that permits spontaneous breathing during ventilatory support. It is a viable option to CMV in many patients requiring ventilatory support. The theory of IMV is that the patient is permitted to breathe spontaneously at a comfortable respiratory rate. Periodically, a ventilator-triggered breath is delivered. The IMV rate can be programmed so that a "guaranteed" baseline support rate is delivered augmenting normal spontaneous breaths. IMV is triggered irrespective of the patient's breath rate. The configuration of a ventilator-triggered breath is based on predetermined criteria as defined above.

Two distinct IMV techniques have been clinically used. Nonsynchronized IMV is the technique in which a ventilator-triggered breath is delivered independent of patient activity. In this mode, it is possible to hyperinflate the lung during a single breath if the IMV cycle occurs during a natural breath. To avoid "breath stacking" (simultaneous pulmonary inflation by spontaneous and assisted means producing excessive pulmonary inflation), synchronized intermittent mandatory ventilation (SIMV) was developed. In this mode, the IMV breath is coordinated with spontaneous breath initiation. This avoids potential hyperinflation associated with nonsynchronized IMV mode. SIMV has become the standard of care in adult respiratory medicine.

Intermittent mandatory ventilation is more physiologic than CMV. Advantages reported with IMV include reduced risk of respiratory alkalosis, lower delivered mean airway pressure, better matching of intrapulmonary ventilation and perfusion, reduced risk of respiratory muscle atrophy, reduced requirement for sedation and muscle relaxation, and improved "weaning" ability. Disadvantages include hypoventilation and carbon dioxide (CO_2) retention, increased work of breathing, respiratory muscle fatigue, and prolonged "weaning."

One value of IMV is in transitioning the patient from CMV support during the "weaning" process. Permitting the patient to assume a portion of its respiratory function and increasing respiratory muscle "work" is important in patients that have been on CMV for an extended time. This role is vital to successful removal of ventilatory support.

Pressure Support Ventilation

Pressure support ventilation (PSV) is a mode in which each spontaneous breath receives a programmed pressure assist to complete inspiration. PSV is maintained at a plateau level following breath delivery until the inspiratory period is completed. The level of pressure support ranges from zero to a complete breath depending on the patient's ability to participate in developing an effective change in transpulmonary pressure producing a breath volume. PSV is a useful strategy for transition from full ventilatory support to "weaning." Using PSV permits increased respiratory muscle work and helps prepare the patient for return to spontaneous breathing. PSV adapts to unusual respiratory pattern or rate better than IMV or SIMV. Limitations of PSV include inability of the patient to initiate PSV (bronchoconstriction, secretions) and equipment limitations that do not permit PSV support.

High-Frequency Ventilation

High-frequency ventilation (HFV) incorporates strategies in which tidal volumes less than or equal to anatomic dead space are delivered at breath rates ranging from 60 to 3000/min. The precise mechanism by which these techniques work is unclear; it is believed that their efficacy is due, in part, to increased kinetic energy in gas molecules facilitating gas diffusion in lower airways. All HFV techniques produce lower peak airway pressure compared to conventional ventilation. It is believed that peripheral airway pressures are higher and mean alveolar pressures are not significantly different from those observed during conventional ventilation.

Three HFV principles have been described (see Fig. 9-2). High-frequency positive pressure ventilation is identical to CMV; however, tidal volumes are small and are delivered at a higher rate than CMV (>60/min). High-frequency jet ventilation (HFJV) uses a small-diameter gas injection catheter to provide pulsatile gas flow at fast rates. Additional gas volume is "entrained" with jet gas to provide the delivered tidal breath volume. HFJV rate appears to be most effective when used between 150 and 400 breaths/min. High-frequency oscillation (HFO) uses very small (1–3 mL/kg) tidal volumes delivered at very high frequency (500–3000 cycles/min). HFO ventilators actively control both inspiratory and expiratory phase.

The role of HFV is still being defined. It has documented value in cases where chest wall movement is not desired, during bronchoscopy procedures, laryngeal surgery, bronchopleural fistula, and newborn (surfactant depleted) respiratory distress syndrome. Areas for further study include methods of cosupport with CMV to reduce atelectasis. Airway injury and drying are concerns with certain HFV modes. Monitoring of lower airway indices is also a limitation.

ADJUNCTIVE TECHNIQUES

The basic ventilator set up may be supplemented to provide support in the period between individual breaths. Maintaining airway pressure at a positive pressure plateau between breaths provides important support in cases of intrinsic pulmonary disease. Interbreath positive airway pressure is maintained by use of PEEP or continuous positive airway pressure (CPAP).

Positive End-Expiratory Pressure

This procedure maintains positive airway and alveolar pressure between ventilator-delivered breaths. Indications for PEEP are respiratory disease characterized by hypoxemia and reduced pulmonary compliance. PEEP is composed of two elements: (1) auto-PEEP, a slight positive airway pressure that is associated with ventilator design and operation and (2) extrinsic PEEP, which is intentionally applied to support airway opening and patency. PEEP is used in cases of surfactant-based pulmonary disease that places alveolar units "at risk" for complete deflation at the termination of each respiratory cycle. Constant opening and closing of an individual alveolus is detrimental to normal lung homeostasis and delays healing of injured tissues. Alveolar units that collapse and expand with each breath do not effectively participate in O_2 exchange. Mechanical cycling of pulmonary tissue above and below alveolar closing volume may induce shearing stress and increase risk of pulmonary tissue injury and gas leak into the pleural space.

Increasing gas flow resistance on the expiratory limb of the ventilator circuit creates PEEP. Methods for producing PEEP include variable resistance spring-loaded valves, fixed-weight ball valves, or a length of tubing placed in a water trap. The scale for PEEP is generally reported in centimeters of water pressure. PEEP application is empirical in that no one level is best for all patients. Each patient must be adjusted to its own PEEP level. This is pragmatically accomplished by serially increasing PEEP by 5 cm water steps at 30-minute intervals and monitoring blood gases and hemodynamic parameters. The PEEP level that produces the highest PaO_2 with the least drop in blood pressure and cardiac output is classified as "best PEEP" for that patient. Fine tuning within a 5-cm water range may be needed to specifically target the best PEEP level.

Problems associated with PEEP include decreased preload to the right and left heart, reduced cerebral perfusion, increased dead space ventilation, and barotrauma.

Continuous Positive Airway Pressure

Continuous positive airway pressure is useful in transition from ventilatory support to spontaneous breathing. CPAP is used to maintain a positive airway pressure during all phases of the ventilation in spontaneously breathing patients. It may be combined with core support modalities including IMV and certain HFV techniques. By exposing the patient to a constant gas flow delivered through the breathing circuit, CPAP helps maintain pulmonary inflation and functional reserve capacity during transition between mechanical support and weaning. CPAP is also helpful in conditioning weak respiratory muscles to facilitate transition to spontaneous breathing.

The key advantage of CPAP is to maintain alveolar inflation during all phases of spontaneous breathing. Constant alveolar inflation results in improved O_2 delivery, CO_2 removal, and better ventilation-perfusion matching. Disadvantages of CPAP are similar to those noted for PEEP.

STRATEGIES TO IMPROVE GAS EXCHANGE AND REDUCE PULMONARY DAMAGE

Mechanical ventilation has risks attendant with its use. The greatest risk is improper ventilatory support producing mechanical lung injury and comorbidity. In the past decade, several new strategies to improve intrapulmonary gas exchange and reduce potential pulmonary injury have been described. There is still emerging information regarding indications and use for "lung protection" strategies. The current strategies will be briefly described below.

High PEEP, Low Tidal Volume

High tidal volume support has been shown to increase parenchymal injury and inflammation in patients with ARDS and ALI. Recent studies indicate that decreased inflammation and increased survival occur when high PEEP levels (10–20 cm H_2O) are used to maintain alveolar inflation. Tidal volume (6–8 mL/kg) and peak airway pressure (30 cm H_2O) should be kept as low as possible to prevent alveolar distention and "volutrauma." Tidal volume should be calculated on ideal body weight rather than actual body weight due in patients with high body condition scores.

Permissive Hypercapnia

Permissive hypercapnia is a strategy that places a higher priority on avoiding pressure-induced tissue injury than maintaining optimal levels of minute ventilation (tidal volume multiplied by rate) and CO_2 elimination. The goal of this strategy is to protect damaged tissue from ventilator-induced injury by permitting $PaCO_2$ to rise above a physiologically normal value. This is helpful in preserving tissue stability in acute inflammatory disease where tissues are fragile, airway resistance is high, and there is nonuniform gas distribution to parenchymal zones.

Permissive hypercapnia appears to reduce ventilatory workload, the pressure cost of breathing, and support rate. Gradual $PaCO_2$ increase over a few hours produces minimal shifts in intracellular pH and is generally well tolerated. As $PaCO_2$ rises, each breath exhales more CO_2 than normal thus increasing elimination efficiency. Studies in humans indicate that pH may be maintained in the range of 7.15 to 7.20 for extended periods without significant comorbidity. Abrupt pH changes are accompanied by bicarbonate loss and will require supplementation to maintain bicarbonate levels in the reference range. Gradual "compensation" for this state occurs over a period of several days normalizing pH. This is achieved by renal bicarbonate retention; this response blunts respiratory drive. Permissive hypercapnia is contraindicated in patients receiving β-adrenergic blocking drugs, those with intracranial pathology, hemodynamic instability, pulmonary hypertension, or severe hypoxemia.

Permissive hypercapnia is initiated by adjusting ventilator rate, tidal volume, minute volume, and peak airway pressure to less than calculated values. The most effective strategy is to gradually reduce tidal and minute volume, thereby decreasing peak airway pressure. Ventilator rate is generally set in normal range and decreased only if volume adjustment does not produce CO_2 retention.

Inspiratory/Expiratory Ratio Modification (Inverse Ratio Ventilation)

Inspiration occupies a shorter duration than expiration in normal breathing. This principle is also used in ventilator support strategies. Ventilators are generally programmed so that the inspiratory/expiratory (I:E) ratio is approximately the same as a normal breath (an I:E ratio of 1:2). In the past decade, evidence indicates that prolonging the inspiratory period improves intrapulmonary gas exchange in diseased lung (see Fig. 9-3). This strategy is useful in patients with respiratory disease characterized by alveolar instability and collapse. Patients with pneumonia or ARDS have demonstrated benefit from this ventilator strategy.

Two strategies have been used to modify I:E ratio. When volume-targeted ventilation is selected, increasing inspiratory time and adding end-inspiratory pause increases I:E ratio and enhances lower airway gas distribution. In this mode, improved gas distribution is due to recruitment of pulmonary regions with long inflation time constants. When pressure-targeted ventilation is used, rapid pulmonary inflation is achieved by selecting a decelerating flow pattern. This maneuver maintains a preset pressure for a longer period during the inspiratory phase. By maintaining peak airway pressure for a longer period during each breath, improved gas distribution occurs for reasons noted above.

The I:E ratio modification has potential physiologic implications. Extending I:E ratio to greater than 4:1 may impair venous return and cardiac output. Gas exchange may actually be impaired at high ratios evidenced by decreased O_2 and increased CO_2 partial pressure values. This strategy should be used only by personnel familiar with pulmonary physiology and experienced with ventilator application.

MONITORING THE VENTILATOR PATIENT

The goal of monitoring during ventilatory support is to evaluate patient response and provide a basis for identifying physiologic changes that may occur during the support period. Data relevant to the output, efficiency, capacity, and reserve of the respiratory system is important to patient management during cardiopulmonary failure. Monitoring techniques may be classified as those that characterize pulmonary gas exchange, ventilatory capacity, and dynamic characteristics.

Gas Exchange

Arterial blood gas analysis is the "gold standard" method for evaluating pulmonary gas exchange. Understanding individual blood gas components and interpreting what values indicate is key to evaluating the ventilator patient. Blood gas indices important to the ventilator patient include pH, PO_2, PCO_2, SO_2, bicarbonate, and base excess. A comprehensive review of each parameter and its importance is reviewed in Chapter 19.

Oxygen uptake and transport is a key concern. The ability of the injured lung to effectively support O_2 uptake is evaluated by PO_2, ScO_2, and alveolar-arterial oxygen difference (see second equation below). The ability of the diseased lung to excrete waste products is represented by PCO_2, which provides a means for the clinician to determine how well the animal is ventilating. Many decisions regarding ventilator settings and patient response are made on the basis of evaluating these parameters.

Oxygenation

Efficiency of O_2 exchange is important to understanding dynamic pulmonary gas exchange at the alveolar level. Efficiency may be computed by evaluating alveolar O_2 tension and the difference in alveolar-arterial O_2 tension. This parameter provides information regarding the estimated O_2 partial pressure at the alveolar level of the lung. Alveolar O_2 tension (P_AO_2) is calculated in the following manner:

$$P_AO_2 = P_IO_2 - (1.25 \times PaCO_2)$$

where P_IO_2 = (barometric pressure − 50) × F_IO_2. F_IO_2 represents the inspired O_2 concentration. Under room air conditions, P_AO_2 is 100 to 110 mm Hg.

This information is also used in estimating the alveolar-arterial O_2 tension difference as follows:

$$P(A - a)O_2 = P_AO_2 - PaO_2$$

where PaO_2 is the partial pressure of O_2 in arterial blood measured from blood gas analysis. Expected value is 10 to 15 mm Hg in room air ($F_IO_2 = 0.21$). A rapid assessment may be performed by calculating the PaO_2/F_IO_2 ratio. This ratio may be rapidly calculated with information obtained from blood gas analysis at a known inspired O_2 concentration. Patients with normal pulmonary function have a ratio of 4 to 5. This decreases with pulmonary disease and intrapulmonary shunting. A minimum of 2 to 3 is required to maintain adequate tissue oxygenation.

The classic methodology for evaluating O_2 efficiency is to calculate venous admixture and shunt. This is described in Chapter 2. Pulse oximetry is a valuable tool for monitoring patient oxygenation at the tissue level. In conjunction with arterial blood gas evaluation, it provides an indicator of the adequacy of O_2 uptake and delivery to tissue beds. As a general rule, trends in oximetry values are of greater significance than the absolute saturation value. A detailed review of pulse oximetry is found in Chapter 8.

Carbon Dioxide

Efficiency of CO_2 exchange is important to maintain physiologic function. There is a direct correlation between $PaCO_2$ and alveolar ventilation. This parameter is maintained in the ventilator patient by controlling ventilation and quieting muscle activity with sedation and/or paralysis. The CO_2 level is affected by both intrapulmonary and extrapulmonary factors. For example, the lung may be capable of excreting CO_2 but hypoventilation may be present due to the action of sedative or anesthetic drugs. Thus, patient evaluation is essential to understanding the origin of CO_2 levels outside reference range.

The diagnosis of inability to excrete CO_2 is based on monitoring exhaled gases by capnography and measuring arterial partial pressures of CO_2. This information is used to calculate the dead space fraction, which indicates the fraction of wasted ventilation. Dead space is calculated as follows:

$$V_D/V_T = (PaCO_2 - P_ECO_2)/PaCO_2$$

where $PaCO_2$ is arterial partial pressure of CO_2 and P_ECO_2 is end expired concentration of CO_2 measured by capnography.

Pulmonary Mechanics

A number of measurements may be performed to evaluate the status of the lung and chest wall in an individual patient. Sophisticated devices and techniques have emerged to provide real-time evaluation of mechanical function. Several techniques for monitoring pulmonary function have been described and are useful in monitoring dynamic changes in pulmonary mechanics. Most indices are based on monitoring airway pressure and volume as defined in the pulmonary compliance relationship. Peak airway pressure may be monitored for changes that indicate altered pulmonary compliance. Although crude, peak pressure gives a composite evaluation of inflation volume, flow resistance in airways, and elastance of the lungs and chest wall. At a constant inflation volume, peak pressure is directly related to airflow resistance and elastic recoil force (elastance) of the lung and chest wall. End-inspiratory plateau pressure (EIP) is helpful in determining pulmonary elastance. EIP is performed by temporarily occluding the expiratory tubing at the end of expiration. When the inflation volume and pressure is held at the termination of a delivered breath, the proximal airway pressure decreases initially and reaches a plateau as intrapulmonary volume distribution is completed. Because no airflow is occurring, airway resistance is negated; therefore, EIP reflects elastance of the lungs and chest wall. This information may be used with peak airway pressure as follows:

$$P_{plateau} \sim \text{elastance}$$

$$P_{peak} - P_{plateau} = \text{airflow resistance}$$

Expiratory Volume and Flow

Newer ventilators have the ability to monitor expired gas volume on a breath-by-breath basis. This feature provides useful information regarding patient status as well as monitoring breathing circuit function. Comparing preset tidal volume and pressure to measured expired volume is useful in determining delivered volume, potential circuit leaks, and pathologic gas volume losses such as bronchopleural fistula or pulmonary rupture due to ventilator support. Sudden changes in expired volume and flow should be investigated to identify the underlying cause.

DISCONTINUING VENTILATORY SUPPORT (WEANING)

The goal of ventilatory support is to allow the patient to emerge from the "crisis" period and resume normal ventilatory function. One of the critical decisions that a clinician makes is when, and how, to discontinue ventilatory support. This is a challenging decision that is based on both science and clinical experience. A

Table 9-3. Weaning Indices/Predictors of Success

Parameter	Normal Range	Weaning Threshold
PaO_2/FIO_2 (100% O_2 support)	>400	200
Tidal volume (mL/kg)	5–7	5
Respiratory rate (min)	14–20	<35
Minute ventilation (L/min)	1–3	>1
Greater Predictive Value		
Maximum inspiratory pressure (cm H_2O)	−40	>−25
Rate/tidal volume	<50/min/L	<75/min/L

cohort of weaning parameters has been defined in human critical care (Table 9-3). These parameters are predictive in that meeting the criteria increases the chances of successful transition. It should be noted that these parameters are guidelines and should be balanced by clinical observation of the patient's ability to undergo transition to spontaneous breathing.

There are two approaches to withdrawing ventilatory support. One involves alternating periods of spontaneous breathing with mechanical support. The other involves a gradual reduction in the fraction of total minute volume supplied by the ventilator. Prior to initiating either strategy, a trial challenge to evaluate the patient's ability to breathe spontaneously should be performed. Several options for interspersed spontaneous breathing and mechanical breathing are available. The simplest form is the T-piece trial. A T-piece breathing system as used in anesthesia is substituted for the ventilator breathing circuit. High-flow O_2 is provided to the patient through the T-piece. The patient is evaluated for a specified time period (0.25–2 h). Evaluation includes physical parameters of respiratory rate, tidal volume, breathing effort, and O_2 tension, PO_2, and SaO_2. If the patient is successful in completing this trial, increased confidence of successful weaning is present. Progressive increase in trial periods may enable the patient to transition to spontaneous breathing without any further support. By permitting a "rest" phase between trials, one is "training" the atrophied respiratory muscles to recover and progressively assume an increased workload.

Synchronized IMV and PSV are also used in weaning. SIMV is commonly used due to the ability to predetermine a baseline respiratory rate and tidal volume. The patient is permitted to augment the baseline support level based on the capability to contribute spontaneous breaths. PSV is designed to be used as a partial ventilatory support role during transition from full support to discontinuation of support. The patient initiates a breath that is supplemented by the ventilator to a predetermined airway pressure value. This strategy is helpful in progressively shifting work of breathing from the ventilator to the patient. In several human studies, T-piece, SIMV, or PSV techniques were equally successful in weaning the patient from ventilator support.

Weaning strategies may include PEEP or CPAP as a component of support. The use of these modalities is based on the requirement for continued pulmonary inflation to maintain functional reserve capacity and reduce inspiratory effort.

PROBLEMS AND COMPLICATIONS

Ventilators disturb normal physiology and may create pathology with inappropriate use and management. Potential problems are associated with cardiovascular, pulmonary, CNS and renal system physiology, visceral organ function, and difficulty or inability to discontinue ventilatory support.

Cardiovascular

Mechanical ventilation is well tolerated in patients with normal cardiac function, autonomic tone, and intravascular volume. Patients may have impaired hemodynamic function if abnormalities associated with the above indices are present. Risk factors contributing to unstable cardiovascular function include decreased venous return to the right heart, compression of atrial and ventricular free walls during positive pressure delivery, and reduced cardiac output secondary to reduced "preload." PEEP may further affect these changes by creating a constant positive intrathoracic pressure gradient during the ventilatory cycle.

Respiratory

Upper airway complications include sinusitis and pharyngitis secondary to impaired drainage and clearance of resident flora. Problems associated with artificial airway presence include laryngeal injury and malacia, tracheal mucosal injury and necrosis secondary to cuff pressure, cuff deflation and loss of airway "seal," endobronchial intubation secondary to tube movement, and airway occlusion with mucus or blood.

Lower airway complications are more commonly noted with positive pressure ventilation. Pulmonary overinflation (volutrauma, barotrauma) is the most common complication reported with positive pressure ventilation. Overinflation injury produces alveolar rupture and communication with the pleural space producing tension pneumothorax. Bronchiolar damage and systemic gas embolism have also been demonstrated. In extreme cases, tracheal rupture may produce pneumomediastinum and subcutaneous emphysema. Overinflation will produce tissue inflammation secondary to stress fractures of the alveolar epithelium and capillary endothelium. This damage produces a water and protein leak into the alveolus evoking an inflammatory response. Inflammation may produce pulmonary edema, surfactant dysfunction secondary to hyaline membrane disease, ALI, and regional inhomogenicity of inflation and perfusion (V/Q mismatch). Ventilator-acquired pneumonia (VAP) is always a concern because normal upper respiratory defense mechanisms (glottic closure, mucociliary escalator transport, and pharyngeal clearance) are bypassed. Infection source may be from the upper airway region, gastric content aspiration, or primary pulmonary infection. The primary source of infection may be hematogenous or airway related. Risk factors for VAP include impaired nutritional status, age, immobilization, immune compromise, and poor hygiene management during support.

Neurologic

Increased intracranial pressure (ICP) has been associated with high airway pressure ventilation. Increased ICP may contribute to secondary cerebral edema and neurologic dysfunction of the thalamic, hypothalamic, pontine, and medullary regions. These changes may contribute to the syndrome noted as "failure to wean." It is important to separate central neurologic origin from peripheral and musculoskeletal origin elements.

Renal

Mechanical ventilation has been recognized to produce changes in renal function characterized by decreased glomerular filtration rate, urine output, and urine sodium levels. Several mechanisms have been shown to be associated with altered renal function. Decreased cardiac output secondary to ventilation alters intrarenal blood flow distribution with the juxtaglomerular zone receiving increased flow facilitating sodium and water retention. Increased sympathetic activation associated with decreased carotid sinus baroceptor function amplifies reduced renal blood flow and sodium retention. Increased renal venous pressure also contributes to decreased renal blood flow. Activation of the renin-angiotensin-aldosterone and antidiuretic hormone mechanisms has been noted during ventilatory support. Atrial natiuretic factor is also released and contributes to water and sodium retention.

Visceral Function

Hepatic dysfunction may occur secondary to reduced hepatic perfusion and O_2 delivery. This is due to decreased portal blood flow and increased hepatic vascular resistance. Increased bile duct pressure has been noted with positive pressure ventilation. Increased biliary pressure is reversed when spontaneous breathing is reestablished.

Gastrointestinal function is affected by positive pressure ventilation. The incidence of gastrointestinal bleeding is increased by 40% in patients supported for more than 3 days. This is due to changes in gastrointestinal perfusion pressure secondary to decreased systemic blood pressure and increased venous pressure.

Difficult "Weaning"

Long-term ventilatory support may be accompanied by a challenging transition from support to spontaneous breath mode. Unfortunately, there are no accurate predictors of success other than trial events. In many cases, weaning is successfully accomplished over a period of several hours. However, there are cases where weaning may be delayed or unsuccessful. These cases provide the greatest challenge and require identifying possible reasons for failure. Three physiologic parameters must work in harmony for weaning to be successful. Each parameter requires careful assessment to determine which component may play a role in the delayed weaning process.

Inadequte Respiratory Center Control

Inadequate respiratory center control may produce delayed weaning. The most common reason for inadequate respiratory center control is residual effects of sedative drugs. Patients that have endured a multiple day sedation protocol have altered neurotransmitter function that may produce adverse effects when recovering from sedation. If long-term sedatives (*i.e.*, pentobarbital) are used, a time window for drug withdrawal must occur prior to final weaning. In general, a 24-hour transition period from pentobarbital should be used to improve weaning. Sedation may be maintained with either diazepam or propofol infusion during the transition period. In cases of prolonged sedation (>1 wk), an increased risk of seizures may occur during emergence. Prophylactic phenobarbital therapy should be initiated and pentobarbital reduced by 50% per day until less than 1 mg/kg/h is infused. It may then be discontinued to facilitate emergence and spontaneous ventilation. Patients with primary intracranial disease may have difficulty weaning from ventilatory support. Primary damage to respiratory control centers in the pons and medulla may produce delayed weaning. These patients may not require sedation but will not wean unless functional recovery of these areas occur. Injury or disease of the anterior cervical spinal column may also produce pontine and medullary pathophysiology that results in delayed weaning. These patients may benefit from airway management alternatives including tracheostomy, which will permit ventilatory support with minimal sedation.

Increased Respiratory Workload

Increased respiratory workload greater than respiratory muscle capacity is a second factor in weaning failure. Increased workload may be associated with increased respiratory rate and effort during weaning, increased metabolic rate due to fever, sepsis, agitation, or pain, low thoracic or pulmonary compliance secondary to injury or disease, lower airway obstruction, secretion retention, undersize endotracheal tube, and excess levels of PEEP or CPAP support during weaning. Nonpulmonary factors include obesity, ascites, pleural fluid, and ventilator circuit resistive load.

Decreased Respiratory Capacity

Decreased respiratory capacity is the third major factor in delayed weaning. The magnitude of pulmonary parenchymal injury may reduce functional lung tissue producing insufficient pulmonary reserve to meet normal gas exchange demands. These cases will require an extended period of support until functional recovery occurs.

Depressed respiratory drive secondary to sedation, alkalosis, and hypothyroidism may also produce decreased respiratory capacity. Impaired signal transmission to respiratory muscles associated with spinal disease or injury, phrenic nerve injury, peripheral neuropathy, or neuromuscular junction alteration may contribute to decreased capacity. Primary muscle weakness associated with malnutrition, electrolyte and acid–base disturbance, or endocrinopathy may also decrease capacity.

Patients that have difficult weaning may require reintubation and short-term support until muscle power is regained. Short periods of spontaneous breathing are done to increase respiratory "work" and retrain dormant muscle groups. Increased work may be generated by use of PEEP or CPAP during these periods. Gradual withdrawal of support by use of intermittent spontaneous breathing periods, PSV, or CPAP may be selected to facilitate weaning.

SUMMARY

Mechanical ventilation requires the knowledge of physiologic principles and the ability to apply them in a clinical environment. Ventilatory support can be rewarding and successful when early recognition of need and therapeutic intervention occurs. Mechanical ventilation provides support during the critical disease period by reducing O_2 consumption needed for vital functions, thereby conserving O_2 for tissue repair and healing.

SUGGESTED READINGS

Haskins SC: Strategies for weaning a patient off ventilatory support. ACVECC Postgraduate Course 2001, pp 26–29.

Hirschl RB, Merz SI, Montoya JP, *et al.*: *Crit Care Med* 23:157, 1995.

King LG: Ventilating the veterinary patient with acute lung injury. ACVECC Postgraduate Course 2001, pp 14–25.

Marini JJ, Wheeler AP: Critical Care Medicine: The Essentials, 2nd ed. Baltimore: William & Wilkins, 1997, p 72.

Marino PL: The ICU Book, 2nd ed. Baltimore: William & Wilkins, 1998, p 421.

Owen A: Pocket Guide to Critical Care Monitoring. St. Louis: Mosby, 1996, p 57.

Spector SA: Critical Care: Clinical Companion. Philadelphia: Lippincott Willams & Wilkins, 2000, p 451.

Stock M, Perel A: Handbook of Mechanical Ventilatory Support, 2nd ed., Baltimore: Williams & Wilkins, 1997.

10
Gastrointestinal Endoscopy

Michael E. Matz

INTRODUCTION

Upper gastrointestinal (GI) endoscopy is a minimally invasive, atraumatic technique that permits direct visualization of the esophagus, stomach, and small intestines. In emergency medicine, upper GI endoscopy plays an important diagnostic role in the evaluation of the upper GI tract following caustic injury and acute GI hemorrhage, and a therapeutic role for the removal of foreign bodies. These endoscopic procedures offer a valuable alternative to surgical intervention.

Once the decision is made to incorporate endoscopy into an emergency practice, it is necessary to develop appropriate endoscopic skills. This requires becoming knowledgeable about normal endoscopic anatomy and familiar with the appearance of common lesions. More importantly, the clinician should receive appropriate hands-on instruction and devote the time and effort required to become proficient in its use.

Before discussing the specific roles of GI endoscopy in emergency medicine, it is important to first review necessary endoscopic equipment and endoscopic technique involved in upper GI endoscopy.

ENDOSCOPIC EQUIPMENT

Both rigid and flexible endoscopes can be useful in upper GI endoscopy. Most rigid endoscopes are approximately 25 cm in length and have an outside diameter of 20 mm (Fig. 10-1). This type of endoscope is inexpensive and easy to use. Rigid endoscopes are most valuable for assisting in the removal of esophageal foreign bodies. Poor visualization, limited maneuverability, and relatively short length, compared to flexible endoscopes, limit the use of rigid endoscopes for other diagnostic or therapeutic procedures in the upper GI tract.

Selection of a flexible GI endoscopy system requires knowledge of the types and sizes of endoscopes available as well as an understanding of the functional components of an endoscope.[1] A number of flexible endoscopes of different makes, lengths, diameters, and functions are available for use in evaluation of the upper GI tract. Most endoscopes used in the practice setting contain fiberoptic bundles that deliver bright light to the endoscope tip and transmit an image to an eyepiece. Video endoscopes use electronics in place of fiberoptic bundles to relay an image to a processor and video monitor. Selection of a flexible endoscopes should be based on specific needs, intended use, and cost. Too often cost

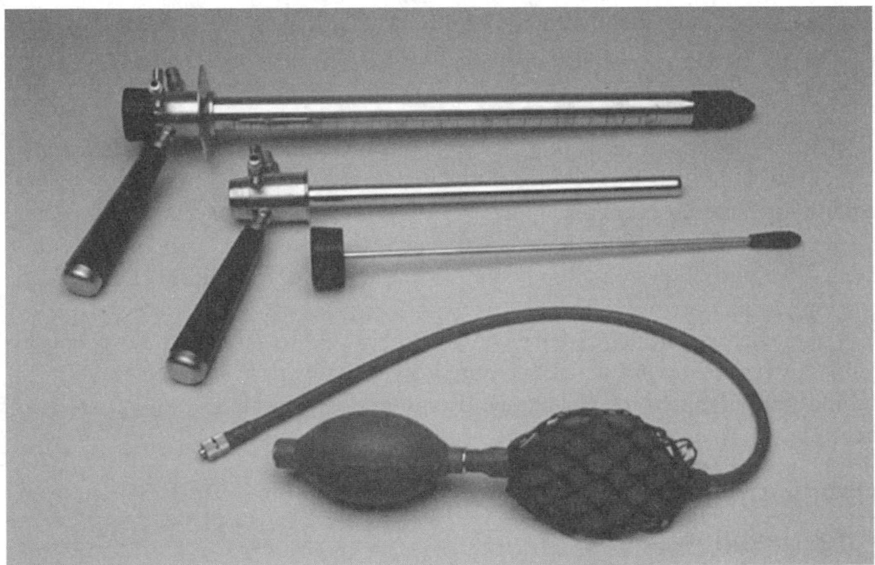

Figure 10-1
Examples of rigid endoscopes used for examination of the esophagus and removal of esophageal foreign bodies. An insufflator (below), attached to the endoscopes, distends the esophagus, allowing for better visualization.

is the major determinant in the selection of a flexible endoscope. Inexpensive flexible endoscopes often have poor optics and handling characteristics resulting in poor diagnostic capabilities and user frustration. Purchasing a good-quality flexible endoscope will improve diagnostic and therapeutic capabilities and result in increased use, offsetting the higher cost of the instrument.

Versatility is important in small animal veterinary medicine as patient size varies. A flexible endoscope to be used for upper GI endoscopy in dogs and cats should possess the following characteristics: a working length of at least 100 cm, ideally 125 cm; an insertion tube diameter of less than 10 mm, preferably less than 8.5 mm; a minimum operating channel diameter of 2.0 mm with an ideal size being 2.8 mm; four-way distal tip deflection with at least 180° to 210° in one direction and 90° to 100° in the other three directions; automatic air-water insufflation; suction capabilities; a forward direction of view; an angle of view of 90° to 120°; a depth of field of 3 to 100 mm; and comfortable handling. Light sources for the endoscope should be halogen, or preferably, xenon. A portable vacuum source is sufficient. A variety of quality veterinary and human endoscopes, new and used, are available.[2]

Additional instrumentation required for endoscopy in the emergency setting include biopsy forceps, cytology brushes, and foreign body retrieval instruments. The author prefers fenestrated ellipsoid biopsy forceps. Foreign body retrieval instruments that are most useful are the rat-tooth forceps, alligator-jaw forceps, polyp snare, and wire basket. Rat-tooth forceps are most often used for small or flexible (*e.g.*, cloth, rubber) objects that have a narrow edge. Alligator-jaw forceps are most useful for grasping smooth, flat objects. Polypectomy snares (minimally 2 cm in diameter) are useful for the retrieval of larger objects, particularly ones with irregular surfaces. These snares are the most versatile instruments for retrieving foreign objects. Basket forceps are used for smooth, circular objects. A laryngoscope and forceps (*e.g.*, sponge, alligator) should be available for any object that is difficult to pull through the upper esophageal sphincter. Long, rigid colonic or mare uterine biopsy forceps or long alligator forceps are utilized for retrieving esophageal foreign bodies through a rigid endoscope. These instruments can also be passed alongside a flexible endoscope to aid in the removal of esophageal foreign bodies.

Another useful instrument is an overtube used to protect the esophageal mucosa when removing sharp or pointed objects. Overtubes can be made from tubing or purchased commercially. Rigid endoscopes can also be used as overtubes.

UPPER GI ENDOSCOPY

Anesthesia

General anesthesia is necessary for upper GI endoscopy. The choice of anesthetic regimen should be made with respect to the animal's general condition and constellation of disease processes. Narcotics (morphine, meperidine, butorphanol) increase antral motility and may increase pyloric and cranial duodenal tone, potentially interfering with the passage of the endoscope into the duodenum and the manipulation of gastric foreign bodies.[3] For upper GI endoscopy the animal is placed in left lateral recumbency and a mouth speculum is placed to protect the endoscope. When upper GI endoscopy is being used for foreign body removal, maintenance of an endotracheal tube is especially important. This will prevent tracheal compression when a large foreign body is pulled retrograde through the esophagus and prevent aspiration of any object that could be accidentally dropped in the pharynx during removal.

Endoscopic Technique

The following is only meant to provide a general description of how to perform upper GI endoscopy (esophagogastroduodenoscopy) using a flexible endoscope. The reader is encouraged to read more detailed descriptions of the procedure.[4–8]

Esophagoscopy

The insertion tube of the endoscope is lubricated and passed through the oropharynx and upper esophageal sphincter. Once the endoscope is in the esophagus, air is insufflated until the esophagus is adequately distended to visualize the lumen. The endoscope is centralized in the esophageal lumen and then slowly advanced toward the gastroesophageal junction. The endoscope should only be advanced when the lumen is visible. Normal esophageal mucosa is smooth, pale, and glistening. Submucosal vessels are not normally visualized in the dog, but are observed in the distal esophagus in the cat. Little or no fluid is normally found in the esophageal lumen. In the proximal esophagus, an impression of the trachea can be seen. Pulsations of the heart and aorta are visualized in the thoracic esophagus. In the distal esophagus of the cat, concentric circular rings are observed because of the presence of smooth muscle. The gastroesophageal sphincter (GES) is usually closed in the normal animal. The bright pink to red color of the gastric mucosa is often visible in the GES, creating a rosette appearance.

Gastroduodenoscopy

Following examination of the esophagus, the endoscope is centered at the GES and gently advanced into the stomach. When properly directed there should be no resistance to advancing the endoscope into the stomach. The larger lumen of the stomach requires that the endoscopist develop a systematic approach to gastroscopy, otherwise lesions will be missed. During initial examination, the stomach should be examined for the presence of ingesta or fluid, ease of distensability of the gastric wall during insufflation, and the appearance of the rugal folds and mucosa. Submucosal vessels are not normally observed except in the cardia.

On entry into the stomach, the rugal folds on the greater curvature are observed. Following evaluation of the rugal folds, insufflation of the stomach is begun. The stomach should be distended until spatial orientation is achieved. Care must be taken not to overdistend the stomach, which can easily and quickly occur in the cat due to its relatively small stomach size. Gastric overdistention can cause respiratory compromise and may activate vagal reflexes that produce bradycardia. Overdistention also can make endoscopic duodenal intubation more difficult by stimulating antral and pyloric contractions. Once spatial orientation is achieved, the endoscope is passed along the greater curvature following the rugal folds until the incisura angularis comes into view. The incisura angularis is a narrow shelf of tissue that separates the pyloric antrum from the lesser curvature of the gastric body and is an important endoscopic landmark. The endoscope is then moved along the greater curvature into the antrum. The antrum contains no rugal folds. The antrum in the cat is small and attached more acutely to the gastric body than in dogs. This makes it more difficult to obtain a direct frontal view of the angularis incisura, a view that is easily achieved in the dog. Manipulation of the endoscope in this area is limited by the small luminal diameter, making it more difficult to advance the endoscope into the antrum. For this reason, the endoscope may retroflex into the gastric body instead of entering into the antrum.

Once in the antrum, the endoscope is slowly advanced toward the pylorus. The pylorus in most dogs is readily visible. The appearance and location of the pylorus will vary. In general, the pylorus has clean margins, is not obscured by excessive folds, and demonstrates rhythmic opening and closing. The pylorus is aligned in the center of the visual field and the endoscope is advanced into the duodenum using slow, steady, gentle pressure. Rapid and forceful advances of the endoscope should be avoided. In some cases, entry into the pylorus is difficult. Closing of the pylorus is a normal physiologic response to gastric distention. If gastric distention is minimized, the pylorus is usually in a more relaxed state facilitating passage of the endoscope. Positional changes (dorsal or right lateral recumbency) of the patient also may facilitate passage. As the endoscopist becomes experienced drug intervention is not needed.

After passage through the pylorus, a blurred image is commonly observed because the endoscope tip is against the wall of the duodenum as it makes a sharp angle away from the pylorus. Turning both control knobs in a clockwise direction to provide a downward and right tip reflection while advancing the endoscope usually facilitates advancement into the duodenum. The duodenal mucosa has a more granular and friable nature than the stomach mucosa. The major duodenal papilla is observed in most dogs and is rarely seen in cats. Careful examination may reveal the minor duodenal papilla in dogs. Peyer's patches are often observed in the nondistended duodenum. After the endoscope reaches its full working length it is slowly retracted.

Thorough examination of the duodenum and stomach is best accomplished as the endoscope is slowly retracted. Diagnostic procedures or therapeutic procedures are performed at this time. When the endoscope is retracted proximal to the incisura angularis, the tip of the endoscope is retroflexed allowing visualization of the fundus and cardia, the latter region being defined by the location of the entrance of the endoscope into the stomach. Torquing the endoscope at this point will provide complete (360°) evaluation of this area. The retroflexion of the scope is corrected and the endoscope is retracted further along the greater curvature. At this point, insufflation of the stomach should be sufficient to cause flattening of the rugal folds facilitating observation of the entire gastric mucosa. Overdistention must be avoided. After retraction of the endoscope into the cardia, all air is suctioned from the gastric lumen and the endoscope is removed.

REMOVAL OF GI FOREIGN BODIES

Removal of foreign bodies is the most common use for GI endoscopy in the emergency setting. In fact, endoscopic retrieval has become the procedure of choice for dealing with retained esophageal and gastric foreign bodies.

Foreign bodies are more often encountered in young animals, with dogs being more often represented than cats due to their indiscriminate eating habits. Ingestion of foreign bodies most often occurs during a pillage through garbage or while playing. Ingestion of a foreign body is often observed or suspected by the owner; however, small animals that present for excess salivation, regurgitation, vomiting, or clinical signs of intestinal obstruction should always be considered as suspects.

The ingestion of foreign bodies should always be confirmed radiographically before considering endoscopy. Depending on the animal's clinical signs, survey radiographs of the thorax and abdomen should be performed. Radiographs of the cervical soft tissues also should be obtained if an esophageal foreign body is suspected. Radiopague objects usually are easily localized (Fig. 10-2). A thorough evaluation of the survey radiographs should be conducted to ensure that additional foreign bodies, which may be less obvious than an easily recognizable

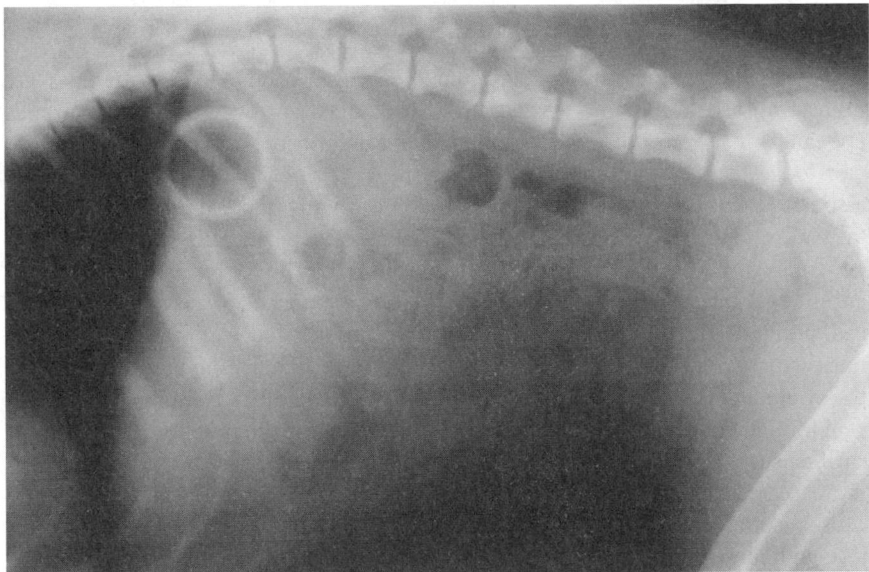

Figure 10-2
Lateral abdominal survey radiograph in a young dog. A round foreign object is noted within the stomach. The object was found to be a hollow rubber ball on endoscopic removal.

radiopaque object, are not present. Diagnostically, radiolucent foreign bodies present more of a challenge. Radiolucent gastric foreign bodies may be suspected if generalized or segmental gastric distention is observed. The presence of gas may help identify the foreign body. Negative (air) or positive (barium) contrast agents can assist in the identification of radiolucent foreign bodies. The size of foreign bodies composed of both radiopague and radiolucent materials may be underestimated on survey radiographs. Survey or contrast radiographs should also be scrutinized for evidence of esophageal or gastric perforation.

The decision to remove a foreign body must be individualized in each case. Most foreign bodies pass through the GI tract without complications. The size, shape, location, and type of foreign body and the degree, duration, and progression of clinical signs are important factors to consider when contemplating intervention versus conservative management. The majority of esophageal and gastric foreign bodies can be removed endoscopically. To determine the feasibility of endoscopic retrieval consider the size, shape, and weight of the object. This will also help determine which retrieval instrument to use. Before attempting endoscopy, the retrieval instrument to be used should be evaluated to see if it can grasp and hold a similar object. Foreign objects that reach the small intestine usually cannot be removed endoscopically unless the objects are located in the proximal duodenum. Endoscopic removal of GI foreign bodies usually minimizes morbidity and mortality, reduces anesthetic and hospitalization time, and decreases patient costs.

Esophageal Foreign Bodies

The most commonly encountered esophageal foreign bodies in dogs are bones and fish hooks. In cats, bones, sewing needles, fishhooks, and hairballs appear to make up the majority of esophageal foreign bodies.[9] Hairballs enter and lodge in the esophagus from the stomach during vomition. Clinical signs associated with esophageal foreign bodies are usually acute and include excess salivation, dysphagia, regurgitation, and anorexia. The severity of clinical signs depends on the type of foreign body, degree and duration of luminal obstruction, extent of damage to the esophageal wall, and the presence or absence of esophageal perforation. Esophageal foreign bodies commonly lodge at areas of anatomic narrowing, which are the areas just caudal to the upper esophageal sphincter, the thoracic inlet, the heart base, or the esophageal hiatus. Removal of esophageal foreign bodies is considered an emergency because the probability of complications such as aspiration pneumonia, esophageal perforation, and mediastinitis increases with time. Foreign body impaction in the proximal esophagus may also cause respiratory distress because of tracheal compression. Removal of esophageal foreign bodies should first be attempted endoscopically, unless evidence of esophageal perforation exists. Surgery of the esophagus should be avoided when possible due to the difficulties with access, healing capability, and associated morbidity. If endoscopy or the expertise to remove the foreign body surgically is not available, the patient should be referred to an appropriate facility.

Either flexible or rigid endoscopes can be used for retrieval of esophageal foreign bodies. Flexible endoscopes provide better visualization and manipulative capabilities for foreign body removal. Retrieval instruments passed through the operating channel of the flexible endoscope can be used to grasp the foreign body. Retrieval instruments for flexible endoscopes that have proven most useful are rat tooth forceps and polyp snares.

Bones are usually difficult to dislodge once they have become embedded into the esophageal wall. In most cases, some degree of mucosal laceration acts as an anchoring site. The degree of laceration is usually directly related to length of time the bone has been lodged (Fig. 10-3). Bones must be separated from the esophageal wall before they can be retrieved. Air insufflation should be used in an effort to distend the walls of the esophagus away from the bone. A flexible retrieval instrument is then anchored to an available site on the foreign object and an attempt is made to retract the bone toward the tip of the endoscope. If the bone fails to move in response to this initial effort, other maneuvers can be attempted. In some cases, a firmly embedded object can be freed from the wall by first pushing it in aboral direction, and subsequently retrieving it in the oral direction. Objects may also be dislodged by gentle rotation. If flexible retrieval instruments are unable to grasp the object tightly enough to allow successful removal, larger instruments such as rigid colonic or mare uterine biopsy forceps can be passed alongside the endoscope to securely grasp the object (Fig. 10-4). Alternatively, a large-bore rigid endoscope can be used to retrieve the object. The rigid endoscope has the advantage of dilating the esophagus just cranial to the foreign body which may dislodge it from the esophageal wall. Long colonic

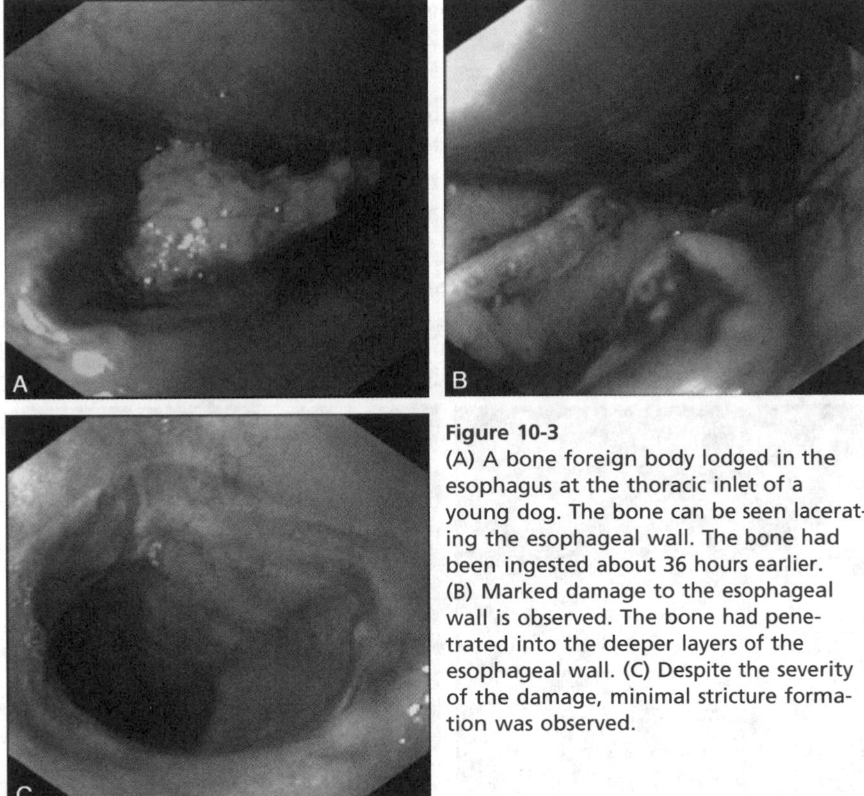

Figure 10-3
(A) A bone foreign body lodged in the esophagus at the thoracic inlet of a young dog. The bone can be seen lacerating the esophageal wall. The bone had been ingested about 36 hours earlier. (B) Marked damage to the esophageal wall is observed. The bone had penetrated into the deeper layers of the esophageal wall. (C) Despite the severity of the damage, minimal stricture formation was observed.

or uterine biopsy forceps can be passed through the rigid endoscope to grasp the foreign body. This method is most useful if the object has sharp points.

Fishhooks embedded in the proximal esophagus may be difficult to visualize and remove, because a hook in this location is bypassed by a forward-viewing endoscope as it is advanced through the upper esophageal sphincter. Fishhooks in this area may more easily be removed with a laryngoscope and alligator-type forceps. Fishhooks located further down the esophagus are easily visualized. Before removal, the depth of esophageal wall penetration should be evaluated, and if a treble barb hook is involved, the number of embedded hooks should be determined. If the hook is free within the esophageal lumen, the point or curve (so the point is directed caudally) of the hook should be grasped to protect the esophagus on removal. When the hook is embedded in the esophageal wall but the point of the hook is protruding into the lumen, the point can be grasped and the entire hook pulled through and removed. If fishing line is attached, it can saw through the esophageal wall during this maneuver. For this reason this technique should only be performed if the hook is superficially embedded in the submucosa or mucosa to prevent a deep esophageal laceration or perforation. If the point of the hook is not visible but appears to be embedded only in the

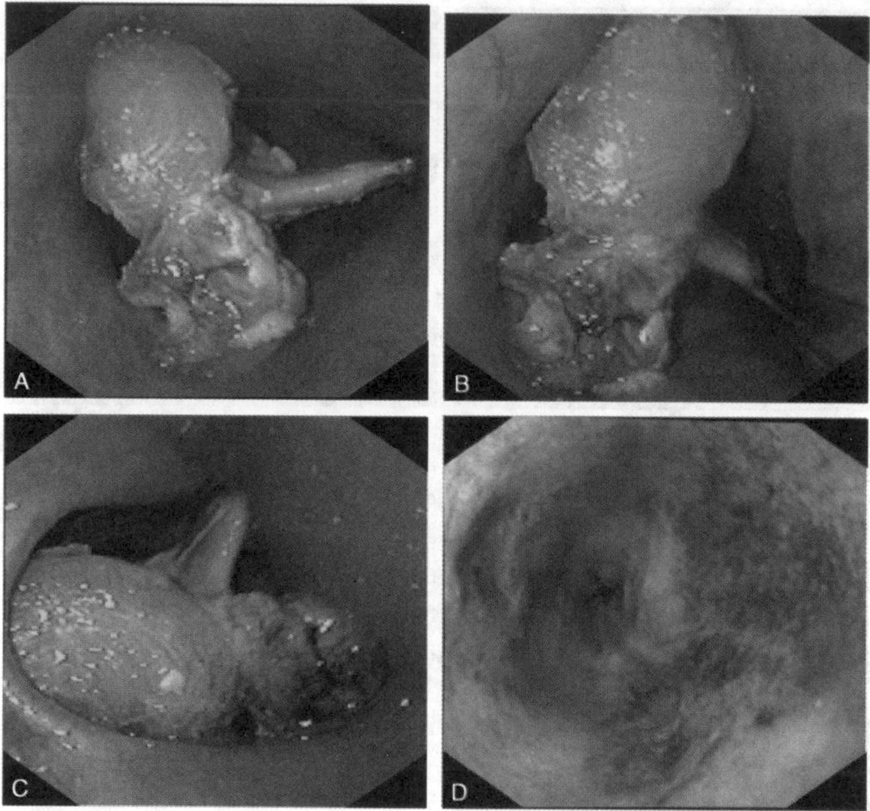

Figure 10-4
(A) A bone foreign body lodged in the esophagus of a dog just proximal to the esophageal hiatus. The bone was wedged in place by the spinous process (vertebral bone) making it difficult to dislodge the bone without risking significant damage to the esophageal wall. (B) A uterine biopsy forceps was passed alongside the flexible endoscope and used to break away the tip of the spinous process. (C) With the tip of the spinous process removed, the bone was freed. It was then rotated to facilitate passage and removed. (D) The esophageal wall after removal. Minimal damage is noted. No additional therapy was needed.

mucosa or submucosa, it can be gently pulled out. The superficial tear created will usually heal without complication. If the hook appears to have penetrated the esophageal wall, it can possibly be removed through a coordinated effort between the surgeon and endoscopist, with the surgeon cutting off the point and barb of the hook and the endoscopist removing the remainder of the hook through the esophageal lumen. This technique avoids having to make an incision into the esophagus. Endoscopic removal of fishhooks embedded near the heart base is discouraged because of the risk of laceration of a major vessel. In a recent study, endoscopic retrieval was successful in 66% of the animals.[10] The only factor found to associated with a successful outcome was the type of fishhook.

Failure rates in animals with treble-bard hooks was significantly higher than failure rates in animals with single-barb hooks.

Multiple extractions are generally necessary to remove hairballs because these objects tend to peel apart when grasped with retrieval forceps (Fig. 10-5). For this reason, removal may best be achieved using a rigid endoscope because the scope can remain in place while pieces of the hairball are withdrawn through its lumen. With a flexible endoscope, the endoscope must be withdrawn each time a piece is grasped and then reintroduced into the esophagus, making the procedure time consuming and laborious. In certain cases, it may be best to push the hairball into the stomach where it can be more easily manipulated with a flexible endoscope. Basket or polyp snare forceps can then be used to remove the hairball from the stomach.

Regardless of the type of foreign body or endoscope used, manipulations of the foreign body should be performed with care to avoid further mucosal damage or esophageal perforation. Tightly wedged foreign bodies should never be forcibly removed because of risk of laceration of the esophageal wall or adjacent vessels. The patient should be monitored closely during removal. During the procedure, insufflated air may be forced around the object into the stomach, leading to gastric distention with resultant respiratory compromise. In addition, manipulation of the object can increase vagal tone resulting in bradyarrhythmias. Once an object is grasped it should be pulled to the end of the endoscope (Fig. 10-6). Preferentially, pointed objects should be grasped and withdrawn with the pointed edge trailing. Alternatively, these objects can be removed with the aid of an overtube to prevent esophageal mucosal damage. The object is then secured in position at the end of the endoscope by holding the pliable stem of the retrieval forceps firmly against the control section with the middle finger as is exits the working channel port. With a flexible endoscope, air is insufflated during gentle, simultaneous withdrawal of the endoscope and object to dilate the esophagus and minimize esophageal mucosal damage. This maneuver is performed under visualization through the endoscope. The object should be gently teased through the upper esophageal sphincter. Excess force should never be exerted. If the object cannot be removed atraumatically in the oral direction, propulsion into the stomach should be considered. Here they may be digested (*e.g.*, bones), better manipulated to an appropriate orientation for removal, or surgically removed. Objects that cannot be removed by forceful traction or propulsed into the stomach require surgical removal.

Following removal of a foreign body or propulsion of a foreign object into the stomach, the esophageal mucosa should be visualized to assess the degree of esophageal damage and check for the presence of tears or perforations. Medical therapy depends on the degree of esophageal damage and is discussed more thoroughly with caustic esophageal injury. If a perforation is present, life-threatening tension pneumothorax may develop. Survey thoracic radiographs also may be valuable in determining whether esophageal perforation has occurred. Perforation usually results in the development of pneumomediastinum or pneumothorax. Extremely small perforations caused by sharp objects (fishhooks, sewing needles) may

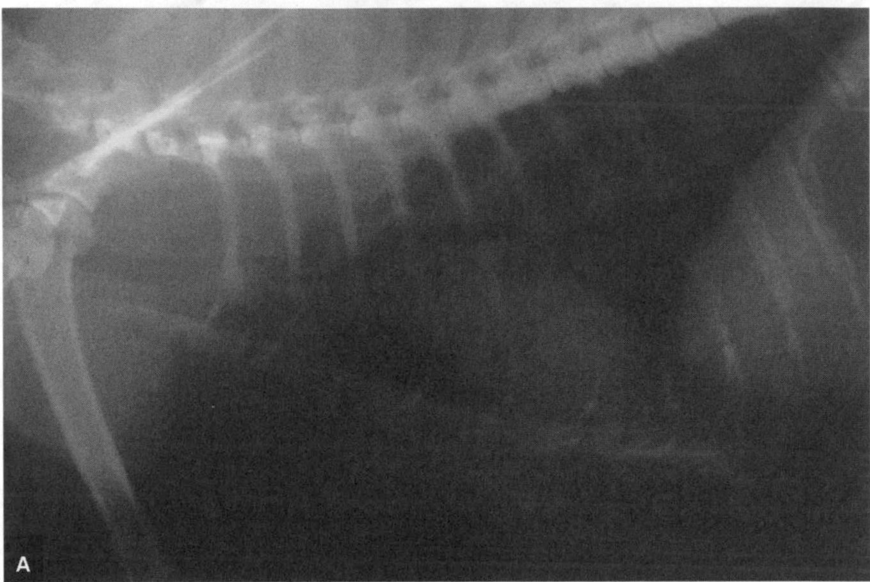

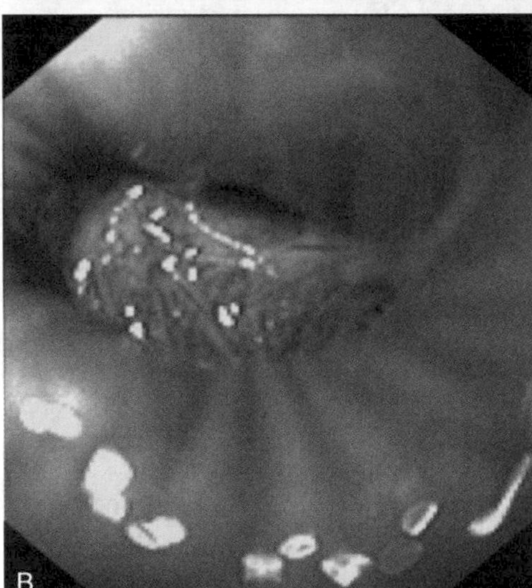

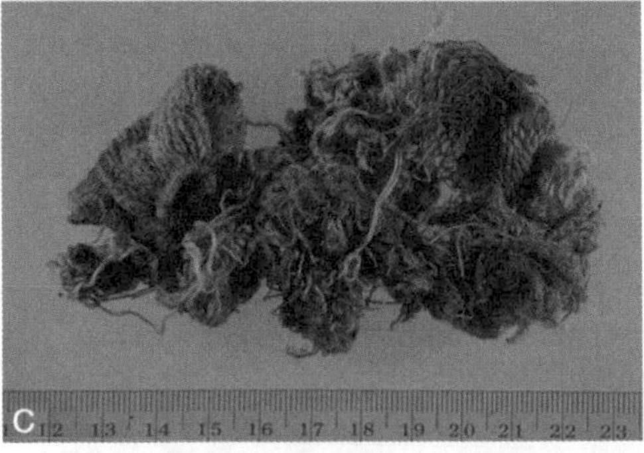

Figure 10-5
(A) Lateral abdominal survey radiograph of a cat with hair ball foreign body. A soft-tissue density is noted extending cranially and caudally from the thoracic inlet. Ventral depression of the trachea by the soft-tissue density is also noted. (B) On endoscopic evaluation the proximal aspect of the hairball was found just inside the upper esophageal sphincter. Fragmentation of the hairball necessitated multiple extractions (C). For this reason, a rigid endoscope was passed in place of a flexible endoscope. This allowed the rigid endoscope to remain in place while multiple fragments were removed with an alligator-type forceps.

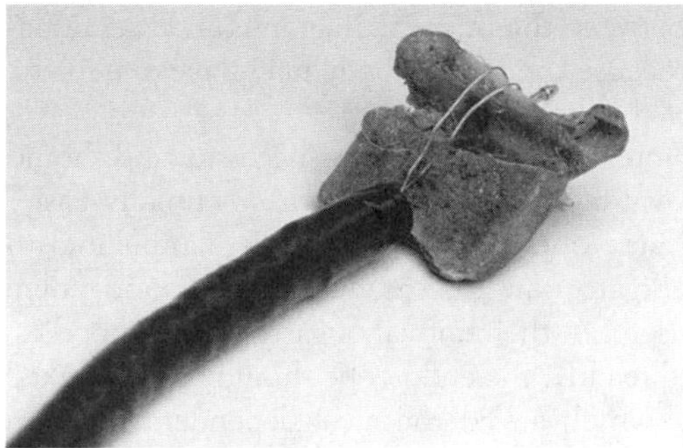

Figure 10-6
Demonstration of the proper positioning of a foreign body against the end of the endoscope for removal.

be managed conservatively with intravenous fluids, broad-spectrum antibiotics, and gastrostomy tube feedings. Large perforations require surgical intervention.

Gastric Foreign Bodies

Gastric foreign bodies are much more commonly encountered in dogs and cats than esophageal foreign bodies. Commonly ingested foreign bodies in dogs include bones, rocks, clothing, plastic and rubber toys, apricot or peach pits, fishhooks, and coins.[9,11] In cats, sewing needles and trichobezoars are commonly encountered.[9,11] Endoscopy is useful to confirm a suspected gastric foreign body, and more importantly, to remove these objects.

The most common clinical sign associated with gastric foreign bodies is vomiting. If the object is small and freely movable, only intermittent vomiting may be observed. Inappetence, lethargy, and mild abdominal tenderness may also be noted. Pain and fever in combination suggest perforation. As opposed to esophageal foreign bodies, removal of gastric foreign bodies is less commonly considered an emergency procedure. Large, sharp, or linear objects should be removed promptly to avoid GI perforation or obstruction. Although sharp objects such as sewing needles have the capability of passing through the GI tract without incident, these objects also have the capability of perforating the intestinal wall and causing peritonitis. Thread attached to a ingested sewing needle, if of significant length, also could lead to intestinal plication if the needle where to become impacted or impaled at the pylorus with the thread moving progressively down the small intestine. Objects suspected of containing lead, zinc (*e.g.*, pennies minted after 1982), or caustic materials (*e.g.*, batteries) must be removed immediately. Clinical signs in these cases may be related to the inherent toxicity of these metals (*e.g.*, seizures for lead, hemolytic anemia for zinc) or chemicals. Foreign bodies that cause acute, severe vomiting (most notably objects lodged in the pylorus) can result in life-threatening metabolic disturbances and should be removed immediately. Objects lodged in the pylorus also are often associated with marked abdominal pain. If in doubt whether an object should be removed, remove the object. Endoscopic removal from the stomach is less invasive and has less potential for complications than surgical removal from the stomach or intestine. Prior to inducing general anesthesia, fluid and electrolyte abnormalities should be corrected. In addition, radiographs may need to be repeated if a significant period of time has elapsed between the initial radiographs and the induction of anesthesia for endoscopy, because the foreign body may have exited the stomach and traversed a portion of the small intestine.

Endoscopic removal of gastric foreign bodies is usually successful and should be attempted before surgery. Removal of gastric foreign bodies is usually easier than esophageal foreign bodies because objects are more easily manipulated in the stomach. Rat-tooth forceps, alligator-jaw forceps, wire basket, and polyp snare have been found to be most useful in the removal of gastric foreign bodies. If the foreign object is not visualized readily, the endoscope should be retroflexed to examine the fundus and cardia, which are in the most dependent position with the animal in left lateral recumbancy. To remove the foreign body, it is grasped, pulled to the end of the endoscope and secured there. The endoscope, forceps, and foreign body are then removed as a unit. Foreign objects should be grasped so that the longest axis of the object is parallel to the endoscope. Sharp edges or points should be aligned so they are trailing (Fig. 10-7). Thick linear objects (*e.g.*, socks) should be grasped at either end to minimize their thickness. Difficulty may be encountered when withdrawing the foreign body from the stomach through the GES. It is essential that the endoscopic forceps being used has a strong grasp on the foreign body. Air should be insufflated to dilate the GES while the foreign body is gently teased through the sphincter. Once the foreign body is brought into the esophagus, air insufflation should be continued to reduce esophageal mucosal damage. Once the object is removed, the stomach and duodenum are thoroughly examined for the presence of additional foreign material and the gastric and esophageal mucosa are inspected for damage. Additional treatment is rarely needed. If gastric mucosal injury is moderate to severe, administration of an H_2-receptor antagonist (cimetidine [Tagamet] 5–10 mg/kg

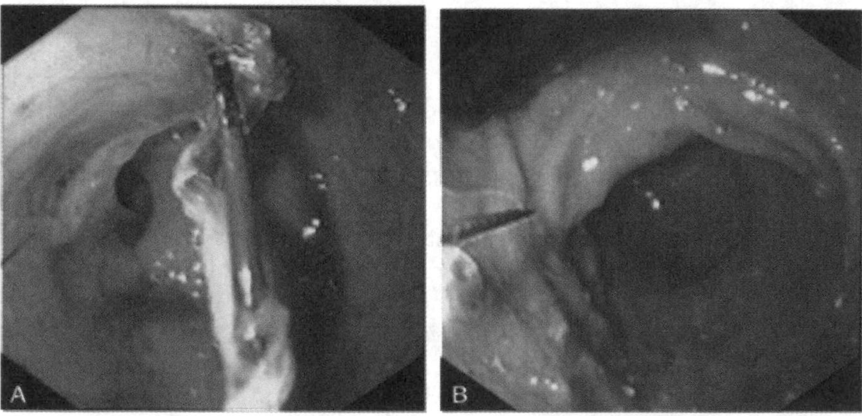

Figure 10-7
A needle foreign body is impaled into the gastric wall near the pylorus in a dog. The needle was pulled from the gastric wall by grasping the thread attached to the needle. Note how the point of the needle is aligned so that it is trailing, preventing or minimizing trauma to the gastric or esophageal wall during removal.

q 6–12 h PO, IM, IV; ranitidine [Zantac] dogs: 2 mg/kg q 8 h PO, IV, cats: 2.5 mg/kg q 12 h IV or 3.5 mg/kg q 12 h PO; famotidine [Pepcid] 0.5 mg/kg PO, SQ, IM, IV) or proton pump inhibitor (omeprazole [Prilosec] 0.7 mg/kg q 24 h PO) is indicated. Patients can generally be discharged within hours following the procedure.

Removal of extremely large or awkward foreign objects endoscopically may not be appropriate. The objects may be difficult to correctly align for passage through the gastroesophageal junction and esophagus resulting in excessive damage during removal (Fig. 10-8). Smooth objects can be difficult to grasp firmly enough to pull through the GES and upper esophageal sphincter. If large amounts of foreign material are encountered, surgical removal should be considered. The increased time taken for removal may increase morbidity and ultimately be more expensive than an exploratory laparotomy and gastrotomy. Esophageal damage caused by repeated removal and reintroduction of the endoscope is also prevented. If endoscopy is used to remove multiple small pieces of foreign material, the procedure can be shortened by inserting an overtube into the stomach and removing the pieces through the tube with the endoscope.[12] This allows the endoscope to be rapidly returned to the stomach each time it is removed. In addition, the sphincters and esophageal mucosa sustain less

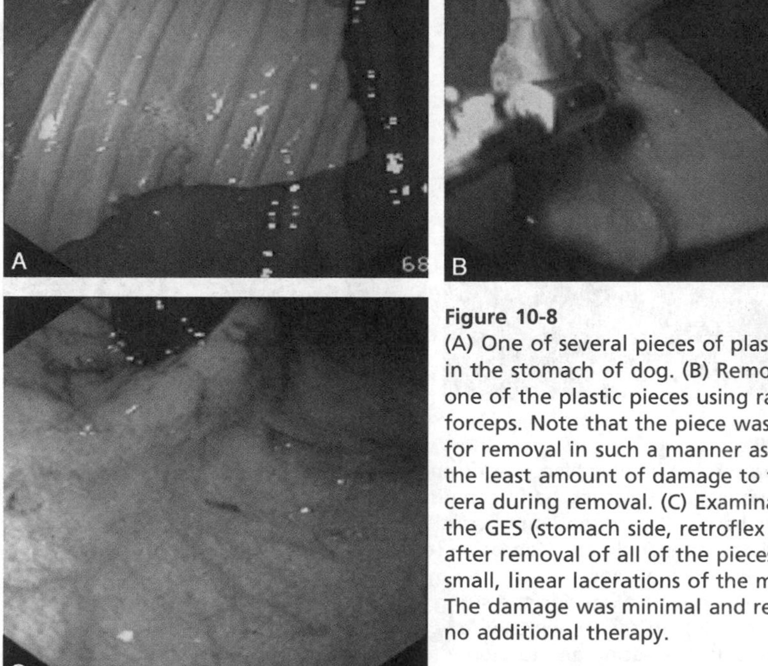

Figure 10-8
(A) One of several pieces of plastic found in the stomach of dog. (B) Removal of one of the plastic pieces using rat-tooth forceps. Note that the piece was aligned for removal in such a manner as to cause the least amount of damage to the viscera during removal. (C) Examination of the GES (stomach side, retroflex view) after removal of all of the pieces showed small, linear lacerations of the mucosa. The damage was minimal and required no additional therapy.

trauma when this method is used. Surgical intervention is also indicated when additional foreign material is suspected to be beyond the stomach. Surgical exploration allows visualization of the entire GI tract for damage or obstruction caused by foreign material.

When a linear foreign body (*e.g.*, string, towel, hosiery) is encountered on entering the stomach, the endoscopist must be sure that the object is not entering the small bowel before attempting removal (Fig. 10-9). Pulling on a linear foreign body that has caused plication of the small bowel may result in severe damage to the bowel wall or perforation. If the object has entered the small bowel it can be grasped where it enters the pylorus and gently pulled a short distance. If

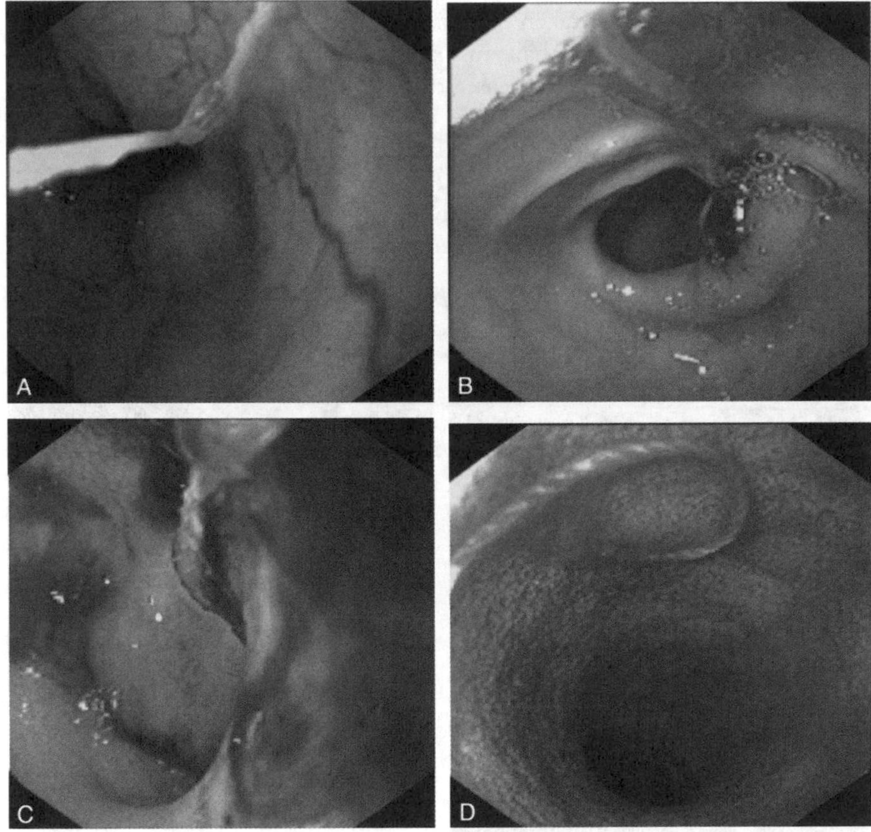

Figure 10-9
(A) A string foreign body is seen passing through the esophagus (note the submucosal vessels) in a cat. The string had been discovered on physical examination wrapped around the base of the tongue on physical examination. No plication of the bowel was noted on abdominal palpation or on survey radiographs (B). The string was followed and is shown passing through the pylorus into the small bowel. The endoscope was next passed alongside the string into the small bowel where mucosal damage was noted (C). Further down the bowel the end of the string was located (D). This end was grasped using an old biopsy forceps and the entire length of the string removed.

the object comes easily, the object is released and regrasped at the pylorus and again pulled a short distance. The procedure is repeated until the entire linear foreign body is within the stomach. In some instances the endoscope can be passed beside the linear object through the pylorus and into the small intestine. The object is then grasped as close to its aboral end as possible and pulled out of the small bowel into the stomach. One end of the linear foreign body is then grasped and the linear foreign body removed from the animal. If the linear foreign body cannot be easily removed from the small bowel, surgical intervention is required. The author has also used endoscopic scissors to cut a string foreign body anchored in the antrum and passing into the small intestine. The string was cut at the pylorus and allowed to pass on its own. Endoscopic management of linear foreign bodies should only be attempted by the most experienced endoscopists. Removal of known linear foreign bodies where bowel plication is noted on physical examination or abdominal radiographs should not be attempted.

Foreign body ingestion can occur at or near the time of ingestion of food. A food-filled stomach may obscure visualization of the foreign body and increase the risk of aspiration during general anesthesia (Fig. 10-10). Allowing the food to empty from the stomach, over an 8- to 12-hour fast, will facilitate the identification and removal of the foreign body and reduce the risk of aspiration. However, fasting will increase the risk of the foreign body entering the small intestine and moving out of the reach of the endoscope. If food does obscure the foreign body, repositioning the animal may allow visualization of the object. In some cases, gastric lavage can be used to facilitate removal of food.

Occasionally, foreign bodies can successfully be removed from the duodenum endoscopically. However, if the object becomes impacted to any degree, it usually is difficult to move it in an aboral direction and an enterotomy is required.

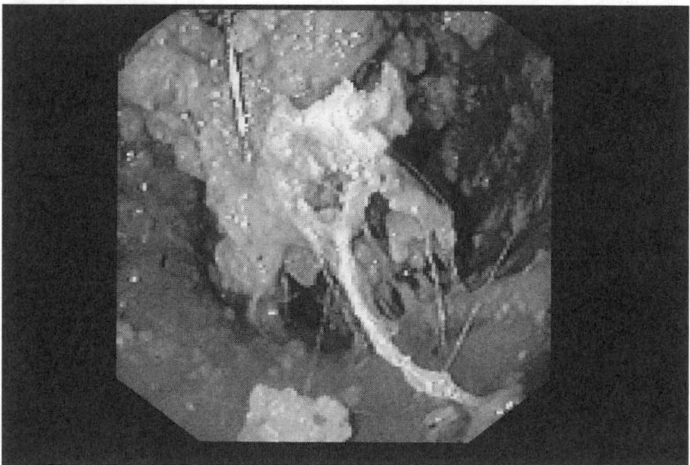

Figure 10-10
Food obscures a needle with string foreign body in a cat. Food makes visualization more difficult and prolongs procedure time. It also increases the potential for aspiration.

The following discussions on caustic esophageal injury and acute GI bleeding are included for completeness. Although these problems are not commonly encountered in small animal practice, the ability to manage these problems is imperative for the emergency clinician.

EVALUATION OF CAUSTIC ESOPHAGEAL INJURY

Ingestion of caustic agents can result in significant esophageal and gastric damage. If the patient survives the acute effects, the reparative response can result in esophageal stenosis. Caustic esophageal injury can be produced by strong alkaline or acidic agents. Common alkalis include sodium and potassium hydroxides, which are found in cosmetics, soaps, washing detergents, button batteries, and drain and oven cleaners. Other common alkalis include sodium and calcium hypochlorite found in bleaches. Common acids include sulfuric and hydrochloric, which are found in toilet bowel cleaners, antirust compounds, battery fluids, and swimming pool cleaners. The degree of injury depends on the agent; its concentration, quantity, and physical state; and the length of exposure.[13] Alkaline injury is usually more severe because of rapid tissue penetration by alkali.[14] In addition, products containing alkalis are often tasteless and odorless and are swallowed before protective mechanisms can be invoked.

Owners often observe animals ingesting caustic agents or suspect ingestion of such substances based on the observation of acute oral lesions, although esophageal injury may be present even when examination of the mouth and pharynx is normal. History of possible ingestion of a button battery requires immediate evaluation. Clinical signs may include persistent salivation, dysphagia, and pain. Stridor may indicate epiglottal or laryngeal involvement. Batteries greater than 15 mm can result in esophageal perforation within 6 hours.[15] Severe esophageal injury may lead to the rapid development of tachypnea, dyspnea, and shock as the result of esophageal perforation and resultant mediastinitis.

When caustic injuries are suspected, upper GI endoscopy is indicated to evaluate the extent of damage and to direct therapy (Fig. 10-11). Before endoscopy survey, thoracic and possibly abdominal radiographs should be obtained. Evidence of esophageal perforation would indicate the need for surgical intervention.

Therapeutic goals are to prevent perforation and to avoid progressive fibrosis and stricture. The magnitude of the treatment depends on the degree of esophageal damage. Mild esophagitis necessitates only short-term withdrawal of food. With moderate to severe esophageal injury, oral feeding should be withheld for 5 to 10 days. In these cases, feeding may be accomplished through an endoscopically placed gastrostomy tube. If the gastric mucosa is also damaged, jejunostomy tube or total parenteral nutrition would be the feeding methods of choice.

Corticosteroid administration has been advocated to limit fibrous tissue production and prevent stricture formation in association with caustic induced esophageal injury. Anecdotal clinical reports suggest that the incidence of stricture formation can be reduced by corticosteroids in children.[16] In a prospective trial in children with caustic esophageal injury, corticosteroids did not prevent

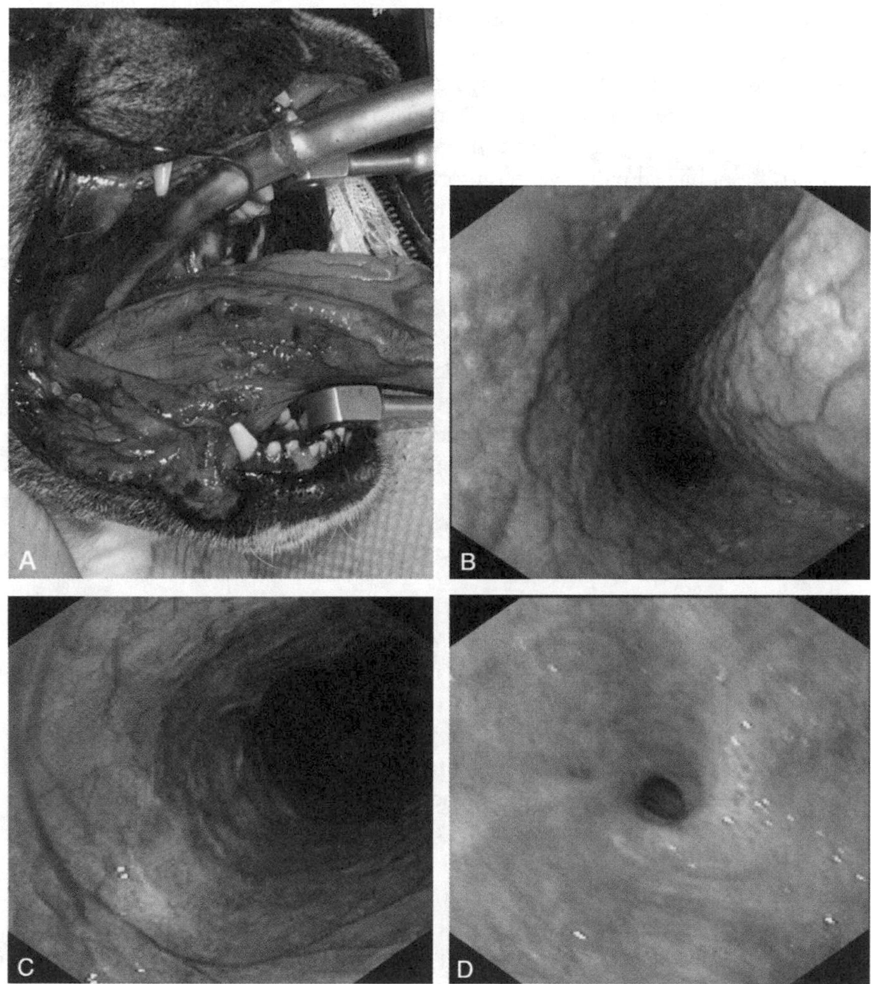

Figure 10-11
(A) Caustic chemical injury to the oral and lingual mucosa in a Boxer. (B) The denuded mucosa in the proximal esophagus (note tracheal indentation) as evidenced by the appearance of submucosal vessels. (C) Similar mucosal damage is present in the caudal esophagus. (D) Stricture formation as the result of the circumferential injury.

strictures.[17] Strictures did develop in all of the children with circumferential injury.

Broad-spectrum antibiotics (amoxicillin/ampicillin, amoxicillin/clavulanic acid, cephalosporins) appear to be indicated if corticosteroids are used because corticosteroids appear to decrease the incidence of local infections. Local infections may increase the granulation response, with a resultant increase in tissue fibrosis and stricture formation. Prophylactic antibiotic therapy is otherwise not indicated in the treatment of esophagitis until specific indications develop.

The use of an H_2-receptor antagonist or proton pump inhibitor is also indicated to reduce gastric acid secretion during healing of the esophagus. Refluxed gastric acid will delay or prevent mucosal healing. Reflux of gastric acid can also be decreased by the administration of metoclopramide (0.2–0.4 mg/kg q 6–8 h PO, SQ, IM or 1–2 mg/kg/d constant rate IV infusion). Opioids should be used to control esophageal pain or discomfort associated with esophagitis. For short-term pain control buprenorphine (Buprenex: 0.005 to 0.03 mg/kg IV, IM, SQ [dog]; 0.005–0.01 mg/kg IM, IV [cat]), butorphanol (Torbugesic: 0.2–1.0 mg/kg q 3–6 h, IM, SQ, IV [dog]; 0.1–1.0 mg/kg q 12 h I IM, SQ, IV [cat]), or morphine (Informorph: 0.1–0.5 mg/kg q 4 h IM, SC [dog]; 0.1 mg/kg q 4–8 h IM, SQ, IV [cat]). Fentanyl transdermal patches (Duragesic: 5–10 kg, 25 mg/h, 10–20 kg 50 mg/h, 20–30 kg 75 mg/h, >30 kg 100 mg/h) can be for long-term pain control. The oral administration of lidocaine gel also may be beneficial for control of esophageal pain. Cases with moderate to severe esophagitis should be reevaluated endoscopically in 5 to 7 days following the initial examination to evaluate esophageal repair.

EVALUATION OF ACUTE GI HEMORRHAGE

Patients with acute GI hemorrhage should be assessed rapidly to determine hemodynamic status, activity of bleeding, and the underlying medical conditions that complicate management. Careful assessment of the vital signs (heart rate, respiratory rate, blood pressure, mucous membranes) are the best way to judge a patient's hemodynamic stability. The first priority in acute GI bleeding is the restoration of cardiovascular stability, after which identification of the source of hemorrhage and tailored therapy can be considered.

If bleeding is active, immediate therapeutic intervention is required endoscopically or surgically. Vomitus containing frank blood or the passage of large fresh clots rectally are obvious indicators of active bleeding (Fig. 10-12). The passage of a nasogastric or orogastric tube to obtain an aspirate of gastric contents or perform gastric lavage may be helpful in determining if the patient is actively bleeding in the upper GI tract.

GI bleeding in small animals most often results from mucosal ulceration. Ulcers can occur in any region of the GI tract, but are most commonly found

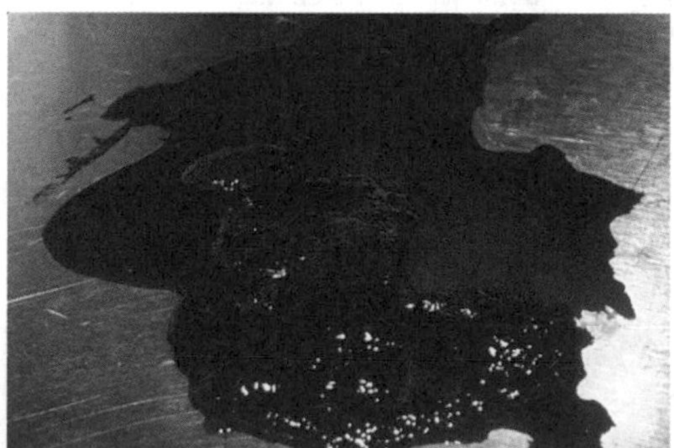

Figure 10-12
Severe hematemesis in a dog with gastric ulcers. The ulcers resulted from administration of ibuprofen. The dog died despite immediate resuscitative efforts.

Table 10-1. Causes of GI Ulceration in Small Animals

Drugs
Nonsteroidal anti-inflammatory drugs
Corticosteroids
Metabolic and endocrine disorders
Liver disease
Renal disease
Pancreatitis
Hypoadrenocorticism
GI neoplasia
Adenocarcinoma
Leiomyosarcoma
Lymphosarcoma
Mastocytosis*
Gastrinoma*
Stress (ischemia)
Shock
Sepsis
Trauma
Major surgery
Neurologic disease
Head trauma
Intervertebral disk disease
Inflammatory bowel disease

* Conditions associated with hyperacidity

in the stomach or proximal duodenum. A variety of drugs and clinical conditions have been associated with gastric or duodenal ulceration (Table 10-1). The majority of these factors cause ulcer formation by damaging mucosal defense mechanisms. Nonsteroidal anti-inflammatory drugs appear to be the most common cause of GI ulcers in small animals, with liver disease being the most common metabolic disease resulting in GI ulceration.[18] Mastocytosis and gastrinoma appear to be the only conditions in which hyperaciditiy is considered to be the primary underlying mechanism for GI ulcer formation. Lower GI bleeding is most often associated with neoplasia.

Endoscopy is indicated when acute, severe upper or lower GI bleeding is suspected (Fig. 10-13). Depending on the circumstances, endoscopy provides information regarding the source of hemorrhage, allows the clinician to assess the likelihood of rebleeding, and can be used as a therapeutic modality. It is both sensitive and relatively safe. Endoscopy should be performed as soon as the patient appears hemodynamically stable. For upper GI bleeding, systemic evaluation of the esophagus, stomach, and duodenum is essential to avoid missing small lesions. Care should be taken to avoid overdistending the stomach with air during insufflation and when inserting the endoscope into the duodenum because perforation may result if an ulcer is present. Careful examination of the proximal duodenum should occur as the endoscope is removed to avoid missing lesions in this area. Lesions can easily be missed on insertion of the endoscope

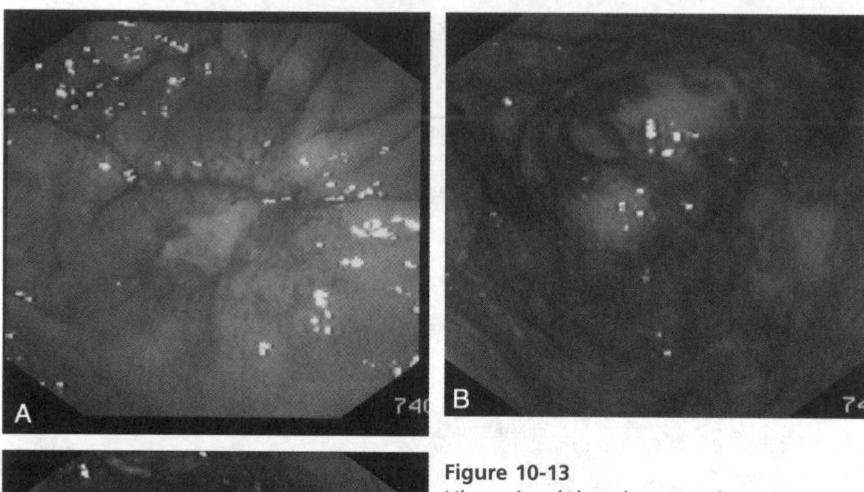

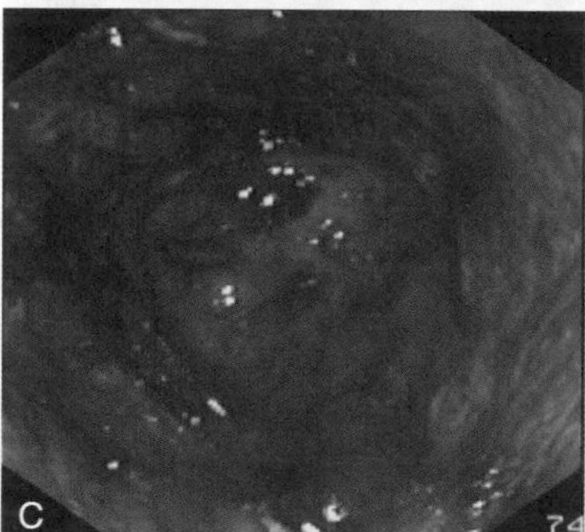

Figure 10-13
Ulceration (A) and severe ulcerative gastritis (B and C) in a dog on aspirin (25 mg/kg q 8 h) for degenerative joint disease. Despite a history of hematemesis (fresh blood) and melena no active bleeding was noted. The dog responded to crystalloid fluid therapy and gastric acid inhibition.

through the pylorus and into the duodenum. Direct colonoscopic examination is the procedure of choice for evaluation of lower GI tract bleeding.

Brush cytology and biopsies should be performed on all ulcers because neoplasia is often associated with gastric ulceration (Fig. 10-14). Samples should be taken only from the rim of the ulcer. Samples taken from the center of the ulcer may result in perforation because the gastric wall is thinnest in this area. Multiple biopsies should be obtained to confidently rule out neoplasia. If the GI wall is noticeably thickened around the ulcer, multiple samples may be taken from the same site to obtain deeper tissue. Biopsies of the superficial aspects of tumors often contain only inflammatory cells and may lead to misdiagnosis.

Severe GI hemorrhage in most cases can be controlled with aggressive fluid and transfusion therapy, together with treatment directed at the underlying cause. Severe bleeding from GI ulcers may be controlled by endoscopically administered hemostatic therapy. Effective hemostasis can be achieved injecting 1:10,000 epinephrine or 98% alcohol (limit 1 mL) through a endoscopic sclerotomy needle into the base of an ulcer. When bleeding fails to respond to these treatments, surgical intervention is required.

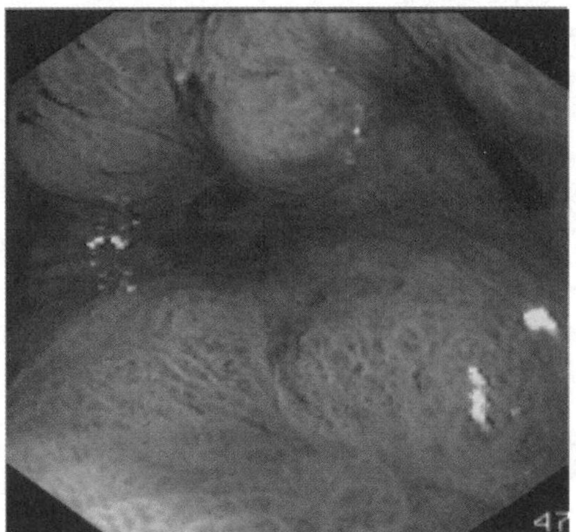

Figure 10-14
Ulceration secondary to gastric adenocarcinoma in an older dog. Note the proliferation of tissue surrounding the ulcer.

REFERENCES

1. Chamness CJ: Endoscopic intrumentation. *In* Tams TR, ed.: Small Animal Endoscopy. St. Louis, Mosby, 1999, p 1.
2. DeNovo RC: Selecting a gastrointestinal endoscope. *In* Bonagura JD, ed.: Kirk's Current Veterinary Therapy XII, Small Animal Practice. Philadelphia: WB Saunders, 1995, p 664.
3. Donaldson LL, Leib MS, Boyd C, *et al.*: Effect of preanesthetic medication on ease of endoscopic intubation of the duodenum in anesthetized dogs. *Am J Vet Res* 54: 1489, 1993.
4. Leib MS: Gastrointestinal Endoscopy. *In* August JR, ed.: Consultations in Feline Medicine. Philadelphia: WB Saunders, 1994, p 119.
5. Guilford WG: Gastrointestinal Endoscopy. *In* Guilford, ed.: Strombeck's Small Animal Gastroenterology. Philadelphia: WB Saunders, 1996, p. 114.
6. Sherding RG, Johnson SE, Tams TR: Esophagoscopy. *In* Tams TR, ed.: Small Animal Endoscopy. St. Louis: Mosby, 1999, p 39.
7. Tams TR. Gastroscopy. *In* Tams TR, ed.: Small Animal Endoscopy. St. Louis: Mosby, 1999, p 97.
8. Tams TR: Endoscopic examination of the small intestine. In Tams TR, ed.: Small Animal Endoscopy. St. Louis: Mosby, 1999, p 173.
9. Ryan WW, Greene RW: The conservative management of esophageal foreign bodies and their complications: a review of 66 cases in dogs and cats. *J Am Anim Hosp Assoc* 11:243, 1975.
10. Michels GM, Jone BD, Huss ST, *et al.*: Endoscopic and surgical retrieval of fishhooks from the stomach and esophagus in dogs and cats: 75 cases (1977–1993). *J Am Vet Med Assoc* 207:1194, 1995.
11. Davies C, Leib MS: Endoscopy case of the month: retrieving multiple gastric foreign bodies in a dog. *Vet Med* 94:26, 1999.
12. Tams TR: Endoscopic removal of gastrointestinal foreign bodies. *In* Tams TR, ed.: Small Animal Endoscopy. St. Louis: Mosby, 1999, p 247.
13. Cello JP, Fogel RP, Boland R: Liquid caustic ingestion spectrum of injury. *Arch Intern Med* 140:501, 1980.

14. Leape LL, Ashcraft KW, Carpelli DG, *et al.*: Hazard to health: liquid lye. *N Engl J Med* 284:578, 1971.
15. Litovitz, TL, Senmitz BF: Ingestion of cylindrical and button batteries: an analysis of 2382 cases. *Pediatrics* 89:747, 1982.
16. Haller JA, Andrews HG, White JJ, *et al.*: Pathophysiology and management of acute corrosive burns of the esophagus: results of treatment of 285 children. *J Pediatr Surg* 6:578, 1071.
17. Anderson KD, Rousse MR, Randolph JG: A controlled trial of corticosteriods in children with corrosive injury to the esophagus. *N Eng J Med* 323:637, 1990.
18. Stanton ME, Bright RM: Gastroduodenal ulceration in dogs: a retrospective study of 43 cases and literature review. *J Vet Intern Med* 3:238, 1989.

11
Thoracoscopy

Ronald S. Walton

INTRODUCTION

Thoracoscopy is as a minimally invasive operative endoscopic procedure designed for visual inspection and surgery in the thoracic cavity. Thoracoscopy is used extensively in human medicine and has seen increased use in veterinary medicine over the last 10 years. Today with efforts to explore and expand minimally invasive surgical techniques, thoracoscopy has evolved into a mainstream diagnostic and surgical tool in most human hospitals. The basic techniques and skills required for thoracoscopy are simple and similar to those of placing a thoracic drain. The ability to easily place a small, highly maneuverable, rigid telescope into the pleural space and provide a magnified view of the thoracic cavity and its organs provides an excellent window for visualization of structure, function, and pathology in the critical patient. New techniques for thoracoscopic surgery appear in the human literature daily. The application of these techniques is limited only by the size of the patient and the skill and imagination of the clinician involved.

INDICATIONS AND USE IN THE CRITICAL PATIENT

The use of minimally invasive technologies is becoming common in intensive and critical care. The primary indication in the veterinary patient is evaluation and visual inspection of the thoracic cavity when standard operative procedures are not indicated or desired. Thoracoscopy is far less invasive than a open thoracotomy and may be a useful tool for critical patients that are not capable of enduring the rigors of an open surgical procedure and postoperative care. The use of thoracoscopy in veterinary medicine has developed as a powerful tool for staging neoplastic disease, preoperative evaluation of lesion's resectibility, direct visualization of pathologic conditions, visually directed biopsy, evaluation and treatment of spontaneous and persistent traumatic pneumothorax, treatment of pericardial and pleural effusion, and evaluation and repair of intrathoracic trauma. The small size of the new telescopes and the ability to introduce them into regions difficult to access with standard techniques provide a view beyond what is possible through direct visualization.

Contraindications

Thoracoscopy requires development of a working space to insert and maneuver the telescope and instruments; an obliterated pleural space is therefore, an absolute contraindication (*i.e.*, after pleurodesis). Certain conditions, such as clotted hemothorax and stiff noncompliant lungs, can make thoracoscopy difficult to perform, and should be approached with more invasive procedures. Pleural adhesions, hypoxemia, severe cardiac instability, and coagulopathies are relative contraindications. Every thoracic diagnostic or surgery case is not a candidate for thoracoscopy. Limitations in three-dimensional orientation, ease of hemorrhage control, and a lack of tactile discrimination have been the early drawbacks to its use in critical patients.

EQUIPMENT

Basic Set

The instrumentation is basically the same as that needed for laparoscopy; one basic instrument set can be purchased for examination of both major body cavities with minimal adjustment required by the operator. The basic equipment for performing thoracoscopy includes a surgical telescope, trocar-cannula units, light source, a basic set of endoscopic manipulation and surgical instruments, and a standard surgery pack. Table 11-1 provides a basic starting set of instruments. The use of a small surgical video camera attached to the telescope and video monitor makes the procedure much easier to perform and enables the operator and assistants to view a simultaneous, enlarged and clear image. Adapters to fit most standard electrocautery units are readily available. Generally bipolar units are recommended. Most of the major electrocautery manufacturers make units designed exclusively for endoscopic utilization.

Preparation

Before the first trocars are placed into the thorax, the patient should be draped for a standard thoracotomy. The scope should be immersed in warm sterile water prior to the procedure to limit fogging. Sterile antifogging solutions (FRED) are available and may further reduce the incidence of optical fogging. The light cable should be attached to the telescope and the surgical video camera should be placed in a sterile camera bag with the assistance of an operating room technician. The video camera should be color balanced according to the manufacturer's instructions. The assembly is now ready for insertion when the telescope and operative ports are placed.

TRAINING AND STAFF CONSIDERATIONS

Continuing education courses are available at several locations worldwide for basic and advanced thoracoscopic techniques. At a minimum, a basic course in rigid endoscopy is recommended before attempting thoracoscopy for the first

Table 11-1. Suggested Endoscopic Instrumentation for Basic Thoracoscopy and Video-Assisted Diagnostic and Surgical Procedures in Small Animals

Basic Thoracoscopy Set
Hopkins telescope 0° or 30°
Fiberoptic light cable
Xenon light source
Operative and camera trocar-cannula sets (3) minimum
Palpation probe
Insulated endoscopic graspers
Insulated endoscopic grasping forceps (Kelly)
Insulated endoscopic scissors
Insulated endoscopic biopsy forceps (double spoon grasping or cutting)
Surgical suction
Basic standard surgery pack with thoracotomy pack available
Surgical towels and drapes
Thoracic drain
Suture material
Gauze
Heimlich valve
Good Additional Items to Basic Thoracoscopy Set
Surgery video camera
Video control unit
Video monitor
Video printer
Camera and light cable sterile cover
Underwater seal drainage system
Portable endoscopy cart
Basic Surgical Thoracoscopy Set
All of above plus:
Suction-irrigation unit
Electrocautery (bipolar)
Endoscopic forceps (DeBakey)
Endoscopic forceps (right angle)
Endoscopic lung retractors
Endoscopic linear stapler
Endoscopic cherry dissector
Endoscopic Kittner dissector
Endoscopic grasping forceps
Endoscopic clip applier
Endo-loop(s) and introducer
Flexible thoracic trocars
Specimen retrieval bag

From Walton RS: Video-assisted thoracoscopy. *Vet Clin North Am Sm Anim*, 51:729, 2001. Used with permission.

time. Learning simple techniques can end hours of frustration. Training and practice of the operative team are essential. The camera operator, surgeon, assistant, and anesthetist must all be synchronized to operate as an effective team. A sound knowledge of anatomy, appropriate preoperative staging, and a comfortable working knowledge of the equipment are prerequisites before you begin to work with diagnostic/surgical thoracoscopy in any patient.

PREOPERATIVE CONSIDERATIONS

Minimum Patient Evaluation

Risk limitation with thoracoscopy is the key to success and complete patient evaluation including biochemical screen, clotting profile, thoracic radiographs, and ultrasound examination within 24 hours of the procedure will limit costly mistakes. Preoperative staging is essential to avoid the serious complications of thoracoscopy, which include penetrating the lung with the trocar, entering the wrong side or location, penetrating viscera of a large diaphragmatic hernia, or entering a clotted hemothorax.

Anesthesia

Various techniques are used from heavy sedation, general inhalant anesthetics, total intravenous anesthesia, to selective lung ventilation techniques. Anesthetic agent selection and technique are based on the condition and systemic derangement present in the patient. General anesthesia is usually recommended. Administration of supplemental high fractional inspired oxygen concentrations (F_IO_2) will compensate for the ventilation-perfusion mismatching, which occurs during a partial pneumothorax. Patient monitoring should include as a minimum pulse oximetry, capnography, blood pressure measurement (direct or indirect), and an electrocardiogram.

Working Space

All thoracoscopic procedures and proper examination of the thoracic cavity require creation of a working space by induction of a pneumothorax. Without this working space, the telescope and instruments cannot be adequately maneuvered and visualization of structures would be negligible. Techniques to establish this working space include controlled partial pneumothorax, selective lung ventilation, and intrathoracic insufflation.

Controlled Partial Pneumothorax

Normal animals tolerate moderate pneumothorax with little systemic compromise. During induction of routine partial pneumothorax, the lungs readily collapse in most patients to provide an adequate working space for rapid diagnostic evaluation.

One-Lung Ventilation

One-lung ventilation (OLV) is performed in many human and veterinary surgical procedures to increase intrathoracic visibility. The technique involves selective bronchial intubation or the use of a bronchial blocker allowing the nonventilated lung to collapse. Collapsing one of the lungs markedly improves the working space and improves access to the pulmonary hilus and heart base. If lung is the tissue to be evaluated or resected, collapse of the operative lung simplifies biopsy sampling, lesion location, and partial or full lobectomy. Normal dogs show increased $PaCO_2$ and shunt fraction and a mild decrease in PaO_2 with OLV techniques. These effects were considered transient or easily overcome by adjustments in mechanical ventilation. Extensive monitoring is an absolute requirement for these techniques in clinical patients.

Thoracic Insufflation

Thoracic insufflation is also technique used to collapse the lungs and improve intrathoracic working space. Low-pressure intrathoracic insufflation with carbon dioxide is used to facilitate collapse of the lungs. Normal dogs tolerate this procedure without significant cardiovascular or pulmonary compromise using intrathoracic insufflation of 5 mm Hg or less. Overinflation of the thoracic cavity sets up the physiology of a tension pneumothorax and could have disastrous consequences. Patients that lack pulmonary compliance and require pleural insufflation to establish a working space, may be better candidates for open thoracotomy rather than thoracoscopy.

Expectations

As with any new technique speed and accuracy come with experience. The view obtained with thoracoscopy, however, is often superior to that obtained with open thoracotomy because any structure within the thorax can be imaged with a magnified well-illuminated view.

Emergency Plan

Thoracoscopy is generally a very safe and easily performed procedure, but you must have a backup plan and ability to perform an emergency thoracotomy. Uncontrollable hemorrhage is the most common indication for emergency thoracotomy. Inadvertent large vessel laceration or dislodging a large clot can obstruct the working area with blood and control may be difficult in the close confines of the thoracic cavity. If you do not have the ability or resources to perfom a rapid thoracotomy, thoracoscopy should not be attempted, especially in a trauma patient.

SPECIFIC TECHNIQUES

Basic Approaches to Thoracoscopic Examination

Two basic approaches to the thorax are routinely used, the paraxiphoid-transdiaphragmatic (PX) and intercostal (IC). The selection of approach is based on the anatomic feature you wish to access. Table 11-2 lists the major anatomic features accessible via thoracoscopy and the recommended approach. A thoracoscopic examination requires the placement of telescope and a minimum of one instrument portal through the thoracic wall or diaphragm to view the thoracic cavity and introduce instruments to manipulate tissues. Figure 11-1 outlines the basic portal placement locations.

The PX (see Figure 11-1A) approach is easiest for the beginning thoraco-

Table 11-2. Thoracoscopic Localization by Major Anatomic Feature

Anatomic Feature	Paraxiphoid Approach	Intercostal Approach
Diaphragm	+/−	+
Individual lung lobes	+	+/−
Ventral aspect	+	+/−
Dorsal aspect	−	+
Both	+/−	+/−
Intrathoracic trachea and bronchi	−	+/−
Thoracic wall	−	−
Intercostal regions	+	+/−
Thoracic duct	+	−
Sternum	+	+/−
Heart	+	+/−
Pericardium	+	+
Base	−	+/−
Apex	+	+/−

Basic structure locator and best approach to visualization. A good approach allowing excellent visualization is indicated by (+) and a less than ideal or unsatisfactory approach indicated by a (−). An approach that is difficult or requires extensive scope maneuver or tissue traction is indicated by a (+/−).

Adapted from Walton RS: Video-assisted thoracoscopy. *Vet Clin North Am Sm Anim*, 51:729, 2001. Used with permission.

scopist to master. The telescope portal is placed through the diaphragm with the patient in dorsal recumbency. This position allows an excellent evaluation of the ventral aspects of both hemithoraces. On penetration of the pars sternalis of the diaphragm, the thorax is examined by advancing the scope cranially. A number of structures may be visualized using this approach; only the length of the scope limits exploration of cranial thoracic structures. For example, the ventral aspects of each lung lobe, ventral aspect of the pulmonary hilus, costal diaphragmatic reflection, sternal diaphragmatic recesses, ventral aspect of the thoracic inlet, and entire subphrenic pericardium can be viewed from this position. Additional portals can also be placed in the intercostal spaces (see Figure 11-1 B,C) and a palpation probe can be inserted to gently retract and manipulate the lung lobes. This technique allows direction of the scope between the lobar fissures, thereby allowing excellent visualization of the visceral pleural surface as well as pulmonary vessels. By insertion of a forceps and scissors, the pericardium can be easily grasped and incised from this position. The dorsal aspects of the lungs and vessels, however, cannot be easily visualized from this position.

The IC (see Fig. 11-1B,C) approach is the most common approach described in the literature. The patient can be positioned in right and left lateral, dorsal recumbency, or in an oblique fashion depending on the structure(s) to be evaluated. Figure 11-1 serves only as a guide to routine placement of the

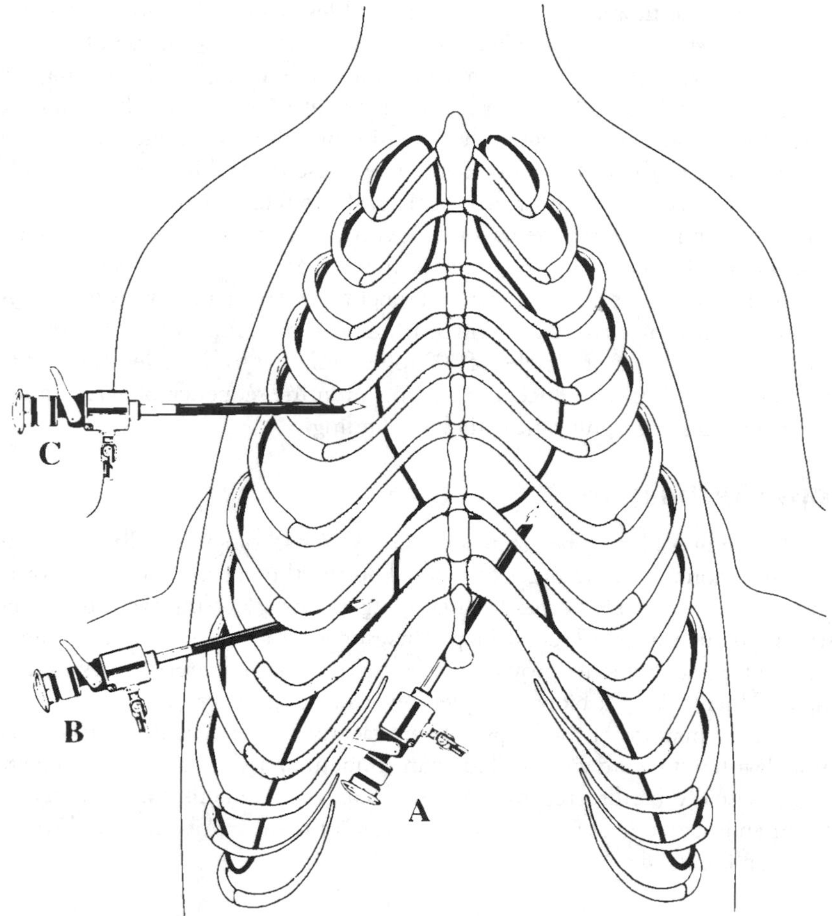

Figure 11-1
Canine thorax (dorsal recumbent) depicting various camera and instrument portal insertion sites. (A) Paraxiphoid, (B) caudal intercostal, (C) cranial intercostal. Adapted from Walton RS: Video-assisted thoracoscopy. *Vet Clin North Am Sm Anim*, 51:729, 2001.

instrument and telescope portals. Portal placement is based primarily on lesion location and ability to access the lesion or anatomic feature in question. With placement of an additional instrument trocar, a palpation probe will allow movement of adjacent lung lobes and visualization of peribronchial tissues, pulmonary arteries and veins, hilar lymph nodes, and all aspects of the pleural surface of the diaphragm.

Diagnostic Evaluation

A complete rapid assessment of the thoracic cavity should be performed each time you perform a thoracoscopic examination. Severe pathology can mesmerize the novice thoracoscopist and additional lesions may be missed. A minimum of one instrument portal in addition to the primary telescope port for insertion of a palpation probes that permit visceral manipulation and examination. Placing the portals too close to a lesion or operative field severely limits the action of the instrument. Placing them to distant will make operation difficult at the extremes of the instrument length. The telescope and instruments should always be directed toward the video monitor. If the telescope is pointed toward the monitor and the instruments away, a condition of paradoxical movement occurs, giving the operator a visual image that appears to move opposite to the direction intended. Instruments may be brought into the field of view and easily oriented by inserting the portals in a triangular pattern. Instrument portals should be placed to create angles of 30° to 60° relative to the telescope and to each other to limit interference. Developing a routine sequence of examination will prevent missing significant pathologic findings.

Biopsy Techniques

Obtaining a biopsy specimen of a variety of pathologic conditions is one of the most common procedures conducted during thoracoscopy. Biopsy instruments come in numerous types from grasping/crushing/cutting types to needle instruments such as the Tru-cut biopsy instrument. Larger specimens obtained with cup-type instruments provide the pathologist with a more representative sample. When taking a biopsy sample, never close the jaws of the instrument unless all the margins of the biopsy site are clearly visible. Small lesions can be biopsied with a standard grasping biopsy instrument or a Tru-cut type instrument and can visually be directed to the lesion. Larger specimens can be obtained with an endoscopic ligature or a wedge section of tissue can be removed with a linear stapling device.

Hemostasis

Effective hemostasis is critically important to a successful thoracoscopic examination. Uncontrolled hemorrhage can rapidly deteriorate the operators' visual field reducing operative accuracy and efficiency. Temporary hemostasis can be achieved by application of gentle pressure at the point of hemorrhage with a palpation probe or other blunt instrument. Vessels can be easily grasped with endoscopic forceps and a ligature or electrocautery used to provide definitive hemostasis. A small intercostal incision can be used to rapidly introduce almost any instrument required to clamp a vessel as needed. Most mild to moderate hemorrhages are not problematic and will resolve with conservative management and the use of a thoracic drain.

Subphrenic Pericardectomy and Pericardial Window

Thoracoscopic partial pericardectomy is now routinely performed in many veterinary clinics worldwide. The techniques range from subtotal pericardectomies to creation of a small pericardial window. The entire pericardium below the phrenic nerve can be accessed easily via the PX approach. The telescope is placed in the PX position (see Fig. 11-1) with the animal in dorsal recumbency. Instrument portals are then placed intercostally under direct visualization. The pericardium can be easily grasped, drained and incised via this technique. Typically the majority of the pericardial fluid is removed prior to surgery. Excessive pericardial fluid limits cardiac function to the extent anesthesia becomes a tremendous risk. Diseased pericardial tissue tends to be markedly thicker and more vascular than normal. Electrocautery and suction must be available with this procedure to control hemorrhage and clear the visual field. The phrenic nerves are prominent landmarks on the pericardial surface and must be spared. After grasping the pericardial tissue, it is easily incised and removed.

Pleurodesis

Animals with chronic pleural effusion and recurrent spontaneous pneumothorax can often benefit from the technique of pleurodesis. This procedure can be performed by manual abrasion of the pleural surface with devices such as an endoscopic cherry dissector or gauze sponge or with instillation of a pleurodesis agent (*i.e.*, sterile talc or tetracycline). This procedure can be accomplished either from the PX or IC approach. The PX approach has the advantage of providing access to both hemithoraces without repositioning the patient. Operative ports can be placed in the right and left fourth or fifth intercostal spaces most of the parietal pleural surface can be easily accessed.

POSTOPERATIVE CARE AND MONITORING

Re-establishment of thoracic integrity and providing an airtight seal is essential at the conclusion of the procedure. This is accomplished by correction of the pneumothorax, withdrawal of the instrument portals, and primary repair of the chest wall and skin defect. These incisions are usually very small (<12 mm) and are easily repaired with interrupted sutures. A two-layer closure is usually adequate. Visual evaluation of the efficacy of thoracic evacuation is performed by application of standard suction to the stopcock valve on the telescope portal cannula with the telescope in place. When a simple diagnostic procedure alone is performed, a thoracic drain is often not required in the postoperative period. A thoracic drain should be placed, after completion of each procedure in which lung tissue is removed or significant effusion or hemorrhage is expected. Visual evaluation and placement of the thoracic drain is possible prior to removal of the telescope portal. The drain can be placed by passing it through an instrument cannula and pulling the cannula over the end of the drain or a drain may be placed through a new intercostal entry in standard fashion. The patient must be closely evaluated in the early postoperative period to ensure that the thoracic cavity is properly evacuated. Intermittent or continuous suction of the drain should be used during the recovery period until the lungs are fully expanded. A postoperative thoracic radiograph should be used to confirm the resolution of pneumothorax. In many patients, the thoracic drain can be removed in the early recovery period; however, the length of time the thoracic drain is maintained depends on the individual pathologic process.

COMPLICATIONS

The overall complication rate with thoracoscopy is small when appropriate procedure planning and patient evaluation are conducted before the procedure. The most common complications that arise during thoracoscopy are severe hemorrhage, puncture or tearing of the pulmonary parenchyma, laceration of a vessel or nerve during biopsy. Damage to the phrenic nerve is particularly easy during pericardectomy or pericardial window formation and can markedly affect diaphragm function. Removal of biopsy specimens directly through small incisions holes in the thoracic wall or cannulas may cause malignant or infected material to contaminate the pleural or abdominal space. Seeding the thoracic wall with infected or neoplastic tissue has been reported in humans as a common complication. Mild to moderate and persistent pneumothorax is also a reported postoperative complication. If they occur, small air leaks typically are at the site of a biopsy. Close evaluation of the biopsy site before completion of the procedure will often reveal a problem area, allowing rapid resolution. Most air leaks occurring in the postoperative period resolve with continuous underwater seal thoracic suction applied for 12 to 24 hours.

SUGGESTED READINGS

Cantwell SL, Duke T, Walsh PJ, *et al.*: One-lung versus two-lung ventilation in the closed-chest anesthetized dog: a comparison of cardiopulmonary parameters. *Vet Surg* 29:365, 2000.

Faunt KK, Cohen LA, Jones BD, *et al.*: Cardiopulmonary effects of bilateral hemithorax ventilation and diagnostic thoracoscopy in dogs. *Am J Vet Res* 59:1491, 1998.

Faunt KK, Jones BD, Turk JR, *et al.*: Evaluation of biopsy specimens obtained during thoracoscopy from lungs of clinically normal dogs. *Am J Vet Res* 59:1499, 1998.

Garcia F, Prandi D, Pena T, *et al.*: Examination of the thoracic cavity and lung lobectomy by means of thoracoscopy in dogs. *Can Vet J* 39:285, 1996.

Jackson J, Richter KP, Launder DP: Thoracoscopic partial pericardectomy in 13 dogs. *J Vet Intern Med* 13:529, 1999.

McCarthy TC: Diagnostic thoracoscopy. *Clin Tech Small Anim Pract* 14:213, 1999.

Potter L, Hendrickson DA: Therapeutic video-assisted thoracic surgery. *In* Freeman LJ, ed.: Veterinary Endo Surgery. St. Louis: Mosby, 1999, p 169.

Walsh PJ: Thoracoscopic versus open partial pericardectomy in dogs: comparison of postoperative pain and morbidity. *Vet Surg* 28:472, 1999.

Walton RS: Thoracoscopy. *In* Tams TA, ed.: Small Animal Endoscopy. St. Louis: Mosby, 1999, p 471.

Walton RS, Hackett TB: Thoracoscopy. *In* Bonagura J, ed.: Current Veterinary Therapy XIII. Philadelphia: WB Saunders, 2000, p 157.

12
Respiratory Care

Marc R. Raffe

INTRODUCTION

Diseases of the respiratory system are commonly diagnosed in clinical veterinary medicine. Clinical management of patients with respiratory disease is based on a working knowledge of respiratory and cardiovascular physiology, complete and accurate physical examination, appropriate diagnostic tests, intensive monitoring, and supportive therapy. Support procedures in management of these patients include oxygen (O_2) administration, procedures to improve and optimize respiratory function, and provision of artificial airway support in selected cases.

OXYGEN$_2$ THERAPY

One of the key goals in patient management is to support O_2 delivery. The process of tissue O_2 delivery may be divided into three stages: (1) external respiration, (2) blood transport, and (3) internal respiration. External respiration is the process of transferring atmospheric O_2 to the blood. This process depends on many factors including airway patency, adequate alveolar O_2 tension, and alveolar gas exchange. The goals for successful external respiration include delivery of physiologic O_2 levels to the alveolus, maintenance of normal alveolar ventilation, and control of normal protective reflexes. These parameters should be maintained within normal limits for efficient O_2 transport and delivery.

Hypoxemia is defined as an arterial O_2 tension less than 80 mm Hg. Clinical signs of hypoxemia may include tachypnea, tachycardia, dyspnea, cyanosis, positional discomfort, and restlessness. Hypoxemia caused by intrapulmonary shunting is common in pulmonary disease; the degree of hypoxemia is determined by evaluating hemoglobin saturation of arterial blood. Physiologic responses to hypoxemia include increased cardiac output, a decrease in O_2 consumption at the tissue level, and local modification of regional pulmonary perfusion to decrease intrapulmonary shunting. Hypoxemia caused by decreased alveolar O_2 tension (V/Q mismatch, which causes regional decrease in alveolar O_2 tensions) is generally O_2 responsive. Absolute intrapulmonary shunting is not O_2 responsive.

In emergent patients, several emergency O_2 delivery procedures have been described. Placement of a high-flow O_2 tube in front of the nares provides immediate "flow-by" O_2 support. An O_2 enclosure may be created from a plastic garbage bag into which a high-flow O_2 line is introduced. A homemade O_2 enclosure can be fashioned from a garbage bag and Elizabethan collar. The plastic bag is secured at the edge of the collar using duct tape or other package sealing tape. The O_2 tubing is placed in the vicinity of the muzzle. A vent is created by a large opening in the top of the "tent" to provide release of pressure and carbon dioxide (CO_2). In small dogs and cats, a pediatric O_2 hood can be used for support. This hood is commercially available as a cuboidal frame covered with polyvinyl plastic. One side of the cube has a flap that seals around the patient. A top vent hole is present to release pressure and permit venting of CO_2. The patient's head or body can be enclosed in the cube and O_2 introduced. For small dogs and cats, an anesthetic induction chamber may be used for an emergency O_2 cage. Long-term use may produce heat retention that may require supplemental cooling methods.

Oxygen masks can be commercially purchased or made from homemade materials. A tight fitting seal around the muzzle allows for optimal delivery of O_2. The rubber diaphragm provided on some designs may be substituted with soft, flexible bandaging material such as Vetwrap (3M Corp) for better mask acceptance and tolerance. Mask acceptance is better if vision is not blocked. Homemade O_2 masks can be fashioned from syringe cases, plastic drinking glasses, or disposable plastic soft drink bottles to provide a variety of sizes. These masks can be adapted with a tie string to encircle the head and maintain mask position.

Nasal cannulae may be used to provide supplemental, low concentration O_2 delivery. Human nasal cannulae ("prongs") are tolerated in quiet dogs and cats and can provide acceptable O_2 delivery. They are secured with single sutures over the zygomatic arch area of both sides of the head.

Administration of O_2 via nasal catheter is a common procedure in critically ill patients (Fig. 12-1). Nasal catheters are constructed from 5 or 8 Fr red rubber feeding catheters, polyvinyl nasal feeding tubes, or modified human nasal catheters (prongs). The catheter is premeasured from the nasal orifice to the medial canthus of the eye; this length is marked with a felt-tipped pen. After the head is tilted up, 1 to 3 drops of a rapid-acting local anesthetic agent (0.5% proparacaine or 2% lidocaine) are instilled in the nostril to desensitize the nasal cavity. The nasal catheter is liberally lubricated with 2% lidocaine lubricant. The dorsal aspect of the nose is pressed upward and backward to facilitate placement. The catheter is inserted downward and medial to pass through the ventral meatus. Once placed to the premarked depth, the catheter is gently looped around the alar cartilage. A single nylon suture or drop of "super glue" on crossed hair tufts is used to anchor the catheter. The glue can be removed with nail polish remover or special glue remover. Several additional sites are used to secure the catheter along the center line of the maxilla and over the dorsum of the head. Following placement, the catheter is attached to an O_2 line that has passed through a humidifier. O_2 flow rate is provided at 100 cc/kg. A maximum of 4 L/min can be administered through a single nasal catheter.

Oxygen cages are valuable in critically emergent dogs and cats. This approach for O_2 administration is preferred in these cases because it reduces patient stress. In addition, environmental factors such as humidity and temperature may be controlled. O_2 cages have the added advantage of being able to regulate the delivered O_2 concentration. Usual settings for an O_2 cage are 30% to 40% oxygen, 70° to

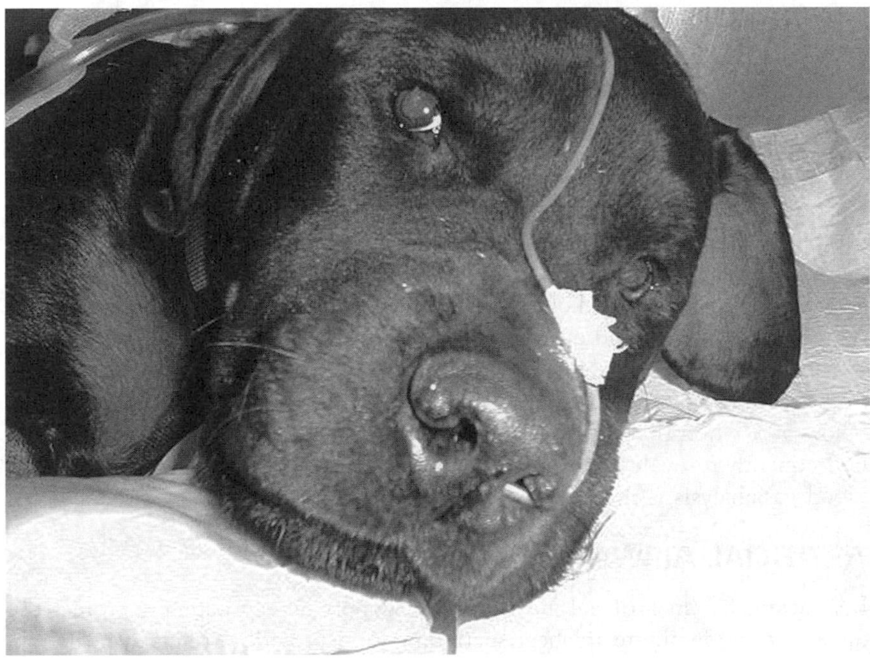

Figure 12-1
Nasal oxygen tube placement.

75°F, and 40% to 50% humidity. In emergency situations, a homemade O_2 enclosure may be fashioned from plastic bag enclosures, or an Elizabethan collar and plastic front shield as previously described. Plastic shrouding of a transport crate will provide sufficient O_2 in extremely fractious but stressed patients. These are temporary solutions until a long-term delivery technique is identified.

Transtracheal O_2 delivery may be used in cases with facial and upper airway injury in which use of a nasal O_2 catheter is contraindicated (Fig. 12-2). The transtracheal catheter is made from a flexible intravenous (IV) catheter with

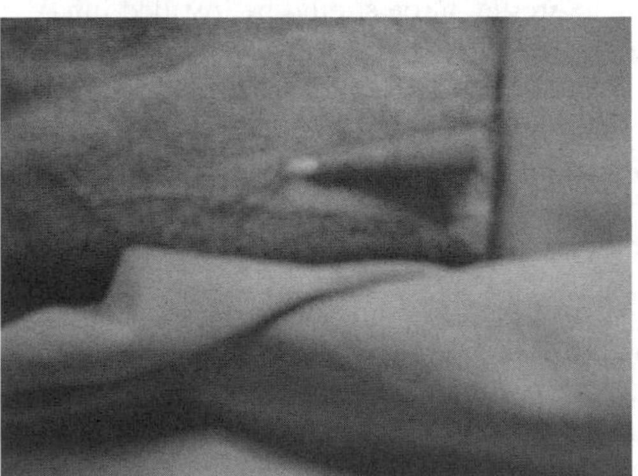

Figure 12-2
Transtracheal O_2 catheter placement.

several side holes cut near the tip. A "through-the-needle" or "over-the-needle" style catheter may be used for O_2 delivery. Generally a 14-gauge × 5-inch catheter is used. Location for tracheal placement is based on individual anatomy. The catheter may be passed through the cricothyroid membrane or moved to the third to fifth inter-ring site as is used for transtracheal wash. The side holes created in the catheter prevent the O_2 from producing a pressure "jet" lesion of the tracheal epithelium. An O_2 flow of 1 to 2 L/min can be used to deliver about 30% to 40% O_2 concentration. The O_2 should be humidified if possible.

Although O_2 is therapeutic, one must be aware of O_2 toxicity. O_2 in excessive amounts over a period of time leads to additional alveolar injury, decreased pulmonary function, and eventual death. There is wide species and individual variation in the susceptibility to O_2 toxicity. In general, small animals should not receive 100% O_2 for longer than 12 to 24 hours. O_2 concentration should be below 50% when therapy is used for extended time periods. The animal should be frequently re-evaluated to determine if O_2 therapy is still indicated. Arterial blood gas analysis is the best method to determine response to O_2 therapy.

ARTIFICIAL AIRWAY MANAGEMENT

Indications for an artificial airway are to support airway patency, protect the upper airway, facilitate tracheal suctioning, and provide artificial ventilation. Tracheostomy and the endotracheal tubes are the two methods of providing artificial airway support. Although endotracheal tubes are often used in humans, tracheostomy tubes are more practical for long-term use in veterinary patients. Orally placed endotracheal tubes are easily damaged by chewing. They can cause irritation in the oral pharynx and induce laryngeal complications. It must be recognized that patients with an artificial airway require 24-hour monitoring and meticulous nursing care.

Bypassing the upper airway eliminates the normal means of warming, humidifying, and filtering the air that is taken into the lungs. In canine patients, it is also important to remember that the respiratory tract is a normal means of heat loss contributing to thermoregulation. Ideally, inspired air should be warmed and humidified to prevent the drying of secretions. This can be accomplished with the use of gas humidification and nebulizer treatments. If humidification or nebulization is not available, sterile saline should be instilled into the tracheostomy or endotracheal tube periodically to help moisten and loosen secretions. It is important to monitor patient hydration status to help prevent the further drying out of pulmonary secretions. Chest physiotherapy and exercise can also prevent the pooling of secretions in the lower airways.

Endotracheal Tubes/Tracheostomy Tubes

Various endotracheal tube and tracheostomy tube designs are available in human medicine. These tubes have been adapted for use in veterinary medicine. Recently, companies have designed tracheostomy tubes specifically for veterinary use due to the differences between human and animal anatomy.

Endotracheal tubes using soft pliable material that conforms to patient anatomy are preferred. Tracheostomy tubes should have an inner cannula that can be removed for easy cleaning. Endotracheal tubes and tracheostomy tubes can be cuffed or cuffless. For positive pressure ventilation, a cuffed tube will be required. The cuff should be a high-volume–low-pressure type to help prevent ischemia and necrosis of the trachea wall.

Tracheostomy tubes require surgical placement. The patient is placed under general anesthesia and positioned in dorsal recumbancy with a rolled towel placed under the cervical region and front limbs caudally extended. Following surgical preparation, a midline incision is performed from the first to the eighth tracheal ring. Separation of connective tissue and sternohyoideus muscle allows tracheal visualization. The endotracheal tube is withdrawn to a position rostral to the incision site. The tracheal interspace between the fourth and fifth tracheal ring is incised. Three techniques for tracheal incision, transverse, longitudinal, and flap, have been described. Following incision, traction sutures are placed in both ends of the incision on the ventral aspect to control the trachea. Hemorrhage and mucus are evacuated from the tracheal lumen. An appropriate size tracheostomy tube is then inserted into the trachea. Following tracheostomy tube placement, the skin is loosely apposed to prevent dissecting subcutaneous emphysema. A sterile wound dressing is applied. The tracheostomy tube is secured around the neck using umbilical tape attached to the suture tabs of the tracheostomy tube. The area is lightly bandaged to prevent soiling.

Recently, a percutaneous tracheostomy technique has been described. This technique uses a set of dilator devices that are used to facilitate placement. Insertion sites may be at either the cricothyroid membrane or at the 5 to 6 interring area. A small surgical wound is created in the superficial tissues over the proposed insertion site. A needle is introduced into the tracheal lumen and a guidewire threaded through the tracheal lumen. The needle is withdrawn leaving the guidewire in place. A series of dilators are sequentially inserted to enlarge the "tract" until the desired trachesotomy tube has a path large enough to be easily inserted. The disadvantage to the technique is that the endotracheal tube used for initial airway management may interfere with the procedure. Caution must be observed that the endotracheal tube is withdrawn proximal to the insertion point before beginning the procedure.

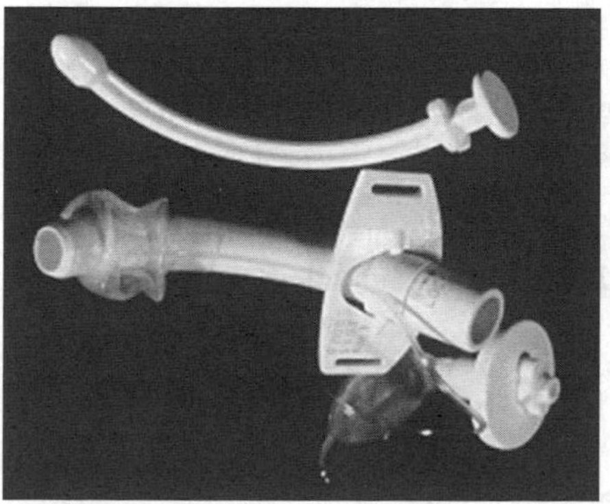

Figure 12-3
Cuffed tracheostomy tube with introducer.

Table 12-1. Steps to Correct Artificial Airway Obstruction

1. Manipulate the tube.
2. Remove the inner cannula, if the tracheostomy tube has one. If not, deflate the cuff to allow the patient to breathe around the tube.
3. Attempt to pass a suction catheter.

Following placement, the tracheostomy tube cuff is inflated if ventilatory support is to be provided (Fig. 12-3). If overinflated, a high-volume–low-pressure cuff can become a high-pressure cuff, which significantly increases the chance of tracheal wall necrosis. For positive pressure ventilation, the cuff is inflated until the air leak disappears. Air is then gradually withdrawn in small increments until there is a slight leak at peak inspiration. For spontaneous ventilation or continuous positive airway pressure, remove small amounts of air until a small expiratory leak is heard. Periodic cuff deflation, whether it is a high-pressure or low-pressure cuff, does not reduce the chances of tracheal necrosis.

Complications associated with artificial airways include cuff leaks, accidental extubation, and obstruction. Obstruction may be due to tube kinking, cuff overinflation herniating and blocking the end of the tube, or buildup of secretions within the tube lumen. Airway obstruction due to mucous plugs occurs more frequently in tubes with a small diameter. These complications can be immediate and life-threatening. To avoid this complication, periodic removal and cleaning of the inner cannula is recommended (Table 12-1). Airway suctioning generally occurs at the same time. There should always be a replacement tube and intubation equipment near the patient.

SUCTIONING

Pulmonary hygiene is an important aspect in caring for the patient with an artificial airway. Suctioning will need to be performed to prevent the accumulation of secretions. Auscultating breath sounds, noting previous amounts suctioned, and monitoring temperature and respirations can help determine how frequently the patient needs to be suctioned. Suctioning causes tracheal irritation and can cause an increase in mucous production, so it should never be done more than 3 to 4 times per day. The procedure for suctioning is outlined in Table 12-2.

The suction catheter should be no more than one half the size of the tracheal tube and made of a soft pliable material to minimize the damage to the mucosal wall. A side port or hole that can be digitally occluded is recommended to prevent injury associated with excess suction pressure. The vacuum of the suction apparatus should be adjusted to −80 to −120 mm Hg. Possible complications from suctioning include hypoxia, dysrhythmias, hypotension, and lung collapse.

The tracheotomy wound is an open surgical site and is subject to complications. Immediate complications include hemorrhage and subcutaneous and mediastinal emphysema. Late complications include bleeding from tracheal irritation and infection. Aseptic technique must be used when working with these patients.

Table 12-2. Airway Suction Procedure

1. **Always** use sterile gloves, suction catheter, bowl, and saline. You will need a suction source, an Ambu bag connected to O_2, and someone to assist. Ideally, the patient is on an electrocardiogram monitor.
2. Bag the patient 4–5 times with 100% O_2 to hyperoxygenate.
3. Insert the catheter, applying no suction, until a slight resistance is met. Pull back slightly, then apply intermittent suction and use a twisting motion as you continue to withdraw the catheter.
4. This process should take no longer than 10–15 sec.
5. Bag the patient 4–5 times with 100% O_2 or until vital signs return to baseline.
6. Repeat process, if needed.
7. Small amounts of sterile saline can be instilled to help loosen secretions and stimulate coughs.
8. The oral cavity can be suctioned with the same catheter, but never reuse it in the trachea.
9. Note amounts, color, consistency, and patient tolerance on the chart. Notify the clinician if there are any significant changes.

The site is treated as any other open surgical incision. It must be kept clean and dry and checked frequently for signs of redness or swelling. The area should be cleaned routinely with a 50:50 solution of 3% hydrogen peroxide solution and sterile water or saline, then rinsed with sterile saline or water alone. Folded sterile gauze pads placed in a manner to provide a cushion around the tracheostomy tube prevents the tracheostomy tube collar from applying pressure and rubbing against bare skin. Care should also be taken in positioning the patient to prevent pulling or placing traction on the tube. A swivel adapter helps to prevent this. There is controversy concerning if and how often a tracheostomy tube should be changed. Normally, a tracheostomy tube is not changed during the first 3 to 4 days after placement unless there is a complication. If replacement is required during this initial period, it should be done by the surgeon or clinician. If there are no problems, the tracheostorny tube should be replaced once a week.

THORACIC DRAINAGE

Thoracocentesis

Thoracocentesis (Table 12-3) is the procedure in which the pleural cavity is drained by temporary insertion of a needle through the intercostal space into the pleural cavity. Thoracocentesis may be considered in emergent patients that demonstrate increased work of breathing in conjunction with diminished breath sounds. It is typically performed prior to diagnostic radiography in severe, emergent cases to effect respiratory system stabilization. The goal is to determine the presence of air, fluid, or blood in the pleural space. Removal of air and fluid from the pleural space permits lung tissue re-expansion and restores normal thoracic physiology. A sample of any collected fluid may be analyzed by clinicopathologic and cytologic techniques to determine its character and possible origin.

Table 12-3. Thoracocentesis (Needle Thoracostomy)

1. Give O_2 via face mask at a minimum of 10 L/min.
2. Allow the animal to assume position of comfort.
   a. Sternal in most cases.
3. Identify **mid-thorax** region for needle placement.
   a. 7th interspace
      i. Midway between shoulder and last rib
   b. About 4 inches below the spine for anticipated air drainage
   c. About 3 inches above the sternum for anticipated fluid drainage
4. **Shave** a 1 × 1 inch area of hair. Quickly scrub with surgical prep.
5. Assemble a thoracostomy unit using a 20-gauge × 1-inch needle, three-way valve, IV extension tubing, and 35-mL syringe. A small hemostat is also useful.
6. Palpate the rib space. Infiltrate the proposed thoracentesis site with 1-2 mL 2% lidocaine in the subcutaneous and muscle tissue.
7. **Insert the needle unit at a 45° angle** beginning just off the front edge of the 8th rib. As needle is advanced, aspirate on syringe. Generally, needle will not go in more than 1 inch when free air begins to be aspirated.
8. **Stabilize needle** at this point. A hemostat clamped around the needle shaft at the skin surface level may be helpful in preventing the needle from advancing.
9. Begin aspirating with the syringe. When syringe is full of air, rotate three-way valve and expel air from syringe. Re-rotate valve to close side port and aspirate again.
10. **IN A LIFE-THREATENING EMERGENCY, SECURE A CUT-OFF GLOVE FINGER OVER THE NEEDLE HUB, CUT A ¼ INCH SLIT HOLE IN THE FINGER COT, AND INSERT INTO CHEST. THIS WILL RELIEVE LIFE-THREATENING PNEUMOTHORAX.**

Thoracocentesis may be performed using a hypodermic needle, butterfly catheter, over-the-needle catheter, or teat cannula as the drainage device. In all cases, the drain unit is attached to a three-way stopcock and syringe unit. A 6- to 12-inch IV tubing extension set is attached between the needle and three-way valve. All components are assembled prior to thoracocentesis to guard against introduction of air into the pleural space.

Thoracostomy Tube

Thoracostomy tube (chest drain) placement (Table 12-4) is considered when either continuous collection of air or fluid occurs in the pleural cavity, necessitating multiple thoracocentesis procedures, or when it is anticipated that continuous pleural space drainage is required for fluid, air, chyle, or purulent exudates. The two options for thoracostomy drainage are mini-chest tube or regular thoracostomy tube placement.

Mini-Chest Tube

A mini-chest tube is recommended under the following conditions: (1) if thoracocentesis has to be done more that twice to relieve the patient of respi-

Table 12-4. Thoracostomy Tube Placement (Chest Drain)

1. Give O_2 via face mask at a minimum of 10 L/min.
2. Allow the animal to assume position of comfort.
   a. Sternal in most cases
3. Identify **mid-thorax** region for needle placement.
   a. 7th interspace
      i. Midway between shoulder and last rib
   b. About 4 inches below the spine for anticipated air drainage
   c. About 3 inches above the sternum for anticipated fluid drainage
4. **Shave** a 6 × 6 inch area of hair. Scrub with surgical prep as per surgical procedure.
5. Assemble a chest drain unit, tubing adapter, three-way valve, IV extension tubing, 35-mL syringe, plastic lock bands, scalpel blade, curved hemostat, needle holders, suture material, tubing clamp, and bandage.
6. Palpate the rib space. Stretch the skin forward as much as possible. Infiltrate the proposed thoracostomy site with 2 to 4 mL 2% lidocaine in the subcutaneous and muscle tissue. Sedation may be needed to facilitate patient cooperation.
7. Create a 1-cm skin wound over the proposed site. Create a subcutaneous tunnel down to the intercostal muscles using blunt tissue dissection.
8. Insert the thoracostomy tube/stylette unit into the dissected path. With gentle pressure, advance the unit until it enters the pleural space. This will be felt as a loss of resistance. Wait approximately 2–3 seconds to let lung tissue collapse.
9. **Stabilize the stylette.** Advance the thoracostomy tube downward and forward approximately 3–5 inches or until all the drain holes in the tube are estimated to be in the chest cavity.
10. Withdraw the stylette. As the stylette is being withdrawn, clamp the tube to prevent inward air flow and pneumothorax.
11. Attach a tubing adapter and three-way stopcock. Secure the adapter to the thoracostomy tube with a self-locking plastic band. Secure the three-way stopcock to the adapter with a single drop of "super glue" placed in the joint.
12. Attach a 60-mL syringe to the drain. Begin aspirating with the syringe. When syringe is full of air, rotate three-way valve and expel air from syringe. Re-rotate valve to close side port and aspirate again until negative pressure (suction) is felt.
13. Place a purse-string suture through the skin and deep tissue around the base of the drain tube. Secure the drain tube with either a criss-cross weaving of the suture and/or a series of fascial sutures near the end of the tube.
14. Confirm chest drain location with thoracic radiography. Bandage the wound site with sterile occlusive dressing and snug, but not tight, body wrap.
15. Attach to continuous drainage system if indicated.

ratory distress, (2) no blood is being aspirated during thoracocentesis, and (3) negative pressure (vacuum) is able to be reached easily with aspiration. Minidrain placement is preferred in patients with pneumothorax. A "mini-chest tube" is made by adding 5 small side holes in a 16-gauge to 5 Fr clear polyvinylchloride (PVC) feeding tube. The side holes should not involve more than one fourth the circumference of the tube. A commercial PVC or polyurethane thoracocentesis catheter (8 Fr, polyurethane "pigtail catheter" [Cook Inc.], or "cavity evacuation catheter" [Arrow, Inc.]) also work well as mini-chest tubes.

The placement procedure is as follows:

1. The site for chest drain placement is identified.
2. A local anesthetic block is created by injecting 2 to 3 mL of 2% lidocaine into the proposed insertion site.
3. The tube is placed through a 14-gauge needle that is first inserted into the pleural space at the identified intercostal space. It is advanced so that 3 to 5 inches of tubing are inside the pleural space.
4. The needle is withdrawn and the catheter fixed to the chest wall with sutures that penetrate the underlying fascia NOT just the skin.
5. An extension set and stopcock are attached and a dressing applied.

Aspiration is performed once every several hours until little air is removed on several tries and the patient remains comfortable without evidence of respiratory difficulty.

Chest Tube

A chest tube (see Table 12-4) should be inserted under the following conditions: (1) if the patient does not appear to improve following thoracocentesis, (2) if significant air or blood is aspirated, or (3) if vacuum cannot be reached within the pleural space with simple aspiration. The chest tube size should be approximately the same diameter as the patient's mainstem bronchus. Following a complete surgical prep of the proposed insertion site, the skin of the lateral chest wall is pulled forward and held by an assistant. A local anesthetic block (2% lidocaine) is created by injecting into the sixth and seventh intercostal nerves, surrounding tissues and pleura. If the animal is anxious, a small amount of sedation is provided (diazepam 0.1 mg/kg, and oxymorphone 0.05 mg/kg IV) while supplemental O_2 is continued. An incision in the skin and subcutaneous tissue in the center of the seventh intercostal space. A hemostat is used to gently dissect a small hole into the pleural space (Fig. 12-4). Air is allowed to enter the space to collapse the lung away from the chest wall. A styleted chest tube is then inserted, confirming that the stylette is pulled back so that it does not project from the tube's tip (Fig. 12-5). The chest tube's tube unit is inserted 3 to 8 inches until all 5 side holes are inside the pleural space (Fig. 12-6). Some commercial chest tubes require several side holes to be made so that at least five are present. The skin is then allowed to return back to its normal position, thus forming a shelf of tissue that will act as a seal, preventing air from entering the pleural space. A tubing adapter and three-way stopcock are inserted into the

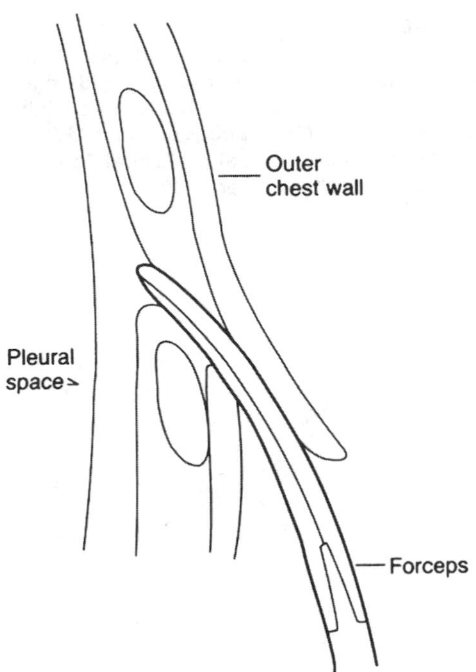

Figure 12-4
Forceps tunneling through chest wall prior to chest drain placement. Note the location of the forceps just cranial to the eighth rib. Note that the forceps is advanced on a 30° angle to penetrate the pleural space. (From Boggs RL, King MW, eds: AACN Procedure Manual for Critical Care, 3rd ed. Philadelphia: WB Saunders, 2001.)

exposed end of the chest drain. The tubing adapter is secured with a self-locking plastic tie wrap (Fig. 12-7B). Aspiration is started with a syringe or underwater seal and suction apparatus. The chest tube is fixed in place using a suture inserted into the periostium of the rib and fascia. A sterile dressing is then applied.

Before a body dressing bandage is applied, it is recommended to take a radiograph to check on the position of the tube and ensure that no kinks have occurred. Supplemental O_2 via a mask, bag, hood/collar, or nasal catheter should

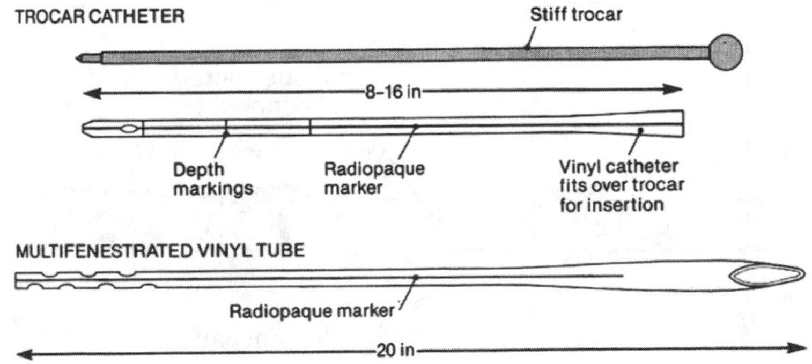

Figure 12-5
Examples of commercially available chest drain systems. (From Boggs RL, King MW, eds: AACN Procedure Manual for Critical Care, 3rd ed. Philadelphia: WB Saunders, 2001.)

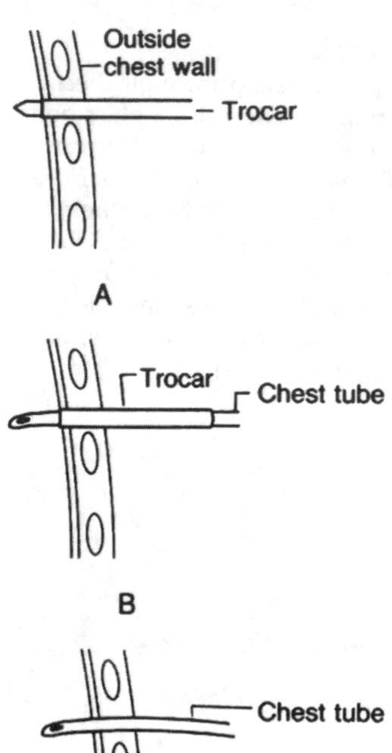

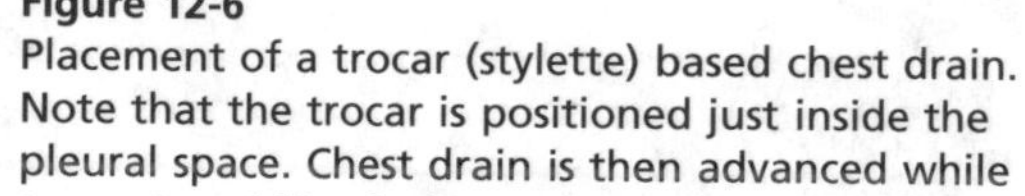

Figure 12-6
Placement of a trocar (stylette) based chest drain. Note that the trocar is positioned just inside the pleural space. Chest drain is then advanced while trocar is stabilized. (From Boggs RL, King MW, eds: AACN Procedure Manual for Critical Care, 3rd ed. Philadelphia: WB Saunders, 2001.)

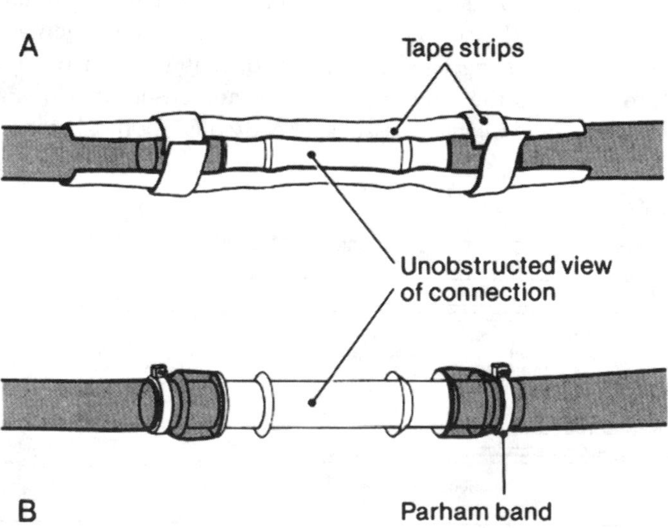

Figure 12-7
Two methods for securing drainage systems connections. Self-locking plastic bands (Parham band) are generally preferred. (From Boggs RL, King MW, eds: AACN Procedure Manual for Critical Care, 3rd ed. Philadelphia: WB Saunders, 2001.)

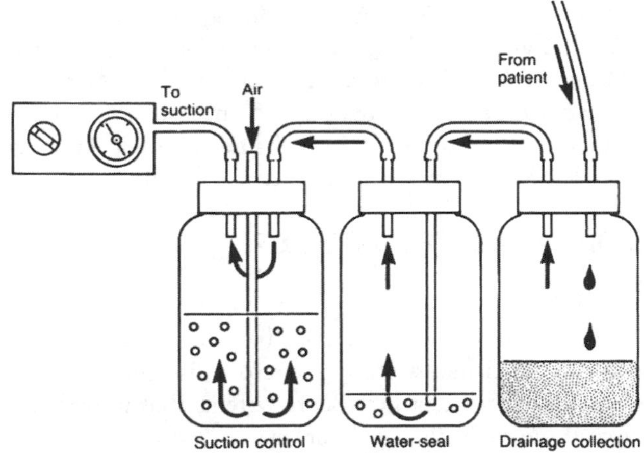

Figure 12-8
Example of a homemade three-bottle chest drain system. (From Boggs RL, King MW, eds: AACN Procedure Manual for Critical Care, 3rd ed. Philadelphia: WB Saunders, 2001.)

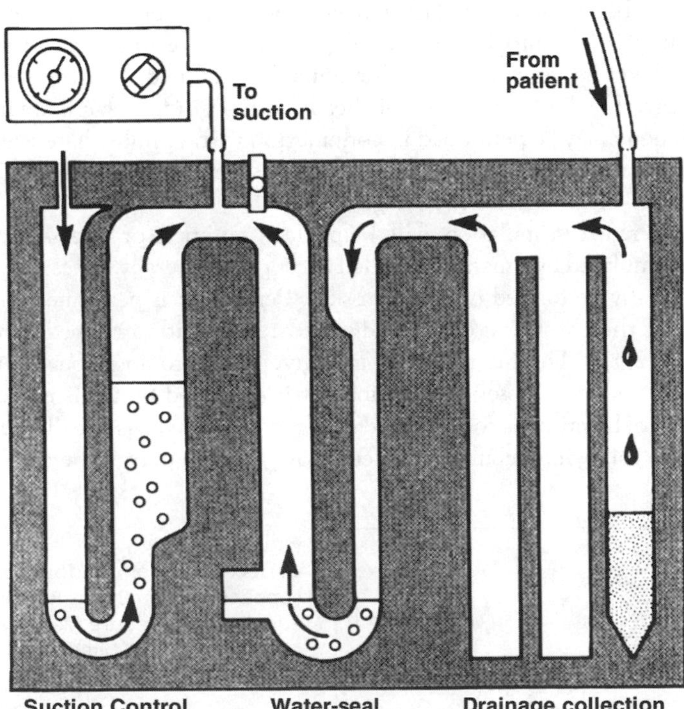

Figure 12-9
Example of a commercially produced water trap chest drain system. (From Boggs RL, King MW, eds: AACN Procedure Manual for Critical Care, 3rd ed. Philadelphia: WB Saunders, 2001.)

be continued and considered a mandatory prerequisite before thoracic radiographs are taken. Homemade chest drain systems or chest evacuation systems (PleuraVac, Deknatei, Inc.; Thoravac, Anderson, Inc.) are preferred (Figs. 12-8 and 12-9). A practical means of providing–15 cm H_2O continuous suction can be done by attaching a section of 5/8 inch diameter tubing in which a 1/4 inch diameter side hole has been cut to a standard suction unit.

RESPIRATORY CARE TECHNIQUES

Physiotherapy

Several maneuvers have been described to assist compromised protective mechanisms in patients demonstrating respiratory disease. The purpose of these maneuvers is to augment mucous transport systems that prevent accumulation and desiccation of mucus in the small airways.

Encouraging deep breathing and early ambulation are two effective methods to decrease retained secretions associated with positional stasis. Mild exercise and pain management (i.e., from thoracotomy) are two commonly used approaches to facilitate deep breathing.

Postural drainage may be helpful in cooperative patients. This technique uses different body positions to facilitate gravity drainage of bronchial secretions. Sequential rotation into lateral, dorsal, and sternal recumbancies both head down and head up are performed. The animal is inclined with the head down position first, then head up, and finally head down position to facilitate drainage. This technique may be performed in conjunction with or immediately after nebulization therapy. This maneuver may be done several times a day for 15 to 30 minutes to assist in secretion drainage.

Cough reflex stimulation will help clear retained or excess secretions. Cough is stimulated by a maneuver called chest physiotherapy. Chest physiotherapy is generally performed using percussion. Percussion is performed by repeatedly striking the chest wall over the diseased region with a cupped hand (Figs. 12-10 and 12-11). The intent of this maneuver is to promote cough reflex and promote clearance of loosened secretions. It is suggested that this procedure be done for 5 to 10 minutes four times daily. This maneuver is usually performed immediately following nebulization (see below). Alternately, a therapeutic mas-

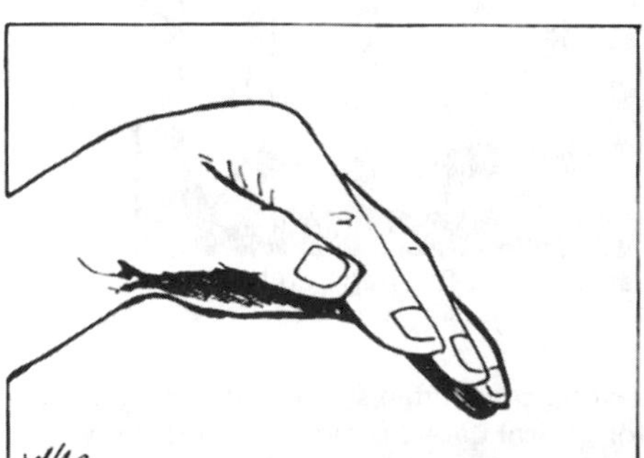

Figure 12-10
Correct hand position for applying cuppage. (From Boggs RL, King MW, eds: AACN Procedure Manual for Critical Care, 3rd ed. Philadelphia: WB Saunders, 2001.)

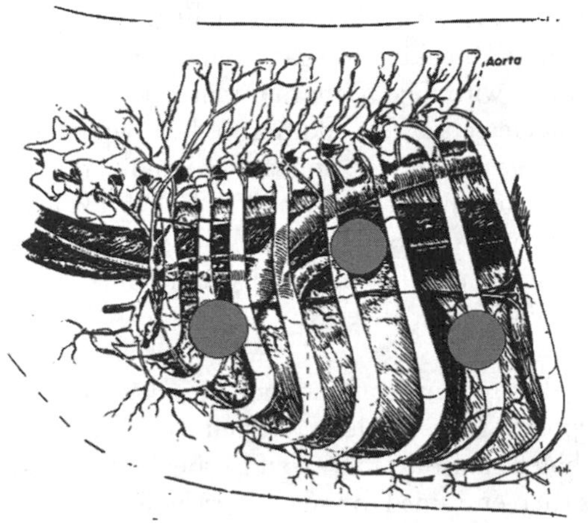

Figure 12-11
Physiotherapy. Circular areas represent primary points for cuppage.

sage vibrator may be used in place of "thumping." Each hemithorax is divided into nine zones for this procedure. The massage unit is placed over one area of the chest and held in place for 60 to 90 seconds and then moved to another area. The vibrating action produces a cough stimulus that facilitates secretion drainage. This technique should also be performed 10 to 15 minutes four times daily.

Humidification

In normal animals, inspired air is warmed and humidified as it passes through the nasal passages. The normal tracheobronchial tree is covered by a mucous layer that continuously moves up the tracheobronchial tree at a rate of 10 to 20 mm/min. One of the valuable effects of humidification is that it maintains hydration of the mucociliary blanket in the trachea. Certain disease states and therapeutic measures may decrease the natural humidification process. Drying of the mucociliary blanket may lead to retained secretions due to decreased clearance. Decreased clearance may produce or further stimulate tracheal inflammation, damage to the respiratory epithelium, increased risk of bacterial infection, and pulmonary parenchymal changes producing atelectasis, increased venous admixture, and decreased functional residual capacity.

Patients with tracheostomy tubes, extended endotracheal tube placement, or those receiving 100% O_2 therapy present the greatest risk for airway dehydration. Supplemental fluids are required to minimize airway dehydration. Systemic fluid administration is helpful; however, it does not directly change mucous viscosity. Humidification of inspired air should be used in "at risk" patients. In-line humidifiers are used to supplement gas humidification.

Two common humidifier designs are the pass-over humidifier and the bubble diffusion humidifier. The pass-over humidifier has gas flowing in an enclosed space over a water reservoir. Moisture is added by evaporation of the water from the liquid surface. A bubble diffusion humidifier has a gas inlet that connects to an internal pipe that is immersed in a liquid reservoir. As gas passes out of the pipe, a diffuser plate permits the gas to be broken into small bubbles and contact the water reservoir. The effect of breaking the gas stream into bubbles is to increase the surface area for contact with fluid. Both humidifier designs may be purchased with or without heating elements. The addition of heat will cause a greater amount of water vapor in the gas. Although unheated humidifiers provide less water entrainment, excessive amounts of heat (>42°C [107.6°F]) may be just as harmful as low humidity. Potential complications using humidifiers include systemic overhydration, tracheal epithelial damage, hyperthermia, electrolyte imbalances, increased venous admixture, atelectasis, and decreased functional residual capacity.

A disposable hygroscopic filter that retains heat and moisture may be used in patients receiving ventilatory support. These devices, referred to as "artificial noses," are designed to recover exhaled moisture that would otherwise be lost to the atmosphere. This moisture is then entrained in the next gas volume delivered to the patient. Such units are economical and simple in design and use. They do, however, clog with pulmonary secretions, have less humidification at high delivered gas flows, and increase "dead space" in the breathing circuit.

Nebulization

Nebulization is used to prevent drying and retention of airway secretions in the tracheobronchial tree. It may also be used as a delivery technique for antibiotics, bronchodilators, decongestants or anti-inflammatory agents. Nebulization increases moisture content by physically adding liquid droplets to inspired gases. Nebulizers fractionate water into tiny particles ranging from 2 to 80 μm in diameter. The lower end of this particle range (<3 μm) is small enough to be distributed to the terminal lung units and alveoli. Larger size particles (>10 μm) "fall out" at various points along the respiratory tract. In general, the larger the particle diameter, the sooner it will be deposited on respiratory mucosa. Two nebulizer designs currently available are jet and ultrasonic nebulizers. An ultrasonic nebulizer will produce higher percent of droplets (90% ultrasonic, 55% jet) in the optimal (<3 μm) particle size. Ultrasonic nebulizers also produce a denser aerosol mist thereby delivering a large fluid volume locally.

In veterinary medicine, saline nebulization in order to thin secretions is probably the most commonly used technique. The patient is nebulized for 15 to 30 minutes three to six times daily. Chest percussion may be used following nebulization to help loosen secretions. Potential complications of nebulization therapy include overhydration, hyperthermia, tracheobronchial irritation, and infection from either bacteria or fungi.

PHARMACOLOGIC THERAPY

Goals for drug therapy in the respiratory patient include control of airway reflexes, secretion control, small airway dilation ("opening up the airway"), inflammation or infection control, and pain management.

Normal airway reflexes include sneezing, pharyngeal closure, coughing, and bronchospasm. Uncontrolled sneezing is usually treated by identifying and managing the underlying cause. In extreme cases, tranquilizers or sedatives may be used to break the sneeze cycle. Pharyngeal swelling (*i.e.*, "croup") may be managed by nebulization and anti-inflammatory drugs. Laryngeal paralysis may be medically managed with tranquilizers or sedatives to reduce symptoms until defined surgical correction.

Coughing is a natural defense against retained secretions and is beneficial when there is an excess of secretions. Nonproductive, "dry" cough due to tracheal irritation ("kennel cough") is not beneficial and may cause global tracheobronchial inflammation. In these cases, cough reflex is best suppressed by medical intervention if the origin cannot be immediately eliminated. Antitussives may be indicated if unproductive coughing occurs. The most common antitussives are opioid class drugs such as butorphanol, dextromethorphan, codeine, and hydrocodone. These drugs should not be used to suppress a moist, productive cough. Corticosteroids will decrease the cough reflex by their anti-inflammatory properties but they are short acting and may predispose to infection. In general, corticosteroids are second-level drugs that are selected after proper hydration and cough reflex suppression is instituted.

Bronchospasm produces a narrowed airway. It will increase airway resistance, work of breathing, and ventilation-perfusion mismatch. Bronchospasm may be produced by a variety of trigger factors including inflammation, mucosal edema, and presence of excess secretions. Bronchospasm is treated with sympathomimetics (β-agonists) or xanthines. A combination of the two drug classes appears to be additive in producing bronchodilation. If bronchodilation is the only therapeutic goal, a sympathomimetic drug with predominant β_2-activity is selected (Table 12-5). The advantages of β_2-agonists are that they are potent bronchodilators largely devoid of side effects associated with activation of β_1- and α-receptor stimulation. Drug tolerance does not occur with repeated administration. Corticosteroids may also be used to reduce bronchospasm. Parenteral administration of hydrocortisone, prednisolone, or dexamethasone is commonly used in refractive bronchospasm. Their selection generally follows trial administration of β_2 agonists.

Antimicrobial therapy should be based on the results of culture and sensitivity tests. Systemic antimicrobial administration is preferred for treatment. Nebulization or intratracheal injection of antibiotics has not been shown to be beneficial and often predisposes to mycotic infections. If nebulization is used, the majority of medication will be deposited in normal lung regions because antibiotic containing droplets will follow the path of least resistance. Antibiotic delivery will be subtherapeutic in affected lung regions that have airway narrowing, increased fluid retention, or consolidation.

One major concern in respiratory patients is their tendency for thickening, accumulation, and retention of airway secretions. Providing airway moisture by systemic hydration or sterile saline nebulization can help liquefy and loosen secretions. Mucolytics such as *N*-acetylcysteine may be nebulized to liquefy secretions. *N*-acetylcysteine is a local tissue irritant and inactivates penicillin class antibiotics. Concurrent nebulization of a bronchodilator is recommended to reduce bronchoconstriction associated with local airway irritation. Expectorants

Table 12-5. Useful Drugs to Nebulize for Pulmonary Pharmacotherapy

Drug Type	Drug	Preparation	Dosage (Nebulizer)	Duration of Effect (h)
Hydration	Sterile water	Sterile water	5–10 mL	4
	Sterile saline	0.45, 0.9% saline	5–10 mL	4
Bronchodilator	Racemic epinephrine	2.25% solution	0.3–0.6 mL	1–2
	Atropine	0.5% solution	0.025–0.075 mg/kg	4–6
	Glycopyrollate	0.2 mg/ml	0.0044 mg/kg	2–8
	Isoproterenol	0.25 (2.5 mg/mL) 0.5 (5 mg/mL) 1.0% 10 mg/mL)	0.05–0.1 mg/kg	2–4
	Isoetharine	0.1–0.2%	0.1–0.2 mg/kg	2–4
	Metaproterenol	l5% (50 mg/mL)	0.25–0.5 mg/kg	2–4
	Albuterol	0.5% (5 mg/mL)	0.1–2.5 mg diluted in 1–2 mL normal saline	4–6
Mucokinetic/Mucolytic	Sterile water	Sterile water	5–10 mL	4
	Sterile saline	0.45, 0.9% saline	5–10 mL	4
	N-acetylcysteine	10% and 20% solution	2.5 mL + 2.5 mL saline	4–8

Modified from Chernow B: Pocket Book of Critical Care Pharmacotherapy 1995 and Marino P: The ICU Book, 2nd ed. Baltimore: Williams & Wilkins, 1999.

are not effective in increasing mucociliary clearance in animals and are not recommended. In most cases, the best therapy for clearing secretions is a combination of proper hydration, physiotherapy, and the normal cough reflex.

In some cases, pain will prevent an animal from taking deep breaths. Pain may also make the patient reluctant to move around or be handled. In these instances, analgesic therapy is indicated to encourage deep breathing and ambulation and reduce postural stasis. If the pain focus is rib injury or a thoracotomy procedure, intercostal nerve blocks or interpleural administration of bupivicaine may be therapeutic. Low doses of systemic opioids may be used for adjunctive analgesia. Opioids should never be withheld because of theoretical concerns about their ability to cause respiratory depression. Multiple studies have demonstrated that this concern is unwarranted in trauma or surgical patients.

SUGGESTED READINGS

Boggs RL, Wooldridge-King M: AACN Procedure Manual for Critical Care, 3rd ed. Philadelphia: WB Saunders, 1993, p 166.

Court MH: Respiratory support of the critically ill small animal patient. *In* Murtaugh RH, Kaplan PM, eds.: Veterinary Emergency and Critical Care Medicine. St. Louis: Mosby, 1992, p 575.

Crowe DT: Support procedures for the critically injured. *Sydney Postgrad Found* 254:174, 1995.

Haskins SC: Management of pulmonary disease in the critical patient. *In* Zaslow IM, ed.: Veterinary Trauma and Critical Care. Philadelphia: Lea & Febiger, 1984, p 339.

Marino PL: The ICU Book. Baltimore: Williams & Wilkins, 1998, 388.

Matthews KA: Veterinary Emergency and Critical Care Manual. Guelph, Ontario: Lifelearn, 1996, p 21.

McKiernan BC: Initial management of wounds and injuries to the chest. *In* Zaslow IM, ed.: Veterinary Trauma and Critical Care. Philadelphia: Lea & Febiger, 1984, p 245.

Taylor NS: Thoracic drainage. *In* Wingfield WW, ed.: Veterinary Emergency Medicine Secrets, 2nd ed. Philadelphia: Hanley & Belfaus, 2000, p 436.

Wheeler SL: Care of respiratory patients. *In* Slatter DM, ed.: Textbook of Small Animal Surgery, 2nd ed. Philadelphia: WB Saunders, 1993, p 804.

13
Fluid and Electrolyte Therapy

Wayne E. Wingfield

Water and electrolytes represent essentials of life. In veterinary medicine these essentials are often required in resuscitation of animals in shock, suffering from dehydration, or affected with diseases resulting in losses or excesses of these essentials.

REGULATION OF WATER AND ELECTROLYTE BALANCE

Water balance within the body plays an important role in the maintenance of plasma osmolality and effective circulating volume. Plasma osmolality is a function of the ratio of body solute to body water; it is regulated by changes in water balance. Water intake is derived primarily from three sources: ingested water, water contained in food, and water produced from oxidation of carbohydrates, proteins, and fats. Water losses occur in the urine and stool, as well as by evaporation from the skin and respiratory tract. Alterations in plasma osmolality of as little as 1% to 2% are sensed by osmoreceptors in the hypothalamus. These receptors initiate mechanisms that affect water intake (via thirst) and water excretion (via antidiuretic hormone [ADH]) to return plasma osmolality to normal.

The major defense against hyperosmolality (accumulation of solute in excess of body water) is increased thirst. Although the kidney can minimize water losses by the action of ADH, water deficits can be corrected only by increased dietary intake. Therefore, symptomatic hyperosmolality will not occur in a patient with a normal thirst mechanism and free access to water, regardless of the patient's ability to conserve body water through renal mechanisms.

Hypo-osmolality can result from excessive body water retention with subsequent dilution of body solutes or from loss of solute in excess of water loss (*e.g.*, diarrhea). Because the kidney daily excretes large volumes of water, persistent water retention resulting in hypo-osmolality occurs only in the presence of decreased renal water excretion. In patients with normal renal function, hypo-osmolality must therefore be due to solute loss in excess of body water loss.

In summary, plasma osmolality is governed by osmoreceptors in the hypothalamus, which influence thirst and the secretion of ADH. ADH increases water resorption and subsequently, urine osmolality, but does not affect sodium transport. Regulation of plasma osmolality is therefore achieved by changes in water balance within the body.

Effective circulating volume is that part of the extracellular fluid (ECF) that is within the vascular space and effectively perfusing tissues. It varies directly with ECF volume and also with total body sodium, because sodium salts are the primary ECF solutes holding water within the extracellular space. Therefore, regulation of sodium balance, by losses/gains in renal sodium ions, and the maintenance of effective circulating volume are closely related.

The kidneys are the primary regulator of sodium and volume balance. With a volume increase (*e.g.*, sodium loading), sodium excretion increases in an attempt to return the volume to normal. Alternatively, volume depletion results in sodium retention. Changes in volume are signals that allow sodium excretion to vary appropriately with fluctuations in sodium intake.

These changes in effective circulating volume are sensed by specific volume receptors, which then activate a series of effectors to result in appropriate volume-correction measures. The primary volume receptors are located in the cardiopulmonary circulation, the carotid sinuses and aortic arch, and the kidneys. Most volume receptors actually sense changes in pressure or stretch as a result of volume expansion or depletion. Stretch receptors in the renal afferent arterioles influence the activity of the renin-angiotensin-aldosterone system, whereas nonrenal sensors primarily govern the activity of the sympathetic nervous system.

Three major effectors alter circulating volume: the sympathetic nervous system, angiotensin II, and renal sodium excretion. Volume depletion, sensed by arterial baroreceptors as hypotension, causes an increase in peripheral sympathetic tone. This increased tone initiates specific compensatory changes, which return volume to normal (Table 13-1). These changes in sympathetic tone, along with changes in effective circulating volume, are mostly compensatory. Appropriate changes in renal sodium excretion are required to restore normal volume balance.

Hypovolemia also causes an increase in renin secretion. The subsequent increase in angiotensin II produces increased blood pressure (as a result of arterial vasoconstriction), as well as renal sodium retention (this is both a direct effect and also the result of increased aldosterone secretion).

Table 13-1. Compensatory Changes

Changes in peripheral sympathetic tone result in the following changes:

- Venous constriction: increased venous return
- Increased myocardial contractility and heart rate: increased cardiac output
- Arterial vasoconstriction: increases systemic vascular resistance and blood pressure
- Increased renin secretion: increases levels of angiotensin II, which is a potent vasoconstrictor
- Increased renal tubular sodium resorption (due to increased levels of angiotensin II and aldosterone)

Although sodium is important in the daily maintenance of effective circulating volume, the other major electrolyte of concern is potassium, which has two major physiologic functions within the body: (1) an important role in normal cell metabolism because the ratio of intracellular to extracellular potassium is a major determinant of the resting membrane potential and (2) important for normal neural, smooth muscle, and muscular function. In the basal state, the distribution of potassium between the cells and ECF is governed primarily by cell membrane Na^+/K^+ adenosine triphosphatase (ATPase), which pumps potassium into, and sodium out of, the cells (against their concentration gradients) in a ratio of 3:2. After a dietary potassium load, catecholamines and insulin promote the cellular uptake of potassium, facilitating its disposition until appropriate measures can be taken to secrete the extra potassium.

Urinary potassium losses are largely a function of its secretion in the distal nephron. Aldosterone and plasma potassium concentration are the major regulators of potassium secretion. After a potassium load, aldosterone secretion is enhanced. Aldosterone stimulates Na^+/K^+ ATPase at the peritubular membrane, thereby increasing cellular potassium concentration and the permeability of the luminal membrane to potassium. Increased potassium secretion results. Plasma potassium concentration also plays an important role in regulating potassium secretion. As ECF potassium levels rise, so does urinary potassium secretion. Other factors that play a more permissive role in potassium secretion include flow rate to the distal nephron and the potential difference generated by sodium resorption.

Magnesium is distributed unevenly throughout ECF, intracellular fluid (ICF), and bone, with the vast majority found in bone and soft tissues. The greatest concentration of Mg is in soft tissues having the highest metabolic activity (brain, heart, liver, and kidney).

Less than 1% of the body's content of Mg is found in the serum. Mg exists in three distinct forms in the serum: a free or ionized fraction, an anion-complexed fraction, and a protein-bound fraction. The ionized fraction (iMg) is the physiologically active fraction normally accounting for approximately 71% of the total sMg concentration. The iMg is the relevant fraction in serum because it is in equilibrium with the intracellular Mg concentration. Little is known about the mechanisms regulating iMg concentration. A variable that can affect iMg sample quality includes large variations in protein concentrations that alter the ratio of iMg to total magnesium. A variety of anions that are either commonly administered or endogenously produced in patients in acute care settings (heparin, citrate, lactate, bicarbonate, phosphate, acetate, and sulfate) may also appreciably reduce iMg (4%–90%) depending on concentration.

Levels of sMg are not routinely determined or monitored in veterinary medicine. Abnormalities in serum magnesium (sMg) are common in critically ill dogs. The significant occurrence of hypomagnesemia and hypermagnesemia observed in critically ill dogs parallels the rates reported in humans. Studies that evaluated the clinical consequences of abnormalities in Mg found that both decreased and elevated levels of sMg are associated with higher morbidity and mortality.[1] Furthermore, disturbances in Mg balance are now commonly recognized in hospitalized veterinary patients[2] and administration of Mg supplements is becoming more common in the CCU.

Determination of sMg concentrations reflects only a small part of the total body content of this ion, the vast majority being located intracellularly. Consequently, the serum concentration and intracellular levels weakly correlate; a normal or minimally low sMg level can occur in the presence of total body Mg deficiency. Therefore, it is important to determine the intercellular concentration of Mg because this may reflect total body stores more closely.

Because of slow equilibration with intracellular stores (days to weeks), the sMg level can be misleading. Acidosis, elevated bilirubin levels, and hemolysis may falsely elevate the sMg value. A circadian rhythm with sMg has been reported with a peak effect around 12:00 PM and the lowest levels from 11:00 PM to 4:00 AM.[3] Also, Mg deficiency severe enough to result in hypocalcemia and cardiac dysrhythmias may be present despite normal serum concentrations.

HISTORY AND PHYSICAL EXAMINATION

When an animal is presented, it is important to first address overall fluid balance. Quickly observing the animal and simultaneously obtaining a thorough and chronological description of the illness are helpful. The history must include information regarding the amount and frequency of abnormal fluid losses (vomiting, diarrhea, wound drainage, etc.) and whether or not polyuria, polydipsia, or anorexia is present. Abnormal breathing patterns and fever are also important indicators of the patient's status. It is useful to know the animal's exact body weight before the onset of illness from the owner or from current medical records. If there is an acute decrease in body weight, this loss can be attributed to water loss. In most cases, body weight will allow a more accurate assessment of dehydration. The exception to weight loss being primarily water loss is in animals with accumulation of third-space fluid (*i.e.*, pyometra, pleural effusions, ascites, peritonitis).

Assuming fluid loss is not life-threatening, a thorough physical examination is performed. If a quick assessment suggests life-threatening complications (abnormal mucous membrane color, abnormal capillary refill time, tachycardia, tachypnea, weak pulse, cool extremities, obvious blood loss), then the first goal of fluid therapy is to save the life of the animal. The thorough physical examination is postponed and fluid therapy to stabilize the patient's condition is started.

During the physical examination you will be observing physical parameters that will guide you to assess the patient's hydration status and thus rehydration requirements. The physical parameters to be evaluated include an accurate body weight, an assessment of skin elasticity, pulse rate and fullness, mucous membrane color and refill time, and respiratory rate and character. Despite these shortcomings, physical examination findings are important and should be used when assessing the degree of dehydration (Table 13-2). Because baseline body

Table 13-2. Physical Examination Findings in Estimating the Percentage Dehydration of an Animal

Estimated Percentage Dehydration	History of Fluid Loss	Dry Oral Mucous Membranes	Panting	Tachycardia	Decreased Skin Turgor	Decreased Pulse Pressure	Shock
<5%	+	–	–	–	–	–	–
5%	+	+	–	–	–	–	–
7%	+	+	+	+	+	–	–
10%	+	+	+	+	+	+	–
12%	+	+	+	+	+	+	+

weights are not often available, the veterinarian must be aware that the assessment of fluid losses is only an estimate; in fact, actual losses frequently are much greater.

Body weight is the best means for assessing fluid volume losses. Baseline weights are often not available or there may be third-spacing where body weight is not decreasing. Losses of lean body mass are never rapid; therefore, acute losses are generally fluid losses and thus are usually an accurate quantitative estimator of deficit volumes.

Changes in skin turgor are assessed in a consistent manner and location. Usually, the lateral thorax is preferred. The skin is pulled up, quickly released, and the time to return to normal is noted. When an animal is 12% dehydrated, the tented area of skin often remains tented for more than 5 to 10 seconds! Skin targer can be misleading in that aged or cachectic animals that normally lose skin elasticity, patients with third-space losses and near-normal body weight, and obese patients which may have normal skin resiliency even when dehydrated.

Third-space losses involve the accumulation of large fluid volumes in cavities such as the pleural or peritoneal space and intestinal or gastric lumen or in tissues around fracture or trauma sites These losses result in diminution of the ECF volume without an actual change in body weight.

Mucous membranes are good indicators of hydration. Color and refill time, as well as moistness, are assessed. The color of the mucous membranes varies considerably. A septic patient often has injected, highly vascular mucous membranes, and a severely hypovolemic patient has pale mucous membranes. Because many factors govern the color of mucous membranes, this feature alone cannot be used to assess hydration.

Capillary refill time has long been promoted as a good indicator of perfusion. Unfortunately, many factors alter refill time (*e.g.*, environmental temperature, sepsis, shock, anemia, fever). In humans, capillary refill time is influenced by age (older patients have delayed refill times) and sex (females have slower refill times).

ESTIMATING FLUID VOLUMES FOR REPLACEMENT THERAPY

The amount of fluid needed for replacement depends on the patient's physiologic status. Of primary concern is the status of the blood volume and later concern is directed to restoration of total body water and electrolytes. Fluid therapy is divided into three phases: (1) the emergency phase, (2) the replacement phase, and (3) the maintenance phase.

THE EMERGENCY PHASE

The distribution of fluids and the response of the body to blood loss are discussed to provide a more logical approach to fluid selection in the animal during the emergency phase of fluid therapy.

Pathophysiology of Shock

The signs and symptoms of acute peripheral circulatory failure or shock depend on the degree of blood volume depletion, the duration of that depletion, and the ability of the body to compensate. Shock is a clinical syndrome with acute perfusion failure and can be classified into four categories: hypovolemic, cardiogenic, distributive, and obstructive. Hypovolemic shock is due to a deficit of vascular volume after endogenous loss of blood, plasma, or electrolyte-rich fluid. In addition, cardiogenic, distributive, and obstructive forms of shock often are complicated by absolute or relative hypovolemia. Although dehydration may result in hypovolemic shock, hemorrhage and internal loss of fluid are equally common causes of hypovolemia. With the fall in intravascular volume, there is diminished venous return to the right side of the heart, low cardiac output, and a drop in systemic blood pressure. Various endogenous responses come into play to counteract this falling blood volume and pressure. A reflex sympathetic vasoconstriction initiates peripheral and splanchnic vasoconstriction and increased peripheral resistance to divert blood to vital organs. This shunting worsens perfusion to peripheral organs and promotes anaerobic metabolism, reflected in the progressive buildup of lactic acid. The peripheral vasoconstriction also causes impairment of renal function, manifested either as oliguria or anuria. In this serious amplification of shock, the volume of urine produced varies in direct proportion to the effectiveness of the compensatory mechanisms and therapy.

Several mechanisms come into play to preserve a physiologic state in acute circulatory failure. Cardiovascular signs are secondary to the decrease in plasma volume, and hypotension usually occurs if the fluid deficit is severe. Severe volume depletion depresses all body systems. ECF sequestration is due to increased microvascular permeability with plasma and protein moving into the interstitium.

Hypovolemia is one of the principal defects contributing to shock in the hospitalized patient. Treatment of this problem involves the administration of crystalloid or colloid solutions to correct the deficiency in the circulation of intravascular volume. Hypovolemia can be seen in shocklike states with or without depletion of intravascular volume. An "absolute" hypovolemia is caused by blood loss (surgery or trauma), by fluid loss (vomiting/diarrhea), and from severe burn injuries. A "relative" hypovolemia can be seen with spinal injury, sepsis, and third-spacing from intra-abdominal sepsis, abdominal surgery, and vasodilatation of the peripheral capillary bed caused by drugs, including anesthetic agents. In sepsis and third-spacing of fluids, interstitial fluid accumulates within the peritoneal cavity, lumen and wall of the small bowel, and wound tissues.

Body Fluid Distribution

The total body water ranges from 55% to 70% of the lean body weight (Fig. 13-1). In the average adult dog total body water is about 60% of lean body weight. Thus, in a 15-kg dog the total body water will equal about 9 liters. This value increases to 75% to 80% in neonates and decreases with increasing body fat levels and age.

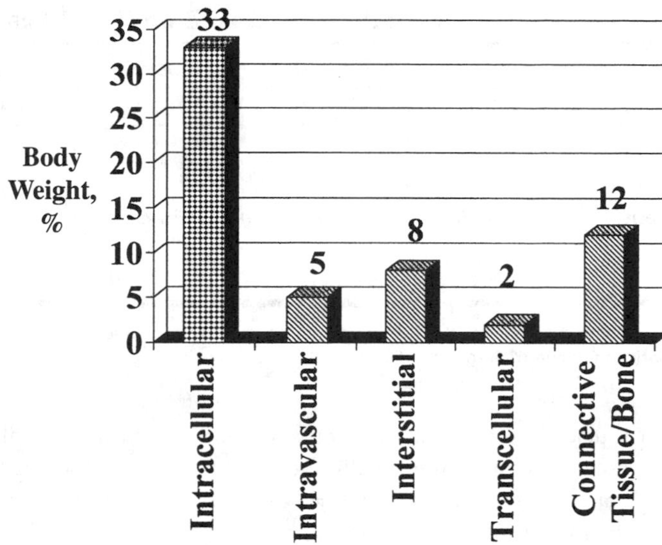

Figure 13-1
Distribution of water in the various compartments expressed as a percentage of body weight.

Total body water is distributed into two main compartments by the cell membrane: (1) the ICF space constitutes 67% of total body water (33% of the lean body weight), and (2) the ECF space contains the remaining 33%. The ECF is further subdivided into two clinically important, water-containing compartments: (1) the interstitial space (8% of the lean body weight) and (2) the intravascular space (5% of the lean body weight). Other minor contributors to the ECF include cerebrospinal fluid (CSF), intraocular fluids, and fluids in the gastrointestinal tract and pleural and peritoneal spaces.

The various fluid compartments of the body do not exist as fixed spaces of water. Because of the nature of the cell membrane, these compartments differ in composition and are in constant exchange with one another. The predominant intracellular cation is potassium. Mg is also present in the ICF in significant quantities. The major ICF anions are the phosphates (*e.g.*, HPO_4^-, $H_2PO_4^-$, ATP) and proteins. In the ECF, sodium is the primary ECF cation and chloride and bicarbonate are the major anions. The concentration of sodium and potassium in these different fluid compartments is maintained by active Na^+/K^+ ATPase in the cell membrane. Although the interstitial and intravascular components of the ECF are in equilibrium across the capillary wall, they too differ somewhat in composition. Proteins contribute significantly to the intravascular anions and are important in the maintenance of vascular oncotic pressure and therefore intravascular volume.

When water is added to one compartment, it distributes evenly across the total body water and the amount of volume added to any given compartment is proportional to its fractional representation of total body water. Thus, if 1 liter

Table 13-3. Hemorrhage Classification Based on Blood Loss

Parameter	Class I	Class II	Class III	Class IV
% Blood loss	<15%	15–30%	30–40%	>40%
Heart rate	+	++	+++	++++
Blood pressure	0	0	—	—
Urine output (mL/kg/h)	0.5–1.0	0.5	0.25–0.5	<0.25
Mentation	Anxious	Agitated	Confused	Depressed

(Modified from Committee on Trauma. Advanced trauma life support student manual. Chicago: American College of Surgeons, 1989, p. 57.)

of free water is placed in the intravascular space, there will be a minimal increase in the intravascular volume after equilibrium occurs. In fact, approximately 30 minutes after rapid volume infusion of free water only one tenth of the volume infused remains in the intravascular space.

Response of the Body to Minimal Blood Loss. In a healthy animal, a 15% loss of blood volume does not require intervention with intravenous (IV) fluids. With a loss of this volume, there is a three-phase compensatory response to mild hemorrhage (Table 13.3).

- **Phase I.** Within 1 hour of mild hemorrhage, interstitial fluid begins to move into the capillaries. This fluid shift continues for 36 to 40 hours. The egress of fluid from the interstitial space leaves an interstitial fluid deficit.
- **Phase II.** The loss of blood volume activates the renin-angiotensin-aldosterone system, which promotes sodium conservation by the kidneys. Because sodium distributes primarily in the interstitial space (80% of sodium is extravascular), the retained sodium replenishes the fluid deficit in the interstitial space.

  Monitoring of the packed cell volume (PCV) will reveal a progressive fall. Within 2 hours, 14% to 36% of the ultimate change in PCV has resulted. Within 8 hours the PCV changes to 36% to 50% of the ultimate change and 63% to 77% will be seen in 24 hours. When any plasma expander, including crystalloids, is infused, a more immediate fall in PCV can be expected. As the IV resuscitation fluids redistribute, the PCV again rises.

  Total serum protein shows similar changes to PCV. Endogenous restoration of depleted intravascular volume occurs through the movement of interstitial fluid into the intravascular space. Catecholamines mediate arteriolar vasoconstriction that diminishes capillary bed hydrostatic pressure favoring influx of interstitial fluid into the vascular tree distal to the arteriolar constriction. Subsequently, the lymphatic flow pattern returns the plasma proteins to the intravascular space. Increases in interstitial pressures caused by crystalloid distribution into the interstitial space may augment lymphatic flow through the "protein-refill" mechanism. This process combined with increased albumin synthesis and spontaneous diuresis secondary to volume repletion explains the return of serum protein levels after crystalloid resuscitation.

- **Phase III.** Within a few hours after mild hemorrhage, the bone marrow begins to increase production of erythrocytes. Unfortunately, their replacement is slow with only 15 to 20 mL cell volume being produced daily. Complete replacement requires a couple of months.

THE REPLACEMENT PHASE

The volume of fluid administered during the replacement phase is based on an assessment of fluid needs for (1) returning the patient's status to normal (deficit volume), (2) replacing normal ongoing requirements (maintenance volume), and (3) replacing continuing abnormal losses (continuing losses volume).

The deficit volume is an estimate based on findings from the physical examination (see Table 13-2) or on known changes in body weight. To calculate the deficit volume, the estimated dehydration is multiplied by the body weight. It must be remembered that it is difficult to replace all deficits in a 24-hour period. An attempt to do so results in urinary losses furthering dehydration. Thus, it is recommended that only 75% to 80% of the deficit volume be replaced during the first 24 hours. Also, do not forget that you must add "daily maintenance volumes" to the calculated deficit volume if the animal is not eating nor drinking.

Example 13-1

A 22-lb (10 kg) dog is assessed to be 7% dehydrated. What volume of fluid deficit should be given during the first 24 hours?

Total deficit replacement volume =
80% of deficit volume + maintenance volume
Deficit replacement volume (mL) =
$\%\ \text{dehydration} \times \text{body weight (lb)} \times 454 \times 0.80$
Deficit replacement fluid volume (mL) =
$0.07 \times 22\ \text{lb} \times 454 \times 0.80 = 560\ \text{mL} + \text{maintenance}$
or
Deficit replacement volume (mL) =
$\%\ \text{dehydration} \times \text{body weight (kg)} \times 1000 \times 0.80$
Deficit replacement fluid volume (mL) =
$0.07 \times 10 \times 1000 \times 0.80 = 560\ \text{mL} + \text{maintenance}$

(Recall that 1 lb water is 454 mL and 1 kg water is 1000 mL.)

Maintenance volumes are normal ongoing losses. Ongoing losses are divided into sensible and insensible losses. Sensible losses can be measured and are water losses in the urine and feces. Insensible losses are normal but are not easily quantitated. These water losses occur during panting or sweating. One third of the maintenance volume is the insensibile volumes and two thirds, the sensible volumes. Traditionally, maintenance

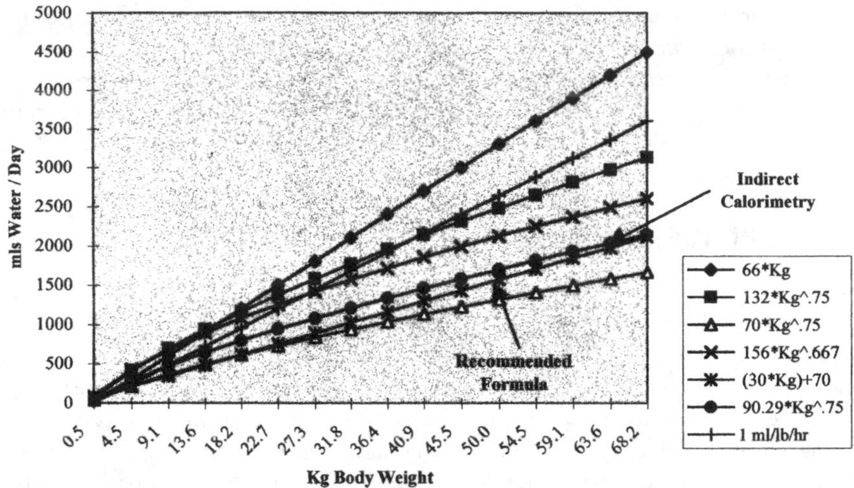

Figure 13-2
Daily water requirements for the dog. The recommended formula is (30 × kg BW) + 70. This formula closely approximates findings of indirect calorimetry (90.29 × $kg^{0.75}$) in the dog.

volumes have been estimated at about 66 mL/kg/d (30 mL/lb/d).[4] Using this volume will underdose some animals and overdose most (Figs. 13-2 and 13-3).

Data are scarce regarding water needs for the dog and cat. We can apply formulas directed to nutritional requirements to estimate water needs. Water and energy requirements are numerically the same (1 Kcal of energy = 1 mL water). Unfortunately, many authors recommend dramatically different fluid and energy requirements.[5,6] Regardless, data from recent research are used to document that energy expenditure or consumption is less than has been previously published. Numerous authors have estimated water needs at 50 mL/kg/d, 132 Kcal × $kg^{0.75}$,[7] 156 × $kg^{0.667}$, (30 × kg) + 70,[8] 70 × $kg^{0.75}$, and so forth. Most of these reports offer no data from which an assessment can be made. More recently, indirect calorimetry is being applied to estimate energy (and thus water) needs for the dog and cat. These studies reinforce that previously recommended formulae overestimate the energy (water) requirements of the dog (see Figs. 13-2 and 13-3). The question regarding energy (water) requirements in sick animals continues to elicit controversy. Traditionally it is taught that illnesses, injuries, and surgery result in the increased need for more energy (water). These teachings are extrapolated from human and rodent data. In the dog, mounting evidence suggests that increased energy requirements are not common in the sick, injured, or surgical dogs.[9] In fact, increased numbers of publications document the lower energy (water) requirements for both the normal[10] and sick or traumatized dog.[11] Additionally, from an evolutionary perspective, it seems logical to expect the dog to preserve available energy (water) with

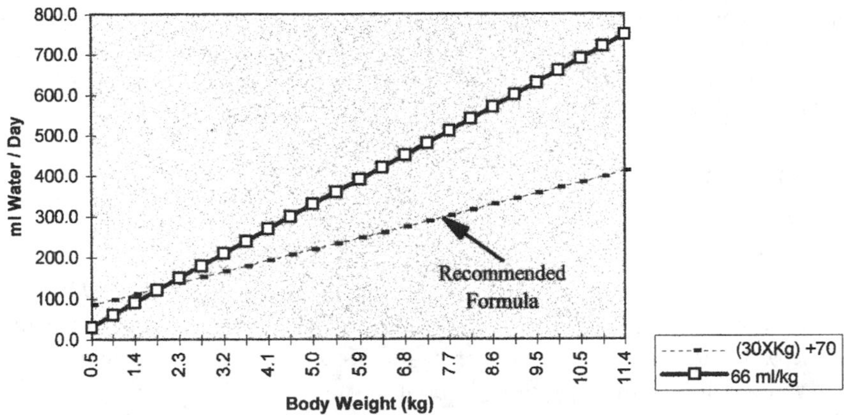

Figure 13-3
Estimating fluid requirements for the cat. The recommended formula is (30 × kg BW) + 70.

illness or injury. The animal's metabolic (water) reserves are already minimal and it makes little sense to increase metabolic requirements to survive. It makes more sense to conserve available energy and to reduce metabolic (thus energy and water) requirements. Studies on dogs in a CCU unit have documented the presence of decreased energy requirements and significant hypothyroidism.[12] Thus, metabolic and water requirements are reduced.

The decision to change the formulae for calculating water requirements will only come with more objective evidence taken from normal and sick dogs and cats. This evidence is currently being collected. At present, the amount of fluid required for daily maintenance is calculated using the following formulae:

Daily basal water requirement (mL) for dogs = (30 × kg BW) + 70
Daily basal water requirement (mL) for cats = (30 × kg BW) + 70

Example 13-2

A 33-lb (15-kg) dog has had a persistent diarrhea for 1 month. There is no vomiting and the animal continues to eat and drink. The patient is 10% dehydrated. How much fluid should be given during the next 24 hours?

Volume (mL) of fluid required =
80% deficit volume + maintenance volume + free-choice water
= [0.10 × 33 × 454 × 0.80] + [(15 × 30) + 70] + free choice water
= [1200] + [520] + free choice water = 1720 mL + free choice water
or
= [0.10 × 15 × 1000 × 0.80] + [(15 × 30) + 70]
= 1720 mL + free choice water

These formulae do not induce diuresis. Thus, if you are dealing with acute or chronic renal failure, toxicities, and the like, where diuresis is indicated, you will need to increase "daily maintenance volumes" by a factor of two or three times.

Example 13-3

A 10-year-old, 5-kg (11-lb), domestic shorthaired cat is admitted with clinical signs of chronic renal failure and dehydration. Laboratory results are blood urea nitrogen (BUN) = 233 mg/dL, creatinine = 9.8 mg/dL, and phosphorus = 10 mg/dL. You have corrected the deficit volume and would now like to induce diuresis to treat the azotemia. How much fluid should you administer over the next 24 hours?

$$\text{Diuresis} = 3 \times \text{maintenance volumes}$$
$$\text{Diuresis} = 3 \times [(30 \times \text{kg}) + 70]$$
$$= 3 \times [(30 \times 5) + 70] = 660 \text{ mL}$$
or
$$\text{Diuresis} = 3 \times [(30 \times 11/2.2) + 70] = 660 \text{ mL}$$

As an alternative to simply multiplying maintenance volumes by 3, one may also use a technique called "ins and outs." This technique requires you to replace volumes equal to the urine output. You will recall that daily maintenance is made up of insensible (not measured) and sensible (measured) water. In most cases, urine will represent the sensible loss. The technique is illustrated in the next example.

Example 13-4

A 10-year-old, 5-kg (11-lb), domestic shorthaired cat is being treated for chronic renal failure. You have replaced the deficit volumes and are now faced with diuresing the cat to treat the azotemia. The urine output over the last 8 hours was 275 mL. How much fluid will you give over the next 8 hours?

$$\text{Ins and outs} = \text{sensible} + \text{insensible losses}$$
$$\text{Insensible losses} = \{[(30 \times \text{kg}) + 70]/3\}/3$$
where one third of maintenance
= insensible losses and 8 h is one third of the day
$$\text{Sensible losses} = \text{urine output}$$
$$\text{Ins and outs} = \{[(30 \times 5) + 70]/3\}/3 + 275 \text{ mL (urine output over the last 8 h)}$$
$$= 24.4 \text{ mL} + 275$$
$$= 299 \text{ mL over the next 8 h}$$

After the next 8 hours, remeasure the urine output and recalculate the ins and outs based on the new urine output.

The need to replace continuing abnormal losses is frequently overlooked. Failure to recognize vomiting, diarrhea, and polyuria as sources of continuing abnormal fluid loss will not allow full correction of deficits. It is impractical to suggest quantitation of each episode of vomiting or diarrhea. Occasionally, a urinary catheter or a metabolic cage is used to quantitate urine volumes (see Example 13-4).

A crude but effective guideline for replacing continuing abnormal losses is to estimate the volume of fluid lost and then double this estimate. The result will be surprisingly close to the actual volume of vomitus, diarrhea, or urine.

Example 13-5

A 3-month-old 22-lb (10-kg) collie puppy has severe, protracted, acute diarrhea. The puppy has been given 20 mL/lb of fluids for shock (the volume used in treating shock is not counted when determining maintenance or deficit volumes) and is now ready for the deficit replacement phase of the fluid regimen. The puppy is assessed to be 7% dehydrated. Within the past few minutes the puppy has had a bout of diarrhea that is estimated to have a volume of 400 mL. How much fluid should be given during the next 24 hours?

$$\begin{aligned}
\text{Volume (mL) of fluid required} &= \text{deficit volume} + \text{maintenance volume} \\
&\quad + \text{continuing losses volume} \\
\text{Continuing losses} &= 2 \times \text{estimated volume lost} \\
&= [0.07 \times 22 \times 454 \times 0.80] \\
&\quad + [(10 \times 30) + 70] + [400 \times 2] \\
&= [560] + [370] + [800] = 1730\ \text{mL} \\
&\text{or} \\
&= [0.07 \times 10 \times 1000 \times 0.80] \\
&\quad + [(10 \times 30) + 70] + [400 \times 2] \\
&= [560] + [370] + [800] = 1730\ \text{mL}
\end{aligned}$$

THE MAINTENANCE PHASE

The last phase of fluid therapy is the maintenance phase. At this point the patient has received enough fluid to compensate for shock and has had a partial replacement of any deficit volume. Chronologically, this phase begins no sooner than 24 hours after fluids are begun. Objective signals that the patient is ready to be placed in the maintenance phase are an absence of clinical signs of shock or dehydration and an increase in the body weight by at least the percentage of dehydration already corrected. If your animal is losing body weight, you are losing excessive water, or water requirements are greater than are being supplied, and you may need to recalculate your fluid volumes.

During the maintenance phase, you will be providing both maintenance volumes and continuing losses volumes.

Maintenance phase = daily maintenance volumes + continuing losses

Administration of Fluids

When giving fluids, the rate of administration is determined first by the patient's initial status. If shock is present, the fluids must be administered rapidly. The use of a pressure bag allows fluids to be administered rapidly and in large volumes.

In correcting deficits, the rate of administration is slower but often difficult, because the animal is likely to be moving about in the cage, and thus the drip rate from the fluid container varies. Although a variety of fluid infusion sets are available, using the technique of counting drops to calculate infusion rates is risky in animals that are awake. Sudden overhydration resulting from a drip rate that accelerated because a patient changed position is not an infrequent event. In small patients a calibrated Burette with a microdrip infusion set can be used. Although the problem of patient movement will not be solved, at least the possibility of inadvertently delivering a very large volume of fluid will be eliminated.

Mechanical infusion pumps provide the most reliable and safest means for delivering accurate fluid volumes. These pumps can be programmed to deliver a broad range of volumes over specific time intervals. The cost of these pumps varies with their quality and the number of extra features.

Parenteral Solutions

A variety of parenteral solutions are available. See Table 29-1 for the compositions of the most commonly used solutions. The content of each solution determines the clinical situation in which it will be most useful.

Dextrose Solutions (D5W)

Because glucose is rapidly metabolized to carbon dioxide and water, the administration of dextrose is physiologically equivalent to administering distilled water. (Note: Distilled water cannot be given IV because it will cause hemolysis.) Thus, the main indication for the use of dextrose in water is to provide free water to replace insensible losses or to correct hypernatremia resulting from a water deficit. When added to crystalloid solutions, D5W is also useful in providing an intracellular carbohydrate source in patients with sepsis. Whenever dextrose is given, it is quickly metabolized to water, and the water will redistribute to the ICF and ECF spaces in volumes commensurate with the water volumes in each compartment.

Dextrose in water should not be used as a maintenance fluid because it will lead to dilution of all electrolytes. For a patient in shock, D5W is not recommended as a replacement fluid; it will be metabolized quickly, and the water generated will be distributed, for the most part, to the ICF space and provide minimal expansion of the intravascular space. Administration of D5W subcutaneously causes electrolyte movement into these tissues and leads to a decreases in circulating blood volume and shock.

Crystalloid Solutions

"Crystalloids" refers to solutions that are isotonic with plasma and contain sodium as their major osmotically active particle. Crystalloid solutions such as Ringer's lactate or 0.9% NaCl (physiologic saline) distribute evenly in the extracellular space when administered intravascularly. Only 25% of the administered crystalloid solution will remain in the intravascular space of the ECF compartment after 1 hour. Equilibrium within the ECF compartments occurs within 20 to 30 minutes after infusion.

Physiologic saline (0.9% NaCl) is often called "normal saline." It contains "normal" levels of sodium ions (154 mEq/L) but abnormally high levels of chloride ions (154 mEq/L) and is considered an isotonic fluid (310 mOsm/L). "Isotonic" implies that the fluid has the osmolality of the extracellular compartments (290–310 mOsm/L). Normal saline is used for acute extracellular volume expansion. It is useful as a replacement fluid in the treatment of hyperkalemia and in the treatment of hyponatremia as seen in hypoadrenocorticism. It should not be used in animals with congestive heart failure because sodium restriction is normally part of that therapy. Physiologic saline is not generally used in animals with liver disease because of the potential for sodium overloading resulting from the animals' inability to metabolize aldosterone.

Half-strength saline (0.45% NaCl) is an excellent maintenance fluid. It is usually combined with dextrose (2.5%) and potassium chloride. The fluids used for maintenance fluids are meant to replace electrolytes normally lost each day. When insensible and sensible (urine) electrolytes are quantitated, an animal will normally lose 40 to 60 mEq/L sodium and 15 to 20 mEq/L potassium. If you continue to use replacement solutions such as Ringer's, 0.9% saline, Ringer's lactate, Normosol-R, or Ringer's acetate, hypernatremia and increased urinary potassium losses (leading to hypokalemia) may result.

In addition, 0.45% saline is the fluid of choice for animals predisposed to sodium retention and those with congestive heart failure or liver disease. Hypernatremia is uncommon in the dog and cat. When the serum sodium does exceed 156 mEq/L, either D5W or 0.45% NaCl with 2.5% dextrose is considered a preferred fluid.

Hypertonic saline (3%, 5%, 7.5%) is considered a possible drug for the treatment of shock. The rationale for use of these solutions is that they induce rapid expansion of the ECF compartment, resulting in water movement from the ICF compartment to the ECF compartment. The drawback to this approach is an expansion of the interstitial space because of the rapid redistribution of crystalloid solutions. Also, intracellular dehydration that occurs may adversely affect cellular function. These fluids should only be given IV and should be administered slowly to avoid inducing pulmonary edema.

Ringer's solution is a crystalloid replacement fluid. It is more of a balanced replacement solution than lactated Ringer's solution (LRS). Because of the ionic concentrations, Ringer's solution is often used as a replacement solution in cases of metabolic alkalosis. When the alkalosis is the result of vomiting from the upper gastrointestinal tract, Ringer's solution supplemented with potassium chloride is an excellent fluid.

In diabetes mellitus, Ringer's solution is a good fluid for replacement. Previously, there was concern about the sodium and potassium content of Ringer's solution. With the polyuria of diabetes, significant sodium, potassium, and water losses must be replaced. Following ionic replacement, one must consider the influence of sodium on the tonicity of the plasma. Because glucose also increases osmolality, there is the theoretical possibility of cerebral edema. Fortunately this does not appear to be an important clinical entity in animals.

In diabetes mellitus, the initial plasma potassium levels are usually elevated as the result of a metabolic acidosis. Remember, potassium is predominantly an intracellular ion and, when elevated, it is usually the result of an exchange whereby hydrogen ions move intracellularly and potassium ions move into the plasma. As fluids and insulin are administered, potassium ions move intracellularly, revealing the true hypokalemia seen with diabetes. Thus, potassium chloride usually is required. Before the patient's electrolyte status is determined, the potassium in Ringer's solution will be adequate and will not exacerbate the extracellular hyperkalemia. As insulin is administered, at least 20 mEq potassium chloride per liter should be added.

Buffered crystalloid solutions include Normosol-R, which contains both acetate and gluconate, and solutions such as Ringer's lactate. With either of these balanced electrolyte solutions, the buffer will supply bicarbonate. Lactate is metabolized by the liver to bicarbonate, and muscles and peripheral tissues metabolize acetate and gluconate to bicarbonate. Buffered crystalloid solutions are useful in the treatment of mild to moderately severe metabolic acidosis.

Ringer's lactate is not an ideal solution for dogs and cats. With a sodium concentration of only 130 mEq/L, it would be considered a moderately hyponatremic solution. In additional, with an osmolality of 272, it is hypo-osmolar to plasma of the dog and cat.

Normosol-R is a reasonably balanced electrolyte solution for dogs and cats. Its osmolality and pH make it close to plasma and the presence of magnesium as a bivalent ion, may be useful in the treatment of critically ill dogs and cats where magnesium is now identified as the most common electrolyte disorder.[13]

Bicarbonate replacement is an issue of continuing controversy. All concede that fluid replacement will likely resolve most acidotic states. Also, empirical usage of sodium bicarbonate will usually overcorrect the acidosis. Bicarbonate administration is associated with movement of potassium into the cells; therefore, potassium deficits must be corrected coincident with sodium bicarbonate therapy. Another risk associated with sodium bicarbonate administration is the resultant expansion of the ECF compartment because of the sodium concentra-

Table 13-4. Clinical Indications for Biocarbonate Administration in Dogs and Cats

1. A bicarbonate concentration <5–7 mEq/L
2. A blood PCO_2 that is not appropriately reduced, resulting in severe acidemia (in this circumstance, the focus should be on improving ventilation)
3. Failure to reduce acid production with insulin or in the presence of another acid load (ethylene glycol intoxication)
4. Presence of significant hypotension with severe acidemia (cardiopulmonary resuscitation)

tion. Other factors often mentioned as potential dangers of sodium bicarbonate therapy include a leftward shift of the oxyhemoglobin dissociation curve, which leads to decreased O_2 delivery to tissues. Also there may be a paradoxical CSF acidosis that compromises cerebral function as the pH of the CSF falls, as a result of rise in PCO_2 and rebound metabolic alkalosis. (It is unlikely a paradoxical CSF acidosis will result so long as the animal is ventilating normally.) Table 13-4 lists indications for bicarbonate therapy in small animals.

The quantity of bicarbonate to be replaced is calculated using the following formula:

$$\text{Bicarbonate deficit} = \text{base deficit} \times 0.4 \times [\text{body weight (kg)}]$$

The error in using this formula comes in thinking you must correct the entire bicarbonate deficit with exogenous sodium bicarbonate. In most cases, crystalloid solutions are being administered concomitantly with sodium bicarbonate; thus, administering the entire deficit causes the pH to increase and an iatrogenic metabolic alkalosis results. Instead of using normal bicarbonate levels to calculate the base deficit, the following formula should be used in the above equation:

$$\text{Base deficit} = (12 - \text{measured bicarbonate})$$

This will avoid excessive bicarbonate replacement. In addition, continual bicarbonate monitoring is mandatory, and when the measured bicarbonate approaches 12 mEq/L, administration of sodium bicarbonate is discontinued. Care must be taken when giving exogenous bicarbonate, because it is very hypertonic (1500 mOsm/L) and rapid administration may lead to high levels of carbon dioxide in the coronary circulation and possible sudden death.

Without question, the use of sodium bicarbonate in the treatment of the ketoacidosis of diabetes mellitus is risky. It is critical to remember that as insulin is given, the ketoacids undergo oxidative metabolism, with the end-products being water and carbon dioxide. Thus, exogenous sodium bicarbonate and insulin in the treatment of diabetes mellitus inevitably leads to an iatrogenic metabolic alkalosis.

Colloid Solutions

Colloid solutions include albumin, fresh-frozen plasma, whole blood, Oxyglobin, and synthetic colloids (hetastarch, pentastarch, dextran-40, and dextran-70). They act primarily to expand the plasma volume. The rationale for using colloid solutions is from the maldistribution of extracellular water, with relative expansion of the interstitial space water, in the face of a plasma volume deficiency with traumatic and septic shock. This maldistribution of interstitial space water will predispose the patient to pulmonary edema and acute respiratory distress syndrome.

With colloid solutions such as the dextrans, the molecules are distributed in the ECF compartment, mainly the intravascular space. The particle sizes of the various dextrans affect the duration of their presence within the intravascular space and therefore the duration of volume expansion. Dextran-40 contains particles with molecular weights ranging from 10,000 to 80,000 D, and dextran-70 contains particles with molecular weights of 40,000 to 100,000 D. The half-life of particles with molecular weights of 14,000 to 18,000 D is 15 minutes, whereas particles with molecular weights greater than 55,000 D have half-lives of several days. As a general statement, only 20% of dextran-40 and 30% of dextran-70 remain in the circulation for more than 24 hours.

Indications for the dextrans include volume expansion and promotion of peripheral blood flow. Studies have shown dextran to improve survival and hemodynamic parameters in shock. The resultant volume expansion after the use of dextrans is at the expense of the intracellular water. For each gram of dextran, 20 to 30 mL water is obligated to the intravascular volume expansion. When used for restoration of blood volume, dextrans are given at a rate of 1.54 g/kg/d for dextran-40 and 1.98 gm/kg/d for dextran-70.

Plasma is another colloid solution and is underused by veterinarians. It is easy to collect and when frozen is considered stable for 2 to 5 years. Plasma contains important proteins (albumin and globulins), which may be useful in liver failure, hemodilution, and hypoproteinemia (as may be seen with chronic gastrointestinal diseases). An important use of fresh-frozen plasma is for specific or multiple clotting factor replacement. It is not used for the routine management of acute volume deficits when crystalloid solutions or commercial synthetic colloids work as well. The usual clinical dose of plasma is 5 to 10 mL/kg. Fresh-frozen plasma should be administered within 6 hours of thawing to obtain the maximum amount of clotting proteins. Compatibility should be evaluated when previous transfusions have been performed.

Giving plasma as a protein source would require very large volumes to raise the intravascular protein concentration. For albumin the equation that accounts for equilibrium in the interstitium is:

$$\text{Albumin deficit (g)} = 10 \times (\text{desired [albumin] (g/dL)} - (\text{patient [albumin] (g/dl)}) \times \text{kg BW} \times 0.3$$

Table 13-5. Empirical Guidelines for IV Supplementation of Potassium Chloride

Serum Potassium Concentration mEq/L	mEq KCl to add to 1 Liter of Crystalloid Fluids
<2.0	80
2.1–2.5	60
2.6–3.0	40
3.1–3.5	28
3.6–5.0	20

Example 13-6

A 3-year-old dog, weighing 10 kg, has a serum albumin of 1.5 g/dL. Calculate how much plasma would be required to raise the albumin to 2.5 g/dL.

$$\text{Albumin deficit} = 10 \times (2.5 - 1.5) \times (10 \times 0.3) = 30 \text{ g}$$

This is equivalent to a liter of plasma (3 g/dL) or 2 liters of whole blood!

Whole blood is the colloid administered most commonly by veterinarians. It has the advantages of availability, ease of collection, and storage. The most common uses of whole blood are for anemia and severe hemodilution. Although anemic patients may not need the plasma portion, whole blood will continue to be used. Anemia is defined as a decrease in red blood cells. The use of packed red blood cells (where the plasma has been removed thereby concentrating the red blood cells) is the most logical means of stretching the usefulness of a unit of whole blood and providing needed blood components.

A unit of whole blood contains approximately 450 mL red blood cells, plasma, white blood cells, and platelets. At the end of 8 hours of storage, very few platelets within the whole blood are hemostatically effective.

Fluid Additives[14]

Potassium chloride is often added to parenteral fluids. Currently, there are no reports in available veterinary literature to estimate the magnitude of potassium losses. The recommended method of providing potassium chloride to parenteral fluids depends on the measured serum potassium of the patient (Table 13-5), the mechanism by which the hypokalemia occurred, and the presence of cardiac or neuromuscular effects. Serum potassium levels above 2.5 mEq/L in asymptomatic animals can often be corrected with oral supplementation. The rate of potassium administration is restricted by two important factors: (1) If given too quickly or not properly mixed,[15] serum potassium increases to danger-

Table 13-6. Guidelines for Selecting the Most Appropriate Fluid for Various Diseases

Condition	Serum					Fluid of Choice
	Na^+	Cl^-	K^+	HCO_3^-	Volume	
Diarrhea	D	D	D	D	D	Normosol-R + KCl or lactated Ringer's + KCl
Pyloric obstruction	D	D	D	I	D	0.9% NaCl + KCl
Dehydration	I	I	N	N/D	D	Normosol-R + KCl, lactated Ringer's + KCl, 0.9% NaCl + KCl, 5% dextrose
Congestive heart failure	N/D	N/D	N	N	I	0.45% NaCl + 2.5% dextrose + KCl, 5% dextrose
End-stage liver disease	N/I	N/I	D	D	I	0.45% NaCl + 2.5% dextrose + KCl
Acute renal failure— oliguria—polyuria	I D	I D	I N/D	D D	I D	0.9% NaCl, Normosol-R + KCl, lactated Ringer's + KCl
Chronic renal failure	N/D	N/D	N	D	N/D	Normosol-R, lactated Ringer's solution, 0.9% NaCl
Adrenocortical insufficiency	D	D	I	N/D	D	0.9% NaCl
Diabetic ketoacidosis	D	D	N/D	D	D	0.9% NaCl (±KCl)

N/D, normal/decreased; I, increased; D, decreased; N/I, normal/increased.

ously high concentrations and may lead to cardiac arrest, and (2) potassium chloride is a strong irritant, often leading to phlebitis. As a general rule, administration of potassium chloride should not exceed 0.5 mEq/kg/h although no recent literature substantiates this rate of administration.

Parenteral solutions of $MgCl_2$ are used to treat hypomagnesemia. Currently, hypomagnesemia is defined as a sMg concentration of less than 1.89 mg/dL. Hypomagnesemia is often seen concurrently with hyponatremia and hypokalemia. It is important in reperfusion injury, in refractory hypokalemia, hypophosphatemia, and hypercalcemia. Supplementing crystalloid fluids is important in animals at risk for hypomagnesemia (ketoacidosis in diabetes mellitus, acute pancreatitis, and chronic diarrheas). The rate of administration is 0.75 to 1.0 mEq/kg/d and $MgCl_2$ is added to the IV crystalloid fluids. Mg-containing fluids are incompatible with solutions containing calcium (do not add $MgCl_2$ to Ringer's or Ringer's lactate solutions).

Fluid Selection in Diseases

In selecting a fluid, it is important to know which electrolytes are lost and to institute replacement therapy based on knowledge of the pathophysiology of the disease. Table 13-6 provides an overview of electrolyte changes and replacement recommendations.

REFERENCES

1. Rubeiz GL, Thill-Baharozian M, Hardie D, Carlson RW: Association of hypomagnesemia and mortality in acutely ill medical patients. *Crit Care Med* 21:203, 1993.
2. Martin, LG, Wingfield, WE, Van Pelt, DR, Hackett, TB. Magnesium in the 1990's: implications for veterinary critical care. *J Vet Emerg Crit Care* 3:105, 1994.
3. Touitou Y, Touitou C, Bogdan A, *et al.*: Serum magnesium circadian rhythm in human adults with respect to age, sex and mental status. *Clin Chem Acta* 87:35, 1978.
4. Garvey MS: Fluid and electrolyte balance in critical patients. *Vet Clin North Am Small Anim Pract* 19:1021, 1989.
5. Burkholder WJ: Metabolic rates and nutrient requirements of sick dogs and cats. *J Am Vet Med Assoc* 206:614, 1995.
6. Kronfeld DS: Protein and energy estimates for hospitalized dogs and cats. Proceedings of the Purina International Nutrition Symposium, January 15, 1991, Orlando, FL, p 5.
7. Nutritional Requirements of the Dog. Bethesda, MD: National Research Council, 1985.
8. Wingfield WE: Fluids and electrolytes. Fluid Therapy Symposium. Eastern States Conference, January 18, 1990, p 1.
9. Ogilvie GK, Salman MD, Kesel ML, *et al.*: Effect of anesthesia and surgery on energy expenditure determined by indirect calorimetry in dogs with malignant and nonmalignant conditions. *Am J Vet Res* 57:1321, 1996.
10. Walters LM, Ogilvie GK, Salman MD, *et al.*: Repeatability of energy expenditure measurements in clinically normal dogs by use of indirect calorimetry. *Am J Vet Res* 54:1881, 1993.
11. Walton RS, Wingfield WE, Ogilvie GK, *et al.*: Energy expenditure in 104 postopera-

tive and traumatically injured dogs with indirect calorimetry. *J Vet Emerg Crit Care* 6:71, 1996.

12. Elliott DA, King LG, Zerbe CA: Thyroid hormone concentrations in critically ill canine intensive care patients. *J Vet Emerg Crit Care* 5:17, 1995.
13. Martin LG, Matteson VL, Wingfield WE, *et al.*: Abnormalities of serum magnesium in critically ill dogs: incidence and implications. *J Vet Emerg Crit Care* 4:15, 1994.
14. Wingfield WE: Potassium and magnesium: the two most important ions in critically ill animals. *Vet Previews* 3:8, 1996.
15. Dhein CR, Wardrop KJ: Hyperkalemia associated with potassium chloride administration in a cat. *J Am Vet Med Assoc* 206:1565, 1995.

14
Transfusion Medicine

Maura T. Green

The intent of this chapter is not to discuss why or when a blood transfusion may be indicated. The goal of this chapter is to address issues and steps required to ensure that one's choice of blood product(s) will afford the maximum benefit and pose the minimum risk to the patient. Methods of blood collection and techniques of component preparation and administration are described.

THE ANTIGENIC NATURE OF ERYTHROCYTES

The antigenic nature of erythrocytes poses the greatest risk to patients in transfusion therapy. The red blood cell (RBC) membrane is coated with proteins and complex carbohydrates that can be antigenic. Some of these antigens are present on the RBCs of all members of a particular species. However, others are allogenic; that is, they are genetically divergent and are present on the erythrocytes of several but not all members of that species.[1] This is the basis for different blood types within a species.

If a patient receives a transfusion of RBCs that possess an antigen that the patient's own RBCs do not carry, those "foreign" RBCs will be recognized as "non-self" and antibody production in the recipient will be stimulated. Antibodies attack the "foreign" infused RBCs by attaching to them at the antigenic site. Erythrocytes with an antibody attached may agglutinate (stick together) and be removed by macrophages in the spleen and liver.[1] This is termed extravascular hemolysis and is usually a delayed reaction.

If the reaction is severe enough due to the presence of preformed alloantibodies in the recipient, or if the antibody is a strong hemolysin, complement may be activated. Complement fixation causes perforations in the RBC membrane, fluid passes into the cell, and the cell is ruptured (lysis). If this occurs in the vasculature, it is termed intravascular hemolysis. This type of reaction is usually an immediate transfusion reaction and can be life-threatening.[1–4]

Blood Types in Dogs

Eight different blood groups have been defined in the canine, but for practical clinical situations, dogs are termed either A negative (A^-) or A positive

(A^+). This nomenclature refers to the Dog Erythrocyte Antigen-1 (DEA-1) locus on the canine RBC. DEA-1 is a three-allele system in which dogs can be either DEA-1.1 positive, DEA-1.2 positive, or negative for both (termed DEA-1 negative or A^-).[1]

Dogs that are DEA-1.1 and DEA-1.2 negative do not possess an antigen at those sites. In the absence of antigenic stimuli, canine recipients of A^- blood will not form antibodies to those RBCs. For this reason A^- donors have been termed "universal" donors. Ideally, a true "universal" donor should be negative for DEA-7, but controversy exists as to whether the anti-DEA-7 antibody can cause a clinically significant reaction.[5]

The A^+ dogs are those whose erythrocytes do possess an antigen at either the 1.1 or 1.2 locus.[1] A^+ donors can safely donate blood to recipients that are also positive for DEA-1.1 because those RBCs will be recognized as "self."[6] The problem arises when an A^- dog is transfused with A^+ blood. Formation of an antibody in the A^- recipient will occur and may result in a delayed transfusion reaction with premature destruction of transfused erythrocytes and a severe hemolytic reaction on subsequent transfusions if the same mismatch occurs.[1,5-7] Blood typing cards for the DEA-1 locus are readily available and affordable.

Dogs that are A^-, patients likely to receive multiple transfusions over time, or any patient for which the blood type is unknown should only receive A^- "universal" blood.[6] Fortunately, because dogs are not born with clinically significant alloantibodies, a mismatch of blood on a first-time transfusion will be temporarily safe but puts the patient at grave risk for future transfusion reactions after 7 to 10 days if the same mismatch occurs.[1,5-7]

Cat Blood Types

Cats have three blood types: A, B, and AB (which is very rare). More than 90% of domestic short hair (DSH) and domestic long hair (DLH) cats in the United States are blood type A; however, the incidence of blood type B in the DSH and DLH cats varies geographically from state to state.[3,8] Seven of 94 DSH cats presented to Colorado State University for transfusion were type B cats. Additionally, the incidence of type B increases up to 45% in some purebred lines.[3,8] To make matters worse, type B cats are born with a strong naturally occurring preformed anti-A antibody; therefore, a severe life-threatening hemolytic transfusion reaction will occur on a first-time transfusion if a type B cat receives type A blood.[3,8] Only 30% of type A cats have naturally occurring anti-B antibodies, which are weak and do not cause a life-threatening reaction but may shorten RBC life span.[1,3] Table 14-1 summarizes the effect of various donor/recipient combinations on erythrocyte life span.

BLOOD TYPING CARDS

Blood typing cards are an extremely useful tool in canine and feline transfusion therapy. An understanding of their role and limitations will aid in clinical application.

Table 14-1. The Effect of Donor/Recipient Combinations on Feline Erythrocyte Life Span[5,12]

Donor Blood Type	Recipient Blood Type	RBC Life Span
A	A	36 d
B	A	2–3 d
A	B	1–3 h (severe hemolytic reaction)

Canine Typing Cards

Canine blood typing cards test solely for the DEA-1.1 antigen. For this reason, these cards are suitable for typing recipients and for identifying A^+ donors. However, they should be used only as a preliminary screening test for A^- "universal" donors.[9]

If a recipient tests strongly positive, that patient can safely receive either A^+ or A^- blood. If a recipient tests negative, the animal should only receive A^- "universal" blood. If, however you are typing a dog as a potential donor, a negative result signifies only that the donor is negative at DEA-1.1; the status of DEA-1.2 is not known, which could potentially sensitize A^- recipients. These donors should be screened further for the DEA-1.2 and DEA-7 locus (Table 14-2). A "universal" donor is a valuable asset to a veterinary clinic and the canine community.

Because agglutination on a typing card signifies a positive result, dogs that are autoagglutinators (IMHA) may show a false-positive result. For this reason canine recipients with autoimmune hemolytic anemia should only receive "universal" blood.

Feline Typing Cards

Cat blood typing cards are more specific and the results are unmistakable. Agglutination at the anti-A site denotes an A blood type cat. Agglutination at

Table 14-2. Clinical Application of Canine Typing Cards

Recipient	Suitable Donor(s)
DEA-1.1 A^+	A^+ or A^-
DEA-1.1 A^-	A^- universal donor*
Donor	**Suitable Recipient**
DEA-1.1 A^+	A^+
DEA-1.1 A^- (This dog could be a universal donor but further screening is necessary).	A^+

* As determined by a complete blood typing.

the anti-B site denotes a B blood type cat. Agglutination at both sites may signify the rare AB type, but more than likely the patient is autoagglutinating as a sequela of disease.

CROSSMATCHING

Crossmatching is the process by which the compatibility of recipient and donor blood is assessed. It is useful in dogs that have received a prior transfusion and in cats on the first transfusion.

Types of Crossmatch

There are two types of crossmatching, major and minor. A major crossmatch, as the name implies, is the most clinically important information for predicting compatibility. Washed donor erythrocytes are mixed with recipient plasma. A minor crossmatch uses washed recipient erythrocytes and the donor's plasma. Incompatibility is signaled by agglutination of the RBCs.[9]

Because dogs have such a low incidence of clinically important, naturally occurring preformed antibodies, the major crossmatch between dogs that have never received a prior transfusion should be compatible.[5,7] These patients should be card typed instead and a crossmatch may be an exercise in futility.

Cats are born with strong preformed alloantibodies; therefore, a crossmatch of incompatible blood (*i.e.*, A → B or B → A) prior to a first-time transfusion will show unmistakable agglutination at either the major or the minor crossmatch (respectively), and is a useful clinical tool although more time consuming than card typing.[8] Both canine and feline patients that have received a previous transfusion should be crossmatched if time allows.

Because agglutination is the end-point of crossmatching, it may be difficult to interpret the results of a crossmatch in samples of dogs and cats that have erythrocyte autoagglutination.[2,6,9]

PRETRANSFUSION CONSIDERATIONS

In keeping with the goal of maximum benefit and minimum risk, attention should be directed toward appropriate product selection. Three considerations are of primary concern:

1. The choice of RBC product, that is, packed red blood cells (PRBCs) versus whole blood
2. The age of the RBC product
3. Whether or not coagulation factors will need to be supplemented

Transfusion requirements are based on the clinical status of the patient, the type of anemia present, and the underlying cause of disease.

A quick and practical method of product selection is to address the following questions:

Table 14-3. Pretransfusion Considerations

Anemia Type	Component Choice
Acute	Whole blood or PRBCs
Chronic	PRBCs
Blood loss	Stored blood products
Hemolysis	Blood product <5 d old
Regenerative	Stored blood products
Nonregenerative	Blood product <5 d old
Normal hemostasis	Whole blood or PRBCs*
Coagulopathy	Whole blood and/or FFP

* PRBCs do not contain clotting factors. PRBCs, packed red blood cells; FFP, fresh-frozen plasma.

1. Is this anemia an acute or chronic condition? If anemia is acute, either whole blood or PRBCs are appropriate. If anemia is chronic, PRBCs are the wiser choice to avoid circulatory overload in a cardiac compensated patient.[6,10]
2. Is this anemia the result of blood loss or RBC destruction? If anemia is the result of hemolysis, the age of the transfused RBCs becomes important. The oldest cells in the donor's blood will be most susceptible to hemolysis.[1,6] A fresh unit of blood or a unit that is less than 5 days old will have a higher percentage of young RBCs, which have a better chance of surviving hemolysis.
3. Is this anemia regenerative or nonregenerative? If bone marrow depression is suspected a unit of blood less than 5 days old is indicated, again because it will contain a larger percentage of young RBCs. RBC life spans and transfusion viability will be prolonged.[1]
4. Is the hemostatic system functional in the patient? Platelet transfusions are impractical in veterinary medicine, but if a coagulapathy is present in the patient, whole blood or fresh- frozen plasma (FFP) can provide stabile or labile clotting factors[6,10] (Table 14-3).

BLOOD COMPONENT COLLECTION AND STORAGE

Anticoagulants

The two most common anticoagulants used are citrate-phosphate-dextrose-adenine (CPDA-1) and acid-citrate-dextrose (ACD). CPDA-1 results in the longest blood shelf life at 35 days. ACD will allow blood to be stored up to 21 days. Approximately 1 mL citrate anticoagulant is used per 7 mL blood collected from a dog or a cat.[6,7,10,11]

Canine Blood Collection

Chemical Restraint: Greyhounds usually do not require chemical restraint. Non-greyhounds can receive a standard dose of atropine sulfate SQ and 2 mg butorphanol IV/dog.

Procedure:

1. When collecting blood for storage, absolute aseptic technique must be used and air should not be allowed to enter the collection bag.
2. When collecting blood for storage, the ratio of blood to anticoagulant must be exact: specifically 450 mL blood ± 10% (*i.e.*, 405–495 mL) per 63 mL anticoagulant (CPDA-1) to ensure maximum cell viability.[11] A triple beam balance or gram scale should be used and collection ended when the total weight of the blood, bag, and anticoagulant equals approximately 537 g.

$$\begin{aligned} 450 \text{ mL blood} &= 450 \text{ g} \\ 63 \text{ mL CPDA} &= 63 \text{ g} \\ \text{Collection bag} &= \underline{24 \text{ g}} \\ & \quad\; 537 \text{ g} \end{aligned}$$

The jugular vein is clipped and surgically prepared. Blood is collected by gravity flow into a standard 450-mL CPDA-1 blood collection bag to the appropriate volume. The bag is rocked gently during collection to ensure adequate mixing of the blood and anticoagulant.[11]

To prevent air from entering the blood bag, the collection line should be cleared of air by turning the bag upside down, removing the needle cover, and allowing a few drops of anticoagulant to exit the needle. The collection line is then immediately clamped and not released until the venipuncture has been accomplished.

If less than a full unit of blood is desired, an appropriate volume of anticoagulant must be removed from the bag prior to collection to avoid citrate toxicity in the recipient.[11] For example, if only one half of a unit is to be drawn, discard one half of the anticoagulant.

$$\tfrac{1}{2} \text{ of } 450 \text{ mL of blood} = 225 \text{ mL}$$

$$\tfrac{1}{2} \text{ of } 63 \text{ mL of CPDA-1} = 31 \text{ mL}$$

At the end of collection, the line should be clamped or tied off before removing the needle from the vein, because air will enter the bag before all the blood has cleared the walls of the line. After the collection line is tied, the blood left in the line is "stripped" using a tube stripper, allowing the blood remaining in the line to mix with the anticoagulant in the bag and then return to the line. The line is then tied or clipped in segments for use in future crossmatches.[11] Note: If your collection method is less than ideal, the storage time should be shortened to 24 hours.

Feline Blood Collection

Chemical Restraint: Cats are routinely sedated with 20 mg ketamine HCl IV/cat.

Procedure: The jugular vein is clipped and surgically prepared. Blood is collected in a 60-mL syringe containing 7 mL ACD or CPDA-1. The maximum quantity of blood to be withdrawn from a donor cat at one time is 53 mL. This method provides only fresh, whole blood, which should be administered within 24 hours.

Stored Feline Blood Units

A method of collection of cat blood for storage in a closed system has been developed at Tufts University. A standard 450-mL CPDA-1 collection bag is used. All the anticoagulant is rolled out of the collection bag into the satellite bag and the line between the two is clamped, leaving only CPDA-1 in the collection line. The volume in the line is 8 mL, enough for a 53-mL unit of feline blood.[6,11] It is imperative that a digital scale be used for collection and that collection is stopped at 85 g.

$$\begin{aligned} \text{53 mL feline blood} &= \text{53 g} \\ \text{8 mL CPDA-1} &= \text{8 g} \\ \text{Collection bag} &= \underline{\text{24 g}} \\ & \quad\ \text{85 g} \end{aligned}$$

PREPARATION OF BLOOD COMPONENTS

To prepare PRBCs a closed collection bag system with one to three satellite bags is required. Some of these systems contain an RBC nutrient solution in one of the satellite bags. These solutions are termed RBC extenders because they lengthen the shelf life of the PRBCs from 35 days to 42 days.[10,12]

PRBCs

The RBCs may be separated by sedimentation, which is more practical for private practice, but usually are centrifuged at 5000*g* for 5 minutes at 6°C (42.8°F). After centrifugation, the outflow seal is broken and the plasma is expressed from the blood bag using a plasma extractor.[7,11] The plasma is allowed to flow into the satellite bag until the white blood cell buffy coat reaches the corners of the original bag (approximately 1 inch from the top). If an RBC extender is being used, all the plasma is removed. The valve to the satellite bag containing the RBC nutrient is opened and the packed cells are immediately reconstituted with nutrient solution. Tie or seal the tubing in at least three places before cutting the tubing to separate the bags.[9]

If an RBC nutrient is not being added, then it is important that some plasma remain to nourish the erythrocytes. Removal of approximately 150 mL plasma from a unit of greyhound blood and up to 250 mL plasma from a non-greyhound unit of blood will result in the PRBCs having a packed cell volume (PCV) of 70% to 80% (for dogs living at an altitude of 5000 feet). A PCV exceeding 80% will increase RBC fragility and may cause hemoglobinuria in the recipient.[12]

The PRBCs are stored at 1° to 6°C (33.8°–42.8°F) and have a shelf life of 35 days in CPDA-1. Frequent mixing is recommended because it helps maintain

Table 14-4. Definitions of Plasma Types

Fresh plasma (FP)	Plasma that is taken off the RBCs within 3-4 h and used within 6 h. vWF, factor VIII, vitamin K-dependent factors, AT III.[1,3,9,10]
Stored plasma (SP)	Plasma that has been refrigerated at 1°–6°C (33.8°–42.8°F) for up to 35 d (using CPDA-1); but has reduced clotting factors.[1,3,9,10]
Fresh-frozen plasma (FFP)	Plasma frozen at −70°C (−148.4°F) within 6 h of collection; optimal clotting factors; may be stored up to 1 y; should be used within 2 h of thawing. vWF, VIII, vitamin K-dependent factors, AT III.[1,3,9,10]
Frozen plasma (FzP)	Plasma frozen >6 h after collection or FFP that is >1 y old; may be stored up to 5 d following thawing. Vitamin K-dependent factors.[1,3,9,10]

adenosine triphosphate (ATP), glucose concentrations in the erythrocyte microenvironment, and 2,3-diphosphoglycerate (DPG) concentrations within the RBC.[7,9–11]

Administration of PRBCs requires dilution with 0.9% sodium chloride (NaCl) to the volume desired. Do not use lactated Ringer's solution, Normosol, or 5% dextrose in water (D5W) for reconstitution.[10] If an RBC extender has been added, further dilution is not required.

Plasma

Plasma is prepared in the above manner. The bag(s) containing plasma are usually frozen for future administration. The types of plasma available are listed in Table 14-4.

Platelets

The preparation and storage of platelets requires special consideration. Specifically:

1. Heparin should not be used as the anticoagulant.[4]
2. Blood must be collected in latex-free plastic bags.[11,13]
3. If platelet-rich plasma (PRP) is desired, the whole blood must be centrifuged at room temperature (25°C [77°F]). Refrigeration will cause platelet dysfunction.[4,6,10-12]
4. A^- recipients should receive platelets from A^- donors to avoid sensitization.[13]
5. Fresh whole blood or PRP should be stored at room temperature, kept on a rocker, and administered within 4 hours and 24 hours of collection, respectively, if platelet function is to be optimal.[12]
6. PRP is prepared by centrifugation of fresh whole blood at 2000g for 3 minutes. The plasma is then expressed into the satellite bag until the RBC layer is entered.[11]

7. For platelet concentrates, a collection bag with two satellite bags is required. PRP is centrifuged an additional 5 minutes at 4000*g*. All but 50 mL of the plasma is expressed into the second satellite bag. The remaining 50 mL is the platelet concentration.[11]

INDICATIONS FOR BLOOD PRODUCT USAGE

Because a transfusion with any blood product carries some risk to the patient and expense to the owner, it is best to replace only the specific component(s) indicated. This practice will reduce transfusion reactions and decrease the demand on the hospital blood bank.[9]

PRBCs

Cardiac Insufficiency. There is less chance of circulatory overload with PRBCs than with whole blood. Whole blood contains approximately 250 mL plasma. This is an unnecessary volume load for a patient with cardiac compromise. Use of 10 mL PRBCs/kg will raise the PCV by 10% versus 20 mL whole blood/kg for the same result. Therefore, the same end-point is obtained in approximately half the volume.[6,9,10]

Chronic Anemia. Cardiac hypertrophy or dilation and increased cardiac output secondary to chronic anemia can result in circulatory overload following a transfusion. Patients with chronic anemia should receive a slow infusion of PRBCs and not whole blood.[6,9,10]

Hemorrhagic Shock. Although whole blood may be used to replace losses due to hemorrhage, PRBCs may be a better alternative. PRBCs play a role in increasing circulating plasma volume by movement of interstitial fluid into the vascular space. The PCV of PRBCs is near 80%; however, 0.9% NaCl is added to achieve a more rapid flow rate.[6]

Liver Disease. PRBCs have less ammonia, adenine, citrate, and sodium when compared to whole blood and are therefore preferred in patients with liver disease.[6,9]

History of Allergies or Prior Transfusion Reactions. Patients who have become sensitized to plasma histocompatibility antigens should only receive PRBCs or, ideally, "washed" PRBCs.[6,9,10]

Blood Products with Short Storage Time

Severe Hemorrhage with Concurrent Coagulopathy. Patients who need RBCs as well as clotting factors due to severe liver disease, disseminated intravascular coagulation (DIC), or the dilutional effect of massive transfusion may be candidates for whole blood with a short storage time.[6,9,10]

Hepatoencephalopathy. Because of the potential for increased ammonia concentrations in stored blood, patients with hepatoencephalopathy that need RBCs should receive RBC products with short storage times.[6,9]

Hemolytic Anemia. Storage decreases erythrocyte viability and survival once they are transfused.[1] Therefore, patients with immune-mediated hemolytic anemia should receive RBCs or whole blood with short (<5 days) storage times to give them the most benefit from the transfusion.[6,9] These RBCs will be destroyed at the same rate as the patient's own RBCs.[1]

FFP

Coagulopathy. Patients with von Willebrand's disease, congenital coagulopathies such as hemophilia A, or severe warfarin toxicity will benefit from the use of FFP. FFP contains the stable vitamin K-dependent factors (II, VII, IX, and X) as well as factors V and VIII and vWF.[4,6,9,10]

DIC. In addition to coagulation factors, FFP contains antithrombin III (AT III), an inhibitor of coagulation. Heparin therapy has been advocated to prevent thromboembolism, but AT III is required for heparin to function as an anticoagulant.

Massive Hemorrhage. After transfusion with multiple units of PRBCs or stored whole blood, clotting factors may become depleted. Clotting factors can be replaced with FFP.[6,7,10]

Frozen Plasma

Frozen plasma is more practical for private practice than FFP. It can be separated from the RBCs by sedimentation, frozen at −20°C (−4°F), and stored for up to 5 years.[6,9,10]

Warfarin Toxicity. Frozen plasma contains the stable vitamin K-dependent clotting factors and can be used to treat severe warfarin toxicity.[6,11]

Liver Diseases. Patients with liver disease have impaired vitamin K utilization. Frozen plasma is indicated when bleeding is present in these individuals or immediately before a liver biopsy if bleeding is expected.[10]

Severe Burns. Frozen plasma is indicated in patients with acute plasma losses as in severe body surface burns.[9]

PRP or Platelet Concentrates

Platelet transfusions may be impractical in veterinary medicine due to the difficulty in acquiring adequate numbers of platelets and their short storage time.[6] There are not enough platelets in 1 U canine blood to functionally raise the platelet count in a thrombocytopenic dog except in the very small patient. Human platelet concentrates contain the platelets from 6 to 10 U blood.[10] Without a cell separator, the veterinarian would need to draw a unit of blood from three to four dogs to functionally treat one standard size dog. In most cases of thrombocytopenia, in which the platelets are being destroyed by an immune-mediated mechanism, the transfused platelets will be rapidly destroyed as well. Platelet transfusions may also be ineffective in cases of splenomegaly, sepsis, DIC, and hypothermia.[4,6,10] The time and expense involved in platelet preparation may be justified in the treatment of very small dogs with thrombocytopenia. The amount of platelets contained in 1 U of PRP or platelet concentrate given to a 15-lb dog would be the equivalent of transfusing a 60-lb dog with 4 U. In small patients, volume overload must be taken into consideration. Therefore, platelet concentrates are preferred to PRP.

ADMINISTRATION OF BLOOD OR BLOOD PRODUCTS

Blood components should be delivered through blood administration filters with a pore size of 170 µm. Nonlatex filters should be used for platelet transfusions. A 40-µm microfilter should be used in autotransfusions to remove microemboli.[6,13]

Blood components should never be mixed with or transfused through lines containing fluid other than 0.9% NaCl. Lactated Ringer's, Normosol, D5W, and hypotonic NaCl are contraindicated.[6,7,10,13]

Red blood cells are generally given in terms of units, that is, one third, one half, 1 or 2 U, to effect but an initial starting dose is 20 mL/kg for whole blood or 10 mL/kg of PRBCs.[6]

Plasma, when given for the purpose of replacing clotting factors, can be administered at a dose of 5 to 20 mL/kg initially. When plasma is necessary for providing clotting factors prior to surgery, it must be given within the hour preceding surgery or during the surgery.[6,10]

Intravenous administration is the preferred route, but if IV catheterization is difficult, whole blood and PRBCs can be given via intraosseous transfusion.

Patients that are severely anemic (PCVs of 12 or below) will frequently arrest if IV catheterization is difficult or stressful. For this reason, jugular catheterization may be contraindicated.

Frequently cats will present with a PCV of 10 or below. One should draw blood from the donor first, have it on site, and perhaps administer at least half the unit via butterfly catheter, before stressing the cat for permanent catheterization.

The rate of administration depends somewhat on the patient and the reason for transfusion. If possible, the blood should be administered slowly over the first 30 minutes to allow the patient to be assessed for transfusion reactions. If no reactions are noted, the rate may be increased such that the transfusion is finished within 4 hours.[9] In life-threatening situations of massive hemorrhage, blood can be infused as quickly as possible. Transfusions should be completed within 4 hours. After that, the unit is considered contaminated by bacteria.

It is not necessary to warm stored RBCs prior to administration except in cases of rapid infusion. Warming RBCs at temperatures in excess of 38°C (100.4°F) will cause lysis and may cause intravascular hemolysis in the patient. Placing the coils of the administration set tubing in a bowl of warm water with a thermometer, to ensure that the temperature does not exceed 38°C (100.4°F), may be a safe method of warming a transfusion but only if it is necessary.

TRANSFUSION REACTIONS

Transfusion reactions can be classified as hemolytic versus nonhemolytic, immune-mediated versus nonimmunologic, or immediate versus delayed. However, because clinical signs in the initial stages of a transfusion reaction can overlap etiologies, it is necessary to differentiate between them so that timely therapy can be instituted.[5,6,8,10]

Hemolytic Reactions

An immune-mediated intravascular hemolytic transfusion due to incompatible erythrocytes can be life-threatening. Initial signs include fever, restlessness, tachycardia, urticardia, and vomiting, progressing to hypotension, shock, DIC, and potentially acute renal failure. Hemoglobinemia and hemoglobinuria occur immediately.[5,6,8,10] At the first sign of a reaction, the transfusion should be stopped. A sample of blood from the recipient and the donor blood bag should be obtained and spun down to check for hemoglobinemia. If hemolysis is evident in the recipient sample and not in the transfusion sample, immune-mediated hemolysis is most likely occurring. A crossmatch should confirm incompatibility. Fortunately, acute immune-mediated hemolytic reactions in the dog are very rare due to a paucity of naturally occurring preformed antibodies in the canine population.[5] Therapy should be instituted relative to the patient's status.

Nonimmune-Mediated Hemolytic Reactions

More common is an acute hemolytic crisis due to nonimmunologic causes. These can include out-of-date units with hemolyzed RBCs, overheating of blood products, diluting of blood products with hyperosmotic solutions, mechanical trauma due to infusion under pressure, or RBC products with a PCV exceeding 80%.[1,6,10] Signs include fever, restlessness, tachycardia, vomiting, hemoglobinemia, and hemoglobinuria. Samples of blood from both the patient and the transfusion should be checked for hemolysis. If hemolysis is evident in the transfusion sample, it indicates that the patient has been transfused with hemolyzed blood, which carries a better prognosis for the recipient. A crossmatch with a fresh sample of blood from the donor should be performed to confirm compatibility. Therapy should be geared toward clinical signs. A crossmatch with another nonhemolyzed unit of blood should be performed and a transfusion begun again if necessary.

Immune-Mediated Delayed Hemolysis

A delayed immune-mediated hemolysis can occur in patients that have been previously sensitized to incompatible RBCs due to a low level of circulating antibodies. A second exposure triggers a response and antibody production increases. Additionally, a patient can become sensitized following a first-time transfusion with premature destruction of transfused erythrocytes.[6] Delayed reactions can occur 2 days to 2 weeks after transfusion.[6,10] The hallmark of a delayed reaction is an unexpected drop in the PCV. Icterus and bilirubinuria may be present. A positive Coombs test will confirm antibody-coated erythrocytes.

Allergic Reactions

Sensitivity to foreign plasma proteins can cause fever, urticaria, facial edema, vomiting, and diarrhea. These reactions are usually mild and not dose related.[10] Most patients respond to the administration of antihistamines. If the symptoms subside, the transfusion can be continued.[6,10]

BACTERIAL CONTAMINATION

Infusion of a unit of blood with bacterial contamination carries a grave prognosis for the recipient. Symptoms include fever, shock, and sepsis.[10] A sample of blood from the unit should be submitted for culture, but a quicker diagnosis may be obtained by microscopic examination of the transfused blood for the presence of bacteria.

REFERENCES

1. Smith JE: Erythrocytes. *Adv Vet Sci Comp Med* 36:9, 1991.
2. Cotter SM: Autoimmune hemolytic anemia in dogs. *Compend Contin Educ Pract Vet* 14:53, 1992.
3. Giger U, Bucheler J: Transfusion of type A and type B blood to cats. *J Am Vet Med Assoc* 198:411, 1991.
4. Meyers KM, Wardrop KJ: Platelets and coagulation. *Adv Vet Sci Comp Med* 36:87, 1991.
5. Giger U, Gelans CJ, Callan MB, *et al.*: An acute hemolytic transfusion reaction caused by DEA 1.1 incompatibility in a previously sensitized dog. *J Am Vet Med Assoc* 206:1358, 1995.
6. Cotter SM: Clinical transfusion medicine. *Adv Vet Sci Comp Med* 36:181, 1991.
7. Greene RT: Blood banking and transfusion therapy. *Compend Contin Educ* 6:134, 1985.
8. Giger U: Feline transfusion medicine. *Probl Vet Med* 4:600, 1992.
9. Miller E, Green M: Canine and Feline Blood Donor Program. Colorado State University, Fort Collins, CO. 1994.
10. Pisciotto PT: Blood Transfusion Therapy. A Physician's Handbook, 4th ed. American Association of Blood Banks, Arlington, VA. 1993.
11. Authement JM: Preparation of components. *Adv Vet Sci Comp Med* 39:171, 1991.
12. Poudre Valley Hospital Blood Bank, Fort Collins, Colorado.
13. Cotter SM, Authement JM: Tufts Transfusion Service Protocol, 1987.

15
Nutrition in Critically Ill Animals

Jeffrey Proulx

PATHOPHYSIOLOGY

Lack of adequate caloric intake shifts the body's neurohumoral mediators so that the balance between anabolism and catabolism is tipped in favor of catabolism. This response to inadequate calories is necessary in order to preserve plasma concentrations of nutrients to supply energy for normal cell function. As a consequence, body weight and, in particular, lean muscle mass and normal organ structure may be compromised because of the need for amino acids to be used as an alternate energy source for the body. Two types of starvation have been recognized. *Simple starvation* is a lack of adequate calories and protein, whereas *stress starvation* is a consequence of systemic inflammation and physiologic stress (critical illness and injury) concurrent with a lack of adequate calories and protein. Interestingly, supplying adequate calories and protein does not always correct the loss of lean body mass characteristic of stress starvation.

Simple Starvation

In animals without injury or illness, several metabolic adaptations result from the lack of nutrient intake.[1] During the postabsorptive phase, the insulin concentration lowers and the glucagon concentration rises, allowing an increase in hepatic glycogenolysis to support euglycemia and triglyceride breakdown from adipose tissue. With continued nutrient restriction, glycogen stores are depleted within 12 to 24 hours and the glucocorticoid concentration rises to support metabolic adaptations to prolonged calorie restriction. Glucocorticoids facilitate protein catabolism with consequent release of free amino acids from muscular tissue. The amino acids, particularly alanine and glutamine, serve as substrate for gluconeogenesis by the liver (in early starvation) and kidneys (in later starvation). In addition, plasma catecholamines in conjunction with glucocorticoids and glucagon, activate hormone sensitive lipase within adipocytes to release free fatty acids. With prolonged starvation, the lipolytic response becomes more pronounced, allowing for protein "sparing." This occurs by induction of hepatic enzymes necessary for the production of ketone bodies from free fatty acids. Organs that are usually obligate glucose users, such as the central nervous system, adapt to using ketone bodies for up to 50% of caloric needs. A balance is maintained between protein and fat catabolism to prevent large fluctuations in blood pH and to preserve the integrity of protein-based structures.

In addition to the "balanced" catabolism described, a second adaptation of starvation during the short term is a lowering of the metabolic rate because of diminished production of thyroid hormone and diminished conversion of thyroxine (T_4) to the active triiodothyronine (T_3).[1] As a consequence, energy stores and protein are conserved for a longer period of time. A longer adaptation to simple starvation includes a reduction in the leptin concentration.[2] Leptin is a hormone produced by adipocytes, with the plasma concentration directly corresponding to whole body adipocyte mass. As adipocyte mass is reduced in starvation, the plasma leptin concentration falls. A low leptin concentration leads to greater production of neuropeptide Y in the arcuate nucleus of the hypothalamus. Neuropeptide Y directly increases the appetite at a hypothalamic site, increases the activity of lipoprotein lipase (increases storage of fat in adipocytes), and increases corticosteroid synthesis. Neuropeptide Y essentially primes the body for reversal of starvation (increased appetite and adipocyte sensitivity for storage) and contributes to the adaptation to starvation by the mobilization of stored nutrients by stimulation of corticosteroid production.

The provision of calories and protein reverses the above processes by restoring glycogen, adipose stores, and anabolism allowing a return to normal cell and organ structure and function.

Stress Starvation

The physiologic stress associated with severe illness or injury often leads to a pronounced catabolic state characterized by hypermetabolism that is compounded by patients that are unable or unwilling to eat.[1] Although fatty acids are the primary source of energy in fully adaptive simple starvation, protein breakdown becomes much more pronounced in the face of the hypermetabolism associated with severe illness or injury. This response is caused by inflammatory cytokines, such as tumor necrosis factor and interleukins, which augment the effects of catecholamines and glucocorticoids associated with stress.[3] In addition, inflammatory cytokines may increase the metabolic rate by instigating mitochondrial dysfunction and, therefore, contribute to inefficient use of oxygen and calories.[4] Inflammatory mediators may also directly regulate or suppress the body's normal responses to starvation by inhibiting signals for body weight control (including appetite).[2] This process is not necessarily reversed by the simple provision of adequate protein or calories.

Starvation Consequences

The effects of starvation are well documented, both clinically and experimentally.[5] Negative energy balance leads to depletion of glycogen stores, skeletal and smooth muscle weakness, gastrointestinal ileus, disruption of the gastrointestinal barrier, and decreases in high turnover cell populations such as leukocytes, gastrointestinal mucosal cells, fibroblasts, and other cells involved in wound healing. Negative nitrogen balance leads to deficiencies in nonspecific and specific immune function, gut mucosal atrophy, loss of visceral and muscular protein with consequent weakness and abnormal function, decreases in albumin, fibrinogen, complement proteins and globulins, and poor wound healing. In general, the induced protein catabolism depletes the body of structural and functional protein, thereby impairing wound healing, immune function, and other normal organ functions. Inadequate nutrition sets the stage for serious complications resulting in sepsis, multiple organ failure, and death. The provision of early nutritional support may prevent some of these deficiencies, hasten recovery from illness and injury, and diminish some of the complications of the critically ill.

Nutritional Support Benefits

Despite the known consequences of calorie and protein restriction, there is much debate over whether providing nutritional support truly influences recovery and outcome in humans as well as in veterinary patients. In human patients, proven benefit of nutritional support has been demonstrated in patients that are unable to eat (simple starvation), in severely malnourished patients scheduled to undergo major surgery, in patients with major trauma, in bone-marrow transplant recipients, and in patients undergoing anticancer therapy.[6]

Enteral or Parenteral Nutrition?

Nutritional support can be instituted by the enteral or parenteral route. In general, enteral nutrition is preferred if the gastrointestinal tract is completely or even partially functional. Enteral nutrition is more physiologic, with nutrients being digested and absorbed by the gut and metabolized by the liver. Direct enteral nutrition also maintains normal gut structure and function.[7] For instance, within 24 hours of anorexia, atrophy of the mucosal lining and diminished digestive and absorptive capacity take place.[8] As a result, it is more difficult to re-institute normal feeding. In addition, with a lack of local nutrients, the gut mucosa becomes leaky, with enterocytes being unable to maintain normal intercellular borders and immune function. Both of these events predispose the gut to translocation of bacteria and toxins and create a greater risk of secondary sepsis.

In addition to the factors stated, providing enteral nutrition is probably more important in animals that have experienced trauma, shock, or general cardiovascular compromise. During the shock state, severe limitation to mesenteric blood flow predisposes to a more severe gastrointestinal insult. The gastrointestinal tract in these types of patients is susceptible to reperfusion injury and greater dysfunction of the gut-barrier, digestive, and absorptive capacities. Providing enteral nutrition increases mucosal blood flow and preserves enterocyte function. Several recent human studies have shown improved outcome and reduction in hospital stay when enteral nutritional support is supplied early, specifically in patients with traumatic injury.[9]

Regardless of whether enteral or parenteral nutrition is used, the goal of nutritional support is to abrogate the catabolic state and to provide essential nutrients in the form of energy, amino acids, and micronutrients. In patients unable to tolerate partial or full enteral feeding, parenteral nutrition is used but will not be as effective in maintaining gut integrity and function.

Immune Enhancing Diets

Recent attention has been given to specific nutrients that may be "conditionally essential" during periods of critical illness and to nutrients that may have immunomodulatory properties.[10] These nutrients include glutamine, arginine, and the omega-3 polyunsaturated fatty acids.

Glutamine is important as a precursor for nucleotide synthesis as a substrate for rapidly dividing cells such as enterocytes, renal tubular cells, lymphocytes, fibroblasts, and endothelial cells. Glutamine is essential for maintenance and integrity of gastrointestinal mucosal structure and function, prevention of bacterial translocation, and maintenance of local immune function.[11] In critically ill animals, glutamine is considered a conditionally essential amino acid because the plasma glutamine concentration markedly declines in the stressed state.[12] Arginine has been shown to be important in wound healing, immunologic function, the metabolism of amino acids, and in the production of nitric oxide. Although arginine is nonessential in humans, it may also be conditionally essential or may have positive pharmacologic effects in critical illness.[10] Omega-3 fatty acids have anti-inflammatory properties that may be helpful in the systemic inflammation associated with trauma and sepsis by changing the balance of eicosanoid synthesis and positively modulating immune function.[10]

In critically ill humans, several studies have shown benefit with the use of arginine and ω-3 fatty acid-enhanced enteral formulations in regard to length of stay and total complications.[13,14] Veterinary diets are supplemented with arginine because of its essential nature in metabolism, but no specific "immune-enhancing" diets exist for dogs and cats.

Clinical Nutritional Support

The general guidelines for the institution of nutritional support include patients with evidence of malnutrition, patients that have lost or are expected to lose 10% of lean body mass, and patients that are anorectic and not expected to be eating within 3 days. Increased nutrient demand due to the catabolic response associated with fever, infection, and neoplasia may require initiation early in the course of illness or injury. Patients with severe trauma, sepsis, or systemic inflammation and patients with nutrient losses through vomiting, diarrhea, draining wounds, or burns should be started on nutritional support once the patient has stable cardiorespiratory values and has normal fluid and electrolyte balance. All patients entering an ICU should be assessed for the potential benefit and route of nutritional support (Figure 15-1). If the gastrointestinal tract is completely or partially functional, a feeding tube should be placed at the time of admission to the hospital. Gastrostomy and jejunostomy tube placement should also be considered in patients undergoing a major surgical procedure.

Parenteral nutrition allows for provision of nutrients through the intrave-

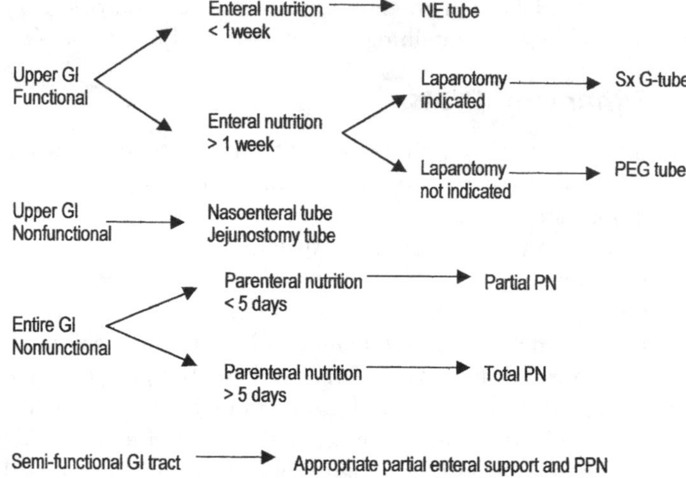

Figure 15-1
Nutritional support route indications. (Adapted from LM Freeman, Tufts University School of Veterinary Medicine Clinical Hospital Notes)

nous administration of variable mixtures of amino acids, lipids, and dextrose, along with vitamins, minerals and electrolytes. Indications for parenteral nutrition include severe vomiting and regurgitation, acute pancreatitis, severe intestinal disease with malabsorptive disorders, or as a supplement to enteral nutrition so that full caloric needs are met. Exclusive use of parenteral formulations for nutritional support should be performed with the understanding of the negative effects on the gastrointestinal barrier function and the development of mucosal atrophy.

Energy and Protein Requirements

Several equations can be used to calculate resting energy requirements (RER), although there are many factors and individual differences in a patient's true metabolic requirement.[15] More important is the use of a consistent, "ballpark" formula in calculating nutritional requirements. The following formulas are adequate for the calculation of RER:

$$<2 \text{ kg: RER} = 70 \times \text{weight (kg)}^{0.75}$$

$$>2 \text{ kg: RER} = [30 \times \text{weight (kg)}] + 70 \text{ or above equation}$$

Calorie supplementation should include RER multiplied by an injury/illness severity factor in order to attempt maintenance of lean body mass and sufficient calories. Previously, severe injury and sepsis were thought to require a doubling of basal requirements, but this has shown to actually result in overfeeding and potential complications of hyperglycemia, hyperammonemia, and hyperlipidemia (especially with parenteral nutrition). General guidelines for estimation of caloric requirement (Illness Energy Requirement [IER]) include calculation of RER and multiplication by the following factors:

× 1.0–1.2 for non-stressed anorexic, cage rested patients

× 1.2–1.5 for post-operative patients

× 1.2–1.5 for trauma and sepsis

Enteral Nutrition

Provision of enteral protein and calories is the preferred route of nutritional support for the ill and injured veterinary patients. Patient factors such as level of consciousness, diagnosis, and status of gastrointestinal function dictate which type of feeding tube and diet are indicated.[16]

Feeding Tubes

A *nasoesophageal tube* (NE tube) is used for short- to medium-term nutritional support (3–14 days). This is an effective and easy method of providing nutritional support in patients with general illness, oral cavity disease, or a simple unwillingness to eat.[17] Patients undergoing NE tube placement and feeding must have a functional gastrointestinal tract, normal level of consciousness, and good airway control.

Nasoesophageal tube placement is inexpensive since no special equipment or general anesthesia is required. After topical anesthesia is applied to the nostril, a 3½ to 10 F red rubber tube is introduced into the ventromedial nasal meatus, and the distal tip is delivered to the caudal esophagus. Pushing the nose upward and holding the head in a flexed position helps to facilitate passage into the esophagus as opposed to the trachea. Mild sedation (narcotic and diazepam) may enhance patient comfort during placement. Tube position should always be verified by radiography. The tube should be secured at the nose and its proximal end capped.

Contraindications include vomiting, functional or mechanical gastrointestinal obstruction, upper airway disease, pneumonia, head and facial trauma, and esophageal disease. In patients with an impaired level of consciousness, the risk of aspiration must be carefully evaluated. Patients that are intubated or mechanically ventilated often tolerate nasal tube feeding if the distal end is passed into the stomach (NG tube). Disadvantages include patient discomfort, epistaxis, sinusitis, vomiting, and reflux esophagitis (especially with NG tubes). The size of the nasoesophageal tube necessitates liquid diets to prevent tube occlusion. The author has also found NE tubes useful in the decompression (air and liquid) in patients with megaesophagus and acute aspiration pneumonia and NG tubes useful in the decompression of the stomach in patients with gastroparesis (*e.g.*, postoperative gastric dilatation-volvulus, primary gastroenteritis).

An *esophagostomy tube* (E-tube) is ideal in a patient that is mentally alert and has minimal systemic disease and normal gastrointestinal function but has difficulty prehending or chewing food (*e.g.*, severe mandibular or maxillary fracture, trigeminal neuropathy) or requires medium to long duration of enteral support. The E-tube is placed by a left mid-cervical surgical approach with the patient intubated and under general anesthesia.[18] The distal end is placed just cranial to the gastroesophageal sphincter and the proximal external end capped and sutured or anchored to the periosteum of the atlas. Because of the insertion site, the placement of a relatively large red rubber or specifically marketed E-tube (12–22 F) allows provision of appropriate blenderized soft food as opposed to the more expensive liquid formulations.

Risks associated with the E-tube use include aspiration pneumonia, reflux esophagitis, and vomiting/regurgitation, tube dislodgement, occlusion, and stoma infection. An incorrectly placed E-tube may result in serious complications such as upper airway dysfunction, broncho-pulmonary trauma, and iatrogenic pneumonia.

Gastrostomy tube (G-tube) placement is indicated for any patient needing medium to long-term, enteral nutritional support. The G-tube bypasses the oral cavity, pharynx, and esophagus. Gastrostomy tubes are well tolerated in anorectic and ill animal patients and are easily managed by owners in the home environment. Gastrostomy tube placement by surgical, endoscopic, or a blind, percutaneous technique has been described.[19,20,21] Although many tubes are available, a pezzar tube (16–22F) is most commonly used. Tube size and direct delivery into the stomach allow use of blenderized diets in a bolus fashion.

Contraindications include persistent vomiting or functional/mechanical obstruction. Gastroesophageal reflux and aspiration are potential complications in patients that do not tolerate feeding. Disadvantages include the necessity of general anesthesia, the potential for infection or inflammation at the stoma, and dehiscence with tube migration and peritonitis. To allow adequate adhesion formation at the stoma site, G-tubes should be left in place for a period of 10 days before removal is attempted. Malnourished and hypoalbuminemic patients may require longer periods because of delayed wound healing.

Jejunostomy tube (J-tube) placement is done during abdominal surgery for conditions in which feeding via oral or upper gastrointestinal feeding tube may or will be precluded. A J-tube should be considered in patients with major dysfunction of the proximal gastrointestinal tract, including the pancreas and biliary system. Disadvantages include the need for surgical placement, risk of stoma infection, tube dislodgement, and peritonitis, and tube occlusion. A J-tube must remain in place for at least 10 days before attempted removal (longer if the patient is malnourished or hypoalbuminemic). The relatively small tube bore size (3½–8F) limits feeding to liquid formulas. Calculated calories should be provided as a continuous infusion because of to the location of delivery. Methods for placement have been described.[22]

Enteral Diets

Enteral formulations produced for human and veterinary patients vary according to a wide range of factors including consistency, caloric density, osmolarity, percentage and type of nutrients, and various additives. In general, enteral diets formulated for human patients may be used for short periods in dogs and cats with special needs. However, enteral veterinary diets are balanced for canine and feline patients and should be used whenever possible. Formula selection should be based on knowledge of the patient needs, including degree of malnutrition, caloric and protein requirements, and digestive and absorptive capacity as well as method of enteral access. The disease process also may be relevant to the type of enteral nutrition provided. For example, patients with renal or hepatic disease have diminished protein tolerance. Veterinary products commonly used in the enteral support of critically ill patients are listed in Table 15-1.

Diet Formulation Enteral formulations are characterized as either polymeric or elemental. Polymeric diets consist of intact protein, polysaccharides, and long-chain triglycerides and are appropriate for most veterinary patients receiving enteral support.

Elemental (or near elemental) diets are composed of oligo-, tri-, and dipeptides or free amino acids, medium chain triglycerides, and mono- or di-saccharides. Available elemental diets are all formulated for humans and are deficient in protein when used in dogs and cats. Patients with severe maldigestive or absorptive conditions may benefit from elemental diets that are more easily assimilated, although there are no current veterinary formulations to accomplish this task. Even though veterinary patients with J-tubes cannot depend on pancreatic enzymes for digestion of intact nutrients, veterinary polymeric liquid diets (as opposed to elemental diets) are well tolerated.

Osmolarity Enteral formulations vary considerably in osmolarity and caloric density. In most veterinary patients, enteral products delivered in to the small intestine via J-tube should be isosmotic (290–310 mOsm) to limit local fluid fluxes, nausea, cramping, vomiting, and diarrhea. Hyperosmolar liquid diets delivered into the esophagus or stomach are well tolerated, although a patient that

Table 15-1. Characteristics of Veterinary Diets Commonly Used for Critically Ill Patients

Product	Calories (kcal/ml)	Protein Content (g/100 kcal)	Lipid Content (% kcal)	Carbohydrates (% kcal)
Canine CliniCare (Abbott)	1	5.5	55	25
Feline CliniCare (Abbott)	1	8.6	45	25
Feline CliniCare RF (Abbott)	1	5.6	57	21
Eukanuba Maximum Calorie (Iams)	2.1	7.4	66	5
Hill's A/D	1.3	8.8	53	12
Hill's P/D blenderized (1 part p/d: 1.5 parts water)	0.9	9.3	56	7

has not eaten or received enteral support in 2 to 3 days may initially require an isosmolar formulation. On a volume or caloric basis, elemental products (products with monosaccharides, free amino acids) have a higher osmolarity due to the large number of particles per unit volume.

Carbohydrates Carbohydrates are provided in enteral products as polysaccharides (corn starch), disaccharides, and monosaccharides. Monosaccharides in elemental formulations add sweetness and increase the relative osmolarity of the product (greater number of molecules per calories).

Protein Dietary protein is supplied in enteral products as free amino acids, protein hydrolysates (di-, tri-, and oligopeptides), or intact protein. Hydrolysates in elemental diets are freely absorbed by enterocytes in a non-energy dependent fashion (faster than free amino acids) and may be of benefit in patients with nutrient malassimilation. Intact proteins theoretically depend on gastric acid secretion and pancreatic exocrine function.

In general, veterinary patients require greater amounts of protein than human patients. Protein requirements in animals are 4g/100 kcals in dogs and 6g/100 kcal in cats. Depending on the product, protein concentration varies <5g/100 kcal to 15 g/kcal. Modular formulations such as amino acid powders (Promod, Ross Laboratories) may be used to supplement human enteral products used in animals.

Patient factors that may dictate special enteral formula selection include renal or liver insufficiency, which necessitates a high-quality, low-protein formulation and a lower concentration of aromatic amino acids (2 g/100 kcal for dogs and 3–4g/100 kcal in cats). Patients in highly catabolic states (e.g., burns, sepsis) require higher protein supplementation (6 g/100 kcal in dogs and 7–8 g/100 kcal in cats).

Lipids The lipid components used in polymeric enteral feeding products contain the long-chain fatty acids, including the essential long chain polyunsaturated fatty acids, linoleic (ω-3), and linolenic (ω-6) acids.

Diets formulated with medium chain triglycerides are ideal for a patient with maldigestion or malabsorption syndrome. Medium-chain triglycerides do not depend on pancreatic lipases, brush-border enzyme activity, or active transport processes but rather are absorbed directly into enterocytes. Medium-chain triglycerides should not be used in diabetic ketoacidotic patients because they are especially ketogenic.

Fiber Fiber is provided in some enteral products formulated for humans at 10 to 13 g/1000 kcal. Normal dietary fiber is composed of minimally digested (10%–15%) insoluble fibers such as cellulose, hemicellulose, and lignin and soluble fibers such as pectins, gums, and mucilages, most of which are digested (90%–99%). Upon ingestion, dietary fiber undergoes fermentation by colonic anaerobes, resulting in the production of short-chain fatty acids such as butyrate, acetate, and propionate. These acids provide an energy substrate for colonocytes, increase bacterial mass, stimulate sodium and water absorption, and may prevent some forms of diarrhea associated with enteral nutrition. Currently, there are no veterinary *liquid* products containing fiber, although over-the-counter products containing psyllium and pectin are available and can be supplemented at 1 g/ 100 kcal.

Diet Delivery

After consideration of the type of diet on the basis of disease process and route of enteral feeding, the diet should be introduced slowly to provide assessment of gastrointestinal function. Tolerance of enteral feeding may be assessed by absence of nausea, vomiting, and abdominal discomfort and bloating, auscultation of gut sounds, and lack of gastric residual fluid (if a gastric tube is in place). In general, the institution of enteral support should parallel the onset of malnutrition, taking into consideration structural or functional deficits of the gastrointestinal tract. In some patients with acute illness and injury, full nutritional support may be instituted within 2 days, whereas a chronically malnourished patient may require a slower introduction.

Delivery factors that will increase tolerance include feeding in frequent but smaller volumes, using an isosmolar formula (required for J-tube), feeding slowly, feeding warmed (room temperature) formula, and starting with 1/4 to 1/3 of the calculated caloric requirement. If feeding is tolerated, the frequency and amount may be increased in a step-wise fashion.

Enteral tube size and location will also dictate the type of diet used and the method of delivery. Smaller bore enteral feeding tubes (NE- and J-tube <12F) necessitate liquid formulations, while larger tubes (E- and G-tube >12F) allow blenderized or homogenized diets to be used. Regardless, all feeding tubes should be flushed with a small volume of water or isotonic crystalloid before and after feeding to prevent clogging. Enteral tubes that are placed in the post-pyloric region require continuous infusion because of minimum gut reservoir capacity. Continuous infusion feeding can also be used with NE, NG, E-tubes, and G-tubes if bolus feeding is not tolerated.

Enteral product volume needs to be considered when calculating total fluid input, especially in patients sensitive to fluid overload (cardiac patients).

Complications

Nausea and Vomiting The rapid introduction of a diet or use of a diet high in osmolarity can cause irritation to the stomach or intestine resulting in cramping, nausea, and vomiting. Gastric or intestinal distension due to lack of forward motility may lead to similar clinical signs. Promotility agents such as metoclopramide or erythromycin may increase forward motility.

Pulmonary Aspiration Aspiration may occur in any patient that is depressed or recumbent, lacks airway control, or has pharyngeal or esophageal dysfunction. The risk is heightened in patients that are actively regurgitating or vomiting and in patients that are fed by NE, NG, or E-tube that is incorrectly placed or has become dislodged. The risk of aspiration may be diminished by placement of a jejunostomy tube, concomitant use of anti-emetic and anti-nausea medication, and frequent gastric or esophageal decompression by suctioning.

Diarrhea Diarrhea may develop during enteral feeding. Diets with high osmolarity that are delivered post-pyloric may draw fluid into the gastrointestinal tract in amounts sufficient to overwhelm absorptive capacity. Concurrent use of antibiotics and antacids alter pre-existing bacterial populations or cause bacterial overgrowth leading to diarrhea. In many enteral formulations, the lack of dietary fiber decreases intraluminal colonic production of short chain fatty acids, thereby decreasing the ability of the colon to absorb sodium and water. Patients with severe illness or injury often have multisystemic organ involvement with derangements in blood flow, oxygen delivery, and interstitial fluid dynamics (interstitial edema), which result in malabsorption, maldigestion, and altered intestinal motility. Such changes predispose the patient to diarrhea.

A potentially dangerous source of infectious diarrhea includes the delivery of contaminated enteral products in aged or mishandled formulas. Open enteral products should be refrigerated and discarded after a few days use.

Tube Placement Problems Inappropriate NE, NG, or E-tube placement may lead to aspiration of enteral products or damage to the airways from inadvertent placement into the bronchopulmonary tree. Gastrostomy and jejunostomy tube placement carries the risk of stoma site dehiscence, infection, or leakage of nutrients and ingesta leading to local infection or peritonitis. All stoma and tube sites should be inspected daily, gently cleansed with dilute povidone-iodine solution, and covered with sterile gauze and antibiotic ointment. Nasal tube placement should not be attempted in patients with facial fractures or in patients with high intracranial pressure (induced sneezing may actually increase intracranial pressure).

Parenteral Nutrition

Parenteral nutrition (PN) may be supplied as partial (usually 40%–60% of calories) or total (100%) of calculated requirements.[23,24] Most formulas include the provision of amino acids, triglycerides, dextrose, electrolytes, vitamins, and trace minerals. Individual formulations are calculated to approximate maintenance fluid requirements. Providing partial intravenous nutrient support is especially beneficial in patients unable to tolerate full enteral support and allows a "bridging" until full calories can be administered enterally.

Partial and Total Parenteral Nutrition

Partial parenteral nutrition (PPN) is used for patients expected to have needs for up to 5 to 7 days. Partial parenteral nutrition provides approximately 50% of caloric needs, and is formulated to provide daily requirements for fluid and electrolytes. Although most parenteral formulations are hyperosmolar, the lowered caloric density of PPN allows administration through a smaller, peripheral vein with little risk of thrombophlebitis.

Total parenteral nutrition (TPN) delivers 100% of estimated caloric and protein requirements, although specific amino acid and micronutrient requirements may not be met. Total parenteral nutrition should be administered to patients that are not expected to be able to tolerate enteral nutrition for a period longer than 7 days. The hyperosmolarity of TPN solutions necessitates that they be delivered through a dedicated central venous catheter. Total parenteral nutrition must be started and discontinued in a stepwise fashion to prevent abrupt changes in plasma nutrients, allowing for an appropriate period of metabolic adaptation (*e.g.*, 50% of calories on day 1, full calorie support on day 2).

Parenteral Nutrition Formulation

The calculation of parenteral formulations is based on the energy, protein, fluid, and electrolyte requirements of the patient. The preferred formulation of PN includes the use of individual amino acid (with or without electrolytes added), lipid, and dextrose solutions. Concerns for sterility and difficulties in compounding dictate that most veterinarians use human hospital pharmacies or referral veterinary institutions for their parenteral formulations. Specific recommendations on storage, administration, and compatibility of additives depend on the pharmacy compounding the parenteral formula. Examples of PPN and TPN formula calculation are shown in Figures 15-2 and 15-3.

Parenteral Nutrition Delivery

Vascular Access Intravenous placement of catheters should be done in a sterile fashion (clip, surgical scrub, and placed with sterile gloves). Catheters should be wrapped with sterile gauze applied over the insertion site. The catheter site should be examined every day, and the catheter removed and cultured if evidence of thrombophlebitis is seen. Protective wraps should be changed if they becomes wet or soiled. PPN and TPN solutions should be delivered through a dedicated line with minimal disconnections. A 24-hour supply of PPN or TPN should be connected at any one time, and IV sets and extension sets should be changed daily. An in-line, 1.2-micron filter should be applied to prevent embolization with the lipid component of the PN solution. Since hyperosmolar solutions can predispose to thromboembolism, catheters made from polyurethane or silicone are least thrombogenic.[25] Patients receiving solutions with osmolality >600mOsm (typically TPN) require central venous administration, while PPN can be delivered peripherally.

Complications

Mechanical complications of PN include catheter-related problems. These include catheter occlusion, accidental removal, and line disconnection. If aseptic integrity is suspected, the catheter should be removed and replaced. Thrombophlebitis may manifest as swelling, redness, and pain at the catheter site. Catheter sites should be examined daily and removed (and possibly cultured) if evidence of thrombophlebitis is seen.

Hyperglycemia is a common complication after initiation of PN, particu-

PARTIAL PARENTERAL NUTRITION WORKSHEET

Resting Energy Requirement (RER)

RER (kcal/day) = 70 × body weight (kg)$^{0.75}$

or for animals > 2 kg: RER = [30 × body weight (kg)] + 70 RER = _____ kcal/day

Illness Energy Requirement (IER)

IER = RER × Illness factor IER = _____ kcal/day

Partial Energy Requirement (PER)

PER = IER × 0.50 PER = _____ kcal/day

Nutrient Requirements

For cats and dogs <10 kg:

PER × 0.25 = _____ kcal/day from dextrose
PER × 0.25 = _____ kcal/day from amino acids
PER × 0.50 = _____ kcal/day from lipids

For dogs 10 to 25 kg:

PER × 0.33 = _____ kcal/day from dextrose
PER × 0.33 = _____ kcal/day from amino acids
PER × 0.33 = _____ kcal/day from lipids

For dogs > 25 kg:

PER × 0.50 = _____ kcal/day from dextrose
PER × 0.25 = _____ kcal/day from amino acids
PER × 0.25 = _____ kcal/day from lipids

Nutrient Solution Volume Requirements

5% dextrose = 0.17 kcal/ml _____ kcal/day dextrose ÷ 0.17 kcal/ml = _____ ml/day

8.5 % amino acids (with electrolytes) = 0.34 kcal/ml _____ kcal/day amino acids ÷ 0.34 kcal/ml = _____ ml/day

20% lipid solution= 2 kcal/ml _____ kcal/day lipid solution ÷ 2 kcal/ml = _____ ml/day

Micronutrient Requirements

Multivitamin: Multi-12 Multiple Vitamins For Infusion (Sabex Inc., QC, Canada) : add 1 vial of each water and fat soluble vitamins per 24 hour dose of PPN

Trace minerals: Multitrace 5 Concentrate (America Regent Lab, NewYork, NY): add 1 ml per 24 hour dose of PPN

Total requirements

_____ ml 5% dextrose
_____ ml 8.5% amino acid with electrolytes
_____ ml 20% lipid solution
_____ ml trace minerals
\+ _____ ml multivitamins

= _____ ml total volume of PPN solution

Administration Rate

_____ ml total volume of PPN solution ÷ 24 hours = _____ ml/hr

Figure 15-2
Partial parenteral nutrition worksheet. (Adapted from: Zsombor-Murray E, Freeman LM: Peripheral Parenteral Nutrition. *Compend Contin Educ Pract Vet* 21:512, 1999.)

larly in patients under physiologic stress associated with trauma, surgery, and sepsis because of the insulin resistance characteristic of inflammatory states. The addition of regular insulin in 0.5 units/kg/day increments typically controls hyperglycemia without decreasing the rate of administration. Hypoglycemia may develop upon abrupt discontinuance of PN, especially if voluntary eating or enteral support is not concurrent with PN withdrawal. Patients receiving TPN should be withdrawn over a 2- to 3-day period to prevent this complication. Alternatively, dextrose can be added to an infusion of crystalloids.

Hypokalemia, hypophosphatemia, and hypomagnesemia may develop on

TOTAL PARENTERAL NUTRITION WORKSHEET

Resting Energy Requirement (RER)

RER (kcal/day) = 70 × body weight (kg)$^{0.75}$
or for animals > 2 kg: RER = [30 × body weight (kg)] + 70 RER = ______ kcal/day

Illness Energy Requirement (IER)

IER = RER × Illness factor IER = ______ kcal/day

Nutrient Requirements

1. **Protein Requirement:**

	canine	feline
standard	4 g/100 kcal	6 g/100 kcal
decreased (hepatic/renal)	2 g/100 kcal	3 g/100 kcal
increased	6 g/100 kcal	6 g/100 kcal

______ g/100kcal protein requirement × (IER/100) = ______ g protein required/day

2. **Lipid and Carbohydrate Requirement:**

In dogs: total required kcal/day are divided equally between lipid and dextrose
In cats: calories supplied by protein is subtracted to figure total required kcal/day to be divided equally between lipid and dextrose [protein calories = _____ g protein required/day × 4 kcal/g]

Dog:
IER × 0.50 = ______ kcal/day from dextrose
IER × 0.50 = ______ kcal/day from lipid

Cat::
[IER - protein calories] × 0.50 = ______ kcal/day from dextrose
[IER - protein calories] × 0.50 = ______ kcal/day from lipid

* certain clinical situations may require a different ratio of lipid to carbohydrate

Nutrient Solution Volume Requirements

1. 8.5% amino acids (with electrolytes) = 0.085 g protein/ml
______ g protein required/day ÷ 0.085 g/ml = ______ml 8.5% amino acid solution/day

2. 20% lipid solution = 2 kcal/ml
______ kcal/day lipid ÷ 2 kcal/ml = ______ ml 20% lipid solution/day

3. 50% dextrose = 1.7 kcal/ml
______ kcal/day dextrose ÷ 1.7 kcal/ml = ______ ml 50% dextrose solution/day

Micronutrient Requirements

Multivitamin: Multi-12 Multiple Vitamins For Infusion (Sabex Inc., QC, Canada) : add 1 vial of each water and fat soluble vitamins per 24 hour dose of PPN

Trace minerals: Multitrace 5 Concentrate (America Regent Lab, NewYork, NY): add 1 ml per 24 hour dose of PPN

Total Requirement

______ ml 50% dextrose
______ ml 8.5% amino acid with electrolytes
______ ml 20% lipid solution
______ ml trace minerals
\+ ______ ml multivitamins

= ______ ml total volume of TPN solution

Administration Rate

______ ml total volume of TPN solution ÷ 24 hours = ______ ml/hr
Day 1: begin with 1/2 rate
Day 2: full rate

Figure 15-3
Total parenteral nutrition worksheet. (Adapted from LM Freeman, Tufts University School of Veterinary Medicine Clinical Hospital Notes)

initiation of enteral or parenteral nutrition, especially after a prolonged catabolic state (also commonly seen in diabetic ketoacidotic patients). This condition is termed "refeeding syndrome" and results from a rapid rise in insulin and a shift of plasma potassium, magnesium, and phosphates into the intracellular compartment. Profound weakness, gastrointestinal ileus, vomiting, diarrhea, and neuromuscular and cardiac rhythm disturbances can result. Hypophosphatemia can manifest as hemolysis as the plasma concentrations falls below 2 mg/dL. Hypomagnesemia in its severest form can result in tetany, seizures, panting, and hypertension. Potassium phosphate, potassium chloride, and magnesium sulfate supplementation may be necessary to treat this disorder. Serum electrolytes, blood gases, and glucose should be measured at least once daily during initiation of PN.

A high ammonia concentration is found in patients with deficient deamination of amino acids if hepatic function is overwhelmed. Arginine deficiency, particularly common in cats, predisposes to hyperammonemia; encephalopathic signs can develop.

Hypertriglyceridemia also can develop with the preponderance of catabolic mediators and insulin resistance associated with stress starvation. High triglycerides may overwhelm hepatic metabolism and lead to steatosis. High triglycerides may necessitate reduction of nutrient delivery or alteration of the formula to a lesser percentage of lipid component. Alternatively, the addition of heparin to the parenteral formula may help clear plasma triglycerides by activating lipoprotein lipase.

The administration of hyperosmolar solutions composed of lipid, amino acid, and dextrose solutions provides an excellent growth media for bacteria. Patients showing clinical signs of infection and sepsis should be actively examined for the likelihood of PN solution contamination or catheter related infection. Cultures of PN solution or catheters should guide antibiotic therapy.

REFERENCES

1. Chandler ML, Greco DS, Fettman MJ: Hypermetabolism in illness and injury. *Comp Cont Educ Pract Vet* 14:1284, 1992.
2. Schwartz MW, Seeley RJ: Neuroendocrine responses to starvation and weight loss. *New Engl J Med* 336:1802, 1997.
3. Monk DN, Plank LD, Franch-Arcas G, *et al.*: Sequential changes in the metabolic response in critically injured patients during the first 25 days after blunt trauma. *Ann Surg* 223:395, 1996.
4. Fink MP: Cytopathic hypoxia in sepsis. *Acta Anaesthesiol Scand Suppl* 41:87, 1997.
5. Border JR: Metabolic response to short-term starvation, sepsis, and trauma. *Surg Annu* 2:11, 1970.
6. Souba WW: Nutritional support. *New Engl J Med* 336:41, 1997.
7. Mainous MR, Deitch EA: The gut barrier. *In* Zaloga GP, ed.: Nutrition in critical care. St. Louis:Mosby, 1994, p 557.
8. Deitch EA, Wintertron J, Li MA, *et al.*: The gut as a portal of entry for bacteremia. *Ann Surg* 205:681, 1987.
9. Moore FA, Feliciano DV, Andrassy RJ, *et al.*: Early enteral feeding, compared with parenteral, reduces postoperative septic complications: the results of a meta-analysis. *Ann Surg* 216:172, 1992.

10. Barton RG: Immune-enhancing enteral formulas: are they beneficial in critically ill patients? *Nutr Clin Pract* 12:51, 1997.
11. Herskowitz A, Souba WW: Intestinal glutamine metabolism during critical illness: a surgical perspective. *Nutrition* 6:199, 1990.
12. Shou J: Glutamine. *In* Zaloga GP, ed.: Nutrition in critical care. St. Louis: Mosby, 1994, p 123.
13. Atkinson S, Sieffert E, Bihari D: A prospective, randomized, double-blind, controlled clinical trial of enteral immunonutrition in the critically ill. *Crit Care Med* 26:1164, 1998.
14. Zaloga GP: Immune-enhancing enteral diets: where's the beef? *Crit Care Med* 26, 1143, 1998.
15. Burkholder WJ: Metabolic rates and nutrient requirements of sick dogs and cats. *J Am Vet Med Assoc* 206:614, 1995.
16. Waddell LS, Michel KE: Critical care nutrition: routes of feeding. *Clin Tech Small Anim Pract* 13:197, 1998.
17. Crowe DT: Clinical use of an indwelling nasogastric tube for enteral nutrition and fluid therapy in the dog and cat. *J Am Anim Hosp Assoc* 22:675, 1986.
18. Rawlings CA: Percutaneous placement of a midcervical esophagostomy tube: new technique and representative cases. *J Am Anim Hosp Assoc* 29:526, 1993.
19. Bright RM, Burrows CF: Percutaneous endoscopic tube gastrostomy in dogs. *Am J Vet Res* 49:629, 1988.
20. Fulton RB, Dennis JS: Blind percutaneous placement of a gastrostomy tube for nutritional support in dogs and cats. *J Am Vet Med Assoc* 201:697, 1992.
21. Mauterer JV, Abood SK, Buffington CA, *et al.*: New technique and management guidelines for percutaneous nonendoscopic tube gastrostomy. *J Am Vet Med Assoc* 205:574, 1994.
22. Orton EC: Enteral hyperalimentation administered via needle catheter jejunostoma as an adjunct to cranial abdominal surgery in dogs and cats. *J Am Vet Med Assoc* 188:1406, 1986.
23. Zsombor-Murray E, Freeman LM: Peripheral parenteral nutrition. *Compend Contin Educ Pract Vet* 21:512, 1999.
24. Remillard RL: Parenteral nutrition. *In* DiBartola SP, ed.: Fluid therapy in small animal practice, 2nd ed. Philadelphia: WB Saunders, 2000, p 465.
25. Pottecher T, Forrler M, Picardat, et al: Thrombogenicity of central venous catheters: prospective study of polyethylene, silicone and polyurethane catheters with phlebography or post-mortem examination. *Eur J Anaesth* 1:361, 1984.

SUGGESTED READING

Mazzaferro E: Esophagostomy tubes: Don't underutilize them! *J Vet Emerg Crit Care* 11: 153, 2001.

16
Cancer Cachexia

Martin J. Fettman

"Cachexia" is derived from the Greek words *kakos* (bad) and *hexis* (condition) and is generally used to describe any condition resulting in progressive wasting of host tissue. Cachexia is often a contributing cause of death in malignancy. Recent studies have demonstrated a strong inverse relationship between body mass and mortality in seriously ill, hospitalized patients. The most prevalent disease categories were acute respiratory failure/multiple organ failure, chronic obstructive pulmonary disease/congestive heart failure/cirrhosis, coma, and cancer. Prognostic variables included serum albumin concentration, amount of weight loss before admission, clinical score, number of comorbid conditions, a diagnosis of cancer, and body mass index (BMI). Patients with a BMI at the 15th percentile or less incurred up to a 57% increase in risk for mortality.

Reduced food intake by cancer patients clearly contributes to body mass loss. Involvement of the gastrointestinal tract in the neoplastic process may directly impair food intake and nutrient assimilation. Extraintestinal cancer causes physical pain and emotional distress that also impair appetite. Aggressive antineoplastic therapy also is associated with nausea, vomiting, and malaise. Some paraneoplastic syndromes include release by the tumor of appetite-suppressing peptides. Healthy individuals typically respond to decreased food intake with an adaptive decrease in metabolic rate, thereby conserving nutrient stores and ameliorating the progression of weight loss. Although this process is multifactorial in origin, suppression of thyroid hormone activity often contributes to adaptive decreases in metabolic rate. In some syndromes of this so-called "euthyroid sick syndrome," function of the hypothalamic-pituitary-thyroid axis may be normal, but peripheral monodeiodination of thyroxine (T_4) to triiodothyronine (T_3) is abnormal, leading to decreased production of T_3 and increased production of reverse T_3 (rT_3). Glucocorticoids released in response to stress can diminish pituitary responsiveness to thyroid-releasing hormone, decrease thyroid-stimulating hormone and thyroid hormone release, reduce numbers of T_3 receptors in target tissues, and inhibit peripheral monodeiodination of T_4 to T_3.

Metabolic derangements in patients with cancer may also include untoward increases in resting metabolic rate, despite reductions in food intake. In those cases where overall metabolic rate is unchanged or decreased, substrate partitioning between metabolic pathways may undergo significant changes resulting in loss of lean body mass or futile cycling of substrates and energy expenditure for nonproductive purposes. Finally, when tumor burden is sufficient, diversion of nutrients away from the host may lead to loss of body mass and growth and metastasis of the neoplasm instead. Thus, the definition of "cancer cachexia" has come to include not only loss of body mass, but also the panoply of changes in endocrine and metabolic function often associated with neoplasia.

ENERGY METABOLISM

Loss of body mass in patients with cancer is caused by negative energy balance. Whether they lose weight primarily because of anorexia or increased energy expenditure is controversial. One might expect an adaptive decrease in metabolic rate in response to prolonged reductions in food intake. However, tumor-induced alterations in intermediary metabolism may also accelerate metabolic rate owing to changes including increased glucose recycling, elevated protein turnover in certain tissue compartments, and increased fat oxidation. Tumor cells themselves may release inflammatory cytokines, as will activated host lymphocytes and macrophages. These cytokines include interleukin-1 (IL-1), interleukin-6 (IL-6), tumor necrosis factor-α (TNF-α), and interferon-γ (IFN-γ). These cytokines, in turn, may directly stimulate host catabolism, or may elicit the release of host glucocounterregulatory hormones (GCRH) that promote catabolic processes.

Increases in energy expenditure of 10% to 20% are documented in both weight-losing and weight-stable human cancer patients compared with either weight-losing or weight-stable controls with nonneoplastic disorders. Cancers associated with elevated energy expenditure have included testicular, hepatic, colonic, gastric, esophageal, pancreatic, salivary, prostatic, gallbladder, ovarian, renal, and non–small-cell lung carcinomas. Controls without increases in energy expenditure principally included arteriosclerosis, peptic ulcer, cholecystitis, anorexia nervosa, Crohn's disease, nonviral hepatitis, and a variety of miscellaneous disorders. In these studies, in addition to overall metabolic rate, rates of fat oxidation are significantly increased in the cancer patients despite counterregulatory decreases in thyroid hormone secretion. In a study specifically evaluating cachectic patients with pancreatic cancer, resting energy expenditure was significantly greater in those with an acute-phase reactant protein (APRP) response than in those without such a response. Spontaneous production of TNF-α and IL-6 by isolated peripheral blood mononuclear cells was also greater in those patients with an APRP response, perhaps accounting for the observed changes in metabolism.

However, other studies have demonstrated wide variability in resting energy expenditure among patients with the same type of malignancy. Dempsey and coworkers reviewed 14 prior studies of energy expenditure in human cancer patients; approximately 50% are hypermetabolic (~120% of normal), 25% are normometabolic, and 25% are hypometabolic (~80% of normal). Their own study of colorectal cancer patients reveals a similar distribution. Some studies have shown that individuals with gastrointestinal cancer are predominantly hypometabolic or normometabolic and that diet-induced thermogenesis is reduced by more than one half in patients losing weight. However, these studies may represent the concurrent effects of tumor-induced increases in metabolic rate and adaptive decreases in metabolic rate by the anorectic or malnourished host with gastrointestinal cancer. In a large study of patients with gastrointestinal, gynecologic, or genitourinary malignancies, 33% were hypometabolic, 41% normometabolic, and 26% hypermetabolic, regardless of tumor site, burden, or histologic diagnosis. It is notable that hypermetabolic patients had a significantly longer duration of disease (33 versus 13 months) than normometabolic patients, although cause and effect could not be discerned from the study.

METABOLIC DERANGEMENTS

Lipid Metabolism

Many specific alterations in intermediary metabolism have been observed in humans and animals with cancer cachexia (Fig. 16-1). In the area of lipid metabolism, body fat content is decreased, owing to increases in the rates of lipolysis and decreases in the rates of lipogenesis. Serum levels of lipids, including triglycerides and free fatty acids, may be increased. These changes may be observed independent of changes in the serum levels of the GCRH and insulin that affect lipid metabolism. For instance, adipose tissue lipoprotein lipase activity is shown to decrease in cancer patients, thereby limiting fat uptake from the blood for storage. Increases in the GCRH, such as glucagon, adrenocorticotropin, and the glucocorticoids would be expected to increase target cell adenylate cyclase activ-

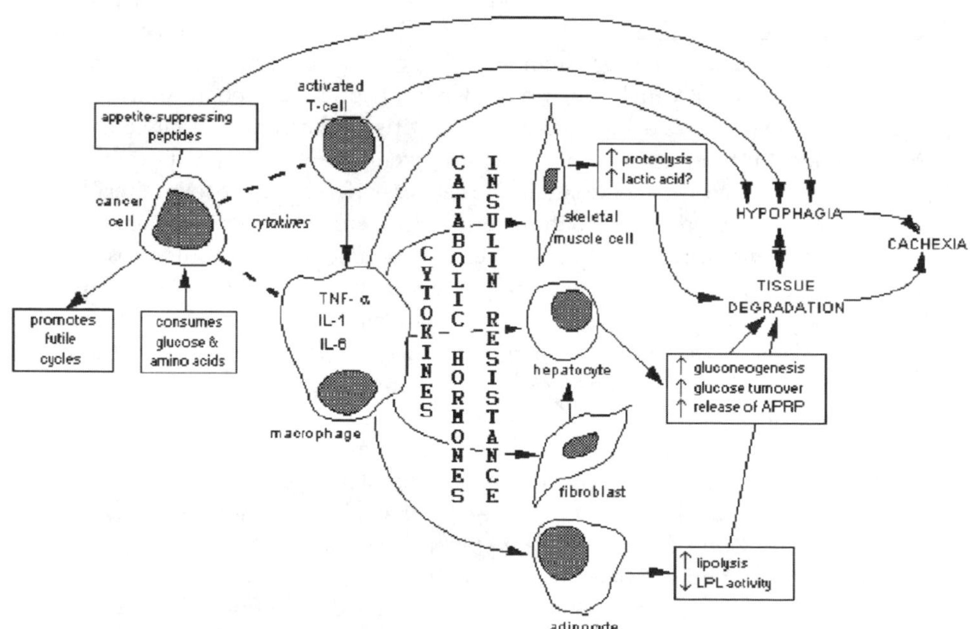

Figure 16-1
Overview of metabolic changes associated with cancer cachexia. (Modified from Douglas RG, Shaw JHF: Metabolic effects of cancer. *Br J Surg* 77:246, 1990.)

ity, cyclic adenosine monophosphate levels, and hormone-sensitive lipase. Decreases in insulin release or increases in insulin resistance, mediated by the GCRH, would contribute to increased lipolysis, as well as decreased lipogenesis. Increased lipid metabolism may also contribute to antagonism of insulin's glucoregulatory actions through the glucose-fatty acid cycle. Cancer patients with weight loss typically display higher rates of free fatty acid release from tissue stores and higher rates of fat oxidation than weight-stable cancer patients or weight-losing patients with nonmalignant diseases. Patients with hepatic metastases also have greater fat oxidation rates than patients with localized malignant disease. It seems unlikely that the malignant tissue itself is responsible for increased fat utilization in cancer patients. Rather, the cytokine and endocrine responses mediate systemic changes toward the preferential use of lipid for energy.

Alterations are also observed in the lipoprotein profiles of dogs with lymphoma. Untreated dogs with lymphoma have significantly higher serum concentrations of very low-density lipoprotein (VLDL), cholesterol, VLDL triglyceride, LDL triglyceride, and high-density lipoprotein (HDL) triglyceride, and significantly lower serum concentrations of HDL cholesterol. With the exception of HDL cholesterol, these parameters are not significantly improved during remission induced by doxorubicin treatment, and triglyceride levels increased further when the patients relapsed and developed overt signs of cancer cachexia.[7]

Carbohydrate Metabolism

Although serum glucose levels may be variable, whole body glucose turnover and glucose recycling through three-carbon intermediates (alanine, pyruvate, lactate) are usually increased in cancer patients. Higher blood lactic acid concentrations are often observed, as well as greater intolerance to exogenous lactate administration (lactated Ringer's solution). Body glycogen mass is often decreased, with the glucose derived from higher resting rates of gluconeogenesis being diverted to incomplete oxidation by the host tissues or by the tumor itself. Under the endocrine conditions of high GCRH and insulin antagonism, it is not surprising that more glucose undergoes incomplete oxidation and subsequent recycling. Both the GCRH and higher free fatty acid levels can obstruct complete glucose metabolism through glycolysis and pyruvate decarboxylation to acetyl-coenzyme A for oxidation by the tricarboxylic acid cycle. Thus, more three-carbon intermediates like lactic acid are released and recycled, resulting in a futile cycle and energy wasting. Weight loss secondary to uncomplicated starvation is associated with reduced rates of glucose turnover, whereas cancer patients with progressive weight loss or the largest tumor burdens typically have the highest levels of hepatic gluconeogenesis and glucose recycling.

When insulin release by the endocrine pancreas is not impaired, it is common to observe resting hyperinsulinemia and exuberant insulin responses to an oral or intravenous glucose challenge. This is similar to what is observed in non-insulin–dependent diabetes mellitus and obesity, or in septic and shock states. The former have been associated with insulin antagonism by higher resting GCRH levels or increased fatty acid metabolism. The latter are associated, as well, with release of insulin-antagonistic inflammatory cytokines from activated mononuclear cells. All of these mechanisms are thought to exist in cancer patients. Increased rates of glucose recycling in cancer patients are linked to rates of body mass loss. One group estimated that if the incomplete oxidation of glucose is substituted by the complete oxidation of fat, it would lead to an increase in energy expenditure of up to 300 kcal/d, and loss of up to 0.9 kg fat per month.

In studies of dogs with lymphoma or with nonhematopoietic malignancies, resting energy expenditure, measured by indirect calorimetry, is not significantly different from healthy controls. However, insulin resistance and hyperlactatemia are evident at rest and following an intravenous glucose tolerance test (IV GTT). More importantly, these changes are not abated when dogs are rendered free of gross evidence of malignancy following chemotherapy or surgery. This indicates that derangements in carbohydrate metabolism observed in cancer patients are not dependent on the presence of a large tumor burden and are likely due to persistent, induced changes in host intermediary metabolism. Conventional chemotherapy (doxorubicin) for lymphoma and surgery for nonhematopoietic malignancies are not sufficient to return host metabolism to normal, and additional therapies may be required to achieve normalization of metabolism.

Protein Metabolism

Whole body protein loss in cancer cachexia patients is manifest by both skeletal muscle atrophy and onset of hypoalbuminemia. Net protein loss and negative nitrogen balance may be observed in individuals who maintain calorie and nitrogen intake. Even in patients who maintain positive nitrogen balance, diversion of amino acids from one metabolic pool to another may result, nonetheless, in muscle wasting or hypoalbuminemia. Reduced levels of whole body protein synthesis, catabolism, and turnover are typically expected in patients with decreased food intake. Instead, tumor-bearing patients appear to lose normal control of protein turnover, consuming lean body mass to release amino acids at an increased rate. These amino acids are then diverted to "non-useful" purposes, including increased protein synthesis by the growing tumor itself, deamination and gluconeogenesis by the liver and kidneys, or synthesis of acute phase reactant proteins by the liver.

A large study of whole body carbon 14-labeled leucine kinetics demonstrated about 50% higher rates of whole body protein catabolism in weight-losing cancer patients than in weight-stable cancer patients or those with benign disease. Whole body protein synthesis is also increased, though to a lesser extent. Fractional synthetic rates of protein in muscle, liver, and albumin are increased, but not enough to compensate for the rates of protein catabolism. Nodal or systemic metastases also progressively increase protein turnover rates. Other studies have shown that depression of muscle protein synthesis is the principal cause for muscle wasting in cancer cachexia. One group reported a six-fold reduction in the rates of muscle protein synthesis, even though whole body protein synthesis is unaffected. A more recent study of cachectic human patients with gastric carcinoma observed a three-fold reduction in the rate of muscle protein synthesis, with no changes in muscle protein breakdown or whole body protein synthesis and breakdown. These studies make the case for substrate partitioning; amino acids that would otherwise be used to maintain muscle mass are instead used by other tissues, including the tumor itself and the liver. Because amino acids are diverted to tumor protein synthesis or hepatic APRP synthesis, whole body protein synthetic rates may undergo little, if any change.

There is also evidence for increased rates of amino acid oxidation, and this proceeds at rates two-fold higher than in healthy controls, even when alternative substrates, like exogenous glucose, are administered. However, some evidence suggests that total parenteral nutrition, including exogenous amino acids, can be as effective in suppressing endogenous protein catabolism in weight-losing cancer patients as it is in weight-stable cancer patients or anorectic patients with benign disease. Supplemental branched-chain amino acids (BCAA), in particular, appear to be taken up preferentially by muscle to supply oxaloacetate and maintain oxidation by the tricarboxylic acid cycle. Catabolism of endogenous muscle proteins is spared by supplying exogenous BCAA, thereby improving nitrogen balance.

Possible mechanisms of cancer cachexia are shown in Figure 16-2.

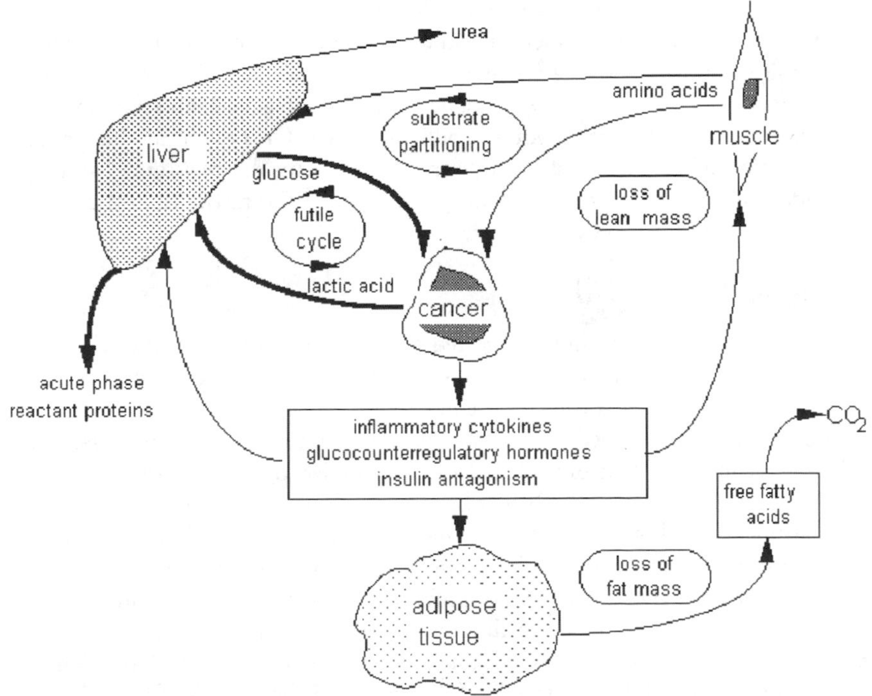

Figure 16-2

Possible mechanisms of cancer cachexia. (Modified from Norton JA, Thom AK: Parenteral nutrition and the patient with cancer. *In* Rombeau JL, Caldwell MD, eds.: Parenteral Nutrition, 2nd ed. Philadelphia: WB Saunders, 1993, chap 26.)

DIETARY THERAPY

Energy Requirements

Resting energy expenditure has been measured in dogs with lymphoma and with nonhematopoietic malignancies and is not different from healthy dogs. Despite substrate partitioning to alternate pathways of intermediary metabolism or to tumor growth, dietary energy requirements do not appear to be increased in dogs with cancer. However, if appropriate antineoplastic therapy and specific nutritional support as described below are unsuccessful in maintaining body mass, increased dietary caloric intake may be indicated. However, alterations in diet composition appear to be more therapeutically useful, at least for canine patients with lymphoma, than changes in overall nutrient/caloric quantity.

Carbohydrate Versus Fat

Two concurrent sets of observations support the use of high-fat rather than high-carbohydrate diets to treat cancer cachexia patients.

1. Cancer patients display insulin resistance, carbohydrate intolerance when challenged with an oral or IV GTT, and hyperlactatemia when challenged with an oral dietary carbohydrate tolerance test.
2. Tumor cells are developmentally immature and do not have large numbers of mitochondria for oxidative metabolism, often outgrow their vascular (and oxygen) supply, and typically produce much lactic acid from anaerobic glycolysis following a carbohydrate challenge. High-fat diets limit the amount of lactic acid produced, ameliorate the degree of insulin resistance, and provide a substrate that is preferentially used by the host, rather than the cancer tissue for oxidative energy metabolism.

Omega-3 Fatty Acids

Several studies have now suggested a role for dietary essential fatty acids (EFA) in the development and progression of cancer in experimental models. Following treatment with the colon carcinogen azoxymethanol, mice fed a diet high in ω-3 EFA developed fewer focal areas of colonic dysplasia than those fed a diet supplemented with ω-6 EFA. In rats treated with azoxymethane, dietary ω-3 EFA supplementation with menhaden oil reduced colon tumor incidence and multiplicity at both the initiation and postinitiation phases of carcinogenesis. Replacing dietary medium-chain triglycerides with marine fish oil high in ω-3 EFA significantly reduced tumor growth rate, host weight loss, and toxicity of both cyclophosphamide and 5-fluorouracil in a murine transplantable colon carcinoma model. Studies with a human breast cancer cell line have demonstrated enhanced cell growth in vitro following addition of ω-6 EFA to the medium, and inhibition of cell growth following ω-3 EFA additions, as well as a reduction in the frequency and severity of metastases in vivo when transplanted to nude mice supplemented with dietary eicosapentaenoic acid (EPA) and docosahexaenoic acid (DHA). In those studies, DHA was more effective than EPA, and the effect was attributed predominantly to alterations in leukotriene synthesis, rather than to eicosanoids. Dietary linseed oil supplementation in rabbits, to increase ω-3 EFA intake, stimulated cell-mediated immunity, as measured by the in vitro T-cell proliferative response to the mitogens phytohemagglutinin and concanavalin A. However, in humans, dietary flaxseed oil (and ω-3 EFA) supplementation had the opposite effect, although indices of humoral immunity are improved.

A long-term study of a high-fat, low-carbohydrate, marine fish oil, and arginine-supplemented diet for canine lymphoma patients has been published. This study was designed to evaluate the hypothesis that the experimental diet would improve metabolic parameters, decrease chemical indices of inflammation, enhance quality of life, and extend disease-free interval (DFI) and survival time (ST) in dogs treated with doxorubicin for lymphoblastic lymphoma. Metabolic parameters examined included blood concentrations of glucose, lactic acid, and insulin during IV GTT and diet tolerance tests, as well as resting energy expenditure measured by indirect calorimetry. Indices of inflammation included blood concentrations of α_1-acid glycoprotein (α_1-AG), TNF-α, and IL-6. Response to chemotherapy was evaluated by host body weight changes, DFI, ST, and clinical performance scores. The dogs were fed isocaloric amounts of a diet supplemented with menhaden fish oil and arginine (experimental diet) or an otherwise identical diet supplemented with corn oil (control diet) before and after remission was attained with up to five dosages of doxorubicin. The ω-3 content of the experimental diet was 7.3% dry matter (DM), with an ω-6/ω-3 ratio of 0.3:1, versus the control diet with an ω-3 content of 1.6% DM and ω-6/ω-3 ratio of 7.7:1. Dogs fed the experimental diet had significantly ($P < 0.05$) higher serum levels of ω-3 fatty acids and arginine when compared to controls. Higher serum levels of DHA and EPA were associated with lesser ($P < 0.05$) plasma lactic acid responses to IV glucose and diet tolerance testing. Increasing DHA levels were significantly ($P < 0.05$) associated with longer ST and DFI for dogs with stage III lymphoma fed the experimental diet. Least squares regression analysis suggested that for each 1 μmol/L increase in serum C22:6, the probability of dying by any given time point decreased by approximately 3.7% in stage III patients fed the experimental diet. For an increase in serum C22:6 concentrations of 1 standard deviation (approximately 11.0 μmol/L), the probability of dying by any given time point decreased by nearly 40%. DHA did not significantly ($P > 0.10$) influence ST or DFI in dogs fed the control diet or in dogs with stage IV lymphoma fed the experimental diet. Diet or serum concentrations of DHA did not influence ($P > 0.10$) clinical performances scores or degree of doxorubicin toxicity.

Conclusions

The derangements that underlie veterinary patients' metabolic responses to cancer and its treatment can have an important effect on clinical outcome. Quality of life, DFI, and even survival can be noticeably improved by early recognition of metabolic abnormalities by the critical care clinician. Therapeutic intervention with management techniques to improve voluntary food consumption, gastrointestinal motility, and digestive function are necessary. Selective administration of specific dietary formulations can favor host metabolism over that of the tumors. Certain nutrients have been demonstrated to have a therapeutic benefit above and beyond standard chemotherapeutic management and intensive medical care. In summary, proactive dietary intervention is a mainstay of critical care for veterinary cancer patients.

SUGGESTED READINGS

Baracos VE: Regulation of skeletal-muscle-protein turnover in cancer-associated cachexia. *Nutrition* 16:1015, 2000.

Cersosimo E, Pisters PWT, Pesola G, *et al.*: The effect of graded doses of insulin on peripheral glucose uptake and lactate release in cancer cachexia. *Surgery* 109:459, 1991.

Cravo ML, Gloria LM, Claro I: Metabolic responses to tumour disease and progression: tumour-host interaction. *Clin Nutr* 19:459, 2000.

Dempsey DT, Feurer ID, Knox LS, *et al.*: Energy expenditure in malnourished gastrointestinal patients. *Cancer* 53:1265, 1984.

Dempsey DT, Knox LS, Mullen JL, *et al.*: Energy expenditure in malnourished patients with colorectal cancer. *Arch Surg* 121:789, 1986.

Den Broeder E, Lippens RJ, van 't Hof MA, *et al.*: Nasogastric tube feeding in children with cancer: the effect of two different formulas on weight, body composition, and serum protein concentrations. *JPEN J Parenter Enteral Nutr* 24:351, 2000.

Douglas RG, Shaw JHF: Metabolic effects of cancer. *Br J Surg* 77:246, 1990.

Dworzak F, Ferrari P, Gavazzi C, *et al.*: Effects of cachexia due to cancer on whole body and skeletal muscle protein turnover. *Cancer* 82:42, 1998.

Emery PW, Edwards RHT, Rennie MJ, *et al.*: Protein synthesis in muscle measured in vivo in cachectic patients with cancer. *Br Med J* 289:584, 1984.

Falconer JS, Fearon KCH, Plester CE, *et al.*: Cytokines, the acute-phase response, and resting energy expenditure in cachectic patients with pancreatic cancer. *Ann Surg* 219:325, 1994.

Fettman MJ: Trace minerals and miscellaneous nutrients. *In:* Adams HR, ed.: Veterinary Pharmacology and Therapeutics, 7th ed. Ames, IA: ISU Press, 1995, p 712.

Fredrix EW, Wouters EF, Soeters PB, *et al.*: Resting energy expenditure in patients with non-small cell lung cancer. *Cancer* 68:1616, 1991.

Galanos AN, Pieper CF, Kussin PS, *et al.*: Relationship of body mass index to subsequent mortality among seriously ill hospitalized patients. *Crit Care Med* 25:1962, 1997.

Hyltander A, Drott C, Korner U, *et al.*: Elevated energy expenditure in cancer patients with solid tumours. *Eur J Cancer* 27:9, 1991.

Knox LS, Crosby LO, Feurer ID, *et al.*: Energy expenditure in malnourished cancer patients. *Ann Surg* 197:152, 1983.

Langstein HN, Doherty GM, Fraker DL, *et al.*: The roles of γ-interferon and tumor necrosis factor-α in an experimental model of cancer cachexia. *Cancer Res* 51:2302, 1991.

Norton JA, Thom AK: Parenteral nutrition and the patient with cancer. *In* Rombeau JL, Caldwell MD, eds.: Parenteral Nutrition, 2nd ed. Philadelphia: WB Saunders, 1993, chap 26.

Ogilvie GK, Fettman MJ, Mallinckrodt CH, *et al.*: Effect of fish oil, arginine, and doxorubicin chemotherapy on remission and survival time for dogs with lymphoma: a double-blind, randomized placebo-controlled study. *Cancer* 88:1916, 2000.

Ogilvie GK, RD Ford, DM Vail, *et al.*: Alterations in lipoprotein profiles in dogs with lymphomas. *J Vet Intern Med* 8:62, 1994.

Ogilvie GK, DM Vail, SL Wheeler, *et al.*: Effects of chemotherapy and remission on carbohydrate metabolism in dogs with lymphoma. *Cancer* 69:233, 1992.

Ogilvie GK, LM Walters MJ Fettman, *et al.*: Energy expenditure in dogs with lymphoma fed two specialized diets. *Cancer* 71:3146, 1993.

Ogilvie GK, LM Walters, MD Salman, *et al.*: Resting energy expenditure in dogs with non-hematopoietic malignancies before and after excision of tumors. *Am J Vet Res* 57:1463, 1996.

Ogilvie GK, L Walters, MD Salman, *et al.*: Alterations in carbohydrate metabolism in dogs with non-hematopoietic malignancies. *Am J Vet Res* 58:277, 1997.

Pisters PWT, Brennan MF: Amino acid metabolism in human cancer cachexia. *Annu Rev Nutr* 10:107, 1990.

Sauer LA, Dauchy RT, Blask DE: Mechanism for the antitumor and anticachectic effects of ω-3 fatty acids. *Cancer Res* 15:5289, 2000.

Shaw JHF, Humberstone DA, Douglas RG, *et al.*: Leucine kinetics in patients with benign disease, non-weight-losing cancer, and cancer cachexia: studies at the whole body and tissue level and the response to nutritional support. *Surgery* 109:37, 1991.

Shaw JHF, Humberstone DM, Wolfe RR: Energy and protein metabolism in sarcoma patients. *Ann Surg* 207:283, 1988.

Shaw JHF, Wolfe RR: Whole-body protein kinetics in patients with early and advanced gastrointestinal cancer: the response to glucose infusion and total parenteral nutrition. *Surgery* 103:148, 1988.

Tisdale MJ: Metabolic abnormalities in cachexia and anorexia. *Nutrition* 16:1013, 2000.

Torosian MH, Bartlett DL, Chatzidakis C, *et al.*: Effect of tumor burden on futile glucose and lipid cycling in tumor-bearing animals. *J Surg Res* 55:68, 1993.

Vail DM, Panciera DL, Ogilvie GK: Thyroid hormone concentrations in dogs with chronic weight loss, with special reference to cancer cachexia. *J Vet Intern Med* 8: 122, 1994.

Vail DM, GK Ogilvie, MJ Fettman, *et al.*: Exacerbation of hyperlactatemia by infusion of lactated Ringers solution in dogs with lymphoma. *J Vet Intern Med* 4:228, 1990.

Vail DM, GK Ogilvie, SL Wheeler, *et al.*: Alterations in carbohydrate metabolism in canine lymphoma. *J Vet Intern Med* 4:8, 1990.

Waterhouse C, Mason J: Leucine metabolism in patients with malignant disease. *Cancer* 48:939, 1981.

Weston PM, King RF, Goode AW, *et al.*: Diet-induced thermogenesis in patients with gastrointestinal cancer cachexia. *Clin Sci* 77:133, 1989.

17
Pacemakers

Eric Monnet

Pacemaker therapy is indicated in veterinary medicine for symptomatic bradyarrhythmias including high-grade second-degree atrioventricular (AV) block, third-degree AV block, sick sinus syndrome, and persistent atrial standstill with a slow ventricular escape rate.[1-5] Pacemaker implantation is indicated when clinical signs such as exercise intolerance, syncope, or congestive heart failure are related to the bradycardia. Pacemaker therapy improves cardiac output and prevents sudden death associated with bradyarrhythmias by maintaining the heart rate above a predetermined rate.

PACEMAKERS AND ELECTRODES
Pacemakers

Several types of pacemaker generators and pacing modalities are available. Pacemaker function is identified by a three-letter code (Table 17-1). The first letter indicates which cardiac chamber is paced, the second letter the cardiac chamber sensed, and the third the electronic response to sensing. The most common pacemaker function used in veterinary patients is "VVI" in which the ventricle is the site of both pacing and sensing, and the pacing impulse is inhibited when a naturally occurring heart beat is sensed. VVI pacemakers have a fixed heart rate unless they are demand pacemakers.[5,6]

Demand pacemakers have a piezzo-electric crystal that allows detection of vibration due to in exercising. Once the piezzo-electric crystal detects vibration it sends information to the pacemaker to increase the heart rate.[5,6] A fourth

Table 17-1. Three-Letter Code System to Identify Pacemaker Function

1st Letter Chamber Paced	2nd Letter Chamber Sensed	3rd Letter Response to Sensing
A (Atrium)	A	I Inhibited
V (Ventricle)	V	T Triggered
D (Dual: A + V)	D	D I&T
	O No sensing	O No response

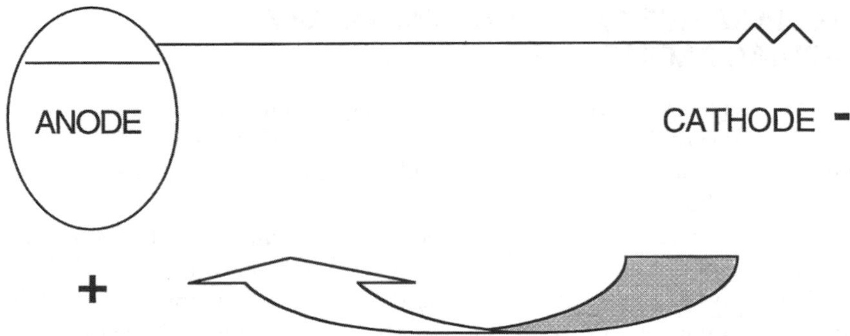

Figure 17-1
Unipolar epicardial electrode. The tip of the electrode is the cathode and the metallic box of the pacemaker is the anode. The electric current has to travel from the cathode to the anode.

letter, "D," identifies such pacemakers. Therefore, unlike fixed pacemakers, demand pacemakers are not limiting the amount of exercise of the patients. Battery life in a pacemaker is usually between 4 to 6 years.

Electrodes

Electrodes may be unipolar or bipolar and can implanted either on the epicardium or the endocardium.[7] With unipolar electrodes the electric current goes from the tip of the electrode (cathode) to the metallic box of the generator (anode) (Fig. 17-1). With bipolar electrodes, the anode and cathode are at the tip of the electrode (Fig. 17-2). Less energy is then required to stimulate a cardiac contraction, which results in a longer battery life. Transvenous electrodes are usually bipolar, whereas epicardial electrodes are usually unipolar. Transvenous electrodes can be used for either temporary or permanent pacemaker therapy.

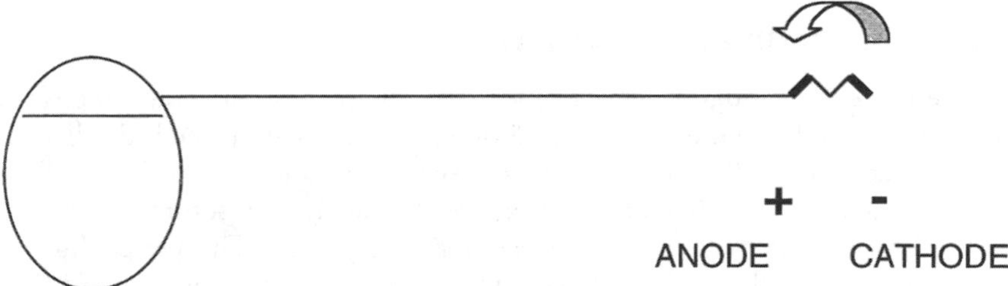

Figure 17-2
Bipolar endocardial electrode. Anode and cathode are at the tip of the electrode. The electric current has to travel from the cathode to the anode.

PREOPERATIVE CARE AND TEMPORARY CARDIAC PACING

Before a permanent pacemaker is implanted, a complete cardiac work-up should be performed with thoracic radiographs, echocardiography, and an electrocardiogram (ECG). Complete blood work should also be done to eliminate any metabolic causes of dysrhythmias.

The heart rate needs to be controlled before implantation of the permanent pacemaker. The natural escape rhythm associated with a third-degree AV block is a slow ventricular rate (30–50 beats/min) (Fig. 17-3). Administration of lidocaine to an animal with this rhythm is contraindicated. Before implantation of the permanent pacemaker, it is also necessary to increase the heart rate either with a temporary external pacemaker or pharmacologically. If a temporary external pacemaker is available, a flow-directed, balloon-tipped, bipolar electrode is introduced into the jugular vein and wedged into the trabeculae of the right ventricle under local anesthesia and light sedation. The transvenous electrode is introduced into the jugular vein through a venous introducer. Transvenous electrode placement can be performed either by monitoring the ECG or using fluoroscopy (Fig. 17-4). Prior to introduction, the transvenous electrode is connected to an external pacing device that is set at 5 V and a rate of 100 beats/min. The transvenous electrode is advanced into the right atrium where the balloon is inflated. The electrode is carried by the blood flow into the right ventricle. The ECG documents capture of the ventricle when the electrode is properly wedged into a trabulae. Fluoroscopy is used to assist with placement of the electrode and confirm its position (see Fig. 17-4).[8] For sick sinus syndrome, the right atrium can be paced instead of the right ventricle. If a temporary external pacemaker is not available, constant intravenous infusion of a β agonist (isoproterenol, 0.01 μg/kg/min) can be used during anesthesia to increase the rate of the escape rhythm, but this method is less reliable.

SURGICAL TECHNIQUE

Intraoperative antibiotic therapy such as first-generation cephalosporin is recommended during pacemaker implantation to reduce the risk of implant infection.

Transdiaphragmatic Approach

Permanent transdiaphragmatic pacemaker implantation is accomplished through a ventral midline celiotomy.[9] Balfour retractors are placed, the liver is gently retracted caudally, and the phrenicohepatic ligament is incised. A midline incision is made in the diaphragm to expose the heart. Stay sutures are placed on the edge of the diaphragm for retraction (Fig. 17-5). The pericardium is opened and retracted with tissue forceps to expose the apex of the left ventricle. A screw-in unipolar epicardial electrode is implanted in the myocardium at the apex of the left ventricle avoiding coronary arteries (Fig. 17-6). The screw-in electrode is turned clockwise into the myocardium with number of turns specified by the manufacturer. Ideally, electrical impedance of the electrode should be

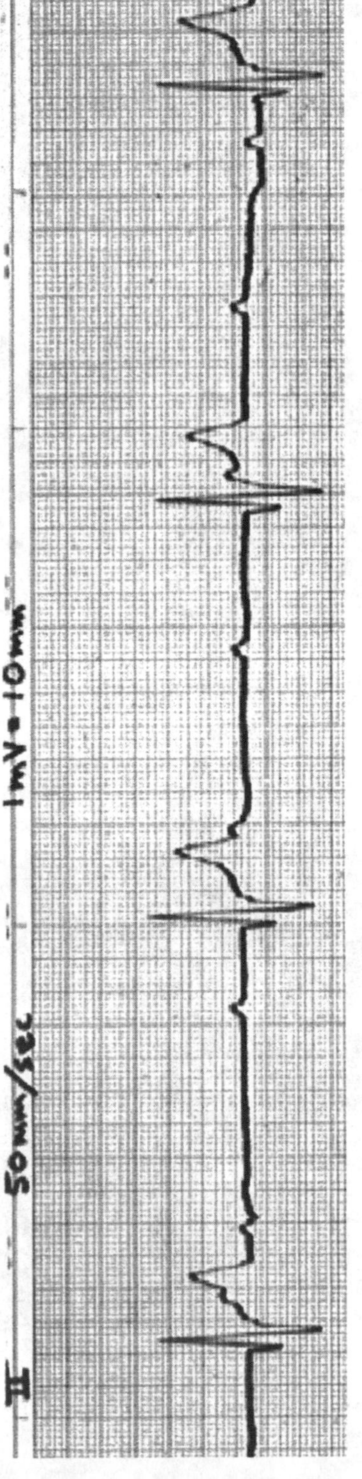

Figure 17-3
ECG of a dog with third-degree AV block. P waves are present and are not associated with a QRS complex.

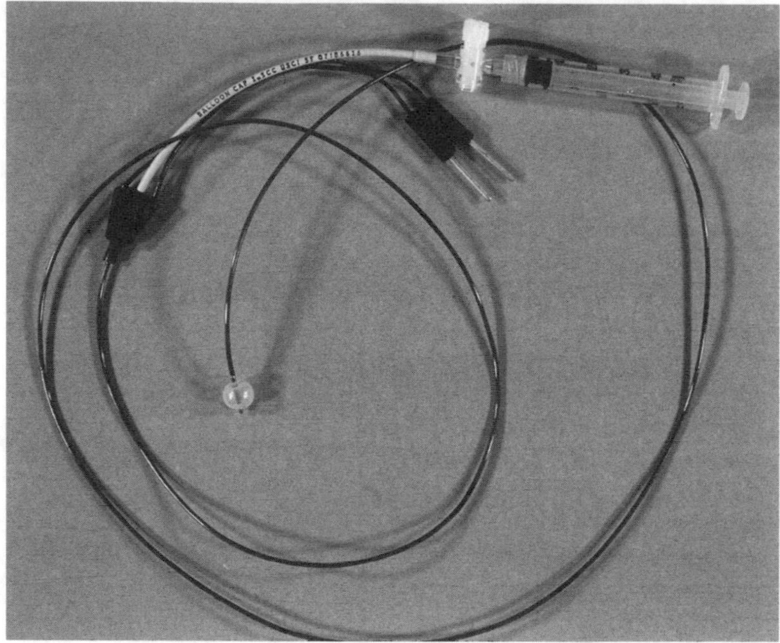

Figure 17-4
Transvenous electrode with the balloon inflated at the tip.

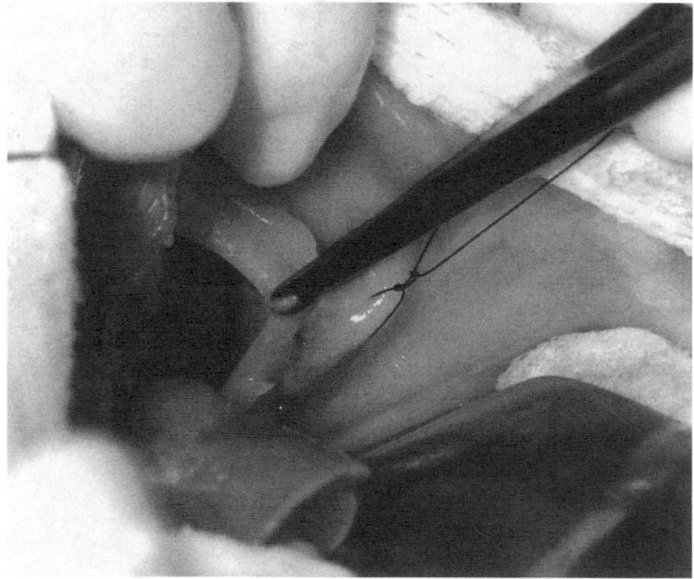

Figure 17-5
The diaphragm and the pericardium have been opened. The apex of the left ventricle is visualized through the incision.

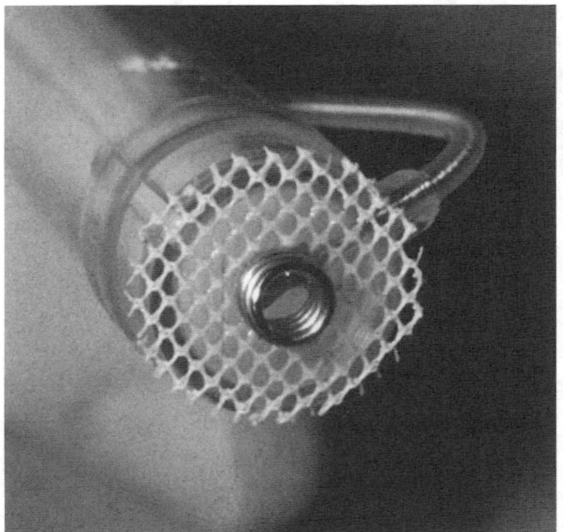

Figure 17-6
Epicardial screw in electrode. The number of turns required to implant the electrode is a specific for each type of electrode.

measured to confirm appropriate implantation of the electrode. Lead impedance at implantation should be between 250 and 1000 Ohms. A broken lead will have an impedance over 1000 Ohms, whereas a leaking lead due to damage to the insulation will have a impedance below 250 Ohms.

The capture voltage (*i.e.*, the lowest voltage at which the heart is paced) also can be determined. The other end of the unipolar electrode is connected and tightly secured with the pacemaker. For the pacemaker generator, a pouch is made between the transverse abdominalis and the internal oblique muscle. As soon as the pacemaker is placed in the muscular pouch the temporary pacemaker is stopped and the permanent pacemaker paces the heart (Fig. 17-7). A subcostal thoracostomy tube is implanted. The diaphragmatic incision, the muscular pouch, and the celiotomy are closed in a routine fashion. Care should be taken not to damage the electrode during suturing.

Transvenous Approach

The transvenous implantation is the less invasive technique and the method of choice.[2,10–13] This technique requires fluoroscopy to confirm electrode placement. After surgical preparation of the left or right lateral side of the neck and the scapular area, the jugular vein is surgically exposed. The jugular vein is isolated and elevated on two silk sutures. A 2–3 mm incision is created with a no. 11 blade between the two silk sutures. The transvenous electrode is then introduced into the jugular vein and advanced into the right ventricle with a curved guidewire under fluoroscopy. Fluoroscopy is used to assist with placement of the electrode and confirm its position. The electrode is screwed into the right ventricular wall according to the recommendations from the manufacturer. The silk sutures are then tied around the electrode. The transvenous electrode is tunneled under the subcutaneous tissue between the scapulae. For the pacemaker generator, a pouch is made in the subcutaneous tissue between the scapulae. The

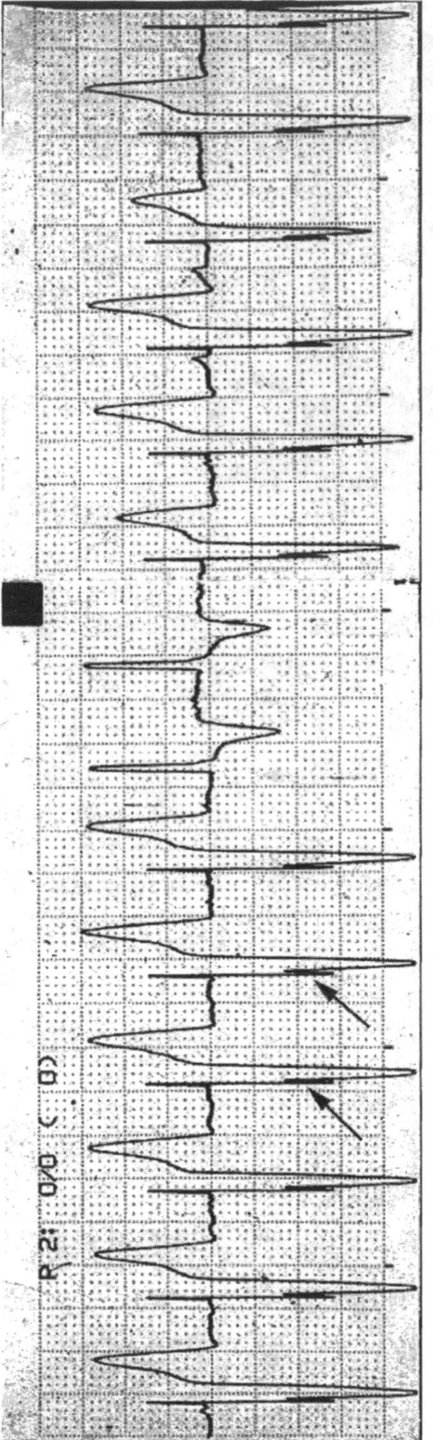

Figure 17-7
Electrocardiogram of a dog with a pacemaker implanted. The pacing spikes are visible on the ECG (black arrows). Normal electrical activities occurred (two QRS complexes in the middle of the tracing). The pacemaker sensed the normal electrical activity and did not send an impulse.

pacemaker is connected to the electrode and implanted in the pouch. For sick sinus syndrome, the right atrium can be paced instead of the right ventricle. Pacing the right atrium allows preservation of the AV synchronization.

POSTOPERATIVE CARE

Pacemakers are usually set at an impulse rate between 80 to 100 beats/min according to the size of the dog and its activity level. After surgery, animals should undergo continuous ECG monitoring for 24 hours to confirm proper function of the pacemaker. The heart rate should not drop below the preset rate of the pacemaker. Ventricular premature contractions often are seen after surgery due to the myocardial trauma from the lead implantation. Lidocaine can be used to suppress ventricular premature contractions but usually is not necessary. The temporary, transvenous lead is left in place for 24 hours as a back-up in case the permanent pacemaker shows problems. The voltage output of the pacemaker is set at two times the measured capture voltage, if known, or at 5 V and 0.5 msec. Lower voltages spare the pacemaker battery.

COMPLICATIONS

Pacing complications are due to failure to capture, failure to sense, failure to capture and sense, or battery failure.[2,3,14,15] Failure to capture is characterized on an ECG by pacemaker spikes not followed by QRS-T complex (Fig. 17-8). Increased lead impedance from fibrous tissue deposition around the lead is the most common cause of this problem. It takes approximately 4 to 6 weeks for sufficient fibrous tissue to develop and create an increase in impedance. The problem is treated by increasing the output voltage. Other causes are a lead fracture, a lead insulation failure, or a lead dislodgment. Failure to sense a nonpaced heartbeat results from a lead fracture, a lead insulation failure, a lead dislodgment, or an increased impedance at the lead-myocardium interface. Failure to sense is recognized on an ECG by the presence of a nonpaced heartbeat between two normally timed paced beats. Sometimes sensitivity threshold can be adjusted to correct the problem. Failure to sense places the animal at risk for competitive tachycardia and ventricular fibrillation. Battery failure is characterized by erratic behavior of the pacemaker (*i.e.*, inconsistent failure to capture, or to sense, or both). Confirmation of a battery failure is usually made after elimination of the other problems. The battery level of newer generation of pacemaker can be measured. A failing pacemaker generator must be surgically replaced.

Pacemakers can be reprogrammed for the rate, the output voltage, and the sensitivity by telemetry. The pacemaker can be interrogated and adjusted with the telemetry unit. If the pacemaker cannot be interrogated a battery failure is suspected.

Pacemaker syndrome results from the selection of a suboptimal pacing mode.[16,17] It is characterized by a reduction of arterial pressure and cardiac output and progression of congestive heart failure. It is most commonly due to a loss of AV synchronization during ventricular pacing or ventriculoatrial (VA) conduction. Atrial contraction contributes to 25% to 30% of ventricular filling. If

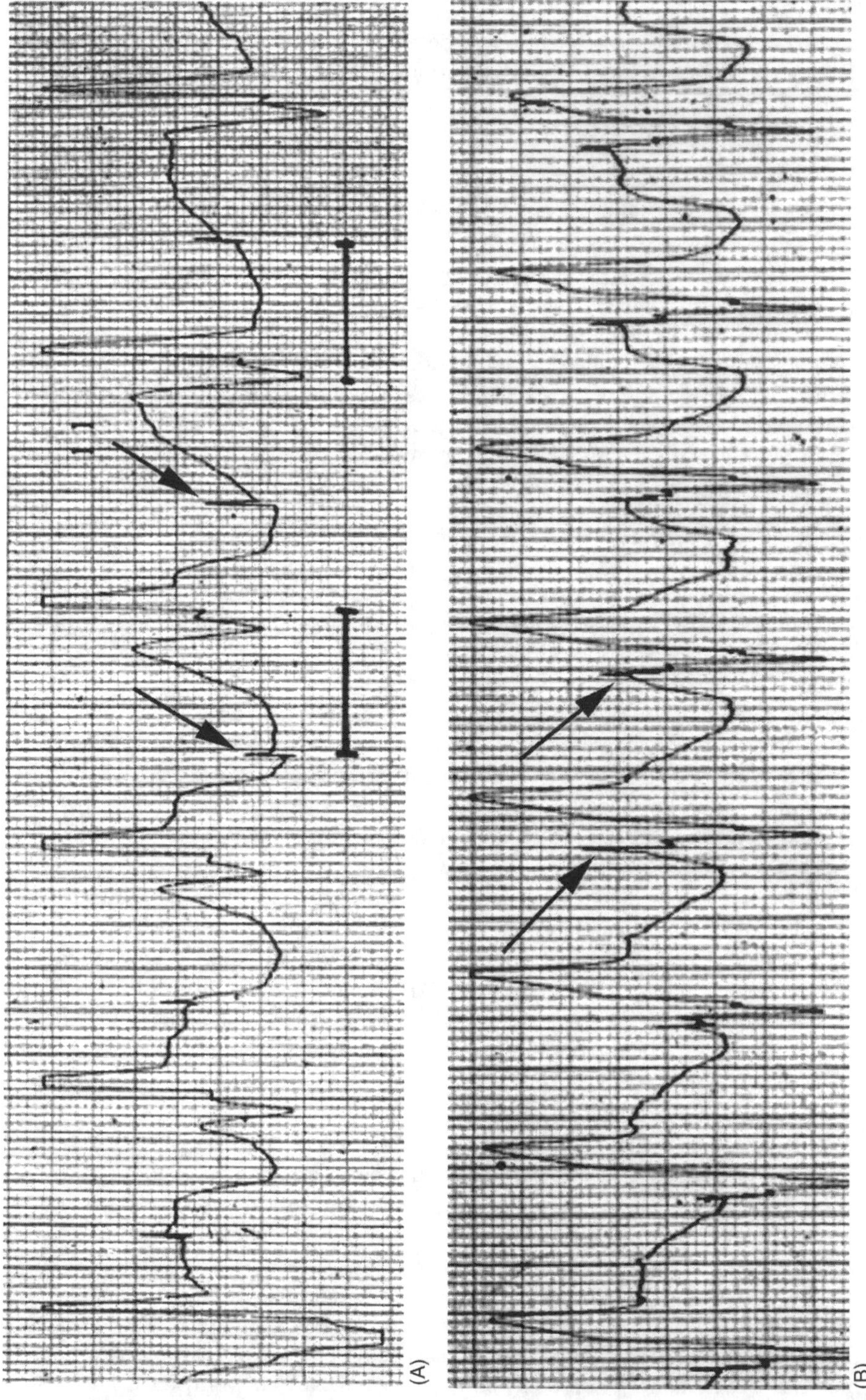
(A)
(B)

AV synchronization is lost, ventricular filling is reduced, cardiac output decreased, atrial pressure increased, and congestion develops. Loss of AV synchronization occurs with ventricular pacing for third-degree AV block and with sick sinus syndrome if the AV conduction is decreased. VA conduction can happen with ventricular pacing and will result in atrial contraction against closed AV valves. It will result in severe atrial dilation and congestion. Pacemaker syndrome can be noticed at the time of implantation when arterial pressure drops more than 20 mm Hg after implanting the pacemaker.

REFERENCES

1. Fingeroth JM: Pacemaker therapy for bradycardias. *Semin Vet Med Surg (Small Anim)* 9:192, 1994.
2. Sisson D, Thomas WP, Woodfield J, *et al.*: Permanent transvenous pacemaker implantation in forty dogs. *J Vet Intern Med* 5:322, 1991.
3. Fox PR, Moise NS, Woodfield JA, *et al.*: Techniques and complications of pacemaker implantation in four cats. *J Am Vet Med Assoc* 199:1742, 1991.
4. Buchanan JW, Dear MG, Pyle RL, *et al.*: Medical and pacemaker therapy of complete heart block and congestive heart failure in a dog. *J Am Vet Med Assoc* 152: 1099, 1968.
5. Moise NS: Pacemaker therapy. *In* Fox PR, Sisson D, Moise NS, eds.: Textbook of Canine and Feline Cardiology, 2nd ed. Philadelphia: WB Saunders, 1999, p 400.
6. Benditt DG, Duncan JL: Activity-sensing rate-adaptive pacemakers. *In* Ellenbogen KA, Kay GN, Wilkoff BL, eds.: Clinical Cardiac Pacing. Philadelphia: WB Saunders, 1995, p 167.
7. Mond HG, Helland JR: Engineering and clinical aspects of pacing leads. *In* Ellenbogen KA, Kay GN, Wilkoff BL, eds.: Clinical Cardiac Pacing. Philadelphia: WB Saunders, 1995, p 1225.
8. Tilley LP, Miller MS,Owens JM: Radiographic aspects of cardiac pacemakers. *Semin Vet Med Surg (Small Anim)* 1:165, 1986.
9. Fox PR, Matthiesen DT, Purse D, Brown NO: Ventral abdominal, transdiaphragmatic approach for implantation of cardiac pacemakers in the dog. *J Am Vet Med Assoc* 189:1303, 1986.
10. Musselman EE, Rouse GP, Parker AJ: Permanent pacemaker implantation with transvenous electrode placement in a dog with complete atrioventricular heart block, congestive heart failure and Stokes-Adams syndrome. *J Small Anim Pract* 17: 149, 1976.

Figure 17-8
ECG of a dog with a pacemaker implanted. The pacing spikes are visible on the ECG (black arrows). Normal electrical activities occurred (two QRS complexes in middle of he tracing). The pacemaker sensed the normal electrical activity and did not send an impulse. (A) Failure to capture. The pacemaker spikes are not followed by a depolarization of the myocardium (black arrows). The electrode was intact because the pacemaker was able to sense the myocardial electrical activity. (B) The output voltage of the pacemaker has been increased to overcome the augmentation of impedance. Each electrical impulse from the pacemaker is capturing the myocardium.

11. Bigler B, Gertsch M, Schupbach P, *et al.*: Implantation of an intravenous pacemaker system in a dachshund with a 3rd grade AV-block and Margagni-Adams-Stokes crises. *Schweiz Arch Tierheilkd* 123:545, 1981.
12. Bellenger CR, Ilkiw JE, Nicholson AI, *et al.*: Transvenous pacemaker leads in the dog: an experimental study. *Res Vet Sci* 49:211, 1990.
13. Flanders JA, Moise NS, Gelzer AR, *et al.*: Introduction of an endocardial pacing lead through the costocervical vein in six dogs. *J Am Vet Med Assoc* 215:46, 1999.
14. Bonagura JD, Helphrey ML,Muir WW: Complications associated with permanent pacemaker implantation in the dog. *J Am Vet Med Assoc* 182:149, 1983.
15. Love CJ, Hayes DL: Evaluation of pacemaker malfunction. *In* Ellenbogen KA, Kay GN, Wilkoff BL, eds.: Clinical Cardiac Pacing. Philadelphia: WB Saunders, 1995, p 656.
16. Ogawa S, Dreifus LS, Shenoy PN, *et al.*: Hemodynamic consequences of atrioventricular and ventriculoatrial pacing. *PACE* 1:8, 1978.
17. Furman S: Pacemaker syndrome. *PACE* 17:1, 1994.

18
Electrocardiography

René Scalf

Electrocardiography is the making of a graphic record that depicts the electrical activity of the heart muscle as detected over time. The electrical activity of the heart is measured by placing electrodes on specific surfaces and measuring electrical potentials between pairs of points. It is also possible to measure potentials from within the esophageal lumen, from within the heart chambers during cardiac catheterization, or from the surface of the heart during thoracic surgery.[1] It has become an indispensable clinical tool that can be used to determine heart rate and rhythm, as well as cardiac arrhythmias and conduction disturbances. Most practicing veterinarians have access to electrocardiograms (ECGs) and are including them in the patient's database.

CLINICAL INDICATIONS

Performing and assessing an ECG gives the veterinarian insight into rhythm and conduction disturbances within the heart, potential electrical abnormalities, the effect of various drugs on the heart, and occasionally anatomic orientation and abnormal chamber size.[1] Therefore, an ECG is indicated in patients not only with primary cardiac pathology but also with certain systemic disturbances, such as hypoadrenocorticism and pheochromocytomas, that can lead to life-threatening arrhythmias. Certain disease states cause severe electrolyte disorders or acid–base disturbances that can alter the depolarization and repolarization of cells and lead to ECG abnormalities.[2] Effective management of heart disease mandates evaluation of an ECG. Patients whose physical examination demonstrates an abnormal heart rate or rhythm should have an ECG performed. Patients presenting in respiratory distress, in shock, or with a history of syncope or seizures are candidates for ECG monitoring. Thus, numerous conditions would benefit from the information gathered from an ECG (Table 18-1). However, it is also important to remember that an ECG must be interpreted in conjunction with all the clinical findings. An animal with severe heart failure or cardiovascular disease may have a perfectly normal ECG.[3] Conversely, a morphologically normal heart can develop lethal arrhythmias.[2] Use the ECG as a piece of the overall puzzle, adding it to existing clinical knowledge, experience, and judgment.

Table 18-1. Clinical Indications for Performing an ECG

Patient history	Syncope Seizures Exercise intolerance
Physical exam findings	Ausculted arrhythmias Heart murmur Gallop rhythms Dyspnea Cyanosis Jugular pulses Shock Muffled heart sounds Pulse deficits
Cardiac monitoring	During anesthesia After anesthesia Preop in older animals During pericardiocentesis
Suspected drug toxicities	Digitalis glycosides Quinidine (Quinidine Sulfate, Key Pharmaceuticals; Quinidine Gluconate, Eli Lilly) β blockers Calcium channel blockers
Serial monitoring in known cardiac patients	Myocardial disease Congenital disease Acquired valvular disease Pericardial disease Heart failure Pacemaker dysfunction Chamber enlargement
Endocrine disorders	Thyrotoxicosis Hypoadrenocorticism Pheochromocytoma
Systemic disorders	Shock Renal disease Pancreatitis Neoplasia Pyometra Trauma
Electrolyte imbalance	Potassium Calcium Magnesium
Acid–base abnormalities	Diabetic ketoacidosis
Radiographic findings	Cardiomegaly

LIMITATIONS OF THE ECG

One should not overinterpret ECGs but rather recognize the limitations set by both the machines themselves and the information provided. ECG machines are designed according to human specifications. For example, the internal electrical filters, which help prevent artifacts on the ECG rhythm strips, are set to strongly attenuate signals above 100 Hz. This is because the majority of the human ECG signal does not occur above 100 Hz. However, feline ECG signals occur mostly at or above 150 Hz and therefore the feline ECG amplitudes are greatly affected by these filters.[2]

The information gathered from an ECG also has built in limitations. For instance, an ECG tells nothing about the mechanical status of the heart. It merely records the electrical stimuli without regard as to whether or not there is a mechanical response.[4] In general, the more severe the ECG abnormalities, the more grave the prognosis.[5] However, this is not a hard and fast rule. Furthermore, an ECG only evaluates the myocardium and records nothing about other important structures within the heart, such as valves and coronary arteries.[5] Finally, in veterinary medicine the wide variations in body conformation among patients makes it difficult to work from a single set of standard measurement values.[5] Not only does body conformation affect values but so does species and breed (consider a toy poodle versus a greyhound ECG or even more dramatic, a Siamese cat versus the greyhound!).

GENERATION OF THE ECG

Depolarization and Repolarization

An ECG records the stimulation (or depolarization) of cardiac cells followed by the relaxation (or repolarization) of cardiac cells. At rest, the surface of cardiac cells are more positively charged than the interior of the cells. This is due to a higher concentration of Na^+ on the outside of the cells. Within these cells there is a higher concentration of K^+. In this state, the resting cells are referred to as "polarized" because they are in a ready state where the electrical charges are stable and there is no electrical flow.[4] During depolarization an impulse triggers Na^+ to rush into the cell and K^+ to depart causing a reversal of the polarized state. Once neutral potential is reached in this reversed state, slow calcium channels open and begin to allow Ca^{++} to enter the cell leading to muscle contraction. Following contraction, Na^+ returns to the outside of the cell and K^+ to the inside. This phase is referred to as repolarization. This information is important to understand when establishing how a directional electrical current is produced in the heart.

Another important key to understanding how an electrical current is produced is related to the properties of cardiac muscle. One of the physiologic properties of cardiac muscle is *conductivity*, which means that activation of an individual cell will produce activity in neighboring muscle cells. Another important property is *automaticity*, which means that cells are capable of initiating their own impulses.[5] Combining the concepts of automaticity, conductivity, and depolarization/repolarization, one can begin to put together how a current is sent through heart muscle.

Specific tissues throughout the heart form a specialized conduction system. The conduction system consists of the sinoatrial node (SA node), internodal tracts, atrioventricular node (AV node), the bundle of His, right and left bundle branches, and the Purkinje fibers. The two important responsibilities of this system are to (1) initiate cardiac depolarization and (2) coordinate the electrical impulse throughout the heart. Based on the property of automaticity, pacemaker cells in the SA node initiate an electrical impulse, which leads to depolarization within the cells in the SA node. Due to the property of conductivity, neighboring cells begin to depolarize. The direction of the wave of depolarization then follows the specialized conduction system. Therefore, the wave should spread down the internodal tract causing atrial contraction. The wave then passes through the AV node to the bundle of His, along the bundle branches, and out through the Purkinje fibers ultimately leading to ventricular contraction. A repolarization wave will follow (Fig. 18-1).

Rules of Current Flow

Depolarization and repolarization create waves of electrical forces with a mean direction after opposite forces are cancelled out. Therefore, at any given moment the majority of electrical current when averaged all together travels in a specific direction. When the direction the electrical force is toward a positive electrode, it will be represented by a positive deflection on the ECG. When the direction is away from a positive electrode, it will be represented by a negative deflection. If the direction is at a 90° angle to the positive electrode there will be little or no deflection recorded (Fig. 18-2). The amplitude of a deflection will be proportional to the thickness of the muscle activated and the proximity of the electrode to that muscle.[5] This information will help in understanding the use of the various lead systems in an ECG.

The Lead System

The primary purpose for obtaining an ECG is to evaluate the electrical activity of the heart. However, because the heart functions within an enclosed three-dimensional compartment, it is difficult to accurately evaluate electrical current direction using only one angle. Consequently, various "leads" are obtained from multiple orientations around the heart. This allows for greater accuracy and localization of problems within the heart.

Knowing that an impulse traveling toward a positive lead creates a positive deflection, and an impulse traveling away from a positive lead creates a negative deflection, one can determine the strongest direction of an electrical wave by moving a positive lead around to various points. Using this premise, Willem Einthoven, a Dutch physiologist, established a fixed lead system that consisted of three bipolar limb leads that formed an equilateral triangle around the heart.[6] When placing the leads on the limbs a true equilateral triangle is no longer formed, but it is close enough for the purposes needed. These leads all lay within

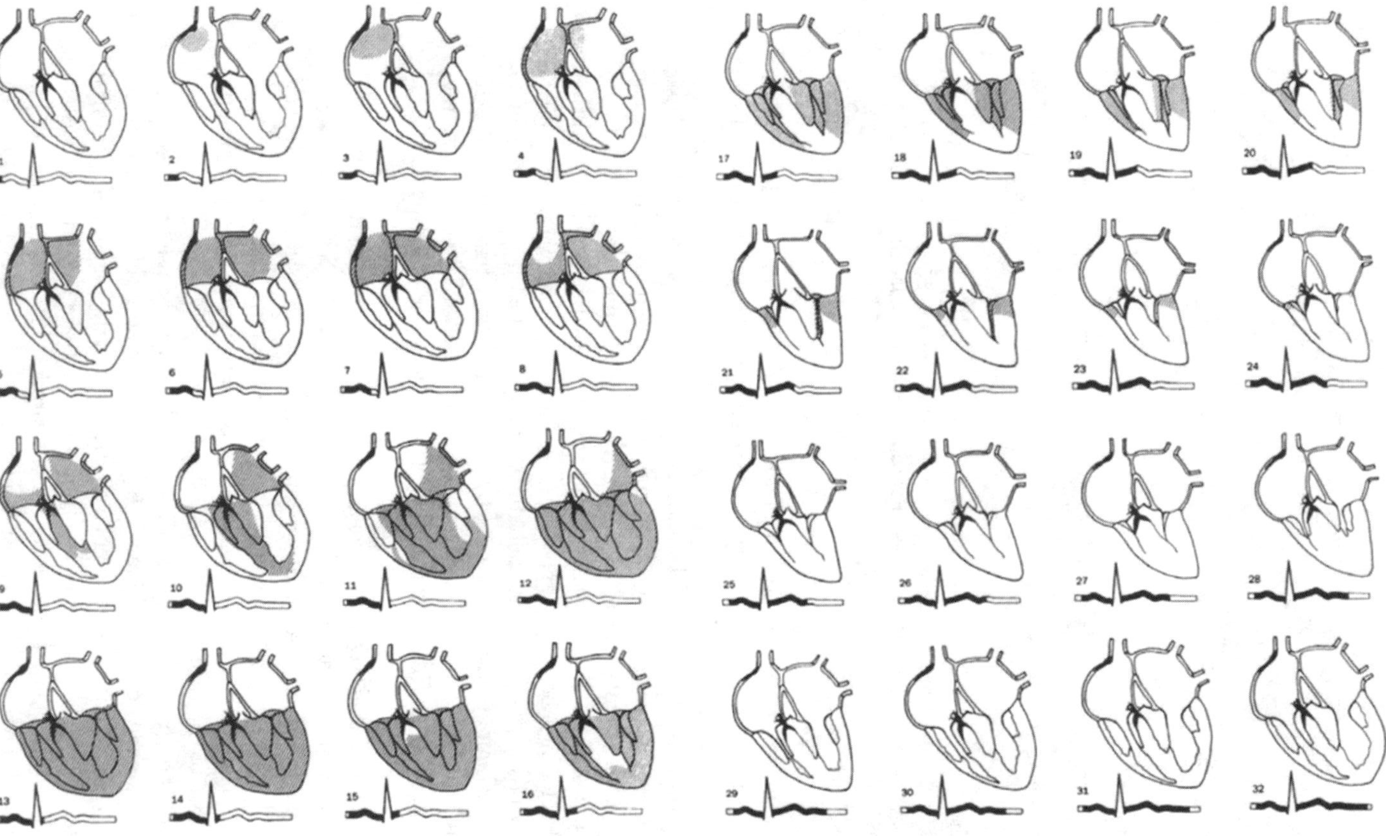

Figure 18-1
Schematic drawings of depolarization and repolarization of the heart and their influence on the ECG. Depolarization is depicted as shaded areas and repolarization is the shaded areas turning white again. (From Hurst JW: Ventricular Electrocardiography, New York: Gower Medical, 1991.)

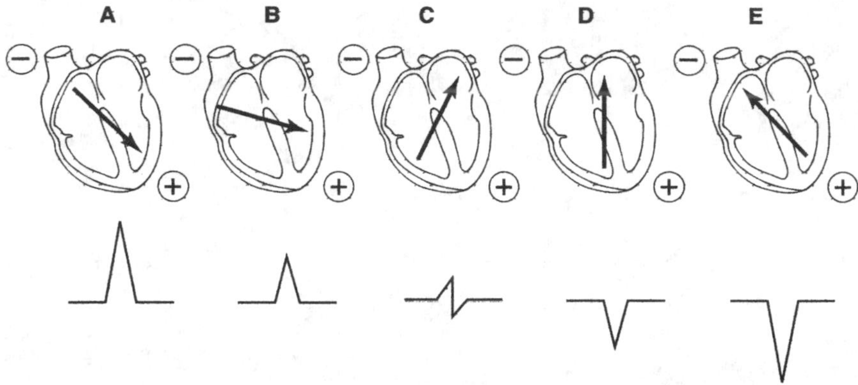

Figure 18-2
The effect of the depolarization wave on the deflection of the ECG. (From Tilley LP: Essentials of Canine and Feline Electrocardiography, 3rd ed. Philadelphia: Lea & Febiger, 1992.)

the frontal plane of the body. Each bipolar lead consists of a positive and a negative electrode, and as a group are referred to as the "standard leads" (Table 18-2).

Expanding on this original lead system, a second grouping of three leads was developed and is referred to as augmented unipolar limb leads. The same electrodes as the bipolar leads are used; however, only one electrode is established as a positive pole and an average of the other two electrodes establishes a neutral reference point (as opposed to using a negative pole).[7] Because a unipolar lead only records one half the voltage of a bipolar lead, the ECG machine will amplify the deflections by doubling their height. This is why they are referred to as "augmented" leads (see Table 18-2). The combination of the standard leads and the augmented leads is referred to as the hexaxial lead system.

The standard leads scan electrical activity over large areas of the heart. This is useful in determining arrhythmias and abnormalities in P-QRS-T deflections. They also play a role in determining mean electrical axis.[5] In contrast, the augmented limb leads scan only specific regions of the heart for directions of electrical activity. Therefore, unipolar leads tend to be most useful in determining the electrical axis of the heart.[5]

A select group of unipolar precordial chest leads can be used to detect ventricular enlargement or bundle branch blocks, or to verify the presence or absence of P waves.[5,8] The chest leads encircle the heart in the saggital or horizontal plane instead of the frontal plane. The three limb leads are left in place to establish a zero reference point at the center of the heart and a fourth unipolar, exploring electrode, is attached to the chest at various locations to evaluate electrical activity. The V_{10} lead is the most frequently used of the precordial leads[5] (see Table 18-2).

Table 18-2. ECG Lead Placement

Bipolar Limb Leads

Name	*Location of Positive Electrode*	*Location of Negative Electrode*
Lead I	Right forelimb	Left forelimb
Lead II	Right forelimb	Left hindlimb
Lead III	Left forelimb	Left hindlimb

Unipolar Limb Leads

Name	*Electrodes Establishing Neutral Reference Point*	*Positive Electrode*
aVR	Left forelimb and left hindlimb	Right forelimb
aVL	Right forelimb and left hindlimb	Left forelimb
aVF	Left forelimb and right forelimb	Left hindlimb

Unipolar Precordial Chest Leads*

Name	*Location of Exploring Electrode*
rV_2	Right 5th intercostal space halfway from sternum to costochondral junction
V_2	Left 6th intercostal space at chondrosternal junction
V_4	Left 6th intercostal space at costochondral junction
V_{10}	7th dorsal spinous process

* In all chest leads the three limb electrodes remain in place to establish a zero reference point (right forelimb, left forelimb, and left hindlimb).[11]

HOW TO OBTAIN A DIAGNOSTIC ECG READING

Positioning and Restraining

When obtaining an ECG reading, it is important to minimize activity surrounding the patient and provide a comfortable surface area for the patient to lie on, using a blanket or padded mat whenever possible. It is imperative that it is a nonconductive surface so as to avoid electrical interference. The patient should be in right lateral recumbency with the limbs perpendicular to the body and slightly separated (Fig. 18-3). Animals in respiratory distress may not tolerate this positioning and the only option may be to record the ECG in sternal recumbency or a standing position. When the animal is not in right lateral recumbency, the ECGs can be used for rhythm and interval interpretation but may not be accurate for amplitude measurements. Young, aggressive, or stressed patients may require chemical restraint, although this is generally not advised. Although wave deflections and electrical axis should not be significantly altered, arrhythmias can be induced by certain drugs, which also must be considered when interpreting results.[5]

Lead Placement

Once the patient is in the proper position, the electrodes are attached using alligator clips directly to the skin, using alligator clips attached to subcutaneous

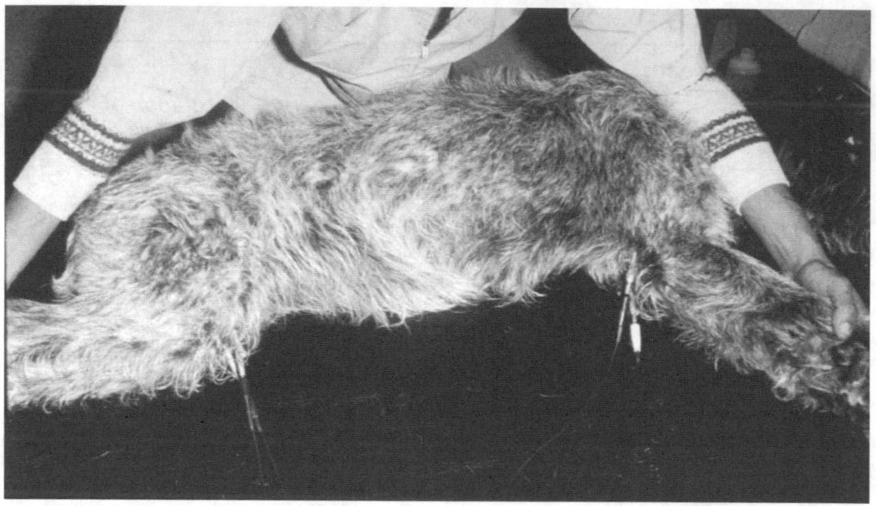

Figure 18-3
Patient in right lateral recumbency with the limbs perpendicular to the body and slightly separated with ECG leads. This is the proper standard position for recording an ECG. (Photograph courtesy of Vicki Matteson, RN.)

wires, via electrode patches, or even metal plates held in place by rubber straps. When using alligator clips directly on skin, it is recommended that the alligator teeth be flattened before they are placed on the patient because the teeth are sharp and induce pain. If it is anticipated that a patient may be in need of a more long-term monitoring of the ECG, then subcutaneous stainless steel wire loops, or electrode patches, are a better choice due to patient tolerance.

For best results, prior to placement of electrodes, the patient's hair should be clipped to allow the most complete contact between the electrode and the skin. When using the alligator clips or subcutaneous wires, shave proximal to the olecranon on the caudal aspect of the forelimbs and over the patellar ligament on the cranial aspect of the hindlimbs.[5] If the patient has respiratory distress or is tachypnic, these sites may have to be moved distally on the limbs. When using the electrode patches, shave either the cranial or caudal area of the carpal and tarsal bones. The patches tend to cause less interference with walking. The use of alcohol, or electrode pastes or gels, will further enhance electrical conduction. Alcohol does evaporate fairly rapidly, so if a prolonged or continuous reading is desired an electrode paste or gel is a better option.[5,9] Most ECG machine electrodes are color coded for placement purposes (Table 18-3). It is important to place these leads in the correct location to evaluate wave deflections.

Recording

Now that the patient is in the appropriate position and the limb leads are attached, it is time to begin recording the ECG. ECGs are recorded on calibrated paper, which is divided by horizontal and vertical lines that are 1 mm apart.

Table 18-3. Lead Color Coding

ECG Lead Color	Placement Location
White	Right forelimb
Black	Left forelimb
Red	Left hindlimb
Green	Right hindlimb
Brown	Chest lead

Every fifth line is indicated with heavier ink. Therefore, the heavier inked squares are 5 × 5 mm. All ECG machines should be calibrated so that complex size can be compared against a standard. This calibration is accomplished using the sensitivity selector. The standard sensitivity is 1 mV = 1 cm, meaning 1 mV of current causes a deflection of 10 small boxes or two heavier inked boxes in height. If the patient being recorded consistently causes the stylus to run off the page, the sensitivity selector can be changed to 1 mV = 0.5 cm. Conversely, if a patient's ECG waves are too small to evaluate the sensitivity can be doubled to 1 mV = 2 cm.

Once sensitivity is established then paper speed should be determined. The two most common choices for paper speed are 25 mm/sec and 50 mm/sec. Most ECGs on dogs and cats are run at 50 mm/sec. However, when running paper speed at 25 mm/sec there is a better opportunity to demonstrate an arrhythmia. At 25 mm/sec every 5-mm box equals 0.2 seconds (200 msec) and every five heavy inked boxes equals 1 second. At 50 mm/sec every 10 heavy inked boxes equals 1 second. This is why it is important to know paper speed when it comes time to determine heart rate and interval duration.

The third point to remember when recording an ECG is to keep the tracing centered on the paper. This is done using the stylus position knob. It may be necessary to make multiple adjustments of the stylus position during the ECG recording and therefore one hand should be kept on the position knob throughout the procedure. Record four or five good complexes in each of the six limb leads at 50 mm/sec and then record a long strip of the lead that produced the largest deflections (usually lead II) at 25 mm/sec.[7] If precordial chest leads are also being run, the recorder will need to be stopped for each placement of the exploring electrode and then restarted.

Continuous Versus Intermittent

Many arrhythmias happen intermittently and therefore checking an ECG periodically will decrease the probability of the arrhythmia being witnessed. Some arrhythmias occur more frequently at slower heart rates (especially premature ventricular contractions) and accordingly may be most likely to be seen when a patient is actually asleep or at least in a very calm state. So, the act itself of moving the patient and placing the ECG leads may be disguising an arrhythmia simply due to the increase in heart rate that ensues with the activity. In

Table 18-4. Continuous versus Intermittent ECG Monitoring

Cases More Suited to Continuous ECG Monitoring
Post-trauma: Especially thoracic trauma
Ruptured bladder/ureter/urethra
Uncontrolled hemorrhage
Head trauma
Postsurgery: Especially splenectomy
Gastropexy due to gastric dilation/volvulus
Any heart surgery
Pacemaker placement
Thyroidectomy
Parathyroidectomy
Pericardectomy
Cases demonstrating unstable arrhythmias that can be immediately life-threatening
Sick sinus syndrome
Multifocal ventricular tachycardia
Third-degree AV block
Paroxysmal tachyarrythmias/bradyarrhythmias
History of syncopy
Severe hypoxia
Pericardial effusion
Pheochromocytomas
Cases More Suited to Intermittent ECG Monitoring
Disease states prone to electrolyte abnormalities
Diabetic ketoacidosis
Hypoadrenocorticism
Renal failure
Certain neoplasias
Urethral obstruction
Patients on long-term cardiac medications
Calcium channel blockers
β blockers
Digitalis glycosides
Angiotensin-converting enzyme inhibitors
Heartworm disease
Hyperthroidism, hypothyroidism
Cushing's disease
Electrocution
Suspected bundle branch blocks

these cases a continuous monitoring of the ECG is more appropriate. On the other hand, when looking for electrolyte abnormalities, bundle branch blocks, or the effectiveness of certain drug therapies, it may be sufficient to check intermittent ECGs (Table 18-4). Hence, it is important to evaluate the purpose of the ECG to determine which is the most effective monitoring protocol, continuous or intermittent.

COMMONLY SEEN ARTIFACTS

Artifacts are distortions of the ECG superimposed over the rhythm of the patient. They are usually due to a technical or mechanical problem and are unrelated to actual cardiac events within the patient. An artifact can severely inhibit one's ability to interpret an ECG.[5] Therefore, it is imperative to recognize and minimize or eliminate these distortions.

Sixty-Cycle Interference

An ECG machine is a piece of electrical equipment that needs to be properly grounded. If it is not, the machine will detect an alternating current from the wires that supply electricity to it, as well as other devices in the room, and record a regular sequence of 60 sharp up-and-down waves per second. This is called 60-cycle interference. There are a number of ways to troubleshoot this problem. First, make sure the power cord is properly grounded by using a three-prong cord into a three-hole wall outlet. Second, make sure all of the electrode clips are clean and securely attached to the patient as well as to the cable going to the machine. A separate electrode may be provided to ground the patient to the machine. This should also be attached securely. Do not use excessive amounts of alcohol in this process. Third, it may be necessary to unplug nearby equipment or turn off fluorescent lights. Electrically heated cages will cause interference and may need to be turned off. Fourth, prevent electrodes from touching together by separating the patient's legs slightly. Finally, make sure there is a rubber mat underneath the patient if you are using a metal surface.

Muscle Tremors

Motion from the patient, either as shivering, muscle twitching, cat purring, or struggling will cause artifacts in the form of irregular motion in the baseline. Therefore, it is essential that the patient be as relaxed as possible. Take time to calm the patient and determine whether it is more beneficial or detrimental to have an owner in the room. Make sure that the electrodes are not causing pain. Sometimes gentle manipulation of the larynx will stop a cat from purring.[5] Also, blowing in a cat's face lightly or waving an alcohol-soaked cotton ball near its nose will deter a cat from purring. If necessary, you can place your hand over the chest wall and apply moderate pressure to minimize trembling temporarily to improve the quality of the ECG recording.[5,9] As a last resort, try decreasing the sensitivity to minimize the artifact.

Wandering Baseline

A wandering baseline is caused by a fluctuation in resistance between an electrode and the patient. The most common cause for this is respiratory patterns and coughing. There are three potential options to correct this problem. First, move the limb leads to below the elbow on the forelimbs and below the stifle on the hindlimbs to minimize chest motion interference. Second, many of these patients will improve greatly if allowed to stand or sit in sternal recumbency instead of lateral recumbency. Although this will affect the evaluation of wave amplitude, it will not affect rate and rhythm interpretation. Finally, try to hold the patient's mouth shut for 3- to 4-second intervals, just long enough to get a decent recording.

Obesity

Obesity will cause a generalized low-voltage QRS complex. The low voltage is due to the increased distance of the heart from the recording electrode.[5]

IDENTIFYING COMPONENT WAVEFORMS OF A NORMAL P-QRS-T COMPLEX

Before evaluating an ECG one should have a basic understanding of the components that make up the P-QRS-T complex including the source of origination and expected duration and deflection.

- *P wave:* The P wave represents atrial depolarization. The width of a P wave delineates the time it takes for an impulse to pass from the SA node to the AV node. In dogs and cats the expected deflection in lead II is positive (Fig. 18-4).
- *PR interval:* The PR interval represents the time in which the electrical impulse is traveling from the SA node through the AV node to the ventricles. It is during this time that the ventricles are filling (see Fig. 18-4).
- *QRS complex:* The QRS complex depicts septal, left, and right ventricular depolarization. Within this complex the Q wave is the first negative deflection, the R wave is the first positive deflection, and the S wave is the first negative deflection following an R wave. If there is no R wave and only negative deflections, this is termed a QS wave. In dogs and cats the overall expected deflection in lead II is positive (see Fig. 18-4).
- *ST segment:* The ST segment represents the early phase of ventricular repolarization. In dogs and cats there should be minimal elevation or depression from the baseline (see Fig. 18-4).
- *T wave:* The T wave represents ventricular repolarization (relaxation). In dogs and cats it may be positive, notched, negative, or biphasic (see Fig. 18-4).
- *U wave:* A U wave is a small deflection that may appear immediately following the T wave. In humans it has been associated with hypokalemia.[5,10]
- *J point:* The J point represents the termination of ventricular depolarization. Usually it appears as a terminal positive deflection within the ST segment.[5]
- *Notching of the QRS:* The QRS is considered "notched" when it displays more than one turning point within the same deflection. For instance, if on the downward side of the R wave there is a momentary deviation in the upward direction that then reverts back to the original direction (down) and continues to the baseline, this is a notched QRS.[11]

ANALYZING THE ECG

When analyzing an ECG it is helpful to get into the habit of following the same steps each time. This will increase familiarity with normal tracings

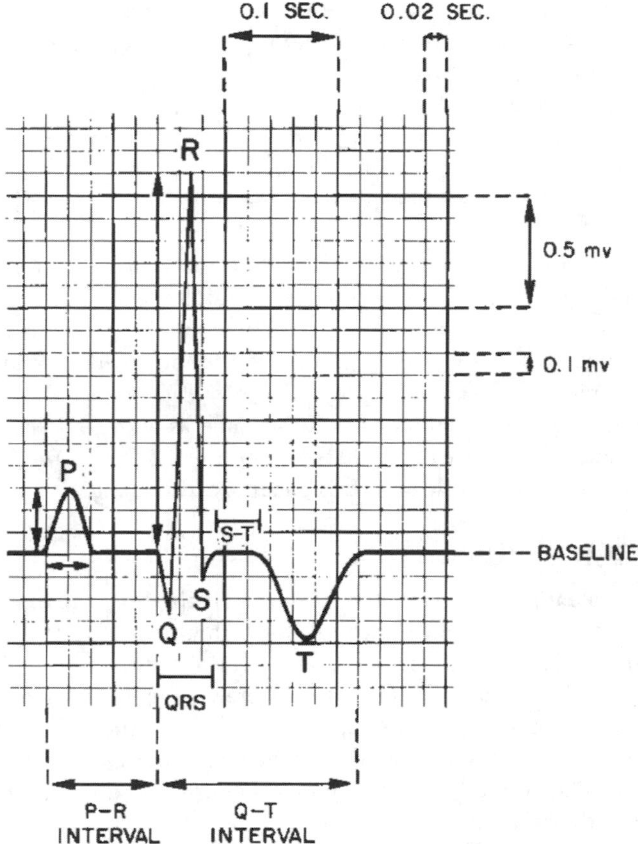

Figure 18-4
Normal ECG complex represented at a paper speed of 50 mm/sec.

and improve recognition of abnormal tracings. The steps include the following: (1) calculate heart rate, (2) interpret rhythm, (3) measure duration and amplitude, (4) identify effects of electrolyte abnormalities, (5) establish mean electrical axis, and (6) identify effects of atrial and ventricular enlargement.

Calculating Heart Rate

Both atrial and ventricular heart rate should be determined using a lead II rhythm strip. There are a variety of ways to calculate a heart rate. Choose the one that is most appropriate based on the following situations.

- When the heart rate is irregular and:

1. The paper speed is 50 mm/second—Starting with the R wave that lines up to the first line of a heavy inked square (the 5 × 5 mm square) count 30 heavy inked squares. This represents 3 seconds in duration. Now count the

number of R waves that occur within this 3 seconds and multiply by 20. This will give you a ventricular rate per minute. You can then do this using the P wave to get the atrial rate.

2. The paper speed is 25 mm/sec—Same as above except multiply by 10 (instead of 20) to get the final rates because 30 squares now equals 6 seconds.

- When the heart rate is regular and:

1. The paper speed is 50 mm/sec—Count the number of small squares (the 1×1 mm square) that occur within one R-R interval and divide that number into 3000 for the ventricular rate. (There are 3000 squares within a 1-minute time span at this paper speed.) Do the same with P-P intervals for the atrial rate.
2. The paper speed is 25 mm/sec—Do the same as above except divide the number into 1500 (instead of 3000) for the rates. (There are 1500 squares within a 1-minute time span at this paper speed.)

Interpreting Rhythm

When evaluating cardiac rhythm, inspect all rhythm strips in every lead recorded. Start with a general inspection for arrhythmias. Do they exist? Are they frequent or do they only occur occasionally? Are they predictable? Is it a regular pattern or irregular? Evaluate the overall complexes for electrical alternans, which is a pattern of alternating amplitudes of the ECG complexes.[12] Most commonly alternans is a variation in height of the QRS complexes.

Second, evaluate the P waves. Are they present? Do they occur at regular intervals? Are they uniform or multiform?

Next, evaluate the QRS complex. Does it have a varying configuration or do they all look the same? Is it wide or narrow? Then evaluate the relationship between the P waves and the QRS complex. Is there a relationship or do they exist independently of each other? Is there a P wave for every QRS and vice versa? Is there a shortened, prolonged, or varying interval between the P and the QRS? Next, evaluate whether the ST segment is elevated or depressed from the baseline. Is there a slurring or coving of the S wave into the T wave? Finally, inspect the T wave. Is the polarity consistent? Are the waves excessively large or small?

Measuring Duration and Amplitude

Measuring duration and amplitude of waves and intervals is the next step in ECG analysis. For this step to be accurate it is necessary for the patient to have been placed in right lateral recumbency with the legs extended at a 90° angle from the body and separated slightly. If this position is not possible, then the measurement of the amplitude will be altered, but duration and interval measurements are still accurate. Calipers are helpful for making the appropriate measurements. When taking measurements do not include the width of the line. Once the width of a wave or interval is known it should be converted into

Table 18-5. Normal Values for Dogs and Cats

	Dogs	Cats
Heart rate (beats/min) Resting to excited	Giant breeds: 60–140 Adult dogs: 70–160 Toy breeds: 80–180 Puppies: up to 220	Asleep (100)–excited (240)
P wave (upper limit)	Width: 0.04 sec Height: 0.4 mV	Width: 0.04 sec Height: 0.2 mV
PR interval	0.06–0.13 sec	0.05–0.09 sec
QRS complex (upper limit)	Width: 0.06 sec Height: 3.0 mV	Width: 0.04 sec Height: 0.9 mV
QT interval (dependent on heart rate)	0.15–0.25 sec	0.07–0.20 sec
ST segment	No > 0.2 mV elevation or depression	No elevation or depression
T wave	Positive, negative, or biphasic	Positive, negative, or biphasic
Mean electrical axis	+40° to +100°	0° to + 160°

(From Kittleson MD, Kienle RD: Small Animal Cardiovascular Medicine, St. Louis, CV Mosby, 1998.)

seconds. The paper speed must be known. (At 50 mm/sec paper speed a 1-mm square = 0.02 seconds and at 25 mm/sec paper speed a 1-mm square = 0.04 seconds.) When measuring amplitudes of waves, the height should be determined in mV (1 mm = 0.1 mV). Table 18-5 lists normal values.

Identifying Effects of Electrolyte Imbalance

Electrolyte imbalance can cause numerous ECG abnormalities. The most important electrolytes related to these abnormalities are potassium (K^+), calcium (Ca^{++}), and magnesium (Mg^{++}).

Potassium is an integral component of electrical conduction at the cell membrane level. Therefore, numerous potential ECG abnormalities may be seen when inappropriate levels of K^+ exist. In the case of hypokalemia, possible abnormalities include a prolonged PR interval or QRS complex (or both), tall P waves, or a flattened or inverted T wave.[13] Sinus bradycardia, first-degree AV block, paroxysmal tachycardia, and AV dissociation are potential arrhythmia's due to hypokalemia.[13] On the other hand, hyperkalemia is associated with peaked T waves, prolonged PR intervals, absent P waves, and prolonged QRS complexes.[13] Arrhythmias that may be noted with excessive K^+ levels include bradycardia, atrial standstill, third-degree heart block, ectopic ventricular beats, and ventricular fibrillation.[13]

Changes in calcium primarily affect QT intervals. In the case of hypocalcemia, the QT interval will be prolonged. In the case of hypercalcemia, the QT interval will be shortened.[14]

Abnormal magnesium levels can cause numerous dysrhythmias. Hypomagnesemia may cause supraventricular tachycardia, torsades de pointes, ventricular tachycardia, or ventricular fibrillation.[13] Hypermagnesemia tends to cause delayed conduction. This will be demonstrated as a prolonged PR interval and may progress to third-degree AV block.[13]

Establishing Mean Electrical Axis

The mean electrical axis (MEA) refers to the average direction of the electrical potential generated by the heart during the entire cardiac cycle.[15] In veterinary medicine this information is used mainly to help determine chamber enlargement and intraventricular conduction defects, such as bundle branch blocks.

There are numerous ways to evaluate MEA. The most accurate (and time consuming) is to measure the net amplitude of the QRS wave in lead I and the net amplitude of the QRS wave in lead III and plot them each on a graph. The graph is meant to be an illustration of the frontal plane of the patient as if it were a 360° circle with the horizontal and vertical axis crossing at the point of the center of the heart. The horizontal axis is labeled with 0° on the right side and 180° on the left side. This would represent lead I in the hexaxial lead system that travels across the heart from the right arm to the left arm. The horizontal axis is labeled with a −90° at the top and +90° at the bottom and represents the aVF lead. The remaining leads are similarly plotted as seen in Figure 18-5. Using this graph, if the net deflection of lead I was a +5 and lead III was a +9, then a point would be drawn representing each of these values on the respective axis (lead I and lead III). A perpendicular line would then be drawn through each of these points, and where the lines intersect would be the direction of the MEA (Fig. 18-6).

A simpler method for determining MEA would be to find the isoelectric lead. Evaluate the six limb leads in the hexaxial lead system and decide which lead has the sum value of deflection equal to zero (deflections equal distance above and below the baseline). This is called the isoelectric lead. If this lead exists then the MEA must be perpendicular to this axis. For instance, if the isoelectric lead is aVL then the perpendicular axis would be lead II. If the net value in lead II is positive then this animal's MEA would be +60°. If two leads are isoelectric, the smaller lead should be used. When no leads are isoelectric then MEA cannot be determined in the frontal plane.[5]

A third method for determining MEA would be using the axis with the largest deflection. This method is based on the assumption that the lead with the largest QRS deflection runs parallel to the MEA. If the deflection is downward then the MEA will follow the axis on the negative side and if it is deflected upward it will follow the positive side. For instance, if the largest deflection is in aVF and deflects upward, then the MEA would be +90°. If there are two leads of equally high QRS deflection, then the axis will generally lie between the two lead axes. To demonstrate, if lead II and aVF were equally deflected in a positive manner, then the MEA would lie between +60° and +90°. Although

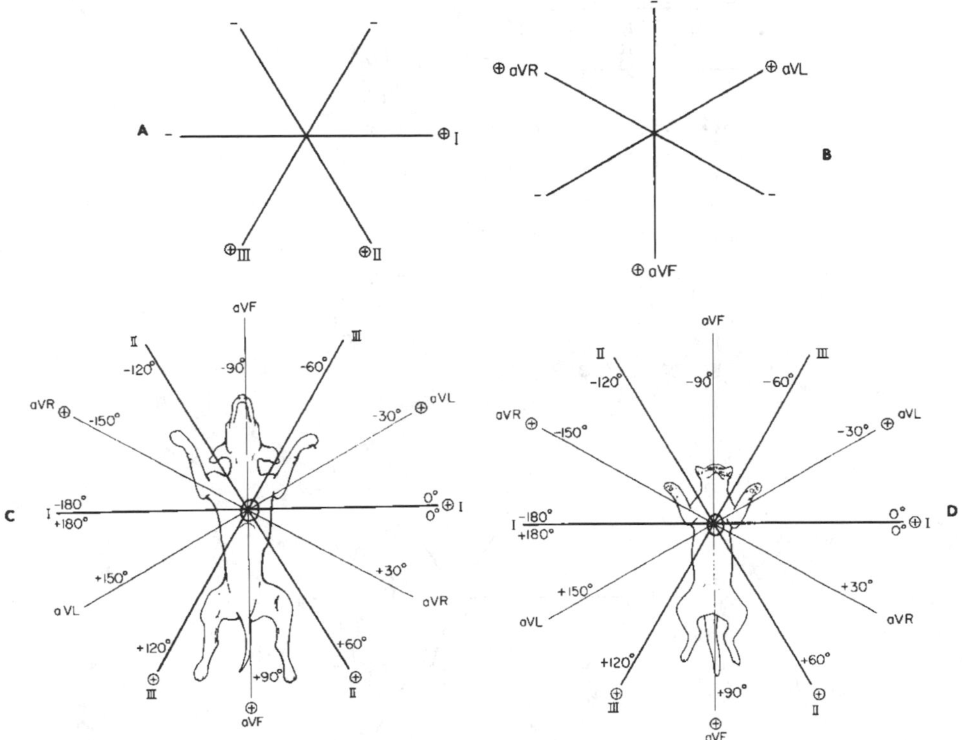

Figure 18-5
The hexaxial lead system for both dogs and cats illustrating the frontal plane of a patient in a 360° circle. **A** is the three standard bipolar leads, **B** is the three unipolar leads. **C** and **D** show these superimposed on each other with the dog and the cat and the degree markings. (From Tilley LP: Essentials of Canine and Feline Electrocardiography, 3rd ed. Philadelphia: Lea & Febiger, 1992.)

these last two methods are not precise, they are generally accurate enough to determine right and left axis deviations.

In dogs and cats a right axis deviation can be associated with right ventricular hypertrophy or right bundle branch blocks. Left axis deviations in dogs and cats can be associated with hypertrophic cardiomyopathy, as well as some other ventricular diseases, left anterior fascicular blocks, and hyperkalemia. However, it is most likely associated with diffuse disease of the myocardium or the left bundle branch or both.[7]

Identifying Effects of Atrial or Ventricular Enlargement

Enlargement of heart chambers can cause alterations in ECG complexes. For instance, left atrial enlargement may cause increased width in P waves, whereas right atrial enlargement may cause an increase in the height of the P

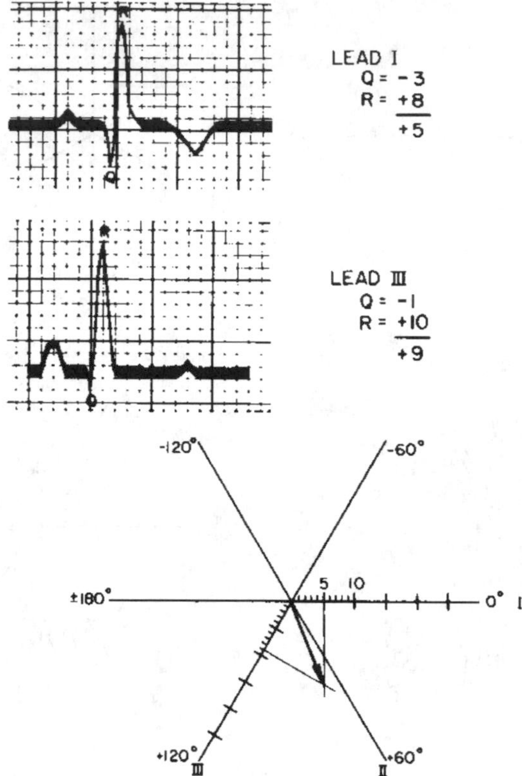

Figure 18-6
Determining mean electrical axis. First determine the net deflection for lead I and lead III as shown above (I = +5, III = +9). Then draw a perpendicular line from each respective lead originating from these net deflection points. Finally, draw a line from the center point of the grid to the point of intersected perpendicular lines. This will approximate the direction of the MEA (in this case about 70°). (From Tilley LP: Essentials of Canine and Feline Electrocardiography, 3rd ed. Philadelphia: Lea & Febiger, 1992.)

wave. A tall, wide, notched P wave is consistent with biatrial enlargement. Left ventricular enlargement can cause a left axis deviation, ST slurring or coving, widened QRS complexes, or increased amplitude of R waves. Right ventricular enlargement is characterized by a right axis deviation and S waves in leads I, II, III, and aVF.[12]

REFERENCES

1. Berne RM, Levy MN: Cardiovascular physiology, 4th ed. St. Louis: CV Mosby, 1981, p 31.
2. Miller MS, Smith FWK Jr, Fox PR: Electrocardiography. *In* Fox PR, Sisson D, Moise NS, eds.: Textbook of Canine and Feline Cardiology, 2nd ed, Philadelphia, WB Saunders, 1999, p 67.

3. Zipes DP: Specific arrhythmias: diagnosis and treatment. *In* Braunwald E, ed.: Heart Disease, 5th ed. Philadelphia, WB Saunders, 1996, p 705.
4. Walraven G: Basic Arrhythmias. Bowie, MD: Robert J. Brady Co., 1980, p 1.
5. Tilley LP: Essentials of Canine and Feline Electrocardiography, 3rd ed. Philadelphia, Lea & Febiger, 1992, pp 1, 82.
6. Fye WB: A history of the origin, evolution, and impact of electrocardiography. *Am J Cardiol* 73:937, 1994, [erratum, 76:641, 1995].
7. Kittleson MD: Electrocardiography: basic concepts, diagnosis of chamber enlargement, and intraventricular conduction disturbances. *In* Kittleson MD, Kienle RD, eds.: Small Animal Cardiovascular Medicine. St. Louis: CV Mosby, 1998, p 95.
8. Smith Jr, FWK, Hadlock DS: Electrocardiography. *In* Miller MS, Tilley LP, eds.: Manual of Canine and Feline Cardiology, 2nd ed. Philadelphia: WB Saunders, 1995, p 47.
9. Glaze K: Basic electrocardiography, part II. *Vet Tech* 17:719, 1996.
10. Taylor EJ, ed.: Dorland's Medical Dictionary, 27th ed. Philadelphia: WB Saunders, 1988, p 535.
11. Hahn AW (chairman), Hamlin RL, Patterson DF: Standards for canine electrocardiography. The Academy of Veterinary Cardiology Committee Report, 1977, p 28.
12. Smith FWK Jr, Tilley LP, Miller MS: Electrocardiography. *In* Birchard SJ, Sherding RG, eds.: Saunders Manual of Small Animal Practice. Philadelphia: WB Saunders, 1994, p 412.
13. Schaer M: Disorders of serum potassium, sodium, magnesium and chloride. *J Vet Emerg Crit Care* 9:209, 1999.
14. Rakita L, Vrobel T, Kaufman ES: Electrocardiography. *In* Ayers SM, senior ed.: Textbook of Critical Care, 3rd ed. Philadelphia: WB Saunders, 1995, p 492.
15. Horan LG, Flowers NC: Electrocardiography and vectorcardiography. *In* Braunwald E, ed.: Heart Disease. Philadelphia: WB Saunders, 1980, p 198.

19
Arterial and Venous Blood Gases

Harold Davis

Blood gases are obtained to determine ventilation, oxygenation, and acid–base status. Arterial blood gases and acid–base status are used to evaluate the progress of therapy and to indicate when adjustments are necessary.

ARTERIAL BLOOD GAS EQUIPMENT AND SAMPLE COLLECTION

Equipment

Until recently blood gas analysis was labor intensive and cost prohibitive in private practice veterinary medicine. Point of care testing (POCT) of blood gases is designed for human hospitals to reduce turnaround time of test results, streamline processes, increase staff efficiency, and reduce overall operating costs. Currently there are two POCT pH and blood gas analyzers that are affordable and easy to run: the i-STAT (I-STAT Corporation, East Windsor, NJ) and the IRMA SL blood analysis system (Diametrics Medical, St. Paul, MN). Both units are hand-held, user-friendly portable units that can operate on battery power. Each test cartridge contains its own electrode or sensor. The advantage of the self-contained electrode/sensor is that protein build-up or drift is eliminated, both of which can affect laboratory results and incur technician maintenance time. Minimal technician time is invested in analyzer maintenance. The initial purchase cost of the POCT analyzers is about one sixth the cost of the bench-top analyzers with many of the same testing capabilities. An alternative to owning an analyzer is to take the blood sample to a human hospital or veterinary facility, which can run those tests. Arrangements perhaps can be made wherein they will run the sample for a minimal fee.

Sampling

Percutaneous

The dead space of a 3-mL syringe is coated with lithium or sodium heparin (1000 U/mL); excess heparin is expelled from the syringe. A cork and alcohol swab are obtained. Commonly used sites include the dorsal pedal artery, femoral artery, and the sublingual artery. The collection site of choice is the dorsal pedal artery because it will be easier to control bleeding when compared to the femoral artery. In the unconscious or anesthetized patient the sublingual artery may be used.

The site is prepped and the artery is palpated. A 25-gauge needle is used. The needle is held at a 45° angle over the site where the pulse is strongest. The skin and arterial wall are punctured in one motion following the path of the artery, or in a two-step fashion: skin first then artery. Watch for a back flash of blood in the needle hub and then gently aspirate the sample. A 1- to 1.5-mL sample size will be needed. Once collected, air is expelled from the syringe and the syringe is capped with the cork. The sample is then mixed and placed in an ice water bath and transported to the laboratory.

Arterial Catheter

Arterial blood gas sample may be collected from an arterial catheter. It is necessary to clear the catheter of heparinized saline. A three-syringe technique is used. The first syringe is attached to an access port in the arterial catheter or extension tubing. Fluid is aspirated into the syringe (~2–3 cc) until all nonblood fluid is removed from the catheter and tubing.[1] The sample collection syringe is attached and sample for blood gas analysis collected. Following collection, the aspirated saline solution is recycled. The final syringe contains 3 ml heparinized saline which is used to flush the line until no evidence of blood remains.

Storage of Samples

Samples stored in an ice bath for up to 4–6 hours show very little change in pH and PCO_2/PO_2. Samples held at room temperature will show significant changes in PO_2 after 12 minutes, and significant changes in acid–base values will occur after 30 minutes.

ARTERIAL BLOOD GAS OVERVIEW

pH

The pH is an inverse logarithmic expression of hydrogen ion concentration. It is a reflection of the balance between HCO_3 (bicarbonate) and CO_2 (carbon dioxide). An increase in hydrogen ions is associated with a decrease in pH and visa versa. The pH can be calculated using the Henderson-Hasselbalch equation:

$$pH = pKa + \log [HCO_3]/[\text{total } CO_2]$$

It is the ratio rather than the absolute values for HCO_3 and total CO_2 that determines pH. As long as the ratio of the equation is 20:1, pH will be 7.40 or normal. The pH decreases or increases when the ratio is less than 20:1 or greater than 20:1, respectively.

The pH is regulated through several mechanisms. In the intracellular and extracellular fluid compartments the two major buffer systems that protect pH are proteins and the HCO_3 buffer system. Other mechanisms include respiratory and renal regulation. Proteins can act as acids or bases. They contain ionizable groups that can release or bind H^+ ions. In the HCO_3 buffer system, carbonic acid is a weak acid and HCO_3 is a weak base:

$$H_2O + CO_2 \leftrightarrow H_2CO_3 \leftrightarrow H^+ + HCO_3^-$$

When extracellular H^+ ions increase they move intracellularly for buffering and K^+ moves out of the cell in exchange for H^+. The respiratory system plays a role in acid–base regulation through the elimination of CO_2. The kidneys regulate acid–base balance through hydrogen and HCO_3 elimination or conservation.

The pH is an indicator of the net H^+ balance. The normal pH range is 7.35 to 7.45. A pH less than 7.35 is known as acidemia (condition in the blood) and the overall process is acidosis. A pH greater than 7.45 is known as alkalemia (condition in the blood) and the overall process is known as alkalosis.

$PaCO_2$

The $PaCO_2$ is the partial pressure of CO_2 dissolved in the plasma of arterial blood and is reported in mm Hg. It reflects the balance between alveolar minute ventilation and metabolic CO_2 production. Alveolar ventilation is the amount of air that reaches the alveoli and participates in gas exchange.

The normal range of $PaCO_2$ is 35 to 45 mm Hg in the dog at sea level. A $PaCO_2$ less than 35 mm Hg is known as hypocapnia or respiratory alkalosis. Hypocapnia (condition in the blood) or respiratory alkalosis is caused by alveolar hyperventilation. A $PaCO_2$ greater than 45 mm Hg is known as hypercapnia (condition in the blood) or respiratory acidosis. Hypercapnia or respiratory acidosis is caused by alveolar hypoventilation.

HCO_3/Base Balance

Two values can be used to assess the metabolic component of acid–base balance. They are HCO_3 or base balance (base excess or deficit). HCO_3 is increased or decreased due to many mechanisms. Base excess/deficit provides a quantitative estimation of surplus acid or base. It is defined as the titratable base or acid, respectively, when titrating to a pH of 7.40 under standard conditions (PCO_2 40 mm Hg and 38°C) and complete hemoglobin saturation.

The normal ranges for HCO_3 and base balance are 18 to 24 mmol/L and 0 ± 4 mEq/L respectively, in the dog. An HCO_3 less than 18 mmol/L or a base deficit less than -4 mEq/L reflects metabolic acidosis and an HCO_3 greater than 24 mmol/L or a base excess greater than 4 mEq/L reflects a metabolic alkalosis.

PaO_2

The PaO_2 is the partial pressure of oxygen (O_2) dissolved in arterial blood and is reported in mm Hg. PaO_2 does not reveal how much O_2 is in the blood (content) but only the pressure exerted by the dissolved oxygen.

The normal range for PaO_2 is 80 to 110 mm Hg assuming the patient is breathing room air at sea level. A PaO_2 less than 80 mm Hg is considered hypoxemia. A PaO_2 less than or equal to 60 mm Hg is the minimum value at which therapy is initiated.

As the altitude increases and barometric pressure decreases, the partial pressure of O_2 in the atmosphere is reduced. At increased altitude PaO_2 decreases. A rough rule of thumb is that the PaO_2 will decrease 4 mm Hg per 1000 feet increase in elevation (Personal communication, Craig Cornell, BS, RVT, VTS [ECC]). An example of this effect is that the normal PaO_2 reported in dogs in Fort Collins, CO is 70.3 to 84.0 mm Hg.[2] Those values were reported at an altitude of 1500 meters (4921 feet) with a mean barometric pressure of 635.8 ± 4.4 mm Hg.

Temperature Compensation

Usually, blood gas samples are analyzed at 37°C; seldom is the patient's temperature the same as the blood gas analyzer. Traditionally we have corrected blood gases to account for the temperature difference, so that we would know the values at the patient's temperature. Temperature-corrected values may be used in those cases where one wants to compare blood gas results over varying temperature changes of the patient. If the clinician is correcting abnormalities based on normothermic reference points, then it is not necessary to correct blood gas values. Hypothermia (37°C reference) results in elevated pH and decreased $PaCO_2$ and PaO_2; the reverse is true for hyperthermia. To correct or not to correct is debatable. Whether you correct or not, one point is important: Sequential blood gases in a patient should be handled in the same way.

ARTERIAL BLOOD GAS INTERPRETATION: A SIX-STEP METHOD

Step 1

Consideration is first given to pH. Is the patient normal, acidemic (pH <7.35), or alkalemic (pH >7.45)?

Step 2

Next evaluate the respiratory component. Is the respiratory component normal or does that patient have a respiratory alkalosis and hypocapnia ($PCO_2 <35$ mm Hg) or a respiratory acidosis and hypercapnia (PCO_2 >45 mm Hg)?

Step 3

Evaluate the metabolic component. Is the metabolic component normal or does that patient have a metabolic acidosis (HCO_3 <18 mmol/L or base deficit <-4 mEq/L), or metabolic alkalosis (HCO_3 >24 mmol/L or base deficit $>+4$ mEq/L)?

Step 4

If possible, we need to determine which component (respiratory or metabolic) is the primary contributor. Generally, the pH will vary in the direction

Table 19-1. Guidelines for Expected Compensation in Acid–Base Disorders[3]

Acid–Base Disorder	Expected Compensation
Metabolic acidosis	Each 1 mEq/L decrease in HCO_3 will decrease PCO_2 by 0.7 mm Hg
Metabolic alkalosis	Each 1 mEq/L increase in HCO_3 will increase PCO_2 by 0.7 mm Hg
Respiratory acidosis	
Acute	Each 1 mm Hg increase in PCO_2 will increase HCO_3 by 0.15 mEq/L
Chronic	Each 1 mm Hg increase in PCO_2 will increase HCO_3 by 0.35 mEq/L
Respiratory alkalosis	
Acute	Each 1 mm Hg decrease in PCO_2 will decrease HCO_3 by 0.25 mEq/L
Chronic	Each 1 mm Hg decrease in PCO_2 will decrease HCO_3 by 0.55 mEq/L

of the primary disorder. The other component is the secondary or compensatory component attempting to restore pH to normal. When both components vary in the same direction, as the pH, both components are primary.

Rather than use the above method of determining the primary or compensatory components of acid–base disorders, some clinicians will determine if expected compensation has occurred before they define the acid–base disorder. They will use guidelines for compensation (Table 19-1) to determine expected compensation and compare that to actual numbers.[3] If the patient meets expected compensation values within ± 2mm Hg or mEq/L, the patient is said to have one acid–base disorder (the primary disorder: metabolic acidosis/alkalosis or respiratory acidosis/alkalosis) and compensation is implied. If the patient does not meet the expected compensation, then it is said to have a mixed acid–base disorder. Given a pH 7.26, $PaCO_2$ 33 mm Hg, and HCO_3 14 mmol/L, according to the expected compensation rule, this patient has a metabolic acidosis. No mention is made of respiratory compensation because according to Table 19-1 it represents appropriate compensation. In another example, given a pH 7.30, $PaCO_2$ 25 mm Hg, and HCO_3 13 mmol/L, it does not meet the expected compensation value; therefore it has a mixed acid–base disorder (primary metabolic acidosis and respiratory alkalosis).

Step 5

Look at the PaO_2; does the PaO_2 show hypoxemia (PaO_2 <80 mm Hg, assuming breathing room air)?

Alveolar-Arterial O_2 Difference

The alveolar-arterial O_2 difference (A-a PO_2) also known as the A-a gradient measures the difference between the O_2 tension in the alveolus (A) and the artery (a).

The equation provides information on the efficiency of the transfer oxygen into the blood. It is an assessment of venous admixture. Venous admixture is the collective term for all the ways in which blood can pass from the right to the left side of the heart without proper oxygenation. Normal A-a PO_2 is 10 mm Hg when the fractional inspired oxygen concentration (FIO_2) is 0.21. (FIO_2 is the fraction of inspired O_2 expressed as a decimal.) A higher A-a PO_2 demonstrates a decreased ability of the lung to oxygenate blood or venous admixture. Evaluation of A-a PO_2 is most accurate and reliable with the patient spontaneously ventilating and the FIO_2 is 0.21.[4] To assess A-a PO_2 the alveolar O_2 (PAO_2) must be calculated. $PAO_2 = PIO_2 - 1.2\ (PaCO_2)$. $PIO_2 = FIO_2\ (P_B = 47)$. PIO_2 is the partial pressure of inspired O_2 expressed in mm Hg; 1.2 is a constant used to take into account the normal respiratory quotient; in this equation $PaCO_2$ is used to represent alveolar CO_2; P_B is barometric pressure; and 47 is the water vapor pressure value. The difference between P_AO_2 and the measured PaO_2 is the A-a PO_2. A simplified version of the alveolar air equation is to add the measured values of PaO_2 and of $PaCO_2$. If the added value is less than 120 mm Hg there is venous admixture; the lower the added value the greater the magnitude of the venous admixture.[5] This assumes that the patient is at sea level, has a normal body temperature, and is breathing room air.

Five Times the Percent Inspired O_2 Rule

When the inspired O_2 concentration exceeds 21%, expected PaO_2 values are different. To determine the expected PaO_2, multiply the inspired O_2 concentration by 5. Thus the expected PaO_2 on 60% O_2 should be at least 300 mm Hg (60×5). The expected PaO_2 value represents the O_2 level achievable in the normal healthy lung. Actual PaO_2 values that fall below the expected value suggest poor lung function.

PaO_2/FIO_2

The PaO_2/FIO_2 ratio is another index of hypoxemia. A ratio less than 300 indicates a severe defect in gas exchange. A value less than 200 meets the criteria for acute respiratory distress syndrome (given the proper clinical conditions).[6] Assuming $PaCO_2$ is reasonably stable, this ratio is a useful assessment parameter in patients with varying PaO_2 and FIO_2 values.

Step 6

Finally we need to look at the total picture. Do these lab values fit the clinical picture and history? Remember numbers alone do not tell the whole story.

Table 19-2. Example Showing the Importance of Considering CaO_2 When Assessing Oxygenation Status

Patient	Hgb (g/dL)	SaO_2 (%)	PaO_2 (mm Hg)	CaO_2 (mL/dL)
1	15	97	100	19.8
2	10	97	100	13.3

Other Considerations for Arterial Blood Gas Interpretations

O_2 Saturation

Oxygen saturation (SaO_2) represents the amount of O_2 bound to hemoglobin and is reported as a percentage. Normal is 95% or greater. It is not possible to achieve 100% when breathing room air.

O_2 Content

Oxygen content (CaO_2) is the total amount of O_2 carried in the blood. A total of 98% to 99% of the O_2 is bound to hemoglobin and the remaining 1% to 2% is dissolved in plasma. Normal CaO_2 is 16 to 20 mL/dL. To calculate CaO_2 use the following formula:

$$CaO_2 = (1.34 \times Hgb \times SaO_2) + (PaO_2 \times 0.003)$$

where 1.34 is the O_2-binding capacity of hemoglobin (mL O_2/g Hgb) and 0.003 is the solubility constant for dissolved O_2 in plasma (0.003 mL O_2/dL/mm Hg PaO_2). When assessing SaO_2, consideration should be given to hemoglobin level. Oxygen can only saturate the hemoglobin that is available. Emphasis should be placed on "available" because the hemoglobin level is not always within normal limits and O_2 can only bind with what is available. A 96% saturation level associated with hemoglobin of 8 g/dL does not deliver as much O_2 as does 96% saturation associated with 15 g/dL hemoglobin. One should not assume that the O_2 content status is normal because the SaO_2 is normal. The importance of evaluating CaO_2 is best illustrated by the example in Table 19-2, in which it is clear to see that errors can be made in assessing oxygenation if CaO_2 is not considered. In the two patients, SaO_2 and PaO_2 are the same, but patient 2's hemoglobin is reduced by one third, resulting in a decreased CaO_2.

VENOUS BLOOD GASES

Venous blood gases are a reasonable alternative to arterial blood gases when one wants to assess acid–base status.[7] It has been reported that venous blood will accurately reflect the acid–base status of dogs with normal circulatory status.[8] If there is concern about the patient's oxygenating ability then arterial gases are required. Venous samples are best taken from the jugular vein. The sample should be free flowing to avoid acid metabolites from venous stasis and muscular activity when the vessel is held off. Pressure on the vessel should be released after the venipuncture has been achieved. One study looking at lingual venous samples collected in normal dogs undergoing routine surgical procedures determined that lingual samples were useful in assessing acid–base status except in low cardiac output states.[9]

There is good correlation between venous and arterial pH. Venous PCO_2 is approximately 3 to 6 mm Hg higher than arterial in stable states. It is a reflection of tissue PCO_2. Venous PO_2 is a reflection of tissue PO_2 and does not correlate with arterial PO_2. Normal range is 40 to 50 mm Hg. Values below 30 mm Hg suggest decreased O_2 delivery. Values greater than 60 mm Hg suggest reduced O_2 extraction by the tissues.

REFERENCES

1. Preusser BA, *et al.*: Quantifying the minimum discard sample required for accurate arterial blood gases. *Nurs Res* 38:276, 1989.
2. Wingfield WE, Matteson VL, Hackett T, *et al.*: Arterial blood gases in dogs with bacterial pneumonia. *J Vet Emerg Crit Care Med* 7:75, 1997.
3. Haskins S, Copland VS, Patz JD: The cardiopulmonary effects of oxymorphone in hypovolemic dogs. *J Vet Emerg Crit Care Med* 1:32, 1991.
4. Van Pelt DR, Wingfield WE, Wheeler SL, *et al.*: Oxygen-tension based indices as predictors of survival in critically ill dogs: clinical observations and review. *J Vet Emerg Crit Care Med* 1:19, 1991.
5. Haskins SC: Monitoring the anesthetized patient. *In* Thurmon JC, Tranquilli WH, Benson GH, eds.: Lumb and Jones' Veterinary Anesthesia. Baltimore: Williams & Wilkins, 1996, p 416.
6. Martin L: All You Really Need to Know to Interpret Arterial Blood Gases. Philadelphia: Lippincott, Williams & Wilkins, 1999, 63–64.
7. Wingfield WE, Van Pelt DR, Hackett TB, *et al.*: Usefulness of venous blood in estimating acid base status in the seriously ill dogs. *J Vet Emerg Crit Care Med* 4:23, 1994.
8. Ilkiw JE, Rose, RJ, Martin ICA: A comparison of simultaneously collected arterial, mixed venous, jugular venous and cephalic venous blood smaples in the assessment of blood-gas and acid-base status in the dog. *J Vet Intern Med* 5:294, 1991.
9. Wagner AE, Muir WW, Bednarski RM: A comparison of arterial and lingual venous blood gases in the anesthetized dog. *J Vet Emerg Crit Care Med* 1:14, 1991.

SECTION III
Monitoring the Critically Ill Animal

20
Cardiovascular Monitoring

Eric Monnet

The principal function of the heart is to transport an adequate amount of oxygen (O_2) from the lung to the peripheral tissue to maintain organ metabolism. Because O_2 delivery is a function of cardiac output (CO) and O_2 content of the blood, evaluation of cardiac function is important for the optimization of O_2 delivery. Cardiac function depends of heart rate, preload, afterload, and contractility. Evaluation of these different parameters is important to obtain a correct CO.

HEART RATE

Heart rate can be monitored by palpating the apex impulse on the chest wall or the arterial pulse, auscultation, recording arterial pulse waves on a monitor, or with an electrocardiogram (ECG).

The CO depends on stroke volume and heart rate although the heart rate does not correlate directly with CO. Heart rates outside the normal range, high and low, are associated with reduced CO. Trends in rate reflect variation of cardiac function. A high resting heart rate or an increased rate with time indicates hypoxemia of the myocardium, deterioration of cardiac function, or hypovolemia. Bradycardia reduces O_2 transportation and allows development of myocardial ischemia that may lead to ventricular dysrhythmias.

Heart rhythm influences heart rate and CO. Ventricular dysrhythmias can elevate heart rate but reduce arterial pressure and CO (Fig. 20-1). Because optimal O_2 delivery is important, control of heart rhythm and rate is important.

Palpation of the apex impulse or the arterial pulse detects cardiac activity but may be inaccurate in the obese patient or patient in shock. Palpation might assist in the detection of dysrhythmias. Auscultation gives an accurate reading of the heart rate. The ECG gives valuable information on heart rate and cardiac rhythm.

ARTERIAL PULSE

Arterial pulse can be palpated from the femoral, lingual, brachial, dorsal pedal, and median coccygeal arteries. The femoral artery is most commonly used. Arterial pulse is the product of left ventricular contraction. Its character depends on stroke volume, rate and force of ejection, and vascular tone. Palpation of the femoral pulse allows quick and easy subjective evaluation of cardiac function.

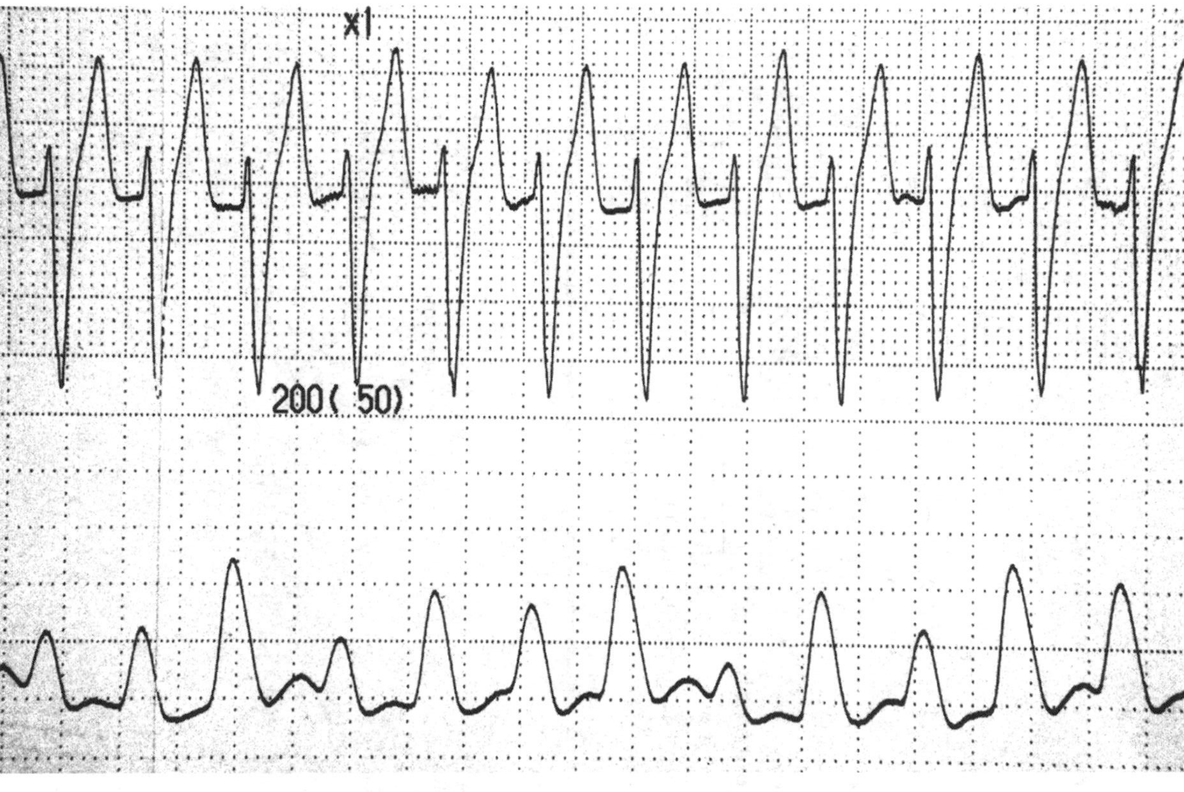

Figure 20-1
Sustained ventricular tachycardia and arterial pressure tracing in a dog. Arterial pressure was significantly affected by the arrhythmia.

Table 20-1. Normal Hemodynamic Variables in Dogs and Cats

Variables	Normal Value	Units
Arterial pressure (systolic/diastolic)	120/80	mm Hg
Mean arterial pressure	80–95	mm Hg
Pulmonary artery pressure (systolic/diastolic)	30/10	mm Hg
Mean pulmonary artery pressure	10–20	mm Hg
Pulmonary capillary wedge pressure	4–9	mm Hg
Central venous pressure	0–5	cm H_2O
Cardiac output	100	mL/min/kg
Arterial oxygen tension (PaO_2)	80–95	mm Hg
Mixed venous oxygen tension (PvO_2)	35–50	mm Hg
Arterial oxygen saturation	96–99	%
Mixed venous oxygen saturation	65–75	%
Arterial oxygen concentration (CaO_2)	17–20	mL/dL
Mixed venous oxygen concentration (CvO_2)	12–15	mL/dL
Oxygen extraction ratio	25–30	%

1 mm Hg = 1/1.36 cm H_2O = 0.736 cm H_20

Palpation of proximal and distal arterial pulses allows a crude estimate of blood pressure. Variation of the quality of the pulse over time gives quick information on the progression of the cardiac function and the response to treatment. The weaker the proximal pulse and the more difficult it is to palpate the distal pulse, the lower blood pressure.

CENTRAL VENOUS PRESSURE

CVP is a reflection of intravascular blood volume, cardiac function, venous compliance, and intrathoracic pressure. Central venous pressure (CVP) is recorded most commonly from a catheter with its tip in the cranial or proximal caudal vena cava or from the proximal lumen (right atrium) of a pulmonary artery catheter. A jugular catheter in the a cat or small dog can give an adequate measurement of the CVP because the tip of the catheter will be close to the right atrium. Both methods yield similar pressure waveforms, and for clinical purposes, CVP and right atrial pressure are considered to be identical.[1] CVP is between 2 and 3 mm Hg (Table 20-1). Because of its simplicity and availability, CVP is commonly measured to guide fluid therapy in critically ill medical and surgical patients.

The normal CVP waveform consists of five phasic events, three peaks (*a*, *c*, *v*) and two descents (*x*, *y*) (Fig. 20-2).[2,3] The *a* wave results from atrial contraction. It follows the P wave on the ECG. The *c* wave is due to the ventricular contraction and bulging of the tricuspid valve in the right atrium. It follows the R wave of the ECG. The *x* wave results from the reduction of atrial pressure at

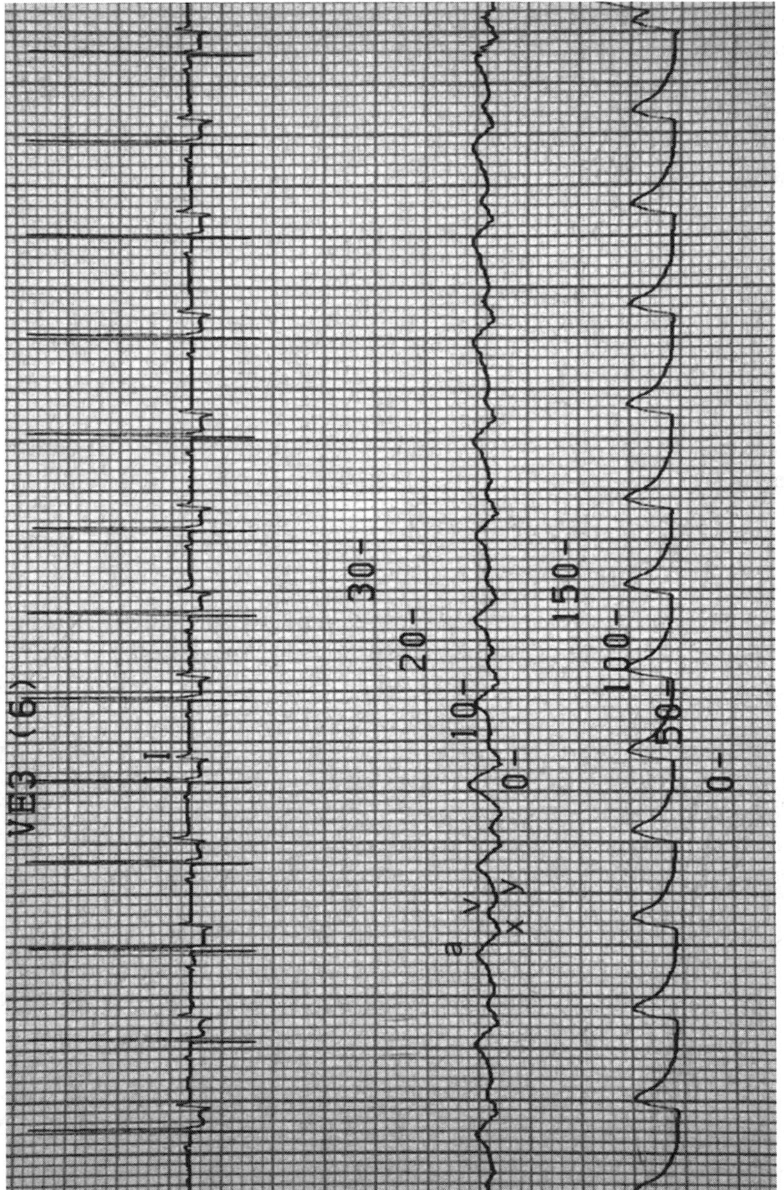

Figure 20-2
Electrocardiogram shows right atrial pressure tracing and arterial pressure tracing in a dog. On the right atrial pressure tracing, the *a*, *x*, *v*, and *y* waves are visible. The *c* wave is usually difficult to see with a water-filled pressure system.

the end of systole due to atrial relaxation. The last atrial peak, *v* wave, results from atrial filling during late diastole. It follows the T wave on the ECG. Finally, the atrial pressure decreases with *y* descent due to right ventricular filling after opening of the tricuspid valve.[4,5]

ARTERIAL PRESSURE

Arterial pressure is a function of CO and vascular resistance.

$$\Delta P = CO \times SVR$$

where ΔP is the mean drop of pressure, CO the cardiac output, and SVR the systemic vascular resistance.

$$\Delta P = P_a - P_{ve}$$

where P_a is the arterial pressure and P_{ve} is the mean venous pressure. Therefore, the first equation becomes:

$$P_a - P_{ve} = CO \times SVR$$

$$P_a = CO \times SVR + P_{ve}$$

This equation is true for a continuous blood flow. It is common to replace ΔP by the mean arterial pressure (MAP). MAP is estimated also with the following equation:

$$MAP = DAP + (SAP - DAP)/3$$

where MAP is the mean arterial pressure, DAP the diastolic arterial pressure, and SAP the systolic arterial pressure.

Arterial pressure reflects overall circulatory status but lacks diagnostic specificity. Arterial pressure falls after hypovolemia from blood or fluid loss, cardiac failure, sepsis, acute trauma, anaphylactic reactions, neural lesions, and terminal stage of systemic diseases. Systemic arterial pressure is commonly affected in critical care patients, especially after trauma or during shock. Reduction of arterial pressure leads to multiple organ failure if not treated. Modifications of arterial blood pressure should be monitored and treated in the critically ill patient to prevent multiple organ failure.

Increased arterial pressure can then be due to an augmentation of vascular resistance (vasoconstriction) or an augmentation of CO. Therefore, an augmentation of arterial pressure is not always equivalent to an augmentation of tissue perfusion. Mucous membranes should be evaluated for their color and extremities for their temperature.

Arterial pressure can be evaluated either with a direct technique (arterial catheter) or with an indirect technique (Doppler or oscillometry). Direct measurement also allows collection of blood samples for blood gas analysis. However, it is more invasive and requires electronic equipment for monitoring.

Direct blood pressure is measured following placement of a catheter in the dorsal pedal artery, the medial auricular artery, or a coccygeal artery in the ventral part of the tail to monitor arterial pressure in the ICU. The femoral artery can be used but its catheterization is associated with potential for complications such as hematoma.

After preparation of the skin with standard sterile technique, an 18- or 20-gauge catheter can be introduced in the artery. A 24-gauge catheter can be used for cats and small breed dogs. Local anesthesia can be performed with a 2% lidocaine local block. After palpation of the pulsation in the artery, the catheter is directed toward the artery. The skin can be penetrated initially by an 18-gauge needle to allow an easier introduction of the catheter through tough skin. If the artery cannot be catheterized percutaneously a cutdown is performed to place the catheter. After catheterization of the artery, a T connector with Luer lock is then attached to the catheter. The catheter with the T connector is secured to the patient with white tape or even glued to the skin. A light bandage is then applied on the catheter. The catheter is then connected to a continuous flushing system pressurized at 150 mm Hg. The catheter is also flushed by hand every 2 hours with 1 to 3 mL heparinized saline.[1,5,6]

Arterial pressure is then measured by connecting the arterial catheter to a pressure transducer zeroed to the level of the right atrium. Short and stiff tubing should be used to connect the catheter to the transducer to minimize resonance in the tubing. Air bubbles should be flushed from the connecting tubing because they will also increase resonance. After connection of the pressure transducer to a monitor, pressure tracings can be visualized and SAP, DAP, and MAP measured (see Fig. 20-2 and Table 20-1). MAP has to be maintained above 60 mm Hg to allow perfusion to the kidney, myocardium, and brain. A dicrotic notch can be seen on the arterial pressure tracing. It is most commonly visible when pressure is measured close to the aorta. The dicrotic notch is due to the aortic valve closure or from reflection of pressure wave.[5]

Indirect measurement can be performed with either a Doppler or an oscillometric technique. Indirect measurement of arterial pressure is not as accurate as direct measurement. The trends in arterial pressure measurement with the indirect techniques can give valuable information on the critical patient's status.[1] Doppler instrumentation, using piezo-electric crystals detects blood flow over peripheral arteries to evaluate the arterial pressure during deflation of a cuff placed proximally on the artery. The oscillometric technique detects motion of the wall of the artery to evaluate the arterial pressure during deflation of a cuff placed proximally on the artery. In both techniques, the cuff placed proximal on the artery interrupts the blood flow. When the blood flow is re-established by deflating the cuff, the arterial pressure can be evaluated. When the pressure in the cuff exceeds SAP, no blood flow or motion of the arterial wall occur. When the cuff is slowly deflated, pulsatile blood flow is re-established. The piezzo-electric crystal detects an audible Doppler signals corresponding to the systolic pressure. The oscillometric device detects oscillation of the wall of the artery and a systolic pressure is determined. Maximum amplitude of the oscillation corresponds to the MAP. DAP is when the amplitude of oscillation does not change. These indirect techniques are accurate and correlate well with direct measurements if a proper cuff width is used. The cuff width should approximate 40% of the circumference of the limb. Narrow cuff widths yield erroneously high values for blood pressure, whereas inappropriately wide cuffs yield erroneously low values.[6] At low pressures the measurements may not be accurate and it might be difficult to identify an artery.[7] Doppler technique accurately measures systolic pressure; the oscillometric technique can measure SAP, DAP, and MAP, as well as pulse rate.

Reduction of arterial pressure in the trauma or shock patient might be delayed by compensatory mechanisms. Arterial pressure decreases after compensatory mechanisms are exhausted. CO may be reduced for periods up to 2 hours prior to any visible changes in arterial pressures. On the other hand, arterial pressure might improve with fluid therapy without a change in CO.

RIGHT-SIDED CARDIAC CATHETERIZATION

Right-sided cardiac catheterization is performed with a pulmonary artery catheter or Swan-Ganz catheter placed in the pulmonary artery. A pulmonary artery catheter usually has three lumens. The most distal lumen is located in the pulmonary artery and the most proximal in the right atrium. A third lumen is located in the right ventricle and it is used for injection of cold saline during determination of CO. If a fourth lumen is present it is used for fluid administration. It allows the measurement of right atrial, right ventricular, and pulmonary artery pressures. Pulmonary capillary wedge pressure (PCWP) can be measured. PCWP is an analog to CVP to evaluate the preload of the left ventricle. CO is also evaluated with the thermodilution technique. Swan-Ganz catheters with fast response thermistors are able to estimate right ventricular systolic and diastolic volumes and right ventricular ejection fraction.[8,9] If the Swan-Ganz catheter has oxymetry capabilities it would also be able to measure O_2 saturation in the mixed venous blood. If systemic arterial O_2 saturation is known, the O_2 extraction ratio can be continuously measured.[10] It is commonly used to differentiate an acute heart failure from fluid volume problems. It is also used to monitor the progress of therapy in patients with shock and after trauma.

Placement of a Swan-Ganz Catheter

A Swan-Ganz catheter is placed through a jugular vein introducer.[3,4,11,12] Jugular vein introducers are placed using the Seldinger technique. An 8 Fr introducer and a 7.5 Fr Swan-Ganz catheter are used for dogs. A 5 Fr introducer and a 4 Fr Swan-Ganz catheter can be used for cats. After sterile preparation of the neck over the jugular vein, sterile towels are used to drape the neck of the patient. An 18-gauge over-the-needle catheter is first placed in the jugular vein. A J-tip guidewire is then advanced through the catheter in the jugular vein. The wire can trigger ventricular premature contractions if it is advanced in the right ventricle. This is possible in small dogs or cats. The over-the-needle catheter is removed. A no. 11 blade is used to puncture the skin around the wire to allow an easier placement of the introducer sheath. The introducer sheath over a vessel dilator is introduced in the jugular vein over the wire. The vessel dilator and the wire are then removed and the introducer sheath sutured to the skin.

Blood is first aspirated from the introducer. The introducer sheath is then flushed with heparinized saline. Each lumen of the Swan-Ganz catheter is flushed with heparinized saline and capped with a three-way stopcock. The distal port of the Swan-Ganz is connected to a pressure transducer zeroed to the level of the right atrium and a pressure monitor. The catheter is advanced through the introducer sheath in the right atrium, the right ventricle, and finally the pulmonary artery while observing the pressure tracing. The position of the catheter tip is identified from the pressure reading and the pressure tracing. First the pressure tracing is showing right atrial pressure tracing with *a*, *c*, and *v* waves (see Fig. 20-2). It then enters the right ventricle. The waveform is recognized by the significant increase in systolic pressure and by the low diastolic pressure (Fig. 20-3). After inflation of the balloon at the tip, the catheter will float through the right ventricular infundibulum and the pulmonary valve to end up in the pulmonary artery (Fig. 20-4). The waveform shows the same systolic pressure as in the right ventricle, but the end-diastolic pressure is significantly increased compared to the right ventricular end-diastolic pressure. After proper placement of the catheter, pres-

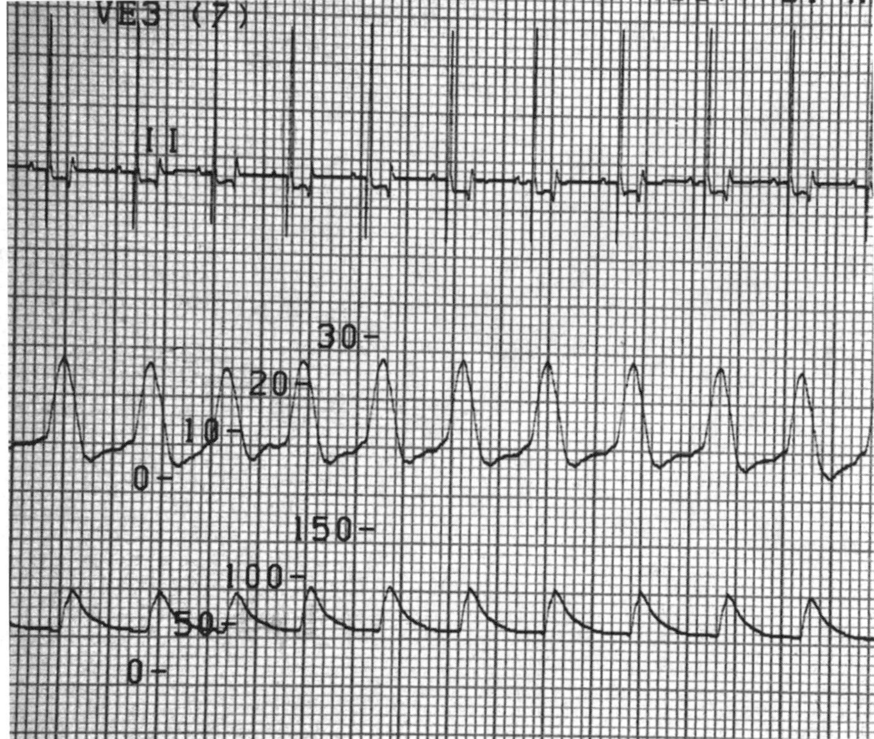

Figure 20-3
Electrocardiogram shows right ventricular pressure tracing and arterial pressure tracing in a dog. Diastolic pressure in the right ventricle is close to zero.

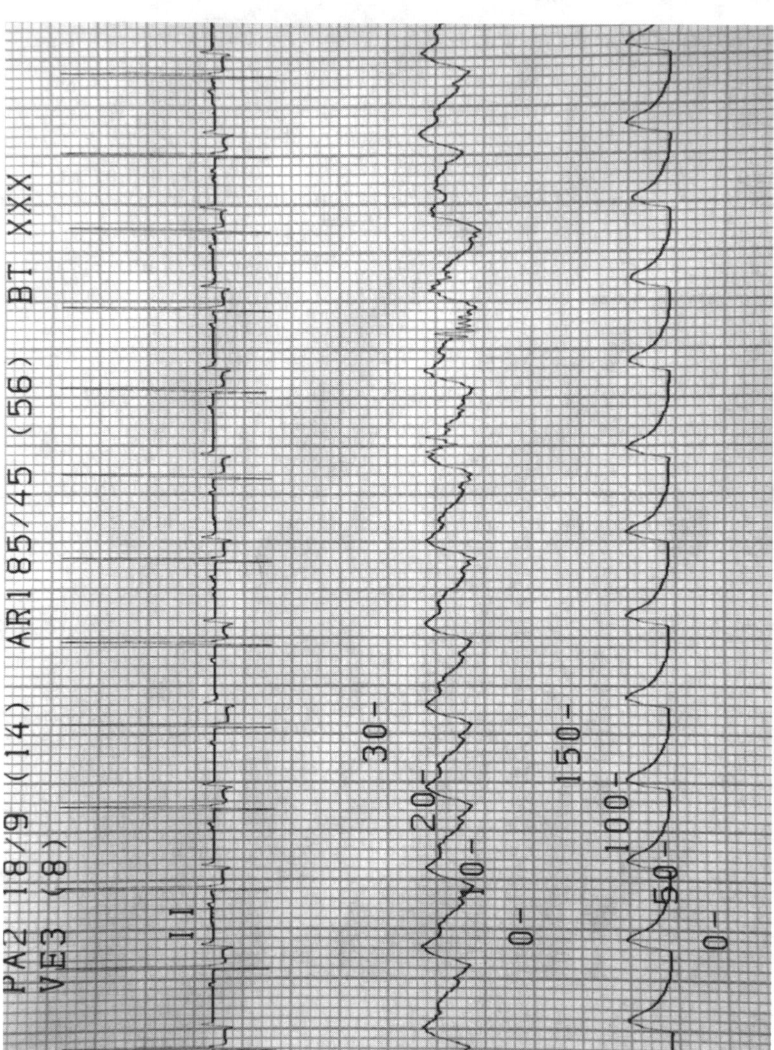

Figure 20-4
Electrocardiogram shows pulmonary artery pressure tracing and arterial pressure tracing in the same dog as in Figure 20-3. Systolic pulmonary pressure is very close to the systolic pressure in the right ventricle. The diastolic pressure in the pulmonary artery is 10 mm Hg.

sure transducers zeroed to the level right atrium can be connected to the different ports of the catheter to measure right ventricular pressures and CVP in addition to the pulmonary artery pressure.

PULMONARY ARTERY PRESSURE

Pulmonary artery pressure is a function of pulmonary vascular resistance and CO. It is measured with a Swan-Ganz catheter. Mean pulmonary artery pressure should be between 10 to 20 mm Hg (see Table 20-1). Pulmonary artery systolic pressure is the highest pressure generated by the right ventricle (see Fig. 20-4). Pulmonary artery diastolic pressure reflects pulmonary vascular resistance.[3] Pulmonary artery elevation mostly occurs with pulmonary parenchymal disease, pulmonary thromboembolism, pulmonary hypertension, and septic shock. Pulmonary artery hypotension is seen commonly in hypovolemic shock.

PULMONARY CAPILLARY WEDGE PRESSURE

The PCWP is measured by wedging the Swan-Ganz catheter with a balloon inflated at the tip of the catheter. The balloon occludes antegrade blood flow to a portion of the pulmonary vasculature. Blood flow ceases between the pulmonary catheter tip and a junction point where pulmonary vein draining the occluded pulmonary vascular region join other veins in which blood still flows toward the left atrium. A static column of blood now connects the wedged pulmonary artery catheter tip to the junction point in the pulmonary vein next to the left atrium. Because the resistance in the pulmonary vein is low, the PCWP measured is similar to left atrial pressure. During wedging of the catheter, the pulmonary artery pressure wave disappears on the monitor and respiratory cycle artifacts are then visible (Figs. 20-5 and 20-6). The PCWP shows the *a*, *c*, and *v* waves from the left atrium. The PCWP is the pressure at the end of expiration. End of expiration on the pressure tracing is different if the animal is breathing spontaneously or if it is breathing with a ventilator (see Figs. 20-5 and 20-6). The pressure monitor may have an algorithm that recognizes respiratory artifact allowing the computer to measure the pressure; however, visual determination from a pressure tracing is more accurate.[2]

The PCWP is also called left ventricular end-diastolic pressure because at the end of diastole the mitral valves are opened. Therefore, the pressure in the left atrium is similar to the pressure in the left ventricle. It is a good measurement of left ventricular preload if the patient does not have mitral valve stenosis or an occlusion of a pulmonary vein. Positive end-expiratory pressure induces an augmentation of the PCWP. The PCWP is between 5 and 10 mm Hg in the normal animal (see Table 20-1). Volume loading, pulmonary edema, mitral valve regurgitation, and congestive heart failure result in an augmentation of PWCP.[12] Serial measurement of the PCWP is mostly valuable to judge the effect of fluid therapy on left ventricular preload.

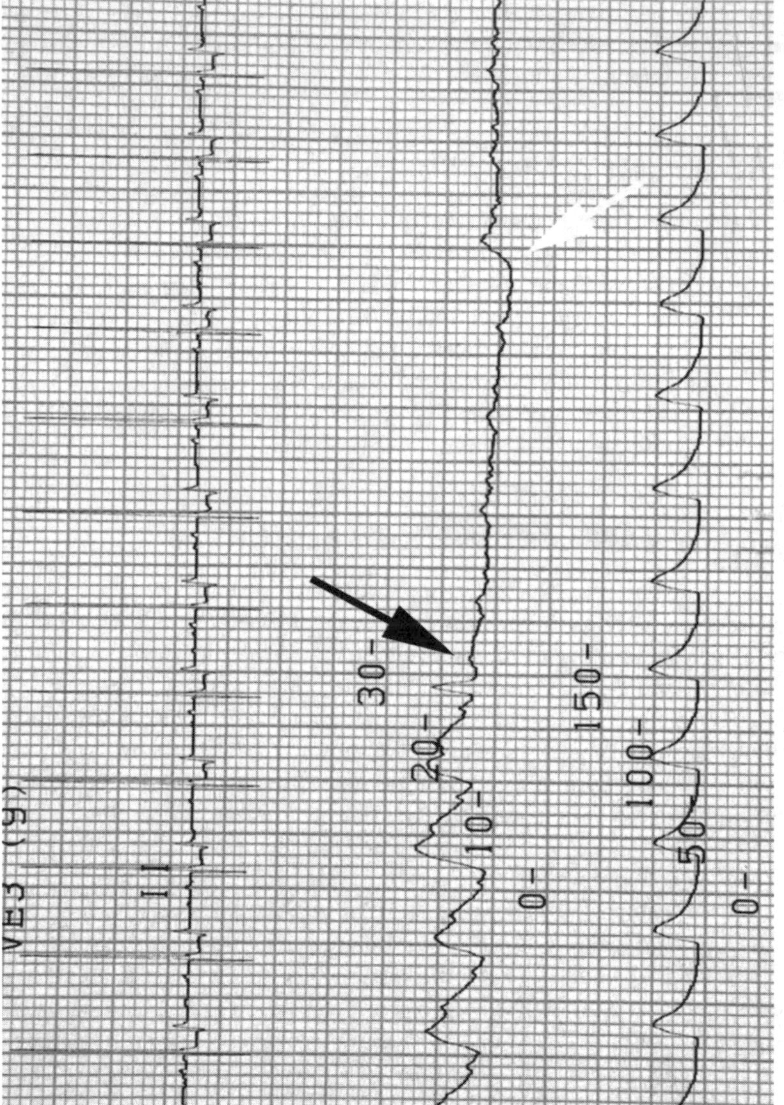

Figure 20-5
Pulmonary capillary wedge pressure in a dog. When the balloon is inflated the waveform from the pulmonary artery disappears (black arrow). Respiratory artifact on is apparent with spontaneous breathing (white arrow).

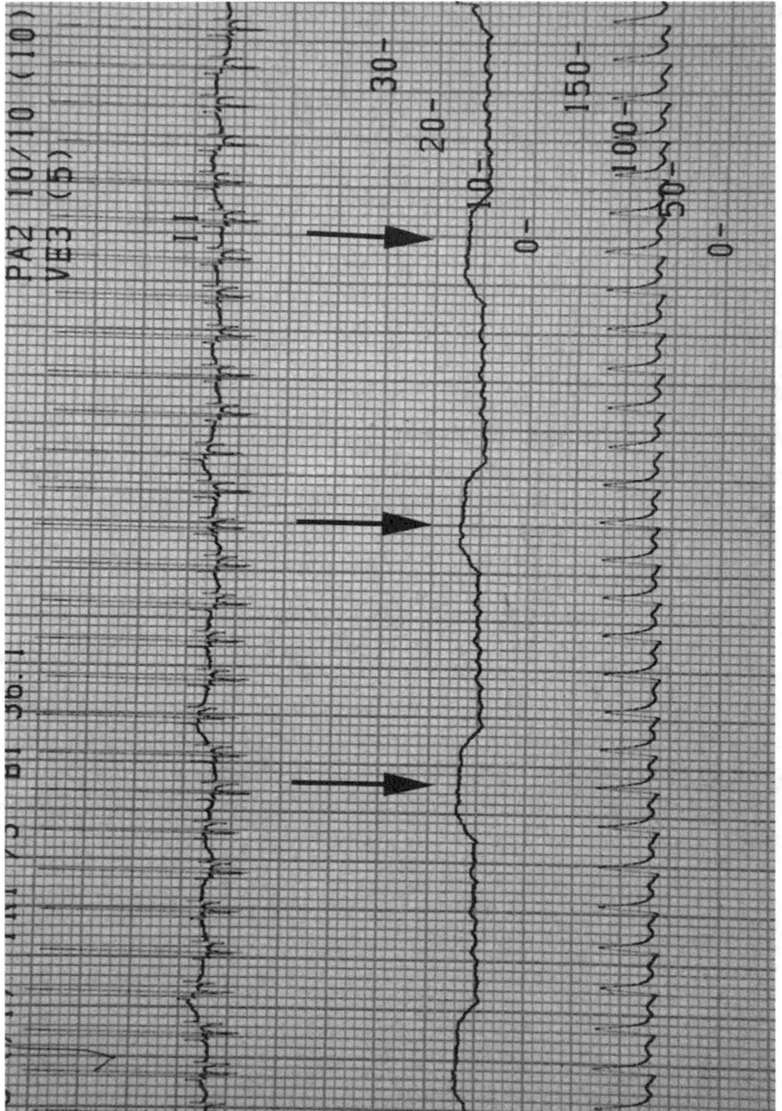

Figure 20-6
Respiratory artifact (black arrows) during pulmonary capillary wedge pressure tracing in a dog with mechanical ventilation.

RIGHT VENTRICULAR SYSTOLIC AND DIASTOLIC VOLUMES

A Swan-Ganz catheter with fast response temperature thermistor and sensing of the heart rate can determine right ventricular diastolic and systolic volumes and right ventricular ejection fraction by thermodilution. These measurements also provide information on right ventricle preload. Frank-Starling curves can be constructed with the stroke volume and the right ventricular end-diastolic volume, which allows a better evaluation of the cardiac function. Right ventricular ejection fraction has been shown as a prognostic indicator for survival in human patients with sepsis and heart failure.[9,13]

CARDIAC OUTPUT

The contractile state of the myocardium can be affected by hypoxemia, metabolic acidosis, electrolytes imbalances, and shock. Contractility is a major determinant of CO, which is the volume pumped by the heart per minute. It is a function of stroke volume (SV) and heart rate (HR):

$$CO = SV \times HR$$

Stroke volume is function of preload, afterload, and contractility. Preload and contractility are two parameters that can be manipulated in the critical care unit for the treatment of hypotension or reduction of perfusion.

The CO is measured by thermodilution. Iced saline is injected as a bolus in the right ventricle. A temperature thermistor at the tip of the Swan-Ganz catheter measures the variation of blood temperature with time after the injection of the saline bolus (Fig. 20-7). CO is the area under the curve of temperature

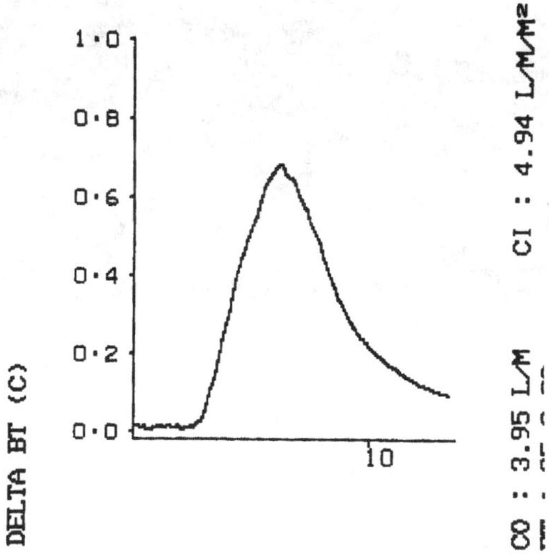

Figure 20-7
Cardiac output. Curve represents the variation in blood temperature in the pulmonary artery after iced saline injection in the right ventricle.

decay over time. Iced saline is recommended over room temperature saline because it induces a more significant variation of temperature in the pulmonary artery. For a dog of 30 kg, it is better to inject a 10-mL bolus of iced saline, whereas for a smaller dog and a cat, 5 mL of iced saline is recommended. Three good quality measurements should be performed and an average taken. The quality of a measurement is made by looking at the tracing of the variation of temperature with time (see Fig. 20-7). The curve should show a steep ascending part followed by exponential descending part. Normal CO is 100 mL/min/kg in the dog (see Table 20-1).

The homogenous mixture of iced saline and blood in the right ventricle depends on the rate of injection of the saline, the volume of the right ventricle, and the presence of arrhythmias. A fast bolus injection in a small ventricle results in a better mixture than if the bolus is performed slowly or in a large ventricle. Insufficiency of the right atrioventricular valves results in regurgitation of iced saline in the right atrium, which will result in reduction of the slope of the ascending curve followed by fluctuation of the descending part. Ventricular premature contractions also result in poor mixture of blood and iced saline. Finally, poor CO cannot be measured accurately because iced saline mixed with blood will not be ejected fast enough to obtain a correct recording of the temperature variation. Measurement of CO can also be influenced by the respiratory cycle. It is recommended to perform the bolus injection of iced saline at the end of expiration.[14]

SUMMARY

Evaluation of cardiac function provides the practitioner with valuable information on the hemodynamic status of a critically ill patient. Cardiovascular monitoring can be as simple as measuring femoral pulse and as sophisticated as measuring the oxygen extraction ratio continuously. Right-sided cardiac catheterization is invasive and should be performed on specific indications. The degree of sophistication has to be adapted to the complexity of the case and the level of technicality of the practice. Monitoring of the cardiac function allows titration of inotropic drugs and fluid therapy.

REFERENCES

1. Haskins SC: Monitoring the critical ill patient. *Vet Clin North Am Small Anim Pract* 9:1059, 1989.
2. Marino PL: Central venous pressure and wedge pressure. *In:* Marino PL, ed.: The ICU Book, 2nd ed. Philadelphia: Lippincott Williams & Wilkins, 1998, 166.
3. Mark JB: *Atlas of Cardiovascular Monitoring*. New York: Churchill Livingstone, 1998.
4. Ganz P, Swan HJC, Ganz W: Ballon-tipped flow directed catherters. *In:* Grossman W, ed.: Cardiac Catheterization and Angiography, 3rd ed. Philadelphia: Lea & Febiger, 1986, p 88.
5. Grossman W: Pressure measurement. *In:* Grossman W, Baim DS, eds.: Cardiac Catheterization, Angiography, and Intervention, 4th ed. Philadelphia: Lea & Febiger, 1991, p 123.

6. Kittleson MD, Olivier NB: Measurement of systemic arterial blood pressure. *Vet Clin North Am Small Anim Pract* 13:321, 1983.
7. Grandy JL, Dunlop CI, Hodgson DS, *et al.*: Evaluation of the Doppler ultrasonic method of measuring systolic arterial pressure in cats. *Am J Vet Res* 53:1166, 1992.
8. Davidson CJ, Fishman RF, Bonow RO: Cardiac catheterization. *In:* Braunwald E, ed.: Heart Disease. A Textbook of Cardiovascular Medicine. Philadelphia: WB Saunders, 1997, p 177.
9. Hurford WE, Zapol WM: The right ventricle and critical illness: a review of anatomy, physiology, and clinical evaluation of its function. *Intensive Care Med* 14:448, 1988.
10. Nelson LD: Mixed venous oximetry. *In:* Snyder JV, ed.: Oxygen Transport in the Critically Ill. Chicago: Year Book Medical Publishers, 1987, 235.
11. Nelson LD, Snyder JV: Technical problems in data acquisition. *In:* Snyder JV, ed.: Oxygen Transport in the Critically Ill. Chicago: Year Book Medical Publishers, 1987, 205.
12. Tuman KJ, Carroll GC, Ivankovich AD: Pitfalls in interpretation of pulmonary artery catheter data. *J Cardiothoracic Anest* 3:625, 1989.
13. Schulman DS, Biondi JW, Matthay RA, *et al.*: Effect of positive end-expiratory pressure on right ventricular performance: importance of baseline right ventricular function. *Am J Med* 84:57, 1988.
14. Marino PL: Thermodilution: methods and applications. *In:* Marino PL, ed.: The ICU Book. Philadelphia: Lippincott Williams & Wilkins, 1998, 178.

21
Respiratory System

E. Christopher Orton

INTRODUCTION

The major function of the cardiopulmonary system is the delivery of oxygen (O_2) to tissues and elimination of carbon dioxide (CO_2) generated by tissue metabolism. Rapid and thorough assessment of cardiopulmonary function is a core skill in critical care medicine that must be firmly grounded by an understanding of physiologic and pathophysiologic processes within the cardiopulmonary system. This chapter reviews these processes and provides the clinician with a logical framework for assessment of animals with cardiopulmonary dysfunction.

O_2 PATHWAY

The O_2 pathway is a clinically useful concept that provides a logical framework for evaluation and treatment of disturbances in the cardiopulmonary system (Fig. 21-1). It reduces O_2 transport to a step-by-step process that begins with atmospheric O_2 and ends with O_2 delivery to tissues. Each step in the pathway is important and must be assessed independently to ensure adequate overall cardiopulmonary function. The steps of the O_2 pathway can be viewed as a clinical checklist for monitoring cardiopulmonary function in critically ill animals.

VENTILATION

Ventilation is the mechanical process that causes gas to flow into and out of the lungs. Not all gas flow into the respiratory system reaches areas of gas exchange, and as a result total ventilation ($\dot{V}_T$) is portioned into alveolar ventilation ($\dot{V}_A$), where gas exchange occurs, and dead space ventilation ($\dot{V}_D$):

$$\dot{V}_T = \dot{V}_A + \dot{V}_D$$

Dead space ventilation includes flow of gas to anatomic areas not normally involved in gas exchange, as well as flow to alveoli that are ventilated but not receiving pulmonary blood flow. The former is referred to as anatomic dead space, while the latter is physiologic dead space. Anatomic dead space ventilation remains constant, whereas physiologic dead space changes depending on the number of functioning alveoli. The ratio of $\dot{V}_A$ to $\dot{V}_D$ changes with the pattern of breathing. For example, an animal that is panting can increase $\dot{V}_T$ and $\dot{V}_D$ several-fold without changing $\dot{V}_A$.

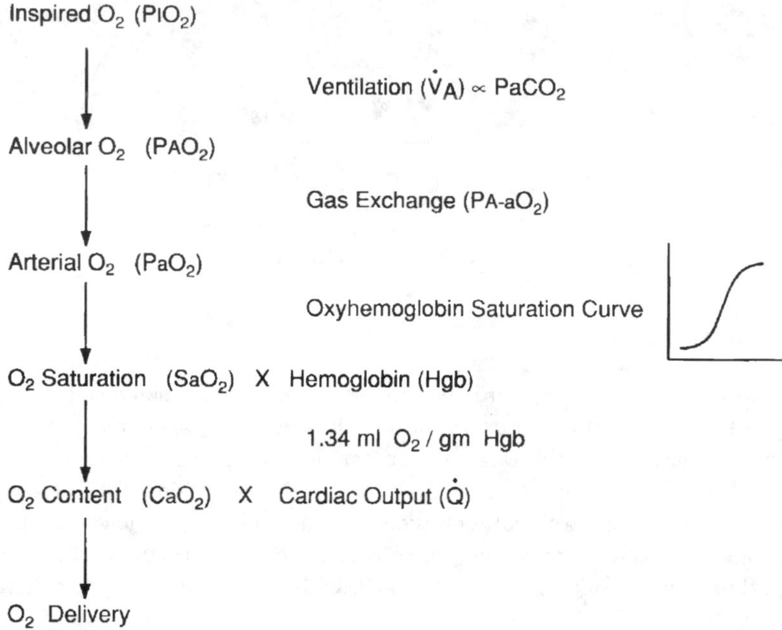

Figure 21-1
The O_2 pathway. Inspired O_2 (P_{IO_2}) in the atmosphere is transported to pulmonary alveoli by the process of alveolar ventilation (V_A) to determine the alveolar O_2 tension (P_AO_2). O_2 then is transferred from pulmonary alveoli to the pulmonary capillary blood by mechanisms known collectively as pulmonary gas exchange to determine the arterial O_2 tension (P_aO_2). The alveolar-arterial O_2 tension difference (A-a PO_2) quantifies the efficiency of the gas exchange process. The P_aO_2 is the principal determinant of arterial hemoglobin (Hb) saturation (S_aO_2) in a relationship described by the oxygen-Hb saturation curve. Arterial O_2 content (C_aO_2) is principally a function of the Hb concentration of blood and S_aO_2. Each gram of Hb is capable of carrying 1.34 mL O_2 when fully saturated with O_2. O_2 delivery ($\dot{D}O_2$) to tissues is a function of C_aO_2 and cardiac output ($\dot{Q}$).

CO_2 Tension

The primary drive for alveolar ventilation is arterial CO_2 tension (P_aCO_2). Under normal conditions, the central respiratory center drives $\dot{V}_A$ to keep P_aCO_2 at 40 mm Hg, regardless of the total volume of CO_2 produced (V_{CO_2}) by the metabolism of the patient. This relationship of P_aCO_2, $\dot{V}_A$, and $\dot{V}_{CO_2}$ is described by the equation (where K is a conversion constant)[1]:

$$P_aCO_2 = \frac{\dot{V}_{CO_2}}{\dot{V}_A} \times K$$

By definition, hypoventilation is present when $\dot{V}_A$ fails to match $\dot{V}_{CO_2}$, and as a result, P_aCO_2 increases (*i.e.*, becomes >40 mm Hg). Conversely, hyperventilation is present when $\dot{V}_A$ exceeds what is necessary to eliminate $\dot{V}_{CO_2}$ causing P_aCO_2 to decrease (*i.e.*, becomes <40 mm Hg).

Alveolar Gas Equation

Because arterial O_2 tension (P_aO_2) cannot be higher than alveolar O_2 tension (P_AO_2), P_AO_2 is important to all subsequent steps in the O_2 pathway. The P_AO_2 is not measured clinically, but is estimated from the alveolar gas equation[1]:

$$P_AO_2 = P_IO_2 - P_aCO_2/R$$

From above equation, it is apparent that P_AO_2 is a function of the inspired oxygen tension (P_IO_2), P_aCO_2 (and thereby $\dot{V}_A$), and the respiratory exchange ratio (R). Thus, R is the ratio of O_2 ($\dot{V}O_2$) to $\dot{V}CO_2$. R can be determined by indirect calorimetry, but this is not routinely done in the clinical setting. In a study of dogs undergoing indirect calorimetry, R was found to be 0.76 in postoperative or post-trauma dogs compared to an R of 0.84 in normal dogs.[2] For purposes of the above calculation, R is generally assumed to be 0.8. The P_IO_2 is determined by the fraction of inspired O_2 (F_IO_2, 0.21 on room air), barometric pressure (P_B, 760 mm Hg at sea level), and the vapor pressure of water (P_{H_2O}, 47 mm Hg at 100% saturation and body temperature):

$$\begin{aligned} P_IO_2 &= F_IO_2\,(P_B - P_{H_2O}) \\ &= .21\ (760 - 47) \\ &= 150 \end{aligned}$$

Thus, the P_IO_2 of room air at sea level is approximately 150 mm Hg. From the above equation, it can be seen that either barometric pressure or F_IO_2 can alter P_IO_2, and in turn, the P_AO_2. Substantial change in barometric pressure is most likely to result from exposure to altitude, whereas F_IO_2 is altered clinically by administration of supplemental oxygen. Increasing F_IO_2 to 40% nearly doubles P_IO_2 and increases P_AO_2 substantially without any change in V_A.

Alveolar ventilation is the other major determinant of P_AO_2. The alveolar gas equation predicts that an animal breathing room air at sea level with a P_aCO_2 of 40 mm Hg would have a P_AO_2 of approximately 100 mm Hg:

$$\begin{aligned} P_AO_2 &= F_IO_2\,(P_B - P_{H_2O}) - P_aCO_2/R \\ &= .21\ (760 - 47) - 40/0.8 \\ &= 150 - 50 \\ &= 100 \end{aligned}$$

The alveolar gas equation predicts that in animals breathing room air, for every 1 mm Hg elevation in P_aCO_2, there will be approximately a 1.25 mm Hg decrease in P_AO_2.

Hypoventilation

Adequate ventilation requires central respiratory centers, spinal pathways, peripheral respiratory nerves, primary respiratory muscles, pleural-pulmonary coupling, and pulmonary mechanical function to be intact or normal. Hypoventilation occurs when any component of this pathway is disrupted or abnormal. Important causes of hypoventilation include depression or injury of the central respiratory center, injury or disease of the neuromuscular apparatus of ventilation, disruption of pleural-pulmonary coupling, or excessive respiratory work resulting from abnormal pulmonary mechanics. The major determinants of respiratory work are airway resistance and lung compliance. Either obstructive airway disorders or restrictive lung conditions, or both, can increase respiratory work and lead to hypoventilation when they are severe.

Assessment of Ventilation

Breathing Patterns

Clinical assessment of ventilation should include observation of breathing. The first indication that a patient is hypoventilating may come from the simple observation that ventilatory excursions are poor. Information about abnormal pulmonary mechanics is gained from observation of the pattern of breathing. Animals adopt a pattern of breathing that minimizes respiratory work. Normal breathing balances the major elastic force, lung compliance, with the major viscous force, airway resistance.[1] Elastic forces in the lung are minimized by a rapid and shallow breathing pattern, whereas resistance forces in the lung are minimized by a slow and deep breathing pattern (Fig. 21-2). Thus, animals with restrictive lung diseases (*e.g.*, pulmonary edema, interstitial pneumonia, pulmonary fibrosis, pleural effusion) will adopt a rapid and shallow breathing pattern, whereas animals with airway obstruction (*e.g.*, laryngeal paralysis, bronchoconstriction) will adopt a slow and deep pattern of breathing. Obstructive breathing patterns are further assessed by observation of the phase of respiration that produces the most ventilatory effort. Upper airway obstruction causes an exaggerated effort during inspiration, whereas lower airway obstruction causes an exaggerated effort during expiration.

Tidal Volume and Minute Volume

Total ventilation is measured directly with a Wright's respirometer attached to an endotracheal tube or tight-fitting mask (Fig. 21-3). Tidal volume is the volume (mL) of gas expired during each breath and is normally at least 10 mL/kg body weight. Minute volume ($\dot{V}_T$) is the total volume of gas expired each minute (L/min). If tidal volume or minute volume is low, there is a good possibil-

Figure 21-2
Work of breathing. Airway resistance work increases with respiratory rate, whereas elastic work decreases with respiratory rate. Animals generally adopt a respiratory rate that balances resistance and elastic work and minimizes the total work of breathing (normal). Restrictive lung diseases that decrease lung compliance and increase elastic work usually are associated with an increased respiratory rate (decreased lung compliance). Obstructive respiratory conditions that increase airway resistance and work usually associated with a decreased respiratory rate (increased airway resistance).

Normal

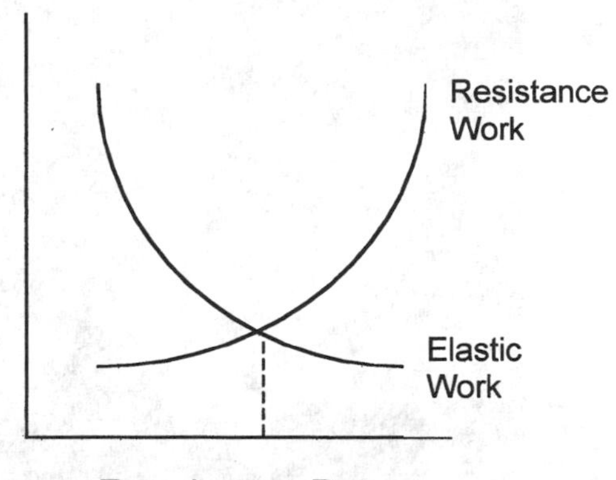

Decreased Lung Compliance

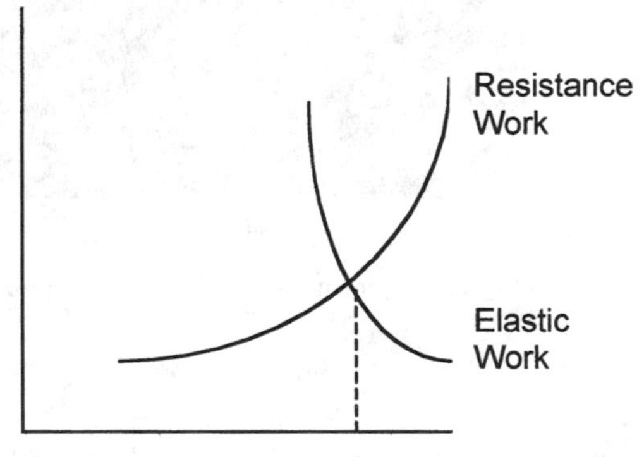

Increased Airway Resistance

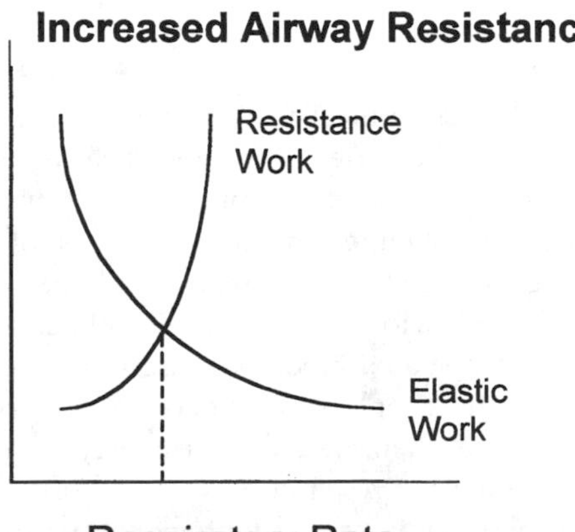

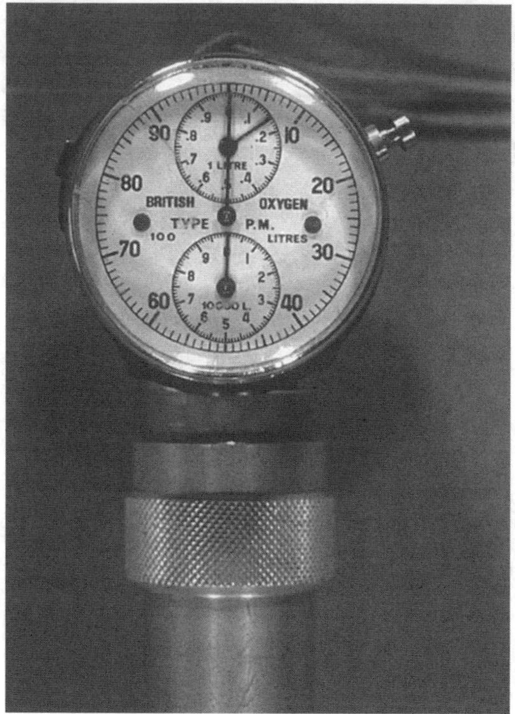

Figure 21-3
Respirometer. A Wright's respirometer can be used to measure tidal volume and minute volume in animals.

ity that ventilation is inadequate. However, because $\dot{V}_T$ includes both $\dot{V}_D$ and $\dot{V}_A$, measurement of an adequate tidal volume or minute volume does not ensure that $\dot{V}_A$ is adequate.

Hypercapnea

Ultimately, the best clinical assessment of alveolar ventilation is to measure P_aCO_2. By definition, the patient is hypoventilating when hypercapnea is present. The most direct method of assessing P_aCO_2 is by arterial blood gas analysis. Arterial blood can be obtained by direct puncture of a femoral or dorsal pedal artery with a 25-gauge needle. The sample should be collected into a 3-mL heparinized syringe, have obvious gas bubbles expelled, sealed with a stopper, and transported to an automated blood gas machine. The sample is placed on ice if measurement of the sample will be delayed. Alveolar ventilation should be considered inadequate when the P_aCO_2 is greater than 45 mm Hg. Hypoventilation causes hypoxemia and respiratory acidosis. Administration of supplemental O_2 corrects the hypoxemia caused by hypoventilation by increasing the P_{IO_2}, but not the respiratory acidosis.

Capnography

Because diffusion of CO_2 in the lung is highly efficient, P_aCO_2 and alveolar CO_2 carbon dioxide tension (P_ACO_2) are essentially equal. The CO_2 tension of expired gas at the end of expiration closely approximates P_ACO_2 and is termed end-tidal carbon dioxide tension ($P_{ET}CO_2$). The $P_{ET}CO_2$ is measured clinically with a capnograph that samples expired gas continuously and reports the peak CO_2 tension at the end of expiration. Measurement of $P_{ET}CO_2$ provides a good clinical estimate of P_aCO_2, and therefore V_A. A disadvantage of capnography is that sampling of expired gases and measurement of $P_{ET}CO_2$ requires that the patient be intubated. The principles and clinical application of capnography are reviewed in Chapter 8.

PULMONARY GAS EXCHANGE

Pulmonary gas exchange is the collective process by which O_2 and CO_2 are exchanged between the alveolus and arterial blood. Exchange of O_2 is complex and depends on diffusion across the alveolar-capillary membrane, matching of alveolar ventilation and perfusion, and the amount of venous admixture to arterial blood. Ideally, P_aO_2 should be nearly equal to P_AO_2 (*i.e.*, 100 mm Hg under physiologic conditions at sea level). Impaired gas exchange is present when P_aO_2 becomes substantially less than P_AO_2. Because P_aO_2 can be measured directly and P_AO_2 can be calculated from measurable values, the degree of gas exchange impairment can be quantified by the alveolar-arterial O_2 difference (A-a PO_2):

$$\begin{aligned} \text{A-a } PO_2 &= P_AO_2 - P_aO_2 = [F_IO_2(P_B - P_{H_2O}) - P_aCO_2/R] - P_aO_2 \\ &= [.21\ (760 - 47) - (40)/0.8] - 98 \\ &= 100 - 98 \end{aligned}$$

The A-a PO_2 should be less than 10 mm Hg for animals breathing room air. The normal A-a PO_2 gradient increases 5 to 7 mm Hg for every 10% increase in F_IO_2.[3]

Impaired Gas Exchange

There are three basic mechanisms of gas exchange impairment: diffusion impairment, shunt, and ventilation-perfusion mismatch.

Diffusion Impairment

Diffusion of O_2 across the alveolar-arterial membrane is directly proportional to the concentration gradient of O_2 across the membrane and the total membrane area, and inversely proportional to the membrane thickness. Under normal conditions, diffusion of O_2 in the lung is highly efficient and generally is complete by the time blood has traversed about one fourth of the alveolar capillary bed.[1] Thus, pulmonary disease must be severe before diffusion will limit gas exchange. The most important clinical cause of diffusion impairment is pulmonary thromboembolism (PTE), which impairs diffusion by drastically decreasing the total membrane area available for O_2 diffusion. The other consequence of PTE is an increase in dead space ventilation ($\dot{V}D/\dot{V}T$). Dead space ventilation can be quantified by measuring the P_aCO_2 and exhaled CO_2 tension (P_ECO_2):

$$\dot{V}D/\dot{V}T = \frac{P_aCO_2 - P_ECO_2}{P_aCO_2}$$

Determination of P_ECO_2 requires collection of expired gases into a collection bag and analysis of CO_2 tension with an infrared analyzer. This determination is rarely performed in veterinary patients. In theory, the increase in dead space ventilation could lead to an increase in P_aCO_2. However, CO_2 diffuses about 20 times more rapidly than O_2 across the alveolar-arterial membrane and is rarely if ever limited by diffusion.

Pulmonary diseases that increase the thickness of the alveolar-arterial membrane (*e.g.*, pulmonary interstitial fibrosis) can cause some degree of diffusion impairment when severe. However, because of the efficiency of O_2 diffusion, this is a relatively unimportant cause of diffusion impairment and hypoxemia in animals at rest.

Administration of supplemental O_2 rapidly corrects hypoxemia caused by diffusion impairment by increasing the concentration gradient of O_2 across the alveolar-arterial membrane. This explains why hypoxemia due to PTE is so responsive to administration of supplemental O_2 and serves as a useful clinical observation that supports a diagnosis of PTE in animals.

Shunt

Shunt occurs when unoxygenated venous blood bypasses viable gas exchange areas of the lung and mixes with oxygenated arterial blood. The resultant venous admixture produces hypoxemia. Shunt can result from either right-to-left cardiac shunt or intrapulmonary shunt. Examples of right-to-left cardiac shunt include ventricular septal defect with suprasystemic pulmonary hypertension (*i.e.*, Eisenmenger syndrome) and tetralogy of Fallot. Pulmonary shunt results from perfusion of completely collapsed or fluid-filled alveoli. Shunt is an important cause of clinically significant hypoxemia. The magnitude of hypoxemia caused by shunt is a function of the ratio of shunt flow to total cardiac output, termed the shunt fraction ($\dot{Q}s/\dot{Q}$). Because venous admixture has no opportunity for gas exchange, hypoxemia arising purely from shunt is unresponsive to administration of supplemental O_2. This physiologic reality distinguishes shunt from other causes of hypoxemia and serves as a useful clinical finding for diagnosing shunt as the mechanism of hypoxemia.

Shunt does not effect the P_aCO_2 until in becomes very severe (Fig. 21-4).[4] Thus, shunt usually does not result in hypercapnia. In fact, animals with shunt often have a low P_aCO_2 as a result of hypoxia-driven hyperventilation.

Ventilation-Perfusion Mismatch

Ventilation-perfusion ($\dot{V}A/\dot{Q}$) mismatch occurs when ventilation and blood flow are not closely matched in gas exchange units. The result is inefficient

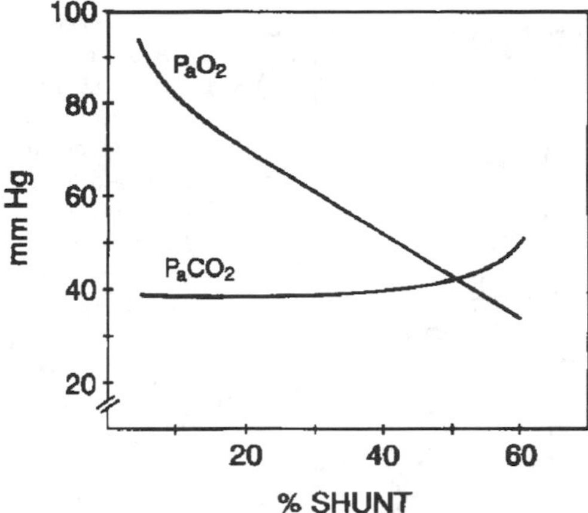

Figure 21-4
Shunt. The influence of shunt fraction on arterial O_2 tension (P_aO_2) and arterial CO_2 tension (P_aCO_2). (From D'Alonzo GE, Dantzger DR: Mechanisms of abnormal gas exchange. *Med Clin North Am* 67:557, 1983.)

gas exchange and hypoxemia. The reason for this inefficiency becomes more clear by considering the extremes of $\dot{V}A/\dot{Q}$ mismatch. For example, if regions of the lung are ventilated but not perfused (*i.e.*, the extreme of high $\dot{V}A/\dot{Q}$), the functional result is a decrease in the total area available for gas exchange and an increase in $\dot{V}D/\dot{V}T$. On the other hand, if regions of the lung are perfused but not ventilated (*i.e.*, the extreme of low $\dot{V}A/\dot{Q}$), the functional result is intrapulmonary shunt (Fig. 21-5). Although these extremes are not reached with $\dot{V}A/\dot{Q}$ mismatch, they illustrate why matching of ventilation and perfusion is important. Low $\dot{V}A/\dot{Q}$ mismatch is a frequent cause of hypoxemia in animals with pulmonary disease. Any pulmonary condition that causes partial alveolar collapse or poor ventilation to a region of the lung will result in low $\dot{V}A/\dot{Q}$ mismatch. Because alveoli are still partially ventilated in the setting of low $\dot{V}A/\dot{Q}$ mismatch, the resultant hypoxemia is responsive to administration of supplemental O_2. In reality, however, pulmonary diseases that cause low $\dot{V}A/\dot{Q}$ mismatch are almost always accompanied by an increase in intrapulmonary shunt, and thus are only partially or poorly responsive to supplemental O_2.

Assessment of Pulmonary Gas Exchange

Alveolar-Arterial PO_2 Gradient

The A-a PO_2 can be calculated by measuring P_aO_2 and P_aCO_2 by blood gas analysis and inserting these values into that for alveolar-arterial O_2 difference. The calculated A-a PO_2 for an animal breathing room air is normally less than 10 mm Hg. A calculated A-a PO_2 of 30 mm Hg or greater in an animal breathing room air suggests that significant gas exchange impairment is present. Because the normal value of A-a PO_2 is affected by FIO_2, the above normal valves do not apply to animals breathing supplemental O_2. Although normal values of A-a

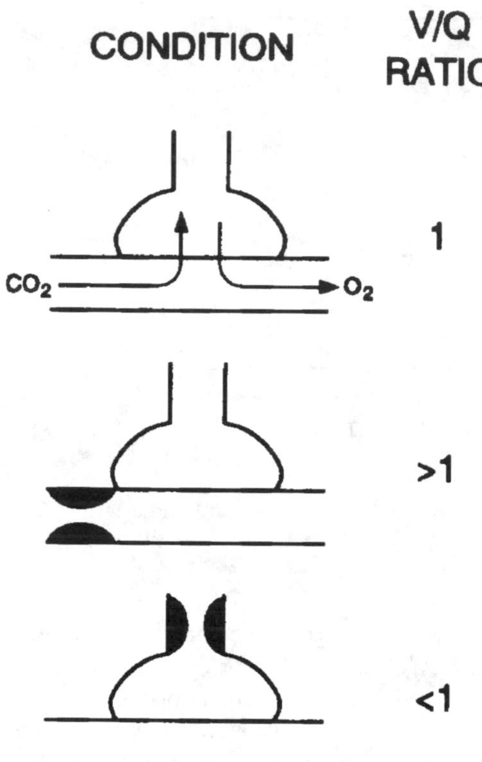

Figure 21-5
Ventilation-perfusion ($\dot{V}A/\dot{Q}$) relationship. Under ideal conditions, ventilation and perfusion to small respiratory units are closely matched (*i.e.*, V/Q = 1). Pulmonary gas exchange becomes inefficient when perfusion, but not ventilation, to respiratory units is impaired (*i.e.*, V/Q > 1), or when ventilation, but not perfusion, to respiratory units is impaired (*i.e.*, V/Q < 1).

PO_2 are reported for various levels of F_{IO_2}, it is often difficult to determine an accurate F_IO_2 in the clinical setting. Thus, blood gas analysis and calculation of A-a PO_2 is most revealing when performed with the animal breathing room air. The A-a PO_2 has been shown to be an important predictor of survival in critically ill dogs.[5]

Shunt Fraction ($\dot{Q}_s/\dot{Q}$)

The magnitude of intrapulmonary shunt can be determined by calculation of the shunt fraction from the O_2 saturation of arterial blood (S_aO_2), mixed venous blood (S_vO_2), and pulmonary capillary blood (S_cO_2) during breathing of pure O_2:

$$\dot{Q}_s/\dot{Q} = \frac{S_cO_2 - S_aO_2}{S_cO_2 - S_vO_2}$$

The S_cO_2 is not measured directly, but is assumed to be 100% during breathing of pure O_2. Ideally, the S_vO_2 sample should be obtained from a catheter placed in the pulmonary artery. Alternatively, the S_vO_2 sample may be obtained from a central venous catheter although this may lead to small errors in the calculation. Shunt is the only mechanism of impaired gas exchange that persists during administration of supplemental O_2; and thus, calculation of the $\dot{Q}_s/\dot{Q}$ is the best way to assess impaired gas exchange in animals receiving supplemental O_2 therapy. A calculated $\dot{Q}_s/\dot{Q}$ greater than 10% is abnormal and indicates clinically important gas exchange impairment in animals breathing supplemental O_2.

O_2 SATURATION AND O_2 CONTENT

O_2-Hemoglobin Saturation Curve

The P_aO_2 actually is a measure of the amount of O_2 dissolved in plasma. Dissolved O_2 is insufficient to meet metabolic requirements. Hemoglobin (Hb) greatly increases the O_2-carrying capacity of blood. Arterial O_2 saturation (S_aO_2) is defined as the fraction or percent of O_2-bound Hb-binding sites to the total available Hb-binding sites in the arterial blood. The P_aO_2 is important because it is the principal determinant of S_aO_2.

The relationship between P_aO_2 and S_aO_2 is described by the O_2-Hb saturation curve (Fig. 21-6). The affinity of Hb for O_2 increases as more O_2 binds to it. This property gives the O_2-Hb curve its sigmoid shape. The shape of the O_2-Hb curve has important physiologic and pathophysiologic implications. The plateau phase of the curve causes Hb to remain saturated over a wide of range O_2 tensions. The S_aO_2 is approximately 97% when the P_aO_2 is 97 mm Hg. The S_aO_2 cannot be increased substantially by higher than normal P_aO_2 values. The steep phase of the O_2-Hb curve allows for efficient O_2 release in the peripheral tissues where O_2 tension normally decreases. A pathophysiologic implication of the steep phase of the curve is that small changes in P_aO_2 can have profound changes on S_aO_2 when severe hypoxemia is present.

The O_2-Hb curve can "shift" to the right or left reflecting changes in the

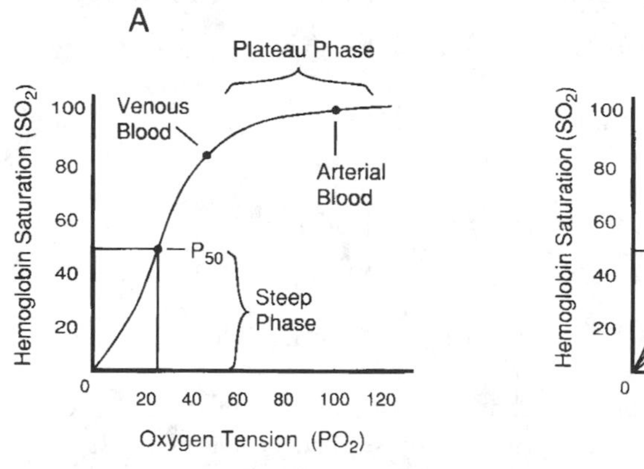

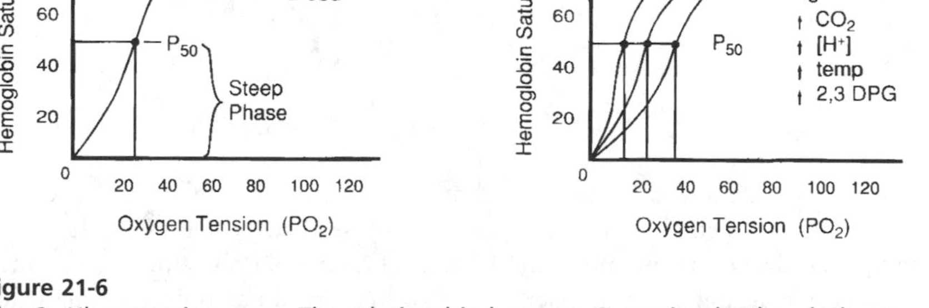

Figure 21-6
The O_2-Hb saturation curve. The relationship between O_2 tension (PO_2) and Hb saturation (S_aO_2) is depicted by the O_2-Hb saturation curve (A). The O_2 tension that corresponds to 50% saturation of Hb is termed the P_{50}. The O_2-Hb curve can shift to the right or left reflecting a change in O_2-Hb affinity (B).

overall affinity of Hb O_2 (see Fig. 21-6). A shift of the curve to the right decreases overall O_2 affinity of Hb, whereas a shift to the left increases Hb O_2 affinity. Conditions that shift the curve to the right include increased CO_2 (Haldane effect), increased hydrogen ion concentration (Bohr effect), increased temperature, and increased 2,3-diphosphoglycerate concentration. Interestingly, conditions that decrease Hb affinity prevail in the peripheral tissues where unloading of O_2 is desirable. Conversely, a decrease in any of the above conditions shifts the curve to the left. Because shifted curves converge in the plateau phase, a shift in the O_2-Hb curve has a more profound effect on the steep phase than on the plateau phase of the curve. For this reason, shifts in the curve have a greater physiologic effect on unloading of O_2 in the peripheral tissues than on loading of O_2 in the lung. Shifts in the O_2-Hb curve are quantified by measurement of the O_2 tension at which Hb is 50% saturated (P_{50}). Even though shifts in the O_2-Hb curve can have an important effect on pulmonary function, they are generally not assessed clinically. Nevertheless, it is useful for clinicians to be mindful of the possibility for such effects in their patients.

O_2 Content

Arterial O_2 content (CaO_2) is the total O_2 present in arterial blood. Each gram of Hb is capable of carrying 1.34 mL molecular O_2 when fully saturated. Thus, the amount of O_2 bound to Hb can be calculated by multiplying 1.34 (mL O_2/g) times the Hb concentration of blood (g/dL) times S_aO_2. Dissolved O_2 can be calculated from the barometric pressure and P_aO_2. At sea level, dissolved O_2 is equal to 0.003 mL O_2/dL of blood/mm Hg P_aO_2 loading pressure. Thus, C_aO_2 is calculated:

$$C_aO_2\ (\text{mL } O_2/\text{dL}) = S_aO_2\ (\%) \times \text{Hb (g/dL)} \times 1.34\ (\text{mL } O_2/\text{g}) + P_aO_2\ (\text{mm Hg}) \times 0.003\ (\text{mL } O_2/\text{dL/mm Hg})$$

For an animal at sea level with a P_aO_2 of 97 mm Hg, an S_aO_2 of 97%, and a Hb concentration of 15 g/dL, the C_aO_2 would be:

$$\begin{aligned} C_aO_2\ (\text{mL } O_2/\text{dL}) &= 0.97 \times 15 \text{ g/dL} \times 1.34 \text{ mL } O_2/\text{g} \\ &\quad + 97 \text{ mm Hg} \times 0.003 \text{ mL } O_2/\text{dL/mm Hg} \\ &= 19.5 \text{ mL } O_2/\text{dL} + 0.3 \text{ mL } O_2/\text{dL} \end{aligned}$$

From this calculation it is apparent that the contribution of dissolved O_2 to overall C_aO_2 is negligible and for clinical purposes can be ignored. Thus, the principal clinical determinants of C_aO_2 are S_aO_2 and Hb. Polycythemia and anemia can have an important impact on C_aO_2. Within limits, polycythemia is an important adaptive mechanism for physiologic (*e.g.*, altitude) or pathophysiologic causes of hypoxemia. Conversely, anemia can substantially decrease C_aO_2, even when pulmonary function is normal.

Cyanosis

Cyanosis is the result of desaturation of Hb. Central cyanosis is caused by central hypoxemia of the arterial blood due to abnormal pulmonary function (*i.e.*, low S_aO_2). Increased O_2 extraction in the capillaries due to low O_2 delivery can cause excessive desaturation of capillary and venous blood and can give the appearance of cyanosis. This is termed peripheral cyanosis. Thus, the presence of cyanosis alone does not distinguish between pulmonary and circulatory dysfunction.

Anemia

The importance of the direct effect that anemia has on C_aO_2 is generally not totally appreciated by veterinary clinicians. In animals with a relatively normal cardiovascular system, deficits in C_aO_2 caused by anemia can be compensated for by an increase in cardiac output. However, if the cardiovascular system is compromised, as is often the case in critical patients, anemia can have an important effect on O_2 delivery.

Assessment of S_aO_2 and C_aO_2

Hemoximetry

The S_aO_2 can be measured directly or calculated from the P_aO_2. The S_aO_2 reported by most automated blood gas machines actually represents a calculated value based on measurement of the P_aO_2 and then calculation from a normalized O_2-Hb saturation curve. Direct measurement of S_aO_2 can be obtained by spectrometric analysis of an arterial blood sample using an automated hemoximeter. Automated hemoximeters measure the amounts of total Hb, O_2-bound Hb, carboxyhemoglobin, and methemoglobin; and can be calibrated to the type of Hb of the species being measured. From these measures, an accurate S_aO_2 and C_aO_2 can be reported. Hemoximeters can also be used to assess shifts in the O_2-Hb saturation curve.

Pulse Oximetry

The most common method of assessing S_aO_2 in veterinary patients is pulse oximetry. Pulse oximetry is a colormetric technique that compares color differences during and between arterial pulse surges in capillary beds, and thereby estimates Hb saturation of arterial blood. The equipment and methodology of pulse oximetry are reviewed in Chapter 8.

O_2 DELIVERY

Oxygen delivery ($\dot{D}o_2$) is the milliliters of O_2 delivered to the peripheral tissues each minute and is the product of C_aO_2 and cardiac output ($\dot{Q}$):

$$\dot{D}o_2(\text{mL } O_2/\text{min}) = C_aO_2(\text{mL } O_2/\text{dL}) \times \dot{Q}\ (\text{dL/min})$$

Thus, when hypoxemia or anemia causes C_aO_2 to be low, O_2 delivery can be maintained by an increase in cardiac output.

Oxygen consumption ($\dot{V}O_2$) is the milliliters of O_2 consumed by tissues each minute and can be calculated by multiplying the difference between C_aO_2 and mixed venous oxygen content (C_vO_2) times $\dot{Q}$:

$$\dot{V}O_2(\text{mL } O_2/\text{min}) = [C_aO_2 - C_vO_2 \text{ (mL } O_2/\text{dL)}] \times \dot{Q} \text{ (dL/min)}$$

From the above relationship it can be seen that in the setting of a low cardiac output, $\dot{V}O_2$ can be maintained by an increase in the $C_aO_2 - C_vO_2$ difference.

Low Cardiac Output

Low cardiac output has a direct adverse effect on O_2 delivery. The causes of low cardiac output in the critical care unit are many and are the subject of other chapters in this textbook. Briefly, low cardiac output can result from deficits in the circulation (*i.e.*, circulatory failure) or the heart (*i.e.*, low output heart failure). Important causes of circulatory failure include hypovolemia, sepsis, and major vascular obstruction. Causes of low output heart failure include myocardial failure, valvular insufficiency, cardiac dysrhythmias, and cardiac tamponade.

Assessment of O_2 Delivery

Measurement of Cardiac Output

Cardiac output is the volume of blood pumped by the heart in 1 minute. Direct measurement of cardiac output is accomplished clinically by the technique of thermodilution. Thermodilution is based on the indicator dilution principle of measuring flow and requires a thermistor-equipped Swan-Ganz catheter (Fig. 21-7). The technique is performed by injecting saline at a known volume and temperature, and then recording the temperature change that results as it passes the thermistor. The area under the time-temperature curve is inversely proportional to the cardiac output. Because normal cardiac output is dependent on the size of the patient, cardiac output is usually reported as cardiac index (CI) normalized to body weight or body surface area. Normal CI for healthy conscious dogs at rest is reported to be 5.4 dL/min/m^2 body surface area.[6] Because of the equipment, expertise, and expense required for Swan-Ganz catheterization, it is not commonly used in clinical veterinary medicine. Swan-Ganz catheterization is indicated for advanced cardiopulmonary supportive care in animals with severe cardiopulmonary compromise.

O_2 Extraction Ratio

The O_2 extraction ratio is the proportion of O_2 consumed ($\dot{V}O_2$) to O_2 delivered ($\dot{D}O_2$):

$$O_2 \text{ extraction ratio} = \frac{\dot{V}O_2}{\dot{D}O_2} = \frac{[C_aO_2 - C_vO_2]}{C_aO_2 \times \dot{Q}} \times \dot{Q}$$

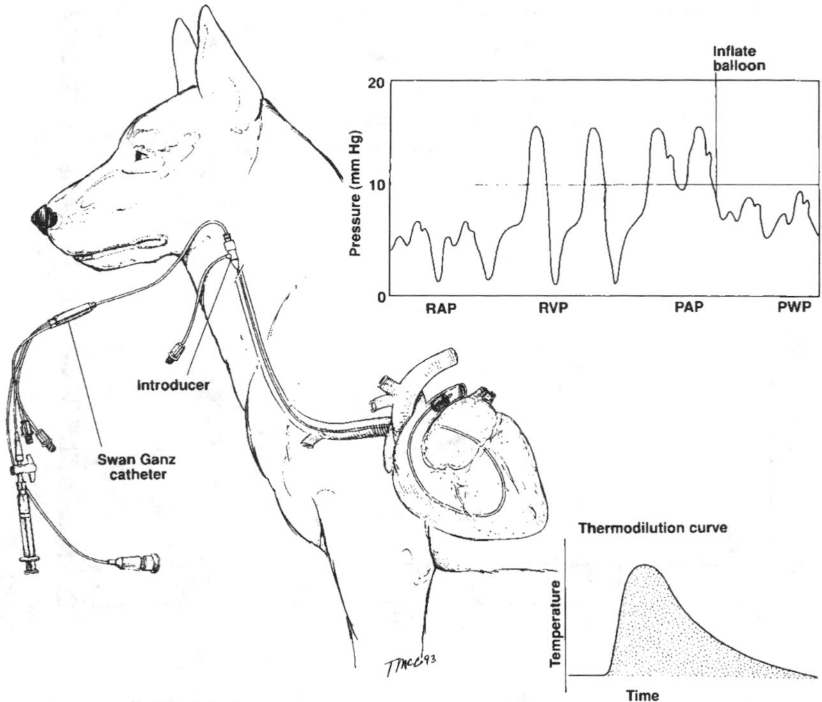

Figure 21-7
Swan-Ganz catheterization. A flow-directed Swan-Ganz catheter is introduced into a jugular vein and floated through the right heart into the pulmonary artery with the aid of an inflatable balloon. The position of the catheter is determined by observing characteristic right atrial pressure (RAP), right ventricular pressure (RVP), and pulmonary artery pressure (PAP). Pulmonary wedge pressure (PWP) is obtained by inflation of the balloon with the catheter placed in the pulmonary artery. Cardiac output is determined by thermodilution during injection of a known volume and temperature of saline and measurement of the change in blood temperature by a thermistor on the tip of the Swan-Ganz catheter. Cardiac output is calculated from the area under the temperature-time thermodilution curve.

Because cardiac output is in both the numerator and denominator, it cancels out. Thus, determination of O_2 extraction ratio does not require actual measurement of cardiac output. Also, Hb concentration is the same in arterial and mixed venous blood. As a result, calculation of O_2 extraction can be simplified to:

$$O_2 \text{ extraction ratio} = \frac{S_aO_2 - S_vO_2}{S_aO_2}$$

Because the O_2 extraction ratio accounts for any deficits in S_aO_2 in the delivery of O_2 to tissues, it becomes primarily a measure of the adequacy of cardiac output. The utility of the O_2 extraction ratio is that it is independent of the patient size and does not require actual measurement of cardiac output. As such, the O_2 extraction ratio is a clinically useful method of assessing the adequacy of cardiac

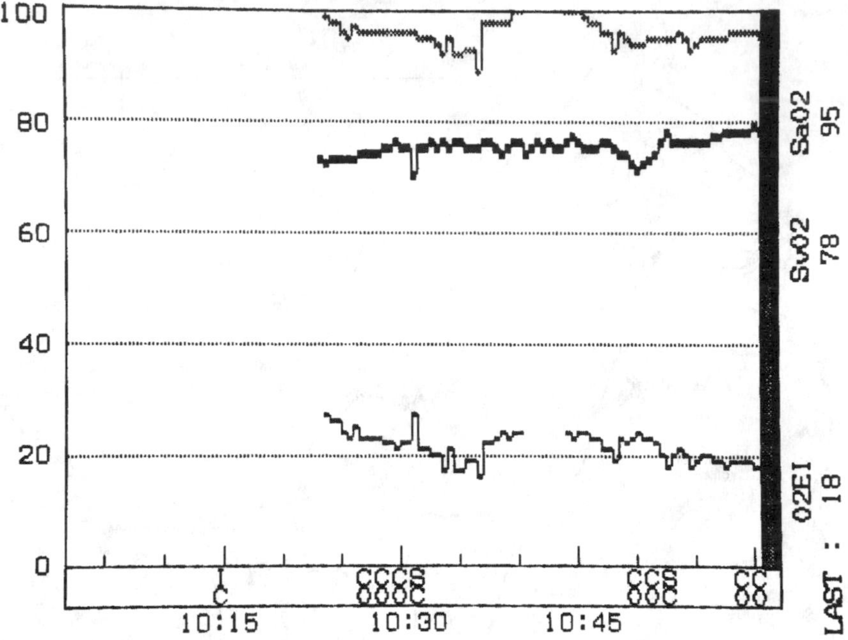

Figure 21-8
Oxygen extraction ratio measured continuously in a dog with a pulmonary artery catheter with oximetry. The first tracing is arterial pulse oximeter, the second is the pulmonary artery pulse oximeter, and the third is the oxygen extraction ratio.

output in veterinary patients. Under normal physiologic conditions at rest, O_2 extraction is about 0.25. When cardiac output becomes inadequate to meet the demands of the patient, O_2 extraction increases. An O_2 extraction ratio of greater than 0.4 suggests that cardiac output is seriously inadequate (Fig. 21-8).

SUMMARY

Adequate cardiopulmonary function depends on several physiologic processes to achieve the ultimate goal of delivering O_2 to tissues. Derangement of any of these physiologic processes can result in inadequate O_2 delivery. The challenge of the veterinary critical care clinician is to quickly and logically determine the pathophysiologic causes of disruptions in O_2 delivery. Fortunately, techniques for determining the nature and magnitude of pathophysiologic disruptions in the cardiopulmonary system are readily available to the clinician with an understanding of these processes.

REFERENCES

1. West JB: Pulmonary Pathophysiology—The Essentials, 2nd ed. Baltimore: Williams & Wilkins, 1982.
2. Walton RS, Wingfield WE, Ogilvie GK, *et al.*: Energy expenditure in 104 postopera-

tive and traumatically injured dogs with indirect calorimetry. *J Vet Emerg Crit Care* 6:71, 1996.
3. Gilbert R, Kreighley JF: The arterial/alveolar oxygen tension ratio. An index of gas exchange applicable to varying inspired oxygen concentrations. *Am Rev Respir Dis* 109:42, 1974.
4. D'Alonzo GE, Dantzger DR: Mechanisms of abnormal gas exchange. *Med Clin North Am* 67:557, 1983.
5. Van Pelt DR, Wingfield WE, Wheeler SL, Salman MD: Oxygen-tension based indices as predictors of survival in critically ill dogs: clinical observations and review. *J Vet Emerg Crit Care* 1:19, 1991.
6. Bennett RA, Orton EC, Tucker A, Heiller C: Cardiopulmonary changes in conscious dogs with induced progressive pneumothorax. *Am J Vet Res* 50:280, 1989.

22
Acute Renal Failure

Sheri J. Ross, Carl A. Osborne, Jody P. Lulich, and David J. Polzin

INTRODUCTION

The goal of this chapter is to provide information that will assist ICU staff in the management of patients with acute renal failure (ARF). For in-depth discussions about etiopathogenesis, diagnosis, and treatment of acute and chronic renal failure, consult appropriate reference material.[1,3,7,11,12]

PATHOPHYSIOLOGY OF ACUTE RENAL FAILURE

Acute renal failure may be defined as a potentially reversible syndrome of diverse etiology characterized by an abrupt and sustained decline in renal function (glomerular filtration, tubular reabsorption, and tubular secretion) producing impaired excretion of metabolic wastes (as indicated by azotemia), impaired ability to maintain fluid, electrolyte, and acid-base balance, and uremia. Acute intrinsic renal failure is commonly associated with ischemic events or exposure to nephrotoxins (including drugs), although it may be caused by other mechanisms including renal infections (ie, leptospirosis, borreliosis, or bacterial UTI associated with urine outflow obstruction), immune mediated diseases, and hypercalcemia (Table 22-1). Many risk factors, which are additive, predispose patients to acute renal failure.

A common event in both ischemic and nephrotoxic ARF is structural and functional damage to renal tubules, giving rise to the term "acute tubular necrosis." ATN may be associated with many different causes, may be mild or severe, and may be associated with varying degrees of alterations in renal perfusion, glomerular filtration, and tubular dysfunction.

Conceptually the syndrome of ARF may be divided into three sequential stages: 1) initiation, 2) maintenance, and 3) recovery. However, in many patients, the transition from one stage to the next may not be clearly evident. In addition, all three stages may not be evident in the same patient.

The first, or *initiation (induction) phase* may last from hours to days and is the period during which the kidneys are exposed to ischemia, toxins, or other causes of dysfunction (Table 22-1). During this period tubular epithelial cells are damaged, and there is a progressive decline in GFR (as evidenced by azotemia) and impairment of tubular function (as evidenced by impaired ability to concentrate urine). A history of exposure to the underlying cause(s) of ARF, nonurinary clinical signs attributable to these causes, and progressive increases

Table 22-1. Classification of Some Causes of Acute Renal Failure Based on Localization of Azotemia

- A. Prerenal
  - 1. Intravascular Volume Depletion
    - a. Shock (hypotensive; heat-stroke)
    - b. Gastrointestinal losses (especially if associated with impaired renal concentrating capacity)
    - c. Renal losses (inappropriate use of diuretics)
    - d. Third space sequestration of fluid (pancreatitis; peritonitis; trauma)
    - e. Hypoalbuminemia
  - 2. Decreased Effective Arterial Volume
    - a. Shock (septic; cardiogenic)
    - b. Antihypertensive drugs
    - c. Prolonged or deep anesthesia
    - d. Reduced cardiac function (congestive failure; arrhythmias; pericardial tamponade)
  - 3. Systemic Diseases
    - a. Pyometra
    - b. Hypoadrenocorticism
    - c. Diseases associated with DIC
- B. Intrarenal
  - 1. Vascular
    - a. Bilateral renal artery obstruction due to thromboembolism
    - b. Vascular lesions in a single functioning kidney
  - 2. Glomerular
    - a. Immune mediated glomerulonephropathy
    - b. Amyloidosis (uncommon)
  - 3. Tubular
    - a. Ischemic (including persistent prerenal causes)
    - b. Nephrotoxic (ie, Heavy metals; Ethylene glycol; Antimicrobials, including aminoglycosides, sulfonamides, amphotericin, etc.; Chemotherapeutics, including methotrexate, azothioprine, cisplatin, etc.; Analgesics, including non-steroidal anti-inflammatory drugs given to hypotensive patients)
    - c. Iodinated radiographic contrast agents given to dehydrated patients
    - d. Endogenous pigments (hemoglobin from intravascular hemolysis; myoglobin from rhabdomyolysis)
    - e. Hypercalcemia
  - 4. Interstitial
    - a. Leptospirosis
    - b. Bacterial infection of kidneys associated with urine outflow obstruction
    - c. Adverse drug reactions
- C. Postrenal
    - a. Obstruction of both ureters (perineal herniation of urinary bladder; iatrogenic surgery) or one ureter (when there is poor function in contralateral kidney)
    - b. Urethral obstruction (uroliths; trauma; neoplasia; etc)
    - c. Reabsorption of urine into circulation (rent in wall of urinary bladder or ureters)

in enzymuria, proteinuria, and cylinduria may also occur. However, the initiation phase of ARF is not often recognized because these abnormalities are not associated with the onset of clinical signs that direct one's attention to the kidneys. This is unfortunate because therapeutic intervention at this phase may reduce the severity of renal damage and dysfunction thereby enhancing the likelihood of recovery.

The second, or *maintenance phase*, may last for days to weeks. It represents the period during which renal parenchymal damage is extensive, and is associated with persistent reductions in GFR and tubular dysfunction associated with oliguria, nonoliguria, and less commonly polyuria. Unlike the initiation phase, polysystemic clinical and serum biochemical manifestations of uremia become obvious. Eliminating inciting factors at this stage will not correct existing damage, but will likely minimize further injury.

The third, or *recovery stage*, may last for weeks to months and is usually characterized by a transition from an oliguric or nonoliguric state to a polyuric state, progressive improvement in GFR resulting in gradual resolution of azotemia, and amelioration of the polysystemic consequences of renal dysfunction. Recovery of adequate function to restore homeostasis without the need for continuous supportive therapy is dependent on regeneration of damaged tubular epithelial cells and compensatory hypertrophy of viable nephrons. Although there is potential for recovery of renal function, in some patients residual impairment in glomerular filtration and renal concentrating capacity may persist indefinitely.

Oliguria associated with formation of a reduced quantity urine may be physiologic or pathologic. Production of a decreased volume of highly concentrated urine in patients with prerenal azotemia is an example of *physiologic compensatory oliguria* designed to maintain body fluid balance (Table 22-2). Azotemia associated with high urine specific gravity values provides evidence that the kidneys are structurally normal and capable of quantitatively adequate function to maintain homeostasis provided the prerenal cause is removed in a timely fashion. However, if the prerenal cause is allowed to persist, ischemic renal disease resulting in acute renal failure may develop. Rapid resolution of azotemia (ie, within 1 to 3 days) in response to replacement of fluid deficits and the onset of a brisk diuresis is the expected response if the patient has prerenal azotemia and physiologic oliguria (Table 22-3).

Following the onset of ischemia or exposure to nephrotoxins (initiation phase of acute renal failure), extensive renal cell damage combined with host responses may result in *pathologic oliguria* (maintenance phase of acute renal failure) and progressive azotemia (see Table 22-2). The magnitude of azotemia can not be used to reliably predict whether the patient is oliguric, nonoliguric, or polyuric, nor is it a reliable index of the duration (acute or chronic) of the underlying disease.

At least four intrarenal mechanisms have been incriminated to explain pathologic oliguria in patients with intrinsic ARF. They include: 1) constriction of renal vessels and contraction of the glomerular mesangium via tubuloglomerular feedback resulting in reduced renal blood flow and decreased glomerular filtration; 2) reduced filtration of water and solute through glomerular capillary walls; 3) obstruction of tubular lumens with swollen and disintegrating epithelial cells, casts, heme pigments, and/or extraluminal compression of tubular lumens secondary to interstitial edema and inflammation; and 4) backleak of tubular fluid across damaged tubular walls into the renal interstitium. Conceptual knowledge of these mechanisms is of value since it facilitates formulation of treatment protocols designed to interrupt them.

Table 22-2. Characteristic Urine Specific Gravity Values Associated with Azotemia in Dogs and Cats[a]

Prerenal Azotemia

Physiologic oliguria
Dogs: U_{SG} > 1.030†
Cats: U_{SG} > 1.035 to 1.040†

Primary Acute Ischemic or Nephrotoxic Azotemia

Initial Oliguria[b]
Dogs: U_{SG} = 1.006 to ~1.029
Cats: U_{SG} = 1.006 to 1.039††
Subsequent Polyuric Phase
Dogs: U_{SG} = 1.006 to ~1.029
Cats: U_{SG} = 1.006 to ~1.039

Obstructive Postrenal Azotemia

Initial oliguria or anuria
Diuresis and polyuria following relief of obstruction
Urine specific gravity values are variable

Primary Chronic Azotemia

Polyuria
Dogs: 1.006 to ~1.029
Cats: 1.006 to ~1.039[c]††
Terminal Oliguric Phase
U_{SG} = 1.007 to ~1.013
Reversible Oliguria Due to Factors Indicing Prerenal Azotemia
Dogs: U_{SG} = 1.006 to ~1.029
Cats: U_{SG} = 1.006 to ~1.039[c]††

[a] From Osborne CA, et al: Pathophysiology of renal disease, renal failure, and uremia. *In* Ettinger SG (ed.): *Textbook of Veterinary Internal Medicine,* vol 2, ed 2. Philadelphia, WB Saunders Co, 1982, p 1758.
[b] Acute renal failure caused by nephrotoxic drugs often is not associated with an initial phase of pathologic oliguria. The term nonoliguric is often used to describe such patients.
[c] Urine specific gravity may become fixed between approximately 1.007 and 1.013 if sufficient nephron function is altered. The specific gravity of glomerular filtrate is approximately 1.008 to 1.012.
† Unless concentrating capacity is impaired by concurrent disease (ie, hypoadrenocorticism, hypercalcemia), parenterally administered fluids, or diuretics.
†† Some cats with primary renal azotemia may concentrate urine to 1.045 or higher.

Not all patients with acute renal failure develop pathologic oliguria. Nonoliguric acute renal failure is common (up to 50% of the patients) and is characterized by azotemia associated with formation of a relatively fixed but inappropriate volume of urine that is intermediate between oliguria and polyuria.

The underlying causes of a nonoliguric state associated with ARF are similar but less severe than those associated with oliguric ARF (see Table 22-1). Nonoliguric ARF is more often associated with nephrotoxic renal failure than ischemic renal failure. Compared to oliguric acute renal failure, nonoliguric and polyuric acute renal failure are often associated with lesser degrees of renal paren-

Table 22-3. Differentiation of Azotemia

Observation	Prerenal*	Intrarenal* Normal hydration	Prerenal and Intrarenal*	Postrenal*
Blood urea nitrogen	↑	↑	↑	↑
Serum creatinine	↑	↑	↑	↑
Serum phosphorous	N, ↑	↑	↑	↑
Serum calcium	N	↑, N, ↓	↑, N, ↓	N
Serum sodium	N, (↑), (↓)	↑, N, ↓	↑, N, ↓	↑, N, ↓
Serum potassium	N	N, ↑, ↓	N, ↑, ↓	N, ↑
Serum chloride	N	↑, N, ↓	↑, N, ↓	N
Blood bicarbonate	↓, N	↓, N	↓, N	↓, N
Urine specific gravity	1.030+ dog 1.040+ cat	1.007 to 1.029 dog 1.007 to 1.039 cat	1.007 to 1.029 dog 1.007 to 1.039 cat	Variable
Urine output	↓, N	↓, N, ↑	↓, N, ↑	↓
Packed cell volume	N, ↑	N, ↓	N, ↑, (↓)	N
Historical polydipsia/polyuria	0	+, (0)	+, (0)	0, (+)
Historical oliguria/anuria	+, (0)	0, (+)	0, (+)	+, (0)
Historical uremic symptoms	0	+, 0	+, 0	0
Debilitation	0	+, 0	+, 0	0
Renal osteodystrophy	0	+, 0	+, 0	0
Kidney size	N	↓, N, ↑	↓, N, ↑	N, ↑
Response of azotemia to rehydration with fluids	Good	Comparatively poor	Partial**	Variable**
Response of oliguria to rehydration with fluids	Dramatic	Variable	Partial**	Variable**

↑ = increased; N = normal range; ↓ = decreased; 0 = absent; + = present, values in parentheses = atypical.
* Values expected prior to the initiation of therapy. ** Magnitude of response is dependent on magnitude of prerenal component contributing to azotemia.

chymal damage, less severe azotemia, fewer complications, and less mortality. In context of fluid and electrolyte imbalances, oliguric renal failure tends to be associated with greater retention of water and electrolytes, while polyuric renal failure tends to be associated with comparatively greater deficits of water and electrolytes.

CLINICAL PRESENTATION

There are many similarities between the clinical manifestations of acute and chronic renal failure (Table 22-4). In addition to localizing the underlying cause(s) of azotemia (see Table 22-3; Fig. 22-1), be sure to distinguish acute onset of acute renal failure from acute decompensation of chronic renal failure (so-called "acute-on-chronic" renal failure) (see Table 22-4). Whereas acute renal failure is potentially reversible if the underlying cause is corrected, chronic renal failure is typically irreversible and progressive. Although patients with acute renal failure may not regain total renal function, if appropriately managed they have the potential to eventually regain adequate renal function to sustain life without need for extensive and prolonged therapy. Structural and functional changes in patients with chronic renal failure are typically progressive and irreversible.

Oliguria has been defined as production of approximately 0.25 to 0.5 ml/kg/hr. This figure is derived from the estimated minimum quantity of urine in which the average daily solute load can be excreted by kidneys with normal concentrating capacity. Urine production of <0.5 to 1.0 ml/kg/hr during IV fluid therapy is suggestive of oliguric renal failure. Production of urine that does not exceed 1 to 2.0 ml/kg/hr following rehydration with IV fluids is suggestive of nonoliguric renal failure.

MONITORING

The kidneys' capacity to produce urine is best assessed in well-hydrated patients with adequate blood pressure. Normal urine production for a healthy adult euvolemic, normotensive dog is 1 to 2 ml/kg/hr (20 to 40 ml/kg/24 hours). Normal urine production for a healthy adult euvolemic, normotensive cat is 1 to 1.5 ml/kg/hr (20 to 30 ml/kg/24 hours). Normal urine production for an healthy adult dog or cat during intravenous fluid therapy is approximately 2 to 5 ml/kg/hr.

Early detection of pathological oliguria is especially important since it influences the quantity and type of parenteral fluids that can be safely given to the patient. The most accurate method to determine and monitor urine volume is with the aid of a transurethral catheter. To minimize the risk of nosocomial bacterial UTI, intermittent urinary catheterization is usually recommended over indwelling transurethral catheterization (see Table 22-7). Alternatives to transurethral catheterization include collection of urine via a metabolism cage, measuring weight gains of a cat's litter pans attributable to urine, or weighing absorbent pads used to collect voided urine. Less reliable methods of assessing urine volume include serial assessment of bladder size by abdominal palpation or ultra-

Table 22-4. Typical Profile of Patients with Acute Primary Renal Failure, Chronic Primary Renal Failure, and/or Acute Decompensation of Chronic Primary Renal Failure

History and Physical Exam	Chronic	Acute	Acute or Chronic
Recent exposure to nephrotoxin or ischemic episode	Unlikely	Probable	Possible
Previously diagnosed renal failure	Possible	Unusual	Usually
Weight loss	Chronic due to tissue loss	Acute due to fluid loss	Tissue and fluid loss
Urine volume	Prolonged polyuria; potential oliguria	Initial oliguria; subsequent polyuria	Oliguria preceded by prolonged polyuria
Severity of signs for comparable degree of azotemia	Less severe due to compensatory adaptations	Marked	Moderate
Radiographs / Ultrasound			
Renal size and shape	Often decreased; may be normal, increased, or unequal in size	Normal to increased	Decreased, may be normal or increased. May reveal radiodense uroliths.
Renal surface contour	Often irregular	Smooth	Often irregular
Osteodystrophy	Often	Absent	Often
Blood Chemistry			
Serum urea nitrogen	Increased	Increased	Increased
Serum creatinine	Increased	Increased	Increased
Serum osmolality	Increased	Increased	Increased

Serum phosphorous	Increased	Increased	Increased
Serum calcium	Usually normal to decreased; may be increased	Variable, dependent on cause	Usually normal to decreased; may be increased
Serum potassium	Normal if polyuric; Increased if oliguric	Increased if oliguric; Normal if polyuric	Normal if polyuric; Increased if oliguric
Blood bicarbonate (metabolic acidosis)	Mild to moderate decrease	Moderate to severe decrease	Moderate to severe decrease
Hemogram			
PCV and Hb	Normal to decreased (nonregenerative)	May initially be normal or increased; then decreased	Normal to decreased (nonregenerative)
Urinalysis			
Impaired renal concentrating & diluting ability	Yes	Yes	Yes
Glucosuria	Very uncommon	Sometimes, primarily with nephrotoxins	Uncommon
Pyuria	Variable	Variable; suggests infectious cause	Variable
Crystalluria	Uncommon	Calcium oxalate with ethylene glycol	Uncommon
Proteinuria	Variable	Variable	Variable
Tubular casts	Uncommon	Granular casts frequently associated with ischemia and nephrotoxins; white cell casts indicate infectious cause	Possible

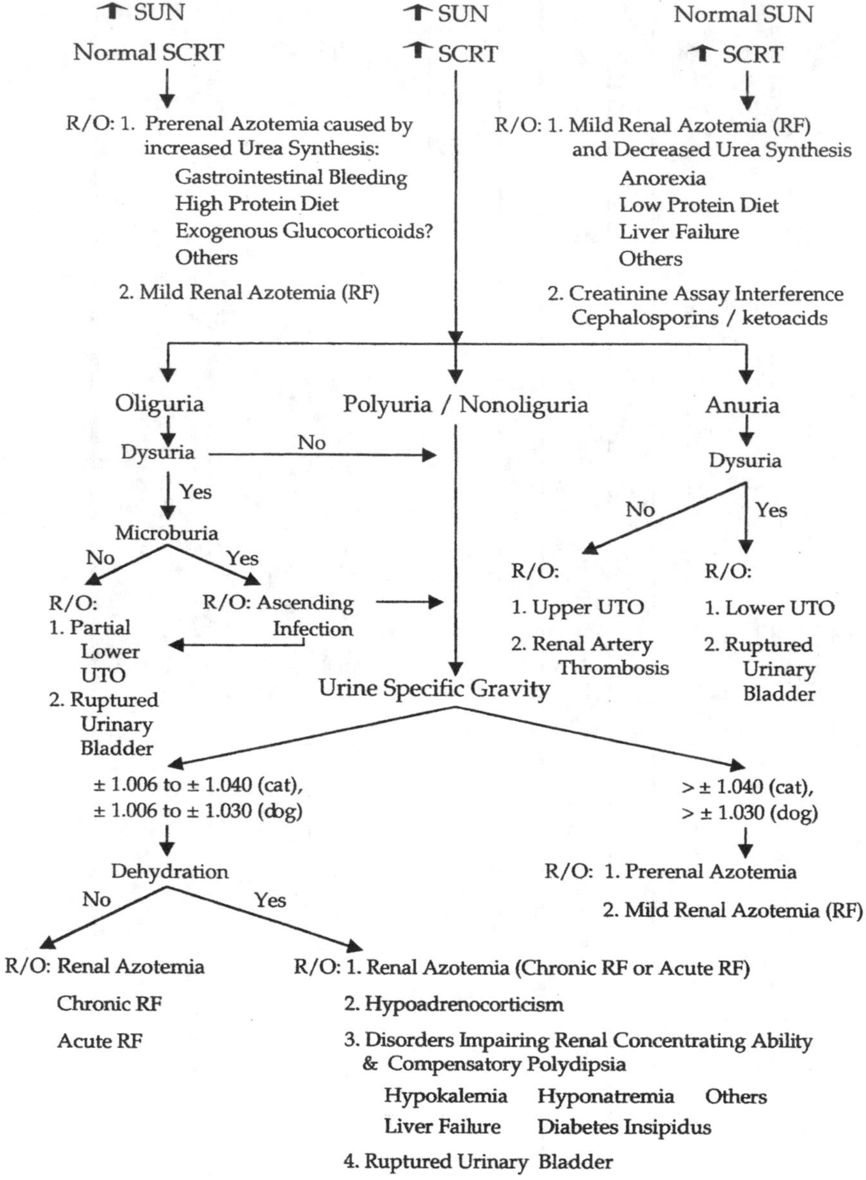

Figure 22-1
Algorithm for diagnosis of azotemic renal failure. SUN = serum urea nitrogen concentration; SCRT = serum creatinine concentration; R/O = rule out; UTO = urinary tract obstruction.

Table 22-5. Potentially Life-threatening Clinical Findings in Renal Failure Patients

I. Life-threatening Abnormalities
  A. Severe dehydration
  B. Iatrogenic overhydration
  C. Severe metabolic acidosis
  D. Severe hypokalemia or hyperkalemia
  E. Severe hypocalcemia
  F. Iatrogenic drug events
II. Non Life-threatening Abnormalities
  A. Severe azotemia
  B. Severe hyperphosphatemia
  C. Moderate anemia
  D. Moderate hypercalcemia

sonography, and visual assessment of the quantity of urine that is voided. These methods are more likely to be reliable when the patient is producing large rather than small volumes of urine. In addition to monitoring fluid balance, accurate measurement of urine volume facilitates evaluation of endogenous creatinine clearance.

Fluid administration must be monitored carefully because patients that remain oliguric following restoration of vascular volume and pressure are at high risk for iatrogenic overhydration (Tables 22-5, 22-6, 22-7, and 22-8). These consequences include systemic hypertension, pulmonary and peripheral edema, and congestive heart failure. Therefore, in addition to monitoring the rate of formation of urine, the fluid therapy prescription may be regularly readjusted on the

Table 22-6. Biochemical Findings in Patients with Polyuric and Oliguric Renal Failure

Factor	Polyuria	Oliguria
Urine Specific Gravity	1.007 to 1.029 dog 1.007 to 1.040 cat	1.007 to 1.029 dog 1.007 to 1.040 cat
Urea nitrogen (serum)	Increased	Increased
Creatinine (serum)	Increased	Increased
Sodium (serum)	Usually normal	Variable
Sodium (total body)	Variable	Variable
Potassium (serum)	Usually normal	Increased
pH (blood)	Normal to decreased	Marked decrease
Phosphorus (serum)	Usually increased	Usually increased
Calcium (serum)	Usually normal to decreased*†	Usually normal to decreased*†

* Unless renal failure is caused by hypercalcemia.

† Occasionally hypercalcemia occurs as a sequelae to primary renal failure.

Table 22-7. Guidelines to Reduce Risk of Catheter-induced Bacterial UTI

1. Urinary catheterization should only be performed by personnel properly trained and experienced with use of proper aseptic, atraumatic techniques.
2. Select indwelling urethral catheters constructed of materials least likely to cause irritation and inflammation of the adjacent mucosa.
3. Thoroughly cleanse the external genitalia, and insert the catheter using aseptic technique.
4. Avoid overinsertion of catheters to minimize damage to urinary bladder mucosa.
5. Avoid open catheters; maintain a closed collection system.
6. Prevent retrograde flow of urine from the collection receptacle by positioning it below the level of the patient.
7. Perform urinalyses every 24 to 48 hours for evidence of infection. Culture urine if infection is suspected.
8. If catheter-induced infection develops and remains asymptomatic, treat the infection following removal of the catheter.
9. Remove the catheter as soon as possible. At the time of catheter removal, perform a urinalysis, quantitative urine culture, and antimicrobial susceptibility test.
10. Avoid giving prophylactic antimicrobial drugs in attempt to prevent UTI unless the duration of catheterization is less than 2–3 days.
11. If UTI is confirmed after the catheter is removed, initiate therapy with an appropriate antimicrobial drug known to be effective against nosocomial hospital pathogens and continue giving for at least 10 to 14 days.
12. If infection with more than one bacterial species occurs, and if the pathogens have different susceptibilities to drug, first treat the bacteria most likely to be virulent. Then select the drug most likely to eliminate the remaining pathogens.
13. Remove and, if appropriate, replace indwelling catheters that are contaminated.

basis of sequential assessment of body weight, skin turgor, PCV, plasma total solids, and central venous pressure (CVP).

Body weight should be monitored with a reliable scale at least twice per day. Rapid gain or loss of 1 kg of body weight represents a corresponding gain or loss of one liter of fluid. The quantity of fluid given should be adjusted so that body weight remains stable. However, if the patient is not receiving sufficient calories, a decline of approximately 0.3 kilograms per day should be allowed for each 1000 kilocalories of unmet energy requirement.

Central venous pressure provides a reliable index of hydration status. In the absence of heart disease, an increase of CVP in a patient with ARF could indicate overhydration. The CVP should not increase more than 2 to 4 cm water above baseline if cardiovascular function is normal. An increase of CVP of 5 to 7 cm above baseline or an absolute CVP of greater than 10 cm water is indicative of excessive rate or volume of fluid administration.[1,3]

In addition to CVP, serum urea, creatinine, electrolyte, and TCO_2 concentrations should be reassessed at appropriate intervals. If the prerenal components are the primary cause of decreased GFR, restoration of fluid deficits will be followed by a rapid onset of diuresis (urine production > 1 mL/kg/hour) and rapid reduction of azotemia.

Table 22-8. Overhydration of Acute Renal Failure Patients

	Vascular Hypervolemia	Interstitial Hypervolemia
Clinical Signs	1. Jugular vein distention, weight gain, pounding pulses, hypertension, radiographic evidence of pulmonary vein or caudal vena cava distention.	1. Serous ocular and nasal discharge. 2. Subcutaneous edema, nonpainful, dependent, pitting. 3. Ascites, hydrothorax etc. 4. Increased respiratory rate +/− crackles. Radiographic evidence of pulmonary interstitial edema.
Risk Factors	1. Iatrogenic fluid overload, especially in oliguric patients. 2. Concomitant heart failure.	1. Iatrogenic fluid overload especially in oliguric patients. 2. Concomitant heart failure. 3. Impaired renal excretion of fluids. 4. Concomitant hypoproteinemia 5. DIC 6. Hypertension
Management	1. The best treatment is prevention. Fluid overload is difficult to manage. 2. Strive to eliminate or correct the underlying disease process. 3. Discontinue and reassess prescription for fluid therapy. 4. Attempt to initiate diuresis. If there is no response, do not use additional diuretics. 5. Attempt to restore fluid balance by peritoneal dialysis or by hemodialysis.	

Diuresis due to increased renal tubular fluid flow rate, but unassociated with a corresponding increase in RBF and glomerular filtration rate, may reduce the serum concentration of urea nitrogen to a greater degree than serum creatinine concentration. This occurs because diuresis decreases the passive renal tubular reabsorption of urea from tubular filtrate. Since tubular reabsorption of creatinine is not affected by changes in tubular flow rate, the magnitude of decrease in serum urea nitrogen concentration is substantially greater than serum creatinine concentration. Therefore evaluation of the serum concentration of creatinine provides a more reliable index of glomerular filtration rate than does SUN concentration. Improved GFR is indicated by increased urine production combined with a decrease in serum creatinine concentration.

Once the patient is adequately rehydrated, fluid balance can be maintained by providing sufficient parenteral fluids to match estimated insensible respiratory losses, and continuous losses via urine, vomiting, and diarrhea. Insensible fluid losses have been estimated to be approximately 20 to 25 ml/kg/day, but may vary with the patient's daily caloric requirements (or body weight), respiratory rate, body temperature as well as room air temperature and humidity. Because estimates of insensible and continuous losses of fluids are subject to error, the patient's body weight and other indices of hydration status should be accurately determined every 12 hours.

THERAPY

Early recognition of acute renal failure is important since therapeutic intervention during the induction stage is most likely to be successful in minimizing renal injury. Formulation of therapeutic strategies designed to interrupt the pathophysiologic events contributing to oliguric renal failure is especially important. In addition, search for underlying cause(s) (see Table 22-1) with the objective of eliminating the patient's exposure to them (see the section on specific therapy). If life threatening complications are present (severe hyperkalemia, acidemia, etc.; Table 22-5) it will be necessary to treat them (supportive therapy) before the underlying causes are identified. Detection and elimination of concurrent reversible prerenal and post-renal disorders that may have precipitated or aggravated a uremic crisis should also be considered.

Since the best cure is prevention, staff in intensive care units should be familiar with risk factors that predispose patients to acute renal failure (see Table 22-1). Recognizing that various risk factors may be additive in terms of predisposing to ischemic or nephrotoxic acute renal failure; try to eliminate or control them before exposing patients to additional diagnostic (intravenous contrast urography) or therapeutic procedures (deep anesthesia or prolonged surgery) associated with ischemia or nephrotoxicity.[1,3,6,11] Advanced age and pre-existing chronic irreversible primary renal disease are risk factors that cannot be eliminated. However, dehydration, fever, sepsis, hypotension, decreased cardiac output, acidosis, hypokalemia, hyponatremia, hypomagnesemia, and hypocalcemia are treatable risk factors. Concurrent use of NSAIDs and other potentially nephrotoxic drugs, and prolonged anesthesia are also examples of risk factors that can be modified (see Table 22-1).

Prior to formulation of a therapeutic prescription for acute renal failure, the following 9 steps should be considered: 1) Collect applicable information. Collect samples of blood and urine before initiating any form of therapy; 2) Identify life threatening clinical findings and manage them accordingly (see Table 22-5). It is often necessary to initiate supportive therapy prior to the availability of diagnostic test results; 3) Localize the underlying cause of azotemia (see Table 22-3, Fig. 22-1); 4) Attempt to identify the underlying cause(s) of renal failure with the goal of eliminating or counteracting them (see Table 22-1); 5) In order to prevent iatrogenic complications associated with treatment, devise a plan to determine if the renal failure is associated with oliguria, nonoliguria, or polyuria; 6) To assist in prognosis, strive to determine if the renal failure is acute or chronic (see Table 22-5); 7) Administer drugs to patients with renal failure only after consideration of their routes and rates of metabolism and elimination, and their potential to induce adverse reactions in the uremic environment.[14] If it is absolutely essential to use potentially toxic drugs that are highly dependent on adequate renal function for metabolism or elimination, make appropriate adjustments in dosage and/or maintenance intervals; 8) Avoid polypharmacy. Do not give any drug with the philosophy that it might help, but can do no harm. Use the fewest drugs at appropriate doses consistent with proper patient care. Use special caution not to overhydrate patients in the oliguric phase of acute renal failure; 9) Formulate a systematic plan to monitor response to therapy. The type and frequency of data collected should be individualized to meet each patient's specific needs. Serially collected data should be recorded on flow charts to facilitate timely assessment of whether the abnormalities are decreasing, increasing, or remaining the same, and the rate of their change. Decreasing or increasing trends may be initially more important in assessing the patient's response to treatment than absolute laboratory values.

Conceptually, treatment of acute renal failure may be divided into three basic components: 1) specific therapy, 2) supportive therapy, and 3) symptomatic therapy.

Specific Treatment

Specific treatment is given to eliminate, destroy, or modify the primary cause(s) of the disease process. Examples of specific treatment include: 1) minimizing further ischemic renal damage by use of appropriate fluids to restore and maintain adequate renal perfusion, 2) eliminating exposure to drugs that are causing nephrotoxic injury, 3) administration of antidotes to counteract nephrotoxins, and 4) use of antibiotics to eliminate bacterial infections or leptospira. Strive to design therapy to interrupt the pathophysiolgic events that, if allowed to persist, will result in acute oliguric renal failure.

Specific therapy will not substantially alter existing renal lesions once acute primary renal failure has become established (so-called maintenance phase). In the latter situation, restoration of renal function depends on spontaneous repair of renal lesions along with compensatory increase in function of remaining viable nephrons. However, specific treatment is important to prevent further nephron damage.

Supportive Treatment

Supportive treatment consists of therapy that modifies or eliminates abnormalities that occur secondary to primary disease. Treatment of the polysystemic metabolic and biochemical dysfunctions that occur as a consequence of generalized acute renal lesions is an example of supportive therapy. Supportive therapy should be designed to minimize retention of metabolic wastes, and alterations (deficits and excesses) in fluid, electrolyte, acid-base, endocrine, and nutrient balance, with the overall goal of sustaining life (ie, "buying survival time") until sufficient nephron repair and compensatory adaptation result in the return of adequate renal function to reestablish homeostasis. Special attention should be directed toward treatment of life-threatening fluid, electrolyte, and acid-base disturbances (see Table 22-5).

Successful specific therapy is often dependent on successful supportive therapy. Although specific therapy of acute renal failure varies with the underlying cause, supportive therapy varies with the severity of associated renal dysfunction. Supportive therapy of acute renal failure should be formulated according to whether the patient has oliguric, nonoliguric, or polyuric primary renal failure.

Symptomatic Treatment

Symptomatic treatment consists of therapy given to eliminate or suppress clinical signs. Examples of symptomatic treatment include use of antiemetics to control vomiting, and use of drugs to enhance appetite.

Fluid Therapy

Because most uremic patients with ARF are initially dehydrated and hypovolemic, therapy with intravenous fluids should be given first priority. Clinical signs of dehydration are reliable evidence that a portion of the azotemia is prerenal in origin, and therefore partially amenable to rapid correction by restoring vascular volume and pressure with replacement fluids. With the overall goal of sustaining the patient's life, the primary objectives of fluid therapy of ARF are: 1) to improve renal perfusion by restoring euvolemia and normotension, 2) to correct electrolyte and acid-base imbalances, and 3) to induce diuresis.

Although fluid therapy (including the type and quantity of fluids, and the route and rate of their administration) is the cornerstone of treatment of ARF, it must be carefully monitored and integrated with other aspects of treatment (Table 22-8).

Initially the intravenous *route* of administration of fluids is recommended because of the large volume of fluid and rapid administration rate often needed to maximize renal perfusion in patients with uremia caused by ARF. We routinely use aseptically placed jugular intravenous catheters because they also facilitate: 1) infusion of hypertonic solutions, 2) intensive diuresis, 3) sequential blood sampling, and 4) measurement of central venous pressure. The subcutaneous route of fluid administration is generally unsatisfactory for initial treatment because poor perfusion associated with clinical dehydration impairs the rate of fluid absorption.

The *type* of fluid chosen for initial replacement therapy should be based on knowledge of deficits and excesses in the patient's fluid, electrolyte, and acid-base balance. Isotonic solutions designed to promote isonatremia (ie, 0.9% saline, Normosol-R, Abbott; Plasma-Lyte 148, Baxter) are often used for initial rehydration of patients with normal serum sodium concentrations. Physiologic saline solution is often the initial choice for hyperkalemic oliguric patients because it is devoid of potassium. A combination of half-strength saline (0.45%) and 2.5% dextrose may be used as replacement solutions for patients with mild hypernatremia due to excessive free water loss or hypotonic losses associated with vomiting and diarrhea.[3] Maintenance fluids designed to replace insensible losses and for maintenance requirements should not be used as replacement fluids since they may cause hyponatremia and overhydration without effectively restoring vascular volume and renal perfusion.

The initial *quantity* of replacement fluids in milliliters is calculated from clinical estimates of dehydration according to the formula:

$$\text{Milliliters of fluid required} = \text{body weight (kg)} \times \text{percent dehydration} \times 1000$$

Allowances for maintenance fluid requirements and continuous fluid losses should also be considered. The volume of fluid that can safely be administered should be determined in context of the patient's urine volume (oliguria, nonoliguria, or polyuria). The rate of urine production (ml/kg/hr) should be carefully monitored. A favorable *response* to fluid therapy is indicated by increased urine production.

Initial replacement fluids should be administered at a *rate* calculated to correct extracellular fluid deficits over a 4 to 6 hour period in order to rapidly restore renal perfusion and thereby prevent ischemia. In patients with profound hypovolemia and hypotension, estimated fluid deficits may be intravenously administered at a rate of up to 90 ml/kg/hr (dogs) or 55 ml/kg/hr (cats).[5] A slower infusion rate is warranted in patients known to have cardiopulmonary dysfunction.

Parenteral fluid therapy should be continued until the patient's clinical status improves so that fluid balance can be maintained by voluntary drinking and eating, and until reduction in the magnitude of azotemia has stabilized for 2 to 3 days. Appropriate monitoring (body weight, skin turgor, and serum biochemical profile) is essential to assure that the patient is able to maintain adequate hydration.

In order to prevent recurrence of dehydration and its undesirable consequences, parenteral fluid therapy should not be abruptly discontinued. Rather, it should be gradually reduced (ie, approximately 25% per day for the next 2 to 3 days). The patient should be appropriately monitored during this period to prevent recurrence of fluid and electrolyte deficits. In some instances, it may be beneficial to supplement fluids consumed in food and water with fluids given subcutaneously as needed to maintain fluid balance.

Care must be used not to induce electrolyte disturbances by inappropriate use of replacement and maintenance fluids. Maintenance fluids (ie, 0.45% saline in 2.5% dextrose: Normosol-M; Plasma-Lyte 56) differ from replacement fluids in that they generally have a much lower sodium concentration (approximately 40 mEq/L in maintenance fluids versus 130 mEq/L in lactated Ringer's solution and 154 mEq/L in physiologic saline solution), and a higher potassium concentration (13 mEq/L in maintenance fluids vs 4 mEq/L in LRS). The reason for this difference is that the daily requirements of sodium and potassium are not directly related to the serum concentration of sodium and potassium. Inappropriate use of rehydration fluids for maintenance fluids for several days is likely to result in hypernatremia. On the other hand, administration of excessive quantities of maintenance fluids or electrolyte free fluids (5% dextrose) may result in hyponatremia.

Electrolyte and acid-base disorders are common in patients with azotemic oliguric acute renal failure. Because they are potentially life threatening, a high priority should be placed on their detection and treatment.

Hyperkalemia

Potassium levels should be monitored closely in the intensive care setting. In patients with ARF, serum potassium varies substantially with the volume of urine produced. Life threatening hyperkalemia may develop during the oliguric phase of acute renal failure secondary to decreased glomerular filtration and decreased tubular secretion. Hyperkalemia may be aggravated as a consequence of widespread cellular damage and/or shifts of intracellular potassium into the extracellular fluid as a result of acidosis. Hyperkalemia is less commonly associated with nonoliguric acute primary renal failure. With the exception of hypoadrenocorticism, it is rarely associated with prerenal azotemia. However, it is very common in patients with postrenal azotemia. The severity of hyperkalemia may also be increased by inappropriate use of potassium-containing fluids and/or drugs such as angiotensin converting enzyme inhibitors. Because acidemia potentiates the severity of hyperkalemia, serum potassium concentration should be interpreted in context of the acid-base status of the patient.

Serum potassium concentrations >6.5 to 7.0 mEq/L can cause cardiac conduction disturbances (bradycardia, atrial standstill, idioventricular rhythm, ventricular tachycardia, fibrillation). If oliguric renal failure is suspected an EKG should be performed to assess cardiac function. However, EKG's are not a reliable substitute for evaluation of serum potassium concentration. Other clinical signs of hyperkalemia include generalized muscle weakness and neurological abnormalities.

Initial therapy of hyperkalemia may be designed to: 1) remove excessive potassium from the body, 2) redistribute potassium from the extracellular to intracellular fluid compartments, or 3) counteract the membrane effects of hyperkalemia. The type of treatment selected for hyperkalemia is determined by the severity of this abnormality and concurrent cardiac and neuromuscular disturbances.

In most circumstances, mild hyperkalemia (potassium concentration 6.0 mEq/L or less) will resolve following initial fluid replacement. Moderate hyperkalemia (potassium concentration 6.0 to 7.5 mEq/L) usually will resolve following administration of potassium free fluids (dilution), correction of acidemia with sodium bicarbonate (redistribution), and improved urine flow (excretion). Treatment with furosemide may also promote kaliuresis. Of these options, sodium bicarbonate is commonly used first because both hyperkalemia and acidemia commonly occur in association with ARF.

Sodium bicarbonate increases extracellular pH and produces cellular exchange of potassium for hydrogen ions. The dosage of sodium bicarbonate may be based on the calculated bicarbonate deficit (refer to the section on treatment of metabolic acidosis). If measured serum bicarbonate concentration is unavailable, sodium bicarbonate may be administered at 1 to 2 mEq/kg IV over 15 to

20 minutes.[3] Beneficial effects usually begin within 10 minutes and may persist for 1 to 2 hours. If pre-existing hypocalcemia is present (especially common in patients with ethylene glycol intoxication), $NaHCO_3$ must be given cautiously because it may lower ionized serum calcium concentration and precipitate a hypocalcemic crisis.

If severe increases in serum potassium concentration (>8 mEq/L) are associated with cardiotoxicity, emergency drugs that decrease potassium concentration (sodium bicarbonate or glucose), or that counteract the effects of hyperkalemia on cardiac conduction (calcium gluconate) may be considered.

Glucose stimulates insulin release and promotes the transcellular uptake of potassium. Therefore, if $NaHCO_3$ is ineffective or inappropriate, 20 to 50% dextrose may be administered at 1.5g/kg IV to increase the intracellular shift of potassium. Alternatively, regular insulin can be given intravenously at 0.1 to 0.25 units in combination with dextrose at 1 to 2 grams per unit of administered insulin.[3] However, administration of insulin offers little benefit over the effects of glucose alone. If insulin is given, blood glucose must be serially monitored to avoid iatrogenic hypoglycemia.

Calcium gluconate directly counteracts the toxic effects of potassium on the heart, but does not lower serum potassium concentration. It may be administered as a 10% solution at a dose of 0.5 to 1.0 ml/kg over 10 to 15 minutes to correct life threatening electrocardiographic abnormalities.[3] Infusion of calcium gluconate may be discontinued when the heart rate increases, or when arrhythmias detected by ECG are controlled. The effects of calcium infusion on the electrocardiogram are rapid in onset, but short-lived (approximately 25 to 35 minutes). Therefore, infusion of calcium should be recognized as a very short term type of supportive therapy designed to correct immediate life threatening cardiotoxic effects.

Caution—Combining calcium solutions with bicarbonate solutions should be avoided since an insoluble precipitate of calcium may form. Also, because rapid injection of calcium solutions may cause hypotension and cardiac arrhythmias, arterial blood pressure should be monitored during calcium administration. If conventional therapy fails to provide an immediate or lasting resolution of the hyperkalemia, peritoneal dialysis or hemodialysis is indicated.

Hypokalemia

Hypokalemia may develop during the diuretic phase of ARF. Administration of fluids devoid of potassium (0.9% saline solution), diuretic therapy (especially hypertonic dextrose), inadequate dietary potassium intake, vomiting, and diarrhea may contribute to the development of hypokalemia. By altering systemic hemodynamics and decreasing GFR, hypokalemia may contribute to further impairment of renal function.

Abnormalities typically noted with hypokalemia fall into four main categories: 1) neuromuscular, 2) cardiac, 3) renal, and 4) metabolic. Irrespective of cause, clinical signs of hypokalemia (anorexia, vomiting, gastric atony, intestinal ileus, skeletal muscle weakness, cardiac arrhythmias, and impaired renal concentrating capacity) may occur if the serum potassium concentration is lower than 2.5 mEq/L.

Potassium supplementation of parenteral fluids given should be based on serial evaluations of serum potassium concentration. The rate of intravenous potassium administration should not exceed 0.5 mEq/kg/hour. Once hypokalemia has been corrected, therapy should be continued to maintain normal serum potassium. This is usually achieved via potassium enriched IV fluids. Supplementing the potassium content of fluids to 10 to 30 mEq/L with KCl is usually sufficient to maintain normokalemia in nonoliguric patients As soon as the patient can tolerate oral therapy, potassium supplements may be given by mouth.

Metabolic Acidosis

Patients with acute renal failure typically have metabolic acidosis due to excessive production and impaired renal excretion of metabolic acids, impaired renal tubular reabsorption of bicarbonate, and impaired production of ammonia by the renal tubules. Consequences of metabolic acidosis associated with acute renal failure include anorexia, vomiting, weight loss, lethargy, and exacerbation of hyperkalemia. Severe acidemia may be associated with reduced cardiac contractility, peripheral arterial vasodilation, and central venoconstriction. Decreases in vascular compliance may predispose patients to pulmonary edema during administration of fluids. Metabolic acidosis may contribute to bone demineralization and progression of renal failure.

Treatment should be formulated by assessing serum bicarbonate (TCO_2) or a venous blood gas profile. If serum bicarbonate or blood gas values are not available, the magnitude of bicarbonate deficit may be estimated according to the following scale: 5 mEq/L in mild uremia; 10 mEq/L in moderate uremia; 15 mEq/L in severe uremia.

Mild metabolic acidosis (serum $HCO_3 > 16$ mEq/L) usually resolves after fluid replacement and the onset of diuresis.

In patients with severe metabolic acidosis (blood pH <7.3, or total CO_2 <15 mEq/L), sodium bicarbonate should be administered intravenously in increasing doses until symptoms are relieved (TCO_2 content about 20 mEq/L) or until evidence of sodium overloading prevents further therapy. The quantity of bicarbonate needed to correct existing deficits in the extracellular fluid may be estimated from the formula:

$$\text{mEq } HCO_3 \text{ required} = \text{kg body wt} \times 0.3 \times \text{base deficit}$$
$$\text{Base deficit} = (\text{desired } HCO_3 - \text{measured } HCO_3)$$

To minimize iatrogenic complications, the immediate goal is not to attempt to restore acid-base balance to normal, but rather to administer sufficient bicarbonate to ameliorate the adverse cardiovascular effects associated with acidosis. This may be accomplished by administering half the dose calculated to correct the bicarbonate deficit slowly over 30 minutes. The remainder of the dose may be given with IV fluids during the next 2 to 4 hours. Serum TCO_2 (or blood gas measurements) and electrolytes should be reassessed following initial replacement and daily to determine whether the deficits have been adequately replaced or whether additional replacement therapy is required. Once acidemia has been corrected, most uremic patients require additional bicarbonate (estimated to be 80 to 90 mEq/kg/day) to offset production of metabolic acids.[3] The dose selected should be adjusted on the basis of serial evaluation of serum TCO_2 concentration or blood bicarbonate concentration.

Caution—Administration of excessive $NaHCO_3$ may result in iatrogenic ionized calcium deficits, metabolic alkalosis, paradoxical CSF acidosis (when severe respiratory disease exists), cerebral edema, hypernatremia, hypokalemia, ECF volume overload, hypertension, and pulmonary edema.

Pharmacotherapy

Persistence of oliguria and azotemia following initial fluid therapy may be related to inadequate correction of prerenal factors that are reducing renal perfusion. Before considering diuretics and/or vasodilators, a volume of fluid equal to approximately 3 to 5% of the patient's body weight may be administered after apparent correction of clinical dehydration. The rationale for this fluid bolus is that 3 to 5% dehydration may be clinically undetectable. In addition, because generalized renal disease may impair renal auto-regulatory mechanisms that normally preserve renal perfusion and glomerular filtration over a wide range of blood pressures, slight overhydration is preferable to ongoing unrecognized dehydration that may exacerbate the severity of renal lesions. If intravenous fluid therapy fails to promote appropriate diuresis after rehydrating the patient (urine output is <1 ml/Kg/hr), the oliguria is likely to be associated with intrarenal causes. Further attempts to induce diuresis by intravenous fluid therapy alone are usually futile and will likely result in iatrogenic overhydration. Therefore, pharmacologic management of oliguria may be considered.

Diuretics (furosemide, mannitol, and/or hypertonic dextrose) and vasodilators (dopamine) are generally advocated for treatment of acute oliguria that persists after (not before) rehydrating the patient. If diuresis is associated with increased GFR, the severity of hyperkalemia, acidemia, and nitrogenous waste product retention is often reduced. Even if GFR does not improve, induction of diuresis may minimize factors related to obstruction of renal tubular lumens, and also reduce the risk of iatrogenic overhydration.

If appropriate diuretics and vasodilators are not given early in the initiation phase of ARF, their efficacy in reducing the functional and morphological alterations often is negligible. On the other hand, prematurely inducing diuresis prior to rehydration can aggravate or prolong renal injury.

Caution—If oliguria persists despite diuretic therapy, care must be taken to avoid iatrogenic overhydration (see Table 22-8).

Furosemide Furosemide (Lasix, Hoechst) is commonly used when fluid replacement alone does not produce adequate diuresis because furosemide is readily available, relatively easy to administer, and because a short course of therapy is associated with minimal risks. By impairing reabsorption of chloride and sodium in the thick ascending limb of Henle's loops, furosemide enhances tubular flow rate and thereby may reduce obstruction of renal tubular lumens. It may also impair glomerulotubular feedback, one of the compensatory mechanisms that may contribute to oliguria by sustaining renal vasoconstriction and reduced GFR. However, diuresis induced by furosemide may not coincide with improved GFR.

An initial dose of 2 to 4 mg/kg is given intravenously. If diuresis occurs, the dose may be repeated every 6 to 8 hours, or may be given at a constant infusion rate of 0.25–1.0 mg/kg/hr for up to 48 hours. However, if urine production remains <1ml/kg/hr after 30 minutes, the original dose may be doubled (4 to 8 mg/kg) and given rapidly. If there is no response, other alternatives should be considered.

Because treatment with furosemide alone often does not cause an increase in GFR, a combination of furosemide with dopamine or mannitol may be more effective in increasing GFR and inducing diuresis than treatment with either of these agents alone. The pharmacologic effects of dopamine and furosemide are synergistic in promoting diuresis.

Caution—Furosemide should not be given to patients that are dehydrated. Likewise, it should not be routinely used in patients with nonoliguric ARF unless they are hyperkalemic or overhydrated. Because furosemide has been reported to exacerbate gentamicin toxicity, it is not recommended in patients with acute renal failure caused by aminoglycosides. Other adverse effects include electrolyte depletion (especially potassium and sometimes calcium), hypotension, gastrointestinal disturbances, ototoxicity, and weakness.

Dopamine Because reduced renal blood flow contributes to the pathogenesis of many forms of ARF, vasodilators have been advocated as a logical choice for therapy. Dopamine (Intropin; Faulding, a precursor of norepinephrine) has become popular because of its potential to selectively promote renal vasodilation without causing changes in peripheral vascular resistance and systemic blood pressure. Beneficial response to intravenous dopamine infusions varies with species (dog > cat), dosage (low > high), severity of renal damage (mild > severe), and duration (short > long) of renal damage.[1] In dogs, constant intravenous infusion of dopamine at low doses (approximately 0.5 to 2 micrograms/kg/min) may be associated with vasodilation of renal vessels, increased renal blood flow and glomerular filtration, and enhanced renal excretion of sodium, thereby facilitating conversion of oliguria to polyuria.[3] Doses between approximately 2 to 5 micrograms/kg/min may increase cardiac output. However, higher doses may cause undesired vasoconstriction, tachycardia, and cardiac arrhythmias.

Dilution of 50 milligrams of dopamine in 500 ml of lactated Ringer's solution or 5% dextrose in water will yield a solution containing 100 micrograms of dopamine per ml. Because of the potential for excessive doses of dopamine to cause vasoconstriction and oliguria, dopamine infusions are administered with the aid of an IV infusion pump. Because dopamine may be inactivated in an alkaline environment, it should not be administered in fluids containing sodium bicarbonate. Combining dopamine infusion (2 to 5 micrograms/kg/min) with furosemide (0.5 to 1 mg/kg/hr) may produce synergistic effects that enhance diuresis. Once adequate diuresis is established, therapy should be continued until renal function can sustain fluid, electrolyte, and acid base balance without drug therapy.

Since administration of dopamine may be associated with cardiac arrhythmias, monitoring cardiac rate and rhythm by EKG is warranted. Dopamine should not be used concurrently with metoclopramide (a dopamine antagonist).

If therapy is not associated with onset of diuresis in the first few hours after the onset of oliguria, further therapy is unlikely to be beneficial. Once oliguria becomes refractory to diuretic therapy, dialysis is often the only effective alternative.

In cats, intravenous infusion dopamine is not associated with a significant increase in renal blood flow and urine output, because cats apparently do not have renal dopamine receptors.[1,3] Although higher doses of dopamine given to cats may be associated with diuresis and natriuresis as a result of stimulation of alpha-adrenergic receptors that increase blood pressure and decrease renal tubular sodium reabsorption, the risk of cardiac side effects also increases. Pending further efficacy and safety studies, dopamine therapy cannot be routinely recommended for treatment of oliguric renal failure in cats.

Mannitol Mannitol is often recommended in initial treatment of oliguric acute renal failure because clinical experience indicates that it is generally more effective than furosemide. The beneficial effects of mannitol have been attributed to: 1) increased vascular volume and renal perfusion, 2) decreased renal vascular resistance, 3) impairment of renin release, 4) enhanced osmotic diuresis promoting excretion of solute and water, 5) increased release of atrial natriuretic peptide, 6) decreased swelling of renal tubular epithelial cells, and 7) reduced obstruction of tubular lumens by casts and epithelial cell debris.

As with all diuretics, mannitol therapy should not be given until the patient is properly rehydrated (nor should it be given to oliguric patients with iatrogenic overhydration). The recommended intravenous dose is 0.5 to1.0 gram/kg of a 10 to 25% solution given slowly (over 10 to 20 minutes). Urine output should improve within 60 minutes if the treatment is effective. If significant diuresis occurs, adjust therapy to provide a constant rate of intravenous infusion at a dose of 1.0 to 2.0 mg/kg/min. Alternatively, mannitol can be given as intermittent boluses of 0.25 to 0.5 grams/kg every 4 to 6 hours during the next 24 to 48 hours.[3] The total dose should not exceed 2 grams/kg as higher doses may increase the risk of neurotoxicity.

If significant diuresis does not develop within approximately 60 minutes of the initial intravenous bolus of mannitol, an additional intravenous bolus of 0.25 to 0.5 grams/kg may be given. If oliguria persists, therapy with mannitol should be discontinued because of unacceptable risks associated with overhydration and mannitol intoxication.

Delay in initiating mannitol therapy following the onset of acute oliguric renal failure decreases the likelihood that it will be effective in inducing diuresis. Mannitol is contraindicated for treatment of oliguria in overhydrated oliguric patients and patients with congestive heart failure because the resulting increase in intravascular volume may precipitate clinical signs associated with iatrogenic overhydration.

Hypertonic Dextrose Inducing osmotic diuresis with hypertonic (10 to 20%) dextrose may be used as an alternative to mannitol. Dextrose solutions are easy to formulate and the effects are similar to those of mannitol. However, osmotic diuresis induced with mannitol therapy may be expected to produce a more consistent response since it is not metabolized or reabsorbed by the tubules.

Hypertonic dextrose may be administered at a dose of 25 to 50 ml/kg as an intermittent slow intravenous bolus over 1 to 2 hours. If effective (urine output = approximately 1 to 3 ml/minute), the dose may be repeated up to 3 times per day. However, a polyionic isotonic solution such as lactated Ringer's solution should also be given to prevent dehydration and electrolyte depletion. A potential advantage of hypertonic dextrose over mannitol is that the urine may be monitored for the appearance of glucose. The onset of glucosuria indicates that the magnitude of hyperglycemia is sufficient to exceed the renal transport maximum for glucose, which in turn should facilitate osmotic diuresis. Thus the infusion may be discontinued prior to the development of volume overexpansion if glucosuria is not detected. However, because detection of glucosuria does not necessarily coincide with an increased rate of urine production, quantitative assessment of urine volume should also be monitored.

Nutritional Support

Nutritional therapy is an important component of supportive care needed by patients with acute renal failure. Acute renal failure accompanied by anorexia and vomiting is associated with hypercatabolism of body proteins and calories. Protein calorie malnutrition exacerbates the severity of many uremic manifestations (including increased production of protein catabolites, negative nitrogen balance, impaired immune function, increased susceptibility to infections, glucose intolerance, electrolyte disturbances, and acidemia). Metabolic acidosis may further exacerbate catabolism of body proteins, which in turn magnifies azotemia, hyperkalemia, hyperphosphatemia, and loss of muscle mass. Inadequate nutrition may also slow recovery by impairing regeneration of renal tissues, and compromising renal compensatory hypertrophy.

Evidence of malnutrition includes hypoalbuminemia, lymphopenia, muscle wasting, and weight loss. In general, anorexic patients will lose approximately 0.3 kg of body mass per 1000 kilocalories of energy required per day. Unfortunately, changes in body weight associated with fluid balance may mask loss of muscle mass and fat stores.

Uncontrolled vomiting and gastroenteritis during the initial phases of acute renal failure may preclude the use of oral or enteral protocols of nutritional therapy. However, if a well-nourished patient with acute renal failure is likely to resume voluntary consumption of food within 3 to 5 days from the onset of a uremic crisis, specialized methods of nutritional support are often unnecessary. In this scenario, the main focus is appropriate treatment of vomiting, gastritis, and disturbances in fluid, electrolyte, and acid-base disturbances. If rapid response allows the patient to resume eating and drinking, nutritional management may be focused on appropriate dietary modifications, including reduced quantities of phosphorus and high quality protein, and provision of adequate nonprotein calories to minimize catabolism of protein for energy. When possible, effort should be made to encourage the oral intake of calories by offering a highly palatable diet. If a nauseated or vomiting uremic patient is given a diet designed for long-term management of renal failure, aversion to that food may develop. Food aversion is most likely to occur if nauseated patients are force fed. To minimize the possibility of aversion to renal failure diets, they should not be offered to patients until the underlying causes contributing to anorexia, nausea, and vomiting are eliminated.[10]

Daily caloric requirements should be primarily supplied in the form of carbohydrates. Nutrient requirements should ideally be supplied by dietary formulations containing essential proteins or amino acids in quantities that will not result in undesirable production of protein catabolites.[9] If vomiting is not a major problem and the patient is alert enough to avoid aspiration of vomited stomach contents, a nasoesophageal tube may be used for short-term administration of liquid renal diets, oral medications, and water. A percutaneous gastrostomy tube (PEG tube) may be more effective for long term management of the inappetant patient. PEG tubes are usually well tolerated by the patient and are usually large enough to accommodate blenderized mixtures of canned prescription renal diets. PEG tubes also facilitate administration of oral fluids and medications.

When uncontrolled vomiting prevents effective use of oral or enteral protocols of nutritional support, parenteral nutrition should be considered. In-depth discussion about enteral and parenteral nutritional management of patients in acute renal failure is beyond the scope of this chapter, but is described elsewhere.[8]

Treatment of Uremic Gastrointestinal Disorders

Uremic anorexia, nausea, vomiting, and diarrhea are common manifestations of ARF. Local factors include ulcerative stomatitis, erosive gastritis (associated with gastric acidity mediated by hypergastrinemia), and uremic colitis. Central factors associated with uremic vomiting include stimulation of the medullary emetic chemoreceptor trigger zone by circulating uremic toxins, and intolerance to some medications.

Oral fluids and food should be withheld until vomiting has been controlled for 24 hours. Discomfort associated with oral erosions and ulcerations may be reduced by application of compounds containing lidocaine (2% lidocaine viscous; Roxane Labs Inc). Oral rinses with 0.12% chlorhexidine solution (CHX-Guard; VRx Products) may be used to reduce bacteria. Hypergastrinemia-induced anorexia, nausea, and vomiting may be interrupted by parenteral administration of H_2-receptor antagonists such as cimetadine (Tagamet; Smith-Kline, French), ranitidine (Zantac; Glaxo-Wellcome), or famotidine (Pepsid; Merck). Because these drugs are dependent on renal excretion for elimination, their dosage should be reduced in proportion to the severity of renal failure. As an alternative to H_2 receptor antagonists, proton pump blockers (omeprazole, Prisolec; Astra, Merck) may be used to impair gastric acid secretion.

Metoclopramide (Reglan; Robbins) may be given intravenously to minimize the action of uremic toxins on the medullary emetic chemoreceptor trigger zone. Metoclopramide also promotes gastric emptying.

Caution—Metoclopramide is a dopamine antagonist and therefore should not be used when dopamine is being given in attempt to promote renal vasodilation. Likewise, because metoclopramide is eliminated primarily via the kidneys, the dosage should be adjusted when given to patients that are uremic.

Patients in the intensive care setting should be monitored for melena, decreasing PCV, and a disproportionate increase in BUN relative to creatinine. All of these parameters may indicate gastrointestinal bleeding. Conventional therapy usually includes an H_2 receptor antagonist and a gastroprotectant such as sucralfate.

Patients in renal failure commonly are intolerant to gastrointestinal side effects of many drugs. In addition, some drugs may contribute to anorexia by impairing taste or smell. Therefore, the manufacturer's recommendations and description of side effects should be reviewed before giving any drug to a patient with renal failure. Because many renal failure patients are intolerant to drugs, they should not be routinely given with the philosophy that they might help but will do no harm.

Nosocomial Infection Prevention and Treatment

Patients with acute renal failure are at high risk for development of nosocomial bacterial infections, especially when hospitalized in intensive care units. Indwelling intravenous and urinary catheters are a common source of this problem. Therefore, urinary catheters should only be used when necessary. When used, quantitative urine cultures should be performed at appropriate intervals with the goal of timely identification of nosocomial infections (see Table 22-7). Treatment of urinary tract infections should be based on antimicrobial susceptibility tests. Likewise, response to therapy should be based on eradication of bacterial pathogens verified by quantitative urine culture. In general, prophylactic use of antimicrobial agents to prevent bacterial infections is contraindicated because it predisposes the patient to infections with resistant pathogens.

Treatment of Refractory Oliguria

Once oliguria becomes refractory to fluid and diuretic therapy, peritoneal or hemodialysis are often the only effective alternatives. Dialysis may sustain the life of the patient until repair of renal lesions and compensatory hypertrophy of viable nephrons allow the return of adequate homeostasis to sustain life without intensive therapy. Dialysis may also be used to treat overhydration, and to remove nephrotoxins including drugs.[2,4] In the interim, fluid therapy should be carefully titrated to provide for insensible and continuous losses without overhydrating the patient.

PROGNOSIS

Early recognition of ARF combined with proper therapy during the initiation phase may minimize the severity of renal parenchymal damage and dysfunction. Once the maintenance phase has been established, the renal lesions can not be reversed by specific therapy. In addition, the magnitude of deficits and excesses in fluid, electrolyte, and acid-base balance associated with the maintenance phase of oliguric renal failure often vary significantly from those associated with the polyuric recovery stage. For example, patients with oliguric renal failure may develop life threatening hyperkalemia and acidemia, whereas patients with polyuric renal failure are typically normokalemic and may even become hypokalemic. In addition, patients in the oliguric maintenance phase of ARF are at high risk for iatrogenic overhydration, whereas patients in the polyuric phase of ARF are predisposed to dehydration, especially if vomiting impairs compensatory polydipsia.

REFERENCES

1. Chew DJ: Fluid therapy during intrinsic renal failure. *In* Fluid Therapy in Small Animal Practice. 2nd ed. DiBartola SP, ed.: Philadelphia, W.B. Saunders, 2000, pp. 410–427.
2. Cowgill LD: Applications of peritoneal dialysis and hemodialysis in the management of renal failure. In, Diseases of the Canine and Feline Urinary System. Osborne CA and Finco DR, eds.: Baltimore, Williams & Wilkins, 1995, pp. 573–596.
3. Cowgill LD, Elliott DA: Acute renal failure. *In* Textbook of Veterinary Internal Medicine. 5th ed. Vol. 2. Ettinger SJ, Feldman EC, eds.: Philadelphia, W.B. Saunders, 2000, pp. 1615–1633.
4. Cowgill LD, Langston CE: Role of hemodialysis in the management of dogs and cats with renal failure. Vet Clin N Amer 26: 1347–1378, 1996.
5. Day TK: Shock syndromes in veterinary medicine. *In* Fluid Therapy in Small Animal Practice. 2nd ed. DiBartola SP, ed.: Philadelphia, W.B. Saunders, 2000, pp. 428–447.
6. Grauer GF: Prevention of acute renal failure. Vet Clin N Amer 26: 1447–1459, 1996.
7. Grauer GF, Lane IF: Acute renal failure: Ischemic and chemical nephrosis. *In* Diseases of the Canine and Feline Urinary System. Osborne CA, and Finco DR, eds.: Baltimore, Williams & Wilkins, 1995, pp. 441–459, 1995.
8. Marks SL: Enteral and parenteral nutritional support. *In* Textbook of Veterinary Internal Medicine. 5th ed. Vol. 2. Ettinger SJ, Feldman EC, eds.: Philadelphia, W.B. Saunders, 2000, pp. 275–283, 2000.
9. Miller CC, Bartges JW: Parenteral nutrition products. In Current Veterinary Therapy. Vol. 12. Bonagura JD, ed.: W.B. Saunders, Philadelphia, 2000, pp. 80–84.
10. Osborne CA, Lulich JP, Sanderson SL: Treatment of uremic anorexia. *In* Current Veterinary Therapy. Vol. 12. Bonagura JD, Kirk RW, eds.: W.B. Saunders, Philadelphia, 1995, pp. 966–971.
11. Polzin DJ, Osborne CA, O'Brien TD: Diseases of the kidneys and ureters. *In* Internal Medical Disorders of the Dog and Cat. 3rd ed. Vol. 2. Ettinger SJ, ed.: W.B. Saunders Co., Philadelphia, 1989, pp. 1962–2046.

12. Polzin DJ, Osborne CA, Jacob F *et al:* Chronic renal failure. *In* Internal Medical Disorders of the Dog and Cat. 5th ed. Vol. 2. Ettinger SJ, Feldman EC, eds.: Philadelphia, W.B. Saunders, 2000, pp. 1634–1662.
13. Raffe M. Medical use of colloids. *In* Current Veterinary Therapy. Vol. 12. Bonagura JD, ed.: W.B. Saunders, Philadelphia, 2000, pp. 66–69.
14. Riviere JE, Vaden SL: Drug therapy during renal disease and renal failure. *In* Diseases of the Canine and Feline Urinary System. Osborne CA, Finco DR, eds.: Williams & Wilkins, Baltimore, 1995, 555–572.

23
Radiology of the Critical Care Patient

Robert T. O'Brien

INTRODUCTION

While other imaging modalities are more advanced and have greater sensitivity for certain conditions, radiography is still the mainstay for the diagnosis of most intra-thoracic and many intra-abdominal critical conditions. This modality has speed, low morbidity, and high detail as some of its many advantages. A thorough knowledge of the indications and contraindications of radiography and the ability to interpret films is essential for all critical care clinicians. This chapter hopes to provide a concise treatise on radiography and radiology of acute and chronic critical conditions.

RADIOGRAPHY

General Radiography

Radiography is the image collection system whereby x-ray photons differentially pass through the patient and reach the film-screen system, producing a latent image. Proper development transforms the latent image to a useful image on the x-ray film. This image is durable, portable, and conveniently stored. Obtaining useful images depends on many factors. The most important factors are either technical or clinical skills. Technical skills include the proper choice of film-screen and grid combination, measurement of patient part, choice of views and positioning of the patient, adaptation of technique chart to account for suspected disease, and processing of images. Clinical skills include proper choice of imaging based on suspected disease, timing of imaging in the clinical course to avoid undue morbidity, interpretation of the images to reach a radiographic diagnosis, integration of the radiographic findings with the clinical signs, and the decision to seek alternate or more advanced radiographic studies.

Technical skills are extremely important and can change the study from a nondiagnostic study to a wonderfully useful set of images. We assume that the patient need only be casually placed on the tabletop and let the photons fly! In reality the art of radiography requires an adept sense of physics, chemistry, and clinical medicine. The physics component requires knowledge of x-ray beam production, attenuation, and scatter. The competent radiographer is a chemist with a keen sense of the state of the developing chemicals and how they can assist with the production of artifacts and useful images.

The "clinical" part of technical skills is perhaps the most important. It involves asking relevant questions about suspected diseases, especially how the disease will affect the necessary exposure or positioning factors; a consideration of views that would decrease morbidity and accentuate disease; and providing advice on alternative pradiographic studies. These are absolutely vital for optimizing radiography in the critical care setting.

Clinical skills concerning radiography are equally demanding and necessary for maximizing the utility of radiography. Is radiography really the best test for a suspected pyometra? Is there a better test than abdominal radiography for a patient with portosystemic shunt? Of course radiography has it's place in both of the previously mentioned diseases in assisting to rule-out many other diseases that could lead to similar signs, but radiography is not the most sensitive nor most efficient imaging study to definitively diagnose either disease.

Where does radiography fit into the most efficient assessment of disease in a critical care patient? That is a vital question that has a moving target for an answer. The dilemma is: "If I don't take radiographs, I can't diagnose the disease" versus "If I take radiographs now I might kill the patient." Both of these situations can be true at any point in time of a clinical course. It is beyond this text to discuss specifics, but the recommendation of the author is that clinicians should reflect on the cost-benefit relationship of radiography with every case being considered for radiography. The following is a brief list of indications for radiography:

- Thorax
  - Dyspnea (including cyanosis)
  - Cough
  - Auscultable cardiac abnormality (murmur, arrhythmia, gallop, muffled beat)
  - Determine evidence of or for staging cardiac failure
  - Evaluate for evidence of intra-thoracic metastasis
  - Regurgitation or vomiting
  - Suspected trauma
- Abdomen
  - Gastrointestinal signs (vomiting, diarrhea, melena, hemoptysis)
  - Suspected masses
  - Dysuria
  - Suspected trauma
  - Urinary tract signs (suspected urolithiasis, rupture, obstruction)
  - Evaluation for free fluid (peritoneal or retroperitoneal)
  - Disconcerting ultrasonographic findings
  - Evaluation for metastasis (perineal, perianal, pelvic limb primary mass; mast cell neoplasia; and hemangiosarcoma)
- Skull or spine
  - Localized neurological signs
  - Suspected trauma
  - Skull (localized respiratory or gastrointestinal signs)
  - Spine (evaluation for metastasis or myeloma)
- Musculoskeletal
  - Localized musculoskeletal signs
  - Suspected polyarthropathy or polyostotic manifestations

Contrast Radiography

Where does contrast radiography fit into the clinical radiography continuum? It can be vital or unnecessary in two closely related cases. In one clinician's hands, a set of survey abdominal radiographs can provide enough information to alert him to a surgical disease. In another clinician's hands, these same films only pose a question requiring a more definitive test. In the following section, contrast radiography is discussed from the view of a clinician seeking a definitive answer from a question posed by abdominal radiographs.

Nothing can be such a big waste of time or as definitive a test as contrast radiography. All of us have been associated with the 6-hour upper gastrointestinal series that yielded a radiological diagnosis of "possible enteritis." But the next case can result in the definitive diagnosis of lucent gastric foreign body in matter of minutes (Fig. 23-1). How can this range of utility be tolerated? Easily. Radiography, especially contrast radiography, is an exceptionally demanding field of imaging requiring keen insight into case selection and utmost expertise of technique. Ask any radiologist for a case example of what makes an "artist."

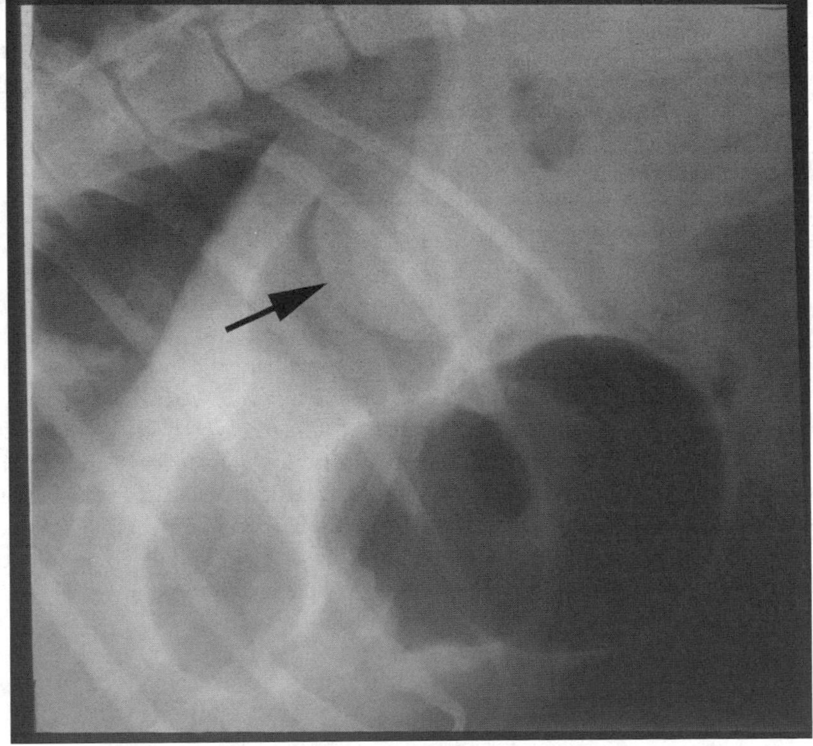

Figure 23-1
Oblique lateral radiograph of 2 year old female spayed Labrador retriever with ball gastric foreign body. Approximately 200 mL of air were added to the stomach by orogastric tube. Note the margin of the ball (black arrow) in the stomach lumen.

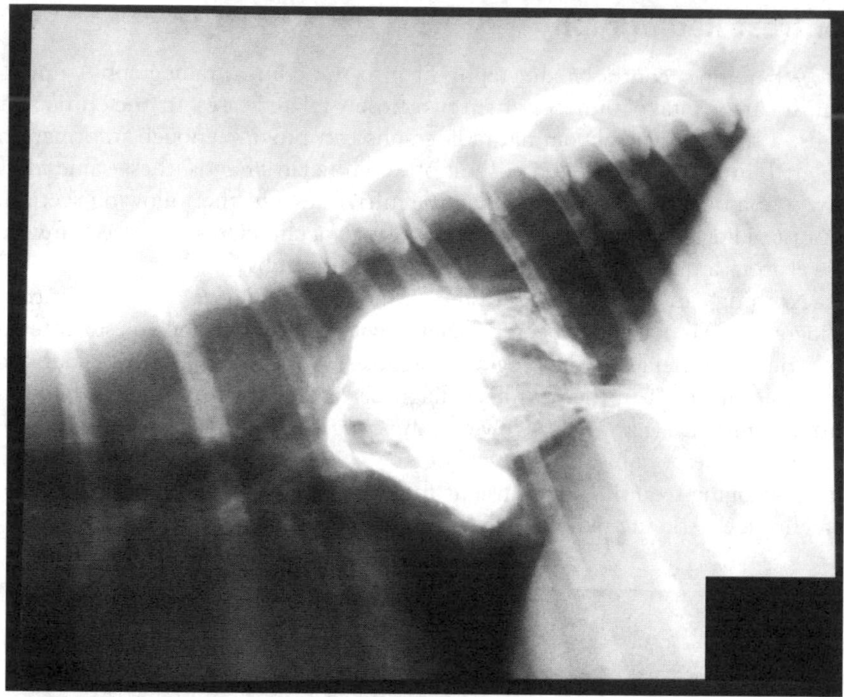

Figure 23-2
Lateral radiograph of thorax of 5 year old male neutered Sheltie with esophageal foreign body. Note barium in caudal thoracic esophagus surrounding the foreign body.

Most of them will remember the case where they properly chose a contrast study that was simple, quick, low in morbidity, and high in sensitivity and specificity for the disease suspected. Let's discuss a few examples where contrast radiography can be useful. I have included dosages and indications. With dosages I have attempted to eliminate the infamous "range of dosages" which leave the reader frustrated as to which end of the range to utilize for a given case. Adjust the dose necessary depending on the suspected disease and various patient factors. A full bladder is defined as "palpably full" or until rebound or resistance is noted on a 10 ml syringe. Too full is the "hard" bladder of a blocked cat. Too full can result in reflux of contrast up the ureters or in bladder rupture.

1. Esophagography (1 mL/10 lb body weight of barium suspension per os)
   a. Suspected esophageal foreign body (Fig. 23-2), stricture, or broncho-esophageal fistula
   b. Verify location of pulmonary mass in relation to esophagus
   c. Possible hiatal hernia or gastroesophageal hernia
2. Pneumogastrography (6 mL/lb body weight of air via orogastric tube)
   a. Lucent foreign body (ball, cloth, hair, toys) (see Fig. 23-1)

3. Positive contrast gastrography (3 mL/lb body weight of iodinated contrast via orogastric tube)
   a. Suspected gastric or duodenal perforation
4. Upper gastrointestinal (UGI) study (6 mL/lb body weight of 20% weight/volume barium suspension via orogastric tube)
   a. Suspected gastrointestinal obstruction, intussusception, or linear foreign body (Fig. 23-3)
5. Pneumocolonogram (dose to effect of full colon of air via rectum by Foley catheter)
   a. Rule out a normal large bowel loop as a distended small bowel loop
   b. Suspected ileocolic or colic-colic intussusception

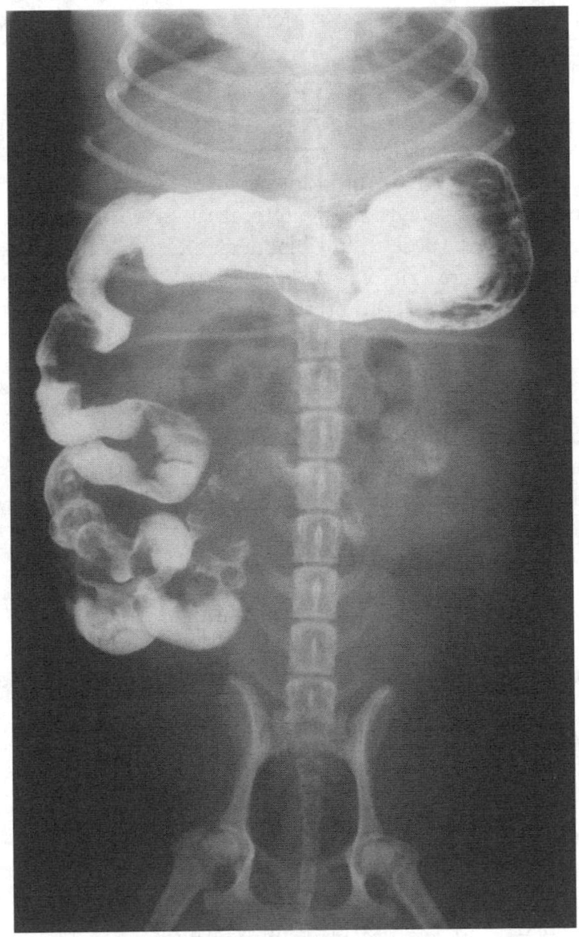

Figure 23-3
Ventrodorsal radiograph of 4 year old female spayed Golden retriever with gastrointestinal linear foreign body. Note plication of small intestines filled with barium.

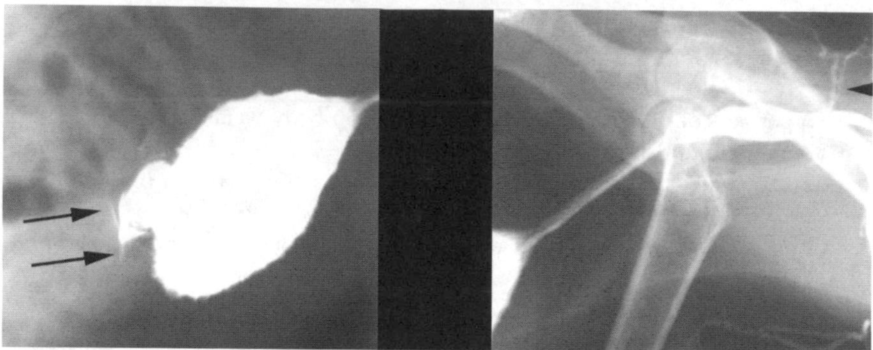

Figure 23-4
Lateral projections of 10 year old male neutered domestic short hair cat with positive contrast cystourethrogram. Note extravasation of contrast through rupture of cranial bladder (black arrows) and caudodorsal urethal (black arrowhead) walls.

6. Excretory pyelogram (EU = IVP)(2.2 mL/kg of iodinated contrast i.v.; 4.4 mL/kg body weight if patient is azotemic)
   a. Determine size or shape of kidneys
   b. Suspected kidney avulsion or ureteral rupture or stricture
7. Positive cystography (dose to full bladder of 25% iodinated contrast)
   a. Suspected rupture (Fig. 23-4)
   b. As a preliminary study to urethrography
8. Double contrast cystography (1mL/10 lbs body weight of 100% iodinated contrast plus air, dosed to full bladder)
   a. Suspected bladder neoplasia, cystitis, polyps, clots, or stones
9. Positive contrast urethrography (1 mL/4.54 kg body weight of 100% iodinated contrast by Foley catheter at the terminal urethra)
   a. Suspected urethral stone, rupture (see Fig. 23-4), or stricture

Positional Radiography

The following guidelines are useful in positional radiography. *Oblique* views can highlight lumps, bumps, and masses (they "cast the biggest shadow"). They can help determine suspected rib origin of an intra-thoracic mass, and they can evaluate the pylorus (UGI or pneumogastrogram), the vesicoureteral junction (EU), the sides of the bladder (double contrast cystography). *Horizontal-beam* views can be helpful in suspected lung lobe torsion (VD with patient in lateral recumbency), suspected pneumoperitoneum secondary to ruptured hollow viscus (VD with patient in lateral recumbency), and determine mobility of pleural effusion (VD with patient erect). *Opposite lateral* views should be taken all the time! In the thorax, they can help determine unilateral lesions, masses, alveolar disease, and pneumothorax. They can also determine symmetry of bilateral lesions. In the abdomen, they can show suspected masses or GI obstruction during contrast studies. Use *compression* views to show suspected intra-abdominal masses or cystic calculi, and to remove superimposed bowel loops over the areas of interest.

RADIOLOGY

Thorax

The thorax is the most commonly imaged body part in critical care patients. The intra-thoracic manifestations of complicated diseases are seemingly endless. At our practice, we routinely take left and right lateral and VD projections. This avoids a common situation when we suspect a lesion requiring the opposite lateral projection. At a bare minimum, take two views: one lateral and one VD/DV projection. Ventrodorsal projections are indicated with suspected pleural effusion: to be most sensitive to small amounts of effusion and, in the face of large amounts of effusion, they most accurately evaluate cardiac size. Dorsoventral projections are best tolerated by dyspneic patients and provide better information on the heart base and caudal lobar pulmonary vessels.

Evaluation of the thorax can be systematic or random. Any method that is complete and applied consistently is a good method. My method follows:

Use a technique that takes into account film exposure factors, the phase of respiration versus body conformation (Is the patient obese?), and any artifacts that may appear.

Use a clockwise approach to the patient starting at the shoulder, then the neck, then the spine including the spinous processes and vertebral bodies and intervertebral foramen. The diaphragm should be next, followed by the abdomen using intra-abdominal contrast to show liver size and gastric size and contents. Then evaluate the sternum, ribs, pleural space, and the mediastinum including the heart (for any enlargement), the pulmonary vasculature, and lungs.

Thoracic Diseases

The following is a simplistic approach to a very complex subject. I hope that by listing the most common differentials that the reader will remember that additional differentials exist and should be tested for when the common diseases are ruled out. Another factor to consider is that a normal radiographic appearance does not exclude severe intrathoracic disease. Two very important and common critical diseases that may have a normal appearance are pulmonary thromboembolic disease and feline asthma complex. Common diseases with their radiologic manifestations are heart failure, which includes left and right heart failure; pulmonary hypertension; lung disease; pleural effusion; and pneumothorax.

Left Heart Failure By far the most common heart disease is left heart failure. The failure may be due to mitral or aortic valve insufficiency secondary to endocardiosis or cardiomyopathy; poor output (cardiomyopathy, arrhythmia, or valvular stenosis); overhydration (zealous fluid therapy in the face of cardiac or renal disease); left-to-right shunting (congenital heart defect); or increased afterload (systemic hypertension).

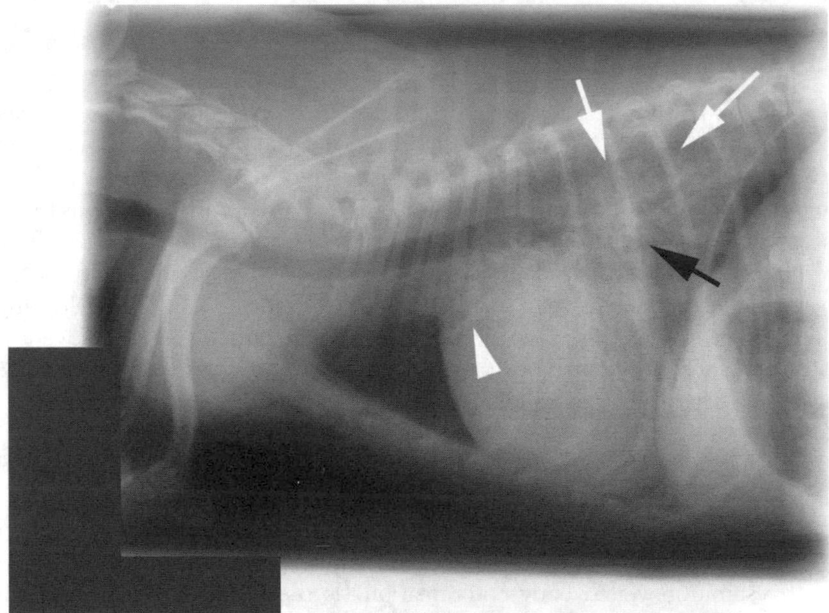

Figure 23-5
Lateral thoracic radiograph of 4 year old Chihuahua with left heart failure secondary to mitral valve insufficiency associated with endocardiosis of the valve leaflets. Note enlarged pulmonary veins (white arrowhead), enlarged left atrium (black arrow), and pulmonary edema (white arrow).

Radiologically, the general signs of left heart failure will show the heart appearing tall on the lateral view (Fig. 23-5). Enlargement of the left atrium can be detected by loss of the 12 to 3 o'clock "waist" of the heart on the lateral projection and a curvilinear lateral displacement of the caudal mainstem bronchi on the orthogonal view. Another general sign will be overall heart enlargement, more than 11 vertebrae, as measured on the vertebral heart scale method. Specific signs of left heart failure are enlargement of the pulmonary veins and pulmonary edema. Enlargement of the pulmonary veins represents left-sided heart failure. Without edema, the failure is referred to as being "compensated." Pulmonary edema, evidenced by an increased pulmonary opacity in the perihilar region, will be noted if the failure is decompensated; the lungs are unable to compensate for the congestion. The pattern is often interstitial to mixed interstitial-alveolar. If severe, the edema may weep into the pleural space, resulting in effusion.

These apply to the dog. Manifestations in the cat have a few key differences. The heart size is better evaluated on the VD view and a maximum width of greater than 4 vertebrae is sensitive for cardiomegaly. The pulmonary veins should be measured where they cross the cranial heart margin on the lateral view. The edema that results from pulmonary congestion may be perihilar (as in the dog), or be patchy and multifocal throughout the lungs.

Right Heart Failure Causes of right heart failure include tricuspid or pulmonic valve insufficiency secondary to endocardiosis, or cardiomyopathy; poor output from cardiomyopathy, arrhythmia, or valvular stenosis; over hydration from zealous fluid therapy in the face of cardiac or renal disease; left-to-right shunting from a congenital heart defect; increased afterload or pulmonary hypertension; or chronic, severe left heart failure.

General radiologic signs of right heart failure include rounding of the heart on both views—increased width of the heart on the lateral and VD/DV views. The pulmonary vessels are usually within normal limits (unless there is concurrent left heart failure). Often the caudal vena cava is enlarged. Free fluid accumulates resulting in pleural effusion (cats more often than dogs) **and** ascites (dogs more often than cats) (Fig. 23-6).

Differentials for a round heart include cardiomyopathy, pericardial effusion, bilateral atrioventricular valve insufficiency, and peritoneal pericardial diaphragmatic hernia.

Pulmonary Hypertension Causes of pulmonary hypertension include heartworm infestation, pulmonary thromboembolism, and congenital or idiopathic hypertension.

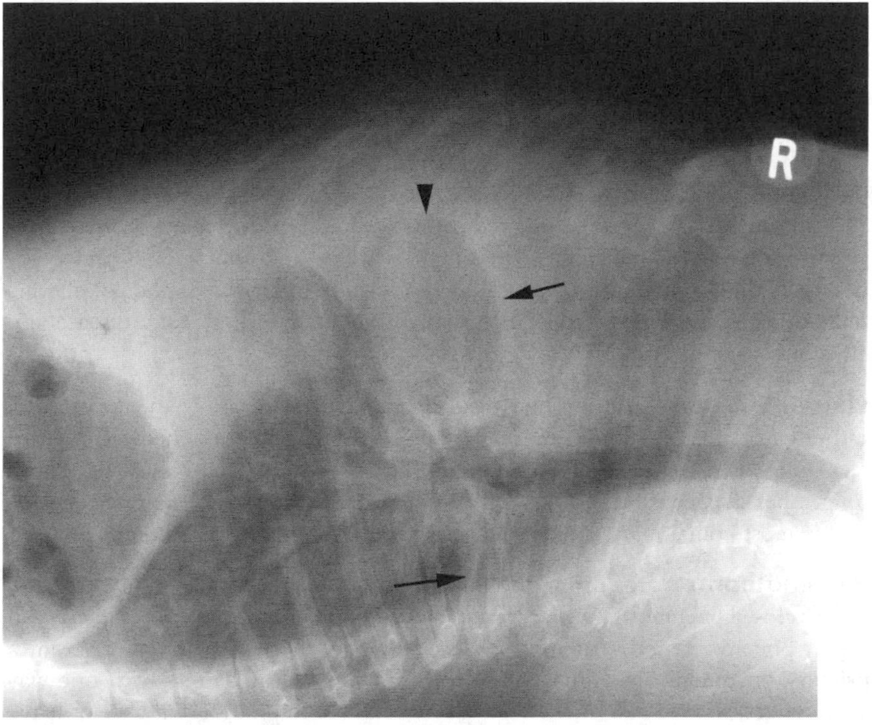

Figure 23-6
Lateral thoracic radiograph of 9 year old male neutered Doberman with cardiomyopathy. Note pleural fissure lines (black arrows), retraction of lung borders (arrowhead), and silhouetting of diaphragm and heart margins.

Radiology of pulmonary hypertension will show enlargement, tortuosity, and blunting of the pulmonary arteries; normal appearing pulmonary veins; and enlargement of the main pulmonary trunk manifest as a "bump" in the heart on the VD view at the 1 to 2 o'clock position. This is supportive evidence of chronic pulmonary hypertension. Lung infiltration will also be evident.

Lung Disease In lung disease, edema will be seen as an alveolar pattern secondary to left heart failure. It can be perihilar in dogs or patchy multifocal in cats. A caudodorsal pattern to edema is seen with various etiologies of noncardiogenic edema, including seizures, neck or head trauma, pulmonary hypertension, thromboembolic disease, ARDS, and systemic vasculopathy.

Pneumonia, caused by bacteria entering the airways, is referred to as bronchopneumonia and is usually manifest as lobar alveolar consolidation of cranial and middle ventral lung lobes. Interstitial pneumonia is seen in neonates with viral etiologies. Fungal pneumonia may manifest as an alveolar or nodular pattern.

Hemorrhage can cause ventral distribution, if subacute. It can also be focal or regional in the site of bleeding, if acute, due to contusions or trauma due to rib fractures. Hemorrhage can be regional in ARDS or bleeding lesions such as hemangiosarcoma metastases.

Neoplasia in an alveolar pattern shows as a primary lung neoplasia in cats. It is often associated with dystrophic mineralization (Fig. 23-7). Lymphoma is often associated with regional lymphadenopathy.

Atypical patchy alveolar patterns in cats can be caused by edema secondary to left heart failure, mycoplasma pneumonia, primary lung neoplasia, or atypical pneumonitis (parasitic, nematodic, allergic).

In lung disease, an unstructured interstitial pattern will show edema manifest as an interstitial pattern in the same locations and etiologies as previously noted. A diffuse interstitial pattern is seen with pulmonary lymphoma, allergic pneumonitis, and forms of ARDS (usually combined with alveolar disease and effusion).

Pleural Effusion Effusion may result from right heart failure in cats or dogs. Other causes include neoplasia (malignant effusion), vasculitis, hemorrhage, infection (pyothorax), or chyle. Rounding of lung lobes, especially the caudodorsal lung lobes as viewed on the lateral projection, is evidence of fibrosis pleuritis and is most commonly caused by chronic chylothorax and pyothorax.

Pneumothorax Free air in the pleural space may originate from inside the chest (closed pneumothorax) or by direct communication through the chest wall (open pneumothorax). Air from a closed pneumothorax can originate from a primary pneumomediastinum or rupture of a lung. If air enters by a one-way valve effect, whereby air enters during one phase of respiration but cannot leave during either phase, a tension pneumothorax can result.

The diagnosis of pneumothorax is the identification of free air in the pleural space (Fig. 23-8). Radiographically the signs include elevation of the heart apex

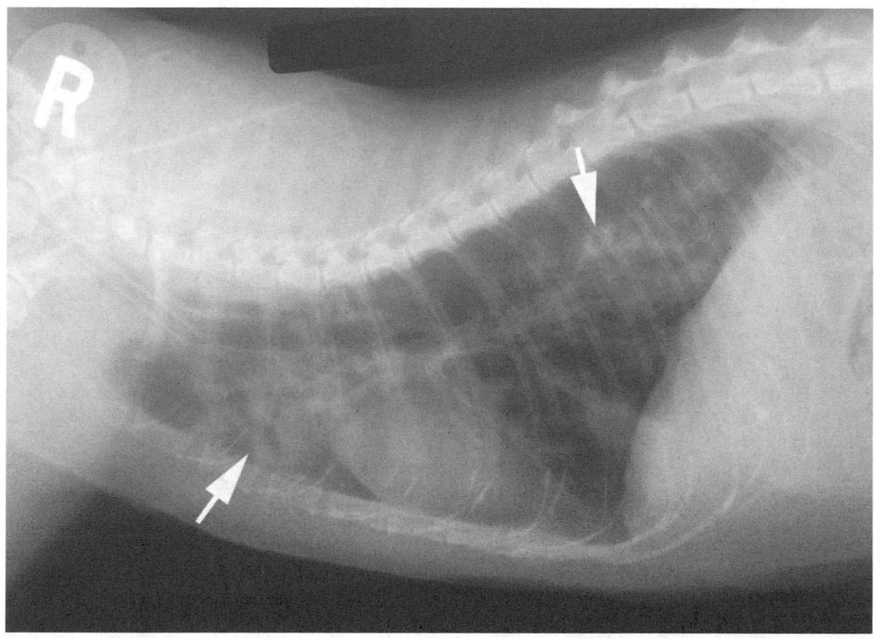

Figure 23-7
Lateral thorax radiograph of 10 year old female domestic short haired cat with pulmonary adenocarcinoma. Note the areas of alveolarized lung (white arrows).

away from the sternum and ability to identify lung margins surrounded by a less opaque region. The elevated heart is due to the lack of support provided to the heart while the patient is in lateral recumbency. With a unilateral pneumothorax, the elevation phenomenon may occur with the pneumothorax in the dependent (down-side pleural space) or nondependent side. Therefore, it is inaccurate to try to predict the side of the pneumothorax based on the elevation effect in opposite lateral radiographs. Elevation of the heart away from the sternum is also seen in a number of other pathologic and anatomic variations. Any cause of a small heart, hyperinflation or mediastinal shift, leads to a similar appearance on lateral projections. Retraction of the lungs can be a subtle finding but is a much more convincing sign than elevation. Lungs retract in the same regions that free air tends to accumulate. This is usually in the tallest part of the chest, which is the caudal-dorsal thorax with patients in lateral recumbency. A lateral view is the best projection if patient clinical condition restricts the radiographic imaging to a single procedure. The ventrodorsal projection is particularly unhelpful in cases of mild pneumothorax because the air rises to the tallest part of the thorax, which is adjacent to the midline and difficult to identify on images. A VD or DV view is helpful to assist with identification of a tension pneumothorax or to identify symmetry of a moderate bilateral or unilateral pneumothorax.

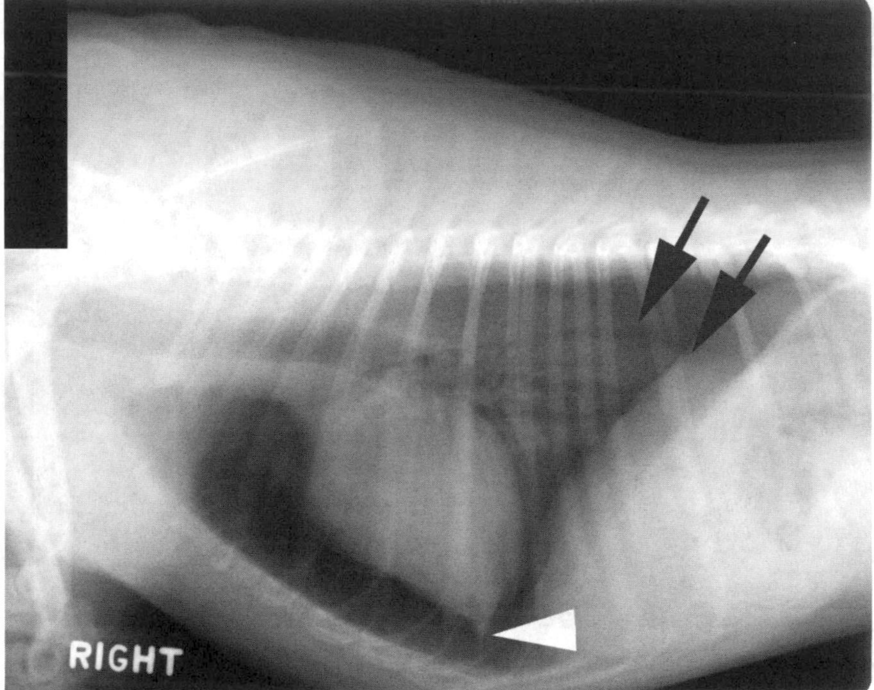

Figure 23-8
A female 2 year old spayed Welsh terrier with pneumothorax. Note retraction of lung margins (black arrows) and "elevation" of heart apex (white arrowhead) away from the sternum.

Abdomen

Evaluation of a set of abdominal radiographs can be very difficult. Inherently, the contrast of the abdomen is poor. Combined with poor technique, nondiagnostic images are easily produced. Abdominal radiographs are taken for evaluation of specific signs or as a test to stage of known disease. A thorough examination of the entire abdomen is essential for the test to be useful. My method for interpreting abdominal radiographs includes the technique of evaluating film exposure factors, the phase of respiration versus body conformation (obese?), and any artifacts. Then in a clockwise fashion examine the thorax, diaphragm, spine with the spinous processes, vertebral bodies, and intervertebral foramen, the retroperitoneum, pelvis with bones and organs, ventral abdominal wall, liver, stomach, spleen, kidneys, urinary bladder, and gastrointestinal tract.

Ventrodorsal radiographs are advantageous because they tend to expand the abdomen and spread the contents over a longer region. Dorsoventral abdominal radiographs tend to bunch the abdominal contents, causing more overlap and superimposition. If the urinary bladder is full, the mass effect will compress adjacent structures and caused decreased abdominal detail. Emptying the bladder and repeating the radiographs will result in a more diagnostic study.

Abdominal Diseases

In abdominal diseases and trauma, there is generally a loss of intra-abdominal contrast, a loss of detail (Fig. 23-9). It can be regional or a focal mass from neoplasia, an abscess, granuloma, a cyst, or a hematoma. Free fluid is one of the causes of loss of contrast. Blood from bleeding masses, systemic coagulopathy, or trauma may be interfering with contrast. Other free fluids such as pus from ruptured gastrointestinal tract or abscess, transudate from right heart failure, hypoalbuminemia, or vasculopathy, urine from a ruptured urinary tract, bile, or chyle may be limiting the contrast. Emaciation, carcinomatosis, and regional peritonitis also cause loss of contrast.

Under many circumstances the evaluation of causes of decreased intra-abdominal detail will benefit from abdominal sonography. Ultrasound and radiographs are complimentary imaging tests. After a confusing sonographic evaluation, radiographs are often beneficial to elucidate the origin of a large mass, cause of large accumulations of gas or minerals, and provide additional information on the gastrointestinal tract. Many patients seem to fly to the ultrasound room prior to radiographs being taken. Although economics and sensitivity issues are

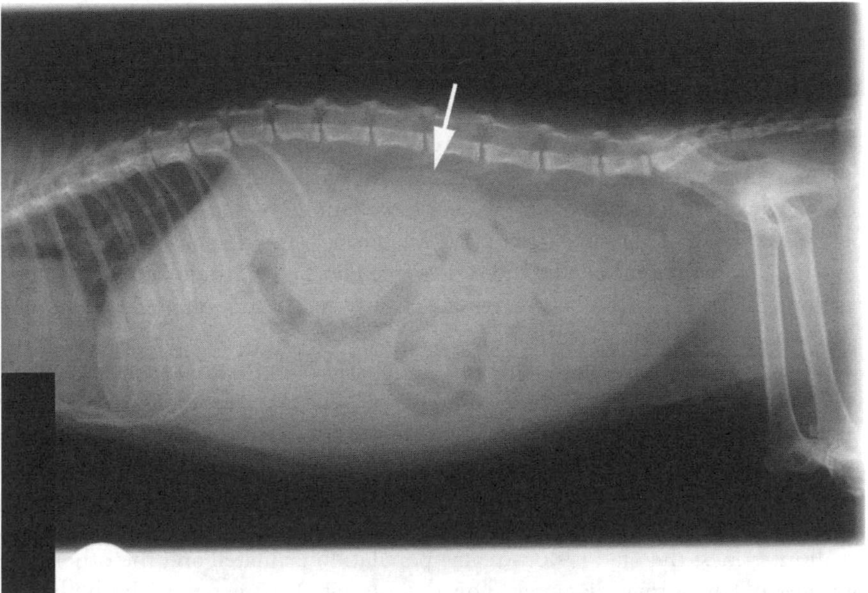

Figure 23-9
Lateral thoracic radiograph of 1 year old Persian cat with peritoneal effusion. Note increased opacity throughout peritoneal space with good retroperitoneal detail (white arrow pointing to margin of kidney in retroperitoneal space).

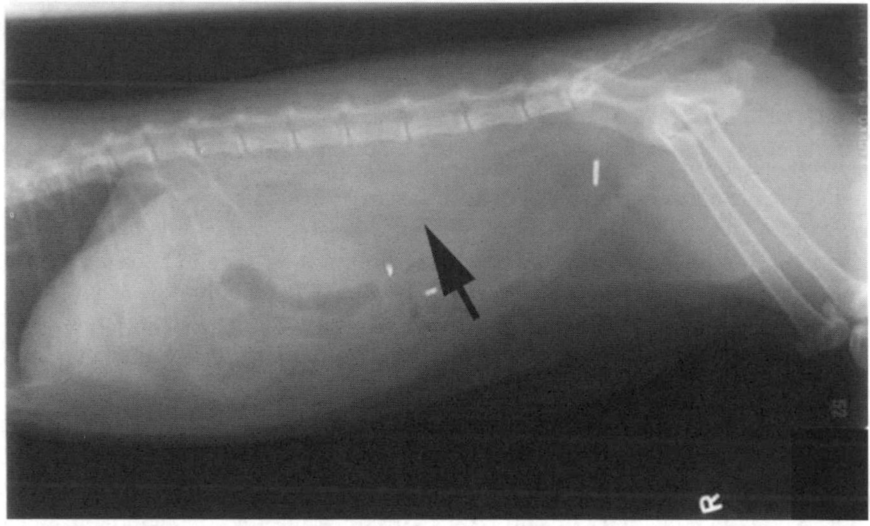

Figure 23-10
Lateral abdominal radiograph of 3 year old male neutered domestic short haired cat with retroperitoneal effusion due to renal failure associated with easter lily toxicity. Note the increased opacity in the dorsal abdomen and loss of retroperitoneal detail (black arrow).

valid, remember that radiographs are a very important part of the evaluation of intra-abdominal lesions.

Retroperitoneal effusion (Fig. 23-10) can be caused by urine from a rupture of a ureter or avulsion of a kidney, trauma, or urolithiasis; by blood from trauma or coagulopathy; or by edema from acute renal failure. In dogs, renal failure may be caused by ethylene glycol toxicity or leptospirosis. In cats, FIP, Easter lily toxicity, and lymphoma can be the causes (see Fig. 23-10). Radiographs of retroperitoneal effusion will show increased opacity in the dorsal intra-abdominal fascial planes that usually contain fat.

Obstruction of the small intestine can be caused by foreign bodies, neoplasia, intussusception, or vascular compromise (Fig. 23-11). Radiology will show dilated small intestines as evidenced by the outside diameter (serosa to serosa) of intestinal loop exceeding the height (on the lateral projection) of an end plate of a lumbar vertebra. Do not utilize the mid-body region, as this is substantially narrower than the end plate region. Usually there are two populations of small intestines; the orad (= upstream) population is dilated and the other, aboral group, has normal diameter. This dichotomy of diameters is the hallmark of small intestinal obstruction. Contrast radiology is often helpful in these cases. An upper GI series can confirm small intestine dilation. Conversely, it can confirm normal or identify the large intestine loops (pneumocolonography) to avoid confusion as a dilated small intestinal loop.

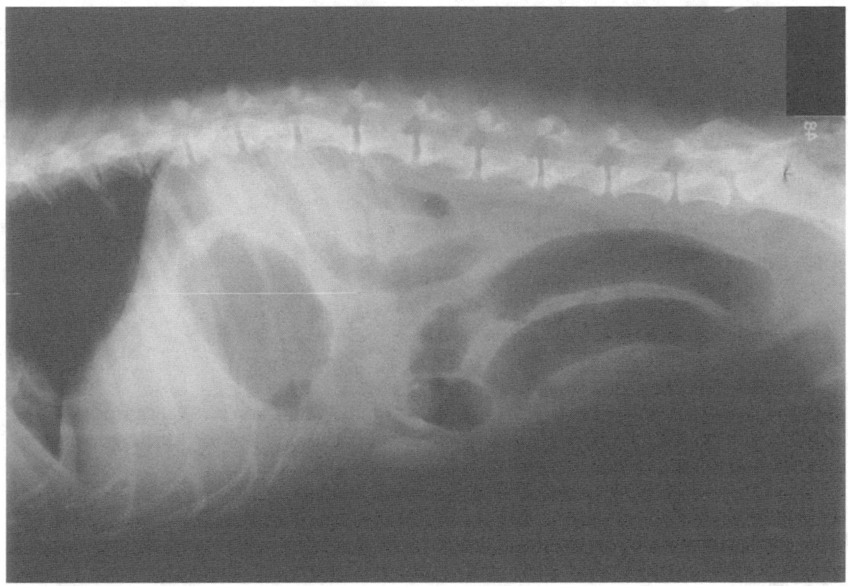

Figure 23-11
Lateral abdominal radiograph of 8 year old male Springer spaniel with small intestinal obstruction. Note dilated intestinal loops and aspiration pneumonia.

Skull and Spine

The skull and spine are usually evaluated for specific localized neurologic signs. Therefore, the evaluation of radiographs can often be biased for location and type of disease. This error in radiology can lead to mistakes of omission. A complete evaluation is just as necessary in these body parts as the thorax and abdomen.

The skull is particularly difficult to evaluate on survey radiographs. Even the seemingly simple diagnosis of fracture can be inordinately difficult. Because of the round shape, fractures of the skull can hide very well. Even with multiple oblique projections, fractures can be occult. Tomographic imaging, especially computed tomography (CT), is much better at detecting skull lesions. Magnetic resonance imaging (MRI) is the most sensitive and specific test for most organic lesions of the brain and spine. In some larger practices, myelography has been replaced by MRI studies. This is especially true of cauda equina syndrome in the lumbosacral region where MRI is more accurate and sensitive than contrast radiographic procedures, including myelography, epidurography, discography, and angiography.

While a discussion of all lesions of the musculoskeletal system is beyond the scope of this chapter, a discussion of the survey radiographic identification of certain spinal lesions seems warranted. The signs of trauma to the spine include

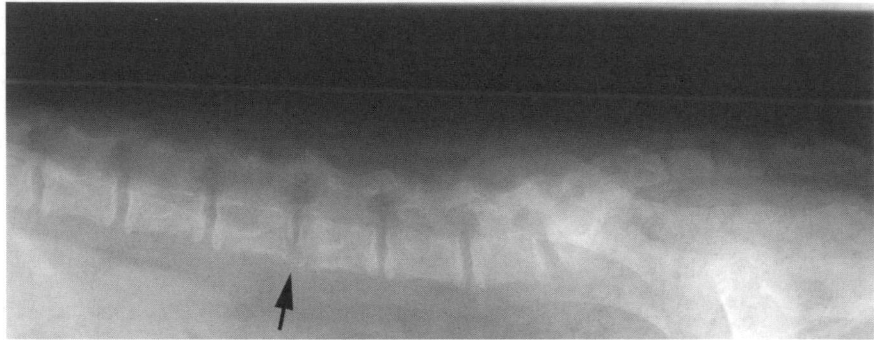

Figure 23-12
Lateral radiograph of lumbar spine of 6 month old Rottweiler with discospondylitis. Note the lysis of adjacent endplate and collapse of the disc space (black arrow) at L4-5.

shortened vertebra, increased opacity, and malalignment of adjacent vertebra. The trauma may be secondary to a large physical force or minimal if there is an underlying pathologic process. Radiographic diagnosis of pathologic bone lesions is based on identification of a change in opacity (increased or decreased) or loss of distinct margins. The underlying process may be inflammatory or neoplastic. If neoplasia is suspected, then additional imaging includes appropriate testing for the primary site or metastases. The most important inflammatory lesion of the spine is diskospondylitis, which manifests as end plate lysis, irregular margination, or subchondral sclerosis of adjacent vertebrae (Fig. 23-12). Although less common in the critical care setting, disk disease is otherwise so common that the signs are worth mentioning. The most common spinal abnormalities include reduced width of the intervertebral disk space, reduced size and increased opacity of intervertebral foramen, and increased focal opacity of the spinal canal.

Musculoskeletal

Musculoskeletal radiographs are lowest on the list of radiographic procedures among critical care patients. They can, however, be very beneficial when additional lesions are discovered. The additional lesions can provide more differentials or evidence to support a particular diagnosis. For example, a concurrent lytic bone lesion in a dog with lobar alveolar infiltration can provide evidence for blastomycosis. Many dogs with systemic diseases have manifestations, including polyarthropathy. This could easily be overlooked as incidental old dog changes, but adds considerably to the evaluation of patients with lupus or tick-borne diseases.

SUGGESTED READINGS

Kornegay JN, Barber DL: Discospondylitis in dogs. *J Amer Vet Med Assoc* 177:4, 1980.
Lord PF, Suter PF, Chan KF, *et al.*: Pleural, extrapleural and pulmonary lesions in small

animals: A radiographic approach to differential diagnosis. *J Am Vet Radiol Soc* 13: 4, 1972.

Moon ML, Greenlee PG, Burk RL: Uremic pneumonitis-like syndrome in ten dogs. *J Am Anim Hosp Assoc* 19:903, 1983.

Myer CW, Bonagura JD: Survey radiography of the heart. *Vet Clin North Am (Small Anim Pract)* 12:213, 1982.

Myer W: Radiography review: The interstitial pattern of pulmonary disease. *Vet Radiol* 21:18, 1980.

Myer W: Radiography review: The alveolar patter of lung disease. *J Am Vet Radiol Soc* 20:10, 1979.

O'Brien RT: Thoracic Radiology for the Small Animal Practitioner. Teton NewMedia, Jackson, WY. 144pp. 2001.

Root CR: Interpretation of abdominal survey radiographs. *Vet Clin North Am* 4:763, 1974.

Thrall DE, Losonsky JM: A method for evaluating canine pulmonary circulation dynamics from survey radiographs. *J Am Hosp Assoc* 12:457, 1976.

24
Echocardiography and Doppler Flow

June A. Boon

BASIC PRINCIPLES OF ECHOCARDIOGRAPHY
Types of Ultrasound
Two-Dimensional Ultrasound

Two-dimensional ultrasound sends out multiple side by side sound waves, which generate a sector or pie-shaped image of the heart. Each beam returns information back to the transducer from reflected surfaces. Based on the speed of sound within the body (1540 m/sec) and the time it takes for the sound to travel to the structure and back to the transducer, the structure's depth is located on the monitor as a white spot. Fluid-filled spaces such as the chambers of the heart or effusions are not cellular enough to reflect sound so nothing is placed on the monitor, and thus, will appear black. As the structures in the heart move so does their relative distance to the transducer and the time it takes for sound to reflect back to the crystals. The location on the monitor is changed accordingly. The result is a moving dynamic image of the heart as it moves throughout the cardiac cycles.

The sound beams leave the transducer as a sheet of sound and are directed though any plane of the heart. There are standard saggital and transverse images, which are landmarks for other imaging planes.[1] In emergency medicine the imaging planes are often modified while searching for masses or ruptured chordae or while performing the exam in nonstandard positions. Knowledge of the standard images will help identify the structures seen under these somewhat adverse conditions.

M-Mode Ultrasound

M-mode ultrasound stands for "motion mode." One sound beam is selected from the two-dimensional sector and the structures that this beam transects are imaged in a diagrammatic fashion. The beam is selected by placing a cursor over the area of interest and only the structures under the cursor are seen on the M-mode. They scroll across a screen; time on the x-axis and depth on the y-axis. The structures change in location depending on how they move relative to the transducer. Left ventricular M-modes will show the septum and free wall thickening during systole and thinning during diastole. The chamber itself will increase and decrease in size during diastole and systole, respectively. In the critical care situation, M-mode echocardiography is important for assessment of cardiac function and size compared to published reference values.[2,3]

Doppler Ultrasound

The Doppler principle states that the frequency of sound changes when the position between the sound source and its receiver changes. Within the heart this means that when the transducer sends out a Doppler beam, the frequency of sound returning to the machine is changed depending on whether the blood cells it encounters are moving away from or toward the transducer. When the Doppler beam interacts with blood cells moving toward the transducer, the frequency of sound returning to the machine is increased. When the Doppler beam interacts with blood cells moving away from the transducer, the frequency of sound returning to the machine is decreased. The difference in frequency is then converted to velocity measurements by the machine.[3,4]

The spectral Doppler flow signal is plotted above a baseline for positive frequency shifts or upward flow. Flow reflecting a decrease in frequency is plotted below the baseline at its respective velocity to represent blood moving away from the transducer. Color flow Doppler simply maps the positive or negative frequency shifts in color. Generally, flow upward is coded in reds and yellows, and downward flow is coded in blues and whites.

Pulsed-Wave Doppler. Pulsed-wave Doppler is specifically used when the interest in flow is specific to a particular locale. A gate is placed at the area of interest and only the flow information from within that area is sampled and recorded. This allows specific locations within the heart to be sampled. Pulsed-wave Doppler, however, is limited in its ability to record high-velocity flow. As its name implies, pulses of sound are sent out. The sound must travel to the gate and be received by the transducer again before a new pulse can be sent out. The deeper the gate is set, and the higher the frequency of sound used, the longer the time interval between pulses. This limits the maximum velocity that can be recorded without aliasing. An aliased signal does allow the magnitude of abnormal flow to be assessed, however, by looking for the extent of the aliased flow within the atrial or ventricular chambers. It is possible to define the perimeter of abnormal flow this way. Continuous wave Doppler cannot do this.[3,4]

Continuous Wave Doppler. Continuous wave Doppler is used to determine the velocity of abnormal flow. It does not specifically record flow at a single point along the Doppler beam but records flow all along the sound beam. The highest velocities are typically the ones of interest, so ambiguous information is generally not a problem. The highest flow is recorded and slower velocities are hidden within the tracing. Only when two different abnormal high-velocity flows occur at the same time in the cardiac cycle, in the same direction, and in close proximity to each other, does continuous wave Doppler become difficult to interpret. Continuous wave Doppler is used to determine pressure gradients across stenotic lesions, shunts, and valvular insufficiencies.[3,4]

Color Flow Doppler. Color flow Doppler provides instant gratification. High-velocity and turbulent blood flow is immediately identified. Shunts, regurgitant jets, and stenotic lesions are quickly located. Assessment of the hemodynamic effect of these problems is not possible with color flow Doppler and spectral Doppler must be used in conjunction with this modality. Color flow Doppler aliases at fairly low velocities so the presence of an aliased signal does not always imply abnormal flow, but it does direct the eye to potential areas of abnormal flow.[4]

Although color flow Doppler is a quick and easy way to identify abnormal flow within the heart, it provides limited quantitative information. Spectral Doppler provides more quantitative information allowing assessment of pressure gradients, pulmonary pressures, the hemodynamic significance of defects, and the evaluation of diastolic function.[3,4]

ECHOCARDIOGRAPHIC FEATURES OF CARDIAC DISEASE IN CRITICALLY ILL PATIENTS

Pericardial Effusion and Cardiac Masses

Pericardial effusion is identified as an echo-free space between the ventricular walls and the pericardial sac (Fig. 24-1).[5,6] This fluid is seen primarily

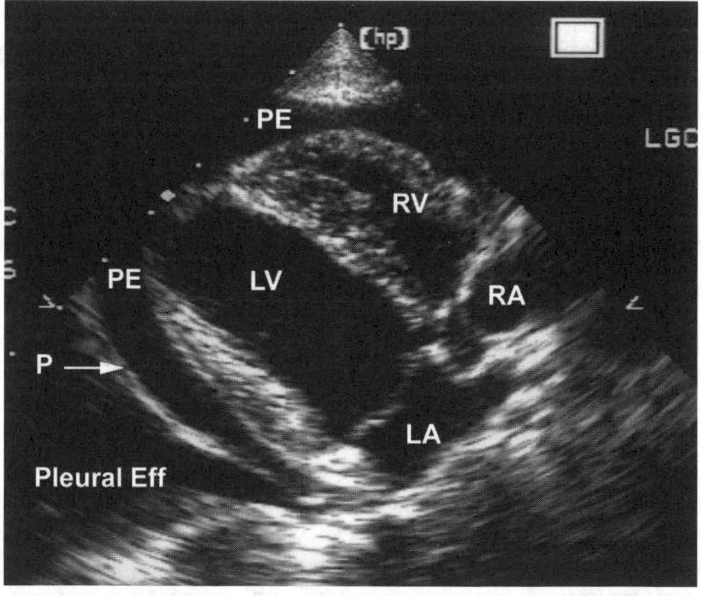

Figure 24-1
Pericardial effusion is an echo-free space surrounding the heart. The inside of the pericardial sac is typically smooth and the fluid typically does not extend much past the ventricular-atrial junction. Pleural effusion does not have the same smooth layering around the heart. This is a right parasternal four-chamber imaging plane. PE, pericardial effusion; RV, right ventricle; RA, right atrium; LV, left ventricle; LA, left atrium; P, pericardium; Pleural Eff, pleural effusion.

around the left and right ventricular chambers. The pericardium attaches to the heart under the atria and pericardial fluid is not seen around the heart base. The inside of the pericardial sac, with the exception of fibrinous pericarditis (rarely seen in the small animal), has a smooth surface. Pleural effusion is seen around the heart base as well as the ventricles, has irregular surfaces, and may contain floating fibrinous tags. Near the top of the sector image on transverse views, there are often echo-free spaces secondary to refractive shadowing and this is sometimes mistaken for effusion. Take care to image various planes to confirm the presence of pericardial effusion. On sagittal and transverse images of the heart, a large left auricle can be seen as an echo-free space between the ventricular chamber and the pericardial sac. This left auricular chamber becomes smaller toward the apex of the heart on long axis views as opposed to larger, and is only present on the right side of the image on transverse views.

End-diastolic collapse of the right atrium with or without early to mid-diastolic collapse of the right ventricular chamber has been used as a diagnostic criterion for cardiac tamponade (Fig. 24-2). This can be seen on long axis four-chamber views, apical four-chamber views, and transverse views of the heart base. The amount of pericardial fluid does not determine whether tam-

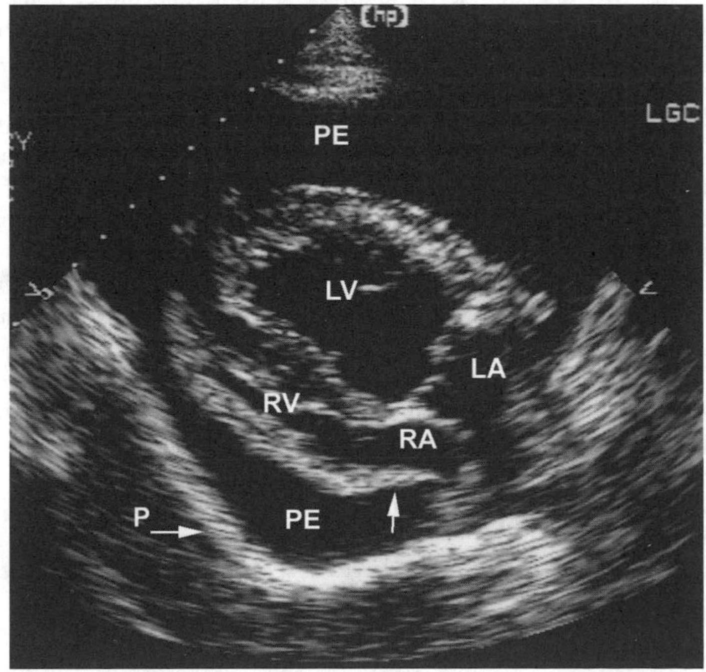

Figure 24-2
Collapse of the right atrial wall (arrow) is a sign of cardiac tamponade. This is a left parasternal modified apical four chamber imaging plane. PE, pericardial effusion; LV, left ventricle; LA, left atrium; RV, right ventricle; RA, right atrium; P, pericardium.

ponade is present or not. Small effusions in the presence of a nonpliable and nondistensable pericardial sac can elevate intrapericardial pressures enough to cause tamponade. Tamponade tends to occur with smaller volumes if the accumulation is acute, versus chronic accumulations where very large volumes can be tolerated before intrapericardial pressures are high enough to cause tamponade.[7]

Recent studies in humans have shown that echocardiographic detection of right ventricular collapse was much more specific for the diagnosis of cardiac tamponade than using the echocardiographic feature of right atrial collapse alone.[8] The presence of ventricular chamber collapse was often seen in patients without clinical evidence of cardiac tamponade. Studies suggest that these patients may have had a mild degree of tamponade with elevated intrapericardial pressures but no obvious jugular distention and other clinical features of cardiac tamponade.

Tumors of the pericardial sac or heart itself are the most common cause of pericardial effusion in the dog.[9] The role of echocardiography, besides confirming the presence of pericardial effusion and perhaps tamponade, is to differentiate, if possible, between idiopathic hemorrhagic pericardial effusion and effusion secondary to cardiac neoplasia. Mesotheliomas are diffuse tumors involving the pericardial sac and pleural spaces. They are typically not detectable by echocardiography and usually cannot be differentiated from idiopathic hemorrhagic effusions.[9,10] Hemangiosarcomas are most often located within or around the right auricular appendage. Hemangiosarcomas are typically heterogeneous in appearance containing many hypoechoic areas. When performing an echocardiographic study for the purpose of ruling in or out the presence of a mass when pericardial effusion is present, obtain images from both sides of the thorax when the animal is in lateral recumbency as well as standing. The slightly different positions of the heart allow tumors, which may not be visible in other planes, to swing into view. Even large masses may be missed if a thorough exam is not performed.[3] The presence of pericardial effusion adds significant diagnostic accuracy in determining the presence or absence of a mass not located inside the auricular, atrial, or ventricular chambers or within their walls. If at all possible, always image an animal with pericardial effusion before pericardiocentesis. Masses located outside the auricular appendage are seen floating within the pericardial sac (Fig. 24-3). Often a thrombus is seen extending from the mass into the pericardial fluid.

Tumors of the aortic body are typically small and do not create clinically significant problems. When they become large and invade the chambers or great vessels of the heart or compress the large vessels of the heart, they cause right or left heart failure. These masses always involve some part of the aorta. If the mass is distal to the aortic arch, or contains small flat tumors extending along the wall of the aorta, echocardiographic examination typically will not be of value. Otherwise ultrasound images will show the masses next to the aorta, between the aorta and one of the atrial chambers, or at times between the aorta, pulmonary artery, and its bifurcation (Fig. 24-4).[11] Pericardial effusions are typically not necessary to see heart base tumor.

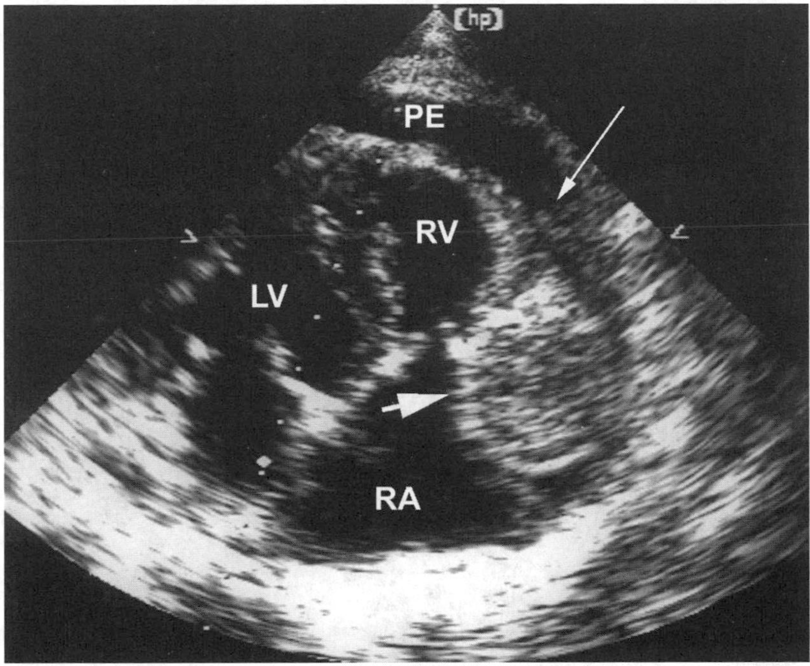

Figure 24-3
Hemangiosarcomas are most often seen within the right auricular appendage (large arrow). A thin strand of clot extending from the auricular appendage as the tumor bleeds into the sac is seen within the pericardial fluid (thin arrow). This is a left parasternal cranial long axis image of the right atrium and auricle. PE, pericardial effusion; RV, right ventricle; LV, left ventricle; RA, right atrium.

Degenerative Mitral and Aortic Valve Disease

Mitral insufficiency is easy to determine without the aid of echocardiography. Echocardiography, however, is necessary to assess ventricular function and the hemodynamic effects of mitral regurgitation.[12] The chronic changes associated with myxomatous degeneration of the mitral valve are easily documented with cardiac ultrasound. The critically ill patient typically will have dilated left ventricular and atrial chambers, increased wall and septal motion, excellent function, large valvular lesions, and mitral valve prolapse (Fig. 24-5). The prolapse may be caused by stretched chordae secondary to dilation of the left ventricular chamber resulting in redundant chordae when the chamber contracts allowing the valves to buckle back into the atrium. Prolapse may also occur as minor chordae are ruptured.[13] When the leaflet edges or chordae float back into the left atrium and point straight back to the base of the heart, or when they fold back on themselves within the left ventricular outflow tract, there is probably rupture of a major chordae. Chronic disease resulting in either rupture or stretch of the chordae will have volume-overloaded left ventricular and atrial

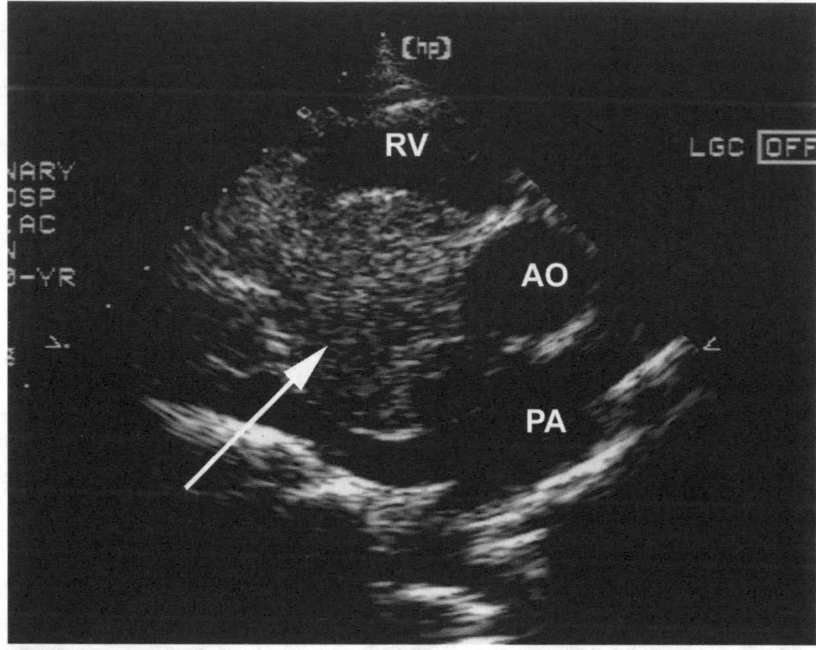

Figure 24-4
Aortic body tumors (arrow) are usually seen associated with the aorta on transverse images of the heart base. They are typically seen between the aorta and atrial chambers or around the aorta and pulmonary artery. This is a right parasternal transverse image of the heart base at the level of the pulmonary artery. RV, right ventricle; AO, aorta; PA, pulmonary artery.

chambers. The degree of volume overload typically correlates with the degree of insufficiency. Using color flow Doppler, a regurgitant jet that encompasses more than 50% of the atrial chamber is classified as severe insufficiency.[14,15] If color flow Doppler shows severe insufficiency with minimal increases in chamber sizes an acute rupture has occurred or systemic hypertension is present.[16]

Myocardial function is typically preserved in these dogs and fractional shortening is elevated secondary to stretch of the myocardial fibers. Fractional shortening that is not elevated suggests mild to moderate myocardial dysfunction. Fractional shortening that is below normal implies significant myocardial dysfunction and secondary cardiomyopathy. Elevated afterload (ie, hypertension) may depress fractional shortening even when intrinsic myocardial function is normal and should be ruled out when function is questionable. Typically systolic ventricular dimensions are normal when myocardial function is preserved. Animals may be in congestive heart failure and have normal myocardial function; they may have myocardial dysfunction and low output failure, without being in congestive heart failure, or they may have both congestive and myocardial failure.[17-19]

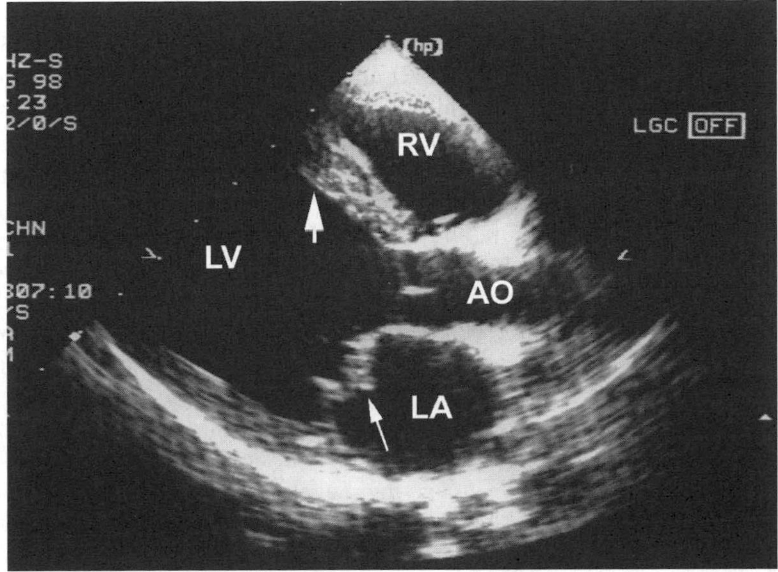

Figure 24-5
Upward septal curvature (fat arrow), an enlarged left atrium, mitral valve lesions, and mitral valve prolapse (small arrow) are commonly seen in patients with myxomatous degeneration of the mitral valve. This is a right parasternal long axis left ventricular outflow view of the heart. RV, right ventricle; LV, left ventricle; AO, aorta; LA, left atrium.

Endocarditis

The mitral valve is the most common site of infection in dogs, followed by aortic, pulmonic, and tricuspid valves. Early lesions, typically smooth and small, may not be detectable with transthoracic echocardiography, but the larger lesions are easily seen. Transesophageal echocardiography brings the detection of even small lesions up to approximately 90%.[20] Large lesions are usually heterogeneous in appearance with hypoechoic and hyperechoic areas within them. It is difficult, and usually not possible, to differentiate the large lesions of degenerative mitral valve disease from infective lesions. Clinical features must be used to make this diagnosis.[21,22] The lesions may cause the valve to become insufficient or stenotic.[21]

Color flow and spectral Doppler can help define stenotic lesions of the mitral valve because the diastolic murmur associated with this lesion is often difficult to hear. Color flow Doppler shows an aliased high-velocity inflow signal, whereas spectral Doppler shows a high-velocity E peak (rapid ventricular filling phase) and slow deceleration creating a fairly square inflow profile. The slow deceleration is referred to as a long pressure half-time, the time it takes for flow velocity to decrease to half its maximum value. The longer the pressure half-time and the more square the flow profile is, the more significant the obstruction.

The diastolic murmurs of aortic insufficiency may also be very soft and color flow Doppler helps identify these problems. A turbulent flow signal is seen moving into the left ventricular outflow tract and chamber during diastole. Diastolic jets that extend past the tips of the mitral valves into the left ventricular chamber and involve more than half the width of the left ventricular outflow tract are considered to be significant insufficiencies. The accuracy of interpreting the severity of aortic insufficiency based on jet size is less than for mitral insufficiency because left ventricular pressure and volume play a role in jet size.[16,22] A fairly square spectral Doppler signal recorded from an aortic insufficiency jet suggests that diastolic left ventricular pressures have not significantly elevated secondary to this added volume (Fig. 24-6A). Regurgitant flows that have a more triangular shape, a rapid pressure half-time, are consistent with elevated left ventricular diastolic pressures (Fig. 24-6B).[16,22] Left ventricular compliance and systemic vascular resistance affect the appearance of these flow profiles. Afterload reducing agents can cause left ventricular and aortic pressures to equilibrate more rapidly creating a triangular flow profile and giving the false impression of hemodynamically significant insufficiency.[24] Stenotic lesions on the aortic valve create aliased high-velocity flow patterns within the aorta and spectral Doppler helps calculate the significance of the obstruction by calculating the pressure gradient. Pressure gradients greater than 90 mm Hg are considered to represent severe obstruction to aortic outflow.[24]

Acute bacterial endocarditis will not have accompanying compensatory dilation or hypertrophy. Chronic changes also include excessive wall motion and elevated parameters of function if the myocardium is not affected.

The infective lesions of endocarditis may spread to the chordae tendinae, the walls of the aorta, and septum, creating abscesses and rupture of adjacent walls. An even greater risk is embolization from large lesions into the coronary arteries, brain, or organs resulting in infarction.[20,21]

Cardiomyopathies

Dilated Cardiomyopathy

The prominent features of dilated cardiomyopathy include left ventricular and left atrial dilation with no compensatory hypertrophy; reduced fractional shortening; diminished aortic, atrial, septal, and free wall motion; and increased E point-to-septal separation (EPSS).[26] Cats that present with dilated cardiomyopathy may not have dilation of the left ventricular chamber despite very poor function.[27] The right side of the heart may also be involved and should be suspected in animals that present in right heart failure. Although the dysfunction seen in dilated cardiomyopathy is diffuse and global, there may be varying degrees of dysfunction throughout the ventricle. Mitral insufficiency can range from mild to severe.

Animals present in either low output failure, congestive heart failure, or both. Low output failure is documented with low aortic flow velocities. Aortic flow velocities are often as low as 0.6 m/sec. Left atrial pressures can be estimated using Doppler and the mitral regurgitant jet. Elevated left atrial pressures de-

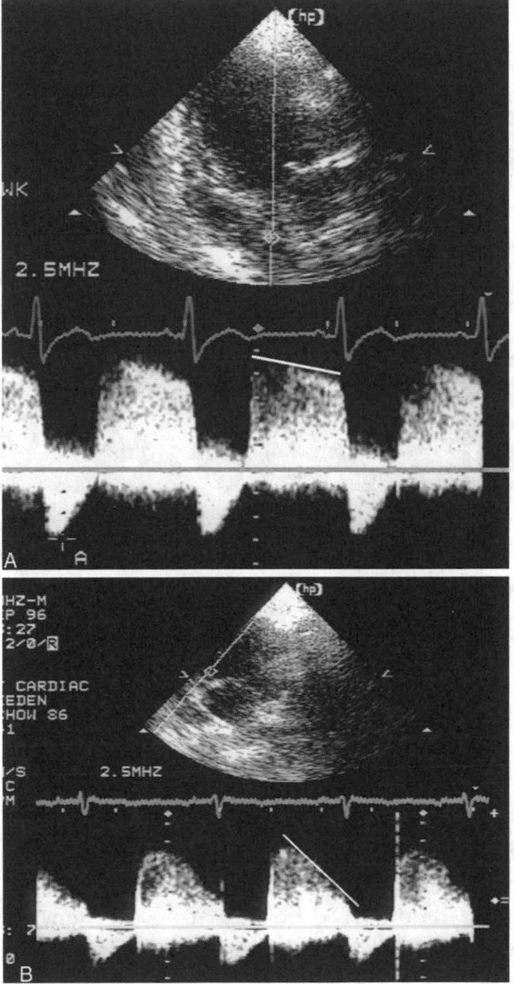

Figure 24-6
Long pressure half-times, the time it takes for regurgitant flow velocity to decrease to half its peak value, are an indication that left ventricular diastolic pressures have not elevated significantly secondary to volume overload from aortic insufficiency. (A) A fairly square shaped regurgitant jet profile with a long pressure half-time. (B) The flow profile shows a rapid deceleration rate, a short pressure half-time, consistent with a rapid increase in left ventricular pressures and concurrent decline in regurgitant flow velocity and volume.

crease the pressure gradient from the left ventricle to the left atrium during systole. As a result, Doppler flow velocities of the mitral regurgitant jet are low. For example, if the mitral regurgitant jet has a velocity of 4.2 m/sec, the calculated pressure gradient after applying the Bernoulli equation ($4V^2$) is 70.5 mm Hg. This means that the left ventricular systolic pressures are 70 mm Hg higher than the left atrial pressures. Therefore, if systolic blood pressure is 100 mm Hg,

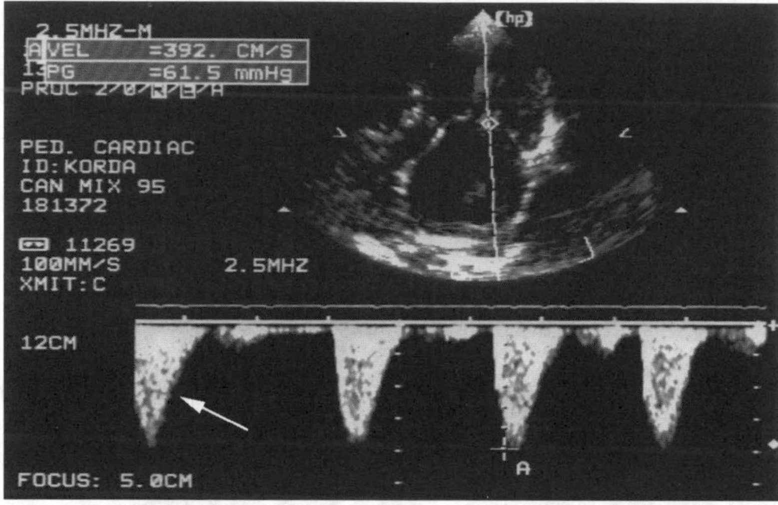

Figure 24-7
Spectral Doppler of mitral regurgitant jets can provide information about left atrial pressures if a good blood pressure can be recorded. The pressure gradient from the left ventricle to the left atrium is calculated from the regurgitant jet velocity. The gradient is 62 mm Hg in this example. The gradient is subtracted from systemic systolic pressures to estimate left atrial pressures. This animal had a systemic blood pressure of 89 mm Hg resulting in estimated left atrial pressures of 27 mm Hg.

the estimated left atrial pressure is approximately 30 mm Hg (Fig. 24-7). These results are, of course, dependent on accurate alignment with flows and an accurate blood pressure measurement.[28-30] In humans, shorter deceleration times for mitral early inflow profiles are correlated to poor prognosis and earlier death. Retrospective studies in dogs have shown that no two-dimensional or M-mode parameter can be used as a prognostic indicator.[31-34]

It is important to state that poor fractional shortening does not always imply poor contractility and dilated cardiomyopathy. Fractional shortening can be affected dramatically by preload. Volume contraction leads to poor stretch of the myocardial fibers resulting in poor shortening. Even fractional shortening in the high teens to low twenties may simply be secondary to decreased preload within the heart. Increased afterload can also decrease myocardial function. Thus afterload may be systemic hypertension or secondary to increased preload within the left ventricular chamber without the muscle mass to handle that volume. A chronic increase in volume without compensatory hypertrophy implies myocardial disease.[19]

Hypertrophic Cardiomyopathy

Concentric left ventricular hypertrophy is the hallmark echocardiographic feature of hypertrophic cardiomyopathy. The hypertrophy may involve just the septum, the free wall, or both. Rarely apical hypertrophy is seen.[35-37] In humans, small left ventricular chamber size correlates with severity of symptoms and func-

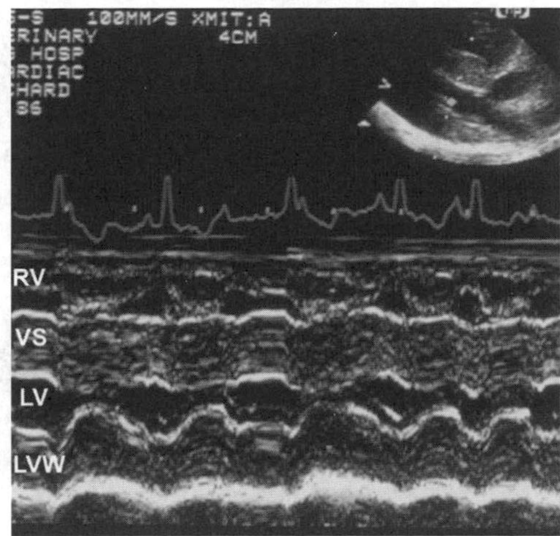

Figure 24-8
Septal systolic thickening is diminished in this cat with severe hypertrophic cardiomyopathy. Despite the elevated fractional shortening that would be calculated from this M-mode, the lack of septal thickening suggests myocardial dysfunction. RV, right ventricle; VS, ventricular septum; LV, left ventricle; LVW, left ventricular wall.

tional limitations.[38] Beware of "pseudo" hypertrophy in the cat that is dehydrated or volume contracted. Re-evaluate the heart after adequate rehydration.

Myocardial function is usually elevated or normal with hypertrophic cardiomyopathy. When the fractional shortening is normal, inspect the septum and free wall. Reduced systolic thickening of the septum and free walls is consistent with myocardial dysfunction regardless of the fractional shortening (Fig. 24-8). In one study, 72% of cats with myocardial failure and fractional shortenings, less than 30% died within 3 months of initial presentation.[36]

The left atrium is dilated in the critically ill cat with heart disease. Although there may be some mitral insufficiency, the left atrial enlargement is secondary to impaired relaxation and decreased compliance of the left ventricular chamber. Mitral insufficiency is secondary to systolic anterior mitral valve motion (SAM). SAM occurs as elevated velocities in the outflow tract pulls the anterior mitral valve leaflet up into the ejection flow. This prevents proper coaptation of the mitral leaflets, corresponding insufficiency, and aggravated outflow obstruction.[39] Although there is dispute over the significance of left ventricular outflow obstruction in feline hypertrophic cardiomyopathy, humans with a systolic pressure gradient of greater than 30 demonstrated significantly more symptomatic patients. Reduced left ventricular chamber size added to the functional limitations of these patients with outflow obstruction.[37,38]

Impaired relaxation may be documented by measuring the isovolumic relaxation time (IVRT). This time period is measured from the end of ventricular ejection using the aortic flow profile to the beginning of ventricular inflow using the mitral inflow profile (Fig. 24-9). Normal cats should have an IVRT of less

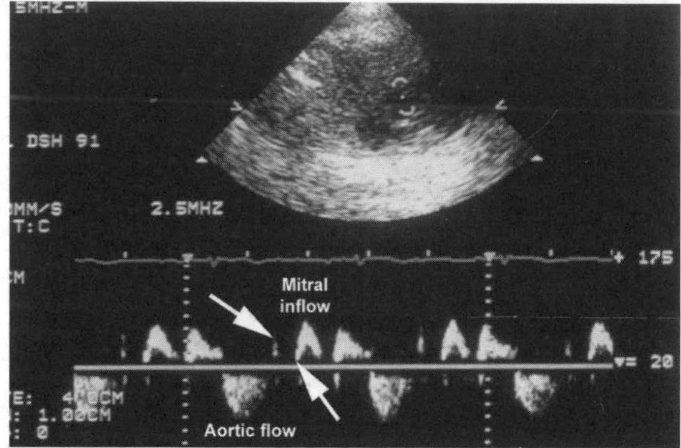

Figure 24-9
The time period from the end of aortic systolic flow to the beginning of mitral diastolic inflow (between arrows) is the isovolumic relaxation time (IVRT). This time period is increased (>60 msec) when there is impaired or delayed ventricular relaxation, often seen in hypertrophic cardiomyopathy.

than 60 msec.[29,40] Because the ventricular muscle takes longer to relax, the early diastolic filling phase (E peak) is reduced secondary to a reduction in the early pressure gradient. Atrial contraction in late diastole contributes more than its usual share of diastolic filling. The resultant E/A ratio is less than 1.5.[29,40] This pattern of left ventricular filling may progress to a pattern representing restrictive physiology (see Restrictive Cardiomyopathy section) with a pseudonormalization phase in between.[29,40] The presence of a large left atrium despite a normal mitral inflow pattern suggests the presence of diastolic dysfunction. Inflow profiles are often not obtained in cats with heart disease because rapid heart rates cause the two phases of ventricular filling to merge.

A potential complication in all forms of cardiomyopathy is thomboembolic episodes. Thrombus is typically first seen within the left auricular appendage and may extend into the main body of the left atrial chamber as it enlarges (Fig. 24-10). An early sign of impending organized thrombus is "smoke" or swirling gray haze within the atrial or even ventricular chambers as the blood becomes stagnant and platelet aggregation or rouleaux begins.[41]

Restrictive Cardiomyopathy

Ventricular inflow restriction causes enlarged atrial chambers seen in restrictive cardiomyopathy. Restrictive physiology may be idiopathic secondary to infiltrative disorders such as amyloidosis and endomyocardial fibrosis, or represent end-stage dilated or hypertrophic cardiomyopathy.[42] Left ventricular chamber size is close to normal. Hypertrophy, if present, is minimal; left ventricular function is normal to mildly reduced. The hallmark echocardiographic finding with restrictive cardiomyopathy is a dramatically enlarged left atrial chamber.[42-44]

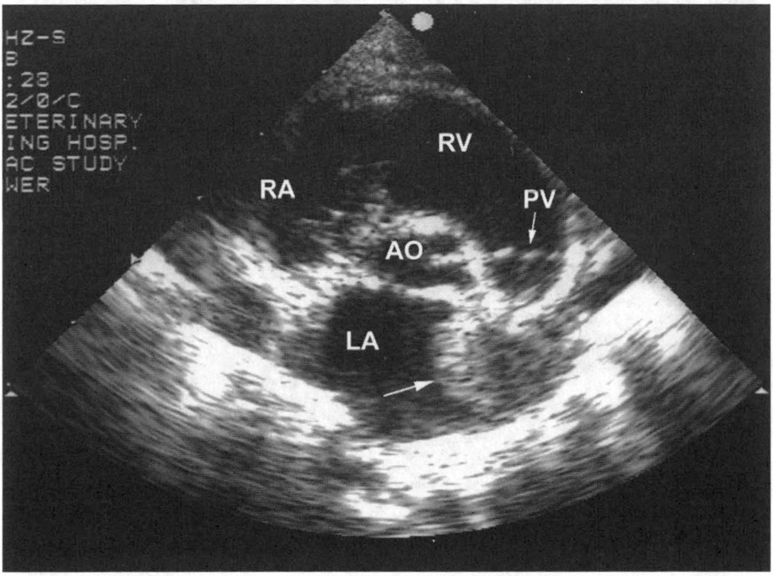

Figure 24-10
Clots within the heart in cardiomyopathies typically form first within the left auricular chamber (arrow). They appear as soft-tissue structures with the appendage and may contain hyperechoic as well as hypoechoic areas. This is a right parasternal transverse image of the heart base at the level of the left atrium. RA, right atrium; RV, right ventricle; PV, pulmonic valve; AO, aorta; LA, left atrium.

"Smoke," the echocardiographic appearance of sluggish blood flow and rouleaux, is often seen within the left atrial chamber. Actual thrombus may be seen and develops within the left auricular appendage.[41] Bright hyperechoic areas within the left ventricular myocardium are suggestive of fibrosis, as is an irregular endocardial surface (Fig. 24-11). The fibrosis is not always seen, and its absence does not rule out the diagnosis of restrictive cardiomyopathy. This disease is often one of exclusion, where other diseases are ruled out and restrictive disease remains.

Color flow Doppler usually shows mild mitral and tricuspid insufficiencies. The degree of insufficiency does not correlate with the significant atrial dilation. Spectral Doppler documents the presence of restrictive physiology. Ventricular filling is completed early in diastole because of reduced ventricular compliance.[43,45] Normal mitral inflow profiles should have an E/A ratio of approximately 2.49 ± 0.28 (mean $\pm$ standard error).[40] With higher left atrial pressures the pressure gradient from the left atrium to the left ventricle is greater and the rapid ventricular filling phase has a greater peak velocity. The atrial component to left ventricular filling is diminished because of high diastolic pressures and restriction to inflow during the latter part of ventricular diastole. The A peak, therefore, is very low or nonexistent.[43] As restrictive physiology progresses it

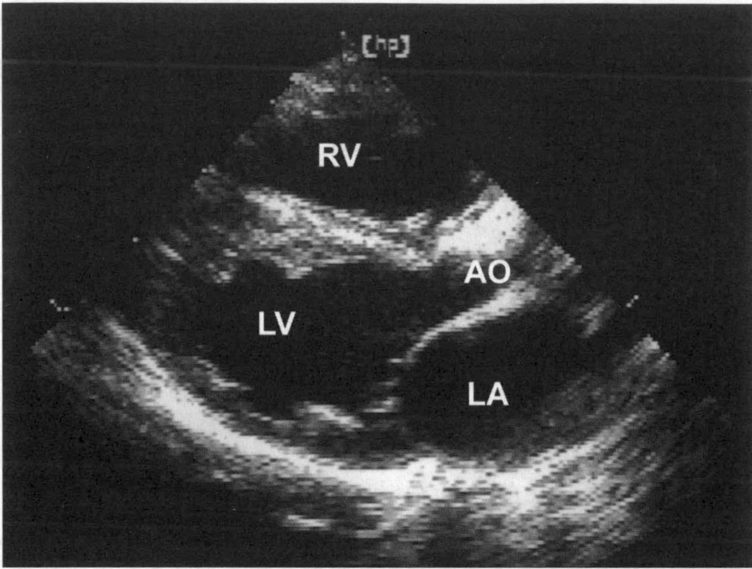

Figure 24-11
Irregular endocardial surfaces and a dilated left atrium are characteristic of restrictive cardiomyopathy. This is a right parasternal long axis left ventricular outflow image. RV, right ventricle; AO, aorta; LV, left ventricle; LA, left atrium.

is possible for compliance to become so reduced that the major driving force for ventricular filling is atrial contraction resulting in reduced early filling and an increased atrial filling component, much like the hypertrophic cardiomyopathy.[43] Deceleration time of early mitral inflow is reduced as ventricular and atrial pressures equilibrate rapidly.[42,43] Spectral Doppler is also used to show changes in left ventricular relaxation. The mitral valve will open early secondary to the high left atrial pressures and the IVRT is reduced in cats with restrictive cardiomyopathy.

Because mitral inflow profiles usually do not show the separate phases of ventricular filling, pulmonary venous flow may be interrogated by placing the pulsed Doppler gate in a pulmonary vein. Venous flow is recorded. Reversal of flow is normal, but reversed flow whose duration is longer than mitral A wave inflow duration is abnormal. This suggests elevated end-diastolic left ventricular pressures.[42] Pulmonary veins are often seen best on apical four- or five-chamber views but can be seen on right parasternal long axis views as well.

Pulmonary Hypertension

Pulmonary hypertension may be seen with chronic respiratory disease, left heart failure, thromboembolic disease, and reverse shunts.[46] Mild to moderate pulmonary hypertension shows subtle signs of right ventricular hypertrophy and

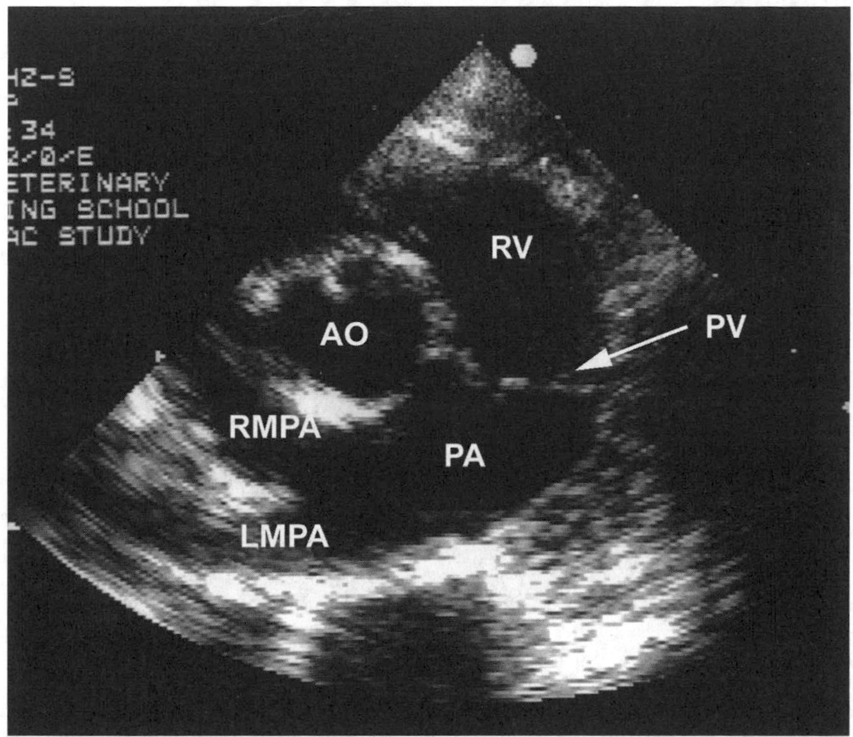

Figure 24-12
Pulmonary hypertension causes the pulmonary artery to dilate from the level of the pulmonic valve all the way into the right and left main pulmonary artery branches. The width of the pulmonary artery at the level of the valve is greater than the diameter of the aorta at the aortic valve level. This is a right parasternal transverse image of the heart base at the level of the pulmonary artery. RV, right ventricle; A, aorta; PA, pulmonary artery; RMPA, right main pulmonary artery; LMPA, left main pulmonary artery.

perhaps some mild main pulmonary artery dilation and a prominent bifurcation.[46,47] Often the tricuspid valve is seen to prolapse secondary to elevated right ventricular pressures. Unless there is tricuspid insufficiency, the presence of pulmonary hypertension can only be suspected. When pulmonary hypertension becomes moderate to severe, right ventricular hypertrophy and dilation is evident, the pulmonary artery is obviously enlarged, and there is almost always some degree of tricuspid insufficiency (Fig. 24-12). Left ventricular chamber size is diminished with increased wall and septal thicknesses secondary to decreased preload. This is another example of "pseudo" hypertrophy. Paradoxical septal motion develops as right ventricular diastolic pressures exceed left ventricular diastolic pressures.[46,47]

The tricuspid insufficiency is used to measure the severity of the hypertension (Fig. 24-13). Spectral Doppler recordings of the tricuspid regurgitant jet are used to measure the pressure gradient from the right ventricle into the right

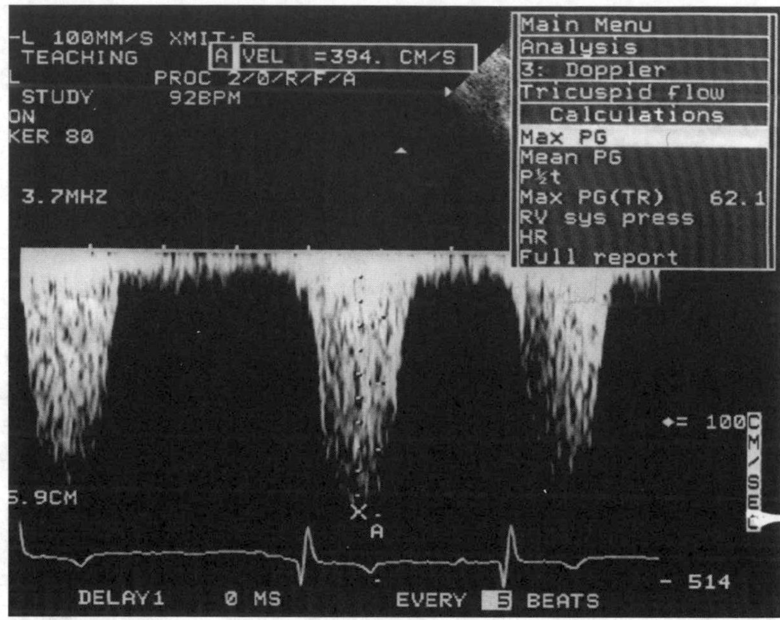

Figure 24-13
Systolic pulmonary arterial pressures can be estimated by using spectral Doppler on tricuspid regurgitant jets. Here the velocity of regurgitant tricuspid flow is 3.94 m/sec with a calculated pressure gradient of 62 mm Hg. Right ventricular pressures must be at least 62 mm Hg. In the absence of pulmonic stenosis this is also the pressure found within the pulmonary vasculature.

atrium. A normal pressure gradient would be about 20 mm Hg (right ventricular pressures of about 20 and right atrial pressures close to 0). As pulmonary pressures elevate, pressures within the right ventricle will elevate to the same degree. For instance, if the velocity of the tricuspid regurgitant jet is 4.0 m/sec, applying the Bernoulli equation ($4V^2$) would result in a calculated pressure gradient of 64 mm Hg. Right ventricular pressures are at least 64, and in the absence of pulmonic stenosis, this also represents pulmonary pressures. These Doppler results are limited by technical expertise in aligning the Doppler beam parallel to flow. Any alignment away form parallel will underestimate the calculated pressure gradient. Use the imaging plane that aligns the Doppler beam best with the regurgitant jet. Volume also affects the velocity of flow with large regurgitant volumes potentially causing overestimation of pressure gradients. Unexplained false-positive diagnosis of pulmonary hypertension has been reported.[46-48]

The pulmonary flow profile may be abnormal when pulmonary hypertension is present. Flow acceleration is more rapid than normal due to the higher systolic pressures that must be generated within the right ventricular chamber. There may also be notching of the flow profile during the deceleration phase; this is often referred to as "the flying W" (Fig. 24-14). This Doppler feature does not differentiate between mild, moderate, and severe pulmonary hypertension and

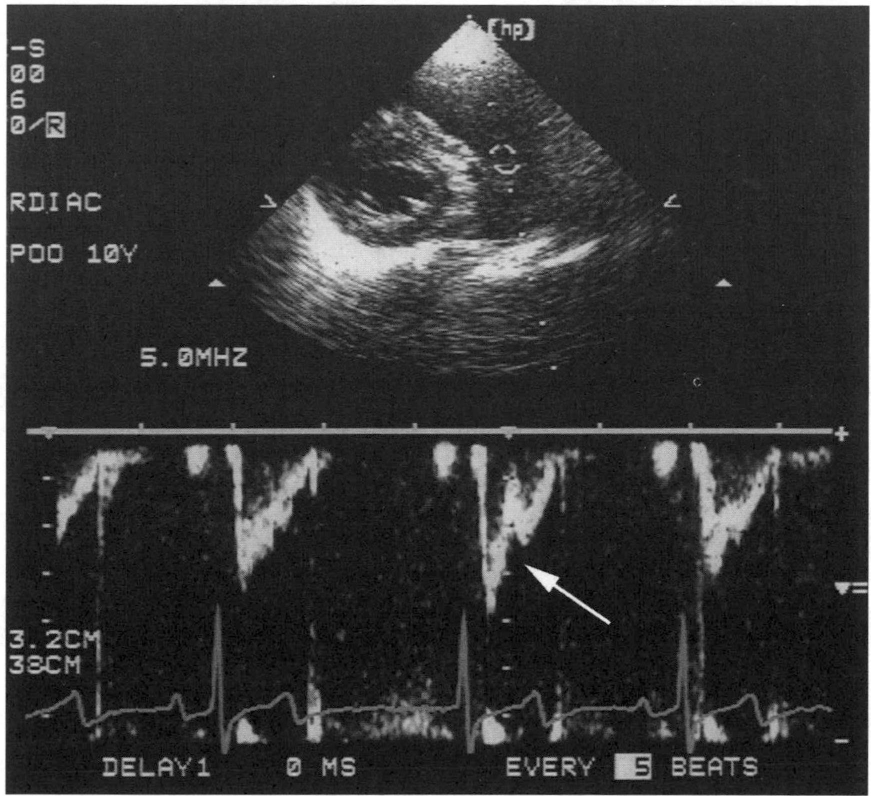

Figure 24-14
Notching, during deceleration on pulmonary flow profiles, is highly suggestive of the presence of pulmonary hypertension. The severity of hypertension cannot be estimated from this flow profile, however.

even animals with significant pulmonary hypertension may not show this characteristic.[46,47,49]

REFERENCES

1. Thomas WP, Graber CE, Jacobs GJ, *et al.*: Recommendations for standards in transthoracic two-dimensional echocardiography in the dog and cat. *J Vet Intern Med* 7: 247, 1993.
2. Boon J, Wingfield WE, Miller CW: Echocardiographic indices in the normal dog. *Vet Radiol* 24:214, 1983.
3. Boon JA: Manual of Veterinary Echocardiography. Baltimore: Williams & Wilkins, 1998.
4. Hatle L, Angelson B: Doppler Ultrasound in Cardiology: Physical Principles and Clinical Application. Philadelphia: Lea & Febiger, 1982.
5. Bonagura JD, Pipers FS: Echocardiographic features of pericardial effusion in the dog. *J Am Vet Med Assoca* 179:49, 1981.

6. Bouvey BM, Bjorling DE: Pericardial effusion in dogs and cats. Diagnostic approach and treatment. *Compend Cont Educ Prac Vet* 13:633, 1991.
7. Berg RJ, Wingfield W: Pericardial effusion in the dog. A review of 42 cases. *JAAHA* 20:721, 1984.
8. Merce J, Sagrista-Sauleda J, Permanyer-Miralda G, *et al.*: Correlation between clinical and Doppler echocardiographic findings in patients with moderate and large pericardial effusion: implications for the diagnosis of cardiac tamponade. *Am Heart J* 138:759, 1999.
9. Berg J: Pericardial effusion and cardiac neoplasia. *Semin Vet Med Surg Sm Anim* 9:185, 1994.
10. Berg RJ, Wingfield WE, Hoopes PJ: Idiopathic hemorrhagic pericardial effusion in eight dogs. *J Am Vet Med Assoc* 185:988, 1984.
11. Thomas WP, Sisson D, Bauer TG, *et al.*: Detection of cardiac masses in dogs by two-dimensional echocardiography. *Vet Radiol* 25:65, 1984.
12. Assi ER, Tak T: Assessment of valvular heart disease. Why echocardiography is an essential component. *Postgrad Med* 104:99, 1998.
13. Shah PM. Echocardiographic diagnosis of mitral valve prolapse. *J Am Soc Echocard* 7:286, 1994.
14. Crawford MH: Valvular heart disease. *Curr Opin Cardiol* 9:143, 1994.
15. Cooper JW, Nanda NC, Philpot EF, *et al.*: Evaluation of valvular regurgitation by color Doppler. *J Am Soc Echocard* 2:56, 1989.
16. Losordo DW, Pastore JO, Coletta D, *et al.*: Limitations of color flow Doppler imaging in the quantification of valvular regurgitation: velocity of regurgitant jet rather than volume determines size of color flow Doppler image. *Am Heart J* 126:168, 1993.
17. Kittleson MD: Left ventricular function and failure. Part 1. *Comp Small Anim Med* 16:287, 1994.
18. Kittleson MD: Left ventricular function and failure. Part 2. *Comp Small Anim Med* 16:101, 1994.
19. Kittleson MD, Eyster GE, Knowlen GG: Myocardial function in small dogs with mitral regurgitation and severe congestive heart failure. *J Am Vet Med Assoc* 184:1253, 1985.
20. Mugge A: Echocardiographic detection of cardiac valve vegetations and prognostic implications. *Infect Dis Clin North Am* 7:877, 1993.
21. Cooke RA, Chambers JB: The role of echocardiography in the diagnosis and management of infective endocarditis. *Br J Clin Pract* 46:111, 1992.
22. Calvert CA: Infective endocarditis. *In* Abbot JA, ed.: Small Animal Cardiology Secrets. Philadelphia: Hanley & Belfus, 2000, p 224.
23. Krivokapich J: Echocardiography in valvular heart disease. *Curr Opin Cardiol* 9:158, 1994.
24. Griffin BP, Flachskampf FA, Reimold SC, *et al.*: Relationship of aortic regurgitant velocity slope and pressure half time to severity of aortic regurgitation under changing hemodynamic conditions. *Eur Heart J* 15:681, 1994.
25. Thomas WP: Doppler echocardiographic estimation of pressure gradients in dogs with congenital pulmonic and subaortic stenosis. Proceedings of the 8th Annual Meeting of the American College of Veterinary Internal Medicine (ACVIM) 1990, p 867.
26. Cobb MA: Idiopathic dilated cardiomyopathy: advances in aetiology, pathogenesis and management. *J Sm Anim Pract* 33:113, 1992.
27. Stepien RL: Feline dilated cardiomyopathy. *In* Abbot JA, ed.: Small Animal Cardiology Secrets. Philadelphia: Hanley & Belfus, 2000, p 258.
28. Nishimura RA, Housmans PR, Hatle LK, *et al.*: Assessment of diastolic function of the heart: background and current applications of Doppler echocardiography. Part I. Physiologic and pathophysiologic features. *Mayo Clin Proc* 64:71, 1989.

29. Nishimura RA, Abel MD, Hatle LK, *et al.*: Assessment of diastolic function of the heart: background and current applications of Doppler echocardiography. Part II. Clinical studies. *Mayo Clin Proc* 64:181, 1989.
30. Nishimura RA, Tajik AJ: Quantitative hemodynamics by Doppler echocardiography: a noninvasive alternative to cardiac catheterization. *Prog Cardiovasc Dis* 36: 309, 1994.
31. Monnet E, Orton EC, Salman M, Boon J: Idiopathic dilated cardiomyopathy in dogs: survival and prognostic indicators. *J Vet Intern Med* 9:12, 1995.
32. Tidholm A, Jonsson L: A retrospective study of canine dilated cardiomyopathy (189 cases). *AAHA* 33:544, 1997.
33. Tidholm A, Svensson H, Sylven C: Survival and prognostic factors in 189 dogs with dilated cardiomyopathy. *AAHA* 33:364, 1997.
34. Werner GS, Fuchs JB, Schulz R, *et al.*: Changes in left ventricular filling during follow-up study in survivors and nonsurvivors of idiopathic dilated cardiomyopathy. *J Card Failure* 2:5, 1996.
35. Bright JM, Golden AL, Daniel GB: Feline hypertrophic cardiomyopathy: variations on a theme. *J Sm Anim Pract* 33:266, 1992.
36. Peterson EN, Moise S, Brown CA, *et al.*: Heterogeneity of hypertrophy in feline hypertrophic heart disease. *J Vet Intern Med* 7:183, 1993.
37. Bright JM: Feline hypertrophic cardiomyopathy. *In* Abbot JA, ed.: Small Animal Cardiology Secrets. Philadelphia: Hanley & Belfus, 2000, p 243.
38. Manganelli F, Betocchi S, Losi MA, *et al.*: Influence of left ventricular cavity size on clinical presentation in hypertrophic cardiomyopathy. *Am J Cardiol* 83:547, 1999.
39. Rakowski H, Sasson Z, Wigle ED: Echocardiographic and Doppler assessment of hypertrophic cardiomyopathy. *J Am Soc Echocard* 1:31, 1988.
40. Bright JM, Herrtage ME, Schneider JF: Pulsed Doppler assessment of left ventricular function in normal and cardiomyopathic cats. *JAAHA* 35:285, 1999.
41. Shen WF, Tribouilloy C, Rida Z, *et. al.*: Clinical significance of intracavity spontaneous echo contrast in patients with dilated cardiomyopathy. *Cardiology* 87:141, 1996.
42. Cetta F, O'Leary PW, Seward JB, Driscoll DJ: Idiopathic restrictive cardiomyopathy in childhood: diagnostic features and clinical course. *Mayo Clin Proc* 70:634, 1995.
43. Gewillig M, Mertens L, Moerman P, Dumoulin M: Idiopathic restrictive cardiomyopathy in childhood. A diastolic disorder characterized by delayed relaxation. *Eur Heart J* 17:1413, 1996.
44. Stepien RL: Feline restrictive cardiomyopathy. *In* Abbot JA, ed.: Small Animal Cardiology Secrets. Philadelphia: Hanley & Belfus, 2000, p 253.
45. Keren A, Popp R: Assignment of patients into classification of cardiomyopathies. *Circulation* 86:1622, 1992.
46. Johnson L: Diagnosis of pulmonary hypertension. *Clin Tech Small Anim Pract* 14: 231, 1999.
47. Johnson L, Boon J, Orton EC: Clinical characteristics of 53 dogs with Doppler-derived evidence of pulmonary hypertension. *J Vet Intern Med* 13:440, 1999.
48. Vachiery JL, Brimioulle S, Crasset V, *et al.*: False-positive diagnosis of pulmonary hypertension by Doppler echocardiography. *Eur Respir J* 12:1476, 1998.
49. Martin-Duran R, Larman M, Trugeda A, *et al.*: Comparison of Doppler-determined elevated arterial pressure with pressure measured at cardiac catheterization. *Am J Cardiol* 57:859, 1986.

25
Critical Care Applications of Abdominal Sonography

Robert H. Wrigley

INTRODUCTION

Sector transducers are generally more versatile for abdominal ultrasonography because the sound beam can be angled around the stomach and bowel gas and between ribs. Linear array transducers can also be used to examine the spleen, left kidney, uterus, bowel, and urinary bladder. A range of ultrasound frequencies, between 3 and 10 MHz, is required, because small animal patients can range from small puppies to giant dog breeds. Before ultrasound examination, the animal should be fasted because food will hinder thorough evaluation of the cranial abdomen. The hair over the ventral body wall and along the costal arches is clipped away. The patient may be restrained in a padded V trough in dorsal recumbency or on its side.

PERITONEUM

Abnormal peritoneal and retroperitoneal spaces are quickly pinpointed if effusion is present.[1] Sonography seems a more sensitive diagnostic tool than radiography to detect mild abdominal effusion. Uncomplicated ascites contains no echoes and outlines the smooth peritoneal surface of the abdominal organs (Fig. 25-1). A small fluid collection adjacent to a single organ hints that the adjacent organ is the source of the fluid. Echogenic fluid, fibrous tag, nodular peritoneal deposits and loculation merit aspiration and cytologic investigation to determine the nature and sometimes the source of the fluid. Ultrasound-guided aspiration may be helpful if only a small volume of fluid is detected (Fig. 25-2).

LIVER

Sagittal hepatic scans are made by placing the transducer just behind the xiphisternum and angling cranially to find the liver and diaphragm. Parasagittal scans are made by moving the transducer to the left and right. Once the transducer comes up against the costal notch, the ultrasound beam is then angled laterally, allowing exploration of the remaining aspects of the liver. Transverse scans are made by placing the transducer in the costal notch, angling cranially and to the left and right. Unfortunately, animal patients will not hold their breath on command, and so the clearest images are obtained only during the inspiratory

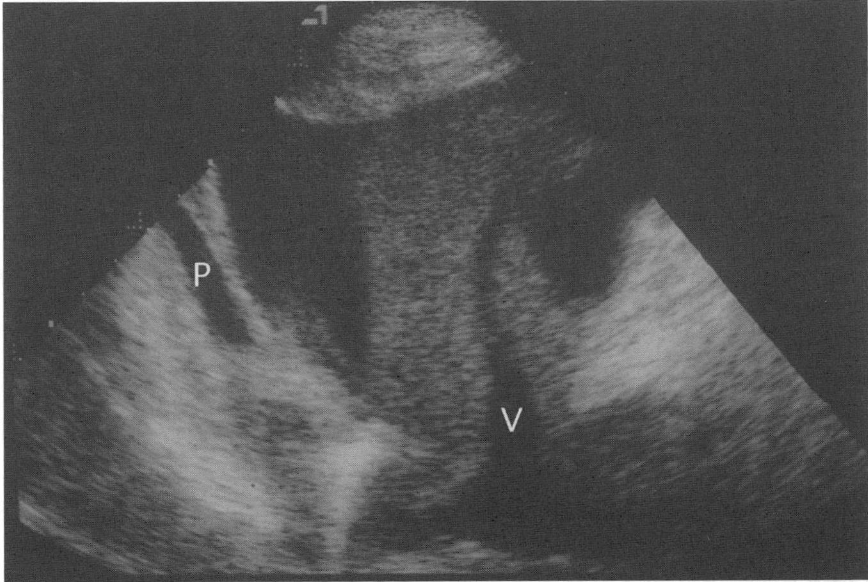

Figure 25-1
Sagittal sonogram of the right liver of a 12 year old dog, presented because the owners had noticed increasing abdominal distention over 1 week and anorexia and vomiting. The sonogram revealed that the abdominal distention was due to the presence of severe abdominal effusion. This outlines the right liver. Also distention of the vena cava and hepatic veins (V) was observed. A pericardial effusion (P) is seen adjacent to the diaphragm. This suggested that the origin of the abdominal effusion could be right-sided heart failure. Also observed is a small outline of fluid in the pleural cavity. Subsequent echocardiography revealed pericardial effusion. Pericardiocentesis revealed an inflammatory exudate. The dog was treated by pericardiectomy and antibiotic therapy. After this treatment, the ascites and clinical signs resolved.

and expiratory pauses. Stomach and bowel gas often prevent evaluation of the caudal and deeper aspects of the liver. The right dorsal liver and adjacent kidney may not be visible until intercostal imaging is done through the overlying thoracic wall. Sometimes laying the animal down laterally or having it stand or sit helps move away overlying gas to allow better visualization of the liver. In deep-chested breeds (setters, Afghan hounds) or in dogs whose liver is small, the liver will be difficult to image[2-7] and intercostal scanning along the dorsal aspects of the caudal third of the chest wall is sometimes helpful. The integrity of the diaphragm should also be evaluated because diaphragmatic hernias are readily visualized by sonography (Fig. 25-3).

Liver size can be evaluated only subjectively and does not seem to be an accurate indicator of true volume.[8] The normal liver parenchyma appears as a finely stippled echo pattern. The larger portal veins are identified by the presence of echogenic walls and confluence with the common portal vein in the caudal right liver. Hepatic veins are recognized by the absence of echogenic walls and confluence with the vena cava just caudal to the diaphragm. Normal hepatic

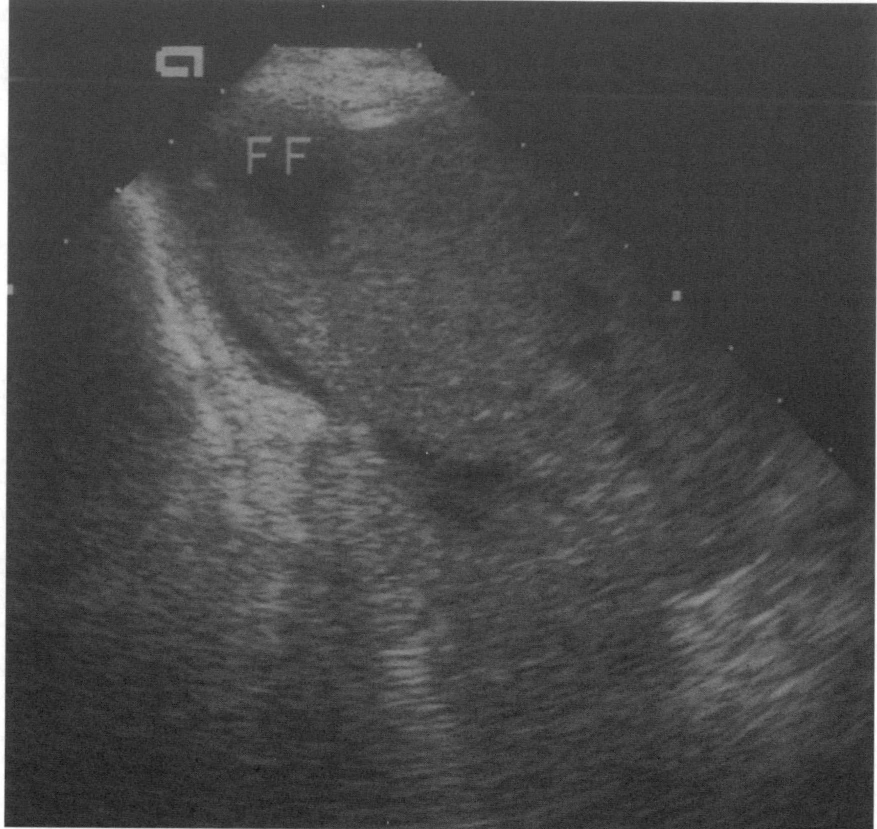

Figure 25-2
Transverse sonogram of the right liver of a 11 year old Husky dog. The dog had fallen off a deck. The owners noticed abdominal distention and the dog seemed in pain especially when the cranial abdomen was palpated. Sonography revealed effusion (FF) in the abdomen most noticeably in the cranial portion adjacent to the right liver. No obvious changes were detected in the liver parenchyma. Ultrasound-guided aspiration of the fluid revealed hemorrhage. An unexpected finding of a large echo-complex mass was found associated with the bowel in the mid-abdomen. The owners elected not to proceed with any therapy and at subsequent necropsy the abdominal effusion arose from a tear through the right lateral liver lobe. The bowel mass was an adenocarcinoma.

arteries are not detected. The gallbladder is usually located slightly to the right of midline in the cranial liver. The gallbladder wall is thin or is not apparent if the insonation angle is poor. In medium-sized dogs the common bile duct is less than 3 mm in diameter, so often normal bile ducts are not visible. The interlobar borders of the liver cannot be seen unless a concurrent peritoneal effusion is present (see Fig. 25-1). The overall parenchymal echo intensity should be compared with the spleen, the normal liver being less echogenic than the spleen. The echo intensity of the right lateral lobe of the liver may be compared

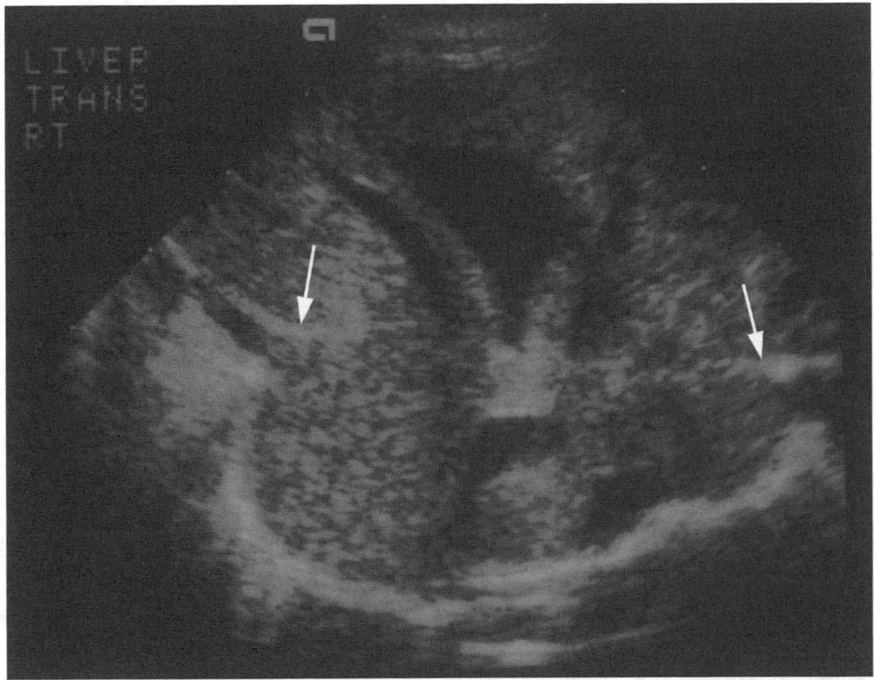

Figure 25-3
Transverse sonogram of the liver region of a Terrier dog that had been hit by a car. Subsequently, the owner noticed increasing respiratory effort and the dog seem to cough excessively. The sonogram reveals a discontinuity of the right diaphragm (between the arrows) with herniation of some right liver into the thorax. Subsequent surgery found three-fourths of the right liver in the chest and the diaphragmatic hernia was repaired.

with the right kidney, though this relationship is less reliable because the normal liver may be as echogenic or more echogenic than the renal cortex.[9] Vascular abnormalities of the liver, apart from central venous congestion and right-sided heart failure, are rare.[10] Heart failure results in a distended vena cava and hepatic veins and ascites (see Fig. 25-1).

Gallstones are rare in small animals, but ultrasonography will occasionally find them in seemingly normal patients. More commonly, echogenic bile (sludge) will be found in the dependent portion of the gallbladder, stemming from fasting, anorexia, or hepatic dysfunction reducing bile outflow. Sometimes the sludge may fill the entire gallbladder, giving the appearance of a hypoechoic mass. The diagnosis of cholecystitis in animals is difficult, because the clinical signs are often vague and serum biochemical tests are nonspecific. Cholecystitis and ascites may cause thickening of the gallbladder wall, sometimes leading to a double-walled appearance. In severe chronic cholecystitis, abscesses and adhesions may be found in the gallbladder and adjacent fossa, resulting in a distorted and disordered appearance. Occasionally the gallbladder may become distended with mucus (mucocele)[11] (Fig.

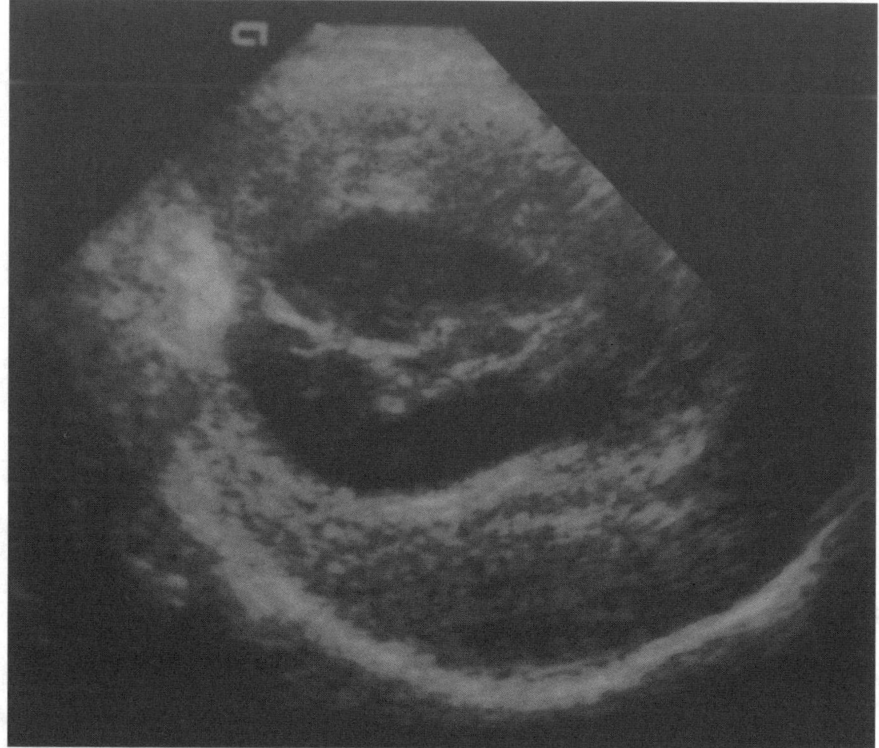

Figure 25-4
Sagittal sonogram of a gallbladder of a spaniel presenting with clinical signs of anorexia, cranial abdominal pain, vomiting, icterus, and fever. The gallbladder is excessively distended but without evidence of bile duct distention. The bile in the gallbladder is abnormally echogenic containing echogenic strands radiating through the bile; these strands did not realign when imaging the dog standing in dorsal recumbency position. These sonographic signs are observed with a gallbladder mucocele. Surgical removal of the gallbladder confirmed the presence of a chronic mucocele and cholecystitis.

25-4). Complications arising from secondary infection, common bile duct obstruction, gallbladder wall necrosis, and rupture have been observed. A characteristic pattern of echogenic strands radiating through the lumen of the distended gallbladder is observed.[11] The echogenic component does not move under gravitation effects of repositioning and the gallbladder remains abnormally distended after eating (see Fig. 25-4). The best treatment is cholecystectomy.

Ultrasonography is a useful diagnostic tool to assess jaundiced animals. Rupture of the gallbladder or biliary system will lead to peritoneal fluid and analysis of a fluid aspirate should lead to the diagnosis (Fig. 25-5). Posthepatic biliary obstruction dilates the gallbladder and bile ducts (Fig. 25-6). However, remember that sonography is unable to detect the dilated bile ducts reliably until several days after obstruction of the common bile duct.[12] So the presence of jaundice, a dilated gallbladder, and visible bile ducts on ultrasonography allows for the

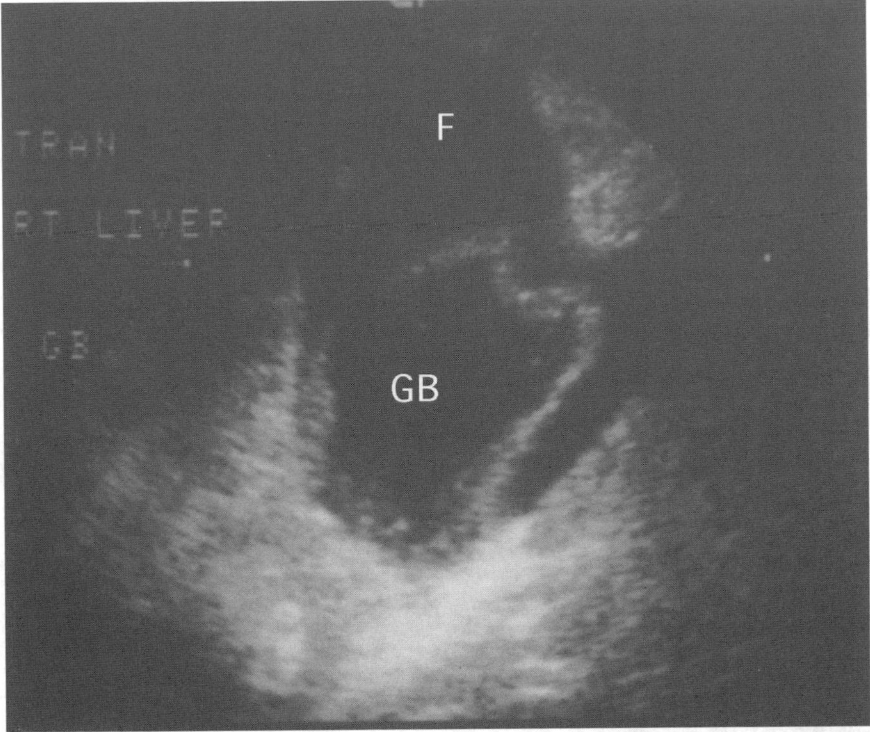

Figure 25-5
Transverse sonogram of the right liver/gallbladder of a Sheltie that had been hit by a car 1 week previously. Initially the dog seemed normal but then had become anorexic, dehydrated, and jaundiced. Sonography revealed peritoneal effusion (F) most pronounced around the liver and the region of the gallbladder fossa. The gallbladder (GB) was not distended and had an irregular flaccid-like wall with a discontinuity of the right wall. Abdominocentesis revealed a yellow fluid. Subsequent surgery confirmed the ruptured gallbladder and presence of bile in the peritoneal cavity. A cholecystectomy was performed and the dog recovered uneventfully.

diagnosis of chronic biliary obstruction (see Fig. 25-6). Thorough evaluation of the common bile duct is required to define the cause of obstruction. Overlying bowel gas is a major problem, often obscuring the common bile duct. Therefore, several examinations may be necessary until the entire duct can be visualized. The detection of only dilated bile ducts is not a reliable sign of biliary obstruction unless accompanied by rising levels of circulating bilirubin. Prior obstruction or inflammation may distend the inelastic bile ducts, leading to persistent enlargement. Serial examinations of jaundiced animals should always be performed and assessed in conjunction with evaluation of bilirubin levels.[4,13]

Focal hepatic lesions may be noted at single or multiple locations. Multiple nodules are most typical of metastatic neoplasia.[2,4,5,7,14] However, multifocal lymphoma and incidental nodular hyperplasia in older dogs may have an identical ultrasonographic pattern (Fig. 25-7). A large single lesion is also a diagnostic

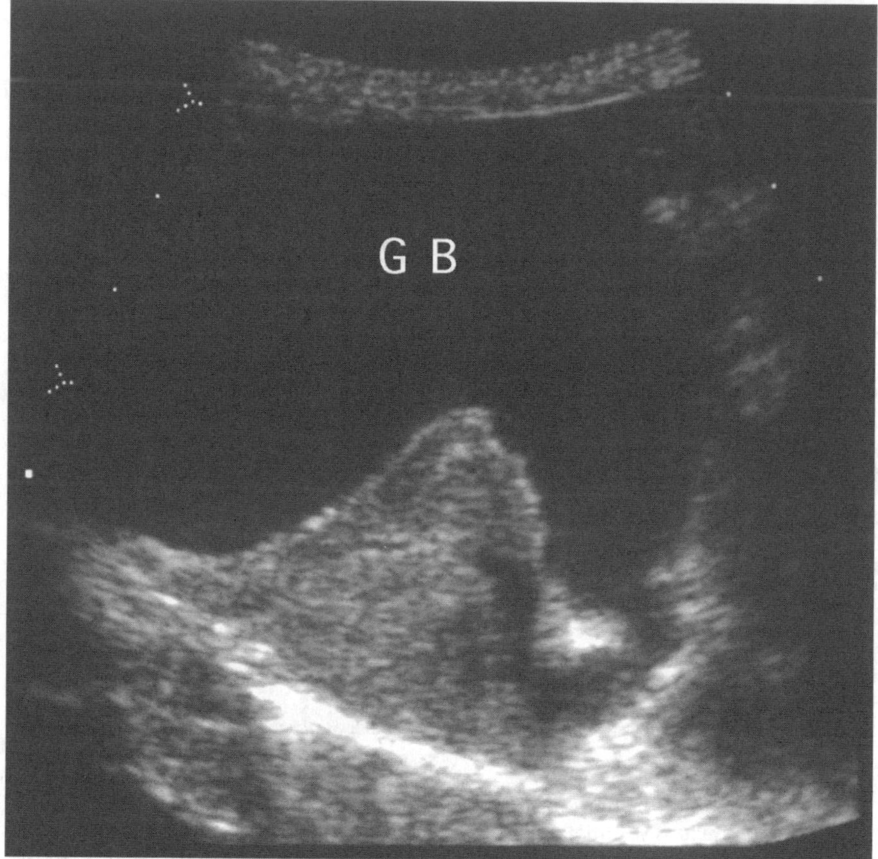

Figure 25-6
Sagittal sonogram of the gallbladder (GB). This 10 year old spaniel presented with the clinical signs of anorexia, vomiting, and icterus. The sonogram shows an excessively distended gallbladder and adjacent bile ducts. These findings indicate the presence of extrahepatic chronic biliary obstruction. At surgery a lesion (adenocarcinoma) was found involving the common bile duct. Despite a cholecystoduodenostomy, the dog died.

dilemma because overlapping echo patterns are seen in primary or metastatic neoplasia, abscesses (Fig. 25-8), hematomas, cysts, and hemorrhagic or necrotic nodular hyperplasia. Overlapping echo patterns also occur with diffuse hepatic disease.[15,16] Disseminated lymphoma, acute inflammation, necrosis, and degeneration may reduce overall echogenicity.[17] Fat infiltration, fibrosis, chronic inflammation, and disseminated neoplasia tend to increase echogenicity.[4] The diagnosis of advanced cirrhosis is aided by the concurrent presence of ascites, which helps define the nodular distortion of the hepatic borders.[4] Advanced cirrhosis tends to show a patchy hyperechoic pattern interspersed between hypoechoic areas due to nodular regeneration.[4,14] Ultrasound-guided needle aspiration or biopsy is required to establish an accurate diagnosis.

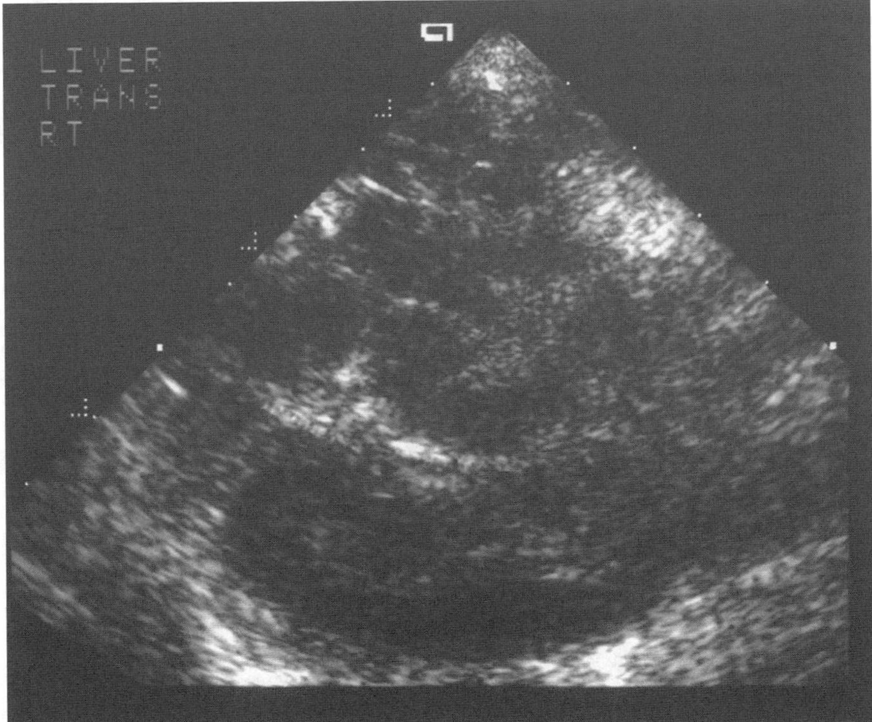

Figure 25-7
Transverse sonogram of the liver of a 11 year old Cocker spaniel diagnosed with diabetes mellitus. The dog was hospitalized because the owners had difficulty regulating the dog's diet and insulin levels. The sonogram shows the liver to have a patchy, almost nodular, hypoechoic appearance with interspersed hyperechoic regions. This sonographic nodular appearance is most commonly associated with widespread neoplasia foci. However, it is important to remember that areas of focal nodular liver regeneration may have this sonographic appearance. Liver biopsies were performed; fibrosis and lipidosis were observed between areas of normal liver tissue. This case illustrates the diverse sonographic appearance of liver disease and neoplasia was not present. Subsequently, the dog's diabetes was stabilized and the owner could manage the dog's treatment at home.

SPLEEN

The canine spleen is located principally in the left abdomen with the ventral portion crossing to the right side, caudal to the costal arch. The spleen lies superficial to the left kidney and abdominal viscera; therefore, ultrasonographic gas artifacts rarely occur. Linear array 5- or 7-MHz transducers are preferable, although sector images and lower frequency transducers also are adequate. The examination is done best with the dog lying in a dorsal or right lateral recumbent position. After the spleen is located, the machine settings should be adjusted to optimize near-field display. The transducer should be moved slowly across the entire spleen in both sagittal and transverse scan planes.

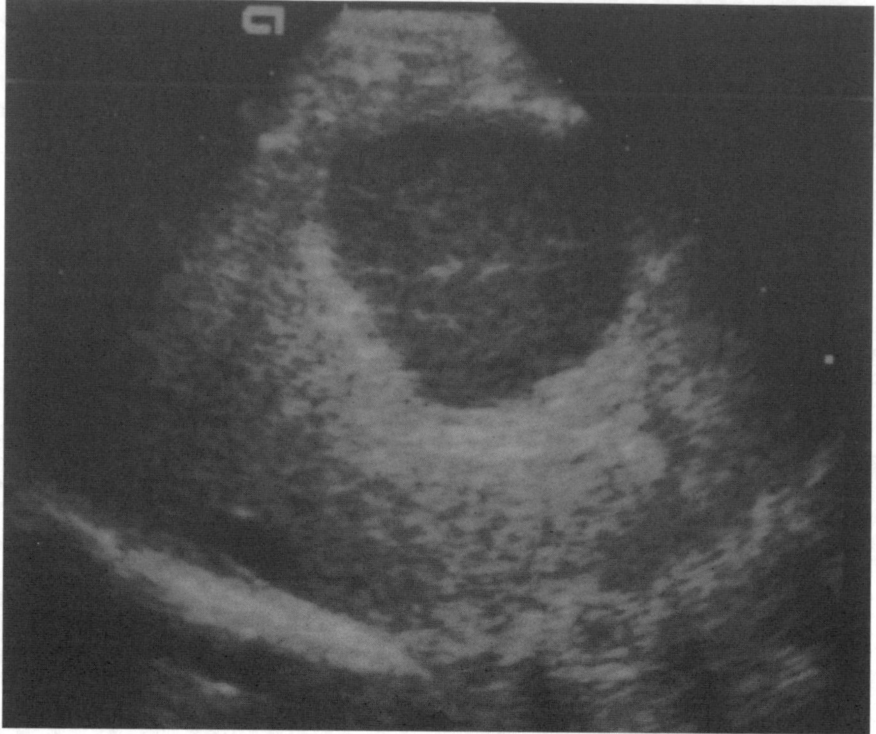

Figure 25-8
Sagittal sonogram of the right liver of a Schnauzer dog presenting with a history of vomiting, anorexia, and a tense painful cranial abdomen. The dog was pyrexic and hematology revealed a marked neutrophilia and left shift. Ultrasonography revealed a hypoechoic circular focus in the right liver. This observation, combined with the clinical findings, was most consistent with a liver abscess. Laparotomy confirmed the diagnosis in the right liver. The abscess was removed by a lobectomy of the right lateral lobe.

Acute crises resulting from injuries or diseases of the spleen (Fig. 25-9) are uncommon in dogs. Only 3 of 600 dogs hit by cars had any evidence of splenic trauma.[18] Hematomas occur more commonly as a consequence of primary splenic diseases, such as hemangiosarcomas (Fig. 25-10), lymphomas, or necrosis of large areas of nodular hyperplasia. Hematomas also seem to arise for no apparent cause,[19] perhaps due to unobserved trauma. Smaller hematomas (<5 cm in diameter) are characterized by focal areas of hypoechoic to anechoic material interspersed through normal parenchyma, localized to one portion of the spleen (see Fig. 25-9). Larger hematomas have a mixed ultrasonographic appearance with septated anechoic and hypoechoic material. Such larger hematomas have well-defined borders with or without encapsulation. Traumatic rupture of the spleen or the capsule over an existing large hematoma will lead to a hemoperitoneum (see Fig. 25-10). If the hemorrhage continues, surgical intervention (including partial or complete splenectomy) is the only treatment for continued hemorrhage due to neoplasia or progressive hematomas.[20,21]

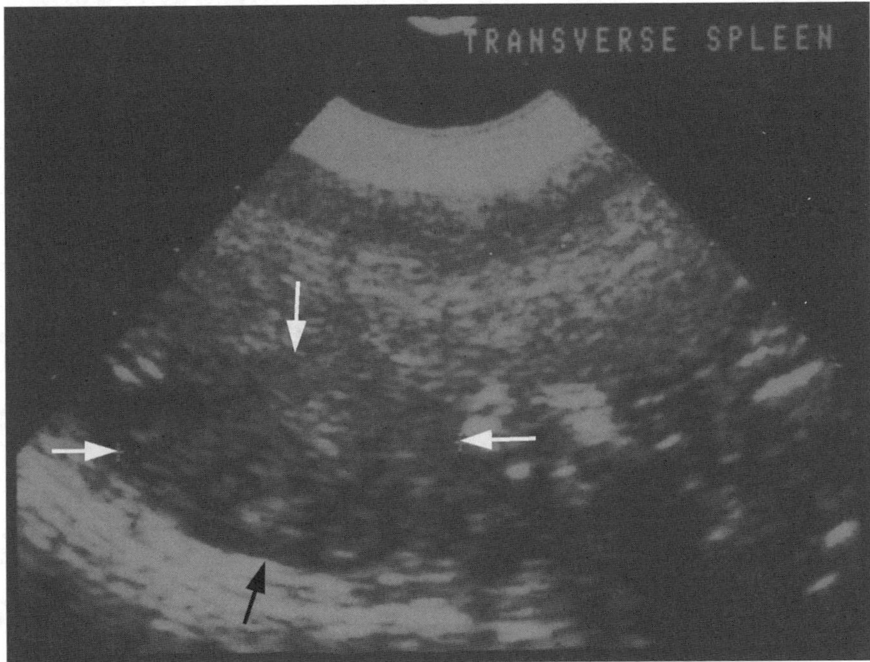

Figure 25-9
Transverse sonogram of the spleen of an Australian shepherd dog that had fallen from a moving vehicle 10 weeks previously. A circumscribed anechoic to hypoechoic mass (arrows) was present adjacent to the mesenteric border of the spleen. Abdominal effusion was not observed. Subsequent histology from a partial splenectomy revealed a splenic laceration and an organizing perisplenic hematoma.

Torsion of the spleen may occlude splenic veins and lead to progressive sequestration of blood. Other vessels in the greater omentum may become involved, leading to secondary pancreatitis and other areas of necrosis. Ultrasonography of a recent or mildly twisted spleen may reveal splenomegaly, dilated veins, and normal parenchymal echogenicity[22] (Fig. 25-11A). Passive congestion and nonspecific causes of splenomegaly such as septicemia, toxemia, erythropoiesis, secondary to drugs, and nodular hyperplasia are all indications for surgery. A similar ultrasonographic pattern also will occur with passive congestion secondary to right heart failure, portal hypertension, and anesthesia.[23] It is important to exclude the presence of concurrent heart or liver disease. Continued obstruction or a more severe degree of torsion leads to a greater degree of vascular congestion and dilation of splenic sinusoids. Few echoes are noted because the entire parenchyma consists of anechoic areas separated by small linear echoes[22] (see Fig. 25-11A). Arterial thrombosis can also lead to splenic necrosis.[24] Initially B-mode sonography will show little change. Color Doppler evaluation is often necessary to demonstrate absence of blood supply (Fig. 25-11B). Rapid surgical intervention is essential to prevent additional vascular compromise and sequelae such as infarct, gangrene, septicemia, and disseminated intravascular coagulation.

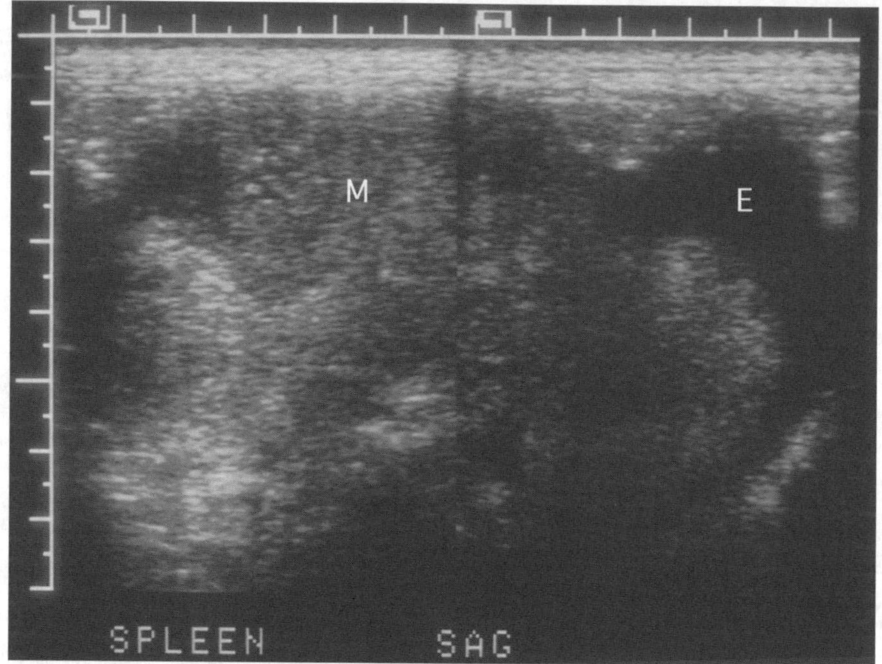

Figure 25-10
Sagittal sonogram of the spleen of an 11 year old Malamute presented for sudden severe collapse. Physical examination revealed pale mucous membranes, abdominal distention, and a mid-abdominal mass. Sonography showed an irregular complex mass (M) protruding from the ventral aspect of the spleen. Mildly echogenic effusion (E) was present in the abdomen especially surrounding the spleen. Hepatic sonography revealed multiple anechoic foci scattered throughout the liver consistent with metastatic foci. The presumptive diagnosis was splenic neoplasia with abdominal hemorrhage and metastasis to the liver. Subsequent necropsy revealed that the abdominal hemorrhage was as a result of rupture of a hemangiosarcoma growing in the spleen. Metastatic nodules were found elsewhere in the spleen, peritoneal cavity, and liver.

Splenic hemangiosarcoma is the most prevalent splenic neoplasm in dogs.[19] The ultrasonographic appearance is complicated by the presence of secondary hematomas and cysts that may be larger than the neoplastic mass. The ultrasonographic features aiding in differentiation of a hemangiosarcoma from a benign hematoma include an ill-defined border to the hemangiosarcoma, echogenic areas in larger tumors, nodules on adjacent visceral surfaces, abdominal effusion (see Fig. 25-10), and hypoechoic metastatic nodes in the liver. Concurrent hemoperitoneum has a high predictive value for splenic neoplasia.[25]

Unfortunately, the ultrasonographic appearances of benign and malignant diseases of the spleen frequently overlap. Large areas of nodular hyperplasia may undergo necrosis and like hemangiosarcoma, lead to intrasplenic hematomas, resulting in confusing ultrasound patterns. Benign lesions tend to have a more defined intrasplenic border and infrequently abdominal effusion. The liver and

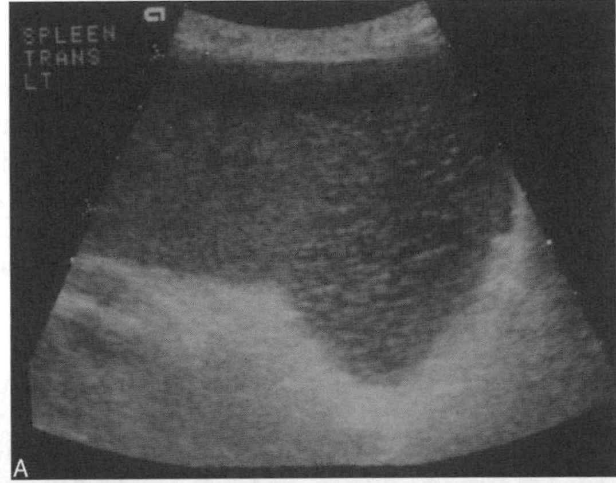

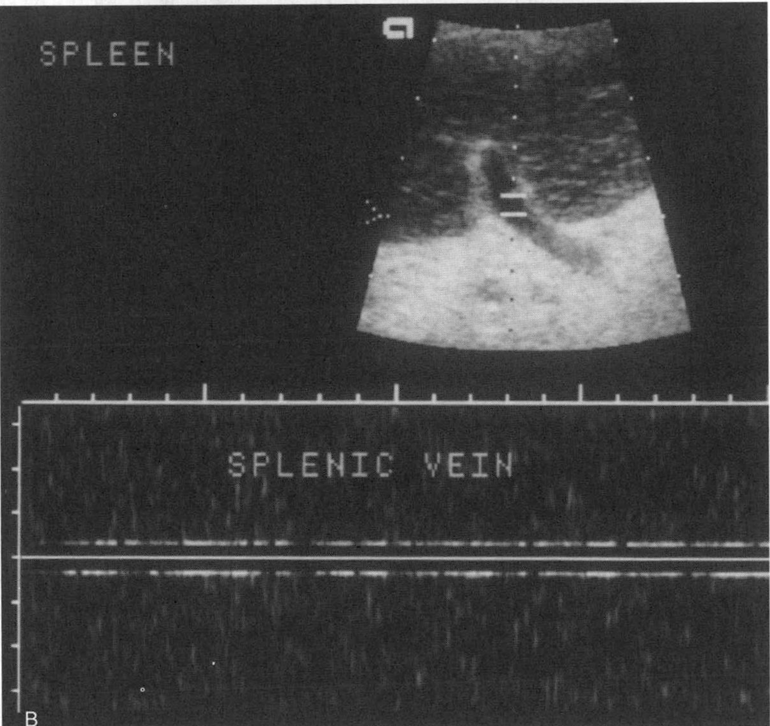

Figure 25-11
(A) Sagittal sonogram of the spleen of a 6 year old Chow presenting with lethargy, anorexia, and collapse. Severe generalized splenomegaly was palpable. The splenic parenchymal echoes were abnormally hypoechoic and bright reflective septi were present interspersed throughout the tissue. The splenic parenchymal echogenicity was less echogenic than the liver. (B) Duplex Doppler interrogation of an abnormally distended splenic vein. No blood flow could be found in the splenic vein. The final sonographic conclusion was splenomegaly due to splenic torsion and severe venous congestion. Abdominal surgery confirmed the diagnosis and the necrotic-appearing spleen was excised.

heart should be examined ultrasonographically if hemangiosarcoma is suspected. Hepatic metastasis may result in hypoechoic foci.

White pulp neoplasia (such as lymphoma), severe congestion, and torsion may all cause a hypoechoic pattern. Hypoechoic splenic nodules, multicentric lymphadenopathy, and nondilated splenic veins all support the diagnosis of multicentric lymphosarcoma. Dilated splenic veins, abruptly ending at the hilus, are more consistent with torsion.

KIDNEY

Ultrasonography of the left kidney is more easily performed because it is situated more caudally than the right kidney. Often the spleen provides an excellent acoustic window to the left kidney. The right kidney is more difficult to image because it lies more cranial and deeper in the abdomen, with more overlying bowel loops. Sagittal and transverse scans of both kidneys should be performed. If a kidney is obscured by gas artifacts, then the transducer can be moved to the side of the abdomen to allow imaging in transverse and dorsal planes.[25-28] The normal pelvic lumen is not visible because the pelvis is a thin, slitlike space between V-shaped walls. The renal pyramids are divided centrally by a hyperechoic renal crest and further divided into papillae by vertical hyperechoic stripes resulting from the summation of echoes from the pelvic diverticuli, interlobar vessels, and renal fat. The corticomedullary junction is outlined by hyperechoic arcuate vessels. The normal canine renal cortex is hypoechoic to both the spleen and liver.[29] In older cats, the cortex may become isoechoic to the liver when imaged with higher frequency transducers.[9] Ultrasound helps determine kidney size, though dehydration and drug-induced diuresis cause variations in the size of the medulla. Normal ureters are too small to image ultrasonographically.[29]

Postrenal obstruction is identified by recognizing hydronephrosis and is characterized by observing splitting of the central pelvic echoes.[30] Progressive hydronephrosis further dilates the pelvis and diverticuli, creating an anechoic pattern radiating into the medulla (Fig. 25-12). A dilated ureter may become visible if the hydronephrosis stems from lower urinary tract obstruction (Fig. 25-13). If a nephrectomy is planned, then excretory urography should be performed to validate the function of the other kidney.[31]

Acute renal disease is difficult to diagnose on B-mode sonography because the kidneys usually still appear normal (Fig. 25-14A). Doppler evaluation of the resistive index of interlobar renal arteries can be helpful because the index may become abnormally elevated[32] (Fig. 25-14B). Ethylene glycol toxicity can be suspected after finding abnormally echogenic renal cortices.[33] Chronic progressive and irreversible parenchymal disease[30,33,34] often leads to fibrosis and scarring of the kidneys. Many parenchymal diseases have similar acoustic patterns.[26,30,33] The kidneys tend to become smaller and more hyperechoic. The normally hypoechoic papillae appear less distinct, and the medulla tends to become isoechoic to the cortex (Fig. 25-15). If the animal is undergoing diuresis at the time of the ultrasonographic examination, then the absence of an obvious hypoechoic

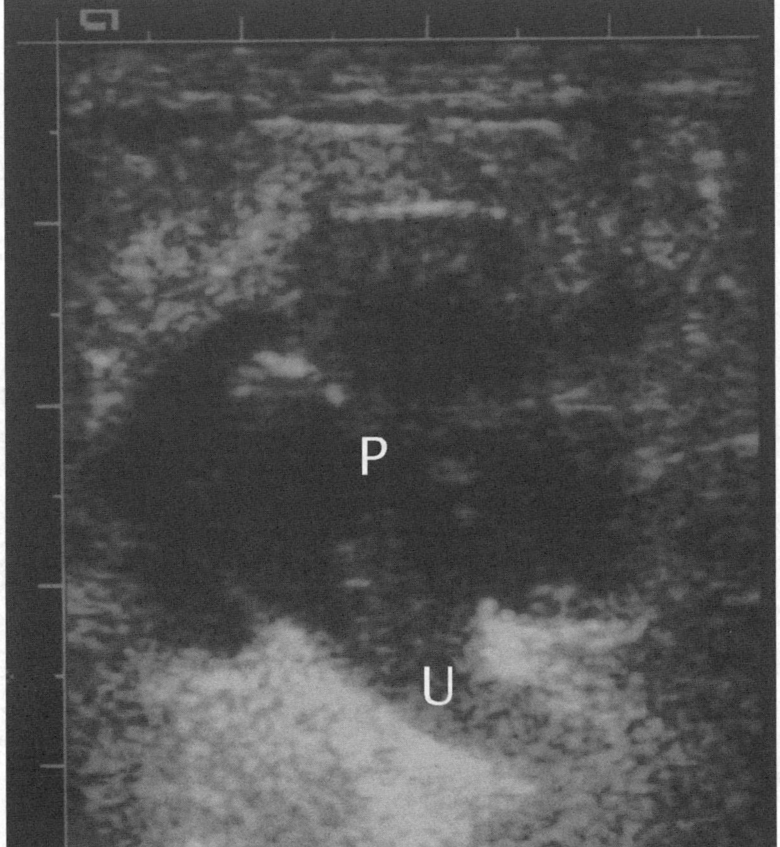

Figure 25-12
Dorsal sonogram of the left kidney. This 11 year old domestic short-haired cat presented with acute clinical signs of fever, anorexia, not drinking, and extreme lethargy. The blood urea nitrogen was 48 mg/dL and creatinine was 2.4 mg/dL. The sonogram showed the presence of distention of the renal pelvis (P) and proximal ureter (U) by echogenic urine. The echogenic urine suggested the presence of severe pyelonephritis, which was confirmed by subsequent urinalysis and supported by an inflammatory leukogram. Subsequent necropsy revealed suppurative pyelonephritis of the left kidney.

medulla is a poor prognostic finding.[29] Ultrasound is a useful technique in the diagnosis of renal calculi. However, chronic renal disease may lead to nephrocalcinosis,[30,35] which, if severe, may also cause acoustic shadowing. Careful attention must be paid to the source of the shadows to differentiate renal calcinosis from a calculus. Pyelonephritis has a variable appearance (see Fig. 25-12), making ultrasonographic diagnosis inaccurate. Single cortical cysts may be incidental findings. Progressive polycystic disease is occasionally seen, more frequently in long-haired cats. Renal neoplasia creates a variable echo pattern. Unless hematuria is present, neoplasia may become advanced before showing clinical signs.

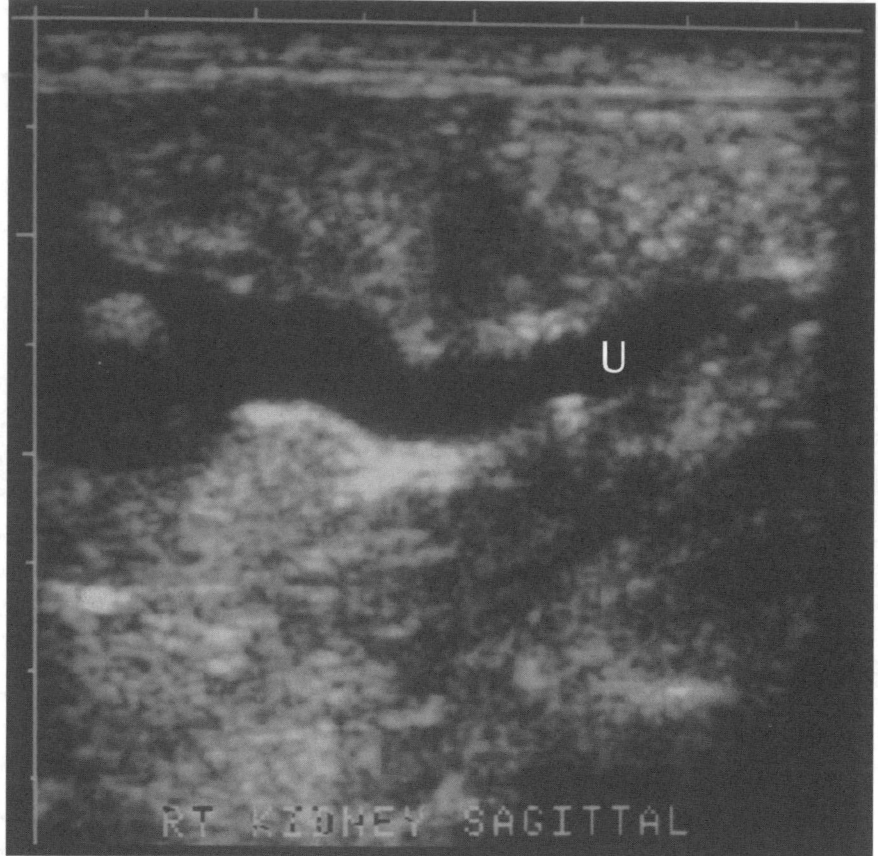

Figure 25-13
Sagittal sonogram of the right kidney of a cat presenting with clinical signs of abdominal pain. The sonogram reveals an abnormal distention of the renal pelvis and proximal ureter (U) by anechoic urine. No cause for this obstructive uropathy could be detected on ultrasound. A subsequent radiograph revealed the presence of a radiopaque calculus in the retroperitoneum consistent with a ureteral calculus. This was confirmed at subsequent surgery, but the calculus could not be dislodged and a nephrectomy had to be performed.

Figure 25-14
(A) Sagittal sonogram of the left kidney of a 7 year old diabetic dog presented for an acute onset of lethargy, vomiting, and weight loss. The owner's house flooded and the dog drank Drano and ate a rotten chicken. Biochemistry revealed a blood urea nitrogen of 90 mg/dL and creatinine level of 8.9 mg/dL. Cystocentesis showed abnormally high levels of protein, glucose, ketones, and blood in the urine. The sonogram of the kidneys showed normal kidney architecture with good corticomedullary differentiation and no evidence of pelvic dilation. (B) Doppler sonogram of the interlobar renal artery. The resistive index (0.8) measured at the interlobar arteries was abnormally elevated. The findings of a normal-appearing kidney on B-mode ultrasound and elevated resistive index are consistent with acute renal failure. The dog was treated with intravenous fluids, diuretics, and antibiotics but despite this therapy, the dog died. At necropsy there was severe tubular vacuolar degeneration with many tubules filled with protein casts indicative of the presence of acute renal failure.

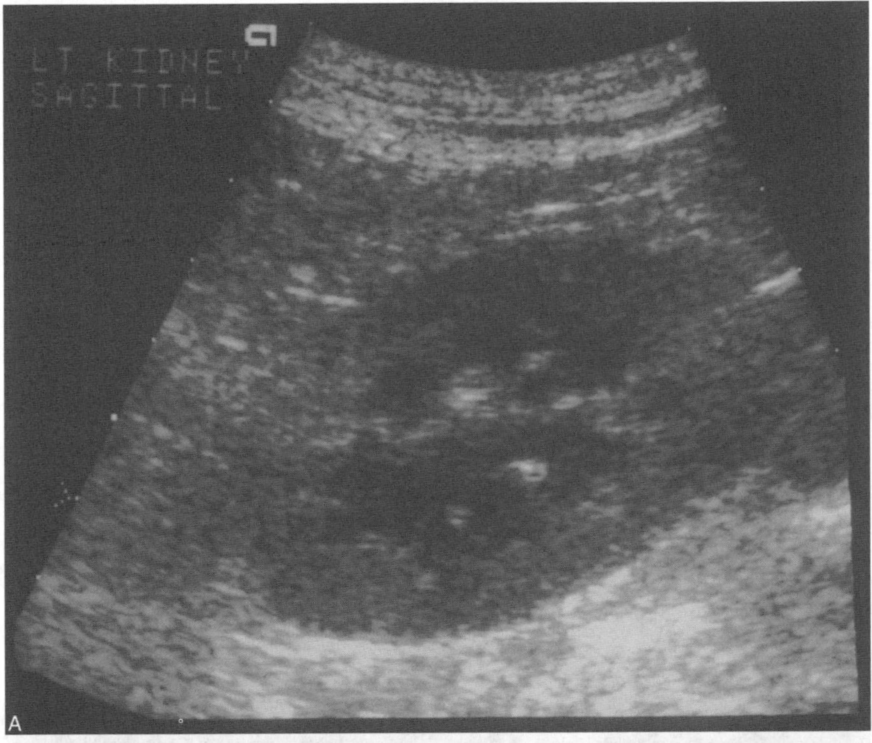
LT KIDNEY
SAGITTAL
A

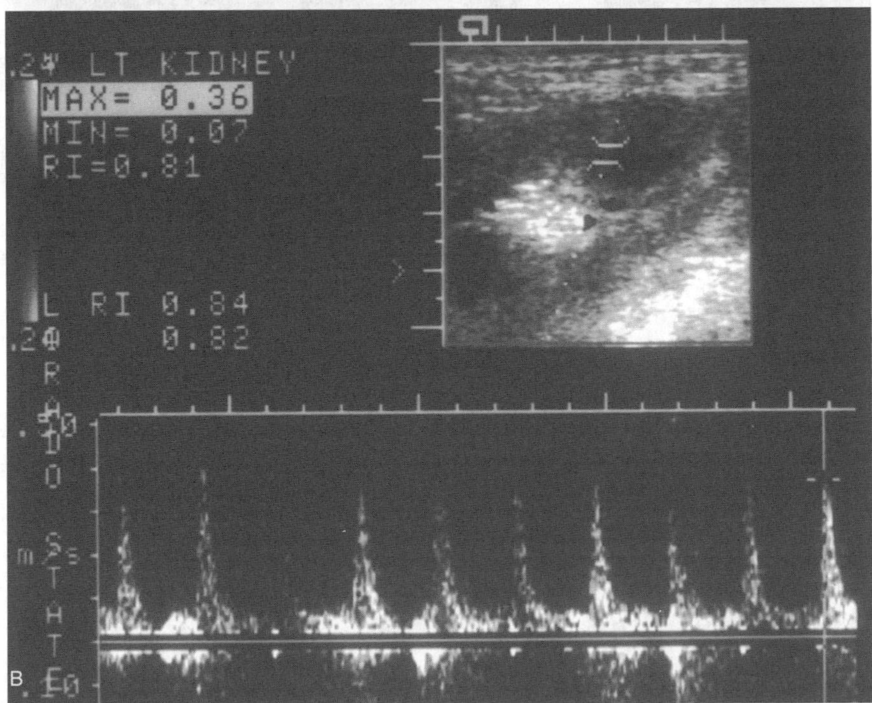
LT KIDNEY
MAX= 0.36
MIN= 0.07
RI=0.81
L RI 0.84
0.82
B

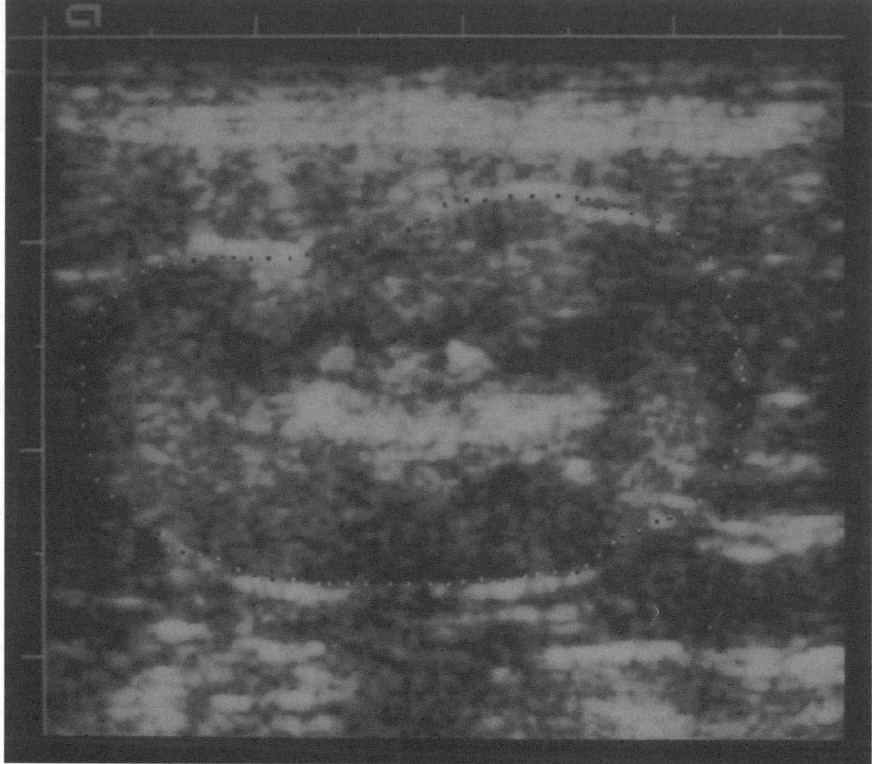

Figure 25-15
Sagittal sonogram of the left kidney of a 13 year old Siamese cat with a history of chronic renal failure that was being supported by dietary modification. Sonography of the left kidney reveals an abnormally small kidney, 3 cm in length. There was irregular distortion to the border of the kidney (outlined by the dotted line). Patchy hyperechoic irregularities were observed through the cortex. There was loss of the normal sonographic differentiation between cortex and the medulla. Similar changes were observed to the right kidney. These sonographic changes are characteristic of advanced chronic primary renal degeneration.

Frequently the entire kidney is replaced by an echo-complex mass.[30,36] A similar pattern can be observed after severe kidney trauma and bleeding. The resultant hematoma tends to be echogenic for the first 24 hours and then becomes variably anechoic and septated (Fig. 25-16). Therefore, correlation to a history of trauma is important. Retroperitoneal effusion can also be readily detected by sonography but differentiation between urine collection from a ruptured ureter and hemorrhage is unreliable. Excretory urography should be used to evaluate the ureters.

URINARY BLADDER

Bladder sonography can be performed in either dorsal or lateral recumbency. High-resolution transducers (7 to 10 MHz), are best suited for examination of

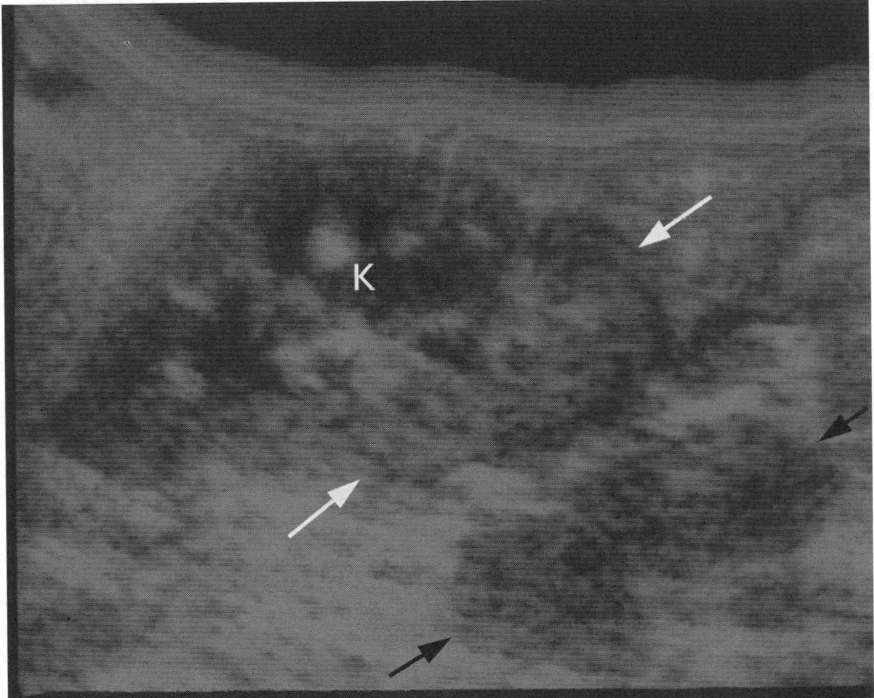

Figure 25-16
Sagittal sonogram of the right kidney of an adult cat presented in shock after likely being hit by a car. The animal's cranial and right abdomen was very painful. Marked hematuria was present. Multiple pelvic fractures were present. Ultrasonography revealed an echogenic mass along the dorsal border of the right kidney (white arrows) and in the right retroperitoneum (black arrows). No owner could be found and because the injuries were severe, the cat was euthanized. At necropsy, there were both retroperitoneal and right kidney subcapsular hemorrhage from the trauma. This sonogram illustrates that a recent blood clot also appears echogenic.

the urinary bladder. Five MHz may be necessary to penetrate to the far wall of a distended bladder in large breed dogs. Linear and curved wide aperture format transducers are particularly useful. A stand-off pad should be used with a sector transducer to improve image quality of the ventral bladder wall. Image contrast settings should be set to high-contrast display and acoustic power and near gain decreased to suppress reverberation echoes generated between the transducer, skin, and abdominal structures.

The sonographic examination is best performed when the bladder is moderately full. A small bladder is more difficult to locate, the wall will be thicker, and image contrast is reduced. The wall of a flaccid bladder can be deviated inward by a distended colon and the acoustic shadow artifacts generated by colonic contents often simulate the appearance of calculi.[37,38] In middle to large dog breeds, a fully distended bladder is less desirable because the needed lower frequency transducer has lower resolution. Free intraluminal abnormalities (ie, calculi, sediment,

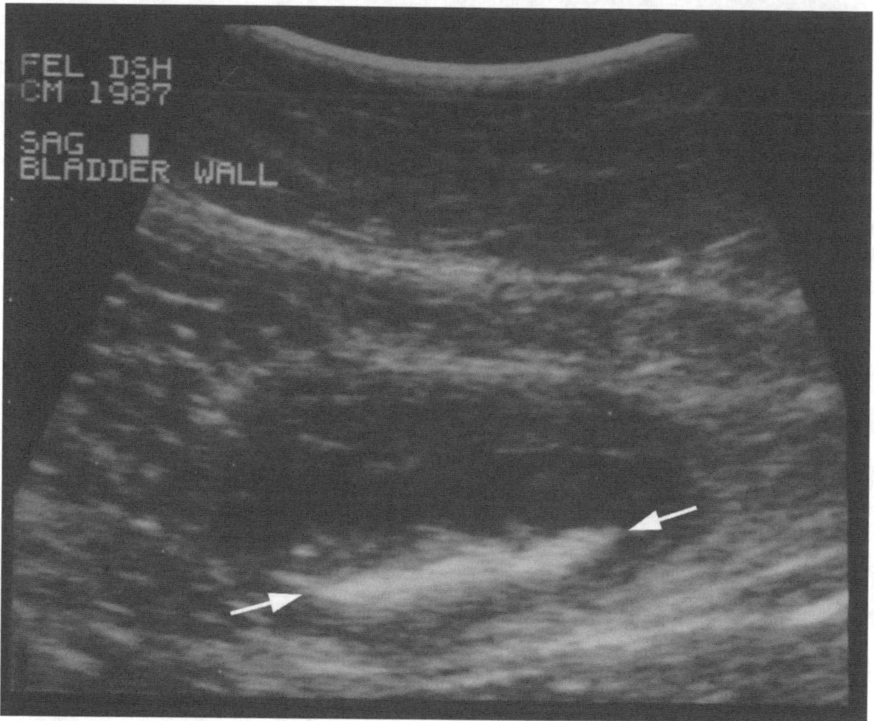

Figure 25-17
Sagittal sonogram of male 3 year old tomcat with recurrent signs of urethral obstruction. The sonogram reveals a small, fairly empty bladder with excessive thickening of the bladder wall due to severe cystitis. In the dependent, down-most portion of the urinary bladder, echogenic sediment (arrows) can be observed. Subsequent urinalysis revealed this to be due to severe calcium oxalate crystal urea. No urinary calculi were detected but this sandy crystalline debris is a likely cause of recurrent cystitis and urinary obstruction in this tomcat.

Figure 25-18
(A) Dorsal recumbent sagittal sonogram of a 3 year old cat presenting with severe hematuria following catheterization 1 week previously for urethral blockage. The sonogram shows a hypoechoic rounded mass in the dorsal portion of a distended urinary bladder. (B) A repeated sagittal sonogram of the bladder but this time made with the cat standing upright. This shows that the hypoechoic mass is free within the lumen of the bladder because it has now migrated to the ventral, more dependent, border. The initial appearance of the mass suggested the possibility of a neoplastic lesion attached to the dorsal bladder wall but the positional study shows that the mass is free within the bladder lumen. This observation, combined with the presence of severe and chronic hematuria, supports the presence of a large blood clot in the bladder. At cystotomy a large blood clot was removed. Severe ulcerative cystitis was the source of the hemorrhage.

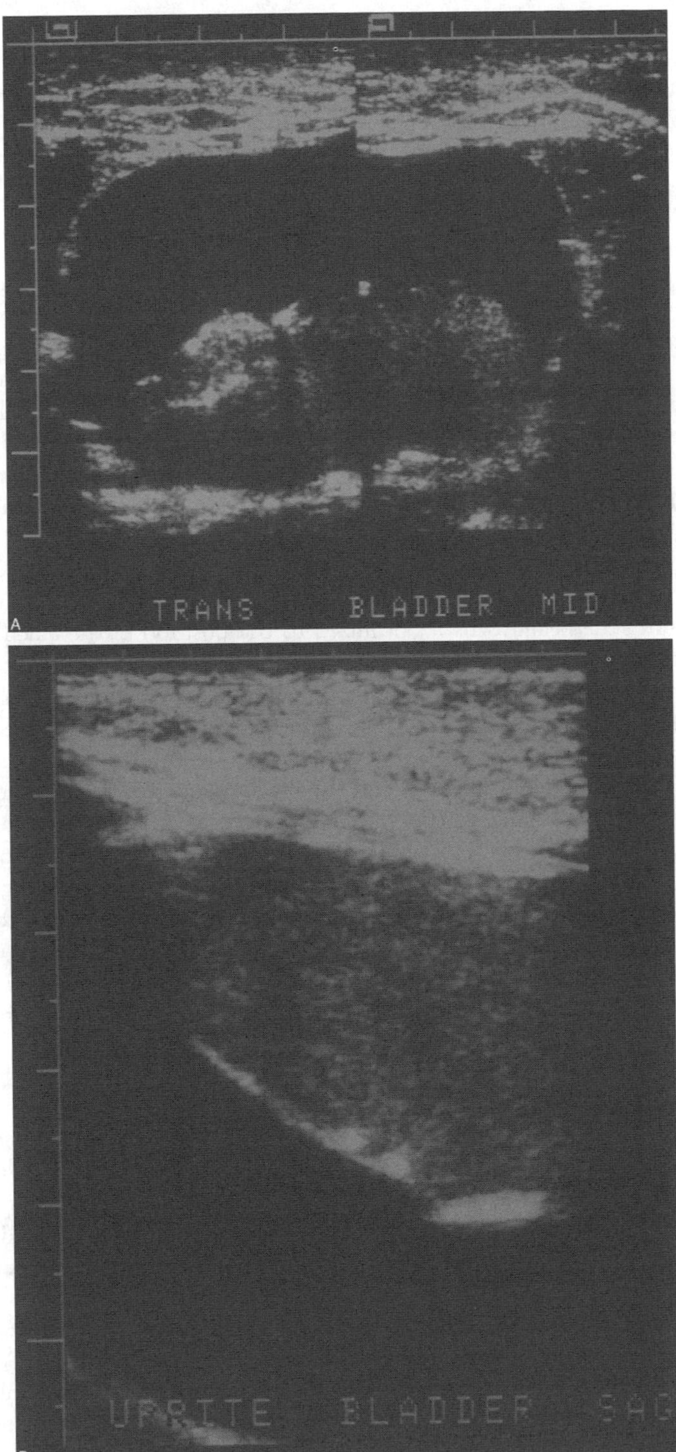
TRANS BLADDER MID
A
UPRITE BLADDER SAG
B

and blood clots) will gravitate to the most dependent side. Ballotment is useful to stir up sediment that swirls across the real-time display. Additional imaging after turning the animal into the opposite lateral recumbency or standing position will show that free intraluminal objects relocate to a new position.

In normal adult cats, the mean bladder wall thickness rarely exceeds 1.7 mm ± 0.56 mm.[39] In normal adult dogs with mild bladder distention the mean wall thickness is 1.6 mm but this thickness does increase with body weight.[40] Normal urine is anechoic. The turbulence created by discharge of urine through the ureteral openings may generate transient jets of echoes in the bladder lumen adjacent to the trigone.[41]

Urinary calculi, cellular and crystalline debris (Fig. 25-17), gas, and blood clots (Fig. 25-18A) are readily detected by sonography. Consideration to the gravitational alignment is especially helpful to differentiate between calculi and blood clots (which fall downward) (Fig. 25-18B) and gas bubbles, which rise upward. The location of cellular or crystalline debris and fresh hemorrhage is more variable. Sedimentation tends to occur but vigorous ballotment will generate swirling echo patterns on real-time display.

Distinct acoustic shadows will be observed deep to calculi that exceed the diameter of the sound beam.[42] Smaller calculi may not generate the characteristic shadows until the beam focus is optimized to the position of the calculi.

Blood clots tend to be associated with the clinical observation of severe hematuria. More commonly a blood clot appears as a hyperechoic nonshadowing mobile mass[43,44] (see Fig. 25-18A). Sometimes the clot may be attached to the wall, covering, or adjacent to, a traumatic injury or a neoplastic mass. Alternately, severe acute hemorrhage can fill the bladder and give rise to a lacy hypoechoic pattern that changes little with ballotment or animal repositioning. A similar appearance can be observed with severe proteinuria and fat droplets.[39]

Sonography is especially useful to detect changes due to cystitis (Fig. 25-19) and neoplasia. However, contrast radiographic techniques are superior to sonography in diagnosing abnormalities of the urachus and ureters. Rupture of the bladder can be suspected when abdominal effusion is present and the bladder poorly visualized. Contrast radiography is more accurate than sonography to detect rupture of the bladder and urethra.

GASTROINTESTINAL TRACT

High-resolution imaging is required to observe the structural detail of the wall of the gastrointestinal tract. Seven- to 10-MHz transducers provide optimum image detail though adjustable focus; 5-MHz transducers can also provide useful information. A 12-hour fast is recommended to allow the stomach to empty of food though gas will frequently remain in the gastrointestinal tract.

Patient positioning may need to be varied during sonography to avoid missing structures obscured by the reverberation artifacts generated by gas. Scanning in dorsal recumbency can be successful, though it is important to remember that stomach and bowel gas will rise toward the ventral abdominal surface and lead

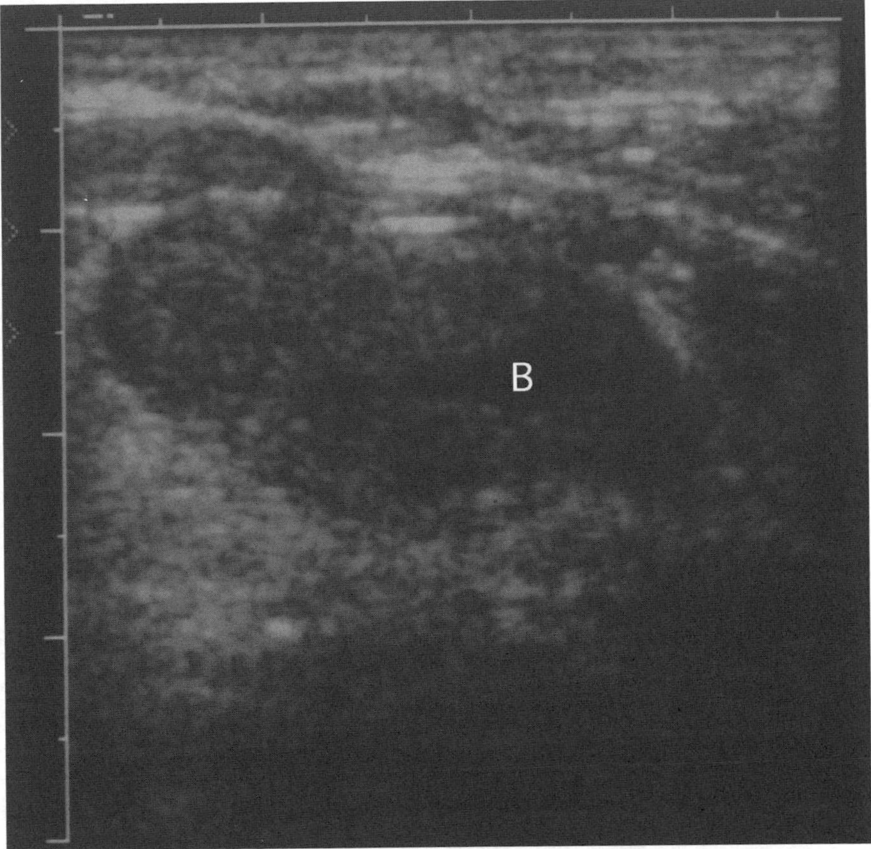

Figure 25-19
Sagittal sonogram of the urinary bladder of a 2 year old cat that had been traumatized by being squashed below a closed garage door. Skin abrasions were present over the caudal abdomen and the cat had severe hematuria. The sonogram reveals a markedly thickened bladder wall due to marked reduction in bladder volume (B). The changes on the sonogram represent traumatic cystitis and hematoma formation. Fortunately, there were no signs of urinary bladder rupture and antibiotics were administered; the cat recovered over the next weeks.

to gas artifacts that can prevent visualization of underlying structures. Positioning the patient in left/right recumbency and a standing position may help to reposition the gas away from the transducer. Also holding the transducer horizontally or pointing it upward is useful as the gas artifacts will be lessened. When a palpable mass is present, it is helpful to locate and digitally stabilize the mass during sonographic evaluation.

Sonography of the stomach in right lateral recumbency aids in visualization of the pylorus, whereas left lateral recumbency helps evaluate the fundus. Subcostal scans should be made in a parasagittal plane (short axis views) and in a transverse plane (long axis view) over the stomach, which is normally positioned along the caudal margin of the liver. Additional intercostal scanning from both the left and right sides is useful when stomach gas is present.

The normal empty stomach has a layered wall in the shape of a cauliflower, rosette, or bull's eye.[45] Five layers of alternating echogenicity are present with the mucosal surface, submucosa and muscular layer being hypoechoic (whiter) and interposed mucosa and muscular layer being hypoechoic (blacker). In dogs, the stomach wall thickness ranges between 3 and 5 mm[45] in thickness and 2 to 2.4 mm in cats.[46] Regular peristaltic contractions (4-5/min) are present in normal dogs. The lumen should be empty though hyperechoic gas generating characteristic reverberation artifacts are frequently present and sometimes anechoic to hypoechoic fluid may be present. Stomach gas reduces the accuracy of the examination because foreign bodies or mural masses may be hidden by the gas induced reverberation artifacts.

Sonography is helpful to evaluate gastric contractility. Reduced contractility such as associated with parvovirus disease and severe pancreatitis may lead to a fluid-filled stomach with reduced contractility. Gastric foreign bodies can be detected and often appear echogenic and generate acoustic shadows.[47,48] A solid object such as a rubber ball will occasionally appear as a round anechoic (nonechogenic) object. However, associated stomach gas may hide foreign bodies so a negative finding is not a reliable observation. Radiographic and endoscopic examinations are more accurate diagnostic techniques to diagnose foreign bodies. Chronic wall thickening is more likely to be revealed by sonography unless hidden behind stomach gas. Gastric wall neoplasia and severe chronic gastritis (with or without ulceration) can be detected. Here the stomach wall will be abnormally thickened and the normal layered appearance is often obscured.[47] Biopsy is needed to differentiate between neoplasia, such as leiomyoma, leiomyosarcoma, adenocarcinoma, lymphoma, and severe chronic gastritis.

Bowel, like the stomach, has a similar five-layered wall between the lumen and the mesentery.[45] Normal canine bowel wall measurements are 4.3 mm for less than 40 kg body weight and 4.8 mm for greater than 40 kg body weight.[49] In normal cats the small bowel is 2 to 2.5 mm thick except for the ileum adjacent to the ileocolic junction, which measures 2.5 to 3.2 mm. Thorough scanning along a grid pattern in both sagittal and transverse planes from the liver to the urinary bladder is necessary to evaluate the bowel. The small bowel has a random alignment, so it is necessary to varying the scan planes to obtain long axis images. The descending duodenum can be identified by locating it along the far right side of the abdomen connecting with the duodenum. The colon has a relatively fixed (question mark) shape and position. Normal small bowel has observable peristaltic contractions whereas the colon is stationary.

In a fasted normal animal there should be no dilated loops of bowel. Sonography can be used to locate loops with abnormal contractility and often these loops are abnormally dilated with fluid, mucus, and gas.[47] Absence of peristalsis of small bowel contents is abnormal and indicates the presence of ileus (Fig. 25-20). Ileus may result from obstructive lesions such as foreign bodies, masses, and intussusception or arise from neuromuscular dysfunction secondary to

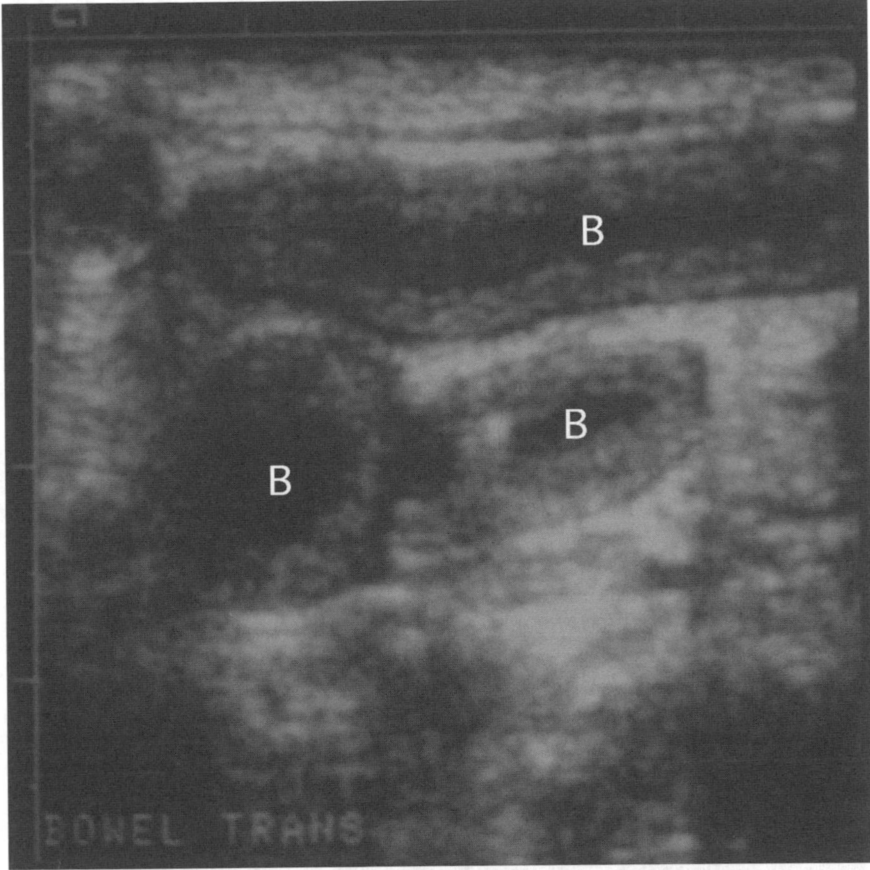

Figure 25-20
Sonogram of small intestine in a 12 week old puppy that presented with hemorrhagic vomiting and diarrhea. Palpation of the abdomen revealed distended loops of bowel. The sonogram shows the presence of multiple loops of fluid-filled bowel (B) in both long and short axis. Little to no peristalsis was present to the bowel. This indicates the presence of ileus. No apparent cause for the ileus was found. Subsequently, viral testing revealed the presence of parvovirus. The gastroenteritis had resulted in functional ileus. Remember radiography and barium contrast studies should always be considered when ileus is detected by ultrasound because concurrent gas may obscure foreign bodies. Also, other causes of bowel obstruction (such as strictures) are unreliably detected by sonography.

trauma, ischemia, pancreatitis, or parvovirus enteritis (see Fig. 25-20). Unfortunately, the concurrent accumulation of gas in the dilated bowel generates reverberation artifacts that can hide the underlying cause of the ileus. If sonography reveals an ileus and no underlying cause can be found, other imaging studies such as contrast radiography or laparotomy must be used to establish a diagnosis.

Foreign bodies will be lodged at the junction of dilated and normal bowel. The foreign body is most frequently hyperechoic (white) and generates far field

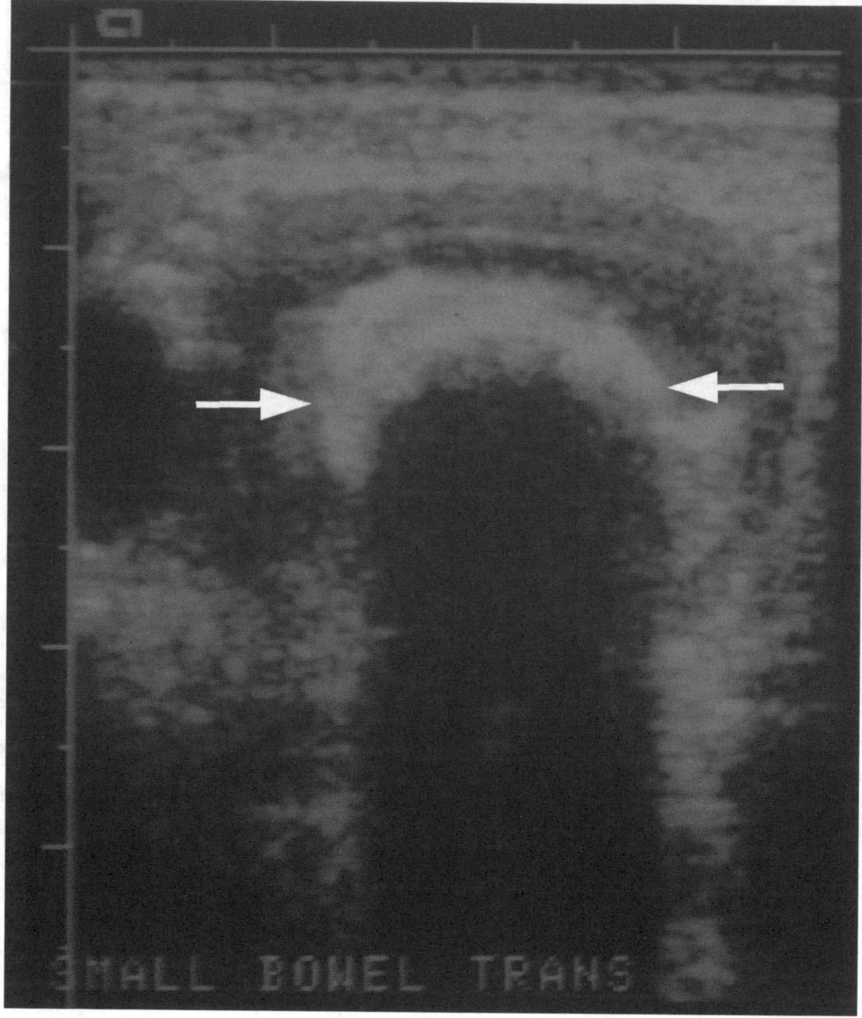

Figure 25-21
Transverse sonogram of small bowel in a 8 year old Australian shepherd dog presented with a 2-day history of severe vomiting. A palpable mass was present associated with distended loops of bowel. Sonography over the mass revealed it to be within a loop of distended small intestine. The mass was hyperechoic and caused far-field shadowing as typically observed with an intestinal foreign body. This was removed at subsequent enterotomy.

acoustic shadowing[47,48] (Fig. 25-21). Linear (string type) foreign bodies are more difficult to recognize. The associated plication tends to distort the alignment of the bowel wall. Intussusception is readily diagnosed by recognizing that the distended bowel loop contains multiple concentric layers of bowel wall (ie, 20 or more) in cross-section[47] (Fig. 25-22). In long section the mass consists of parallel alternating hyperechoic and hypoechoic layers. Also, invaginated mes-

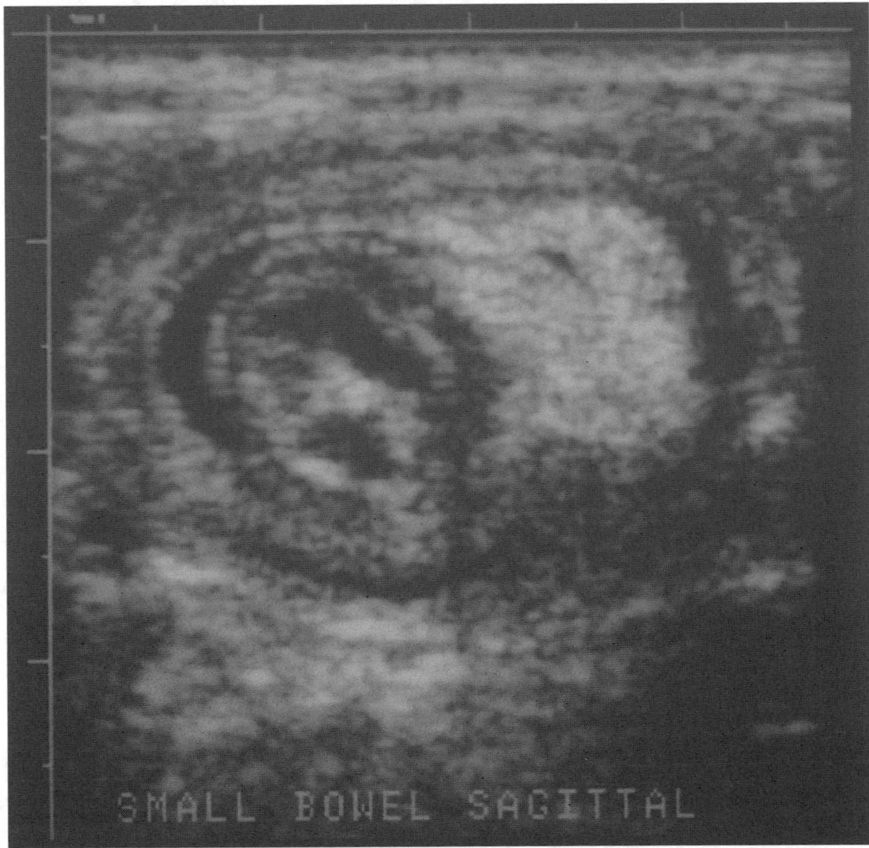

Figure 25-22
Sonogram of bowel in the right mid-abdominal quadrant. This young 9 month old Basset hound presented with a week-long history of vomiting and diarrhea. Distended bowel was palpated in the abdomen and a sausage-like mass was detected in the right mid-abdominal quadrant. Sonography over the mass revealed a loop of intestine inside another loop of bowel. This appearance is typical example of a cross-section through an intussusception. Subsequent surgery revealed this to be a ileocolic intussusception with small bowel present in the ascending colon.

entery can appear as a hyperechoic band and dilated (anechoic) veins may be present.

Mass lesions due to bowel neoplasia, focal granulomas, or abscesses secondary to bowel perforation tend to result in asymmetrical thickening of a segment of bowel. Neoplasia tends to infiltrate the bowel wall and cause loss of the normal layered appearance. Dilated bowel and items adjacent to a mass indicate the need for surgery. If there are sonographic signs of obstruction, then thin-needle sonographic-guided aspirates often help establish the specific diagnosis. Enlarged mesenteric lymph nodes appear as oval to round hypoechoic nodules in the adjacent mesentery. Thin-needle aspiration should also be made of lymphadenopathy because reactive and metastatic neoplasias have similar sonographic appearances.

PANCREAS

A normal pancreas is difficult to visualize because it has an echogenicity slightly less or equal to the surrounding mesenteric fat. Gas in overlying loops of bowel will cause reverberation artifacts that obscure the image of the pancreas. Gas-filled stomach/bowel and a deep narrow chest conformation makes the examination more difficult. In dogs, the left limb of the pancreas often lies deep to or adjacent to the stomach and is less frequently visualized than the right limb of the pancreas, which extends from the liver to the level of the right kidney on the medial side of the duodenum. In cats, the stomach lies more to the left side of the abdomen and the left limb of the pancreas tends to be more readily visualized.

High-resolution transducers, 7 to 10 MHz, should be used to image the pancreas. The patient may be placed in dorsal recumbency and the area of the abdomen, just caudal to the stomach/liver and ventral to the caudate liver lobe, should be scanned thoroughly. Laying the animal in right lateral recumbency and scanning along the right costal arch with the sound beam horizontal is sometimes more successful. It is especially helpful to locate the pylorus and then scan to the right lateral side of the abdomen to locate the duodenum. Once the duodenum is identified, search along its medial side through the mesentery for the pancreas. Frequently, the pancreaticoduodenal vein will be found lying in or against the pancreas.

Acute pancreatitis is more successfully diagnosed by sonography than by radiographs. The pancreas enlarges and the changed hypoechoic echogenicity makes it more readily detectable by sonography.[50] Other useful concurrent observations are a distended gallbladder and proximal common bile duct. The duodenal wall may become thickened and noncontractile (ileus). Peripancreatic effusion may develop.[51] Animals often show pain and splinting of the abdominal wall muscles as the transducer is pushed into the right cranial quadrant of the abdomen. Serial follow-up sonograms should be made to monitor the resolution or progression of the findings. Mild to moderate pancreatitis may show fewer sonographic abnormalities. Acute necrotizing pancreatitis will show a greater degree of pancreatic enlargement and a more hypoechoic change with secondary signs of extrahepatic cholestasis and ileus.

A pancreatic pseudocyst (walled-off focal pancreatic necrosis) is less common in animals than people.[52] Pancreatic abscesses can also develop in the later phase of pancreatitis. Sonography will reveal a focus of echogenic fluid.[53]

Recurrent pancreatitis has a more heterogenous echo pattern due to areas of fibrosis, nodular distortion, and hyperechoic inflammatory response in the adjacent mesenteric fat. Multiple episodes of pancreatitis lead to further heterogeneity in the echo pattern. Sometimes these focal areas (pseudo-mass lesions) are difficult to differentiate from masses arising from pancreatic neoplasia.[54] Less severe sonographic changes of the pancreas and peripancreatic tissue are seen in dogs with transient subtle clinical signs associated with pancreatitis. The pancreas may be detected as a distinct, well-defined slightly hypoechoic structure surrounded by slightly more hyperechoic mesentery. This observation combined with the absence of peripancreatic effusion, duodenal atony, and absence of signs of extrahepatic cholestasis, all make for a better prognosis.[51]

Pancreatic neoplasia is less common. Hypoglycemia secondary to a functional islet cell tumor is a diagnostic challenge because the insulinomas are often small and are infrequently seen with sonography. Adenocarcinomas can be detected but often the diagnosis is difficult due to the small size of the primary mass. Insulinoma and adenocarcinomas frequently metastasize and the secondary neoplastic nodules may be detected in adjacent mesenteric and hepatic lymph nodes and the liver. Histologic confirmation is needed because sometimes lymphomas or enlarged reactive lymph nodes have a similar sonographic appearance.

BLOOD VESSELS

Sonography is useful to detect thrombi in the aorta, vena cava and portal veins.[55] Acute thrombi may not be echogenic and so B-mode imaging is not as reliable as color Doppler imaging. Arterial thrombi are most common in the terminal abdominal aorta (saddle thrombus) (Fig. 25-23). Echocardiography should also be performed to evaluate for a cardiac origin. Venous thrombi are less common. Neoplasia of the adrenals and kidneys can lead to invasion of the vena cava and lead to a thrombus (Fig. 25-24). A gunshot injury to the abdomen is best first evaluated by radiography. Subsequent sonography can be useful to evaluate for hemorrhage (Fig. 25-25). Portal vein thrombi can develop and tend to lodge in the bifurcation of the intrahepatic portion of the portal vein.[55]

CANINE REPRODUCTIVE TRACT—FEMALE

Sagittal and transverse scans should be made in a thorough grid pattern from the pubis to the level of the kidneys.[56] Linear transducers are sufficient to image the body of the uterus and palpable uterine enlargements. Sector transducers are more useful to image between the loops of bowel, improving the chances of locating the uterine horns and ovaries. The normal uterus in a bitch who has never been pregnant is often less than 1 cm in diameter. Overlying bowel gas frequently prevents ultrasonographic visualization of the normal uterine horns. A fluid-filled urinary bladder aids in imaging the body of the uterus.

The adjacent aorta and vena cava are similarly sized hyperechoic structures. Careful evaluation of tubular structures dorsal to the bladder is necessary. Evidence of pulsatile walls and blood flow or a compressible nature help differentiate the adjacent vessels from the body of the uterus. The lack of an echogenic center and peristalsis also helps set the uterus apart from the adjacent bowel. Color Doppler ultrasound is helpful in this evaluation.

Between conception and the 15th day of pregnancy the uterus may enlarge slightly and appear more hypoechoic.[57] However, gestational vesicles will frequently not be noted until about the 20th day of pregnancy. Initially, the gestational vesicle appears as an anechoic, fluid-filled, cyst-like structure containing a small fetus. Cardiac contractility at a rate of more than 200 beats/min may be

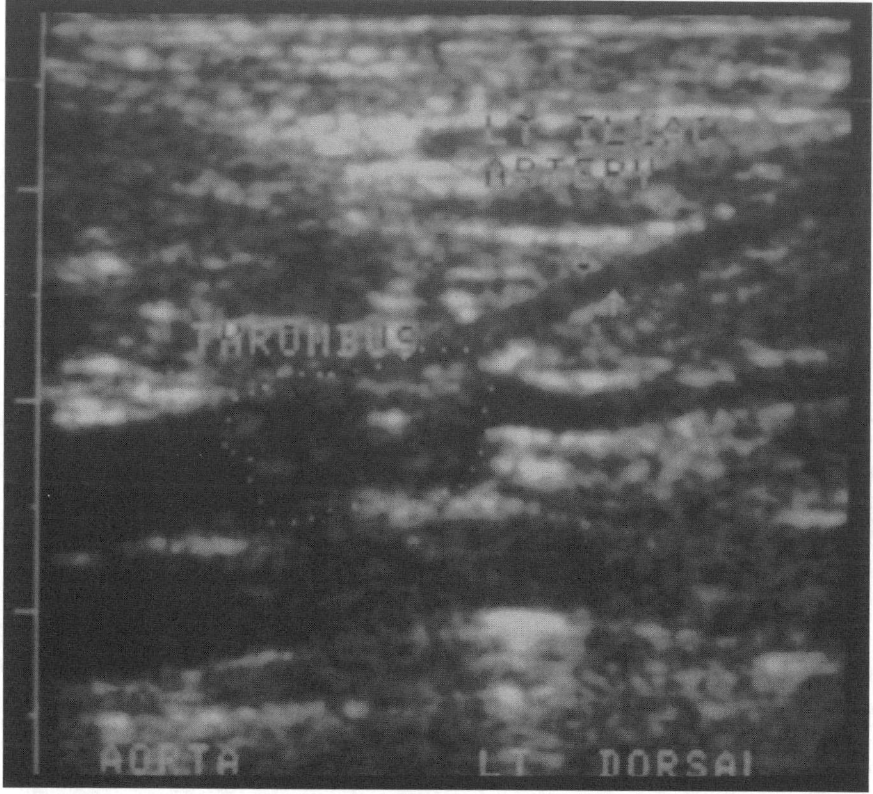

Figure 25-23
Dorsal sonogram of the terminal abdominal aorta in a 9 year old dog. The dog was normal that morning, but the owners noticed it suddenly yelped and could no longer walk on its left hind leg. On physical examination, there was no arterial pulse in the left hindlimb and no motor control of the leg. The ultrasound revealed an echogenic thrombus lodged in the terminal caudal portion of the abdominal aorta just cranial to the iliac bifurcation. Color Doppler examination could not demonstrate blood flow distal to the thrombus in the left external iliac artery. The dog was treated with aspirin and over the next 2 days and began to regain function to its left hindlimb. Echocardiography did not reveal a source for the thrombus and subsequently the dog made a full recovery. Note: It is important to remember that acute thrombi may not be echogenic and are not visible on B-mode sonography. Color Doppler sonography of blood vessels is most useful to rule out the presence of acute nonechogenic thrombi.

detected as early as the 28th day of pregnancy. Between days 30 and 40 the head and appendages become visible, and in the last trimester the bony structures and thoracic and abdominal organs become apparent.[56,57]

Fetal demise is difficult to confirm before mid-pregnancy. The absence of the heartbeat or fetal movement after the 30th day of gestation indicates fetal death. Such findings as disproportionately small embryos in one horn of the uterus or fetuses that fail to grow and lack movement or heart rates less than

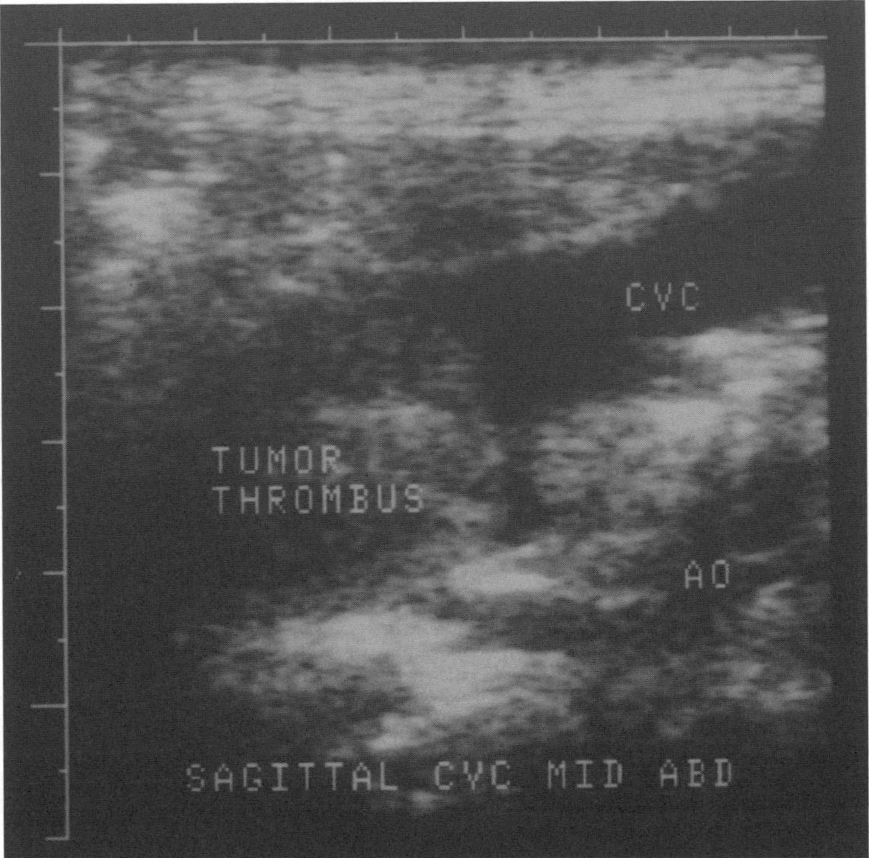

Figure 25-24
Sagittal sonogram of the mid-abdominal vena cava. This 8 year old Brittany spaniel presented with steady weight loss (7 months) and then developed hematuria and edema of the hindlimbs. Sonography of the abdomen revealed a large complex mass replacing the architecture of the right kidney, most consistent with renal neoplasia. The abdominal vena cava (CVC) caudal to the level of the right kidney was abnormally distended. An echogenic thrombus was visible in the vena cava at the level of the right kidney. Similar thrombi have also been observed in the vena cava secondary to adrenal neoplasia. AO, aorta.

twice the maternal heart rate[58] all support the likelihood of impending fetal demise.[56] On subsequent re-examination, fetal resorption is characterized by a disordered gestational vesicle containing disorganized fetal remnants.[59] Fetal maturation at the time of parturition is best determined by radiography. Visualization of tooth bud sockets and beginning of ossification of the paws will be observed at full term. Sonography is more helpful to evaluate fetal viability. Fetal heart rates should be evaluated and normally they are about two times the mother's rate (Fig. 25-26). Slowed fetal heart rates indicate fetal distress and warrant continued monitoring or intervention.

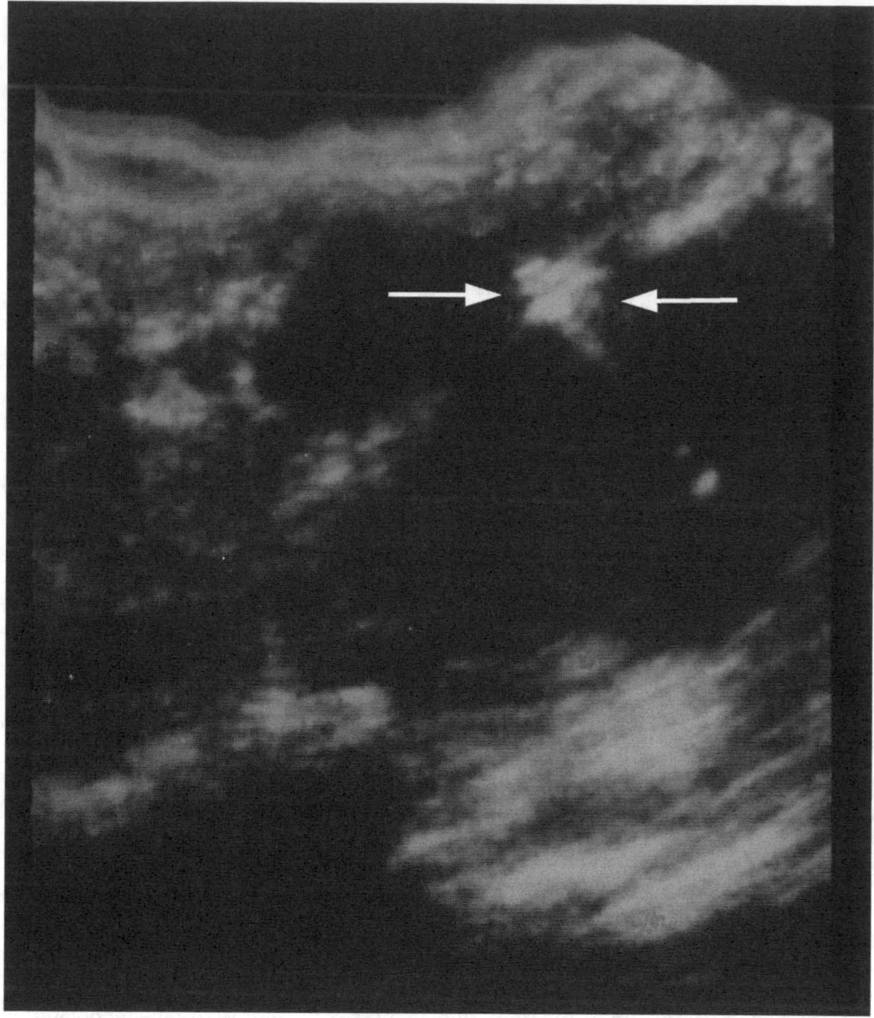

Figure 25-25
Sagittal sonogram of the caudal portion of the abdomen in a farm dog suspected of being shot. A radiograph showed the presence of a large rifle bullet in the caudal retroperitoneum. Sonography located the bullet (arrows) by finding a hyperechoic structure with ring down artifacts deep to it. The bullet was surrounded by a large volume of anechoic fluid. The dog became progressively weaker and developed signs of hypovolemic shock. Subsequent surgery found the bullet had lacerated iliac vessels and resulted in a large hematoma.

Endometritis may be present in seemingly healthy bitches. If the cervix is closed, then the entire uterus becomes distended with purulent fluid. Pyometra, mucometria, and hydrometra are readily distinguished from loops of bowel by the absence of peristalsis and pregnancy[56,60] (Fig. 25-27). Both horns of the uterus frequently become distended and appear as convoluted fluid-filled tubes. The

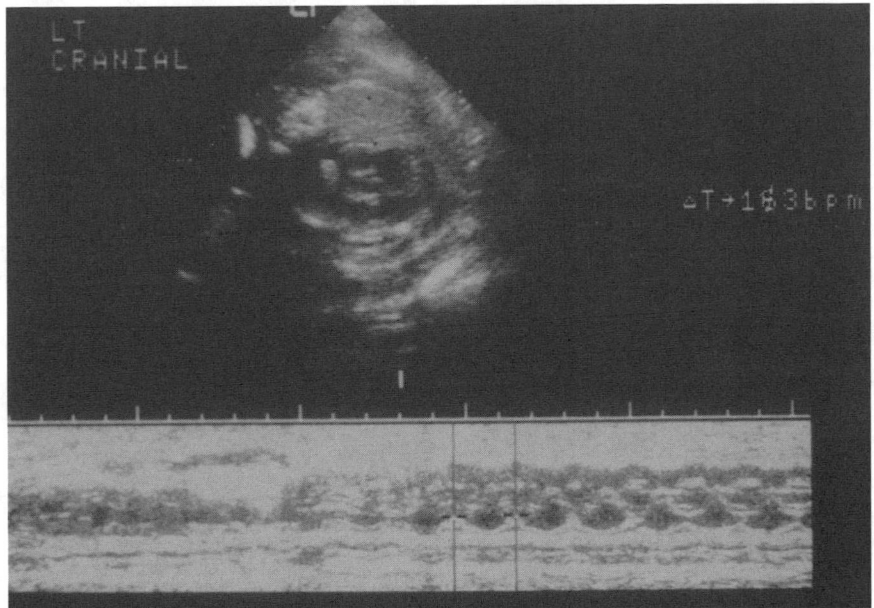

Figure 25-26
Sonogram and M-mode tracing of canine fetus. The 5 year old Collie bitch was at least 60 days pregnant and presented with a bloody vaginal discharge but without clear signs of impending parturition. Multiple viable feti were found. This fetus was in distress because the heartbeat (AT) had slowed to 163 beats/min, whereas the other feti had heart rates greater than 260/min.

tortuous, twisting nature of the distended uterus may result in the false impression of multiple cysts until the transducer is turned through different scan planes, allowing appreciation of the tubular nature of the distended uterus. If the cervix remains open, the uterine diameter often is smaller, and the diagnosis is simplified by the presence of a concurrent purulent vaginal discharge.

Pregnancy in cats may be diagnosed earlier by ultrasound, because gestational sacs are detectable at 11 days and fetuses at 15 days after conception. Cardiac motion is visible as early as 16 days of gestation.[61] Available body and head diameter growth curves allow accurate assessment of gestational age and prediction of parturition date.[62]

PROSTATE

The prostate is the major accessory sex gland in dogs. Benign prostatic hypertrophy is a normal middle-age change in intact male dogs. The variable clinical signs and the limitations of digital rectal examination have made prostatic disease a diagnostic challenge. The canine prostate has a variable location. As the prostate enlarges, it often moves cranially, lying in the caudal abdomen. In dogs, the intra-abdominal position allows for ultrasonic evaluation of the gland via transabdominal approach. If the gland is not readily visible, then transrectal

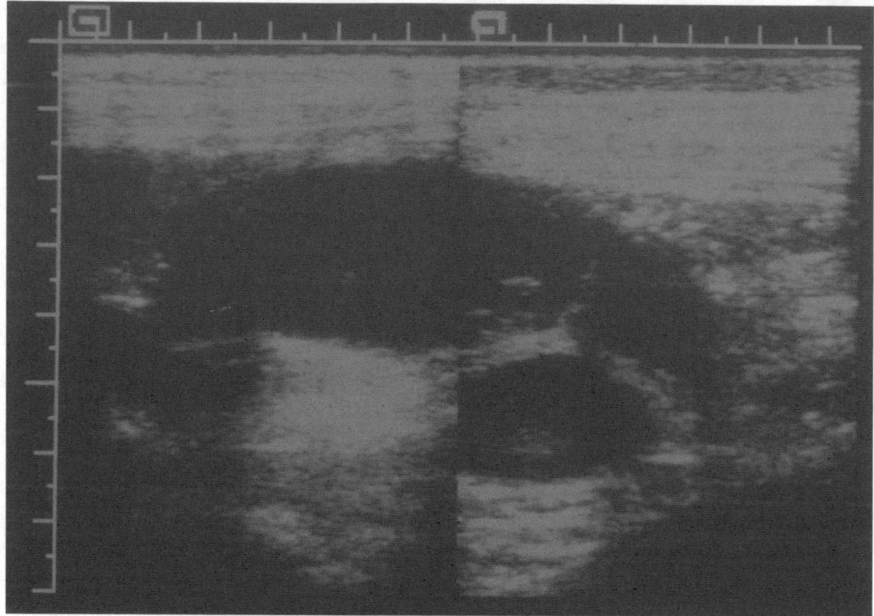

Figure 25-27
Sonogram of the caudal abdomen of a vomiting, lethargic 5 year old Labrador who had been bred more than 3 months ago but not had any puppies. The sonogram reveals the uterus to be abnormally filled with echogenic fluid. This is the characteristic appearance of distended uterine horns due to pyometra.

digital pressure may help move the prostate more into the abdomen during sonography.[63-67]

Sagittal scans are made by placing the transducer beside the prepuce while the penis is held aside. A full urinary bladder helps locate the prostate, because the trigone defines the cranial border of the prostate. The transducer is then angled caudally to image into the pelvic canal. Transverse scans are made by placing the transducer against the bony brim of the pubis and angling caudally into the pelvic canal.

The normal prostate has a bilobar symmetrical spherical shape. The normal margin is smooth, continuous, and rounded. Normal prostatic tissue has a homogenous, coarse echogenicity. Small, circumscribed anechoic foci may be present in older dogs, stemming from retention cysts associated with normal benign hypertrophy. Complicated benign hypertrophy results from superimposed cystic hyperplasia, squamous metaplasia, prostatitis, abscesses, and neoplasia. Clinical correlation with rectal examination aids in differentiating sterile cysts from abscesses. Prostatitis has a variable echo appearance, depending on its chronicity. Acute prostatitis tends to result in a diffusely hypoechoic prostate. However, chronic infection may lead to fibrosis, causing a patchy, increased

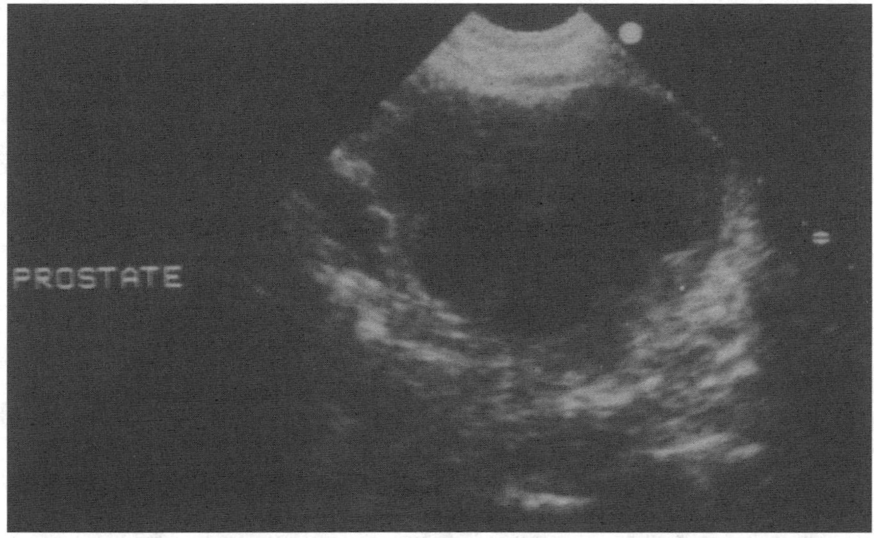

Figure 25-28
Transverse sonogram of the prostate in an intact male Doberman dog. The dog seemed ill to the owner and attempted to urinate frequently. A fever was present. Digital examination of the prostatic region was very painful. Ultrasonography of the prostate revealed irregularly lobulated, multiple, fluid-filled cavities within the prostate. Subsequent surgery confirmed the presence of prostatic abscesses.

echogenicity and abscesses. Unfortunately, this pattern is also seen with prostate neoplasia.[65-67]

Prostatic abscesses are characterized by many large, irregularly shaped anechoic cavities (Fig. 25-28). Echogenic-dependent sediment may be seen. The echogenicity of the adjacent prostatic parenchyma is usually increased because of the chronic inflammation and surrounding fibrosis. Small abscesses similar to retention cysts may appear. In this case, ultrasound-guided aspiration may be required to confirm the diagnosis.[15,64-66] Periprostatic cysts may occasionally develop from extraparenchymal retention cysts or as a remnant of the müllerian ducts. Such cysts may grow large and typically look like a second urinary bladder.[68]

Clinical signs resulting from prostatic neoplasia in dogs are variable and may be visible only in the advanced stages. The prostate is enlarged and typically has an asymmetrical, irregular nodular border. Disruption of the outer margin may be noted. The most common ultrasonographic pattern is caused by fibrosis and mineralization leading to hyperechoic areas that tend to coalesce and shadow. Because canine prostatic neoplasia is often quite advanced at the time of first examination, metastases to the sublumbar lymph nodes may be recognized as variable-sized circular hypoechoic masses dorsal to the urinary bladder.[64-66] Biopsy is required to confirm the presence of neoplasia.[66]

REFERENCES

1. Feeney DA, Johnston GR, Walter PA: Abdominal ultrasonography—1989: general interpretation and abdominal masses. *Semin Vet Med Surg Small Anim* 15:1225, 1985.
2. Cartee RE: Diagnostic real time ultrasonography of the liver of the dog and cat. *J Am Anim Hosp Assoc* 17:731, 1981.
3. Feeney DA, Johnston GR, Walter PA: Two-dimensional, gray-scale ultrasonography: general interpretation and abdominal masses. *Vet Med Surg Small Anim* 15: 1225, 1985.
4. Lamb CR: Ultrasonography of the liver and biliary tract. *In:* Kaplan PM, ed.: Problems in Veterinary Medicine. Philadelphia: JB Lippincott, 1991, p 557.
5. Nyland TG, Hager DA: Sonography of the liver, gall bladder and spleen. *Vet Clin North Am Small Animal Pract* 15:1123, 1985.
6. Whiteley MB, Feeney DA, Whiteley LO, Hardy RM: Ultrasonographic appearance of primary and metastatic canine hepatic tumors: a review of 48 cases (1981–1986). *J Ultrasound Med* 8:621, 1989.
7. Wrigley RH: Radiographic and ultrasonographic diagnosis of liver disease in dogs and cats. *Vet Clin North Am Small Anim Pract* 15:21, 1985.
8. Godshalk CP, Badertscher RR, Rippy MK, Ghent AW: Quantitative ultrasonic assessment of liver size in the dog. *Vet Radiol* 29:162, 1988.
9. Yeager AE, Anderson WI: Study of association between histologic features and echogenicity of architecturally normal cat kidneys. *Am J Vet Res* 50:860, 1989.
10. Bailey MQ, Willard MD, McLoughlin MA, *et al.*: Ultrasonographic findings associated with congenital hepatic arteriovenous fistula in three dogs. *J Am Vet Med Assoc* 10:17, 1988.
11. Besso JG, Wrigley RH, Gliatto JM, Webster CRL: Ultrasonographic appearance and clinical findings in 14 dogs with gallbladder mucocele. *Vet Radiol Ultrasound* 41:261, 2000.
12. Nyland TG, Gillett NA: Sonographic evaluation of experimental bile duct ligation in the dog. *Vet Radiol* 23:252, 1982.
13. Finn ST, Park RD, Twedt DC, Cutris CR: Ultrasonographic assessment of sincalide-induced canine gallbladder emptying: an aid to the diagnosis of biliary obstruction. *Vet Radiol* 32:269, 1991.
14. Nyland TG, Fisher PE: Evaluation of experimentally induced canine hepatic cirrhosis using duplex Doppler ultrasound. *Vet Radiol* 31:189, 1990.
15. Konde LJ, Lebel JL, Park RD, Wrigley RH: Sonographic application in the diagnosis of intra-abdominal abscess in the dog. *Vet Radiol* 27:151, 1984.
16. Stowater JL, Lamb CR, Snelling SH: Ultrasonographic features of canine hepatic nodular hyperplasia. *Vet Radiol* 31:268, 1991.
17. Lamb CR, Hartzband LE, Tidwell AS, Pearson SH: Ultrasonographic findings in hepatic and splenic lymphosarcoma in dogs and cats. *Vet Radiol* 32:117, 1991.
18. Kolata RJ, Johnston DE: Motor vehicle accidents in urban dogs: a study of 600 cases. *J Am Vet Med Assoc* 167:938, 1975.
19. Wrigley RH, Konde LJ, Park RD, *et al.*: Clinical features and diagnosis of canine splenic hematic hematomas. *J Am Anim Hosp Assoc* 25:371, 1985.
20. Wrigley RH: Ultrasonography of the spleen: life-threatening splenic disorders. *In:* Kaplan PM, ed.: Problems in Veterinary Medicine. Philadelphia: JB Lippincott, 1991, p 3.
21. Slatter DH: Textbook of Small Animal Surgery. Philadelphia: WB Saunders, 1985, p 1213.

22. Konde LJ, Wrigley RH, Lebel JL, *et al.*: Sonographic and radiographic changes associated with splenic torsion in dogs. *Vet Radiol* 130:41, 1989.
23. Nyland TG, Hager DA: Sonography of the liver, gall bladder and spleen. *Vet Clin North Am Small Anim Pract* 15:1123, 1985.
24. Schelling CG, Wortman JA, Saunders HM: Ultrasonic detection of splenic necrosis in the dog. *Vet Radiol* 29:227, 1988.
25. Wrigley RH, Park Rd, Konde LJ, *et al.*: Ultrasonographic features of splenic hemangiosarcoma in dogs: 18 cases (1980–1986). *J Am Vet Med Assoc* 8:1113, 1988.
26. Cartee RE, Selcer BA, Patton CS: Ultrasonographic diagnosis of renal disease in small animals. *J Am Vet Med Assoc* 176:426, 1980.
27. Feeney DA, Johnston GR: Urogenital imaging: a practical update. *Semin Vet Med Surg* 1:144, 1986.
28. Konde LJ: Sonography of the kidney. *Vet Clin North Am Small Anim Pract* 15:1149, 1985.
29. Konde LF, Wrigley RH, Lebel JL: Ultrasonographic anatomy of the normal canine kidney. *Vet Radiol* 25:173, 1984.
30. Walter PA, Feeney DA, Johnston GR, O'Leary TP: Ultrasonography evaluation of renal parenchymal diseases in dogs: 32 cases (1981–1986). *J Am Vet Med Assoc* 191:999, 1987.
31. Konde LJ, Wrigley RH, Lebel JL, *et al.*: Sonographic and radiographic changes associated with splenic torsion in dogs. *Vet Radiol* 30:41, 1989.
32. Morrow KL, Salman MD, Lappin MR, Wrigley RH: Comparison of the resistive index to clinical parameters in dogs with renal disease [abstract]. *Vet Radiol Ultrasound* 37:193, 1996.
33. Adams WM, Toal RL, Breider MA: Early renal ultrasonographic findings in dogs with experimentally-induced ethylene glycol nephrosis. *Am J Vet Res* 50:1370, 1989.
34. Walter PA, Johnston GR, Feeney DA, O'Brien TD: Applications of ultrasonography in the diagnosis of parenchymal kidney disease in cats: 24 cases (1981–1986). *J Am Vet Med Assoc* 92:92, 1988.
35. Barr FJ, Patteson MW, Lucke VM, Gibbs C: Hypercalcemic nephropathy in three dogs. *Vet Radiol* 30:169, 1989.
36. Konde LJ, Wrigley RH, Park RD, Lebel JL: Sonographic appearance of renal neoplasia in the dog. *Vet Radiol* 26:74, 1985.
37. Biller D, Kantrowitz B, Partinton R, Miyaqbayshi T: Diagnostic ultrasound of the urinary bladder. *J Am Anim Hosp Assoc* 26:397, 1990.
38. Berry CR: Differentiating cystic calculi from colon. *Vet Radiol* 33:282, 1993.
39. Finn-Bodner ST: The urinary bladder. *In:* Cartee RE, ed.: Practical Veterinary Ultrasound. Philadelphia: Lea & Febiger, 1995, p 219.
40. Geisse AL, Lowry JE, Schaeffer DJ, Smith CW: Sonographic evaluation of urinary bladder wall thickness in normal dogs. *Vet Radiol Ultrasound* 38:132, 1997.
41. Spaulding KA, Stone E: Color Doppler evaluation of ureteral flow dynamics in the dog as influenced by relative specific gravity. Proceedings of the Annual Scientific Meeting of the American College of Veterinary Radiology, Chicago, 1993.
42. Voros W: Ultrasound of urinary bladder calculi in dogs. *Canine Pract* 19:29, 1993.
43. Feeney DA, Walter PA: Ultrasonography of the kidneys, adrenal glands and urinary bladder. Proceedings of the American Institute of Ultrasound in Medicine Animal Ultrasound Course, 1989.
44. Ackerman N: Radiology and Ultrasound of Urogenital Disease in Dogs and Cats. Ames, IA: Iowa State University Press, 1991, p 1.

45. Penninck DG, Nyland TG, Fisher PE, *et al.*: Ultrasonography of the normal canine gastrointestinal tract. *Vet Radiol* 30:272, 1989.
46. Goggin, JM, Biller DS, Debey BM, *et al.*: Ultrasonographic measurement of gastrointestinal wall thickness and the ultrasonographic appearance of the ileocolic region in healthy cat. *J Am Anim Hosp Assoc* 36:224, 2000.
47. Penninck DG, Nyland TG, Kerr LY, *et al.*: Ultrasonographic evaluation of gastrointestinal diseases in small animals. *Vet Radiol* 31:134, 1990.
48. Tidwell AS, Pinninck DG: Ultrasonography of gastrointestinal foreign bodies. *Vet Radiol Ultrasound* 33:160, 1992.
49. Delaney FA, O'Brien RT: Ultrasound evaluation of small bowel thickness vs. weight in normal dogs. *Vet Radiol Ultrasound* 40:658, 1999.
50. Nyland TG, Mulvaney MH, Strombeck DR: Ultrasonic features of experimentally induced acute pancreatitis. *Vet Radiol* 24:260, 1983.
51. Saunders HM: Ultrasonography of the pancreas. *Prob Vet Med* 3:583, 1991.
52. Rutgers C, Herring DS, Orton EC: Pancreatic pseudocyst associated with acute pancreatitis in the dog: ultrasonographic diagnosis. *J Am Anim Hosp Assoc* 21:411, 1985.
53. Salisbury SK, Lantz GC, Nelson RW, Kazacos EA: Pancreatic abscess in dogs: six cases (1978–1986). *J Am Vet Med Assoc* 193:1104, 1988.
54. Edwards DF, Bauer MS, Walker MA, *et al.*: Pancreatic masses in seven dogs following acute pancreatitis. *J Am Anim Hosp Assoc* 26:189, 1990.
55. Lamb CR, Wrigley RH, Simpson KW, *et al.*: Ultrasonographic diagnosis of portal vein thrombosis in four dogs [abstract]. *Vet Radiol Ultrasound* 37:121, 1996.
56. Wrigley RH: Ultrasonography of the spleen: life-threatening splenic disorders. *In:* Kaplan PM, ed.: Problems in Veterinary Medicine. Philadelphia: JB Lippincott, 1991, p 3.
57. Cartee RE, Rowles T: Preliminary study of the ultrasonographic diagnosis of pregnancy and fetal development in the dog. *Am J Vet Res* 45:1259, 1984.
58. Johnston SD, Smith FO, Bailie NC, *et al.*: Prenatal indicators of puppy viability at term. *Compend Contin Educ Pract Vet* 1:13, 1983.
59. Barr FJ: Pregnancy diagnosis and assessment of fetal viability in the dog: a review. *J Small Anim Pract* 29:647, 1988.
60. Fayrer-Hosken Ra, Mahaffey M, Miller-Liebl D, Caudle AB: Early diagnosis of canine pyometra using ultrasonography. *Vet Radiol* 32:287, 1991.
61. Dividson AP, Nyland TG, Tsutsui T: Pregnancy diagnosis with ultrasound in the domestic cat. *Vet Radiol* 27:109, 1986.
62. Beck KA, Baldwin CJ, Bosu WTK: Ultrasound prediction of parturition in queens. *Vet Radiol* 31:32, 1990.
63. Cartee RE, Rowles T: Transabdominal sonographic evaluation of the canine prostate. *Vet Radiol* 24:156, 1983.
64. Feeney DA, Johnston GR, Klausner JS, Bell FW: Canine prostatic ultrasonography—1989. *Semin Vet Med Surg Small Anim* 190:1027, 1987.
65. Feeney DA, Johnston GR, Klausner JS, Bell FW: Canine prostatic ultrasonography—1989. *Semin Vet Med Small Anim* 4:44, 1989.
66. Finn St, Wrigley RH: Ultrasonography and ultrasound-guided biopsy of the canine prostate. *In:* Kirk RW, ed.: Current Veterinary Therapy X. Philadelphia: WB Saunders, 1989, p 1227.
67. Olson PN, Wrigley RH, Thrall MA, Husted PW: Disorders of the canine prostate gland: pathogenesis, diagnosis, and medical therapy. *Compend Cont Educ Pract Vet* 9:613, 1987.
68. Stowater JL, Lamb CR: Ultrasonographic features of paraprostatic cysts in nine dogs. *Vet Radiol* 30:232, 1989.

26
Emergency Use of Magnetic Resonance Imaging in Animals

Patrick R. Gavin, Rodney S. Bagley, and Russell Tucker

INTRODUCTION

Quick and complete evaluation of animals that are critically ill is mandatory. Often, these evaluations require some type of imaging to assess vital anatomic structures. Radiographs and ultrasound are the current mainstays of emergency imaging; however, advanced imaging studies such as computed tomography (CT) and magnetic resonance imaging (MRI) are being used with increasing frequency.[1-6] MRI technology provides for exceptional imaging of anatomic detail, especially of soft tissues throughout the body. Although access to MRI, even for humans, is still limited on an emergency basis, the benefits of such imaging should increase its use for both humans and animals in the future.

The MRIs are produced from manipulation of hydrogen nuclei (protons) within the body.[7,8] Basic MRI techniques have been described in recent veterinary literature and will not be covered here.[8] This chapter focuses on the use of MRI in emergency situations.

TECHNICAL CONSIDERATIONS

Virtually all animals undergoing MRI are required to remain motionless for long periods. Most machines produce significant noise that would startle the animal. Positioning, a critical aspect of obtaining good image quality, is difficult in an unrestrained patient. Movement during imaging sequences will result in artifacts that make interpreting the images impossible. Practically, all of these factors mean that the animals must be under general anesthesia or at least heavily sedated. MRI procedures create no pain and, therefore, the level of anesthesia required can remain rather minimal. Truly comatose animals may be imaged without the aid of anesthesia. Physiologic stability of the animal is obviously a factor in determining if any imaging study can proceed. Initial emergency management and treatment of critical animals is discussed elsewhere in this text.

Patient monitoring equipment normally used in a ICU or surgery suite is not often compatible with MRI equipment due to the strong magnetic field required by the latter. Monitoring equipment compatible with MRI is available and requires an additional capital investment. Because most MRI in humans is performed without anesthesia, many human facilities may not have this equipment available. The desirability to further instrument the patients while imaging is somewhat offset by the increased anesthetic time the instrumentation setup requires. Most machines have the ability to monitor pulse and respiration rate; however, these monitoring systems are not intended for critical patient monitoring. Instrumentation setup for procedures such as an electrocardiogram (ECG) is considerably more difficult due to the high magnetic field. Standard monitoring items such as esophageal stethoscopes may be used; however, the noise produced during imaging makes their use problematic. Additionally, due to the physical size and tubular construction of most MRI units, it is difficult to have close physical animal monitoring. Although the anesthetist may be in the same room with the animal, ease of access to view, for example, respiration, administer drugs through intravenous tubing, or observe the pupils is limited. Pragmatically, this means that patient monitoring is less than ideal compared to other, more physically unrestricted areas. Rapid imaging protocols that reduce anesthetic time, therefore, are the goal.

Magnetic resonance imaging uses a high magnetic field. Any magnetic objects, such as collars, must be removed. Although small identification chips can cause an artifact in the images, they are usually not a problem. It is suggested that animals be radiographed prior to the MRI if there is any doubt about magnetic objects being present. The worst offenders are BBs and steel shotgun shot. Other metals, such as lead, do not pose a problem. Iron-containing objects are highly magnetic and will cause an artifact rendering a useless image with a radius of approximately 10 cm from the steel shot. Therefore, if the steel shot is in the lumbar region and the head is the area of interest, it will not pose a problem.

Magnetic resonance imaging is a technical endeavor requiring a trained operator for successful imaging. Pulse sequences used in MRI are numerous, have advantages and disadvantages concerning resolution and image contrast, and require varying times. Some sequences can be performed rapidly (<1 minute), whereas other sequences take considerably longer (>10 minutes). With the emergency patients, wherever possible, rapid sequences should be performed. Often, there is a paradox between image resolution and image sensitivity.[7] Pulse sequences with the most sensitivity for pathologic change often have less anatomic resolution. Again, efforts should be focused on sequences that allow for a rapid, accurate diagnosis rather than the acquisition of multiple images. An experienced operator or radiologist should be consulted to obtain the most appropriate imaging sequences for the individual problem being examined.

CLINICAL USE OF MRI

CNS Imaging

For animals, the most experience with MRI has been gained in imaging the central nervous system (CNS).[9,10] Similar to other imaging modalities, a complete and thorough physical and neurologic assessment is imperative to determine the location and extent of the problem. Because MRI provides for superior anatomic evaluations, some anatomic abnormalities that have no associated clinical significance will be imaged. Clinical signs are the basis on which any abnormality seen with MRI is determined to be clinically significant. Clinical evaluation of the CNS should be reviewed and understood to most accurately correlate image abnormalities with clinically significant lesions.

Intracranial Imaging

Imaging of the intracranial structures is indicated in any severe or rapidly progressing clinical syndrome associated with intracranial signs. These are most often animals with severe seizures or alterations in mental status such as stupor or coma. Animals that are systemically ill from any cause may have alterations in consciousness. Therefore, a thorough evaluation of all body systems should be performed before advanced imaging.

Once the clinical signs and severity of the impairment are determined, the animals are prepared for imaging. Animals should be placed under general anesthesia following guidelines for neuroanesthesia. Comatose animals may be imaged without anesthesia, but still may require ventilatory support to prevent increases in $PaCO_2$, which can secondarily increase intracranial pressure (ICP). If the animal requires anesthesia, diuretics (mannitol and furosemide) and hyperventilation may be used to aid in decreasing ICP.

Anesthetized animals are generally scanned in either a sternal or dorsal recumbent position. In some situations, scanning may also be performed in a lateral recumbent position. This may be necessary if there is a suspicion of an associated cervical instability. Regardless of position, having the animal straight in the bore of the magnetic is important. Asymmetrical imaging of the animal often results in images that are difficult to interpret, leading to erroneous diagnoses.

The receiver coils most often used for dog intracranial MRI studies are human knee coils. Smaller wrist coils are preferable for smaller dogs (*e.g.*, toy breeds) and cats, whereas larger coils, including human head coils and neck coils, may be needed for the largest dogs. Some head coils are not open on both ends. This makes scanning of intubated animals difficult due to the presence of the endotracheal tube. Sternal (prone in humans) positioning is favored due to less pulmonary compromise. Because the MRI software is intended for human patients who are most often supine (dorsally recumbent), the operator must be certain to enter the patient positioning parameters correctly to avoid errors in labeling.

In general, at least two imaging planes are obtained. Transverse (axial) images perpendicular to the length of the axis of the head and brain are considered the most useful. This position is called "coronal" in human patients due to anatomic differences.[7] Various equipment manufacturers, the operating software, and the magnetic field strength will influence parameters of the image sequences. The desirable signal from the animal is always counterbalanced by the system's electronic noise. Adequate signal-to-noise ratios must be maintained for good imaging. This becomes a paradoxical problem of requiring thicker slices for smaller animals to get significant signal. For most animals, the brain can be imaged with slices 3 to 5 mm thick with an interslice gap of about 10%. Typical sequences used are proton density and a T2-weighted series obtained at the same time, called a dual-echo spin-echo technique. T1-weighted images before and after the intravenous (IV) administration of gadolinium (Gd) contrast agent are used.[10] This element is chelated to render it nontoxic (*e.g.*, Gd-DTPA or gadopentate) and administered at a dose of 0.1 mmol/kg body weight given as an IV bolus. Larger dosages are not necessary. Additional imaging sequences include the use of gradient-echo series and various inversion recovery sequences to null out signals from fat or cerebrospinal fluid (CSF).[7]

A recent series of articles described MRI signal characteristics of common diseases of the brain.[6,9] The abnormalities visualized can generally be placed into four categories including trauma, tumors, infarction, and inflammatory/infectious abnormalities. Although most MRIs can depict lesions as small as 0.5 mm in diameter, microscopic, metabolic, or physiologic derangements are not evaluated. Importantly, many dissimilar intracranial diseases result in a common group of pathophysiologic sequelae. The sequelae that most commonly result in evident signal changes with MRI include edema, hemorrhage, and increases in abnormal cell populations. Although these pathophysiologic changes result in anatomic abnormalities, the image characteristics associated with these changes are often not specific for a single disease process.

In our hospital, a standard series of images are obtained in most instances of intracranial MRI. These include transverse images of the brain with proton density, T2-weighted, and T1-weighted before and after administration of Gd contrast agents. Additional images are performed on an individual basis depending on the results of the standard series of views. Fat suppression can be accomplished by fat saturation techniques or inversion recovery techniques.[7] Lesions in the periventricular area are better seen with a fluid attenuation inversion recovery (FLAIR sequence) to remove signal from the CSF.[7] In comatose animals, rapid sequences with reasonable resolution can be performed in approximately 1 minute.

Intracranial trauma is a common cause of acute, severe neurologic signs. Currently in most human hospitals, CT is usually used for the evaluation of the patient with acute intracranial trauma. This is generally based on the fact that acute hemorrhagic lesions may be evident earlier with CT compared with MRI. On CT, acute hemorrhage usually becomes opaque within an hour as the clot retracts. This opacity lasts a few days and then fades to normal and eventually lucency. A few hours after the injury, however, MRI sensitivity for image detection exceeds CT.[7] Traumatic lesions usually evident with MRI include hemorrhage and edema. Trauma to the calvarium is less evident, but it is most easily viewed by determining a break in the contour of the calvarium. Evaluating the fat signal from the diploic cavities of the skull can be useful in determining abnormalities of the skull. Additionally, the soft tissues external to the skull (*e.g.*, the temporalis muscles) can be evaluated for signs of exogenous injury.

Brain herniation can be appreciated on MRI in animals. With subfacial herniations, cerebral tissue is found underneath the falx cerebri and possibly extending into the opposite supratentorial space. With transtentorial herniation, the parahippocampal gyri are found dorsal to the colliculi (dorsal midbrain) and ventral to the tentorium cerebelli. This results in a flattened appearance of the colliculi. These two types of herniation are best appreciated on transverse, T2-weighted or proton density images.

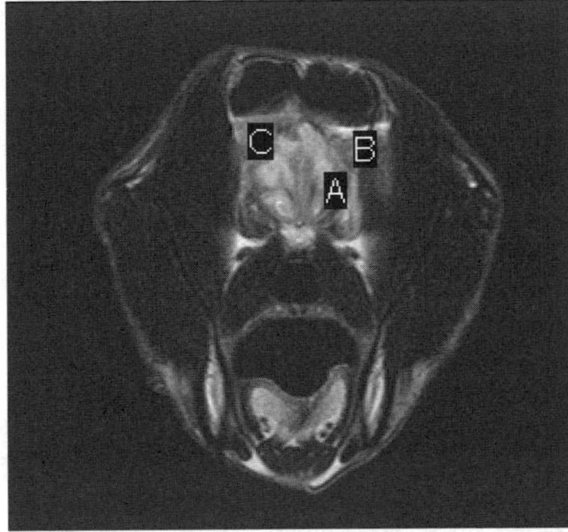

Figure 26-1
T2-weighted images of cranial trauma from a dog fight. **A**, Cerebral edema in the olfactory bulbs and/or hemorrhage. **B** and **C**, Hemorrhage with different signal intensities in the left and right frontal sinus, respectively.

Intracranial abnormalities associated with external head trauma often center around hemorrhage, hematoma formation, or perilesional edema (Fig. 26-1). Imploded fragments of bone may be seen as hypointense lesions from the dark cortical bone. Intracranial edema is noted on T2-weighted images as hyperintense and on T1-weighted images as hypointense. Vasogenic edema commonly conforms to the larger white matter tracts of the cortex (internal capsule, corona radiata).

The appearance of hemorrhage with MRI can be confusing and complex because its imaging characteristics depend on the location of the blood (*e.g.*, parenchymal, subdural, extradural), the oxygen content of the blood (*e.g.*, arterial versus venous), and the time delay between imaging and the hemorrhagic event.[7,14] On MRI, hemorrhage less than 12 to 24 hours in duration will not be differentiated from vasogenic edema. In the circulating blood, hemoglobin exists between the oxyhemoglobin state and the deoxyhemoglobin state. The iron in both oxyhemoglobin and deoxyhemoglobin is in the ferrous Fe^{++} state. When hemoglobin is removed from the high-oxygen environment of the circulation, the iron undergoes oxidation to the ferric state (Fe^{+++}), forming methemoglobin. Continued degradation forms ferric hemichromes (hemosiderin). As red blood cells break down, the various forms of hemoglobin have changing paramagnetic properties influencing the appearance of the clot on the various images (T1- and T2-weighted). Besides the form of hemoglobin present, the signal intensities of a blood clot may vary depending on the operating field strength and the type of image sequence. Hemorrhage may also vary in appearance pending on where the bleed occurred; for example, in the brain, subdural versus intraparenchymal versus subarachnoid. Table 26-1 is a guide for parenchymal hematomas.

Tumors of the brain may be either primary or metastatic. Tumors often result in a disruption of the blood–brain barrier and allow leakage of the contrast

Table 26-1. Parenchymal Hematoma Signal Intensity Changes with Iron Metabolism

Stage	Time	Compartment Hemoglobin	Intensity Relative to Gray Matter T1	T2
Hyperacute	<24 h	Intracellular Oxyhemoglobin	Isointense	Isointense
Acute	1-3 d	Intracellular Deoxyhemoglobin	Dark	Dark
Subacute Early	3+ d	Intracellular Methemoglobin	Bright	Dark
Late	7+ d	Extracellular Methemoglobin	Bright	Bright
Chronic	14+ d	Intracellular Hemosiderin	Isointense	Dark

material into the interstitial space. Recent reviews of the MRI appearance of brain tumors have been published.[6-10] Features of primary brain tumor have been reviewed. Meningiomas most commonly appear as a broad-based, extra-axial (arising outside and pushing into the parenchyma) contrast-enhancing mass on MRI. These tumors may be hemorrhagic or calcified. The MRI appearance of gliomas is varied and enhancement after contrast administration may not be present. A tumor arising within the parenchyma of the brain is characteristic. Choroid plexus tumors, because of the concentration of blood vessels within the tumor, often markedly enhance after contrast administration. Pituitary tumors may be found in the sellar or suprasellar location (Fig. 26-2).

The secondary effects of brain tumor on the intracranial nervous system may also be present. The difference of appearance of the lesion on the T2-weighted images versus the contrast-enhanced T1-weighted images give an appreciation of the degree of perilesional edema. Gliomas (glioblastoma multiforme) tend to be associated with hemorrhage more often than other primary CNS tumors; however, any tumor may disrupt vascular integrity. Metastatic tumors may be more apt to be associated with hemorrhage either because of their more aggressive behavior (hence the metastasis) or because the vasculature is the route of the metastasis. Metastatic hemangiosarcoma is an example.

Cerebrovascular infarction is less commonly described in animals as compared to humans.[11] The apparent prevalence of this condition in animals, however, is much greater than previously thought before the advent of MRI. As with other intracranial diseases, the MRI characteristics of primary cerebrovascular disease usually center around edema and hemorrhage. Enhancement of these lesions following contrast administration is variable. If significant time elapses

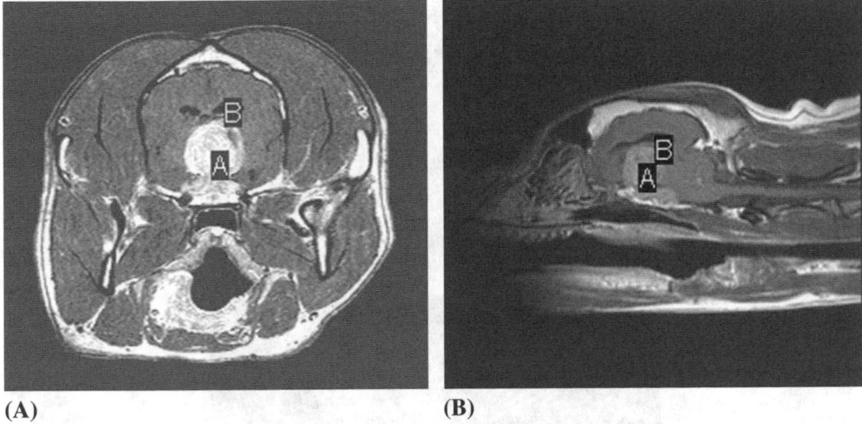

Figure 26-2
(A) A transverse image after contrast. **A**, pituitary tumor; **B**, left lateral ventricle. (B) sagittal image postcontrast. **A** and **B** label same structures.

between the acute event and subsequent imaging, an area of ring enhancement at the periphery of the lesion can be seen. Enhancement may not be seen for several days to a few weeks. The white matter tracks in the periventricular region and the cerebral gray/white matter junction are most commonly affected (Fig. 26-3). Numerous etiologies for the infarctions have been tested, including endocarditis and other cardiac conditions. The authors have noted that many of these patients have significant glomerular nephritis and presumed clotting dysfunction.

Primary brain inflammation (encephalitis or meningitis) may also result in rapid clinical deterioration. A multifocal or diffuse disease process is often seen

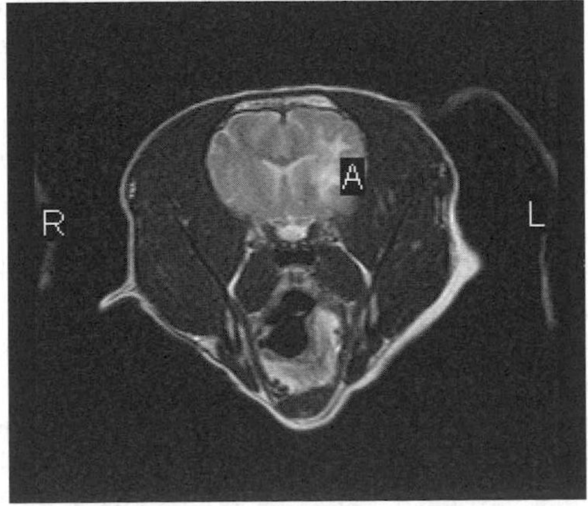

Figure 26-3
T2 transverse image, midcerebrum with white matter edema, left side **A.** This area did not enhance after administration of contrast agent.

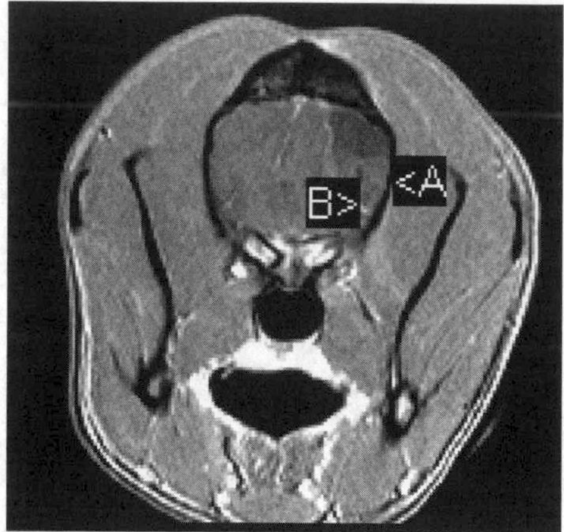

Figure 26-4
T1 postcontrast transverse image of an epidural abscess. A, The sediment in the abscess (dog imaged in sternal recumbency). B, Contrast-enhanced meninges. There is a midline shift. (Image courtesy of Veterinary Diagnostic Imaging and Cytopathology, Clackamas, OR.)

on MRI.[12] In some instances, contrast enhancement is present in the dura, suggesting more of a meningitis or epidural abscess (Fig. 26-4).

All of the aforementioned intracranial disease processes may result in brain herniation as a severe or terminal consequence.

Spinal Cord Disease

Acute spinal cord disease may result in severe paresis or paralysis that may require emergency spinal imaging. Historically, imaging of the spinal cord has been with myelography. MRI, however, is far superior in imaging the spinal cord parenchyma and the associated spinal canal.[9] In our hospital, sagittal T2-weighted sequences of the affected area are acquired initially and provide the most information as a screen for spinal disease. Additional series of transverse or dorsal images are obtained at the level of interest. A heavily T2-weighted fat-suppressed signal yields a typical myelographic appearance of the spinal cord, but it is rarely of significant help compared to conventional T2- and T1-weighted studies. The images of the myelogram can be fused to form three-dimensional volumes, which can be rotated for additional visualization of the subarachnoid column at oblique angles (Fig. 26-5).

The most common emergency conditions of the spinal cord include vertebral body fracture, intervertebral disk herniations, fibrocartilaginous emboli, and tumors. Myelitis and diskospondylitis are also evident on MRI.

When an animal has suffered an exogenous spinal trauma, vertebral body fracture or luxation may occur. Although MRI may not provide the best view of bone, the impact of the fracture on the spinal cord is often most evident (Fig. 26-6). Similar to intracranial trauma, injury to the spinal parenchyma associated

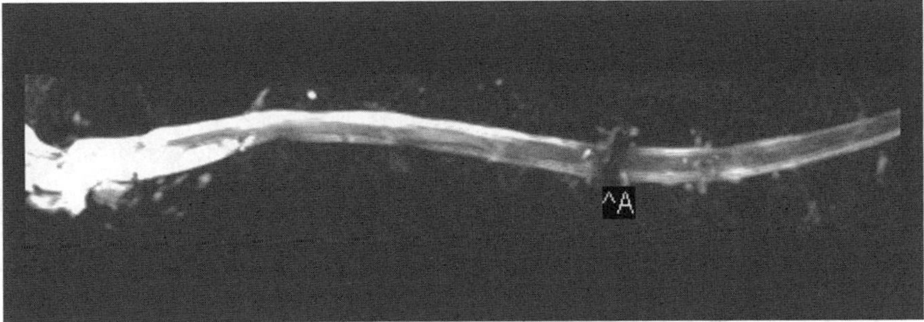

Figure 26-5
Volumetric rendering of an MRI myelogram of the cervical spine with loss of the subarachnoid ventral and dorsal columns from a disc herniation at C5-6 (A).

with a vertebral fracture or luxation often results in edema and hemorrhage. Edema is most easily seen on T2-weighted sequences where it will appear hyperintense. Similar to what is seen histologically in experimental studies of spinal trauma, the imaging changes are initially most severe in the gray matter of the spinal cord. The hyperintense spinal cord, therefore, often follows the orientation of the gray matter "butterfly" pattern centrally within the spinal cord. The central canal may be enlarged proximal to the lesion suggesting an associated hydromyelia.

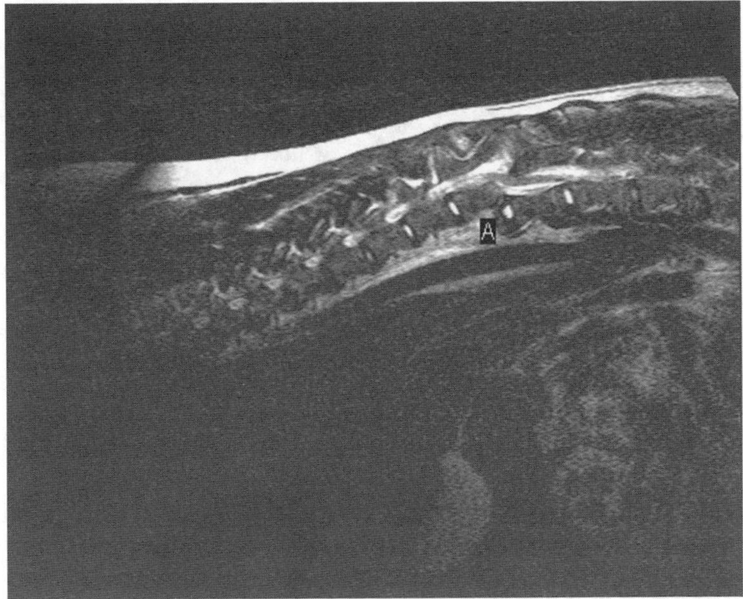

Figure 26-6
T2-weighted sagittal image of T12-13 fracture/luxation. A is next to the caudal endplate of T12. The spinal cord can be seen winding through the area. This dog went home walking normally following surgical stabilization.

Intraspinal hemorrhage may also occur with a variety of spinal injuries. Depending on the stage of hemorrhage, this change may appear similar to edema. Severe spinal disease can also result in malacia. Due to the associated increase in water content of malacia, this process may also appear hypertintense. Although MRI is excellent at determining the location and the extent of these changes, there are no currently recognized pathognomonic imaging features that suggest irreversible myleomalacia. In some instances, the spinal cord can be seen to be discontinuous, strongly suggesting a severed spinal cord. In this situation, a hopeless prognosis is often rendered.

Manipulation of the animal that has sustained an exogenous spinal injury and may have an unstable vertebral segment should be performed with caution. Similarly, manipulations for and during imaging should be performed cautiously to prevent additional iatrogenic spinal cord injury. If the animal is appropriately immobilized using a backboard or similar device, the animal may be imaged in this fixed position and in lateral recumbency using a spinal coil.

Intervertebral disk herniations are some of the most common lesions seen in animals with acute spinal cord disease. The degeneration and desiccation of the intervertebral disk and loss of hydration in the nucleus pulposus is usually easily seen with T2-weighted sequences. Intervertebral disk extrusions or protrusions are often hypointense relative to the spinal cord, indicating loss of hydration or mineralization of the disk material (Fig. 26-7). Influences on the epidural and subarachnoid space are readily appreciated on the transverse image planes with loss of signal from the subarachnoid and epidural space (Fig. 26-8).

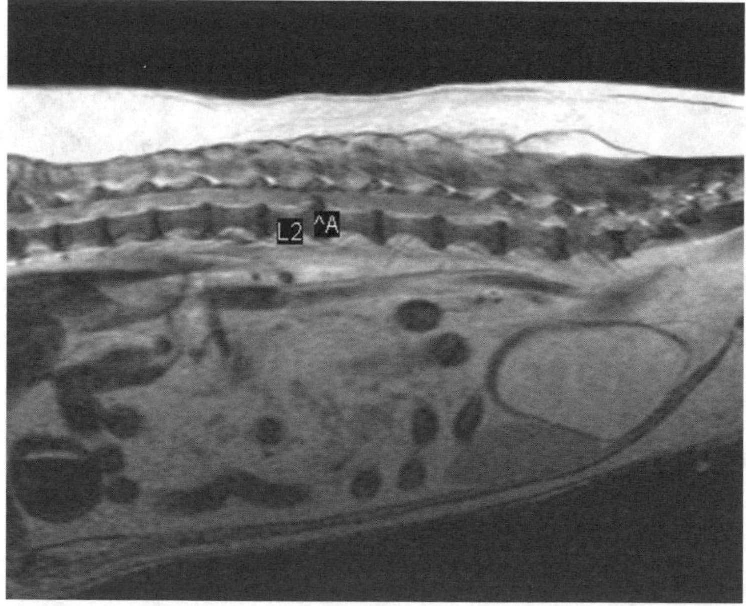

Figure 26-7
Sagittal T2 image with herniated intervertebral disc at L2-3 (A).

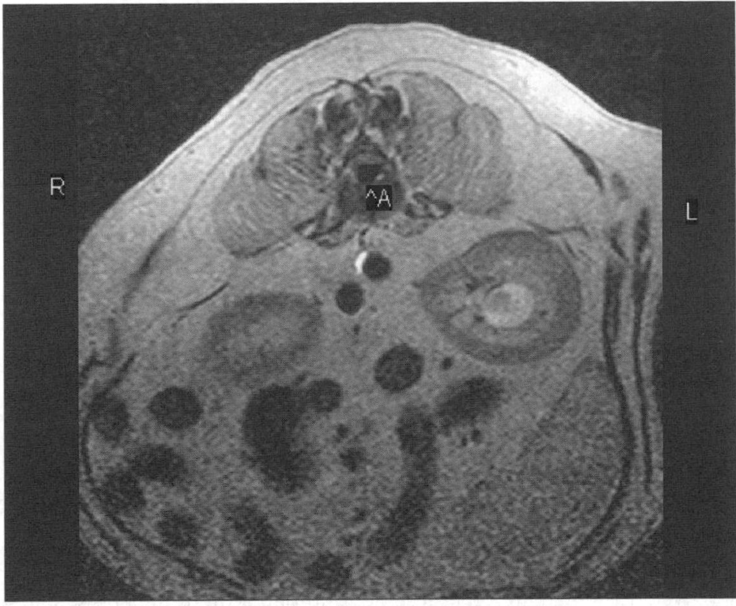

Figure 26-8
Transverse image of disc herniation at L2-3 indicating a left lateral surgical approach to the disk material (A).

Often, spinal cord edema or enlargement of the central canal of the spinal cord are seen cranial to the disk herniation. MRI provides the great benefit of accurately diagnosing the site and extent of the disk material accumulation. This greatly facilitates the surgical approach especially if a hemilaminectomy is performed.

Disease of the spinal cord vasculature is another common cause of acute, severe spinal cord damage. An area of increased signal intensity is seen on a T2-weighted sequence, indicating edema, hemorrhage, inflammation, or malacia within the parenchyma of the spinal cord. There is no evidence of any extradural spinal compression. Often there is a loss of the subarachnoid space due to cord swelling. These lesions will not undergo contrast enhancement if studied within the first few days of the initial history (Fig. 26-9). The authors have seen an acute disk herniation that was histopathologically confirmed with disk material within the spinal cord that mimicked a fibrocartilaginous embolism (FCE) (Fig. 26-10). Therefore, if an FCE lesion is seen immediately dorsal to the intervertebral disk base, this possible differential diagnosis should be considered.

Tumors of the spinal cord may also result in acute spinal deterioration.[13] Between direct imaging of the spinal cord and associated structures and MRI myelography, the typical distinctions of intramedullary, extramedullary intradural, and extramedullary extradural lesions can be identified. Most tumors of the spinal cord, meninges, or vertebral bodies undergo contrast enhancement. Lymphoma and myeloma may not undergo contrast enhancement.

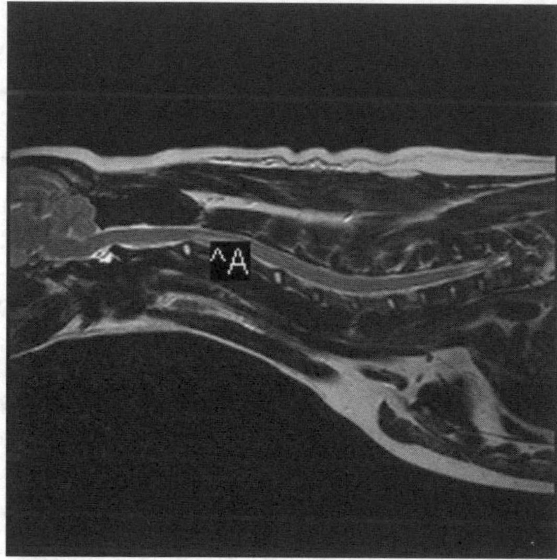

Figure 26-9
Sagittal T2-weighted image of cervical spine. Dog had acute tetraparesis. Spinal cord edema is labeled A in the C3 region. This area did not enhance with contrast and was considered an FCE. The dog recovered with conservative therapy.

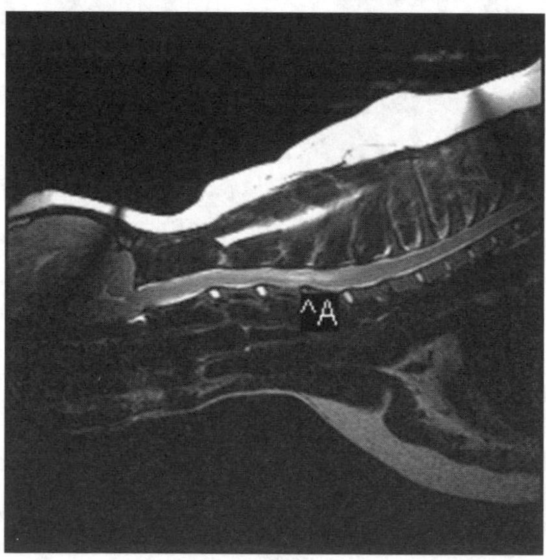

Figure 26-10
Transverse T2-weighted image of cervical spine. Dog had acute tetraparesis. Histopathologically confirmed disk material was obtained from the edematous cord region at C4-5 (A).

Non-CNS Studies

Emergency MRI for non-CNS disease is generally related to acute hemorrhagic disorders. Such hemorrhagic studies above the diaphragm of an emergency nature are generally of the nasal cavity. Most common lesions seen are tumors and chronic inflammation. A distinction can be made between masses of the nasal cavity, fluid accumulation from an obstructive lesion, and primarily lytic lesions associated with fungal rhinitis and foreign bodies (Fig. 26-11).

Thoracic MRI studies of the heart and lungs are possible, and motion artifacts can be relieved from cardiac or respiratory gating. Excellent studies of the heart and mediastinum are possible. Lesions of the lung can be readily appreciated. CT is superior for visualization of small metastases to the lung. Due to the need to physiologic gate these studies, it is generally suggested that studies of the thorax not be performed on an emergency basis.

Emergency MRI studies below the diaphragm generally involve acute abdominal fluid accumulation. Veterinary patients are anesthetized for MRI, which stops gastrointestinal motility, and with minimal abdominal movement during respiration, the abdominal MRI series has excellent resolution. Portosystemic shunts and the associated hepatic encephalopathy may be seen on an emergency basis and the shunts can be diagnosed via MRI angiography (Fig. 26-12).[15] All major abdominal viscera, including the adrenals, pancreas, kidneys, liver, spleen, gallbladder, urinary bladder, prostate, and ovaries can be readily visualized on MRI. Tumors of the organs and intra-abdominal metastases of these tumors are readily visualized. MRI angiography is an easily accomplished study.

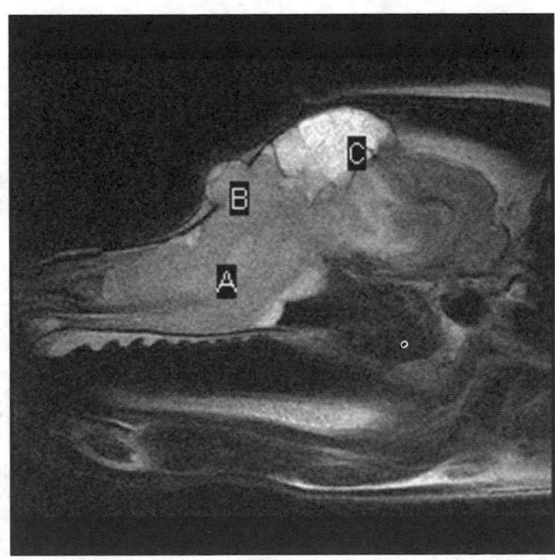

Figure 26-11
T2-weighted sagittal image of a nasal tumor (A) eroding through the nasal bone (B) and causing an obstructive sinusitis (C). (Image courtesy of Veterinary Diagnostic Imaging and Cytopathology, Inc. Clackamas, OR.)

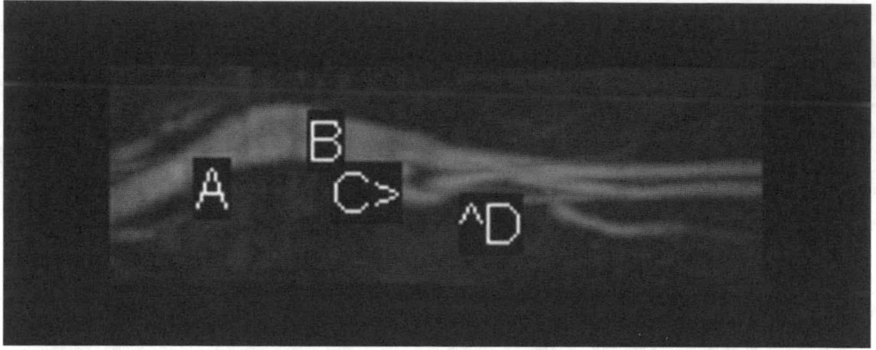

Figure 26-12
Volumetric rendering of an abdominal MR venogram. A, level of the diaphragm; B, vena cava; C, shunt; and D, portal vein.

REFERENCES

1. Jones JC, Cartee RE, Bartels JE: Computed tomographic anatomy of the canine lumbosacral spine. *Vet Radiol Ultrasound* 36:91, 1995.
2. Adams WH, Daniel GB, Pardo AD, *et al.*: Magnetic resonance imaging of the caudal lumbar and lumbosacral spine in 13 dogs (1990–1993). *Vet Radiol Ultrasound* 36:3, 1995.
3. Kippenes H, Gavin PR, Tucker RS, *et al.*: Magnetic resonance scanning techniques and image characteristics in evaluation of canine spinal tumors [abstract]. *Vet Radiol Ultrasound* 39:580, 1998.
4. Karkkainen M, Punto LU, Tulamo RM: Magnetic resonance imaging of canine degenerative lumbar spine diseases. *Vet Radiol Ultrasound* 34:399, 1993.
5. Turrel JM, Fike JR, LeCouteur RA, *et al.*: Computed tomographic characteristics of primary brain tumors in 50 dogs. *J Am Vet Med Assoc*, 188:851, 1986.
6. Kraft SL, Gavin PR, DeHaan C, *et al.*: Retrospective review of 50 canine intracranial tumors evaluated by magnetic resonance imaging. *J Vet Intern Med* 11:218, 1997.
7. Stark DD, Bradley WG Jr: Magnetic Resonance Imaging, vol 1, 3rd ed. St. Louis: Mosby, 1999.
8. Tidwell AS: Advanced imaging concepts: a pictorial glossary of CT and MRI technology. *Clin Tech Small Anim Pract* 14:65, 1999.
9. Adams WH: The spine. *Clin Tech Small Anim Pract* 14:148, 1999.
10. Tucker RL, Gavin PR: Brain imaging. *Vet Clin North Am Small Anim Pract*, 26: 735, 1996.
11. Bagley RS, Anderson WI, de Lahunta A, *et al.*: Cerebellar infarction caused by arterial thrombosis in a dog. *J Am Vet Med Assoc* 192:785, 1988.
12. Thomas WB: Nonneoplastic disorders of the brain. *Clin Tech Small Anim Pract* 14: 125, 1999.
13. Kippenes H, Gavin PR, Bagley RS, *et al.*: Magnetic resonance imaging features of tumors of the spine and spinal cord in dogs. *Vet Radiol* 40:627, 1999.
14. Gavin PR: Imaging dogs with brain tumors. Proceedings 12th Annual ACVIM Forum. San Francisco, CA, June 1994, p 922.
15. Seguin B, Tobias KM, Gavin PR, Tucker RL: Use of magnetic resonance angiography for diagnosis of portosystemic shunts in dogs. *Vet Radiol Ultrasound* 40:251, 1999.

27
Severity of Disease and Outcome Prediction

Lesley G. King

INTRODUCTION

Systems that place a numerical score on disease severity are widely used in human medicine,[1-4] and are beginning to be created and studied in veterinary medicine. In the emergency room and ICU, a variety of systems are available that potentially have multiple purposes. Some are used to globally classify the degree of physiologic derangement in any critically ill animal regardless of the diagnosis; others are designed for application to specific situations, for example trauma. These systems give us a method to objectively classify the severity of disease, in other words, predict the outcome of survival or mortality.

This information must be used with care. In general, scoring systems in veterinary medicine should not be used to make clinical decisions about individual patients because the statistical information is not accurate enough for this purpose. Many of our veterinary systems have not yet been adequately validated; they do not give a level of predictive accuracy that compares with the systems available for human medicine. Veterinary scoring systems should be used to categorize patients into groups with similar disease severity, which then can allow for group comparisons for clinical trials or for quality control within and between institutions.

SCORING SYSTEMS FOR SMALL ANIMALS

A variety of scoring systems have been developed in small animal emergency and critical care.[5-12] Equations have also been developed for use in large animals, but are beyond the scope of this chapter.[13-16] The statistical accuracy of these systems can be assessed by evaluating the area under the receiver operating characteristic curve, sensitivity and specificity, odds ratios, and positive and negative predictive indices.

The predictive accuracy of logistic regression equations is usually estimated using receiver operating characteristic (ROC) curves, which demonstrate the tradeoff between the true positive rate (sensitivity) and the false positive rate (1 minus specificity) at varying predictive cut-points. The area under the ROC curve (AUC) represents the probability that a randomly selected "survivor" has a greater probability of survival than a randomly selected "nonsurvivor," and is therefore a measure of the predictive value of the equation. The higher the AUC value (closer to 1), the more accurate the equation. In human outcome prediction equations, AUC values are commonly obtained as high as 0.85 to 0.90.

The Survival Prediction Index

The survival prediction index (SPI) is a method of scoring disease severity of critically ill dogs in the ICU.[5-7] The system uses parameters that are independent of diagnosis and are part of the routine monitoring and evaluation of patients in the ICU. Data for this calculation can be collected early during hospitalization and before interventions being tested in clinical trials. This system was developed using logistic regression analysis, with data from an estimation sample of 499 dogs, collected in four different small animal CCUs in the United States, and validated using data from a randomly generated validation sample of another 125 dogs.[6] A backward elimination procedure was used to remove variables that did not contribute to the prediction of survival, resulting in a final equation that includes seven variables. For the purposes of data analysis, survival was defined as being alive after 30 days, with day 1 defined as the day of admission to the ICU.

To calculate the SPI, the physiologic variables are recorded within 24 hours of admission to the CCU. When multiple measurements of a variable are obtained, for example, packed cell volume, the most abnormal value in that 24-hour period is included in the calculation. SPI is calculated as follows:

$$\begin{aligned}\text{logit}(P) = {} & 0.3273 + 0.0108(\text{mean arterial pressure}) \\ & - 0.0102(\text{respiratory rate}) - 0.2183(\text{creatinine}) \\ & + 0.0164(\text{packed cell volume}) + 0.3553(\text{albumin}) \\ & - 0.1184(\text{age}) - 0.8069(\text{medical/surgical})\end{aligned}$$

where medical/surgical is equal to 1 if the animal is from a medical service and 0 if it is from a surgical service. The numerical values are entered into the linear equation to give a value for logit P, which is the log odds of survival. An exponential equation is used to solve for P, the predicted probability of survival.

$$SPI = P = \frac{e^{\log it(p)}}{[1 + e^{\log it(P)}]}$$

The predicted probability (SPI) value thereby obtained is within the range from 0 to 1, with 0 indicating the most severe disease and 1 indicating no mortality risk.

The AUC for the veterinary SPI equation estimation sample was 0.76, and that of the validation sample was 0.71. The estimated positive and negative predictive values at the optimal cut-point were 75.6% and 64.7%, respectively. The estimated sensitivity and specificity at this cut-point were 83.3% and 53.3%, respectively.[6]

The lower AUC values obtained in the veterinary equation may be attributed to the relatively small numbers of animals used compared to many thousands of patients in comparable human studies. The predictive accuracy of this equation is not great enough for this system to be used for prediction of outcome in individual patients, but it is high enough to provide a useful statistical tool for risk stratification in clinical research studies.

Preliminary studies of this tool suggest that it may prove to be more accurate in the subset of dogs admitted to the ICU with a medical problem (AUC = 0.75), compared with surgical admissions (AUC = 0.70).[6] Another study evaluated the utility of serial estimations of the SPI on days 1 and 3 of ICU hospitalization.[7] We hypothesized that data obtained later during hospitalization, closer to the time of the actual outcome, might provide a more accurate prediction. In a group of 64 dogs, the AUC was higher using day 3 measurements (AUC = 0.70) than that obtained using day 1 measurements (AUC = 0.65), but the increase in the AUC value was not statistically significant.[7] A pilot study is underway to generate a similar SPI equation for critically ill cats in the ICU.

Survival Prediction in High-Risk Canine Laparotomy Patients

A prediction equation was developed using a group of 169 dogs admitted to the ICU following laparotomy.[8] Seven numerical variables were tested: packed cell volume, total protein (TP), platelet count, albumin, alkaline phosphatase, bilirubin, and age. The overall mortality rate of this group of dogs was 18%. Of the parameters tested, only age, total protein, and platelet count were significantly different between survivors and nonsurvivors.[8] The following equation was generated based on that data:

$$\begin{aligned}\text{Logit (P)} = {} & -0.6727 + 1.247(\text{AGE}) \\ & - 1.103(\text{platelet 1}) - 1.436(\text{platelet 2}) \\ & - 1.999(\text{TP1}) - 2.579(\text{TP2})\end{aligned}$$

where: age 5 years or younger, AGE = 0; age over 5 years, AGE = 1; platelet count less than 201,000, platelet 1 = 0 and platelet 2 = 0; platelet count between 201,000 and 400,000, platelet 1 = 1 and platelet 2 = 0; and platelet count above 400,000, platelet 1 = 0 and platelet 2 = 1; total protein less than 5.6 g/dL, TP1 = 0 and TP2 = 0; total protein between 5.6 and 6 g/dL, TP1 = 1 and TP2 = 0; and total protein greater than 6 g/dL, TP1 = 0 and TP2 = 1.

$$\text{Probability of mortality} = P = \frac{e^{\log it(P)}}{[1 + e^{\log it(P)}]}$$

Unfortunately, the accuracy of prediction by this equation is not reported. Further studies are needed to test this and other equations.

Animal Trauma Triage Scoring System

Trauma scoring is another numerical characterization of disease severity. Scoring systems applied to more uniform patients (*i.e.*, those with similar categories of disease) might be expected to be more accurate than those derived from and applied to a heterogeneous group. The Animal Trauma Triage (ATT) scoring system assigns scores to clinical findings in 6 categories on a 0 to 3 scale, where 0 indicates slight or no injury and 3 indicates severe injury, using the criteria listed in Table 27-1.[9] The six scores are added together to give a total

Table 27-1. The Animal Trauma Triage Scoring System[9]

Grade	Perfusion	Cardiac	Respiratory	Eye/Muscle/ Integument	Skeletal	Neurological
0	mm pink & moist CRT –2 sec Rectal temp ≥37.8°C (100°F) Femoral pulses strong or bounding	HR: C – 60–140 F – 120–200 Normal sinus rhythm	Regular resp rate with no stridor No abdominal component to resp	Abrasion, laceration; none *or* partial thickness Eye; no fluorescein uptake	Weight bearing in 3 or 4 limbs, no palpable fracture or joint laxity	Central: conscious, alert →sl dull; interest in surroundings Periph: normal spinal reflexes; purposeful movement and nociception in all limbs
1	mm hyperemic *or* pale pink; mm tacky CRT 0-2 sec Rectal temp ≥37.8°C (100°F) Femoral pulses fair	HR: C – 140–180 F – 200–260 Normal sinus rhythm or VPCs <20/min	Mildly ↑ resp rate & effort, ± some abdominal component Mildly ↑ upper airway sounds	Abrasion, laceration: Full thickness, *no* deep tissue involvement Eye: corneal Laceration/ulcer, not perforated	Closed appendicular/rib fx or any mandibular fx Single joint laxity/ luxation incl. sacroiliac joint Pelvic fx with unilateral intact SI-ilium-acetab Single limb open/ closed fx at or below carpus/tarsus	Central: conscious but dull, depressed, withdrawn Periph: abnormal spinal reflexes with purposeful movement and nociception intact in all 4 limbs

2	mm v pale pink & v tacky CRT 2-3 sec Rectal temp <37.8°C (100°F) Detectable but poor femoral pulses	HR: C → 180 F → 260 Consistent arrhythmia	Moderately ↑ resp effort with abdomin component, elbow abduction Moderately ↑ upper airway sounds	Abrasion, laceration: full thickness, deep tissue involvement, and arteries, nerves, muscles intact Eye: corneal perforation, punctured globe or proptosis	Multiple grade 1 conditions (see above) Single long bone open fx Above carpus/tarsus with cortical bone preserved Nonmandibular skull fx	Central: unconscious but responds to noxious stimuli Periph: absent purposeful movement with intact nociception in 2 or more limbs *or* nociception absent *only* in 1 limb; ↓ anal and/or tail tone
3	Mm gray, blue, or white CRT 0.3 sec Rectal temp ≥37.8°C (100°F) Femoral pulse not detected	HR: C ≤60 F ≤120 Erratic arrhythmia	Marked respiratory effort *or* Gasping/agonal respiration or irregularly timed effort Little or no detectable air passage	Penetration to thoracic/abdo cavity Abrasion, laceration: full thickness, deep tissue involvement, and artery, nerve, or muscle compromised	Vertebral body Fracture/luxation except coccygeal Multiple long bone open fx above tarsus/carpus single long bone open fx Above tarsus/carpus with loss of cortical bone	Central: nonresponsive to all stimuli; refractory seizures Periph: absent nociception in 2 or more limbs; absent tail or perianal nociception

Table 27-2. ASA Classification of Physical Status[10]

Category	Physical Status	Example
I	Normal healthy patient	No discernable disease
II	Mild systemic disease	Fracture without shock, skin tumor, localized infection
III	Severe systemic disease	Fever, dehydration, anemia, cachexia
IV	Severe systemic disease that is a constant threat to life	Uremia, toxemia, severe hypovolemia, heart failure, sepsis
V	Moribund patient not expected to survive 24 h with or without surgery	Extreme shock, terminal malignancy, severe trauma

ATT score, with a highest possible score of 18. This system defined the end point as survival 7 days following presentation.[9]

This scoring system was tested retrospectively in a group of 76 dogs and 25 cats with a survival rate of 77.2%, and prospectively in a group of 62 dogs and 26 cats with a survival rate of 85.2%. In both groups, there was a significant difference between ATT scores of survivors and nonsurvivors. Odds ratio analysis of the prospectively collected data demonstrated that each increase of 1 in the ATT score resulted in 2.3 times decreased likelihood of survival.[9]

American Society of Anesthesiologists Anesthetic Scores

The American Society of Anesthesiologists (ASA) classification of the physical status of the patient (Table 27-2) is a different scoring system that can be applied prior to initiation of anesthesia.[10] This simple classification system forces the anesthetist to evaluate the patient's condition, may be valuable in selection of anesthetic drugs, defines the extent of monitoring needed for the patient, and should be part of every anesthesia record.[10]

Small Animal Coma Scale

The Glasgow Coma Scale is a routine part of the assessment of human patients with head trauma. An analogous small animal coma scale has been proposed for use in dogs with craniocerebral trauma.[11,12] This numerical scoring system defines categories of neurologic function and assigns numerical scores that reflect the patient's status (Table 27-3). The three categories of neurologic function included are level of consciousness, brainstem reflexes, and motor function. Scores of 1 to 6 are assigned in each category, from worst to best status, with a total possible score between 3 and 18. A score of 3 to 8 is thought to represent the worst prognosis, 9 to 14 a poor to fair prognosis, and 15 to 18 a good prognosis.[11,12] This system has not been objectively tested in a large group

Table 27-3. The Small Animal Coma Scale[11,12]

Points	Motor Activity	Brainstem Reflexes	Level of Consciousness
6	Normal gait, normal spinal reflexes	Normal pupillary light responses and oculocephalic reflexes	Occasional periods of alertness and responsive to environment
5	Hemiparesis, tetraparesis or decorticate activity	Slow pupillary light responses and normal to reduced oculocephalic reflexes	Depression or delirium, capable of responding to environment but response may be inappropriate
4	Recumbent, intermittent extensor rigidity	Bilateral unresponsive miosis with normal to reduced oculocephalic reflexes	Semicomatose, responsive to visual stimuli
3	Recumbent, constant extensor rigidity	Pinpoint pupils with reduced to absent oculocephalic reflexes	Semicomatose, responsive to auditory stimuli
2	Recumbent, constant extensor rigidity with opisthotonus	Unilateral, unresponsive mydriasis with reduced to absent oculocephalic reflexes	Semicomatose, responsive only to repeated noxious stimuli
1	Recumbent, hypotonia of muscles, depressed or absent spinal reflexes	Bilateral, unresponsive mydriasis with reduced to absent oculocephalic reflexes	Comatose, unresponsive to repeated noxious stimuli

of patients, but it may prove helpful in categorizing groups of patients in the future.

APPLICATIONS AND INDICATIONS OF SCORING SYSTEMS

All veterinary scoring systems are developed for the same purpose: to categorize patients into groups with similar severity of disease. This type of scoring system may have some utility for triage of patients to objectively and prospectively allocate resources of staffing and equipment. In individual animals, however, it is arguable whether these systems provide additional information over that obtained by the thoughtful evaluation of an experienced clinician.

The real value of all scoring systems is their use in categorizing groups of patients for research studies. Scoring systems such as the APACHE scoring system are used extensively in human medicine to classify patients into groups for clinical trials.[1,2] To document that a management strategy is associated with an improved outcome when two groups are compared, it is important to objectively demonstrate that the two groups had a similar severity of disease to start with. Similarly, these scoring systems can also be used if a specific test result is being studied to determine its relationship with the severity of disease. Objective characterization of the severity of disease also allows comparison of actual outcomes between institutions and within institutions over time.

LIMITATIONS OF SCORING SYSTEMS

The study of scoring systems in veterinary medicine is still in its infancy. Because they are often derived from relatively small groups of patients in comparison to similar human systems, veterinary scoring systems and prediction equations are not as accurate as those of human medicine. Although they provide useful information for statistical use for clinical research studies, they should not be used alone to make clinical decisions about management of individual patients. Further study needs to be done to refine these systems, to include many more patients in both estimation and validation samples, and to generate more accurate equations and scoring systems.

REFERENCES

1. Knaus WA, Draper EA, Wagner DP, *et al.*: APACHE II: a severity of disease classification system. *Crit Care Med* 13:818, 1985.
2. Knaus WA, Wagner DP, Draper EA, *et al.*: The APACHE III prognostic system: risk prediction of hospital mortality for critically ill hospitalized adults. *Chest* 100: 1619, 1991.
3. Le Gail JR, Lemeshow S, Saulnier F: A new simplified acute physiology score (SAPS II) based on a European/North American multicenter study. *JAMA* 270:2957, 1993.
4. Lemeshow S, Teres D, Klar J, *et al.*: Mortality probability models (MPM II) based on an international cohort of intensive care unit patients. *JAMA* 270:2478, 1993.
5. King LG, Stevens MT, Ostro ENS, *et al.*: A model for prediction of survival in critically ill dogs. *J Vet Emerg Crit Care* 4:85, 1994. (Correction in *JVECC* 5:6, 1995.)
6. King LG, Wohl JS, Manning AM, *et al.*: The survival prediction index: a multicenter study to validate and re-estimate a model of risk stratification for clinical research trials. *Am J Vet Res*. In press.
7. King LG, Fordyce H, Campellone M, *et al.*: Serial estimation of survival prediction indices does not improve outcome prediction in critically ill dogs with naturally occurring disease. *Am J Vet Res*. In press.
8. Hardie EM, Jayawickrama J, Duff LC, *et al.*: Prognostic indicators of survival in high-risk canine surgery patients. *J Vet Emerg Crit Care* 5:42, 1995.
9. Rockar RA, Drobatz KJ, Shofer FS: Development of a scoring system for the veterinary trauma patient. *J Vet Emerg Crit Care* 4:77, 1994.
10. Thurmon JC, Tranquilli WJ, Benson GJ, *et al.*: Considerations for general anesthesia. *In* Lumb WV and Jones EW, eds.: Veterinary Anesthesia. Baltimore: Williams & Wilkins, 1996, p 22.
11. Shores A: Development of a coma scale for dogs: prognostic value in cranio-cerebral trauma. Proceedings of the 6th annual ACVIM Forum, 1988, p 251.
12. Shores A: Small animal coma scale revisited. Proceedings of the 10th annual ACVIM Forum, 1992, p 748.
13. Reeves MJ, Curtis CR, Salman MD, *et al.*: Multivariable prediction model for the need for surgery in horses with colic. *Am J Vet Res* 52:1903, 1991.
14. Hoffman AM, Staempfli HR, Willan A: Prognostic variables for survival of neonatal foals under intensive care. *J Vet Intern Med* 6:89, 1992.
15. Furr M, Tinker MK, Edens L: Prognosis for neonatal foals in an intensive care unit. *J Vet Intern Med* 11:183, 1997.
16. Lofstedt J, Dohoo IR, Duizer G: Model to predict septicemia in diarrheic calves. *J Vet Intern Med* 13: 81, 1999.

SECTION IV
Cardiovascular Disorders

28
Cardiopulmonary Arrest

Wayne E. Wingfield

INTRODUCTION

Cardiopulmonary arrest is defined as the abrupt, unexpected cessation of spontaneous and effective ventilation and systemic perfusion (circulation). Cardiopulmonary resuscitation (CPR) provides artificial ventilation and circulation until advanced life support can be provided and spontaneous circulation and ventilation restored. CPR is divided into three support stages: basic life support, advanced life support, and prolonged life support.

PATHOGENESIS

Cardiopulmonary arrest is usually the result of a cardiac dysrhythmia. This arrest may be the result of primary cardiac disease or diseases that affect other organs. In animals, arrest most frequently occurs with diseases of the respiratory system (pneumonia, laryngeal paralysis, neoplasia, thoracic effusions, and aspiration pneumonitis), as a result of severe multisystemic disease, trauma, and following cardiac dysrhythmias. Predisposing causes of cardiopulmonary arrest include vagal stimulation, cellular hypoxia, acid-base and electrolyte abnormalities, anesthetic agents, trauma, and systemic/metabolic diseases.

CLINICAL PRESENTATION

Warning signs of cardiopulmonary arrest include changes in the respiratory rate, depth, or pattern; a weak or irregular pulse; bradycardia; hypotension; unexplained changes in the depth of anesthesia; cyanosis; and hypothermia. The diagnosis of arrest includes absence of ventilation and cyanosis ("respiratory arrest"), absence of a palpable pulse (the pulse will disappear when the systolic pressure is <60 mm Hg), absence of heart sounds (heart sounds will disappear when the systolic pressure is <50 mm Hg), and dilation of the pupils.

TREATMENT

Readiness for patients at risk for arrest also includes preparing an emergency drug card for each patient. An example of this card can be found at the following internet address:

http://www.cvmbs.colostate.edu/clinsci/wing/emdrugs.html

The emergency drug card lists drug volumes required based on dosage, species, and body weight of the patient. In the emergency, the veterinarian is only required to know which drug to give. With an emergency drug card, the dosage is already calculated, thus accelerating the approach to resuscitation.

A well-stocked "crash cart" is essential. Items for the crash cart are listed in Table 28-1. The crash cart should be checked daily and missing items replaced.

Table 28-1. Recommended Minimum Contents for a Crash Cart

Crash Cart Item	Number/Size or Dosage	Action
Cuffed endotracheal tubes	3–12 mm, 2 each	Airway
Oxygen	Anesthetic machine	Oxygen
Laryngoscope	Small and large blade	Airway
Gauze	1 roll	Tie endotracheal tubes in place
Syringes	3, 6, 12, and 20 mL (6 of each)	Drug administration
Needles	14, 16, 18, 20, 22, and 25 gauge, 6 of each	Drug administration
IV catheters	16, 18, and 20 gauge (3 of each)	Drug administration
Intraosseous catheters or bone marrow needles	18 and 20 gauge (2 of each)	Drug administration
Thoracocentesis setup	60-mL syringe, 3-way stopcock, IV extension set, and 20-gauge, 2.5-cm needle	Thoraco- or pericardiocentesis
Electrical defibrillator	Adult, pediatric, and internal paddles (4 J/kg)	Defibrillation or cardioversion
Epinephrine	0.2 mg/kg IV or 0.6 mg/kg IT	α- and β-agonist
Naloxone	0.03 mg/kg IV or 0.06 mg/kg IT	Opiate antagonist
Sodium bicarbonate	0.25-1 mEq/kg IV	Alkalinizing agent
Magnesium chloride	2 g over 2 min	Chemical defibrillator
Bretylium tosylate	10 mg/kg IV	Chemical defibrillator, ventricular antiarrhythmic
Lidocaine	2-4 mg/kg IV bolus followed by 50–100 μg/kg CRI	Class 1B ventricular antiarrhythmic
Atropine sulfate	0.04 mg/kg IV or 0.12 mg/kg IT	Parasympatholytic

IV, intravenous; IT, intratracheal; CRI, constant rate infusion.

A checklist of crash cart contents is also useful to ensure consistency. This checklist should be dated, initialed, and completed by a designated technician. Desirable features in the crash cart include mobility, organization, and only emergency drugs. Too often a plethora of drugs are put in containers such as a fishing tackle box. These contain too many drugs for ease of convenience during resuscitation.

BASIC LIFE SUPPORT

The ABCs of basic life support are **A**irway, **B**reathing, and **C**irculation (Fig. 28-1).

Airway

The first step is establishment of the unresponsiveness and assessment of the airway. Quickly check the airway for foreign materials (bones, blood clots, fractured mandible, vomitus). Occasionally clearing the airway is achieved by maneuvers such as the Heimlich maneuver. Rarely a surgical or needle tracheostomy is required. Position the animal in *ventral* recumbency in preparation for endotracheal intubation. Accurately place the endotracheal tube with the use of a laryngoscope. Correct placement is best achieved with an end-tidal carbon dioxide (CO_2) monitoring. If the endotracheal tube is accidentally placed in the esophagus, little or no CO_2 is present in the expired gas. The concentration of expired CO_2 changes when blood flow to the lungs changes and is an indirect indicator of stroke volume and systemic blood flow. When ventilation is controlled, end-tidal CO_2 is linearly related to stroke volume even during low blood flow rates as occur during CPR.[1] Experimentally, dogs with the highest levels of end-tidal CO_2 also had the highest rate of survival from cardiac arrest.[2] The higher CO_2 excretion in survivors likely indicates better tissue perfusion during CPR.

Breathing

Once the airway is cleared and established, and the animal is assessed to be not breathing, two long (1.5 second), artificially ventilated breaths are administered with 100% oxygen (O_2). If spontaneous breathing does not occur, continued artificial ventilation is provided at a rate of 12 to 20 breaths per minute and an airway pressure of 20 to 30 cm H_2O. Again, end-tidal CO_2 can be used to monitor ventilation during low flow conditions. During low blood flow states a doubling of the minute ventilation decreases end-tidal CO_2 by 50%, whereas when minute ventilation decreases 50%, end-tidal CO_2 doubles.[3] Errors in interpretation may occur if both ventilation and perfusion are not constant.

Another new technique for supplying O_2 during CPR is with continuous flow insufflation through a plastic catheter whose tip is placed above the tracheal bifercation.[4] Using an O_2 flow of 0.2 L/kg/min, dogs were successfully maintained until spontaneous ventilation returned. Although the dogs in this study did not have cardiac arrest, this technique may be effective in delivering O_2 to arrested dogs.

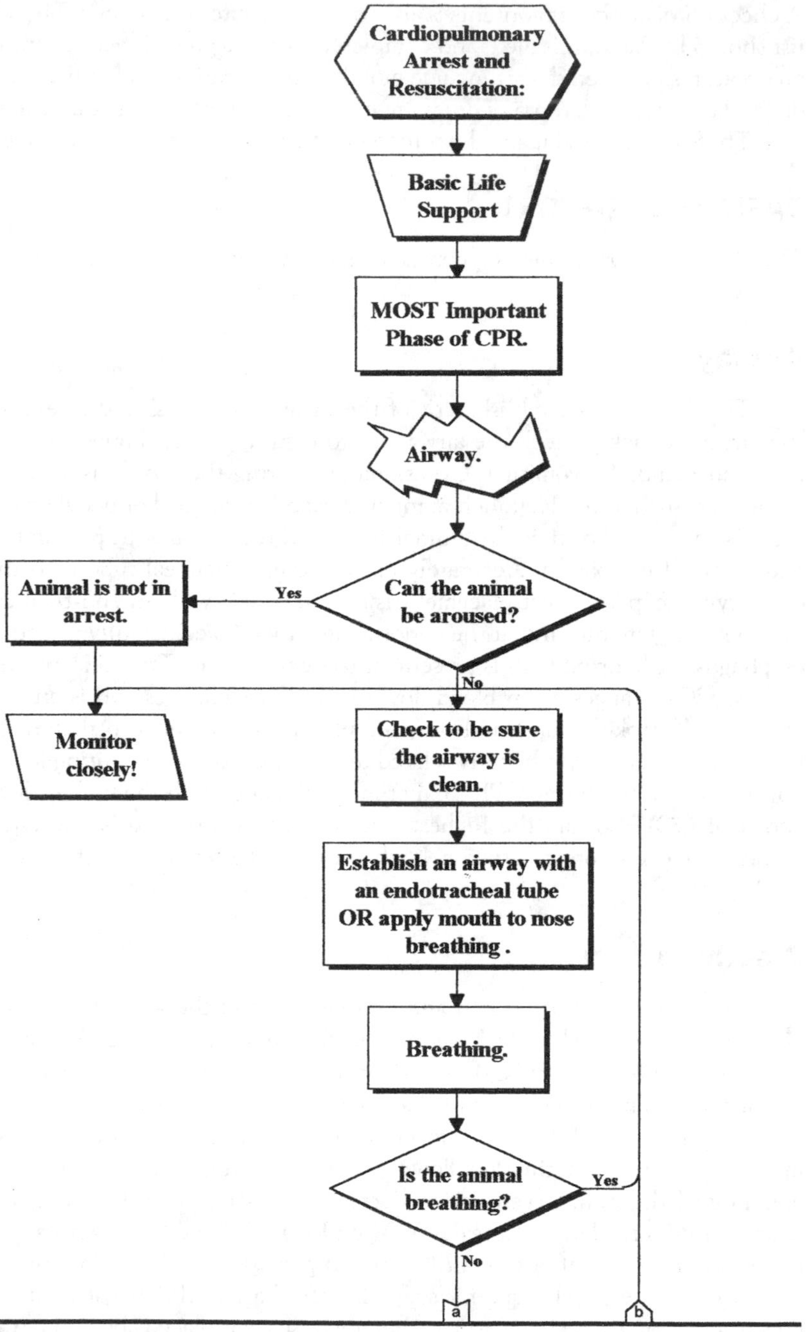

Cardiopulmonary Arrest and Resuscitation:

Basic Life Support

MOST Important Phase of CPR.

Airway.

Can the animal be aroused?

Yes

Animal is not in arrest.

Monitor closely!

No

Check to be sure the airway is clean.

Establish an airway with an endotracheal tube OR apply mouth to nose breathing .

Breathing.

Is the animal breathing?

Yes

No

a

b

Figure 28-1
Flow sheet for basic life support in animals.

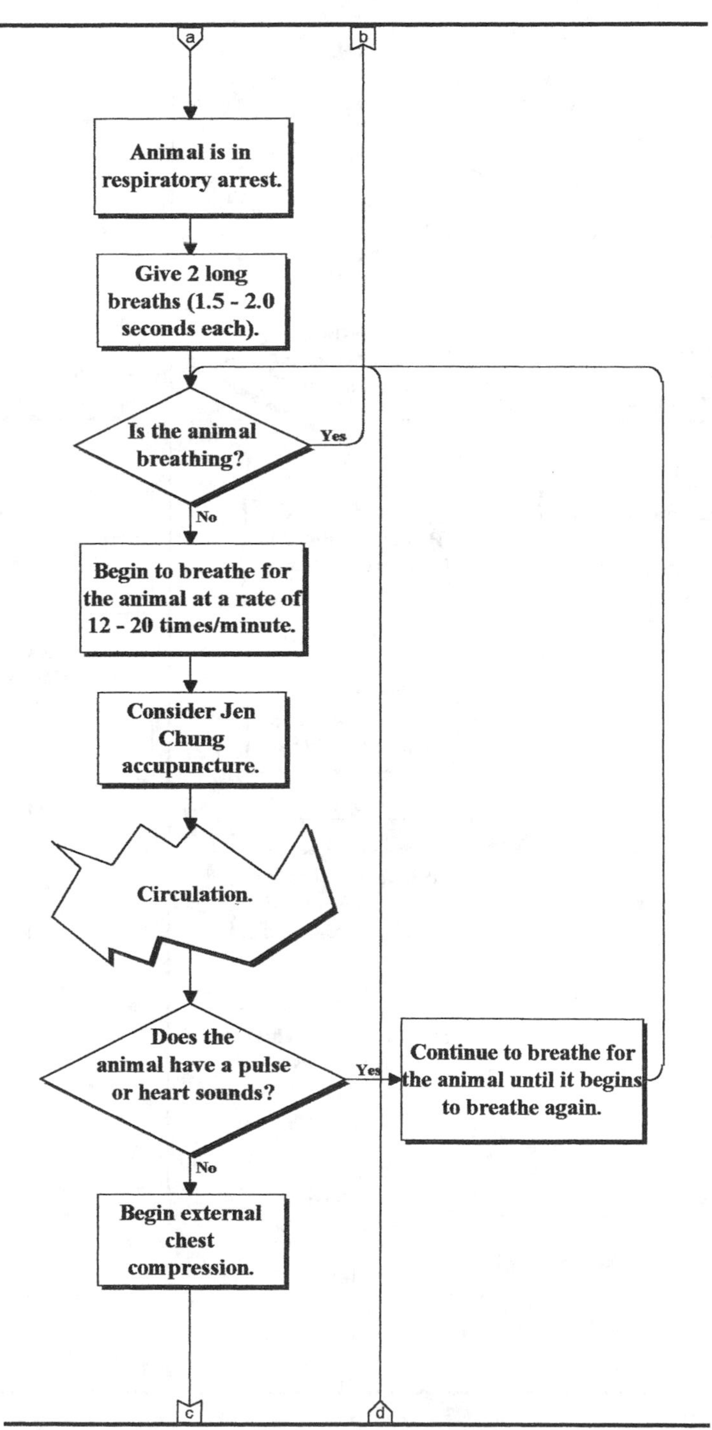
a
b
Animal is in respiratory arrest.
Give 2 long breaths (1.5 - 2.0 seconds each).
Is the animal breathing?
Yes
No
Begin to breathe for the animal at a rate of 12 - 20 times/minute.
Consider Jen Chung accupuncture.
Circulation.
Does the animal have a pulse or heart sounds?
Yes
Continue to breathe for the animal until it begins to breathe again.
No
Begin external chest compression.
c
d

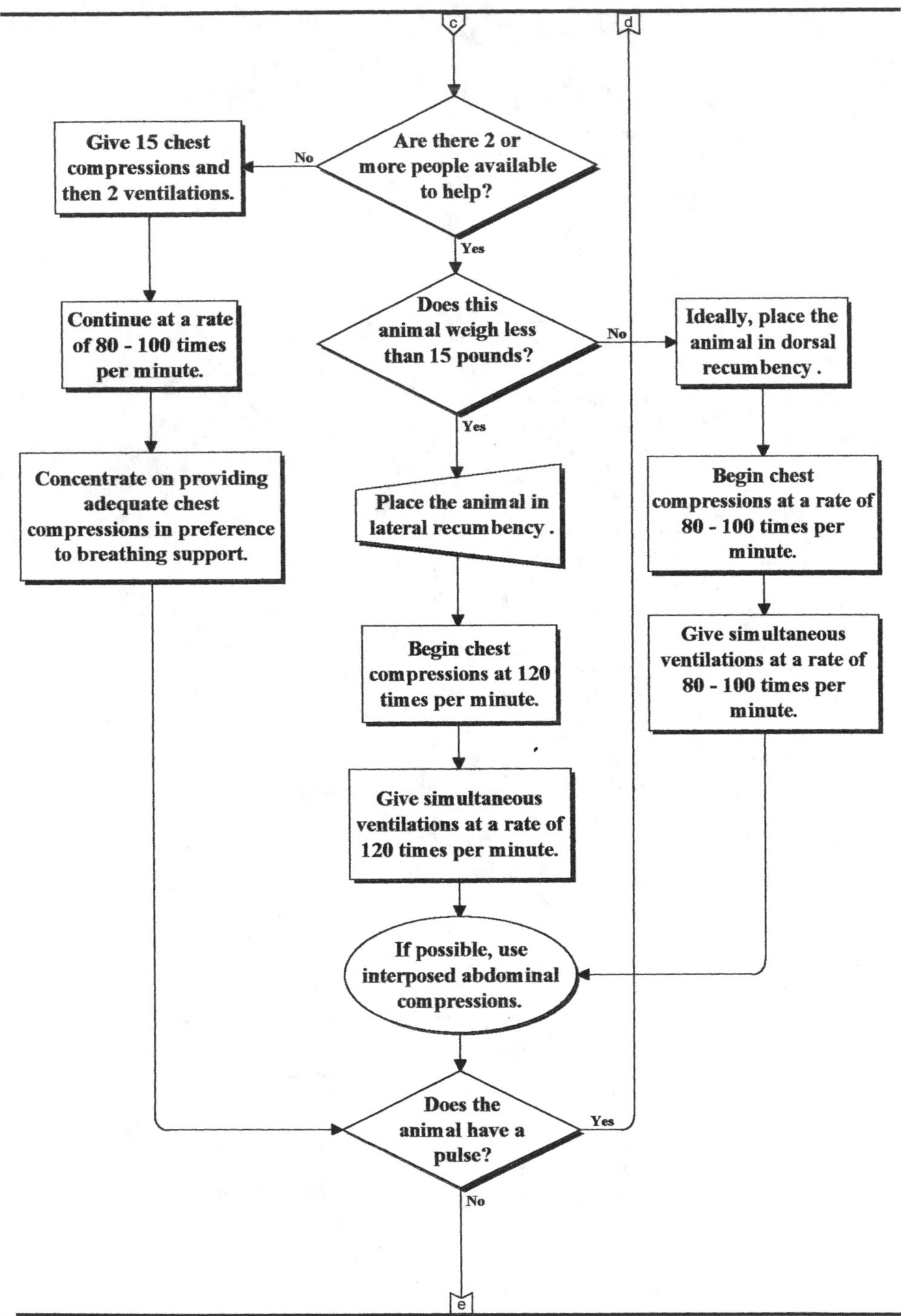

Figure 28-1 *Continued*

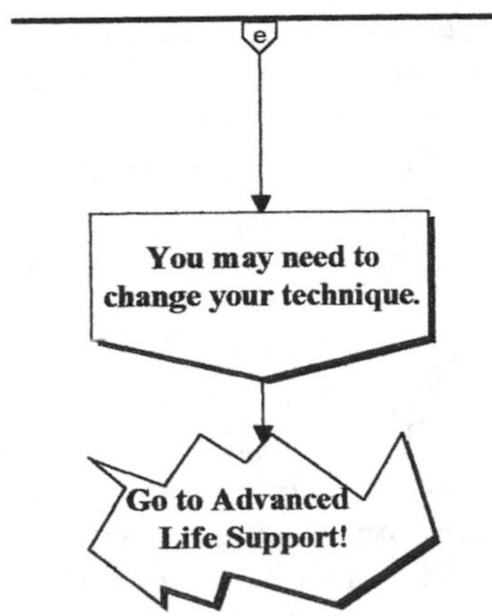

Use of acupuncture to stimulate respiration has been reported.[5] Placing a needle in acupuncture point Jen Chung (GV26) may reverse respiratory arrest under clinical conditions. The technique involves using a small (22-28 gauge, 1-1.5 inch) needle in the nasal philtrum at the ventral limit of the nares. The needle is twirled strongly on the maxillary periosteum and moved up and down while monitoring for improvement in respiration. This is a simple technique and can be used quickly.

For more than 30 years, emergency ventilation has been considered an essential component of basic life support. It would seem logical that ventilation has the potential to improve the success of resuscitation from cardiac arrest by improving tissue oxygenation and acidosis, but this benefit has only recently been studied.[5a]

When blood flow stops, ventilation does not affect tissue conditions. Ventilation does affect oxygenation and arterial and venous CO_2 and pH and may affect intracellular environment in the presence of low rates of blood flow. Ventilation may be unnecessary during the first few minutes of CPR, but under conditions of prolonged untreated cardiac arrest, it affects return of spontaneous circulation and is important for survival.[6] Chest compression alone and spontaneous gasping provides some pulmonary ventilation and gas exchange. However, blood oxygenation can be improved with supplemental O_2.

Sources of ventilation during cardiac arrest include compression-induced ventilation where gas is expelled from the lungs and is "passively inhaled" following elastic recoil of the chest wall during the relaxation phase.[6-11] In multiple animal studies, compression-induced ventilation alone has proved substantial.[6,7,11] However, measured minute ventilation and arterial oxygenation decrease after 4 to 10 minutes of CPR with or without assisted ventilation. This develops because of progressive chest compression-induced atelectasis and thoracic deformity.[7] In addition to compression-induced ventilation, spontaneous respiration, usually in the form of agonal or gasping breathing, commonly occurs during cardiac arrest in both animals and humans further contributing to total ventilation and outcome.[6,10,11]

Instead of using the ABC sequence, in Belgium the approach to witnessed arrests is usually "**CAB**" (**C**irculation, **A**irway, **B**reathing). Rescue breathing is delayed several seconds to minutes to enable prompt provision of chest compression. Survival outcomes with CAB appear to be similar to, if not better than, those reported with ABC CPR.[12-16]

What are the adverse effects of mouth-to-mouth (mouth-to-nose) ventilation? When no endotracheal tube is in place, assisted ventilation maneuvers often are associated with gastric insufflation and aspiration pneumonitis.[17] Another consideration is whether there are important differences between exhaled gas and ambient air. Although air has 21% O_2 and 0.03% CO_2, exhaled gas contains a mean O_2 concentration of 16.6% to 17.8% and a mean CO_2 concentration of 3.5% to 4.1% during one- and two-rescuer CPR.[18] Expired gas is thus slightly hypoxic and hypercarbic. This hypercarbia may have adverse cardiovascular effects including inhibition of rate and force of cardiac contraction.[19,20]

Undoubtedly chest compression with ventilation has been documented to save lives.[21] Nevertheless, applying mouth-to-nose ventilation likely prevents CPR from being done in many animals in arrest. The available evidence does lend credence to the suggestion that providing positive-pressure ventilation in the *early minutes* of resuscitation may not be as crucial as previously assumed. However, there are no convincing data to suggest ventilation is not of high priority when the resuscitation continues more than 5 minutes.[21] Clearly, provision of chest compression without ventilation is far better than not attempting resuscitation at all.[13]

The use of blood gases, particularly arterial, has been a long-standing practice for monitoring ventilation. After 9 minutes of low blood flow states, central venous blood more closely reflect the status at the tissue level.[22] This contrasts with the situation in ventricular fibrillation, when minimal changes in both arterial and mixed venous blood gases occur. Because there is little blood flow during CPR, the larger arteries do not reflect the situation at the tissue level. In fact, a decreasing arterial pH and O_2 level and an increasing CO_2 level may indicate a higher cardiac output and better tissue perfusion. Arterial blood gases can be used to assess perfusion only when ventilation is held constant and used to assess ventilation when perfusion is held constant. Both of these tasks are difficult to achieve during CPR. Mixed venous pH, O_2, and CO_2 levels are more useful because they more closely reflect the tissue environment and are less affected by minute ventilation.[23]

Circulation

The weak link in CPR is the inability of chest compressions to achieve adequate blood flow to the vital organs. In the original report on CPR published in 1960,[24] the ability to achieve a palpable pulse was mistakenly interpreted as indicating that chest compression could achieve adequate systemic blood flow. Blood flow in both systemic and regional (*e.g.*, coronary) circulations is less than one fourth of prearrest levels during closed chest compressions. The difference in arterial and venous (peak) pressures is negligible. It is the arteriovenous pressure *difference* that is the principal determinant of systemic and regional blood flow. The difference between aortic diastolic and right atrial diastolic pressure, called coronary perfusion pressure, is the pressure gradient that drives coronary blood flow. Studies in human CPR outcomes show that a coronary perfusion pressure of at least 15 mm Hg is necessary for satisfactory outcome.[25] This also explains why CPR has had such a poor success rate.

Mechanisms of Blood Flow During CPR

The advent of modern CPR began with Kouwenhoven's description of external chest compressions in 1960,[24] and until recently, many of the theories and techniques behind its use went unquestioned.[26] Recent studies into various methods of improving the outcome of resuscitation efforts have brought forth new information that questions some of these long-standing but unproven theories. The goal of external chest compression CPR is to maximize the generated blood flow. Restoration of native cardiac activity and preservation of brain function are directly related to these flows.

Cardiac Pump Theory. During artificial "systole" (external chest compression), the ventricles are compressed to a greater extent than the atria. Presumably cardiac compression generates higher pressure in the ventricles than elsewhere in the thorax. This results in the production of an atrioventricular (AV) gradient and subsequent closure of the AV valves. Chest compression results in squeezing of the heart between the ribs, reducing ventricular volume and causing ejection of blood into the systemic arteries. During chest relaxation or "diastole," intracardiac pressure falls and ventricular pressure decreases below atrial pressure, leading to opening of the AV valves and ventricular filling from the systemic venous reservoir.[26-31] If this mechanism of blood flow is correct, stroke volume should be determined by the amount of cardiac deformation (determined by the force of chest compression).[26,31] Prolongation of compression beyond the time necessary to squeeze the heart will have no effect on stroke volume because ejection ceases as soon as sternal displacement is maximal. With a fixed amount of rib displacement, increases in the rate of compression will increase flow because a fixed stroke volume is pumped into the arteries per unit time. Evidence supporting the cardiac pump theory has been demonstrated in dogs weighing less than 7 kg.[32] In these small dogs, cardiac compression is readily achieved and has been demonstrated radiographically. However, in larger animals direct cardiac compression may be more difficult to achieve. Supporters of the cardiac pump theory have demonstrated (via the use of ultrasonic transducers implanted in the ventricular wall) that external chest compressions produced changes in ventricular shape that were characterized by decreasing cardiac diameter parallel to the force of compression.[26,31] However, although alterations in ventricular shape were demonstrated, changes in ventricular volume that would prove the cardiac pump mechanism were not documented.

Thoracic Pump Theory. One of the first findings that led to questioning of the cardiac pump theory was that closed-chest CPR failed to generate measurable blood pressure in several patients with flail chest, a condition that should permit direct cardiac compression more readily.[26,29] Only when the chest was stabilized by external binding could blood pressure be generated. Patients who developed ventricular fibrillation during cardiac compression were able to produce a cardiac output adequate to preserve consciousness by repeatedly coughing and phasically elevating intrathoracic pressure.[27,29,30] This observation of "cough CPR" initiated much research into whether direct cardiac compression or elevation of intrathoracic pressure was responsible for blood flow during CPR.

By Boyle's law, the more the thoracic volume is compressed, the more intrathoracic pressure will increase. The thoracic pump theory proposes that blood flow generated by external thoracic compression is the result of phasic changes in intrathoracic pressure, without direct compression of the heart.[26,27,29-31] Displacement of the sternum and direct cardiac compression are irrelevant, whereas the development of intrathoracic pressure is critical. In this theory, all the blood-containing structures within the thorax are considered to be elastic and collapsible by external pressure. The systemic veins are easily collapsed, whereas the aorta and its major branches tend to resist collapse. External chest compression from any direction results in a generalized increase in intrathoracic pressure. The subsequent increase in intravascular pressure is transmitted from the intrathoracic to the extrathoracic arteries. Because of the competent venous valves, collapse of the veins at the thoracic inlet and a highly compliant extrathoracic venous system, pressure is not transmitted to the extrathoracic veins. This results in an AV pressure gradient for extrathoracic blood flow. During "diastole," intrathoracic pressure falls below extrathoracic venous pressure and blood returns to the lungs. In this model of blood flow, the heart acts as a passive conduit and plays no role as a blood pump. Because increases in intrathoracic pressure decrease the size of vessels leaving the thorax, flow limitation will occur.[29,31] This results in a relatively constant flow per unit time. Therefore, flow should be dependent on the duration of compression per cycle rather than on the rate of compression.[27] This fact has been well documented in several canine models of cardiac arrest in which increasing the rate of compression at a constant duty cycle (duration of compression) did not increase myocardial or cerebral blood flow.[26,31] However, increasing the duration of compression from 15% to 50% while maintaining a constant compression rate resulted in a significant increase in cardiac output.[26,31]

Guidelines. Numerous investigations into the mechanism of blood flow during CPR have confirmed that the majority of forward blood flow results from a generalized rise in intrathoracic pressure and not from direct cardiac compression.[26,28,29,31,32] Depending on ventral-dorsal thoracic diameter, the presence or absence of cardiac enlargement, thoracic compliance and patient size, the cardiac pump mechanism may or may not contribute to generation of forward blood flow during closed-chest CPR.[26]

Because of the controversy surrounding blood flow during CPR, the 1986 American Heart Association guidelines[33] for CPR have increased the recommended rate of chest compression from 60 to 100/min in human patients. This change represents a compromise between advocates of the thoracic pump mechanism and those who support the cardiac pump theory. Based on the theory behind the thoracic pump, acceleration of compression rate should have no effect on net cardiac output and in this setting, duration of compression is deemed to be more important (with at least a 50% duty cycle). At a rate of 60/min, a pause between chest compressions is required to achieve a 50% duty cycle. This is difficult to achieve and often tiring for the rescuer. A faster rate of approximately 100/min allows a 50% duty cycle to be more readily achieved and satisfies those proponents of the cardiac pump theory who recommend faster chest compressions.

One way of potentially increasing blood flow would be to increase the amount of chest compression force and displacement. There appears to be a minimum amount of chest compression force that must be applied to generate blood flow.[31] It is likely, therefore, that ineffective CPR occurs in many instances because inadequate chest compression force is applied. There is little chance that ischemia will be relieved, or that drugs will be delivered adequately, if insufficient blood flow is generated.

Newer CPR Techniques

Based on the different mechanisms of blood flow during CPR, several alterations in CPR technique have been proposed.

Simultaneous Compression-Ventilation CPR (SCV CPR)

If phasic increases in intrathoracic pressure can generate blood flow during CPR, then for any given degree of thoracic displacement, any manipulation that augments intrapleural and intrathoracic pressure should increase forward blood flow.[26,32,34] Application of external thoracic compression and simultaneous ventilation at high airway pressures (40-60 cm H_2O) has been shown to significantly increase intrathoracic pressure when compared to conventional closed-chest CPR (CC CPR).[26,35] This technique has produced greater increases in arterial and aortic blood pressure, carotid blood flow, and cardiac output in both human and animal studies when compared to conventional CPR techniques.[26,35] Regional cerebral and coronary blood flow have also been demonstrated to be enhanced using SCV CPR in a canine model.[32]

Interposed Abdominal Compression (IAC)

If abdominal compression is applied, there is an increase in blood flow analogous to the intrathoracic pressure pump. Intrathoracic pressure also increases during abdominal compression.[26] It may also redirect blood flow from the caudal half of the body, resulting in increased venous return and an apparent increase in central blood volume.[26,36] Compression of arterial vessels may cause an increase in systemic vascular resistance and thus contribute to the increased blood pressures observed with abdominal compression.[26,36,37] In addition it is presumed that abdominal compressions applied between thoracic compressions may lead to compression of the aorta, producing greater retrograde aortic flow into the chest[38] and thus augmentation of coronary flow.

Studies involving the use of IAC CPR have yielded conflicting results. In 33 human, adult, nontraumatic cardiac arrest patients, IAC CPR significantly increased end-tidal CO_2 as compared to standard CPR and was associated with an increase in the return of spontaneous circulation (end-tidal CO_2 has been shown to have a positive correlation with coronary perfusion pressure and success of resuscitation).[39] Elevation of diastolic arterial pressure and mean arteriovenous pressure gradients with IAC CPR has also been demonstrated.[40] In animal models, cardiac output, systemic O_2 uptake, and both cerebral and myocardial blood flow were substantially enhanced by this technique when compared with standard CPR.[26] However, in another study involving 30 dogs, there was no difference in initial resuscitation success, 24-hour survival, or neurologic deficit of the survivors, when IAC CPR was compared to conventional CPR.[41] As of yet, no long-term studies have shown an increased survival using this method.

The use of continuous abdominal compression via the use of military antishock trousers (MAST) has also been evaluated.[36,37,42,43] These inflatable trousers cause an increase in peripheral vascular resistance with a resultant increase in aortic systolic and diastolic pressures during resuscitation.[36,37] Once again, however, MAST-augmented CPR has not been demonstrated to increase the survival rate from cardiac arrest[43] and cannot be recommended at this time.

Open-Chest CPR (OC CPR)

It is generally accepted that the generation of forward blood flow is greater with OC CPR than with standard external chest compressions. Numerous studies have documented significant improvement in mean aortic pressure, cardiac output, coronary and cerebral perfusion pressures, and rate of successful resuscitation with open-chest cardiac massage.[26,44,45] Mean circulation time is also shorter with direct cardiac massage.[26] The lower coronary and cerebral perfusion pressures with CC CPR versus OC CPR are thought to be due to the generation of higher right atrial and intracranial pressures with a closed thorax.[26] Interestingly, no reports are available in the literature to document improved outcome using OC CPR versus CC CPR in veterinary clinical patients.

Of 3982 human patients undergoing cardiac surgery over a 30-month period, 29 patients (0.7%) had a sudden cardiac arrest. Of these 29 humans, 13 patients (45%) were successfully resuscitated with CC CPR, 14 (48%) with OC CPR, and 2 (7%) died despite CC CPR and OC CPR.[46]

Despite the fact that blood flow and blood pressures are improved with OC CPR, the impracticalities of using this technique in many situations limit its usefulness. However, in several situations direct cardiac compression via OC CPR is indicated[26,45]: (1) cardiac arrest in the presence of significant thoracic wall trauma, (2) cardiac arrest during surgery when the thorax is already open, (3) arrest during abdominal surgery when the thorax can be entered via the diaphragm, (4) in cases of suspected uncontrolled intrathoracic hemorrhage, and (5) in the face of failure of adequately applied CC CPR. This last indication remains controversial and ill-defined. One author suggests that the thorax be opened in animals greater than 15 kg in whom external CPR has not produced return of spontaneous circulation within 2 to 5 minutes, or in any animal in which CC CPR does not reverse mucous membrane color from cyanotic to pink within 2 minutes.[45] Whether or not to perform OC CPR remains the decision of the primary caregiver. However, this decision should be made early in the arrest period, because OC CPR is more effective in improving the rate of successful resuscitation if efforts at ineffective closed-chest resuscitation are not continued for long periods.[26,45]

ADVANCED LIFE SUPPORT OR ADVANCED CARDIAC LIFE SUPPORT

Advanced cardiac life support (ACLS) includes drugs and definitive therapy to enhance cardiac performance and promote blood flow (Fig. 28-2).

Defibrillation and Drugs

Electrical Defibrillation

Direct-current cardioversion is the single most effective resuscitative measure for improving survival in cardiac arrest.[47-50] In a study of 1667 human cardiac arrest patients with ventricular fibrillation, survival decreased linearly with increasing time to defibrillation.[51]

Total disorder of the ventricles of the heart, accompanied by incoordination of contraction, is known as ventricular fibrillation. For centuries, ventricular fibrillation was recognized as a terminal event from which there was no recovery. In 1899, Prevost and Battelli reported on extensive investigations into electrical methods of treatment of fibrillation in dog hearts. They were able to show that powerful electric shocks applied directly to the heart could convert ventricular fibrillation into a sinus rhythm. No clinical application of this technique was reported until 1947, when Beck successfully resuscitated a 16-year old boy from ventricular fibrillation by applying alternating-current electric shock directly to the heart. Following this, directly applied cardiac electrical shock became common in human operating rooms. The need for conversion of ventricular fibrillation without opening the chest soon became obvious and external electrical defibrillators were developed in the mid-1950s independently by Zoll and Kouwenhoven, and have since received wide clinical application.

Underlying the rationale of electrical defibrillation is the fact that a massive electrical shock will cause complete depolarization of all the individual myocardial fibers. When all the cells within the re-entrant circuit are depolarized, a condition of electrical homogeneity is established, which is inimical to re-entry. This is because ongoing re-entry requires that at all times some part of the chamber not be depolarized, so that this part can be next in line to be activated.[52] To be successful, an electrical shock must produce a period of electrical homogeneity that persists for a sufficient time (>130 msec).[53]

The minimum amount of energy required to defibrillate the heart is called

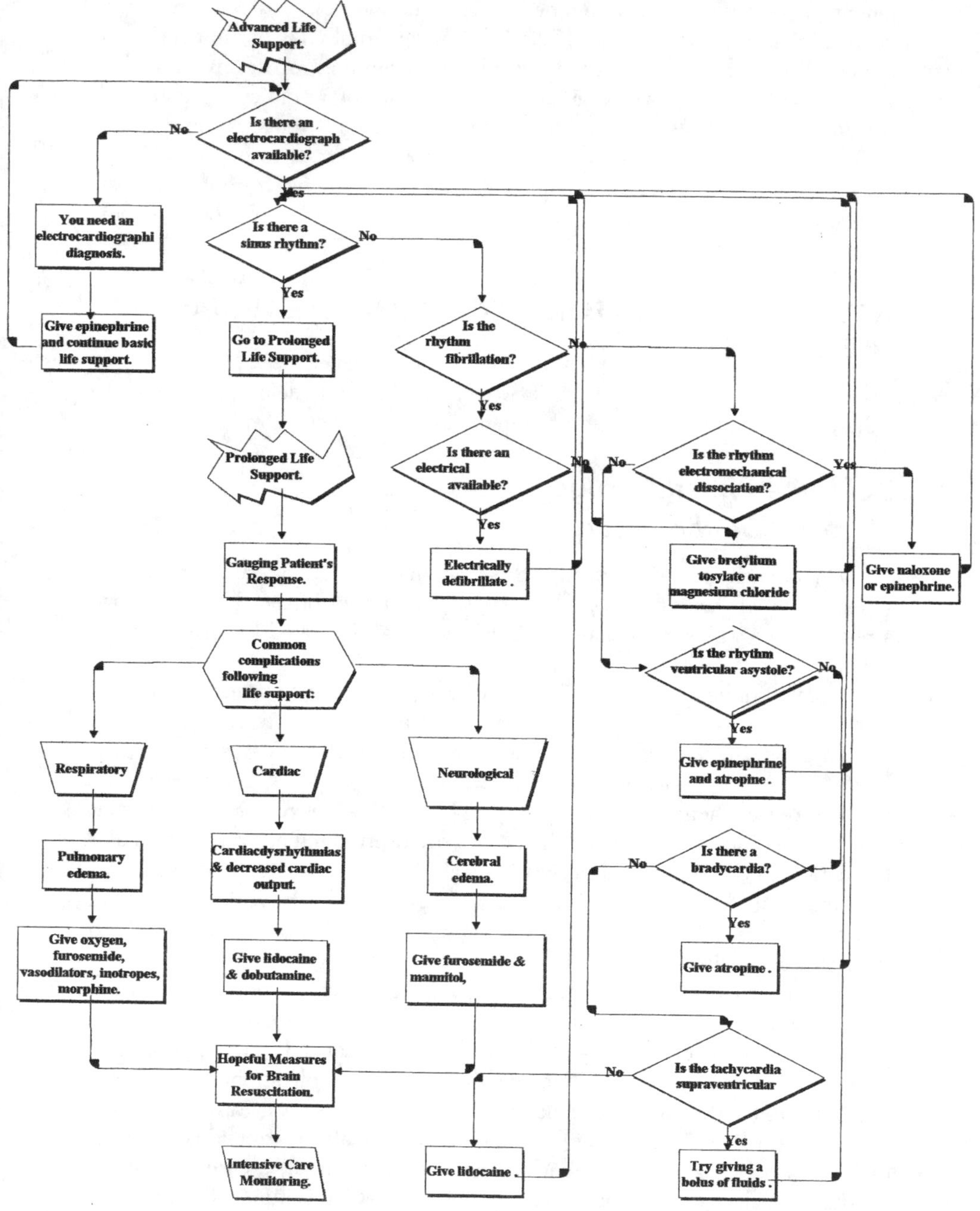

Figure 28-2
Flow sheet for advanced and prolonged life support in animals.

the *defibrillation threshold*. This defibrillation threshold is not a single value but rather is a sigmoidal dose-response relationship. The greater the energy in a shock, the more likely it is to defibrillate a given heart.[54] There is marked variability from animal to animal in the energy threshold, mainly because of interanimal differences in *transthoracic impedence*. This impedence has several important determinants: the size of the animal, electrode size, electrode-thoracic wall contact pressure and couplant ("electrode paste"), and phase of the respiratory cycle. Increases in transthoracic impedence during lung expansion are especially important in animals receiving mechanical ventilation and those receiving basic life support.

Impedence declines with multiple shocks partly because of the edema and tissue hyperemia in the electrical current's pathway.[55] Because current, and not energy, is the determinant of successful defibrillation, recently developed defibrillators automatically deliver more energy when impedence is found to be high. Current required for defibrillation increases with heart and body weight, but excessive current impairs the contractile force of the myocardium. Therefore, defibrillation with the minimum peak current is obviously desirable. Hypoxia, hypothermia, pH, and ionic and catecholamine levels in the circulation are known to affect the amount of current required for defibrillation.[56] Other factors besides transthoracic impedence can influence defibrillation threshold. Lidocaine reversibly increases defibrillation threshold by as much as 50%.[57] Beta agonists and aminophylline, on the other hand, lower the defibrillation threshold. The incidence of defibrillation is inversely proportional to the duration of fibrillation.[59] In Figure 28-3, the duration of fibrillation is seen to be proportional to the maximum achievable success of defibrillation, and up to a certain point is directly related to the energy requirement for conversion. Energy is defined as the ability to do work. In a practical sense, it is the power multiplied by the time it is delivered; the unit used is the joule (J) or watt-second. This defibrillation energy requirement is approximately 4 to 5 J/kg.[59]

Emergency defibrillation should be used to treat rhythms such as ventricular fibrillation or rapid ventricular tachycardia that have caused the animal to be pulseless and unresponsive. In this situation, *speed* should be given the highest priority. This is due to the fact that the strongest determinant of survival is the interval between the onset of a cardiac arrest and the delivery of an effective electrical shock. If ventricular fibrillation is witnessed in the monitored animal, defibrillation precedes basic life-support techniques.

The electrode paddles should be well coated with gel, particularly around the edges. Although salt-containing electrode paste is usually used, ultrasound gel or surgical lubricant may also be used with equal success.[60]

The paddles are applied firmly to the thoracic wall with about 25 lb of pressure. This compresses the thorax, leading to a shorter electrode distance and lower thoracic impedence. Placement across the thorax likely makes little difference in the dog and cat. The paddle surface is generally as large as the heart and only 28% of the fibrillating myocardial cells must be depolarized to cease fibrillation. In the larger dog, one may try and position the paddles so defibrillation occurs from the base to apex of the heart.

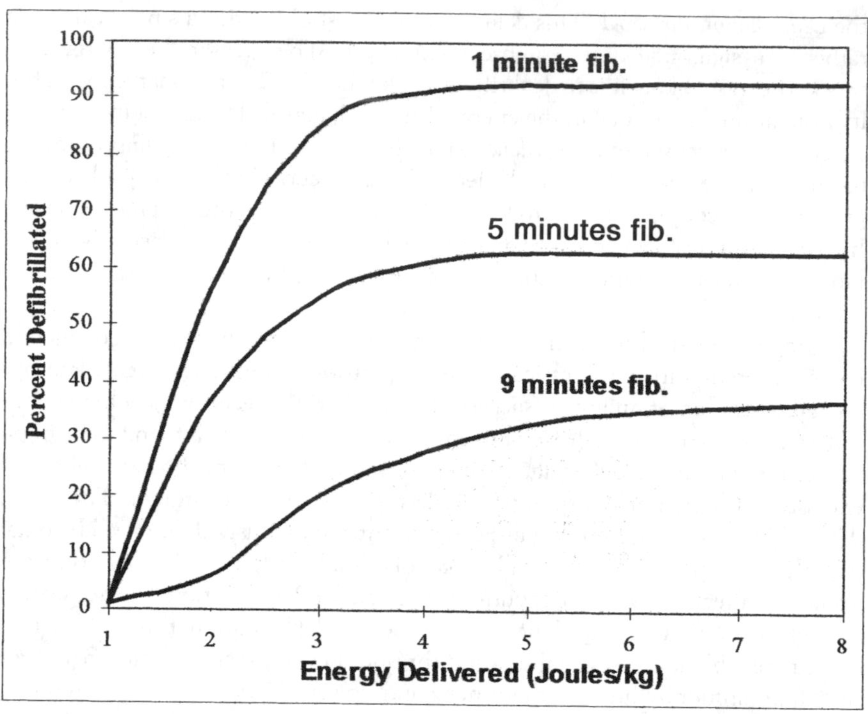

Figure 28-3
Curves showing estimated success of defibrillation versus delivered energy after 1, 5, and 9 minutes of fibrillation in dogs receiving closed-chest cardiac massage and artificial ventilation with epinephrine. (From Yakitis RW, Eqy GA, Otto CW, *et al.*: Influence of time and therapy on ventricular fibrillation in dogs. *Crit Care Med* 8:157, 1980.)

Extreme care must be taken to avoid having the paddles touch each other and that there is no bridging gap between the electrodes by conductive gel. Once the paddles are in place, the defibrillator is charged. Prior to discharging the capacitors, the operator of the paddles MUST ensure no person is in contact with either the animal, the table top, nor a wet floor. Once a quick inspection has been made, the operator then loudly announces "ALL CLEAR!". After a second glance at the scene, the operator may now discharge the defibrillator.

If the first attempt fails to convert to a hemodynamically rhythm, a second shock with near equal energy should be delivered. If the first two shocks fail to defibrillate the animal, a third shock with increased energy is immediately delivered. When all these attempts fail, the veterinarian should look for confounding factors such as inadequate electrode pressure, improper electrode positioning, and insufficient electrode-patient interface (*i.e.*, inadequate gel amounts). Defibrillation may also fail when thoracic impedence is high due to pneumothorax. Table 28-2 lists other confounding variables that may interfere with defibrillation. Attempts should be made to correct these variables. Epinephrine can be used to lower the fibrillation threshold.

Table 28-2. Variables Affecting Successful Defibrillation

Body weight
Metabolic acidosis
Metabolic alkalosis
Hypoxia
Hyper- and hypokalemia
Hyper- and hypomagnesemia
Digitalis intoxication
Antiarrhythmic drugs
Acute reperfusion injury
Myocardial ischemia

No data are available in the veterinary literature for clinical experiences with defibrillation. In humans, success rates are high for electrical conversion of ventricular dysrhythmias immediately after their onset. In the research dog, 80% of induced ventricular tachycardia and ventricular fibrillation are converted with a single 200-J shock. Cumulative effectiveness is 95% after a second 200-J shock, and 99% to 100% after a third 300-J shock.[61] The amplitude of the fibrillation waveform correlates with the time interval from initial cardiac arrest and is a powerful predictor of outcome.[62] Human data indicate a fall off in survival of 6%/min of untreated ventricular fibrillation, such that no survival would be expected after 15 minutes.[63] Only 6% survival is seen in persons with very low amplitude ("fine") ventricular fibrillation.

Open-Chest Defibrillation

Open-chest defibrillation involves direct application of the electrodes to the epicardium. The electrode paddles should be 6 to 8 cm in diameter, covered with saline-soaked gauze. One paddle is applied on the base of the heart overlying the right atrium, and the second paddle is placed on the apex of the heart overlying the left ventricle. The electric shock should not be administered in the presence of any explosive anesthetic agents. The shock is delivered under the control of the veterinarian holding the paddles and should follow the same safety guidelines outlined above for closed-chest defibrillation. Much less energy is required for open-chest defibrillation. Shocks varying from 10 to 60 J may be given. Epicardial burns may occur and will result in myocardial complications after resuscitation.

Anecdotal reports persist regarding spontaneous defibrillation. These reports most frequently are associated with the cat and small dog. Although it is theoretically possible for spontaneous defibrillation to result when a small heart is involved, the reason may well be good perfusion of the coronary arteries during cardiac compression (internal or external). This perfusion, the smallness of the heart, and the use of myocardial stimulant drugs may be sufficient, in rare circumstances, to convert fibrillation into a sinus cardiac rhythm. Spontaneous defibrillation is rare and unpredictable and should play no role in the expectation of resuscitation.

Chemical Defibrillation

Chemical defibrillating drugs have unproven efficacy in veterinary medicine. Unfortunately, many veterinarians do not have electrical defibrillators and thus chemical defibrillating drugs may be their only option. Several drugs are mentioned in the literature as useful for terminating ventricular fibrillation. Although frequently mentioned, acetylcholine with potassium chloride is an unlikely choice for defibrillation. This is because of the lack of availability of acetylcholine as an injectable product. No clinical reports of successful chemical defibrillation using acetylcholine with potassium chloride are available in the clinical veterinary literature.

Bretylium tosylate (10 mg/kg IV) is labeled for use in ventricular tachycardia and fibrillation. It will decrease the fibrillation threshold, but this must be balanced against the apparent loss of hemodynamic recovery following defibrillation. Bretylium possesses antiadrenergic and hypotensive actions associated with depletion of norepinephrine from peripheral adrenergic nerve endings. Thus, animals treated with bretylium may not be able to recover as well from fibrillation-defibrillation episodes because of less effective autonomic reflexes.[64]

Lidocaine has been offered as a possible chemical defibrillating agent in the past. Although lidocaine may possess an antifibrillatory effect under experimental conditions, the clinical relevance of such an effect is questionable. If cardiac arrest occurs, lidocaine has limited utility and may be deleterious secondary to diminished countershock efficacy or lidocaine-induced asystole.[65-67]

Magnesium is the most recently investigated chemical defibrillator drug. Hypomagnesemia is commonly seen in sick animals[68] and results in ventricular dysrhythmias. Most evidence points to a problem with potassium rather than magnesium as the cause, but magnesium infusion will occasionally convert ventricular dysrhythmias to normal sinus rhythms. Currently, use of magnesium chloride (or sulfate) should be considered in the treatment of refractory ventricular fibrillation. The dosage used is 1 to 2 g infused IV over 2 minutes. An alternative dosage is 25 to 40 mg/kg given as an IV bolus.[69]

Adrenergic Drugs

Physiologic Effects. The α-adrenergic agonists have the advantage of peripheral vasoconstriction. This results in an increased diastolic pressure, and thus increased coronary blood flow,[65,70,71] and vasoconstriction of the extracerebral carotid blood flow resulting in increased intracerebral blood flow Drugs commonly used for their α-agonist effects include epinephrine, phenylephrine, and methoxamine.

The β-adrenergic agonists increase the vigor of ventricular fibrillation and offer a positive inotropic effect on the heart. Disadvantages of these drugs include increased myocardial and cerebral O_2 demand, increased occurrence of significant dysrhythmias, and increased heart rates. Drugs used for their β-agonist effects include epinephrine and isoproterenol.

A study to determine the relative importance of α- and β-adrenergic receptors during resuscitation demonstrated that α-receptor stimulation with a concomitant diastolic pressure elevation is more important to the success of resuscitation than β-receptor stimulation.[70] Dogs pretreated with propranolol and then given phenylephrine during resuscitation as well as those given no pretreatment and then epinephrine during resuscitation experienced a 100% return of spontaneous circulation following 5 minutes of asphyxial arrest. However, of those dogs pretreated with phenoxybenzamine and then administered isoproterenol, only 27% were successfully resuscitated. The model demonstrated that the primary usefulness of epinephrine in resuscitation was due to its α-adrenergic effects rather than its effects as a β-receptor agonist.

Coronary and Cerebral Blood Flow. In 1963, studies demonstrated that early administration of epinephrine during CPR resulted in improved recovery rates and postulated that this was due to the increase in aortic diastolic pressure and improved myocardial perfusion.[1] Numerous studies in both humans and animals have confirmed these findings.[65,70,71] Due to its α-adrenergic effects, epinephrine produces an intense vasoconstriction that prevents a significant amount of runoff in peripheral arteries, thus preventing arterial collapse and maintaining arterial pressure.[71] Epinephrine results in an increase in aortic diastolic pressure without an elevation in right atrial pressure. The subsequent increase in coronary perfusion pressure may be as high as 25 to 30 mm Hg when epinephrine administration is combined with SCV CPR.[71]

Cerebral perfusion pressure is also reasonably well preserved by the administration of epinephrine during resuscitation.[70-72] Cerebral O_2 delivery can be maintained without reaching maximal O_2 extraction levels, implying that O_2 delivery is above that necessary to maintain aerobic metabolism.[65] Epinephrine improves blood flow to the brain by preventing or reversing carotid artery collapse while at the same time causing vasoconstriction of the extracerebral carotid vessels, thereby resulting in increased cerebral perfusion pressure.[71] Currently, many new drugs are being used in the treatment of the postischemic-anoxic encephalopathy frequently seen following cardiac arrest.[73]

Epinephrine Versus Pure α-Agonists. If the beneficial effects of epinephrine administration during resuscitation are due to its α-adrenergic effects, then the use of pure α-agonists may offer some promise. Numerous studies have been performed using various α-agonists at varying dosages to determine their effectiveness relative to that of epinephrine in supporting cerebral and coronary blood flow[72,74-78] In several swine models of cardiac arrest, epinephrine produced significantly better cerebral blood flow than equipressor doses of either methoxamine or phenylephrine.[72,74,79] This may be explained in part by the distribution of adrenergic receptors in the cerebral vasculature. Although α-tone may be required to prevent arterial runoff and preserve diastolic pressure, the cerebral microvasculature is dependent on β-stimulation for dilation.[72] Therefore, to allow perfusion at the tissue level, β-adrenergic stimulation may be necessary. Because both methoxamine and phenylephrine lack any significant β-adrenergic activity, their α-adrenergic activity results in cerebral constriction and shunting of blood away from the tissue. Another study, also involving the use of a swine model, demonstrated that epinephrine resulted in better regional myocardial blood flow, increased coronary sinus O_2 content, and improved O_2 extraction ratio when compared with phenylephrine.[75] In 102 human patients suffering from prehospital cardiac arrest due to ventricular fibrillation, conversion rate (the percentage of patients developing a pulse during resuscitation) and successful resuscitation (defined as the conveyance of a patient to the emergency department with a pulse and rhythm) were significantly better with epinephrine than with methoxamine.[76] Although there was only a trend toward greater survival to discharge ($P < 0.07$), most investigators agree that epinephrine is the adrenergic drug of choice in CPR, with improved cerebral and myocardial blood flows versus pure α-agonists.[76]

Dosage. Until recently, the dosage of epinephrine recommended by the American Heart Association during CPR was 0.02 mg/kg, administered IV.[48] However, use of high-dose epinephrine (0.2 mg/kg) has been shown to improve myocardial and cerebral blood flow, O_2 extraction, and the success of resuscitation in both human and animals suffering from cardiac arrest.[48,65,72,74,75,80] In 50 human patients, return of spontaneous circulation occurred in 12% of patients given the standard dose of epinephrine versus 36% of patients administered the higher dose ($P < 0.05$).[81] No statistically significant effect on long-term survival was seen.

Several investigators have questioned the use of high-dose epinephrine, reporting potential problems of hyperglycemia, hyperkalemia, cardiac dysrhythmias, and myocardial necrosis. However, administration of high-dose epinephrine in swine did not produce increased arrhythmias or cardiovascular instability and may have had beneficial effects on mean arterial pressure and cardiac output after resuscitation.[82] Likewise, in four human patients in whom administration of standard doses of epinephrine had been unsuccessful, high-dose epinephrine resulted in the establishment of a perfusing rhythm without any central nervous system, myocardial, or metabolic alterations.[83] These findings would appear to support the continued investigation of high-dose epinephrine in the setting of cardiac arrest and its use in clinical cases resistant to the lower dosages.

Effects of Vagal Tone on Resuscitation from Pulseless Electrical Activity

Cardiac arrest presenting with pulseless electrical activity (PEA), formerly referred to as electromechanical dissociation (EMD), occurs in 9% to 18% of prehospital and 67% of inhospital cardiac arrests in people.[84-89] In dogs and cats, PEA is the most common arrhythmia (22.3%) seen with in-hospital cardiac arrest.[90] The parasympathetic nervous system appears to play a role in the pathophysiology.[91] In a study of surgical vagotomy and complete loss of vagal tone, in experimentally induced PEA in dogs, 75% had a return to spontaneous circulation.[92] From this study, one can speculate that pharmacologic vagolysis with atropine would improve circulation in PEA. Unfortunately, a vagolytic dosage of atropine has not been identified for the patient in cardiac arrest. At present, we use an IV dosage of 0.12 mg/kg (three times the vagolytic dosage listed by the American Heart Association).

Sodium Bicarbonate

The use of sodium bicarbonate in CPR has been vigorously debated. Proponents of bicarbonate administration describe the metabolic acidosis and its deleterious effects commonly seen during cardiac arrest.[65] Recently however, the acid-base status of patients in cardiac arrest has been more accurately documented.[93] A respiratory acidosis exists in the venous circulation due to tissue production of CO_2 and poor delivery of this blood to the alveolar-capillary membrane. Simultaneously, alkalosis is present in the arterial circulation due to the high ratio of pulmonary ventilation compared to perfusion associated with the low flow rates during CPR. Improving blood flow during CPR and adequately ventilating the patient should result in normalization of the patient's acid-base status and thus negate the need for aggressive bicarbonate administration.

Numerous adverse effects of bicarbonate administration have been documented, including the production of hypernatremia and hyperosmolality, hypokalemia resulting in increased incidence of arrhythmias, decreased plasma ionized calcium levels, a leftward shift in the oxyhemoglobin dissociation curve (with decreased O_2 delivery to the tissues), and a paradoxical central nervous system acidosis.[48,65,94] Many of these deleterious effects are related to the production of CO_2, following metabolism of exogenous bicarbonate, which diffuses more readily across cell membranes and aggravates intracellular acidosis.[94]

Current recommendations for correction of acid-base abnormalities during CPR are conservative with regard to bicarbonate administration. In patients that are not acidotic before cardiac arrest, acidosis may be controllable by adequate ventilation and cardiac compression.[48,94] The decision to administer bicarbonate should ideally be based on the measurement of blood pH and PCO_2, and repeated infusion of bicarbonate in the absence of acidosis is contraindicated.[94] In patients with pre-existing conditions in which acidosis is common, bicarbonate should be administered carefully at a dose (mEq) equal to the base deficit (mEq/L) multiplied by the body weight (kg) multiplied by 0.25 (volume of distribution in the extracellular space).[94] Administration of additional sodium bicarbonate may be harmful when effective spontaneous circulation has been restored.

Glucose

It has been well established that conditions that promote metabolism of glucose to lactate in ischemic brain tissue result in increased levels of cellular damage.[65,95] Preischemic hyperglycemia or administration of glucose during resuscitation results in increased tissue and plasma glucose levels, providing the substrate for anaerobic glycolysis. During the ischemic episode lactic acid then accumulates to toxic levels, resulting in cellular damage and permanent neurologic abnormalities. Studies done in adult cats administered 5% dextrose solutions during resuscitation demonstrated that neurologic recovery was significantly worse in glucose-treated cats and the risk of postischemic brain damage increased with increasing blood glucose levels.[96,97] In a retrospective study of human patients suffering cardiac arrest, poorer neurologic outcome was reported in patients with a high blood glucose level at the time of hospital admission.[96] A canine model of cardiac arrest failed to demonstrate any significant difference in neurologic score between glucose and nonglucose treated dogs.[98] However, in all animals surviving more than 2 hours, the initial glucose level was significantly lower than in animals that died, indicating that prearrest glucose levels may be a predictor of mortality in cardiac arrest. These studies provide the rationale of *avoiding* the administration of glucose during CPR unless hypoglycemia is suggested or present.

Calcium and Calcium Channel Blockers

The routine use of calcium in cases of cardiac arrest has recently fallen into disfavor. Calcium entry into cells has been implicated as the trigger for a multitude of cellular reactions that may lead to cell death, including vasospasm, mitochondrial uncoupling, membrane degeneration, and the production of cytotoxic compounds.[65,99-103] Activation of phospholipase A_2 results in arachidonic acid accumulation with the subsequent production of free fatty acids (FFA). These FFA act as detergents and disrupt cell phospholipid membrane integrity. The production of endoperoxides and leukotrienes contributes to the formation of O_2-derived free radicals that further the degree of cellular damage. Postischemic myocardial contractile dysfunction ("stunned myocardium") and neuronal death have both been attributed to the accumulation of intracellular calcium during the ischemic episode.[99] The use of calcium during CPR can only be recommended in cases of known hypocalcemia or in cases of cardiac arrest complicated by hyperkalemia, hypermagnesemia, and calcium channel blocker overdose.[65,99] Close electrocardiographic monitoring of the patient must occur during calcium administration.

Because of the deleterious effects of intracellular calcium accumulation during ischemia, much effort has been directed toward the use of calcium channel blocking agents in the prevention of these postischemic problems. Administration of calcium antagonist drugs at the onset of severe myocardial ischemia has been shown to be followed by an increase in blood flow to the ischemic areas with a decrease in the area of myocardial damage.[104] Calcium channel blockers protect both the performance and the cellular and subcellular structure of the myocardium subjected to ischemia during hypothermic cardiopulmonary bypass.[65,104] The increase in diastolic resting tension that normally follows reperfusion can be avoided with the administration of calcium blocking drugs.[97] Calcium channel blockers also raise the threshold of the ischemic myocardium to ventricular fibrillation.[65,99,104] This antifibrillatory action is thought to be due to, at least in part, the antagonism of enhanced adrenergic input to the heart that follows myocardial ischemia.[104] Several of the newer calcium channel blockers such as lidoflazine and nimodipine have resulted in improved neurologic recovery after cardiac arrest in both dogs and baboons when administered immediately following the return of spontaneous circulation.[100,101,103]

Fluid Volume Loading

For years, one of the mainstays of advanced life support has been the aggressive administration of shock doses of IV fluids. The administration of IV fluids has resulted in an increased carotid blood flow and, in some cases, the arterial pressure generated by external chest compression. It seems only reasonable that volume expansion should increase forward blood flow and therefore improve the success of resuscitation. However, more recently this theory has come into question because it has been documented that there is a positive correlation between coronary perfusion pressure and success of resuscitation.[105,106] The major determinant for myocardial blood flow is *coronary perfusion pressure*, defined as the aortic diastolic pressure minus the right atrial diastolic pressure.[106] To increase coronary perfusion pressure, the gradient between these two diastolic pressures must increase, with either an increase in aortic pressure or decrease in right atrial pressure. An investigation into the potential adverse effects of volume loading during CC CPR in dogs demonstrated that the administration of 1 liter of either 0.9% saline or 10% dextran as rapidly as possible in dogs weighing 20 to 50 kg resulted in a significant increase in total forward blood flow.[107] However, blood flow to the cerebral hemispheres, cerebellum, brainstem, and ventricular myocardium all decreased significantly. These changes in critical regional flow were accompanied by disproportionate increases in right atrial and intracranial pressures (relative to aortic pressure), which reduced the average pressure gradient across the coronary and cerebral circulations. These changes were thought to be somewhat influenced by a spontaneous fall in systemic vascular resistance. It is possible that volume expansion would have different effects on regional blood flow during CPR if vascular resistance was pharmacologically supported. In the face of these findings conservative fluid administration during CPR should be the norm, unless volume depletion is a contributing cause to the cardiac arrest.

Magnesium

Hypomagnesemia is reported with refractory cardiac arrhythmias, often potentially lethal when in combination with digitalis toxicity.[108-110] Several reports have shown a possible antiarrhythmic role for therapeutic magnesium even when serum magnesium is normal in the patient with digitalis toxicity,[110,111] ventricular tachycardia,[112] and torsades de pointes.[113,114] In human cardiac arrest victims, all patients with hypomagnesemia and hypermagnesemia died, whereas normomagnesemia was positively correlated with successful resuscitation.[115] In experimental studies with dogs, magnesium administered before electrical countershock resulted in significantly higher return of spontaneous circulation.[116]

Brain injury during and after ischemia is thought to be the result of two phenomena: decreased cerebral blood flow secondary to vasospasm and release of toxic substances within neuronal cells.[117] During ischemia, the sodium—potassium pump fails, causing efflux of potassium and intracellular accumulation of sodium and calcium. This may cause vasospasm, uncoupling of oxidative phosphorylation, and generation of superoxide radicals and other substances toxic to the brain tissue.

Magnesium is a physiologic calcium antagonist and may block calcium channels in brain tissue and prevent subsequent vasospasm and generation of toxic intracellular mediators. Magnesium may block continued calcium leakage into the cell that occurs during reperfusion or magnesium may interfere with calcium-mediated reactions that occur during reperfusion.[118] These mechanisms may explain published reports describing magnesium as a chemical defibrillator.[118]

PROLONGED LIFE SUPPORT

Recurrence of either respiratory or cardiopulmonary arrest is the biggest concern following resuscitation.[119] In most cases the recurrence of arrest will occur within the first 4 hours of the first episode.

After arrest, cerebral resuscitation becomes the next most important complication. Due to the low flow state to the brain during CPR, ischemia and hypoxia will lead to cerebral edema. As the heart begins to reperfuse tissues, significant injury products may be released to the systemic circulation.[120]

In normal brain, autoregulation will maintain a global cerebral brain flow of about 50 mL/100 g brain per minute, despite cerebral perfusion pressures (*i.e.*, mean arterial pressure minus intracranial pressure) between 50 and 150 mm Hg. When cerebral perfusion pressure drops below 50 mm Hg, cerebral blood flow decreases and the viability of normal neurons seems threatened by cerebral perfusion pressure less than 30 mm Hg, global cerebral blood flow less than 15 mL/100 g/min, or cerebral venous PO_2 of less than 20 mm Hg.[121]

During complete cerebral ischemia, calcium shifts, brain tissue lactic acidosis, and increases in the brain free acids, osmolality and extracellular concentration of excitatory amino acids (particularly glutamate and aspartate) set the stage for *reoxygenation injury*.[120] Postresuscitation cerebral injury appears to consist of four components: (1) perfusion failure (*i.e.*, inadequate O_2 delivery), (2) reoxygenation chemical cascades to cerebral necrosis, (3) extracerebral derangements, including intoxication from postanoxic viscera, and (4) blood derangements due to stasis.[121]

Perfusion failure seems to progress through four stages[120]:

1. Multifocal no reflow occurs immediately and seems to be readily overcome by normotensive or hypertensive reperfusion.
2. Transient global "reactive" hyperemia that lasts 15 to 30 minutes.
3. Delayed, prolonged global and multifocal hypoperfusion event from about 2 to 12 hours after arrest; global cerebral blood flow is reduced to about 50% of baseline, whereas global O_2 uptake returns to or above baseline levels and cerebral venous PO_2 decreases to less than 20 mm Hg, reflecting mismatching of O_2 delivery to O_2 uptake.

4. After 20 hours, either normal global cerebral blood flow and global O_2 uptake is restored or both remain low (with coma), or there is a secondary hyperemia, postulated to be associated with reduced O_2 uptake, followed by brain death.

Reoxygenation, though essential, also might provoke chemical cascades (involving free iron, free radical, calcium shifts, acidosis, excitatory amino acids, and catecholamines) that result in lipid peroxidation of membranes. Extracerebral derangements can worsen cerebral outcome. Studies in dogs have shown a delayed reduction in cardiac output after cardiac arrest despite controlled normotension. Pulmonary edema can be prevented by prolonged controlled ventilation. Blood derangements include aggregates of polymorphonuclear leukocytes and macrophages that might obstruct capillaries, release free radicals, and damage endothelium.[120]

Careful monitoring is most important during the first 4 hours after arrest. All patients require O_2 administered via an O_2 cage, nasal insufflation, or facemask. If CPR is successful, one needs to support the heart during the postresuscitation phase. This support is directed to inotropic support (dobutamine or dopamine), possibly using vasodilator and vasopressor drugs (sodium nitroprusside) and antiarrhythmic drugs (lidocaine). These drugs will be useful in reducing the pulmonary edema usually seen after arrest. Additionally, furosemide is usually administered to further reduce pulmonary edema.

Cerebral hypoxia and ischemia result during CPR. The end result is cerebral edema. Treatment for cerebral edema includes mannitol and furosemide. Corticosteroids have not been effective in reducing cerebral edema and are not currently recommended. Additional drugs that may be tried to improve cerebral resuscitation are listed in Table 28-3.

One should always be concerned about irreversible cerebral injury after arrest. Daily neurologic evaluations and assessment are required. Record your findings each day to note the progress of your patient. Clinical features to observe following arrest include: reactivity of the pupils, increased responsiveness, breathing patterns, motor responses, and motor postures.

No studies are currently available in animals but studies in humans indicate

Table 28-3. Theoretically Useful Drugs for Cerebral Resuscitation after Cardiopulmonary Arrest

Calcium channel blocking drugs: Reverse cerebral vasospasm prevents the lethal intracellular calcium influx.

Barbiturates: Mild calcium antagonists, decrease arachidonic acid and free fatty acid levels in neurons, decrease metabolic demands of the brain. To date, there is no conclusive evidence to support the use of barbiturates. Additionally, the sedation that results makes sequential neurologic assessment impossible.

Iron-chelating drugs: Free radical scavengers. Experimental at this point but very hopeful results for the future.

that certain groups of patients do not survive. Such patients include those with oliguria, metastatic cancer, sepsis, pneumonia, and acute stroke.[122] Very likely animals with these conditions also will not survive.

Do-not-resuscitate (DNR) orders must be initiated by the pet owner. Good client communications will be useful anytime an animal is hospitalized. It is wise to advise owners that arrest occurs suddenly and unexpectedly. Ask the owner "how far should we go if the pet arrests." Record the response and abide by the owner's wishes. A simple coding system can be used to identify DNR animals. A bright yellow, blank sign hung on the cage door works effectively to identify the owner's wishes.

The decision to stop CPR must be tempered with common sense, client communication, and experience of the resuscitators. Our experience suggests that the mean duration of CPR is generally about 20 minutes.

PROGNOSIS

After more than 30 years of widespread use of CPR, the re-evaluation of its benefits in terms of survival and the quality of life shows it to be a desperate effort that will help only a limited number of patients.[119,123,124] For sure, early electrical countershock has proven a lifesaving effect in ACLS.[125] None of the other therapeutic interventions currently supplemented by ACLS providers in human medicine has any proven efficacy over basic life-support skills of early basic CPR.[125] For most, CPR is unsuccessful.

REFERENCES

Basic Life Support

1. Idris AH, Staples E, O'Brian D, *et al.*: End-tidal carbon dioxide during extremely low cardiac output. *Ann Emerg Med* 23:568, 1994.
2. Blumenthal SU, Voorhees WD: The relationship of carbon dioxide excretion during cardiopulmonary resuscitation to regional blood flow and survival. *Resuscitation* 35:135, 1997.
3. Barton CW, Callaham ML: Possible confounding effect of minute ventilation on $ETCO_2$ in cardiac arrest. *Ann Emerg Med* 20:445, 1991.
4. Barnas GM, Smalley AJ, Miller J, *et al.*: Efficacy of several modes of continuous flow insufflation for resuscitation of a canine model of acute respiratory arrest. *Ann Emerg Med* 27:617, 1996.
5. Janssens L, Altman S, Rogers PAM: Respiratory and cardiac arrest under general anesthesia: treatment by accupuncture of the nasal philtrum. *Vet Rec* 22:273, 1979.

5a. Hallstrom A, Cobb L, Johnson E, *et al.*: Cardiopulmonary resuscitation by chest compression alone or with mouth-mouth ventilation. *N Eng J Med* 342:1546, 2000.

6. Idris AH: Reassessing the need for ventilation during CPR. *Ann Emerg Med* 27: 569, 1996.
7. Chandra NC, Gruben KG, Tsitlik JE, *et al.*: Observations of ventilation during resuscitation in a canine model. *Circulation* 90:3070, 1994.
8. Idris AH, Banner MJ, Wenzel V, *et al.*: Ventilation caused by external chest compression is unable to sustain effective gas exchange during CPR: a comparison to mechanical ventilation. *Resuscitation* 28:143, 1994.

9. Idris AH, Wenzel V, Tucker KJ, *et al.*: Chest compression ventilation: a comparison of standard CPR and active-compression/decompression CPR. *Acad Emerg Med* 1:A1, 1994.
10. Noc M, Weil MH, Tang W, *et al.*: Mechanical ventilation may not be essential for initial cardiopulmonary resuscitation. *Chest* 108:821, 1995.
11. Berg RA, Wilcoxson D, Hilwig RW, *et al.*: The need for ventilatory support during bystander CPR. *Ann Emerg Med* 26:342, 1995.
12. Berg RA, Kern KB, Hilwig RW, *et al.*: Assisted ventilation does not improve outcome in a porcine model for single-rescuer bystander cardiopulmonary resuscitation. *Circulation* 95:1635, 1997.
13. Van Hoeyweghen RJ, Bossaert LL, Mullie A, *et al.*: Quality and efficiency of bystander CPR. *Resuscitation* 26:47, 1993.
14. Bossaert L, Vanhoeyweghen R: Belgian Cerebral Resuscitation Study Group: bystanders cardiopulmonary resuscitation (CPR) in out-of-hospital cardiac arrest. *Resuscitation* 17(suppl):S55, 1989.
15. Simoons ML, Kimman GP, Ivens EMA, *et al.*: Follow up after out of hospital resuscitation. Read before the XIIth Annual Congress of the European Society of Cardiology, September 16–20, 1990, Stockholm, Sweden.
16. Pepe PE: Acute respiratory insufficiency. *In:* Hardwood-Nuss A, Linden CH, Luten RC, *et al.*, eds.: The Clinical Practice of Emergency Medicine. Philadelphia: JB Lippincott, 1996, p 636.
17. Wenzel V, Idris AH, Banner MJ, *et al.*: The composition of gas given by mouth-to-mouth ventilation during CPR. *Chest* 106:1806, 1994.
18. Walley KR, Ford LE, Wood LD: Effects of hypoxia and hypercapnia on the force-velocity relation of rabbit myocardium. *Circ Res* 69:1616, 1991.
19. Hongo K, White E. Orchard CH: The effect of mechanical loading on the response of rat ventricular myocytes to acidosis. *Exp Physiol* 80:701, 1995.
20. Shapiro BA: Should the ABCs of basic CPR become CABs? *Crit Care Med* 26: 214, 1998
21. Becker LB, Berg RA, Pepe PE, *et al.*: A reappraisal of mouth-to-mouth ventilation during bystander-initiated cardiopulmonary resuscitation: a statement for healthcare professionals from the ventilation working group of the basic life support and pediatric life support subcommittees, American Heart Association. *Ann Emerg Med* 30:654, 1997.
22. Tucker KJ, Idris AH, Wenzel V, *et al.*: Changes in arterial and mixed venous blood gases during untreated ventricular fibrillation and cardiopulmonary resuscitation. *Resuscitation* 28:137, 1994.
23. Idris AH, Staples E, O'Brian D, *et al.*: Effect of ventilation on acid base balance and oxygenation during low blood flow states. *Crit Care Med* 22:1827, 1994.
24. Kouwenhoven WB, Ing, Jude JR, *et al.*: Closed chest cardiac massage. *JAMA* 173: 1064, 1960.
25. Paradis NA, Martin GB, Rivers EP, *et al.*: Coronary perfusion pressure and the return of spontaneous circulation in human cardiopulmonary resuscitation. *JAMA* 263:1106, 1990.
26. Schleien CL, Berkowitz ID, Traystman R, *et al.*: Controversial issues in cardiopulmonary resuscitation. *Anesthesiology* 71:133, 1989.
27. Weisfeldt ML, Halperin HR: Cardiopulmonary resuscitation: beyond cardiac massage. *Circulation* 74:443, 1986.
28. Ditchey RV, Winkler JV, Rhodes CA: Relative lack of coronary blood flow during closed-chest resuscitation in dogs. *Circulation* 66:297, 1982.

29. Rudikoff MT, Maughan WL, Effron M, *et al.*: Mechanisms of blood flow during cardiopulmonary resuscitation. *Circulation* 61:345, 1980.
30. Babbs CF: New versus old theories of blood flow during CPR. *Crit Care Med* 8: 191, 1980.
31. Halperin HR, Tsitlik JE, Guerci AD, *et al.*: Determinants of blood flow to vital organs during cardiopulmonary resuscitation in dogs. *Circulation* 73:539, 1986.
32. Babbs CF, Tacker WA, Paris RL: CPR with simultaneous compression and ventilation at high airway pressure in 4 animals models. *Crit Care Med* 10:501, 1982.
33. American Heart Association: Standards and guidelines for cardiopulmonary resuscitation and emergency cardiac care. *JAMA* 255:2905, 1986.
34. Henik RA, Wingfield WE, Angleton GM, *et al.*: Effects of body position and ventilation/compression ratios during cardiopulmonary resuscitation in cats. *Am J Vet Res* 48:1603, 1987.
35. Chandra N, Rudikoff, Weisfeldt ML: Simultaneous chest compression and ventilation at high airway pressure during cardiopulmonary resuscitation in man. *Circulation Suppl* 59: II-203, 1978.
36. Einagle V, Bertrand F, Wise RA, *et al.*: Interposed abdominal compressions and carotid blood flow during cardiopulmonary resuscitation [abstract]. *Ann Emerg Med* 17:154, 1988.
37. Barriot P, Riou B, Viars P: High versus low inflation pressures of medical antishock trousers (MAST) in severe hemorrhagic hypovolemia [abstract]. *Ann Emerg Med* 19:213, 1990.
38. Halperin HR, Weisfeldt ML: New approaches to CPR. Four hands, a plunger, or a vest [editorial]. *JAMA* 267:2940, 1992.
39. Ward KR, Sullivan RJ, Zelenak RR, Summer WR: A comparison of interposed abdominal compression CPR and standard CPR by monitoring end-tidal pCO_2 [abstract]. *Ann Emerg Med* 17:12, 1988.
40. Howard M, Carrubba C, Foss F, *et al.*: Interposed abdominal compression-CPR: its effects on parameters of coronary perfusion in human subjects. *Ann Emerg Med* 16):31, 1987.
41. Kern KB, Carter AB, Showen RL, *et al.*: Twenty-four hour survival in a canine model of cardiac arrest comparing three methods of manual cardiopulmonary resuscitation. *J Am Coll Cardiol* 7:859, 1986.
42. Zaayer TW, Mackersie RC: Quantitative effects of external counterpressure on the work of breathing [abstract]. *Ann Emerg Med* 19:166, 1990.
43. Mattox KL, Bickell W, Pepe PE, *et al.*: Prospective MAST study in 911 patients [abstract]. *Ann Emerg Med* 19:167, 1990.
44. DeBehnke DJ, Angelos MG, Leasure JE: Comparison of standard external CPR, open-chest CPR, and cardiopulmonary bypass in a canine myocardial infarct model [abstract]. *Ann Emerg Med* 19:173, 1990.
45. Short CE: Principles and Practices of Veterinary Anesthesia. Baltimore: Williams & Wilkins, 1987, 576.
46. Anthi A, Tzelepis GE, Alivizatos P, *et al.*: Unexpected cardiac arrest after cardiac surgery. Incidence, predisposing causes, and outcome of open chest cardiopulmonary resuscitation. *Chest* 113:15, 1998.

Advanced Life Support

47. Schneider AP II, Nelson DJ, Brown DD: In-hospital cardiopulmonary resuscitation. A 30-year review. *J Am Board Fam Pract* 6:91, 1993.

Defibrillation

48. Emergency Cardiac Care Committee and Subcommittees, American Heart Association: Guidelines for cardiopulmonary resuscitation and emergency cardiac care. *JAMA* 268:2171, 1992.
49. Barton CW, Manning JE. Cardiopulmonary resuscitation. *Emerg Med Clin North Am* 13:811, 1995.
50. DeBehnke DJ, Swart GL: Cardiac arrest. *Emerg Med Clin North Am* 14:57–82, 1996.
51. Larson MP, Eisenberg M, Cummins RO, *et al.*: Predicting survival from out of hospital cardiac arrest: a graphic model. *Ann Emegr Med* 22:1652, 1993.
52. Kim YH, Yashima M, Wu TJ, *et al.*: Mechanism of procainamide-induced prevention of spontaneous wave break during ventricular fibrillation: insight into the maintenance of fibrillation wave fronts. *Circulation* 100:666, 1999.
53. Chen PS, Shibata N, Dixon EG, *et al.*: Activation during ventricular defibrillation in open-chest dogs. Evidence of complete cessation and regeneration of ventricular fibrillation after unsuccessful shocks. *J Clin Invest* 77:810, 1986.
54. Davy J-M, Fain ES, Dorian P, *et al.*: The relationship between successful defibrillation and delivered energy in open-chest dogs: Reappraisal of the "defibrillation threshold" concept. *Am Heart J* 113:77, 1987.
55. Sirna SJ, Kieso RA, Fox-Eastham KJ, *et al.*: Mechanisms responsible for the decline in thoracic impendence after direct current shock. *Am J Physiol* 257:H1180, 1989.
56. Geddes LA, Baker LE: Response to passage of electric current through the body. *J Assoc Advanc Med Instrument* 5:13, 1971.
57. Guarnieri T, Levine JH, Veltri EP, *et al.*: Success of chronic defibrillation and the role of antiarrhythmic drugs with the automatic implantable cardioverter/defibrillator. *Am J Cardiol* 60:1061, 1987.
58. Ruffy R Monje E, Schechtman K: Facilitation of cardiac defibrillation by aminophylline in the conscious, closed-chest dog. *J Electrophysiol* 2:450, 1988.
59. Yakaitis RW, Ewy GA, Otto CW, *et al.*: Influence of time and therapy on ventricular fibrillation in dogs. *Crit Care Med* 8:157, 1980.
60. Sirna SJ, Ferguson DW, Charbonnier F, *et al.*: Electrical cardioversion in humans: factors affecting transthoracic impedence. *Am J Cardiol* 62:1048, 1988.
61. Waldecker B, Brugada P, Zehender M, *et al.*: Dysrhythmias after direct-current cardioversion. *Am J Cardiol* 57:120, 1986.
62. Weaver WD, Cobb LA, Dennis D, *et al.*: Factors influencing survival after out-of-hospital cardiac arrest. *J Am Coll Cardiol* 7:752, 1986.
63. Larsen MP, Eisenberg MS, Cummins RO, *et al.*: Predicting survival from out-of-hospital cardiac arrest: a graphic model. *Ann Emerg Med* 22:1652, 1993.
64. Tacker WA, Niebauer MJ, Babbs CF, *et al*: The effect of newer antiarrhythmic drugs on defibrillation threshold. *Crit Care Med* 8:107, 1980.
65. Schleien CL, Berkowitz ID, Traystman R, *et al*: Controversial issues in cardiopulmonary resuscitation. Anesthesiology 71: 133, 1989.
66. Wesley RC Jr, Resh W, Zimmerman D: Reconsiderations of the routine and preferential use of lidocaine in the emergent treatment of ventricular arrhythmias. *Crit Care Med* 21:305, 1991.
67. Echt DS, Gremillion ST, Lee JT, *et al.*: Effects of procainamide and lidocaine on defibrillation energy requirements in patients receiving implantable cardioverter defibrillator devices. *J Cardiovasc Electrophysiol* 5:752, 1994.
68. Martin LG, Matteson VL, Wingfield WE, *et al.*: Abnormalities of serum magnesium in critically ill dogs: Incidence and implications. *J Vet Emerg Crit Care* 4:15, 1994.

69. Baty CJ, Sweet DC, Keene BW: Torsades de pointes-like polymorphic ventricular tachycardia in a dog. *J Vet Intern Med* 8:439, 1994.

Adrenergic Drugs

70. Yakaitis RW, Otto CW, Blitt CD: Relative importance of alpha and beta adrenergic receptors during resuscitation. *Crit Care Med* 7:293, 1979.
71. Michael JR, Guerci AD, Koehler RC, *et al.*: Mechanisms by which epinephrine augments cerebral and myocardial perfusion during cardiopulmonary resuscitation in dogs. *Circulation* 69:822, 1984.
72. Brown CG, Werman HA, Davis EA: The effect of high-dose phenylephrine versus epinephrine on regional cerebral blood flow during CPR. *Ann Emerg Med* 16:37, 1987.
73. Gisvold SE, Sterz F, Abramson NS, *et al.*: Cerebral resuscitation from cardiac arrest: treatment potentials. *Crit Care Med* 24:S69, 1996.
74. Brown CG, Davis EA, Werman HA, Hamlin RL: Methoxamine versus epinephrine on regional cerebral blood flow during cardiopulmonary resuscitation. *Crit Care Med* 15:682, 1987.
75. Brown CG, Taylor RB, Werman HA, *et al.*: Myocardial oxygen delivery/consumption during cardiopulmonary resuscitation: a comparison of epinephrine and phenylephrine. *Ann Emerg Med* 17:17, 1988.
76. Olson DW, Thakur R, Stueven HA, *et al.*: Randomized study of epinephrine versus methoxamine in prehospital ventricular fibrillation. *Ann Emerg Med* 18:41, 1989.
77. Brillman JA, Sanders AB, Otto CW, *et al.*: Outcome of resuscitation from fibrillatory arrest using epinephrine and phenylephrine in dogs. *Crit Care Med* 13:912, 1985.
78. Brillman JA, Sanders A, Otto CW, *et al.*: Comparison of epinephrine and phenylephrine for resuscitation and neurologic outcome of cardiac arrest in dogs. *Ann Emerg Med* 16(1):27, 1987.
79. Lindner KH, Ahnefeld FW, Pfenninger EG, *et al.*: Effects of epinephrine and norepinephrine on cerebral oxygen delivery and consumption during open-chest CPR. *Ann Emerg Med* 19:55, 1990.
80. Brunette DD, Jameson SJ: Comparison of standard versus high-dose epinephrine in the resuscitation of cardiac arrest in dogs. *Ann Emerg Med* 19:29, 1990.
81. Maha RJ, Yealy DM, Menegazzi JJ, *et al.*: High-dose epinephrine in prehospital cardiac arrest: a preliminary report of 50 cases [abstract]. *Ann Emerg Med* 19:7, 1990.
82. Crespo SG, Spivey WH, Kelly JJ, *et al.*: The effect of high-dose epinephrine on post-resuscitation cardiac output, catecholamines, and electrolytes in swine [abstract]. *Ann Emerg Med* 19:7, 1990.
83. Martin D, Werman HA, Brown CG: Four case studies: high-dose epinephrine in cardiac arrest. *Ann Emerg Med* 19:159, 1990.
84. Edgren E, Jeklsey S, Sutton K, *et al.*: The presenting ECG pattern in survivors of cardiac arrest and its relation to the subsequent long-term survival. *Acta Anaesthesiol Scand* 33:265, 1989.
85. Vanags B, Thakur RK, Stueven HA, *et al.*: Interventions in the therapy of electromechanical dissociation. *Resuscitation* 17:163, 1989.
86. Stueven HA, Aufderheide T, Waite E, *et al.*: Electromechanical dissociation: six years prehospital experience. *Resuscitation* 17:173, 1989.

87. Stueven HA, Waite EM, Troiano P, *et al.*: Prehospital cardiac arrest—a critical analysis of factors affecting survival. *Resuscitation* 17:251, 1989.
88. Sutton-Tyrrell K, Abramson NS, Safer P, *et al.*: Predictors of electromechanical dissociation during cardiac arrest. *Ann Emerg Med* 17:572, 1988.
89. Vincent JL, Thijs L, Weil MH, *et al.*: Clinical and experimental studies on electromechanical dissociation. *Circulation* 64:18, 1981.
90. Rush JE, Wingfield WE. Recognition and frequency of dysrhythmias during cardiopulmonary arrest. *J Am Vet Med Assoc* 200:1932, 1992.
91. Brown DC, Lewis AJ, Criley JM, *et al.*: Asystole and its treatment: possible role of the parasympathetic nervous system in cardiac arrest. *J Am Coll Emer Physicians* 8:448, 1979.
92. DeBehnke DJ: Effects of vagal tone on resuscitation from experimental electromechanical dissociation. *Ann Emerg Med* 22:1789, 1993.
93. Weil MH, Rackow EC, Trevino R, *et al.*: Difference in acid-base state between venous and arterial blood during cardiopulmonary resuscitation. *N Engl J Med* 315: 153, 1986.

Other CPR Drugs

94. Van Pelt DR, Wheeler SL, Wingfield WE: The use of bicarbonate in cardiopulmonary resuscitation. *Comp Cont Ed* 12:1393, 1990.
95. Browning RG, Olson DW, Stueven HA, *et al.*: 50% dextrose: antidote or toxin? *Ann Emerg Med* 19:113, 1990.
96. Nakakimura K, Fleischer JE, Drummond JC, *et al.*: Glucose administration before cardiac arrest worsens neurologic outcome in cats. *Anesthesiology* 72:1005, 1990.
97. Hossman KA: Resuscitation potentials after prolonged global cerebral ischemia in cats. *Crit Care Med* 16:964, 1988.
98. Gaver JW, Browning RG, Olson DW, *et al.*: The effect of dextrose on outcome of cardiac arrest in a canine model [abstract]. *Ann Emerg Med* 19:166, 1990.
99. Hughes WG, Ruedy JR: Should calcium be used in cardiac arrest? *Am J Med* 81: 285, 1986.
100. White BC, Winegar CD, Wilson RF, *et al.*: Possible role of calcium blockers in cerebral resuscitation: a review of the literature and synthesis for future studies. *Crit Care Med* 11:202, 1983.
101. Winegar CP, Henderson O, White BC, *et al.*: Early amelioration of neurologic deficit by lidoflazine after fifteen minutes of cardiopulmonary arrest in dogs. *Ann Emerg Med* 12:13, 1983.
102. Shapiro HM: Post-cardiac arrest therapy: calcium entry blockade and brain resuscitation [editorial]. *Anesthesiology* 62:384, 1985.
103. Steen PA, Gisvold SE, Milde JH, *et al.*: Nimodipine improves outcome when given after complete cerebral ischemia in primates. *Anesthesiology* 62:406, 1985.
104. Resnekov L: Calcium antagonist drugs—myocardial preservation and reduced vulnerability to ventricular fibrillation during CPR. *Crit Care Med* 9:360, 1981.
105. Sanders AB, Atlas M, Ewy GA, *et al.*: Expired PCO_2 as an index of coronary perfusion pressure. *Am J Emerg Med* 3:147, 1985.
106. Ditchey RV, Lindenfeld J: Potential adverse effects of volume loading on perfusion of vital organs during closed-chest resuscitation. *Circulation* 69:181, 1984.
107. Sanders AB, Kern KB, Fonken S, *et al.*: The role of bicarbonate and fluid loading in improving resuscitation from prolonged cardiac arrest with rapid manual chest compression CPR. *Ann Emerg Med* 19:21, 1990.

108. Whang R, Oci TO, Watanabe A: Frequency of hypomagnesemia in hospitalized patients receiving digitalis. *Arch Intern Med* 145:655, 1985.
109. Flink EB: Hypomagnesemia in the patient receiving digitalis. *Arch Intern Med* 145: 625, 1985.
110. Sellers RH, Cangiano J, Kim KE, *et al.*: Digitalis toxicity and hypomagnesemia. *Am Heart J* 79:57, 1970.
111. French JH, Thomas RG, Siskind AP, *et al.*: Magnesium therapy in massive digoxin intoxication. *Ann Emerg Med* 13:562, 1984.
112. Iseri LT, Chung P, Tobis J: Magnesium therapy for intractable ventricular tachyarrhythmias in normomagnesemic patients. *West J Med* 138:822, 1983.
113. Tzivon D. Keven A, Cohen AM, *et al.*: Magnesium therapy for torsades de pointes. *Am J Cardiol* 53:528, 1984.
114. Ramee SR, White CJ, Svinarich JT, *et al.*: Torsades de pointes and magnesium deficiency. *Am Heart J* 109:164, 1985.
115. Cannon LA, Heiselman DE, Dougherty JM, *et al.*: Magnesium levels in cardiac arrest victims: relationship between magnesium levels and successful resuscitation. *Ann Emerg Med* 16:1195, 1987.
116. Cairns CB, Persse D, Niemann JT: Effect of magnesium on cardiac resuscitation outcome after prolonged arrest [abstract]. *Ann Emerg Med* 21:601, 1992.
117. Siesjo BK: Cell damage in the brain: a speculative synthesis. *J Cereb Blood Flow Metab* 1:155, 1981.
118. Tobey RC, Birnbaum GA, Allegra JR, *et al.*: Successful resuscitation and neurological recovery from refractory ventricular fibrillation after magnesium sulfate administration. *Ann Emerg Med* 21:92, 1992.

Prolonged Life Support

119. Wingfield WE, Van Pelt DR: Respiratory and cardiopulmonary arrest in dogs and cats: 265 cases (1986–1991). *J Amr Vet Med Assoc* 200:1992, 1992.
120. Brown SA, Hall ED: Role of oxygen-derived free radicals in the pathogenesis of shock and trauma, with focus on central nervous system injuries. *J Am Vet Med Assoc* 200:1849, 1992.
121. Safer P: Cerebral resuscitation after cardiac arrest: research initiatives and future directions. *Ann Emerg Med* 22:324, 1993.
122. Niemann JT: Cardiopulmonary resuscitation. *N Engl J Med* 327:1075, 1992.

Prognosis

123. Kass PH, Haskins SC: Survival following cardiopulmonary resuscitation in dogs and cats. *Vet Emerg Crit Care* 2:57, 1993.
124. Pepe PE, Abramson NS, Brown CG: ACLS—Does it really work? *Ann Emerg Med* 23:1037, 1994.
125. Cummins RO, Ornato JP, Thies W, *et al.*: The American Heart Association Emergency Care Committee's Subcommittee on Advanced Cardiac Life Support. Improving survival from sudden cardiac arrest. The "chain of survival" concept. *Circulation* 83:1932, 1991.

29
Hemorrhage and Hypovolemia

Marc R. Raffe and Wayne Wingfield

INTRODUCTION

The mammalian cardiovascular system is small relative to body weight, with a sharp response to stresses placed on the patient. This appears to be well suited for daily needs and conservation of energy expenditure, but it is not robust during periods of supraphysiologic demand that may be required in response to acute blood loss or hypovolemia. When cardiovascular reserve capacity cannot meet the body's demands, failure of the hemodynamic system occurs and places the patient at exceptional risk. Decreased circulating blood volume adversely affects hemodynamic performance, producing reduced tissue perfusion and oxygen (O_2) delivery. Decreased tissue O_2 delivery and metabolic waste removal has profound systemic effects that occur in a relatively short time. Rapid recognition and intervention are required to prevent serious patient risk and adverse outcome. This chapter reviews key concepts and therapy in patients demonstrating hemorrhage or hypovolemia.

A discussion of body water distribution and physiologic response to blood loss is found in Chapter 13.

PATHOGENESIS

Tissue O_2 delivery must be balanced with tissue O_2 demand at any moment in time. Under normal conditions, tissue O_2 consumption is constant; a robust O_2 "reserve" is available on the hemoglobin molecule to meet moment-to-moment changes in tissue O_2 demand. Tissue O_2 delivery is predominantly influenced by cardiac output and arterial O_2 content. In hemorrhage or hypovolemia, a critical imbalance in O_2 supply and demand occurs. Biologic safeguards have evolved in an attempt to protect O_2 delivery as a core physiologic goal. In severe cases, protective mechanisms are inadequate to protect O_2 delivery triggering a sequence of events designed to preserve key functions at the expense of global homeostasis.

The sequence of "protective" actions begins when regional blood flow and O_2 delivery are mismatched and do not meet the immediate metabolic needs of the tissues. This imbalance in O_2 demand and supply is initially addressed by increased O_2 extraction of blood at the expense of maintaining systemic O_2 reserves. Imbalance in supply and demand is tolerated for short times because increased O_2 extraction can meet tissue O_2 demands for a brief period. The O_2

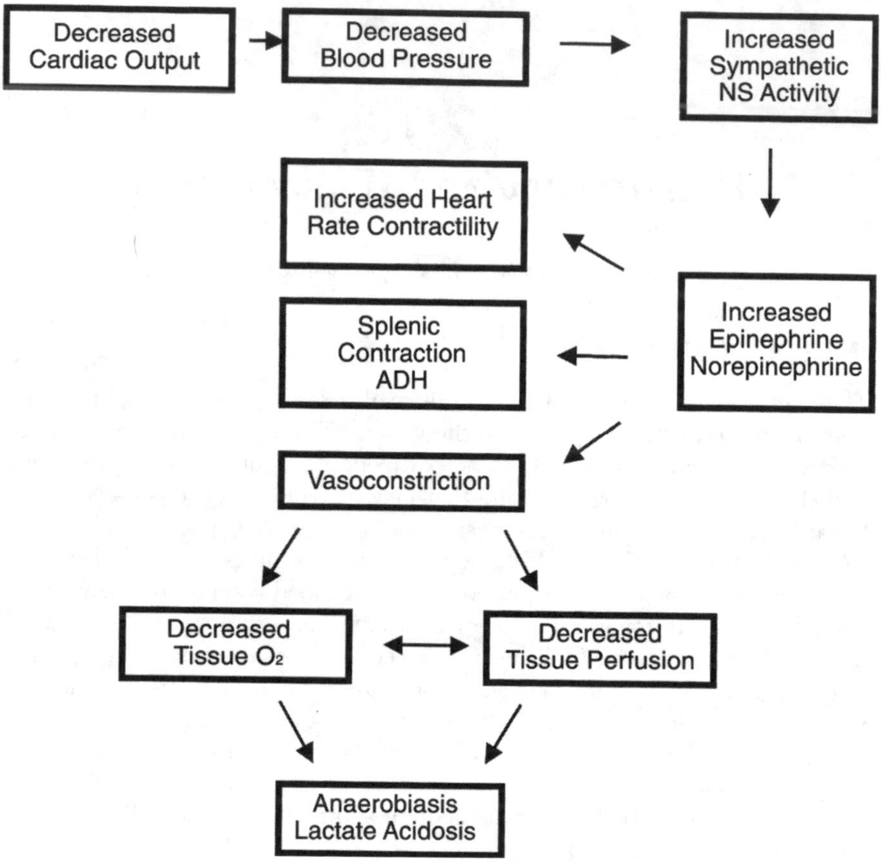

Decreased Cardiac Output
Decreased Blood Pressure
Increased Sympathetic NS Activity
Increased Heart Rate Contractility
Increased Epinephrine Norepinephrine
Splenic Contraction ADH
Vasoconstriction
Decreased Tissue O_2
Decreased Tissue Perfusion
Anaerobiasis Lactate Acidosis

Figure 29-1
Basic cycle of shock.

debt is repaid and homeostasis is restored if perfusion supply and O_2 delivery are stabilized by compensatory mechanisms or therapeutic intervention. If stabilization does not occur, O_2 demand continues to exceed supply, overwhelming compensatory mechanisms and producing physiologic activation of the shock cycle (Fig. 29-1).

Hemorrhage or hypovolemia results in decreased circulating fluid volume producing decreased blood pressure parameters. Specialized stretch receptors located in the aorta and carotid bodies detect a fall in blood pressure evoking a neurohumoral response mediated by the vasomotor center of the medulla oblongata. This response integrates autonomic activation characterized by increased sympathetic nervous system activity and humoral release from the adrenal medulla of epinephrine and norepinephrine. The composite physiologic response is vasoconstriction, increased heart rate, and increased myocardial contractility. This primary response is augmented by extrinsic responses including activation of the renin-angiotensin-aldosterone axis, release of antidiuretic hormone from the posterior pituitary, and release of adrenocorticotropic hormone. These responses increase fluid conservation to stabilize circulatory volume and optimize metabolism by recruiting additional energy substrates. Regional autoregulation preserves perfusion to key body organs including the heart, brain, and kidney at the expense of the liver, gastrointestinal tract, and muscle. Capillary blood flow is regionally affected by activation of pre- and postcapillary sphincters diverting blood from regional tissue networks. This is a key step in progression of the shock syndrome. Reduced capillary blood flow and O_2 delivery produces a mismatch in oxygen supply/demand and triggers a change to anaerobic metabolism at the cellular level. The mismatch is defined as *shock*. Capillary sphincter reactivity is altered producing precapillary sphincter dilatation and "pooling" of blood in microcirculation. Increased hydrostatic pressure produces fluid translocation to the interstitium further reducing circulating fluid volume.

Cell membrane integrity is compromised producing release of intracellular neuropeptides and inflammatory mediators including tumor necrosis factor, interleukin-1, interleukin-6, platelet-activating factor, and nitric oxide. These constituents, when introduced into the systemic circulation, evoke inflammation, further amplifying the shock syndrome. There does not appear to be a predictable time sequence during the initial phase of hypovolemia or hemorrhage that initiates release of these mediators.

Shock syndrome is subcategorized into three distinct stages. The *compensatory stage* is when endogenous response is adequate to stabilize the patient without further intervention. *Early decompensatory stage* is when compensatory mechanisms are inadequate to stabilize the patient. Maldistribution of blood flow and initiation of anaerobic metabolism occur, producing the classic signs of shock syndrome. This stage is amenable to intervention and resuscitation. *Terminal decompensatory phase* is when prolonged tissue hypoxia produces autoregulatory escape and hemodynamic collapse. Sympathetic and neurohumoral response is exhausted, producing a patient that is unresponsive to resuscitation measures.

CLINICAL SIGNS

Shock is a symptomatic syndrome that is diagnosed by recognizing clinical signs reflecting regional perfusion maldistribution. The magnitude and intensity of clinical signs reflect the degree of effective blood volume loss present in an individual patient. Mild to moderate blood loss produces minimal clinical signs reflected as elevated heart rate, increased blood pressure, increased respiratory rate, and normal to intense mucous membrane color. These patients are difficult to distinguish from the normal patient due to normal mentation and activity level. Indication of ongoing shock response may be gained by eliciting a history that includes a known insult that triggers the shock syndrome.

Early shock is characterized elevated heart rate, increased respiratory rate, altered mentation, subnormal or increased body temperature, diminished mucous membrane color intensity, increased capillary refill time, and coolness of extremities. Blood pressure may be either elevated or decreased based on magnitude of circulating fluid volume loss. Oliguria or anuria may be noted.

Terminal shock is characterized by low heart rate, decreased blood pressure and cardiac output, prolonged capillary refill time, pale or cyanotic mucous membrane color, decreased core body temperature, depressed mentation, cold distal extremities, and anuria.

DIAGNOSTIC EVALUATION

No specific diagnostic tests are available to confirm the diagnosis of shock. Early measurement of key parameters is helpful to create a database for later comparison. Parameters that are useful in documenting initial patient status and are helpful for monitoring purposes are listed in the section on patient monitoring.

THERAPY

Immediate resuscitation is indicated in cases demonstrating clinical signs of shock. Core therapeutic intervention includes support of hemodynamic function with fluid administration, O_2 support, and additional measures directed at underlying cause of shock. The universal goal of resuscitation is to maintain O_2 uptake and delivery to vital organs thereby sustaining aerobic metabolism. Therefore, the first priority in resuscitation therapy is to preserve blood flow (cardiac output) while correcting erythrocyte deficits. This strategy is one on which fluid resuscitation has been based for the past three decades.

O_2 Support

All resuscitation strategies are based on improving O_2 transport and delivery to tissues. One of the primary ways to improve O_2 delivery is to increase O_2 uptake at the lung. Increasing inspired O_2 concentration will, in most cases, meet this goal. Techniques for providing O_2 support are reviewed in Chapter 12.

Fluid Resuscitation

Mortality in hypovolemic shock is directly related to duration of the ischemic insult. Early replacement of circulating volume deficits is the key to successful patient management. The ability to infuse fluids rapidly to the central vascular compartment is critical. Several key decisions are made at the initiation of therapy, which dictates how therapy is administered.

Vascular Access

Studies have shown that central vein access is not critical for resuscitation. Vascular catheter dimensions, not vein size, determine the rate of fluid administration (Figure 29-2). Short catheters permit a higher fluid flow; therefore, they are preferred in resuscitation protocols. This is not a trivial issue; several studies comparing catheter diameter and length have reported significant differences in maximum fluid flow rates based on catheter diameter and length. The Hagan-Pouiselle equation indicates that flow rate is logarithmically proportional to catheter lumen diameter. Large-diameter catheters have a significantly higher maxi-

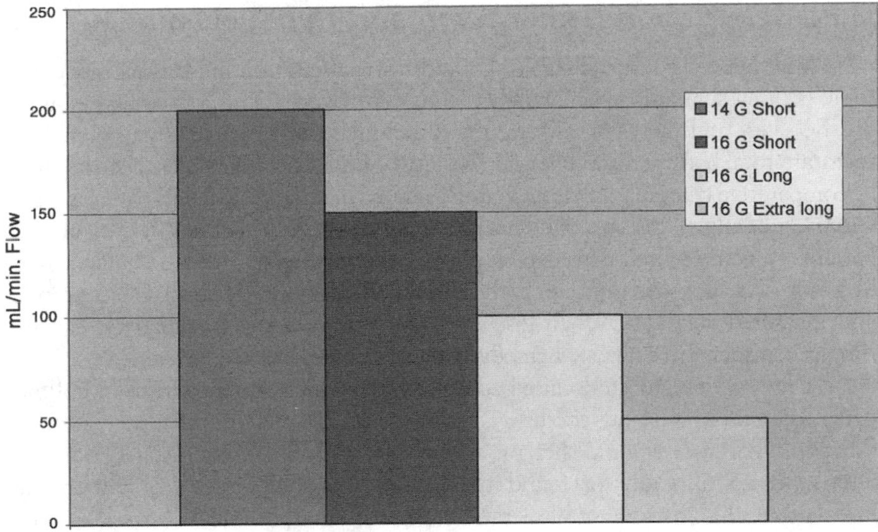

Figure 29-2
Relationship of catheter diameter and length to maximum flow rate (mL/min). (Adapted from Marino PL: The ICU Book. Lippincott Williams & Wilkins, 1998.)

mum flow rate; therefore, they should be selected for shock resuscitation. **The general rule in resuscitation is bigger is better.** Central vein catheterization requires catheters that are a minimum of 4 inches in length; peripheral veins may be catheterized with 2-inch catheters. Due to factors associated with the Hagan-Pouiselle equation, changes in catheter length have a linear effect on flow rates. A 4-inch catheter will have a maximum flow rate that is only one half that of a 2-inch catheter. Because central catheters are two to four times the length of peripheral catheters, flow rates may be reduced by as much as 75% compared to peripheral placement sites.

A minimum of two catheters should be placed for patient resuscitation. Multiple catheters permit higher resuscitation flow rates and provide an additional site for resuscitation drug administration. Multiline manifold systems are not useful in resuscitation. They do not permit higher flow rates because the limitation to higher fluid flow rate is the catheter lumen diameter.

High-volume rapid resuscitation may be facilitated by use of catheter introducers. These are short-length devices with large lumen diameter (>5 F) that are used for introduction of endovascular catheters such as a pulmonary artery or Swan-Ganz catheter. These devices require preplacement of a guidewire (Seldinger technique), which acts to ensure intravascular placement. Maximum flow rates are significantly higher with these devices. Fluid viscosity also plays a role in maximum fluid flow rate. Cellular fluids including blood and packed red blood cells (RBCs) will have a lower maximum flow rate compared to acellular fluids. Protein-based blood derivatives (fresh-frozen plasma) have an equivalent maximum flow rate to saline-based fluid solutions.

Fluid Selection in Hemorrhage and Hypovolemia

Whether to use crystalloids or colloids as resuscitation fluids is more than a topic of discussion, it is a passionately fought controversy! The controversy centers on the safest and most effective means to achieve the proper plasma volume to maintain total body perfusion. A wide variety of human patients have been studied in comparative trials ranging from young trauma to older critically ill patients with variable underlying diseases and conditions. Many of these studies in critically ill patients have presented considerable bias.[1] Most of the studies are characterized by a lack of homogeneity of their patient population and study designs, end-points, and measured variables. When discussing the use of these two fluid types, one should consider the expense, hemodynamic effects, risks, and outcome.

A review of eight randomized clinical trials comparing the effects of colloid versus crystalloid solutions on survival showed a 5.7% relative difference in mortality in favor of crystalloid therapy.[2] However, in trauma patients, a 12.3% difference in mortality rate was found in favor of crystalloids, and a 7.8% difference in favor of colloids in mortality rate in nontrauma patients. The confidence intervals for these studies were large and one must question whether the studies were appropriately assigned to trauma or nontrauma groups.[3]

In an analysis of these trials the pooled data demonstrated a 13.4% mortality rate humans treated with crystalloids and a 21.25% mortality rate for those treated with colloids (not statistically significant at a $P = 0.01$ level).[4] In this same study, when the trials were subdivided into the apparent severity of the underlying processes, again no statistically significant difference was noted between the two treatment groups, although there was a tendency to a higher mortality in patients with more severe illness treated with colloids.[5]

Colloids are more expensive than crystalloids (Table 29-1). With colloids costing anywhere from 20 to 60 times that of crystalloids, this is an important part of the decision for the veterinarian contemplating their use. Users of colloids suggest the cost per patient more than justifies this expense. As in all controversies, the use of these fluids should be based on the intended goals.

The object of resuscitation in hypovolemia is to maintain perfusion to vital organs and to increase oxygen transport, as well as other vital substances. With all IV fluids there is some loss of fluids and solute from the intravascular space into the interstitial space, which subsequently has to be cleared by lymphatic drainage. Furthermore, there is a solute load with potential adverse effects, which must be cleared. To avoid fluid overload and its sequelae, fluid replacement in shock requires careful monitoring. Careful selection and administration of an appropriate fluid are essential. Resuscitation must be tailored to the current and pre-existing disease conditions of the animal.

There are several points of agreement for initial management of hemmorhagic shock:

1. Most resuscitation protocols are based on use of an asanguineous fluid.
2. Asanguineous fluids are preferred for initial resuscitation unless massive bleeding is present.

Table 29-1. Electrolyte Concentrations (mEq/L) of Crystalloid Solutions

Solution	NA^+	K^+	Cl^-	Ca^{++}	Mg^{++}	Buffer mEq/L	Calories Kcal/L	Osmolality mOsm/L
Dextrose 5% in water	—	—	—	—	—	—	170	278
Dextrose 2.5% in 0.45% saline	77	—	77	—	—	—	85	280
Ringer's lactate solution	130	4	109	3	—	Lactate 28	9	272
Ringer's solution	147	4	156	4.5	—	—	—	309
Normosol-R* (Multisol-R)	140	5	109	—	3	Acetate 27 Gluconate 23	15	294
Dextrose 5% in Ringer's lactate	130	4	109	3	—	Lactate 28	179	525
Normal saline (0.9%)	154	—	154	—	—	—	—	308
Dextrose 50%	—	—	—	—	—	—	1700	2525
Dextrose 5% in saline (0.9%)	154	—	154	—	—	—	170	—
Potassium chloride	—	2000	2000	—	—	—	—	4000
Magnesium chloride	—	—	1970	—	1970	—	—	2951

* Normosol-R®, Abbott Laboratories, Animal Health, 1410 North Sheridan Road, North Chicago, IL 60064.

3. Saline-based fluids have a short intravascular retention time and must be supplemented to sustain their initial resuscitation effect.

Asanguineous fluids include isotonic saline and derivatives, colloids, and hypertonic saline.

Crystalloids. Crystalloid fluids are mixtures of sodium chloride (NaCl) and other physiologically active solutes. They are generally isotonic with plasma and have sodium as their major osmotically active particle. The distribution of sodium determines the distribution of infused crystalloid fluids. Sodium is the major solute in the extracellular space and 75% of the extracellular space is extravascular. Therefore, infused sodium will reside primarily outside the vascular compartment.

During phase I hemorrhage there is an interstitial fluid deficit that must be replaced during early fluid therapy. In fact, the goal of fluid therapy for mild hemorrhage is to fill the interstitial space, not the vascular space. This is the rationale for using crystalloid (sodium-containing) fluids for the resuscitation of mild hemorrhage. Sodium-containing fluids are well suited for the replacement of ECF losses (dehydration) and for replacement of blood volume. Their use is directed to replacement of the interstitial fluid deficits seen in hemorrhage. The significance of this deficit has been questioned. Nevertheless, crystalloid solutions have been effective in the resuscitation of animals with acute hemorrhage and they continue to be popular resuscitation fluids for trauma victims.

Isotonic saline and its derivatives (lactated Ringer's, Plasmalyte 148, Normosol R) are classically used in shock resuscitation. They meet many of the criteria described for resuscitation fluids including ready availability, option for high flow rate delivery due to low viscosity, and cost effectiveness. Resuscitation administration rates are reported to be 90 mL/kg/h for dogs and 55 mL/kg/h for cats. In clinical shock, the first hour dose may be "front-end loaded" and administered in as short as a 15-minute period. High flow rates may be achieved by use of large-bore catheter systems, pressurized fluid delivery systems, and multiple catheters.

Several concerns have been documented following saline-based fluid resuscitation. Crystalloids have been shown to quickly redistribute to extravascular spaces. Approximately 70% to 75% of administered isotonic crystalloids move to the interstitial space within 1 hour after administration. This is acceptable in cases with pre-existing dehydration contributing to hypovolemia but does not maintain vascular repletion achieved by initial infusion. When blood volume loss exceeds 15%, intravascular volume is not adequately supported due to transcompartmental fluid redistribution following administration. Hyperchloremic metabolic acidosis has been noted after administration of large volumes of normal saline. Certain buffers, notably acetate, may cause hypotension following high flow rate administration. Caution must be exercised in cases with pre-existing heart disease or low plasma protein levels. These cases will deteriorate with aggressive fluid administration due to underlying disease pathophysiology. If initial patient parameters indicate packed cell volume (PCV) less than 22%

or total protein (TP) less than 3.5 g/dL, blood products should be the primary resuscitation fluid.

Hypertonic Saline. Hypertonic saline produces rapid hemodynamic improvement following acute administration. Acute shock due to blood loss is a primary indication for hypertonic saline therapy. Several reports indicate that hemodynamic indices were better restored following this resuscitation strategy compared to isotonic fluid administration. The response appears to be enhanced by coadministration of a colloid solution.

The dose of hypertonic (5%–7%) saline is 4 mL/kg over 5 minutes as a one-time bolus (Table 29-1). The physiologic response that hypertonic saline produces appears to be a composite of effects. Plasma volume expansion is reported to occur following hypertonic saline administration. Studies in hemorrhage models indicate that a single hypertonic saline dose produces an equivalent resuscitation end point to four times the volume in isotonic saline. It is hypothesized that blood volume expansion occurs by recruiting water from RBCs and tissue spaces. Coupled with this information are reports that pulmonary vagal reflexes are activated to produce plasma volume expansion, increased cardiac output, and increased mean arterial pressure. These responses produce improved hemodynamic indices and tissue O_2 delivery with smaller resuscitation volumes. Hypertonic saline also has immunomodulatory effects that may protect organs from oxidative injury. Enhanced cell-mediated immune function was also noted. This observation support reports of reduced pulmonary pathology and cerebral edema in shock patients managed with hypertonic saline.

Colloids. Colloids are large-molecular-weight substances that do not readily pass across capillary walls. The colloid particles retained in the vascular space exert an osmotic force that maintains transcompartmental water balance and keeps fluid in the blood vessels. Because colloids are more effective than crystalloids in increasing vascular volume, colloid resuscitation should be more useful with severe bleeding. The most commonly used colloid solutions are listed in Table 29-2.

Both naturally occurring and synthetic colloids are commercially available. All colloids have clinical efficacy in shock management. Plasma substitutes such as dextran and hetastarch, with larger molecules than crystalloid or electrolytes solutions, are claimed to remain in the intravascular space longer and preserve higher levels of intravascular water. Such claims assert that colloids maintain blood volume longer than nonprotein solutions. Other clinicians strongly support the contention that crystalloids have an equal capability of raising intravascular volume, remain in the intravascular space long enough to be of practical value, and have other distinct advantages over colloids. These claims have led to a long-standing controversy over the relative merits of crystalloids versus colloids. This conflict has not been resolved over the last 20 years despite the work of many researchers.

Table 29-2. Commonly Used Colloids in the Treatment of Shock

	6% Hetastarch	Dextran-40	Dextran-70	Oxyglobin	Plasma
Colloid oncotic pressure	32.6	61.7	40	43.3	17.4
Unit size	500 mL	500 mL	500 mL	125 mL	Variable
Potency*	1.3:1	2:1	~2.1	—	1:1
Bleeding	0.001	0.010	0.010	—	0.001
Duration of action	24–36 h	4–6 h	24 h	30–40 hrs	24 hrs–14 d
Unit cost	$61.56	$22.77	$16.80	$125	$80

* Potency is the increase in vascular volume (mL) per mL infused colloid.

Adding to the confusion, hypertonic and hyperoncotic solutions have been investigated for use as volume expanders (7.5% NaCl, 6% Dextran, and similar formulations). Relatively small volumes of these formulations dramatically expand intravascular volume with minimal complications.[6] However, little is known about the long-term effects of massive fluid shifts from compartment to compartment in critically ill patients on life-support systems and with multiple cardiotropic IV medications. In general, colloids are considered during the initial resuscitation period or when TP is less than 3.5 g/dL or albumin less than 1.5 g/dL.

Plasma protein (albumin) transfusion is used in cases in which low plasma protein concentration is due to acute loss or hemodilution.. Albumin accounts for approximately 80% of intravascular colloid oncotic pressure under normal conditions. Approximately 40% of albumin is in the intravascular space; 60% is proportionately distributed between the interstitial and intracellular spaces. Interstitial albumin is continuously returned to systemic circulation by lymphatic drainage. Approximately 10% of interstitial albumin remains tissue bound and unavailable for mobilization. In humans, each gram of albumin is responsible for retaining 25 mL fluid in the compartmental fluid space. In acute volume loss, albumin is translocated to the vascular space. Serum levels will be maintained at the expense of interstitial stores. Albumin has several functions unrelated to its colloidal properties. It contributes to transport medium for drugs, hormones, metals, and enzymes. It may also act as a free radical scavenger and binds inflammatory mediators, reducing their activity. It is also protective against edema formation in "leaky" capillary syndrome associated with inflammatory diseases.

Plasma is administered at a dose of 10 mL/kg over a 3- to 6-hour period. Peak oncotic action occurs within 30 to 60 minutes following administration due to translocation of interstitial fluid into the intravascular space. In severe dehydration, supplemental crystalloid infusion is indicated to prevent intravascular hyperoncotic syndrome. The intra-vascular half-life of albumin is approximately 16 days.

Several complications have been associated with albumin administration. Pulmonary edema has been reported; however, studies refute this claim. Hypocalcemia has been reported following administration. This may be a reflection of several factors including properties of the administered anticoagulant and total volume of albumin infused. Allergic reactions characterized by hypotension and prekallkrein activation occur; however, the incidence is low in several reports.

Dextrans are mixtures of glucose polymers of various sizes and molecular weights that are produced by the bacterium *Leuconostoc mesenteroides* or lactobacillus grown on a sucrose medium. The molecular weight of the polymer varies according to growth characteristics and production purification. Currently, dextran 70 is commercially available. Dextran 70 has an average molecular weight of 70,000 with a range of 25,000 to 125,000. It is available as a 6% solution in normal saline. The dose of dextran 70 is 10 to 20 mL/kg/24 h. Up to 15 mL/kg can be given in the first hour for shock management.

Infusion of dextran 70 produces plasma volume expansion and improved hemodynamic performance. Part of the improved performance is a result of improved microcirculatory blood flow. Rheologic effects of dextran include decreased interaction between the endothelium and cellular elements of the blood, reduced viscosity, decreased RBC aggregation and rigidity, and decreased platelet adhesiveness. Three hours after infusion of dextran 70, about 70% of the administered dose is present in the vascular space. Approximately one third is present at 24 hours after infusion. Small dextran molecules are directly filtered in the kidney. Larger molecules are stored in hepatocytes and reticuloendothelial cells until metabolized into carbon dioxide and water.

Anaphylactoid reactions have been reported in humans and sporadically noted in dogs. The reason for the anaphylactoid reaction is dextran-producing bacteria in the gastrointestinal tract. Severe reactions can occur; however, the incidence is reported to be 0.03% of the human population. A dose-related primary hemostatic defect has been noted following dextran administration. The defect is multifactorial but is primarily associated with reduced platelet adhesion and aggregation mediated with factor VIII (von Willebrand) activity. Dextran also lowers clotting factor activity secondary to hemodilution, coats blood vessel walls and cellular elements, and impair elasticity and tensile strength of fibrin clots. Bleeding may occur more readily in patients known to have coagulation abnormalities. To minimize this risk, an administration ceiling of 20 mL/kg/d is recommended. Interference with measuring serum glucose by certain assays as well as interference with crossmatching blood may be noted.

Hydroxyethyl starch (Hetastarch, HES) is a modified amylopectin molecule. HES, like the dextrans, is a mixture of molecular weights ranging from 10,000 to 1 million with a mean molecular weight of 69,000 D. The oncotic pressure of the solution is 32 mm Hg and it has an osmolality of 310 mOsm/L when compounded as a 6% solution in normal saline. The pharmacokinetics of HES are a 50% retention time in the vascular space 48 hours after administration and 33% of the administered dose is still present in the intravascular space 8 days after administration. Small-molecular-weight units less than 50,000 are renally filtered; larger weight units are entrapped in the liver, spleen, and reticuloendothelial system and metabolized with time to glucose. HES has been shown to be an effective volume expander in numerous studies. Intravascular volume is greater than infused volume within 3 hours following administration and may persist as long as 24–36 hours. Studies in humans indicate an equivalent response following HES administration to that documented with plasma protein fraction. The HES dose is 10 to 30 mL/kg/24 h. Up to 15 mL/kg can be given in the first hour for shock management.

Complications reported following HES administration include an increased incidence of bleeding tendencies. Studies in humans indicate a HES related dilution of plasma fibrinogen and antithrombin III levels. Increased partial thromboplastin times and decreased factor VIII activity are noted. A case report of a subclinical von Willdebrand carrier demonstrating increased bleeding tendencies has been reported. Serum amylase levels have been shown to transiently increase following HES administration in humans. A low incidence of anaphylactoid reaction (0.085%) following HES has been reported.

Hemoglobin-based O_2 carriers (HBOCs) have been studied as a replacement for RBC therapy. Most current generation products are polymerized on a carrier molecule that has intrinsic colloid effect. This property, in association with the demonstrated O_2-carrying ability of these products, makes them attractive as resuscitation fluids. Currently, polymerized bovine hemoglobin (Oxyglobin) is available on the veterinary market. It combines qualities of colloid effect and O_2-carrying ability noted for this product group. It is currently approved for use in severe anemia; it has also been evaluated for shock resuscitation with mixed results. The dose schedule for Oxyglobin is 5 to 15 mL/kg in dogs and 5-10 mL/kg in cats.

Side effects with administration may include mucous membrane, scleral, and urine discoloration, mild gastrointestinal effects including nausea, vomiting, and diarrhea, increase in central venous and systemic blood pressure, and transient arrhythmias. Interference with certain laboratory measurements may also occur. Increases in the serum enzymes aspartate aminotransferase (AST), alanine aminotransferase (ALT), and serum protein will be noted. Prothrombin time (PT) and activated partial thromboplastin time (APTT) cannot be accurately measured using optical methods but magnetic, mechanical, and light-scattering methods are unaffected by Oxyglobin. Urinalysis following Oxyglobin will show inaccuracies in dipstick measurements of glucose, ketones, and protein.

The fact that Oxyglobin is stable at room temperature for 3 years, is compatible with all blood types, and is a potent carrier of oxygen, makes it a solution that may become more important in emergency and critical care medicine. The solution is currently used in diseases where it can provide temporary support at best. Hopefully, future O_2-carrying fluids will have a longer duration of action and will be more clinically useful.

Blood. Transfusion of blood components can be lifesaving in hemorrhagic shock patients. Goals for blood product transfusion include improved O_2-carrying capacity, improved colloid support, and coagulation support.

The indications for erythrocyte **(RBC) resuscitation** include PCV less than 22% in dogs or 12% to 15% in cats, estimated blood loss that is greater than 30% (30 mL/kg in dogs, 20 mL/kg in cats), ongoing hemorrhage associated with injury or surgery, and poor response to shock therapy in documented blood loss. The goals of RBC replacement are to restore a critical mass of RBCs to support hemodynamic function and O_2 transport to tissue beds. Products that provide RBC support include stored whole blood, fresh whole blood, and packed (concentrated by removal of plasma fraction) RBCs.

In acute hemorrhage, **whole blood** may be used to restore circulating blood volume and O_2-carrying capacity, intravascular colloid support, and coagulation factors. Fresh whole blood is the primary transfusion option if no stored blood products are available. Crossmatching the recipient to the donor is performed to ensure immunocompability; however, universal donor (CEA1 A-)

blood is used in emergency cases. Infusion rates for compatible blood are as follows:

1. Acute, life-threatening blood loss: 1 to 10 mL/kg/min up to 90 mL/kg in dogs or 75 mL/kg in cats.
2. In general, 20 mL/kg of whole blood will raise the hematocrit 10%.

In cases where blood is not crossmatched, the potential for immunoreaction (host versus graft) must be considered. To minimize this side effect, *all* transfusions are accompanied by intravenous (IV) administration of 0.5 mg/kg diphenhydramine (Benadryl) and 2 mg/kg dexamethasone phosphate or prednisolone analogues to suppress "minor" antigen response. A lower infusion rate (0.25 mL/kg/hr) is selected for the first 15 minutes and observation for transfusion reaction is noted. Transfusion reaction may be noted as the following signs: pyrexia, tachycardia, dyspnea, hypotension, shock, urticaria, pruritis, and hemolysis.

The major indication for selection of **packed RBCs** is correction of acute blood loss anemia. Like whole blood, crossmatching the recipient to a donor is performed to ensure immunocompatability; however, universal donor (DEA-1 A-negative) blood can be used in emergency cases. *All* transfusions are accompanied by administration of 0.5 mg/kg diphenhydramine (Benadryl) IV and 2 mg/kg dexamethasone phosphate or prednisolone analogue IV. Infusion rate protocols for compatible packed RBC units are as follows:

1. Emergency blood loss: 1 to 5 mL/kg/min up to 90 mL/kg in dogs or 75 mL/kg in cats.
2. In general, 10 mL/kg of packed RBCs will raise the hematocrit 10%.

Transfusion reactions are similar to those noted under whole blood above.

Fluid Selection for Treatment of Hemorrhage and Hypovolemia

In shock, therapy should be directed toward restoring the blood volume with an ideal resuscitation fluid. The ideal fluid is one that can carry O_2. The available crystalloid and colloid solutions are limited due to their inability to carry O_2. Whole blood is a complete and physiologic volume expander that is limited by its poor shelf life, fluctuations in availability, allergic reactions, and high cost. Although crystalloid and colloid solutions cannot carry O_2, their usefulness is increased by their availability and relative low risks.

Hemodynamic resuscitation is accomplished more rapidly with colloids because these solutions expand vascular volume more efficiently than crystalloid solutions. Crystalloid solutions equilibrate across the vascular membrane so that 10% to 25% of the solution remains in the plasma at the end of the infusion. However, in all forms of shock it is important to recall that there is an initial fluid shift from the interstitial to intravascular space. In essence, there is an interstitial dehydration that needs to be corrected early in shock. Thus, crystalloids serve an important role in resolution of this dehydration. Crystalloid solutions also dilute plasma proteins with consequent reduction in colloid osmotic pressure allowing for fluid movement into the interstitial space.

With these effects in mind, if the goal in fluid therapy is to replenish interstitial dehydration, then crystalloid solutions are the treatment of choice. If the goal in resuscitation is to increase the plasma oncotic pressure and effectively move fluid from the interstitial compartment into the plasma compartment, then the clinician should select a colloid solution. Advantages of hetastarch over other synthetic colloid solutions include a lower incidence of side effects and allergic reactions, stability on prolonged storage, immediate availability, and no dependence on animal blood donation. Hetastarch produces physiologic effects comparable to dextran and clinical studies have shown that hetastarch is at least as effective as dextran as a plasma expander. High-molecular-weight dextrans do not seem more likely to cause bleeding than hetastarch when recommended doses are used, but dextrans do promote histamine release (hetastarch does not) that can cause anaphylactoid reactions.

When shock occurs, blood proteins (albumin), whose osmotic gradient keeps fluid inside the capillary, are diluted by the flow of interstitial water into the intravascular space. If hypo-osmotic crystalloid is administered, a deterioration of the already diluted intravascular osmotic gradient occurs, and the lung tissue could pull water in from the hypoproteinemic serum, precipitating or worsening pulmonary edema.[7] The rationale for pure colloid solutions presumes that an increase in serum colloid osmotic pressure would increase the osmotic gradient in the serum so that cell free fluid would drift from the interstitial tissues into the intravascular space, promoting a drier lung in shock conditions. Because interstitial water ends up in the intravascular space as a result of increased osmotic activity, administering colloid should also give the added benefit of intravascular repletion greater than the sum effect of the infused volume.

However, the albumin content in lung interstitial tissue contains about 70% of the albumin in plasma. Thus, the increase in serum osmotic activity from infused colloid is very small, possibly too small to elicit a meaningful effect. Under normal conditions, the pulmonary lymphatic system clears albumin and fluid rapidly from interstitial tissues. Hypoproteinemia producing hypo-osmotic blood is quickly counterbalanced by a transient increase in lung lymphatic flow, decreasing the amount of albumin in lung interstitial tissue and promoting reequilibration of the osmotic gradient. Although it is theoretically tempting to postulate that serum of low colloid oncotic pressure promotes pulmonary edema in the presence of shock, no convincing studies demonstrate it, and several studies show that severe hypoproteinemia alone does not cause pulmonary edema.

Regardless of the type of fluid administered, a very fast rate of infusion will fill the right ventricle more completely, resulting in increased stroke volume and increased cardiac output. Studies of numerous kinds of volume expanders have shown few practical differences in outcome. As left ventricular pressures increase, increased pressure will also reflect back into the pulmonary vessels, eventually precipitating wet lungs. Pulmonary function tests in human trauma patients after

Table 29-3. Estimates of Volumes (mL/kg) in the Dog and Cat

	Dogs	Cats
Total body water	717 ± 17	596 ± 50.5
Erythrocyte (RBC) volume	36.9 ± 6	17 ± 3.2
Plasma volume	50.7 ± 4.3	44.3 ± 5
Whole blood volume	88.7 ± 8.3	60.1 ± 9.3

injury are found to be identical in groups of patients given high volume colloids or crystalloids.

The only acceptable end-point is mortality; that is, how many die when resuscitated with one program versus the other. Obviously, the difference in mortality is small. If the differences were large, say 50% or so, the argument would have been put to rest a long time ago.

RESUSCITATION VOLUMES

When a patient is excessively hypotensive and has clinical signs of shock, the blood volume must first be restored. Today it is recognized that shock (no matter which etiologic type) will progress from an initial hypodynamic, to a hyperdynamic, and finally another hypodynamic phase. Thus, if you wait for the classical clinical signs of shock to appear before administering IV fluids, the animal may slip into the terminal phases of shock with little likelihood of successful resuscitation. If you recall the phrase "anticipate shock," you should start all patients requiring in an intravenous catheter with a portion (1/4) of a shock volume before proceeding to the second phase of fluid replacement (replacement phase).

Traditionally for the dog, a shock volume is said to be 90 mL/kg/h (40 mL/lb/h) and for the cat, 44 mL/kg/h (20 mL/lb/h). But the numbers are derived from "whole blood volume" in the dog and a "plasma volume" in the cat (Table 29-3). Shouldn't we use the same criteria in determining shock volumes? Anecdotal experience shows the dog's traditional shock volume (90 mL/kg/h) is rarely required for resuscitation from the insult. More than likely, consideration should be given to recommending a plasma volume (50 mL/kg/h) as the shock volume for the dog and cat. Regardless of the controversy, the volume of fluid required is based on the patient's weight and you should be prepared to administer a shock volume each hour when crystalloid solutions are being used.

The patient's response determines the approximate volume to be given.

Combination Fluid Therapy

Fluid combinations are the most effective method of shock resuscitation. Isotonic and hypertonic saline may be combined with colloids to provide effective resuscitation with a lower resuscitation volume compared to isotonic saline as a monotherapy. Inclusion of colloids reduces isotonic fluid volume requirements by 40% to 60%; this may be useful in animals with a greater body weight. Although studies have shown that hypertonic solutions in combination with colloids provide a total resuscitation response, it is prudent to remember that both solutions rely on water translocation from the interstitial space to produce their effect. For this reason, most authors still advocate inclusion of isotonic solutions to replete the interstitial water volume translocated into the vascular network.

Sympathomimetic Therapy

Sympathomimetic therapy is indicated when fluids alone do not produce satisfactory hemodynamic response and tissue perfusion. The goal of sympathomimetic therapy is to improve cardiac output and systemic tissue perfusion while maintaining blood pressure at acceptable levels.

Dobutamine is the sympathomimetic of choice due to its physiologic actions that include direct positive inotropic response in the heart and systemic vasodilatation. These responses produce improved cardiac output and tissue perfusion while maintaining blood pressure. The dobutamine dose is 5 to 15 μg/kg/min. It is a drug that requires constant rate infusion due to its short intravascular half-life.

Dopamine exhibits both direct and indirect hemodynamic actions. It produces its physiologic actions by direct inotropic effects on the heart coupled with a dose-related constriction in capacitance vessels. High doses may produce increased blood pressure at the expense of improved blood flow. Dopamine may be used at 1 to 3 μg/kg/min for increased renal and visceral perfusion. In cases where direct cardiac support is required, 5-10 μg/kg/min may be required. It is a drug that requires constant rate infusion due to its short intravascular half-life.

Dopexamine has properties that are similar to dobutamine. It increases cardiac output and tissue perfusion without increased vascular constriction and blood pressure. It is administered at 5 to 20 μg/kg/min as a constant rate infusion.

General Medical Therapy

A variety of additional therapies have been investigated for shock management. Many therapies have shown promise in experimental studies that did not translate into successful clinical shock management. There is currently no consensus on value of additional therapeutic strategies in shock management. Potential therapies are briefly described below.

Analgesia

Pain may amplify the physiologic mechanisms that are initiated in response to shock. Many of the physiologic responses to pain and shock are similar and may be difficult to distinguish because both syndromes initiate a supraphysiologic stress state. In unstable patients, pain management is most effectively produced with opioid analgesics. Opioids produce an excellent therapeutic response with minimum hemodynamic consequence. Full agonists (morphine, oxymorphone) or partial agonists (buprenorphine, butorphanol) may be used for pain management. (See Chapter 7 for further information.)

Antimicrobial Therapy

Disruption of visceral organ perfusion carries a risk of barrier breakdown and enteric organism invasion. Endogenous flora varies with individual patient; both gram-positive and gram-negative bacteria may produce secondary effects that amplify the shock cycle. There is general agreement that antimicrobial therapy is indicated in these cases. In general, monotherapy with a "broad-spectrum" antibiotic to inhibit gram-positive and gram-negative bacteria as well as anaerobic flora is selected. Currently, cephalosporins appear to be the preferred monotherapy due to their efficacy and relatively low organ toxicity (Table 29-4).

Anti-inflammatory Agents

Glucocorticoids and nonsteroidal anti-inflammatory drugs have been extensively investigated in the shock syndrome. Although they have repeatedly shown promise in experimental studies, they have not shown consistent efficacy in clinical shock syndromes. Their use in hemorrhage and hypovolemia is not currently recommended.

Alkalinization

Alkalinizaiton has not been shown to be effective in shock states. Correction of underlying perfusion disturbances and restoring tissue homeostasis appear to be the best strategy for correcting acid–base imbalances noted in shock states.

MONITORING

Shock is a "symptomatic" disease; monitoring the shock patient is based on physical findings and key observations coupled with quantitative information regarding hemodynamic function and key organ viability. Despite all the advances in monitoring technology, none replace simple monitoring parameters and sound, fundamental patient evaluation. The parameter list below is not a comprehensive list of all monitoring techniques and technologies, but represents the most accurate, cost-effective options for patient monitoring in the resuscitation period. All observations and measurements should be recorded on a flow chart to determine the patient's progress.

Physical Parameters

Physical parameters are the cornerstone of evaluating the shock patient. Clinical impressions gained from physical parameter interpretation are the basis

Table 29-4. Antimicrobial Therapy in the Shock Patient

	Gram-Negative	Gram-Positive		Anaerobic
		Staph spp.	*Strep* spp.	
Penicillins				
Penicillin, Ampicillin Amoxicillin	−	±	+	+ Except *B. fragilis* and Actinomyces
Oxacillin, Methicillin Nafcillin, Cloxacillin	−	+	±	
Carbenecillin Ticarcillin Azlocillin Piperacillin Mezlocillin	+	+	±	
Cephalosporins				
First-generation	±	+	+	−
Second-generation	±	+	+	±
Third-generation	+	±	+	+
Imipenem/Cilastin	+	+	+	+
Aminoglycosides	+	+	−	−
Fluoroquinolones	+	+	−	−
Aztreonam	+	−	−	−
Metronidazole	−	−	−	+
Clindamycin	−	+	+	+

+ = Effective against this organism
− = Not effective against this organism
± = Variable effectiveness
Staph indicates *Staphylococcus;* strep, *Streptococcus.*
(Adapted from Haskins SC: Therapy for shock. *In* Bonagura J, ed.: Current Veterinary Therapy XIII. Philadelphia: Saunders, 2000.)

for management of the shock patient. Key physical parameters include the following:

1. Hemodynamic
   - Pulse rate
   - Pulse character and strength
   - Pulse rhythm
   - Mucous membrane color
   - Capillary refill time
2. Respiratory
   - Rate
   - Effort
   - Rhythm

- Mucous membrane color

3. Level of awareness
    - Alert
    - Depressed
    - Stuporous
    - Obtunded

Physiologic Monitoring

Serial monitoring of O_2 transport and delivery is key to management of the patient undergoing resuscitation for hemorrhage or hypovolemia. Clinically, no direct method exists to evaluate these parameters. In general, the clinician substitutes surrogate indices that evaluate hemodynamic performance and tissue O_2 delivery. Hemodynamic performance is monitored based on evaluation of preload, inotropy, and afterload.

Preload is clinically evaluated using central venous pressure (CVP) measurement. CVP provides information on intravascular volume status and ventricular function. Normal CVP levels are 0 to 5 cm water. Values in shock patients are generally less than zero. If a shock patient has a CVP greater than 10 cm water before resuscitation, cardiogenic shock is a likely cause. CVP should increase with fluid resuscitation. Generally, an end point of 10 to 12 cm water is used for resuscitation. If crystalloids are the dominant resuscitation fluid, anticipate a decline in CVP in approximately 1 hour. Additional fluid volume administration may be needed in these cases. In advanced centers, placement of a pulmonary artery catheter is used for resuscitation guidance. This catheter may be used to monitor CVP and pulmonary capillary wedge pressure, an indirect measure of left atrial pressure.

Inotropy is evaluated using cardiac output and blood pressure. Cardiac output may be monitored in advanced centers using a thermodilution technique following placement of a thermistor-tipped catheter in the pulmonary artery. In general practice, blood pressure is monitored in lieu of cardiac output. Blood pressure is the mathematical quotient of cardiac output and systemic vascular resistance. Direct blood pressure monitoring is preferred in critical cases. In addition to absolute values, the ability to observe the blood pressure waveform may provide valuable insight into volume status and cardiac performance. Blood pressure measured by indirect techniques (Doppler, oscillometry) are inaccurate due to poor detection capability associated with low perfusion. Inotropy may also be indirectly inferred from urine output.

Afterload may be calculated from data collected during measurement of cardiac output. If this is not feasible, indirect measurement of peripheral perfusion changes using toe web temperature are used as a "rough" assessment of afterload status. Toe web temperature within 8°F of core body temperature indicates normal afterload and perfusion. Temperature differences greater than this indicate poor perfusion and increased afterload.

Urine output is a valuable monitoring tool. Physiologically, urine production requires a minimum mean blood pressure of 60 mm Hg for renal perfusion and glomerular filtration. Urine output should be 1 mL/kg/h. Urine production less than this value may be used to indicate that additional resuscitation is required.

Oxygen delivery may be inferred from interpolation of several physiologic parameters. Pulse oximetry may be used to allow continuous monitoring of hemoglobin saturation (SaO_2) at a specific location. This information is helpful in determining whether O_2 delivery to the microcirculation is adequate. To be of value, pulsatile blood flow should be detected; most units will not provide a reading without pulsatile flow detection. Regional perfusion differences in shock may limit value of the information obtained. In general, perfusion to rostral regions is maintained at the expense of caudal regions. Therefore, monitoring SaO_2 in the head and neck region may not accurately reflect tissue perfusion in the caudal body regions. For this reason, caudal detection sites are preferred to provide a more global evaluation of the patient.

Paired blood gas samples coupled with pulse oximetry may be used to calculate O_2 extraction. See Chapter 2 for additional information.

Laboratory Measurements

Laboratory measurements provide a "trend" monitor of resuscitation response. They are not diagnostic or prognostic; they serve only to assist evaluation of global physiology and response to therapy.

Packed cell volume (PCV) and total protein (TP) are used to monitor resuscitation. These measurements are not sensitive in hemorrhage states; trend values "lag" for several hours following the acute crisis due to hematopoietic reservoirs. Additionally, loss of PCV and TP is proportional; therefore, no change in hematocrit is expected until fluid resuscitation is administered. The American College of Surgeons has issued a policy statement indicating that "use of hematocrit to estimate acute blood loss is unreliable and inappropriate." The value in PCV/TP monitoring is during the resuscitation period. A dilutional response in both parameters accompanies fluid resuscitation. A significant dilution effect in PCV will assist the clinician in selecting the appropriate resuscitation fluid. An optimal PCV should be between 28% and 35% in the postresuscitation period. PCV less than 22% should be regarded as a "transfusion trigger." TP values should not fall below 3.5 g/dL or albumin less than 2.0 g/dL in any case.

Blood glucose is monitored during initial presentation. Due to the stress response associated with the hemorrhage/hypovolemia period, it is expected that hyperglycemia will be present. Hypoglycemia indicates a coexisting reason for shock; this is generally related to infection/sepsis.

Blood gases are monitored to provide information regarding O_2 and acid–base status. The reader is referred to Chapter 19 for further information.

Blood lactate and pyruvate have been used as indicators to evaluate resuscitation therapy. Good evidence supports the value of monitoring the blood lactate/pyruvate ratio during resuscitation. Under normal conditions, pyruvate is a key substrate for cellular energy production. Pyruvate undergoes conversion to secondary substrates in the Kreb cycle and electron transport pathways enhancing energy production. Perfusion disturbance forces conversion of cellular energy production from aerobic to anaerobic glycolysis. This interconversion results in inefficient glucose utilization and lactate production. Restoring tissue perfusion and O_2 delivery promotes restoration of aerobic metabolism. Lactate can either be converted back to pyruvate or oxidized in the citric acid cycle for energy consumption. Lactate utilization consumes hydrogen ions that increase during the anaerobic period. Several studies in human and veterinary medicine have confirmed the value of monitoring lactate as a biochemical marker for evaluating tissue perfusion. Hemorrhage and hypovolemia are clinical presentations in which lactate measurement is a useful parameter.

Resuscitation end points in hemorrhage/hypovolemia:

- CVP: 12-15 cm water
- Pulmonary capillary wedge pressure: 10-12 mm Hg
- Cardiac output: >2.0 L/min
- O_2 uptake (VO_2): >100 mL/min/m^2
- Blood lactate: <4 mmol/L
- Base deficit 0 ± 2 mmol/L

PROGNOSIS

One of the enigmas in resuscitation is that correct therapy may be implemented with poor results. The reason for inconsistent resuscitation response is an active area of investigation. Core hemodynamic function may be restored; however, secondary injury associated with the reperfusion complex (see below) may exacerbate cell injury and ultimately produce an adverse outcome for the patient. Two key factors have been repeatedly shown to dictate patient prognosis. First, time from insult to resuscitation is the most critical variable. Delay in implementing therapy places the patient at risk for progression into irreversible shock. Therefore, early, aggressive intervention is key for successful outcome. The second key factor is patient response to therapy. Patients who favorably respond to initial resuscitation measures have a guarded prognosis; nonresponders have a poor prognosis.

RESUSCITATION CONTROVERSIES

Resuscitation is a science that is constantly evolving as our understanding of cell response to O_2 stress states improves. There are many areas of active investigation; several seem to have clinical significance to the resuscitation practitioner.

Resuscitation-Induced Hemorrhage

The prevailing opinion favors aggressive fluid volume resuscitation; however, an emerging body of evidence suggests volume resuscitation to normal hemodynamic indices increases uncontrolled bleeding. This observation is important for two reasons. One is that blood pressure is not the appropriate end point for resuscitation of hypovolemic shock. Second, therapeutic end points that are appropriate for the normal body may not be normal in injury states. Currently, an emerging body of evidence supports the concept of "hypotensive resuscitation." In this strategy, fluid resuscitation is provided but blood pressure parameters are maintained at levels higher than presentation and lower than normal until bleeding is controlled. Several studies indicate improved patient outcome with this strategy; however, this is an evolving area of investigation.

Postresuscitation Injury

Successful resuscitation does not guarantee survival. Hypoxemia-associated injury to major organs may continue after clinically successful resuscitation. The gastrointestinal tract and brain are the two organs most susceptible to damage. Two processes, no reflow and reperfusion injury, are believed to be involved.

No-Reflow Phenomenon

Microcirculatory defects may persist despite successful clinical resuscitation. Several mechanisms for this response have been proposed including calcium-induced vasoconstriction, leukocyte plugging, and vascular compression secondary to tissue edema formation. Persistent gastrointestinal hypoperfusion may lead to intestinal pathogen translocation and development of sepsis. The incidence and intensity appear to be correlated with the duration of flow disturbance during shock. At present, no specific therapy is available for management.

Reperfusion Injury

Tissue injury may be amplified in the postresuscitation period due to accumulation of toxic metabolites that are systemically redistributed during the reperfusion period. Systemic distribution creates tissue damage at remote locations. Toxic O_2 metabolites have been implicated in this process. Two potential sources of enhanced oxidant production include neutrophil activation and superoxide and hydroxyl radical formation. All organs are affected; the brain is particularly susceptible to reperfusion injury. A variety of therapies including antioxidants, corticosteroids, calcium channel blockers, free radical scavengers, and iron chelators have been studied for efficacy with inconclusive results. The critical element in managing reperfusion injury remains prevention.

Conclusions

In the emergency resuscitation of trauma patient with shock, the primary problem is low intravascular volume; secondary problems involve expansion or contraction of the interstitium depending on the patient's fluid status.[8] The majority of patients suffer from either relative or absolute volume deficits and there is an urgent need to replenish ECF volume. In the later stages of shock, the permeability of the capillaries gradually increases and a large quantity of fluid moves into the interstitial space. This further decreases blood volume with a secondary fall in the cardiac output, which further suppresses tissue perfusion. Under these dynamic circumstances, control of these interrelated clinical factors is difficult and the clinician's evaluation of different fluid regimens becomes nearly impossible.

Based on the available information in the noncritically ill patient, crystalloid solutions provide adequate replacement therapy. In patients with shock, it appears colloid solutions are a better alternative to massive infusion of crystalloids because they restore plasma volume without the excessive salt and water administration that can lead to overexpanded interstitial water and pulmonary edema. If the choice is which colloid to use in a hypovolemic patient, and if side effects are not the issue, then the human literature would support the use of hetastarch. Unfortunately, veterinary medicine must also factor in the economics of therapy. Without convincing evidence of a difference in survival, it is difficult to recommend routine use of colloid solutions.

When rapid expansion of plasma volume is needed, colloids are clearly superior to crystalloids.[9] In fact, crystalloid volumes are 3 to 12 times larger than colloids to produce the same increment in plasma volume. Additionally, the time required for resuscitation with crystalloids is reported to be twice that of colloids. Colloids are also superior to crystalloids in their ability to improve cardiac output and O_2 transport.

Pulmonary edema should not be a problem with either type of fluid if proper precautions and hemodynamic monitoring are used. Although crystalloids should produce pulmonary edema more readily than colloids, the risk appears to be small.

When pulmonary capillaries have an increase in permeability, the colloids leak from the vascular space and promote interstitial edema formation. Studies vary on the importance of this point and likely it is irrelevant which fluid you use. Close monitoring must be provided. Outcome data from human beings shows there is no difference in survival from hypovolemic shock when using colloids or crystalloid fluids for resuscitation.

In summary, if the goal is to expand the plasma volume, colloid solutions seem to be the logical choice. If the goal is to replenish the entire extracellular space, crystalloids are the fluids of choice. Fortunately for the small animal veterinarian, large volumes of crystalloids can be rapidly instilled and thus are the stalwarts of treatment for hypovolemia. If colloids are used for resuscitation, it is important to remember that the plasma volume expansion is not just due to the infused volume. More often the volume expansion occurs as a result of fluid shifts from the interstitial and intracellular spaces thus requiring additional free water and crystalloids for replacement.

REFERENCES

1. Thijs LG: Fluid therapy in septic shock. *In* Sibbald WJ, Vincent JL, eds.: Clinical Trials for the Treatment of Sepsis. Berlin: Springer-Verlag, 1995, p 167.
2. Velanovich V: Crystalloid versus colloid fluid resuscitation: a meta-analysis of mortality. *Surgery* 105:65, 1989.
3. Rubeiz GL, Thill-Baharozian M, Hardie D, Carlson RW: Association of hypomagnesemia and mortality in acutely ill medical patients. *Crit Care Med* 21:203, 1993.
4. Bissoni RS, Holtgrave DR, Lawler F, *et al.*: Colloids versus crystalloids in fluid resuscitation: an analysis of randomized controlled trials. *J Fam Pract* 32:387, 1991.
5. Touitou Y, Touitou C, Bogdan A, *et al.*: Serum magnesium circadian rhythm in human adults with respect to age, sex and mental status. *Clin Chem Acta* 87:35, 1978.
6. Holcroft JW, Vasser MJ, Turner JE, *et al.*: 3% NaCl and 7.5% NaCl/dextran 70 in the resuscitation of severely injured patients. *Ann Surg* 206:279, 1987.
7. Virgilio RW, Rice CL, Smith DE, *et al.*: Crystalloid versus colloid resuscitation: is one better? A randomized clinical study. *Surgery* 85:129, 1979.
8. Mandell DC, King LG: Fluid therapy in shock. *Vet Clin North Am Small Anim Pract* 28:623, 1998.
9. Mattox KL, Maningas PA, Moore EE, *et al.*: Prehospital hypertonic saline/dextran infusion for post-traumatic hypotension. *Ann Surg* 213:482, 1991.

BIBLIOGRAPHY

Day TK: Shock syndromes in veterinary medicine. *In* DiBartola S, ed.: Fluid Therapy in Small Animal Practice, 2nd ed. Philadelphia: Saunders, 2000, p. 428.

Driessen B, Jahr JS, Lurie F, *et al.*: Inadequacy of low-volume resuscitation with hemoglobin-based oxygen carrier hemoglobin glutamer-200 (bovine) in canine hypovolemia. *J Vet Pharmacol Ther* 24:61, 2000.

Haskins SC: Therapy for shock. *In* Bonagura J, ed.: Current Veterinary Therapy XIII. Philadelphia: Saunders, 2000, p. 140.

Hughes DR: Clinical use of blood lactate concentration in the critically ill patient. Proceedings of IVECCS VI, 1998, p. 529.

Mitchell RN, Cotran RS: Hemodynamic disorders, thrombosis, and shock. *In* Cotran RS, Kumar V, Collins T, eds.: Pathologic Basis of Disease, 6th ed. Philadelphia: Saunders, 1999, p. 113.

Mizock BA, Falk JL: Lactic acidosis in critical illness. *Crit Care Med* 20:80, 1992.

Schertel ER, Tobias TA: Hypertonic fluid therapy. *In* DiBartola S, ed.: Fluid Therapy in Small Animal Practice, 2nd ed. Philadelphia: Saunders, 2000, p. 496.

Walton RS: Shock. *In* Wingfield WW, ed.: Veterinary Emergency Medicine Secrets, 2nd ed. Philadelphia: Hanley & Belfus, 2001, p. 28.

SUGGESTED READING

Diagnosis and treatment of shock syndromes. *In* Ayres SM, Grenvik A, Holbrook PR, Shoemaker WC, eds.: Textbook of Critical Care, 3rd ed. Philadelphia: Saunders, 1996, p. 85.

Hemorrhage and hypovolemia. *In* Marino PL, ed.: The ICU Book, 2nd ed. Baltimore: Williams & Wilkins, 1998, p. 207.

30
The Management of Acute Heart Failure

Anthony P. Carr

INTRODUCTION

Acute heart failure is a dramatic emergency that requires rapid and appropriate intervention by the clinician to prevent the death of the patient. This means that the signs of heart failure must be recognized and therapy tailored to the individual requirements of that patient. It is vital to recognize that these patients are frail; they are often incapable of withstanding stressful events such as restraint and positioning for radiography, placement of an intravenous catheter, or even being presented to a veterinary clinic. By recognizing this the veterinary care team can avoid becoming the patient's worst enemy. In some cases it may mean that empiric therapy needs to be started to stabilize the patient without having a definitive diagnosis.

Heart failure has been categorized in various ways. One can differentiate between left and right sided heart failure, between backward and forward failure, as well as between high output and low output states. In most patients there are a combination of these categories present, whereby clinical judgement is needed to determine which category (ies) are the most vital to address. Categorization is helpful in that it can make it easier to understand the basis for the failure present and thereby guide in the selection of therapies to initiate.

PATHOGENESIS

There are a variety of reasons for heart failure. In dogs the predominant causes are valvular insufficiency through endocardiosis or myocardial failure secondary to dilated cardiomyopathy (DCM). In cats, generally myocardial disease (hypertrophic, dilated, or restrictive cardiomyopathy) is the cause for heart failure. In cats signs tend to be acute in nature; in dogs there tends to be a history of signs consistent with heart disease (cough, exercise intolerance). Acute signs of heart failure can occur in a compensated patient as a result of a stressful event such as anesthesia or excessive exercise. Common to heart failure is the inability to provide adequate cardiac output to meet the demands of the tissues.

Often cardiac disease is chronic in nature so that compensatory mechanisms have already come into play. The many mechanisms involved with compensating cardiac insufficiency are complex and not completely understood. Some mechanisms that have been investigated include activation of the renin-angiotensin-aldosterone system and increased activity of the sympathetic nervous system.

These mechanisms can compensate for decreased cardiac output but there are negative consequences. Fluid retention with volume expansion occurs. This increases cardiac output by increasing preload; however, at a certain critical level, it also leads to signs of congestion (pulmonary edema or ascites) through backward failure. Heart rate and contractility are increased by the sympathetic nervous system activity. This increases myocardial oxygen demand and can predispose to arrhythmias. In addition, the periphery is vasoconstricted which maintains blood pressure but also increases afterload which results in decreased cardiac output.

In certain situations forward failure can predominate. This is common in dilated cardiomyopathy and those cases of heart failure induced by an arrhythmia. In this situation poor cardiac output is too low to meet the demands of peripheral tissues. Hypothermia, azotemia, prolonged capillary refill time, hypotension, and poor pulse quality can be present. Treatment is then directed at improving perfusion by the use of judicious fluid therapy and positive inotropes. The most difficult cases to treat are where congestion and low output failure are present as treatment for one can make the other worse.

EPIDEMIOLOGY

Acute congestive heart failure can occur in any breed of dog or cat at any age. In dogs mitral valve endocardiosis and dilated cardiomyopathy are the most common causes of congestive heart failure (CHF). Endocardiosis most commonly occurs in older (>10 years old) small breed dogs such as miniature Poodles, miniature Schnauzers, Pomeranians, and others. Cavalier King Charles Spaniels have a high incidence of mitral valve endocardiosis and clinical signs can develop at an earlier age. Dilated cardiomyopathy generally occurs in large breed dogs at an earlier age. Breeds highly predisposed to DCM include Irish Wolfhounds, Dobermans, Great Danes, and Boxers. Some smaller dogs such as Cocker Spaniels and English Bulldogs can also be affected.

Hypertrophic cardiomyopathy currently is the most common form of cardiomyopathy in cats. Cardiomyopathy in cats usually occurs in middle-aged cats, with males more commonly affected than females. Older cats can also develop secondary cardiomyopathies such as through hyperthyroidism, hypertension, or acromegaly.

CLINICAL PRESENTATION

History and Presentation

Cats can have minimal signs prior to presentation; most dogs do have a history suggestive of heart disease. In cats, thromboembolism may be the first presenting complaint with acute posterior paresis/paralysis.

Exercise intolerance and weakness may be present. In some cases collapse episodes may have occurred.

Signs of respiratory problems such as cough, dyspnea, or tachypnea may have been noted. In cats, open mouth breathing may have been noted.

With chronic disease, inappetance and weight loss may have occurred prior to presentation.

Diagnostic Evaluation

Physical Examination

A thorough physical examination is vital in any emergency patient. Often the findings of the exam combined with the history can lead to a high index of suspicion of heart failure as the predominant clinical problem.

- Visual inspection: Signs of respiratory distress may be present such as dyspnea, tachypnea, cough, or open mouth breathing. The patient may be standing with elbows abducted to recruit accessory respiratory muscles. Muscle mass loss may also be present. Some patients will be recumbent and collapsed. Coughing up of blood-tinged fluid must be considered an indication of severe heart failure and has negative prognostic implications.
- Mucous membranes: Cyanotic and or pale mucous membranes may be noted. Capillary refill time may be increased.
- Body temperature: Hypothermia is common in cats with acute heart failure; in dogs it usually only seen with low output failure states.
- Jugular vein: Distension of the jugular vein or a jugular vein pulse can be an indicator of increased pressure in the right atrium. This can be seen with right-sided heart failure such as occurs with tricuspid disease, heartworm infestation, and pericardial effusion.
- Auscultation: In most cases a heart murmur can be ausculted in dogs and cats with heart failure. The character of the murmur (timing, intensity, and point of maximal intensity) should be delineated. Crackles may be heard with pulmonary edema although this is less commonly heard in cats. Auscultation may reveal that the heartbeat is irregular through arrhythmias. Generally heart rate will be markedly elevated. In cats, a gallop may be heard. Muffling of normal sounds may indicate pericardial or pleural effusion. The latter is common in cats with heart failure. Percussion of the thorax can reveal if damping is present which is suggestive of fluid in the thorax.
- Pulse quality: While ausculting, the pulses need to be felt to detect pulse deficits. Poor and rapid pulses are common.
- Abdominal palpation and ballottement: Fluid may be present; abdominocentesis should be performed to confirm its presence and to determine the nature of the fluid.

Blood Pressure

Blood pressure measurement is definitively indicated in those patients that have signs of low output failure. This is also an important parameter to monitor therapeutic efficacy. Both oscillometric and Doppler based monitors are available. The oscillometric devices have the advantage of determining both the diastolic and systolic pressure. Direct blood pressure measurement via an arterial catheter is also possible though less commonly used. In truly critical patients this does have the benefit of continuous monitoring and is preferable if available.

ECG

The main value of an ECG tracing is determination of heart rate and rhythm. Though an ECG can be suggestive of heart enlargement, the lack of sensitivity and specificity of these changes significantly limit their diagnostic value. Arrhythmias are common in patients with heart failure. Not all arrhythmias require specific therapy since many will resolve with treatment of the underlying heart failure. Certain situations however necessitate intervention. Good examples are supraventricular tachycardias such as atrial fibrillation or atrial tachycardia. In these cases, the high heart rates prevent adequate ventricular filling and cardiac output is significantly compromised. Sustained ventricular tachycardias may also need to be addressed, especially if signs of low output failure are present. In some cases where atrial tachycardia is suspected, use of ocular or carotid pressure with ECG monitoring may allow a definitive rhythm diagnosis to be established.

Radiology

Radiology is still the cornerstone of emergency diagnosis of acute heart failure in both cats and dogs. It allows visualization of the heart, lungs, and other thoracic structures. This is a stressful event and it is necessary to determine if a patient can tolerate the procedure. Some signs that can be seen in heart failure patients include cardiomegaly, pulmonary edema, and pleural effusion. It is important to make sure that the clinical signs noted match the radiographic diagnosis.

Echocardiography

Echocardiography is a valuable tool in diagnosing cardiac disease. In cats it is usually a necessity in order to determine what form of cardiomyopathy is present. Since emergency treatment for heart failure will rarely change based on an echocardiogram, it is possible to delay this procedure until the patient has stabilized. In dogs, this diagnostic method is important in those cases where pericardial effusion is suspected.

Laboratory Evaluation

Certain laboratory abnormalities can be detected in patients with heart failure, especially if a low output failure state is present. Azotemia, hyponatremia, and occasionally elevated liver values can be found at presentation. More importantly, medications used to treat heart failure can cause changes to occur in electrolytes and renal values so that routine laboratory testing is recommended in patients that are being treated for heart failure.

TREATMENT

General Therapy

In most patients with acute heart failure basic general therapy is indicated.

- Quiet: Because of cardiac insufficiency, it is not possible for the patient to adapt to increased demand. Stress through anxiety, fear, and restraint has to be minimized. In most cases placing the animal in a cage in a quiet area and avoiding manipulating the patient excessively is all that is required. Rarely will a sedative (in dogs, morphine 0.1 mg/kg IV, IM) be needed to achieve this goal.

- Oxygen: All patients with acute heart failure will benefit from oxygen supplementation. This will minimize anxiety on the part of the patient and can significantly reduce the frequency of arrhythmias in many. Oxygen can be delivered in many ways. Initial flow rates of 0.05 to 0.1 L/kg/min should be adequate. Humidification of the oxygen delivered is vital if therapy is extended for any length of time.
    - Mask
    - Nasal oxygen catheter
    - Oxygen cage or tent

- Thoracocentesis: Thoracocentesis is indicated whenever significant thoracic fluid accumulation is suspected or confirmed. This is a relatively rare occurrence in dogs but quite common in cats with cardiomyopathy. This procedure has both diagnostic and therapeutic value. A sample of the fluid removed should undergo fluid analysis and cytological evaluation. Thoracocentesis is usually performed between the 7th and 10th intercostal space at the costochondral junction on one or both sides of the thorax after the area has been shaved and aseptically prepared. Most times sedation is not required. Use of a three-way stopcock and an extension set can make the procedure easier to perform.
- Abdominocentesis: Significant accumulation of abdominal fluid is rare in cats with heart disease but it is common in dogs with right-sided congestive heart failure. This procedure also has diagnostic and therapeutic indications. Usually it is only required in patients where massive distension of the abdomen has occurred that is impairing respiration and decreasing patient comfort.

Congestive (Backward) Heart Failure

Congestion is usually reduced either through the use of diuretics or vasodilators (especially venodilators). In animals with cardiac disease, increased preload is one of the compensatory mechanisms used to sustain cardiac output. As a result, overly aggressive preload reduction can lead to a very rapid decline in preload and, therefore, cardiac output.

Furosemide Injections

Furosemide at 2–4 mg IV or IM in dogs (in cats 1–2 mg/kg is usually adequate) repeated every 3 to 4 to 8 hours as needed (in severe cases repeated every hour) till congestion is under control is usually the first therapy initiated. In heart failure, perfusion is poor so that SQ and PO routes of administration result in delayed absorption. Intravenous administration is the most rapid but can be stressful for the animal. Intravenous injection can also significantly reduce preload leading to a drop in cardiac output, this is especially important to consider in those patients with signs of congestive failure and low output failure. Furosemide should only be used as needed for control of congestion. When used aggressively monitor for signs of such as a cool periphery, weakness and lack of appropriate urine output. In those cases where low output signs are present judicious fluid therapy may be needed (half maintenance rate with low sodium fluids such as D5W or half strength saline/dextrose) as a concurrent therapy.

Nitroglycerine

Nitroglycerine acts as a venodilator, reducing preload by putting blood into the abdominal circulation. An antithrombotic effect may also be present which make it attractive in cats at risk for thromboembolism. Wear gloves to apply as it is absorbed through skin. It is available as a 2% ointment that is applied to non-haired skin 3 to 4 times daily, 1/4 inch in a cat, in dogs 1/4 inch per 5 to 10 kg. Patches are also available that are dosed at 0.1 mg/hr patch per 10 kg of body weight.

Nitroprusside

This medication is a potent venous and arteriolar dilator. Nitroprusside must be given as a constant rate infusion. Because of its short half life, it is possible to titrate the dosage to effect with blood pressure monitoring. This medication should not be used unless blood pressure can be monitored. It should be reserved for the most severe fulminant heart failure cases. Initial dosage is 1 mcg/kg/min, this can be increased by 1 mcg/kg/min every 5 to 10 minutes until mean arterial blood pressure is stabilized at around 70 mmHg, but a total dose of 10 mcg/kg/min should be not be exceeded. Ideally pulmonary wedge pressure should also be monitored in these patients. If hypotension is encountered, the infusion rate is reduced. Cyanide toxicity can occur at infusion rates over 2 mcg/kg/min so that the duration of therapy should be as short as possible—depending on the dosage used, possibly less than 24 hours.

Hydralazine

Hydralazine is a potent arteriolar dilator useful for short-term management of congestive heart failure. Arteriolar dilation results in decreased systemic vascular resistance which can markedly improve forward cardiac output in patients with significant regurgitation. In patients with myocardial dysfunction, this medication is less beneficial. The main adverse side effect is significant hypotension that can lead to decreased perfusion of vital organs, especially the kidney. Blood pressure measurement is the ideal way to assess the success of this therapy and to guide in dosage selection. Therapeutic goals are to improve clinical signs (usually in patients with refractory or difficult to treat heart failure) and to bring mean arterial blood pressure down to 60 to 80 mmHg. It is possible to monitor just using clinical signs, however this can at times miss significant hypotension. If blood pressure can be measured, the initial dosage is 1 mg/kg in patients not already receiving an ACE inhibitor (0.5 mg/kg in those on an ACE inhibitor).

Within 1 hour decreases in blood pressure should be seen that will peak at 3 hours post pill. If blood pressure decreases then this is the dose of hydralazine to give every 12 hours. If blood pressure does not decrease, then another 1mg/kg can be given. If it too is not effective, another 1 mg/kg can be given (maximal cumulative dose of 3 mg/kg). In dogs on an ACE inhibitor, dosage increases should be only 0.5 mg/kg at a time to avoid profound hypotension. If blood pressure cannot be measured, then initial dosages should be low (0.5 mg/kg) and dose should be adjusted every 12 hours using clinical parameters.

ACE Inhibitor

ACE inhibitors are balanced vasodilators (venous and arterial) that reduce preload and afterload. Action onset will be delayed because oral absorption will be poor in congestive heart failure (CHF). Enalapril 0.25 to 0. 5mg/kg SID or BID or benazapril 0.25 to 0.5 mg SID can be used. Do check renal values 3 to 5 days into therapy as renal insufficiency can rarely occur.

Low Output (Forward) Failure

Synthetic Caitecholamines

Inotropic support therapy with synthetic catecholamines requires having the facilities to monitor therapy (*i.e.*, blood pressure and continuous ECG) and deliver therapy (infusion pumps). This therapy can be quite helpful with low output failure such as seen in Dobermans with DCM. This form of therapy is rarely needed in cats. Potential adverse side effects include arrhythmias and increases in heart rate. Higher dosages of dopamine (>10 mcg/kg/min) can also result in vasoconstriction, which would increase afterload and thereby decrease cardiac output. This usually is deleterious to the patient's condition, other than in those cases where severe hypotension is seen such as with cardiac shock. Dobutamine (1–15 mcg/kg/min, usually start at 3–5 mcg/kg/min) and dopamine (2–10 mcg/kg/min) are most commonly used and must be given as a constant rate infusion (CRI). Initially lower dosages are used and titrated upward if necessary. If side effects are seen, the rate of administration is reduced. If atrial fibrillation or other tachyarrhythmias are present, medical therapy of the rhythm disturbance is necessary before beginning inotropic support since heart rate will increase with therapy. Dobutamine is the preferred drug since it causes fewer arrhythmias and does not cause vasoconstriction as dopamine does. However, the cost can be considerably higher depending upon whether generic or trade name products are used. The synthetic catecholamines lose efficacy in 24 to 72 hours.

Digoxin

The positive inotropic effects of digoxin are relatively weak, but it has the benefit that advanced monitoring equipment is not needed. The digitalis glycosides also have the advantage that they can also aid in controlling supraventricular tachycardias such as atrial fibrillation. Caution must be used in the face of ventricular tachycardias as digitalis can lead to worsening of the arrhythmia.

Toxicity can occur easily as the therapeutic range is small. Hypokalemia exacerbates toxicity.

Bipyridines (amrinone, milrinone)

This group of compounds has both inotropic and vasodilating properties. Experience with their use in small animal medicine is limited. Amrinone is available as an intravenous agent. Initial dosage in dogs is 1–3 mg/kg i.v. bolus followed by a CRI of 10 to 100 mcg/kg/min.

Arrhythmia Control

Often oxygen therapy and therapy of heart failure will improve the environment of the heart thereby helping to control irregular heartbeats. Certain arrhythmias do require specific intervention. In some cases the arrhythmia alone may be causing the signs of congestive heart failure. This can occur with extremely rapid heart rates such as is seen with sustained atrial tachycardia.

Atrial Fibrillation/Atrial Tachycardia

The rapid heart rates associated with atrial fibrillation and atrial tachycardia result in inadequate ventricular filling and poor cardiac output. The predominant goal of therapy is to control the heart rate. Ideally heart rate in the hospital should be below 160 to 180 BPM. With atrial tachycardia, a vagal maneuver such as ocular pressure or carotid massage may be able to achieve conversion to a normal sinus rhythm. If this maneuver fails or atrial fibrillation is present with a high ventricular response rate, medical attention is necessary. Digoxin (0.22 mg m^2 BID, or 0.0055 to 0.01 mg/kg BID, double dose for first 24 hours if needed for rapid onset of action) is an ideal initial agent to control atrial fibrillation as it also has some positive inotropic effects, whereas many of the other agents used actually depress cardiac output. Care must be exercised in Dobermans as they are very sensitive to the drug and can easily develop toxicity. Digoxin also can worsen ventricular arrhythmias. Checking blood levels 7 to 10 days after initiating therapy is recommended. Diltiazem (0.5 to 1.5 mg/kg TID, start low, titrate upward to effect) will also help to slow heart rate with minimal cardiodepressant effects at lower dosages. Beta blockers could also be used, but their cardiodepressant effects usually do not allow them to be used in patients with tenous cardiac output as is the rule with acute heart failure.

Ventricular Tachycardia

The decision whether to treat a ventricular arrhythmia is a difficult one. In patients with acute heart failure, VPCs would not be unexpected. It must be decided whether the arrhythmia has serious negative consequences to the patient. A large number of VPCs or a sustained ventricular tachycardia with rates exceeding 160 BPM are probably significant enough to warrant therapy in a patient with CHF. The main goal of therapy is to reduce the clinical signs of the arrhythmia, such as poor cardiac output. It is less likely that the commonly used medications (Class I agents such as lidocaine, procainamide) can prevent sudden cardiac death. Other agents, such as beta-blockers, are thought to prevent sudden death. Their use in cases of acute heart failure is exceedingly difficult since they decrease cardiac output considerably. As a result, in emergency situations the most commonly used agent is still intravenous lidocaine. This has minimal cardiodepressant effect and can often resolve ventricular arrhythmias. An initial intravenous bolus of 2 mg/kg can be given. This can be repeated several times at 5 to 10 minute intervals to a maximum total dose of 8 mg/kg. If this therapy is effective in reducing the number of ventricular ectopic beats, a constant rate infusion can be started (25 to 100 mcg/kg/min) which is titrated to effect. Procainamide can be used in place of lidocaine but has more cardiodepressant effects so that caution must be used when using this medication. Hypokalemia and hypomagnesemia make ventricular arrhythmias more likely and less responsive to therapy so these parameters should be monitored in patients with refractory ventricular arrhythmias.

PROGNOSIS

The prognosis for patients with acute congestive heart failure will vary with the underlying cause of the failure and if the acute episode was merely an exacerbation of chronic disease. In general, dogs with mitral valve disease can survive up to 1 year with therapy, dogs with dilated cardiomyopathy usually succumb more rapidly, and Doberman Pinschers often only have 1 to 2 months after onset of signs of congestive heart failure.

Suggested Readings

Beardow AW: The diagnostic and therapeutic approach to the patient in acute congestive heart failure . *Clin Tech Small Anim Pract* 15: 70–75, 2000.

Fox PR: Critical care cardiology. *Vet Clin North Am Small Anim Pract* 19:1095–1125, 1989.

Goodwin JK, Strickland KN: The emergency management of dogs and cats with congestive heart failure. *Vet Med* 93: 818–822, 1998.

Kittleson MD: Management of heart failure. *In* Kittleson MD, Kienle RD, eds: Small Animal Cardiovascular Medicine. St Louis, Mosby, 1998 pp 136–148.

Marks SL, Abbott JA: Critical care cardiology. *Vet Clin North Am Small Anim Pract* 28: 1567–1593, 1998.

Marks SL: Emergency management and critical care. *In* Tilley LP and Goodwin JK, eds: Manual of Canine and Feline Cardiology, 3rd ed. Philadelphia, WB Saunders, 2000 pp 425–436.

Wohl JS, Clark TP: Pressor therapy in critically ill patients. *J Vet Emergency and Crit Care* 10: 21–34, 2000

31
Arrhythmias in Critical Care

Marc R. Raffe and Elizabeth O'Toole

INTRODUCTION

Cardiac rhythm disturbances are frequently noted in critically ill animals. Disturbance in rate, regularity, or site of cardiac impulse generation is classified as an arrhythmia. Arrhythmias may be associated with primary cardiovascular dysfunction or may be secondary to systemic disease. The challenge the critical care clinician faces is to identify the arrhythmia and understand its hemodynamic consequences. It is important that the clinician recognize which arrhythmias require prompt, aggressive medical intervention versus arrhythmias that are tolerated until correction of the underlying cause occurs. The goal of this presentation is to review arrhythmias commonly encountered in critically ill patients and present medical options for acute management and stabilization.

MECHANISMS OF ARRHYTHMIA FORMATION

All cardiac tissues depolarize and conduct electrical impulses. The sequence of electrical impulse spread occurs in an orderly fashion. Cardiac cells depolarize and in turn depolarize cells next to them. Cells that have depolarized are refractive to a second depolarization event for a specific time period. Because of this characteristic, depolarization occurs in an orderly process in one direction and terminates.

Specialized cells called "pacemakers" initiate the depolarization process. Pacemaker cells have the ability to spontaneously depolarize at a repeatable rate governed by intrinsic properties and external influences. Pacemaker cells have been identified in the atrium (sinoatrial [SA] node), atrioventricular (AV) node, and His Purkinjie (HP) system. Under normal conditions, depolarization rate is highest for the cells in the SA node. The generated electrical signal begins the hierarchal sequence of depolarization. Subservient pacemakers are depolarized as part of this sequence preventing initiation of secondary, uncoordinated, depolarization. Arrhythmias are noted when this sequence is altered due to local or regional changes in electrical conductivity or myocardial tissue disease. Two primary mechanisms for arrhythmia formation have been described; these are disorders of impulse conduction and disorders of electrical impulse formation.

Conduction Abnormalities

Conduction abnormalities result in either slow rate (brady) or fast rate (tachy) arrhythmia formation.

Bradyarrhythmias are noted when temporal delay or complete block of electrical impulse spread delays normal depolarization sequence. Conduction abnormalities are noted as a delay or "block" in ECG signal appearance relative to surrounding complexes. Delays in impulse generation from the SA node and conduction to the atrial tissues do not cause perceptible ECG abnormality. Complete SA nodal block unmasks lower pacemaker activity; this is reflected as an ECG appearance devoid of P wave activity. Slowed conduction through the AV nodal region results in prolongation of the P-R interval on the ECG. The specific site of delay may be the proximal AV bundle, AV node, or bundle of His. Intermittent blockade results in loss of the QRS-T complex producing second degree block. Complete blockade in the AV nodal region produces a third degree block.

Tachyarrhythmias are associated with abnormal myocardial tissue or accessory conduction pathways. Regional depolarization speed is altered when abnormal cardiac tissue is present. In general, abnormal tissue slows the velocity of signal conduction through the diseased area. This delay in the depolarization process may be long enough to permit surrounding tissue to partially or completely repolarize, making healthy tissue capable of responding to a second depolarization stimulus. The process by which normal cardiac tissue is capable of supporting a secondary stimulus is called "reentry", reflecting reentrance of the delayed stimulus into normal cardiac tissue. Reentry occurs in a time period shorter than would be expected with the normal depolarization sequence. Therefore, the reentry process initiates a premature beat. Reentry may be a single event following a normal cardiac depolarization or may produce a sequence of depolarization events that are independent of normal depolarization process. Repetitive reentry events that occur faster than sinus depolarization are the basis for many tachyarrhythmias.

Impulse Formation Disorders

Disorders of impulse formation encompass enhanced or depressed impulse formation by normal pacemaker cells and abnormal impulse formation by nonautomatic cells.

Depressed automaticity is a decrease in the discharge rate of the automatic cells in the SA node. Both primary cardiac and extracardiac factors have been shown to influence automaticity. Sinoatrial nodal disease produces intermittent or complete inability to initiate impulse generation. This is clinically noted as "sick sinus syndrome". Extrinsic factors in depressed automaticity include increased parasympathetic activity, electrolyte abnormalities (hyperkalemia), endocrine disorders (hypothyroidism), body temperature (subnormal), and anesthetic drugs (opioids, alpha-2 agonists, halothane).

Enhanced automaticity is an increase in the discharge rate of the automatic cells. Both primary (SA) and subservient (AV, HP) pacemakers may be stimulated to discharge at a faster than normal rate. A variety of extracardiac influences including increased sympathetic activity, electrolyte abnormalities (hypercalcemia), endocrine disorders (hyperthyroidism), body temperature (elevated), and anesthetic drugs (ketamine, isoflurane, pentobarbital, thiopental) have been shown to enhance SA nodal automaticity. Differential activation of pacemaker sites may produce uncoupling of the SA node and subservient pacemakers predisposing to premature depolarization or dissociative rhythms.

Abnormal automaticity is a result of cells that are not normally automatic, or subservient pacemaker sites, depolarizing at a rate faster than normal and functioning as a primary pacemaker. This is a key mechanism in critically ill patients. Abnormal automaticity is due to myocardial ischemia and hypoxia. Tissue damage resulting from ischemia results in altered excitability and impulse conduction velocity. Premature depolarization results and may give rise to tachyarrhythmias. Clinical conditions that increase risk for developing abnormal automaticity include vascular occlusion, blunt trauma, myocardial dilatation or hypertrophy, and extracardiac factors (vascular occlusion secondary to gastric dilatation-volvulus syndrome).

Triggered activity is similar to abnormal automaticity in that nonautomatic tissue attains the ability to self depolarize. Triggered activity is distinct from abnormal automaticity in that it must be linked to a preceding normal action potential. Two types of triggered activity have been described; early afterdepolarization (EAD) and delayed afterdepolarization (DAD). Both are related to membrane potential oscillation following a normal depolarization. EADs are not fully understood but have been associated with antiarrhythmic drugs (quinidine, procainamide, bretylium, sotalol) that increase transmembrane potassium flux. EADs are usually associated with a long Q-T interval. Membrane oscillations may be noted as a "U" wave on surface ECG. Torsades des pointes is an arrhythmia that is noted with EADs. DADs have been described with digitalis class drugs. Both EADs and DADs appear to be more frequent in slow pacemaker rate conditions.

ARRHYTHMIAS OF NORMAL RATE

Premature Ventricular Contractions

Pathogenesis

Premature ventricular contractions (PVC) are one of the most common rhythm disturbances diagnosed in critically ill dogs and cats. Premature ventricular contractions occur when an area of myocardium below the AV node and outside the His bundle becomes hyperexcitable and reaches depolarization threshold prior to the SA and AV pacemakers. The depolarization wavefront propagates across individual myocardial cells without using the normal conduction system; this results in a relatively slow electrical transmission velocity through the ventricles. PVCs occur in association with a variety of stimuli and can be produced by direct mechanical, electrical, or chemical stimulation of the myocardium (Fig. 31-1). PVC's may also be secondary to enhanced automaticity, triggered automaticity or reentry.

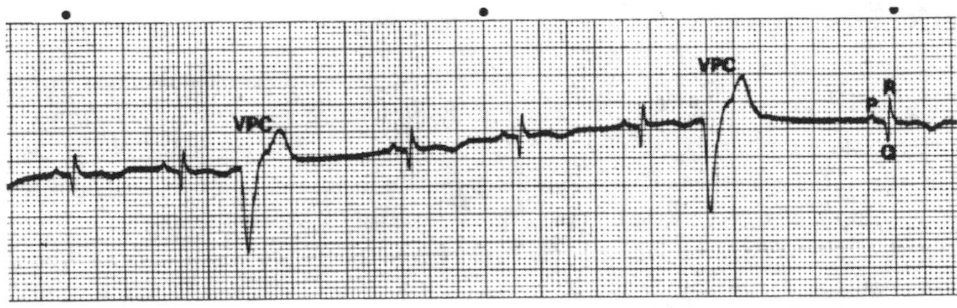

Cat

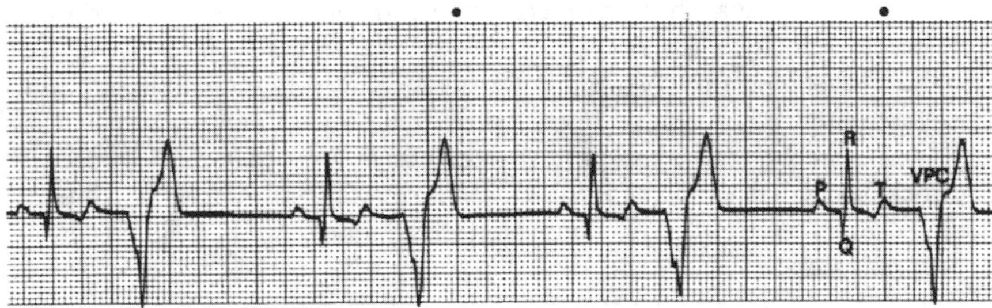

Dog

Figure 31-1
Ventricular premature complexes are cardiac impulses initiated within the ventricles instead of the sinus node. Mechanisms include increased automaticity and reentry. VPCs have direct effects on the cardiovascular system and secondary effects on other systems because of poor perfusion. VPCs are also associated with weakness, exercise intolerance, syncope, and sudden death. (From Tilley, LR and Burtnick, NL: Electrocardiography for the Small Animal Practitioner. Teton NewMedia, 1999.)

Premature ventricular contractions may occur as isolated complexes, couplets, triplets, or "runs" of sustained or nonsustained ventricular tachycardia (VT). The incidence and frequency of PVCs are potentiated by sympathetic nervous system activation, hypoxia, ischemia, acid-base disturbance, electrolyte imbalance, and medications.

Clinical Presentation

The clinical presentation of the animal will depend upon the primary clinical disorder associated with PVCs. PVCs have been observed with gastric dilitation volvulus, pancreatitis, SIRS, respiratory insufficiency, trauma, pain, hypotension/shock, intracranial lesions, cardiac neoplasia, splenic hemangiosacroma, and traumatic myocarditis. Premature ventricular complexes are also commonly observed in animals with cardiac disease, in particular large breed dogs (Doberman Pinchers and Boxers) and cats with cardiomyopathy. Cats may also exhibit PVCs with congestive heart failure, hyperthyroidism, systemic thromboembolism, infarction, and aging.

ECG Findings

Ventricular complexes are relatively easy to recognize on the electrocardiogram. They are characterized by temporally premature complexes that demonstrate wide and bizarre QRS-T conformations and AV dissociation (P waves are not associated with the QRS-T complex). Fusion beats and compensatory pauses are the hallmark of ventricular ectopy. A fusion beat occurs when an ectopic ventricular beat collides with a normal sinus-generated beat below the AV node. This collision results in a QRS-T complex that is a fusion of the 2 individual beats. Fusion beats are observed less commonly in the cat than the dog. A compensatory pause occurs when the premature ventricular ectopic focus fires and prematurely depolarizes the AV node; the sinus-generated P wave of the next sinus beat encounters the AV node in a absolute refractory state and is blocked. Therefore, the R-R interval produced by the two sinus complexes adjacent to the PVC is equal to twice the normally conducted R-R interval. An accurate electrocardiograph diagnosis of PVC is important as aberrantly conducted supraventricular arrhythmias (SVT) conducted may mimic PVCs in electrocardiographic appearance.

Diagnostic Evaluation

Once the diagnosis of PVCs has been established, every effort should be made to identify the underlying disorder. A thorough evaluation of the patient's medication history, metabolic status (CBC, biochemical profile, urinalysis, electrolyte status and acid-base analysis), and cardiorespiratory function should be performed. Correction of the underlying disorders should occur prior to initiation of a specific anti-arrhythmic therapy.

Short duration "rhythm" strips maybe insufficient to correctly diagnosis the presence and frequency of PVCs. Therefore these patients may require evaluation with a continuous ECG monitor (Holter, telemetry).

Treatment

Therapeutic decisions depend upon: 1) whether there is hemodynamic instability due to the arrhythmia; 2) whether PVCs are contributing to clinical signs; and 3) whether an increased risk of sudden death may be present.

PVCs not associated with hemodynamic compromise or clinical symptoms are generally benign and do not require specific anti-arrhythmic therapy. Premature ventricular contractions that are associated with hemodynamic instability (low cardiac output, hypotension, oliguria, syncope, weakness, poor capillary refill time, pallor, and dyspnea) or in patients with severe underlying heart disease require therapy. Heart rate appears to be the most important factor in determining hemodynamic stability. ECG features which imply electrical instability include presence of an R on T phenomena, paroxysms of rapid VT, sustained VT with a rate > than 160 bpm, and polymorphic PVC's. The goal of therapy is to reduce ectopic ventricular activity rather than completely suppress the ectopic focus.

Initial management should be directed at identifying and treating coexisting disorders (*i.e.*, shock/hypotension) that may contribute to PVC development. **Non-cardiac based therapy may include the administration of intravenous fluid, blood products, supplemental oxygen, analgesics, and correction of electrolyte imbalances.**

Primary antiarrhythmic therapy for PVCs consists of an intravenous bolus of lidocaine (1–4 mg/kg repeated a maximum of 3 times in a 10 minute period). If successful in converting the rhythm to sinus rhythm or in significantly slowing the ventricular rate, a constant rate lidocaine infusion (CRI) at 30 to 80 ug/kg/min is initiated. If lidocaine is unsuccessful, procainamide, (2–15 mg/kg) administered intravenously over 20–30 minutes may be used. If both medications are unsuccessful, β-blockers (esmolol: 500 ug/kg slow IV bolus, propranolol: 0.02–0.06 mg/kg slow IV bolus), quinidine (5–10 mg/kg slowly IV), or magnesium sulfate (30 mg/kg slow IV bolus, then 210 mg/kg infused over 24 hours) is selected. In refractive cases, amiodarone (5 mg/kg IV bolus) may be attempted prior to DC conversion.

A significant number of critically ill patients are documented to have low serum levels of potassium and magnesium. Clinically, hypomagnesemia has been associated with cardiac arrhythmias in human ICU patients; this has been observed experimentally in the dog. Magnesium sulfate supplementation, either as an intravenous bolus (30 mg/kg slowly IV up to 95 mg/kg in a 24 hour period) or CRI (5 mg/kg/hr), can reduce the severity and frequency of arrhythmias. Antiarrythmic medications tend to be more efficacious at high normal serum potassium concentration (4–5 mEq/l); concurrent Mg supplementation maybe required to obtain this serum concentration (see chapter 14). Mg replacement therapy should be reduced in the presence of abnormal renal function.

Prognosis

Prognosis depends upon the underlying disease process. PVCs secondary to systemic disease tend to be self-limiting and will spontaneously resolve in 3 to 10 days. The overall prognosis for these patients is good if the underlying disease process has stabilized or is improving. The prognosis for patients with structural heart disease is poor and is related to the ventricular dysfunction. In human medicine, an increased mortality has been reported in patients with asymptomatic PVCs receiving anti-arrhythmic medication (encainide, flecainide, and moricizine).

Accelerated Idioventricular Rhythm

Ventricular arrhythmias that are initiated after a pause (*i.e.*, they are not premature beats), are regular, are approximately equal to sinus rate (70–150 bpm), and are classified as idioventricular tachycardia or accelerated idioventricular rhythm (AIR) (Fig. 31-2). They are also referred to as "slow ventricular tachycardia" reflecting ECG complex morphology associated with this rhythm disturbance.

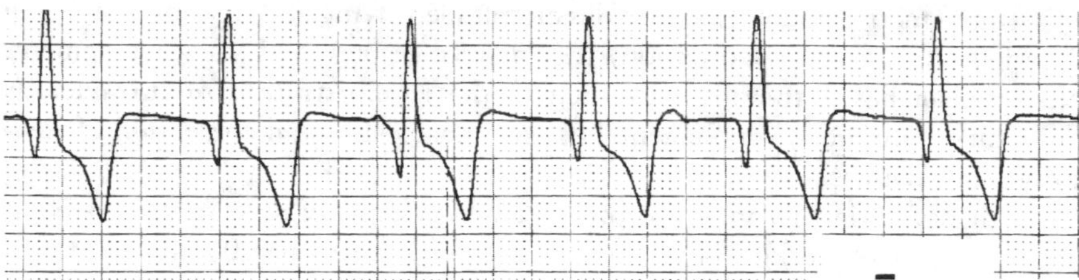

Cat

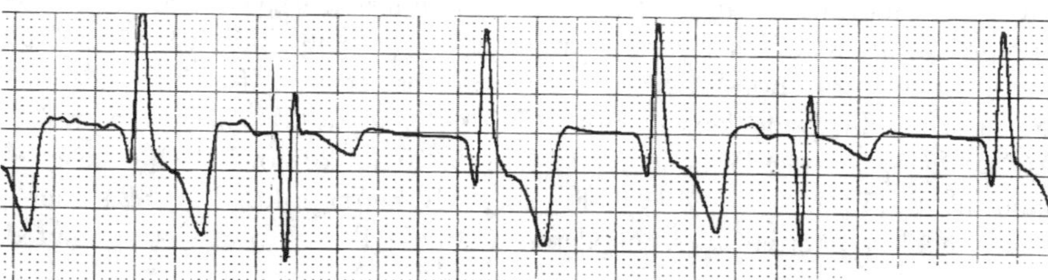

Dog

Figure 31-2
Accelerated bioventricular rhythm is a unique form of ventricular tachycardia characterized by complex morphology dependent on pacemaker locations. Both AV nodal and ventricular origin pacemakers may initiate this rhythm.

Pathogenesis

AIR is due to enhanced secondary pacemaker automaticity. Clinically, AIR is noted when the SA node depolarization rate slows down to approximately the same rate as a ventricular or junctional pacemaker. This results in the cardiac rhythm being controlled by two competing pacemakers (sinus and ectopic idioventricular).

Clinical Presentation

This arrhythmia is typically associated with traumatic myocarditis. However, it may be observed with conditions which predispose to sinus bradycardia and AV block. In humans, it is associated with heart disease (acute myocardial infarction), digitalis toxicity, reperfusion of a previously occluded coronary artery, and following cardiac resuscitation.

ECG Findings

Because the arrhythmia is secondary to a slowing of the sinus rate, SA or AV block, or acceleration of the ventricular rate is noted. Morphology of the QRS complex depends on the origin of the ectopic pacemaker. If the ectopic pacemaker is at the AV junction, QRS complex tends to have a normal configuration with negative P waves that may precede, be superimposed on, or follow the QRS complex. If the ectopic pacemaker is in the ventricles, the QRS complex will be wide and bizarre, similar in appearance to a PVC. Fusion beats are frequently noted at the beginning and end of an arrhythmia episode.

Diagnostic Evaluation

A detailed history, complete physical examination, CBC, biochemical profile, and blood gas analysis is warranted.

Treatment

This arrhythmia is generally benign and therapy is rarely indicated due to the slow ventricular rate and paroxysmal incidence. Attention should be focused on identification and correction of any cofactors (*i.e.*, hypoxia secondary to pulmonary contusions or general anesthesia). Often simply increasing the sinus rate with atropine suppresses the accelerated idioventricular rhythm.

Therapy may be considered under the following criteria: 1) a hemodynamically unstable patient; 2) when accelerated idioventricular rhythm occurs with ventricular tachycardia; 3) when the accelerated idioventricular rhythm begins with a premature ventricular complex that has a short coupling interval; or 4) if ventricular fibrillation develops as a result of the accelerated idioventricular arrhythmia. Specific antiarrhytmic therapy is the same as described for ventricular tachycardia.

Prognosis

Prognosis is good as this arrhythmia is self-limiting and has little effect on hemodynamic stability.

Bundle Branch Block

Pathogenesis

Delayed ventricular conduction occurs when one or more of the His bundle branches do not support impulse conduction. Conduction delay occurs because complete ventricular depolarization in the region with His bundle block requires cell-to-cell depolarization. Cell to cell depolarization produces temporal dispersion and results in a wide and bizarre QRS complex on electrocardiogram. Aberrant ventricular conduction is more likely when a short coupling interval between a sinus and supraventricular impulse produces a premature beat that reaches a bundle branch in its refractory period.

Left bundle branch block has been associated with cardiac trauma, neoplasia, fibrosis, cardiomypathy and congenital defects (subvalvular aortic stenosis) in the dog and cat. The left bundle branch is thick and extensive; significant damage to the left ventricle must occur to produce a LBBB. LBBB has the potential to progress into more severe arrhythmias or complete heart block (Fig. 31-3). Right bundle branch block has been associated with cardiac trauma, cardiac neoplasia, chronic valvular fibrosis, chronic infection with Chagas's disease, heartworm disease, acute thromboembolism, cardiomypathy, congenital heart disease and hyperkalemia (most commonly observed in cats with urethral obstruction) (Fig. 31-4).

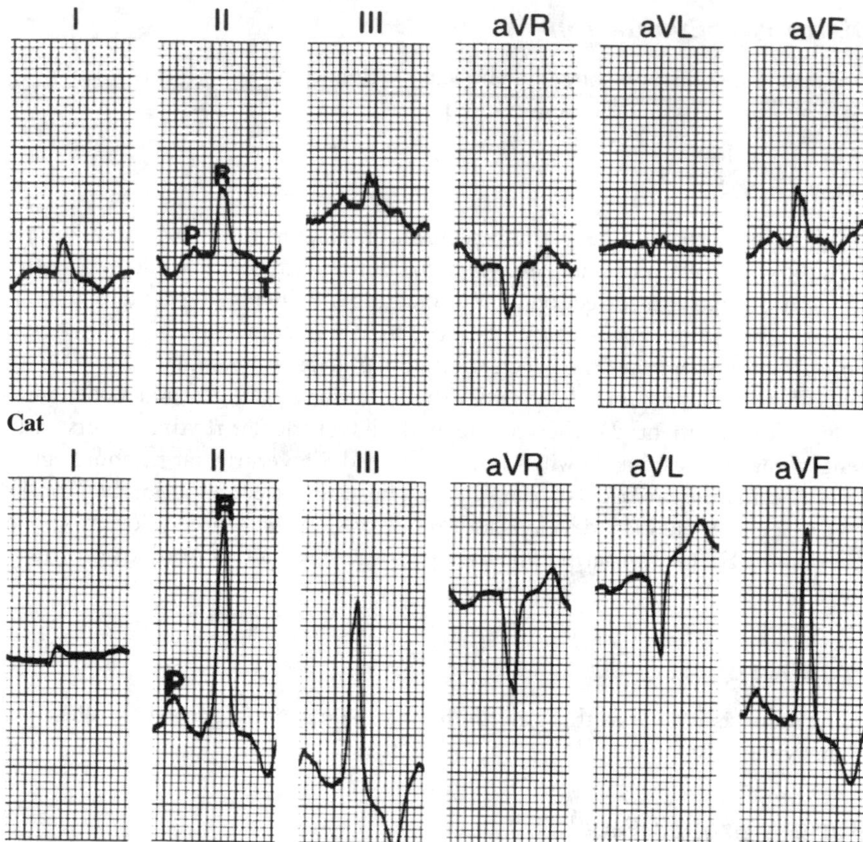

Figure 31-3
Left bundle branch block is a conduction delay or block in both the left posterior and left anterior fascicles of the left bundle. A supraventricular impulse activates the right ventricle first through the right bundle branch. The left ventricle is then activated late, causing the QRS to become wide and bizarre. (From Tilley, LR and Burtnick, NL: Electrocardiography for the Small Animal Practitioner. Teton NewMedia, 1999.)

Clinical Presentation

Left (LBBB) and right (RBBB) bundle branch blocks rarely cause clinical signs.

ECG Findings

There are several ECG features which help to identify BBB. The QRS is prolonged (>0.08 sec in the dog; >0.06 sec in cats) in LBBB and RBBB. In LBBB, the QRS is positive in leads I, II, III and AVF. In RBBB, there is a right

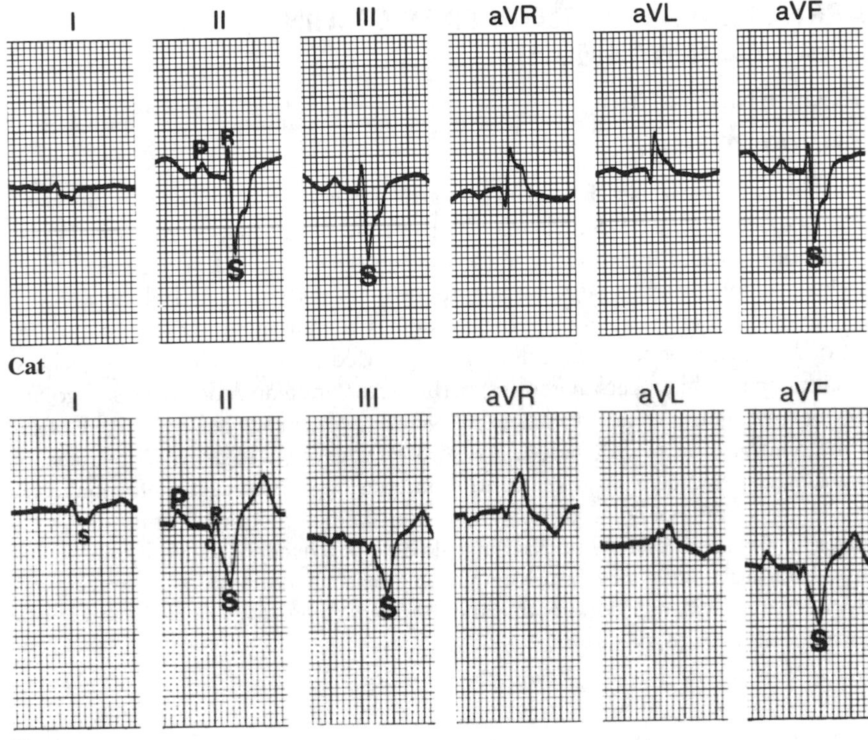

Figure 31-4
Right bundle branch block is a conduction delay or block in the right bundle. Branch resulting in late activation of the right ventricle. The block can be complete or incomplete. (From Tilley, LR and Burtnick, NL: Electrocardiography for the Small Animal Practitioner. Teton NewMedia, 1999.)

axis deviation with large wide S waves in leads I, II, III, and AVF. The BBB may be continuous (permanent failure of conduction) or intermittent (transient failure of conduction).

Diagnostic Evaluation

Attention should be focused on identification of any underlying disorders or structural heart disease. A detailed history, complete physical examination, CBC, biochemical profile, electrolyte status, heartworm test (dog and cat), thyroxine concentration (in cats), thoracic radiographs, and echocardiogram are warranted.

Treatment and Prognosis

Specific antiarrhythmic therapy is not required. Therapy and prognosis are dependent upon the underlying cause.

ARRHYTHMIAS OF SLOW RATE ORIGIN (BRADYARRHYTHMIAS)

Sinus Bradycardia

Pathogenesis

Sinus bradycardia (SB) occurs when the SA node discharges at a rate slower than expected (Fig. 31-5). SB may be the result of decreased rate of impulse generation, slowed intranodal conduction, or exit block. SB may be associated with a physiologic response, secondary to medications, or as a pathologic process. Physiologic SB is a normal response to increased parasympathetic tone and decreased sympathetic tone (*i.e.*, during sleep). Medications including β-blockers, calcium channel blockers, narcotics, barbiturates, inhalant anesthetics, digoxin, IV contrast agents, or anticholinesterases have been associated with SB. Conditions predisposing to SB include gastrointestinal (*e.g.*, intestinal obstruction, obstructive jaundice, vomiting), central nervous (*e.g.*, meningitis, elevated ICP, intracranial tumors), genitourinary (*e.g.*, urethral obstruction), respiratory (*e.g.*, lower airway obstruction) and pharyngeal (*e.g.*, brachycephalic syndrome) disorders. Infiltrative neoplastic or inflammatory disease, hypothermia, electrolyte imbalance (hyperkalemia), and endocrine disorders (hypothyroidism, hypoadrenocortism) also predispose to SB.

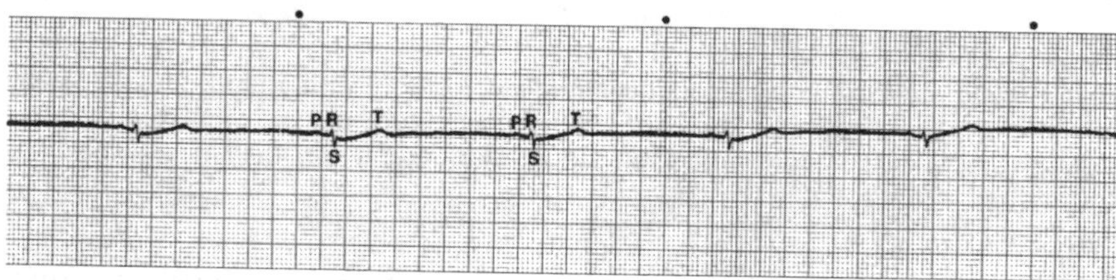

Cat

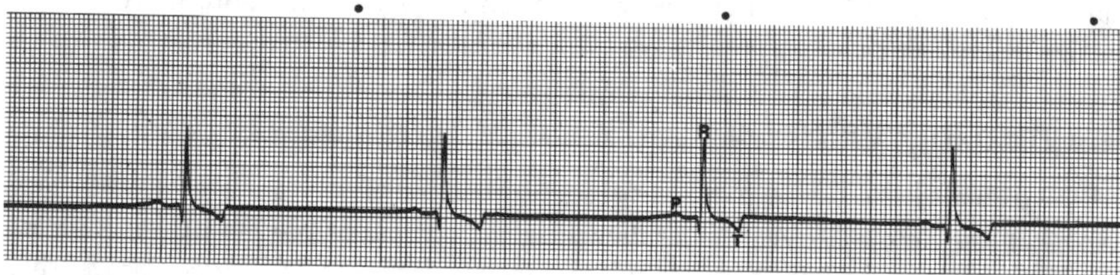

Dog

Figure 31-5
Sinus bradycardia is a regular sinus rhythm with a heart rate below normal discharge rates. Heart rates of 60–70 bpm may be normal for large breed dogs. In cats it is often associated with a serious disorder that warrants treatment. (From Tilley, LR and Burtnick, NL: Electrocardiography for the Small Animal Practitioner. Teton NewMedia, 1999.)

Clinical Presentation

SB is rarely associated with clinical signs. Exercise intolerance, lethargy, anorexia, or episodic weakness has been reported in cases demonstrating SB and intercurrent cardiac disease.

ECG Findings

SB is diagnosed when heart rate is less than 140 bpm in a cats, less than 60 bpm in a large breed dog, or less than 90 bpm in a small breed dog.

Diagnostic Evaluation

Once a slow heart rate has been identified on thoracic auscultation, a 12 lead ECG or lead II strip is used to confirm SB.

Treatment

The majority of animals with SB are asymptomatic and do not require specific therapy. Management of drug-associated SB consists of removal or hastening elimination of the primary medication, supportive therapy (intravenous fluids, alleviation of hypothermia, correction of electrolyte imbalances and use of specific antidotes).

Treatment of symptomatic SB is directed to the underlying cause. Intervention may be required in cases under general anesthesia or sedation. Decreasing the depth of sedation/anesthesia may correct SB. If this maneuver is unsuccessful, a parasympatholytic drug such as atropine sulfate (0.02 to 0.04 mg/kg IM or IV) or glycopyrrolate (0.005 to 0.1 mg/kg IM or IV) is administered to increase heart rate and maintain cardiac output.

Sinus Arrest or Block

Pathogenesis

Sinus block is recognized by a pause in the normal sinus rhythm. The block is due to a conduction disturbance during which an impulse formed within the sinus node fails to depolarize the atria or does so with a delay. Sinus arrest is defined as a complete loss of SA node automaticity (Fig. 31-6). Either condition may produce loss of atrial depolarization and ventricular asystole if secondary pacemakers do not initiate depolarization. Sinus arrest and block are associated with vagal stimulation, medication (digitalis, β-blockers, class 1a anti-arrhythmics), sinus node disease (sick sinus syndrome), and vagovagal reflexes. Brachycephalic breeds with respiratory deformities appear to be at increased risk. It is relatively uncommon in cats.

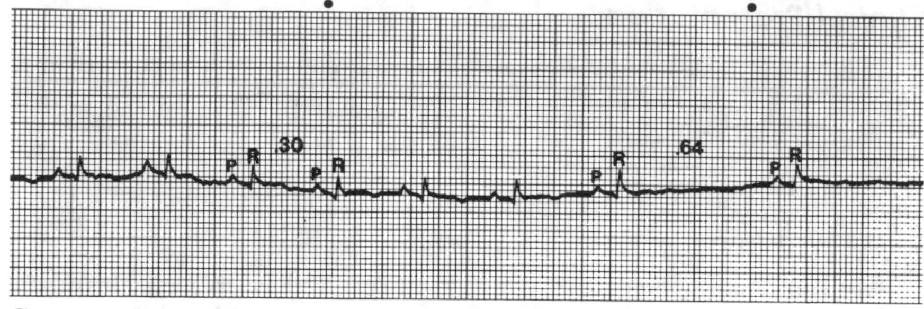

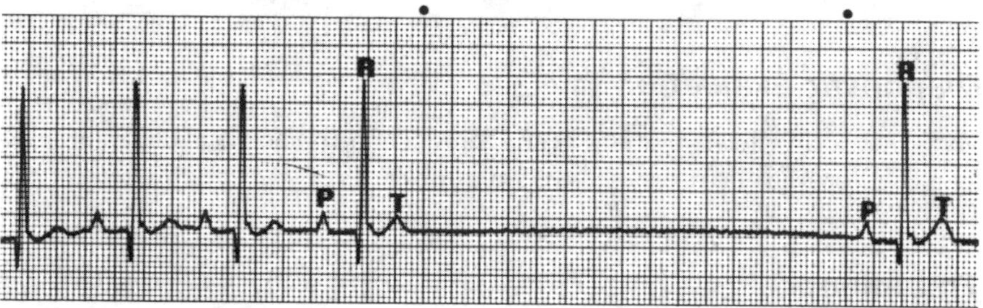

Figure 31-6
Sinus arrest is a normal sinus rhythm interrupted by an occasional prolonged failure of the sinoatrial node to initiate an impulse. Sinus block is a conduction disturbance in which normal sinus rhythm is interrupted by an occasional prolonged failure of the impulse generated by the sinoatrial node to reach the atria. With prolonged pauses, episodes of low cardiac output may occur. (From Tilley, LR and Burtnick, NL: Electrocardiography for the Small Animal Practitioner. Teton NewMedia, 1999.)

Clinical Presentation

Syncopal episodes characterized by weakness, lethargy, collapse, and temporary loss of consciousness are noted with prolonged block periods.

ECG Findings

Periods of electrical inactivity may be equal to a regular P-P interval (SA block) or greater than two P-P intervals (SA arrest). Sinus rhythm predominates; however junctional and ventricular escape beats may be present. In the presence of a sinus arrhythmia, differentiation of sinus arrest from sinus block may be difficult without the use of a 12 lead diagnostic ECG or direct sinus node recordings.

Diagnostic Evaluation

Diagnostic evaluation should be directed towards identification and correction of the underlying disorder.

Treatment

Therapy for symptomatic animals is the same as described for sinus bradycardia. Terbutaline (2.5 mg PO T.I.D.) or isoproterenol (0.04 to 0.08 ug/kg/min CRI) may also be used for short-term therapy. Artificial pacing is the therapy of choice in animals with symptoms that are unresponsive to medical management.

Prognosis

Prognosis is good if the underlying cause is determined and effectively managed. Pacemaker implantation is highly successful in cases that have no intercurrent heart disease.

Atrial Standstill

Pathogenesis

Atrial standstill occurs when the atria fail to depolarize following a SA nodal generated impulse (Fig. 31-7). The atria do not respond appropriately (absence of P waves) and the impulse spreads through specialized internodal pathways to the AV node. Atrial standstill may be related to AV nodal disease or associated with metabolic disorders including hypoadrenocorticism, urinary obstruction, renal failure, or severe metabolic acidosis. It may also be due to inher-

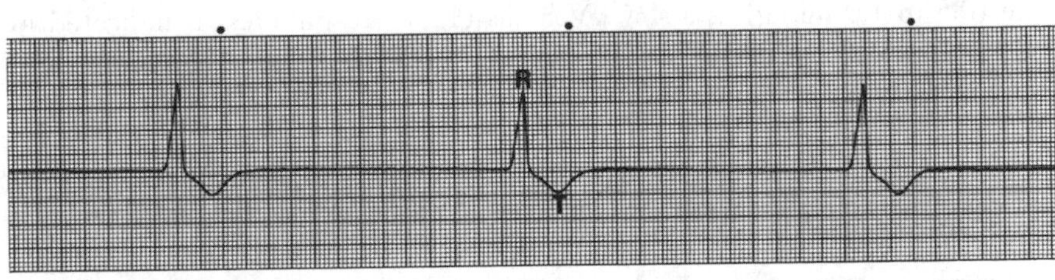

Cat

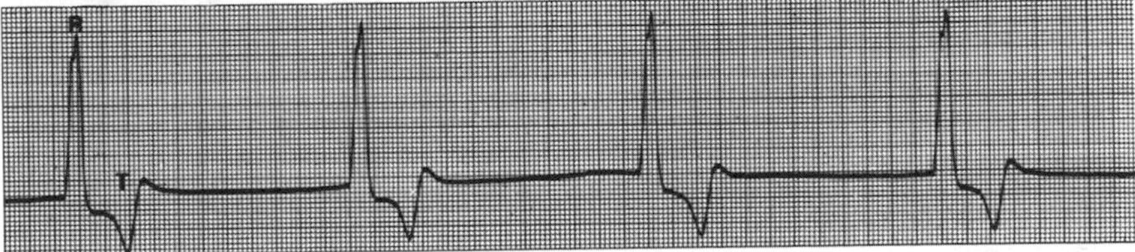

Dog

Figure 31-7
Atrial standstill is characterized by an absence of P waves and by a regular escape rhythm with a supraventricular-type QRS. The condition can be temporary (associated with hyperkalemia or drug induxed), terminal (associated with severe hyperkalemia or dying heart), or persistent. Hyperkalemic patients with atrial standstill have sinus node function, but impulses so not cause atrial myocyte activation. Persistent atrial standstill is caused by inherited atrial myopathy. (From Tilley, LR and Burtnick, NL: Electrocardiography for the Small Animal Practitioner. Teton NewMedia, 1999.)

ited atrial myopathy in the dog or atrial distension secondary to cardiomyopathy in the cat.

Clinical Presentation

Episodic weakness and syncope are noted in the history. There may be no current symptoms exhibited on physical examination.

ECG Findings

Atrial standstill is characterized by a slow regular rhythm (heart rate <60 bpm) and the absence of a P wave in any ECG lead. QRS complexes have normal morphology if the animal has persistent atrial standstill. But they may become wide in severe hyperkalemia or bundle branch blocks.

Diagnostic Evaluation

Diagnostic evaluation should be directed toward ruling out the presence of hyperkalemia. Once hyperkalemia has been ruled out, patient evaluation should be directed towards identifying structural heart disease using echocardiography and thoracic radiographs.

Treatment. Emergent therapy is required in animals with ECG changes secondary to hyperkalemia (see chapter 14). Administration of 10% calcium gluconate (0.5 to 1.0 ml/kg) as a slow IV bolus (10 to 20 minutes) is indicated in life-threatening situations. Once the cardiac rhythm has stabilized, therapies that lower the serum potassium concentration, such as intravenous glucose (0.5 to 1 g/kg), may be initiated. Regular insulin (0.06 to 0.2 U/kg) or sodium bicarbonate (1 to 2 mEq/kg) may be administered if the serum potassium does not satisfactorily decrease with the intravenous glucose. Definitive therapy should also be initiated once the animal is stable (intravenous fluids and corticosteriod therapy for hypoadrenocortism).

Prognosis

The prognosis for atrial standstill is good if the underlying disease is identified and is responsive to therapy. Animals with persistent atrial standstill will require a pacemaker as pharmacologic therapy is of limited value in these animals.

Sick Sinus Syndrome

Pathogenesis

Sick sinus syndrome (SSS) is a term used to describe a constellation of ECG abnormalities associated with the sinoatrial node. These abnormalities result from inadequate impulse formation or conduction in the SA node and surrounding tissue in conjunction with an inappropriate autonomic tone (Fig.

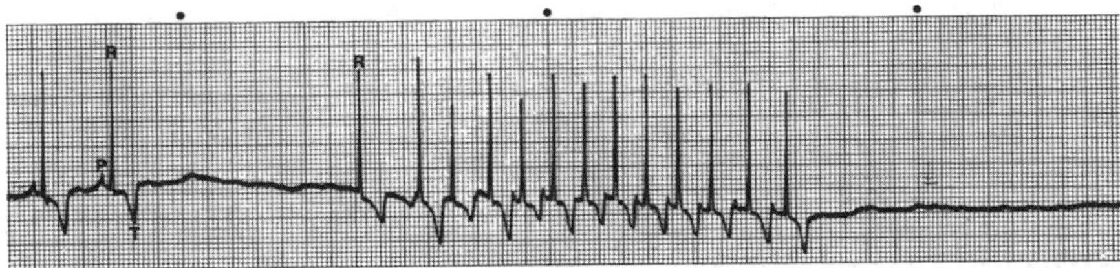

Figure 31-8
Sick sinus syndrome is a term given to a number of ECG abnormalities of the sino-atrial (SA) node including severe sinus bradycardia and severe sinus block. The majority of these patients also have coexisting abnormalities of the AV junction and/or bundle branches. (From Tilley, LR and Burtnick, NL: Electrocardiography for the Small Animal Practitioner. Teton NewMedia, 1999.)

31-8). The anatomic basis of SSS may reflect total or subtotal destruction of the sinoatrial node, areas of nodal-atrial discontinuity, inflammation or degenerative changes of the nerves and ganglia surrounding the node, and pathological changes in the atrial wall. Occlusion of the SA nodal artery may also be important. This syndrome has been noted in Cocker Spaniels, West Highland White Terriers, and female miniature schnauzers. SSS has not been documented in the cat.

Clinical Presentation

Syncope is the most common complaint and is associated with pauses of at least 8 seconds in length.

Diagnostic Evaluation and ECG Findings

The diagnosis of SSS is based on signalment, history, and abnormal electrocardiographic findings. ECG abnormalities may consist of the following; 1) severe and persistent sinus bradycardia (not induced by drugs); 2) severe sinus bradycardia alternating with rapid ectopic supraventricular tachycardia (atrial fibrillation or flutter); 3) AV junctional escape rhythm with or without slow and unstable sinus activity; and 4) sinus block with or without escape beats. During long periods of sinus block, latent AV junctional pacemakers may fail to pace the heart and periods of cardiac standstill will result. These ECG features may be captured on a lead II ECG rhythm strip, but extended Holter monitoring (24 to 48 hours) may be required to make the diagnosis.

Treatment

Medical therapy is usually unsuccessful. Theophylline can be useful to reduce the time between pauses. In animals with the bradycardia-tachycardia syndrome, pacing for the bradyarrhythmias combined with drug therapy for the tachyarrhythmia is required.

Prognosis

Prognosis depends on therapeutic response. Animals with severe bradyarrhythmias tend to demonstrate significant clinical improvement when artificially paced.

Atrioventricular Block

Atrioventricular (AV) block exists when there is a delay or complete block of atrial impulse conduction at a time when the AV node is not physiologically refractive. AV block may be associated with either intrinsic disease of the conduction system or extrinsic factors acting on the conduction system. In the critical care setting, the majority of these arrhythmias are due to extrinsic factors.

First-degree Artioventricular Block

Pathogenesis. First-degree AV block occurs when there is a delay of the atrial impulse conduction through the AV node producing a long P-R interval. Every atrial impulse is conducted through to the ventricles (Fig. 31-9). It has

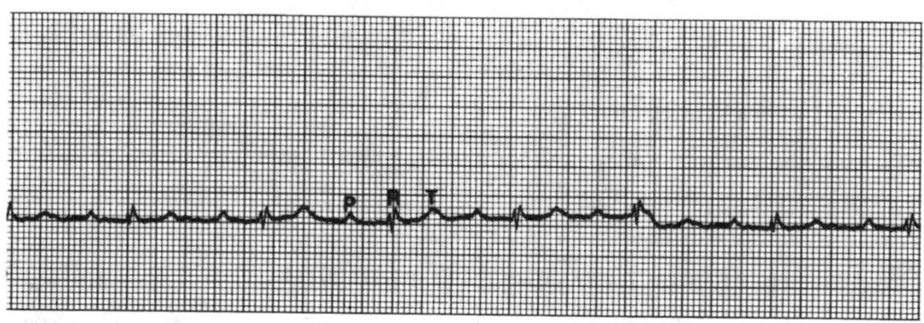

Cat

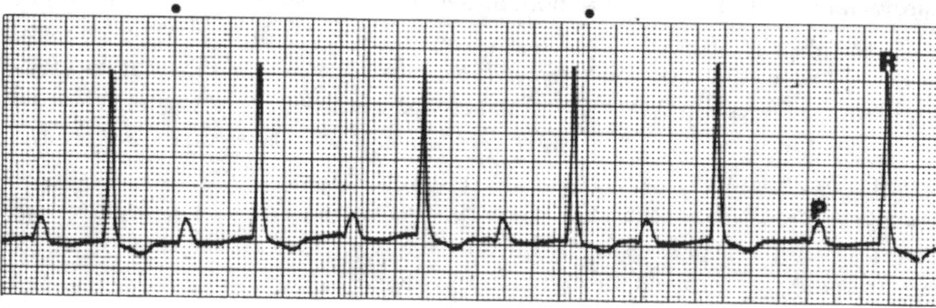

Dog

Figure 31-9
First degree atrioventricular block is a delay in conduction of a supraventricular impulse through the atrioventricular junction and bundle of His. (From Tilley, LR and Burtnick, NL: Electrocardiography for the Small Animal Practitioner. Teton NewMedia, 1999.)

been associated with older patients (especially Cocker Spaniels and Dachshunds), young puppies and brachycephalic breeds. It is also observed with potassium imbalance, reflex vagal stimulation or high vagal tone, hypothyroidism, protozoal myocarditis, and certain medications (digitalis, propranolol, quinidine and procainamide). In cats, first-degree heart block is the most common ECG abnormality noted with idiopathic myocardial failure.

Clinical Presentation. First-degree AV block is generally asymptomatic.

ECG Finding. First-degree AV block is an electrocardiographic diagnosis. There is a regular sinus rhythm and a P wave for every QRS-T complex. The only abnormality observed is prolongation of the P-R interval (dogs > 0.13 sec, cats > 0.09 sec) in the presence of a normal sinus rhythm.

Diagnostic Evaluation. A detailed history, complete physical examination, CBC, and biochemical profile are warranted in each case. Attention should be focused on identification and correction of the reversible causes. Medications, electrolyte imbalances, and increased vagal tone are common causes.

Treatment. Therapy is not necessary in most cases. If the AV block is due to certain medications (*i.e.*, anti-arrhythmic drugs), their dosage should be re-evaluated.

Second-degree Atrioventricular Block

Second-degree atrioventricular block is characterized by intermittent failure of AV conduction.

Pathogenesis. Second-degree atrioventricular block may be subclassified into Mobitz I (Wenckebach) and Mobitz type II AV block. The two types differ in the location of the AV nodal conduction disturbance; Wenckebach block occurs in the AV node and Mobitz type II within or below the bundle of His (infranodal).

Mobitz type I is secondary to disorders with increased vagal tone (see sinus bradycardia) or medications which depress AV nodal conduction (*i.e.*, morphine derivatives, digitalis, B-blockers and calcium channel blockers) (Fig. 31-10). **Mobitz type II** is associated with organic heart disease. Mobitz type II is often associated with conduction system disease (idiopathic fibrosis, hereditary HP stenosis in Pugs, myocarditis secondary to Lyme's disease, ehrlichiosis, or cardiac neoplasia) or electrolyte abnormality (Fig. 31-11). Medications such as low dose intravenous atropine, digitalis, diltiazem, propranolol, and lidocaine may all result in either Type I or II second-degree heart block. Second-degree atrioventricular block is often observed in cats with hyperthyroidism or cardiomypathy.

Clinical Presentation. Animals present with exercise intolerance, weakness, syncope, or congestive heart failure.

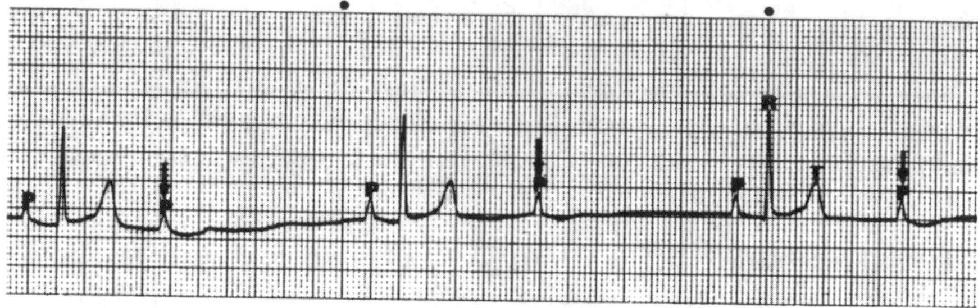

Figure 31-10
Second degree atrioventricular block is characterized by an intermittent failure or disturbance of AV conduction. One or more P waves are not followed by QRS-T complexes. Second degree block can be classified as Mobitz type I (Wenkebach) and Mobitz type II. Thje classification cam be further defined by QRS duration; and type B (lesion below the His bundle) with a wide QRS complex. (From Tilley, LR and Burtnick, NL: Electrocardiography for the Small Animal Practitioner. Teton NewMedia, 1999.)

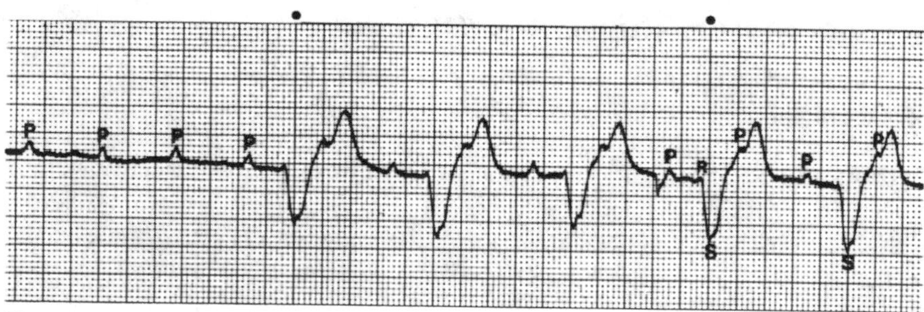

Cat

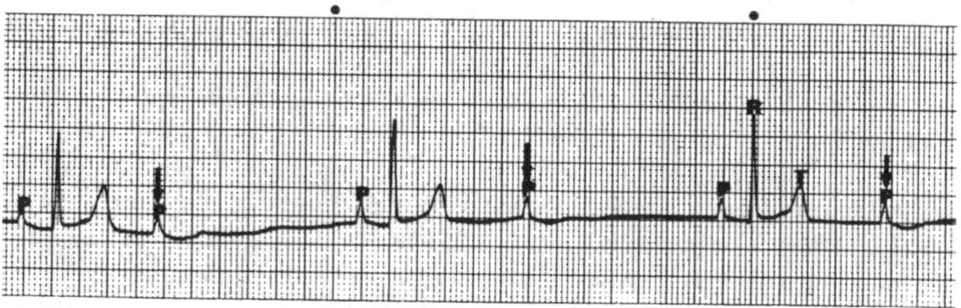

Dog

Figure 31-11
Second degree AV block, Mobitz type II can be more frequent and severe because the block is unpredictable. (From Tilley, LR and Burtnick, NL: Electrocardiography for the Small Animal Practitioner. Teton NewMedia, 1999.)

Diagnostic Evaluation. A history and complete physical exam is performed to identify if an underlying cause may be present. Laboratory test may include a CBC, biochemical profile, serum thyroxine concentration (cats), and serum tick titers. Diagnostic imaging may include thoracic radiographs and or cardiac ultrasound.

ECG Findings. Conduction abnormalities may be noted on a lead II ECG rhythm strip, but Holter monitoring may be needed to establish a diagnosis.

Mobitz type I block is characterized by a progressive prolongation of the P-R interval with successive beats until a P wave is blocked. The QRS complex is normal duration as the conduction disturbance is above the His bundle bifurcation. This may be a normal ECG finding in young dogs; those with increase vagal tone or a sinus arrhythmia.

Mobitz type II block is characterized by block that has a constant P-R interval. A fixed ratio of conducted to non-conducted impulses through the AV node is noted (2:1, 3:1, 4:1 AV block). The QRS complexes often demonstrate abnormal morphology because the conduction block occurs below the His bundle bifurcation. High-grade or advanced second-degree heart block occurs when two or more consecutive P waves are blocked.

Clinically, it is important to differentiate between the two subclasses of second-degree block. Mobitz type II is a more serious condition as the frequency and severity of the AV block is increased.

Treatment. Therapy for Mobitz type I is usually not indicated. Electrolyte status should be evaluated and medications that prolong AV nodal conduction discontinued. Periodic ECG monitoring is advised to monitor the severity of the AV block.

Mobitz type II second-degree AV block may require therapy if the animal is symptomatic. Suppression of ventricular escape complexes is contraindicated. Medical management with sympathomimetic agents (*i.e.*, isoproterenol 0.02 to 0.04 ug/kg/min or dopamine 2 to 7 ug/kg/min) or parasympatholytic drugs (atropine sulfate 0.02 to 0.04 mg/kg or glycopyrrolate 0.005 to 0.01 mg/kg) may be attempted; however, they rarely enhance AV conduction and reverse clinical signs. Judicious use of furosemide (1 to 2 mg/kg IV or IM) may be warranted if there is pulmonary edema or ascites. Definitive therapy for long-term management is a permanent cardiac pacemaker.

Prognosis. The prognosis is related to the underlying disorder. Dogs with idiopathic heart block and pacemaker implantation tend to do well. The prognosis in animals with structural heart disease is guarded to poor.

Third-degree Atrioventricular or Complete Heart Block

Complete AV heart block occurs when all atrial impulses are blocked at the atrioventricular node or His bundle. An independent ventricular pacemaker coordinates ventricular depolarization. As a result the atria and ventricles are controlled by independent pacemakers (Fig. 31-12).

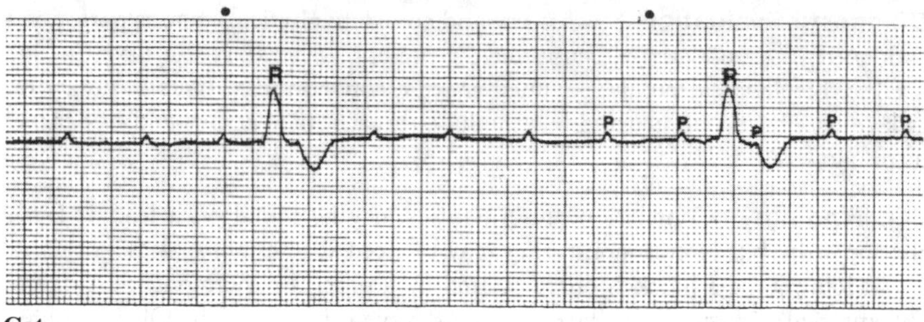

Cat

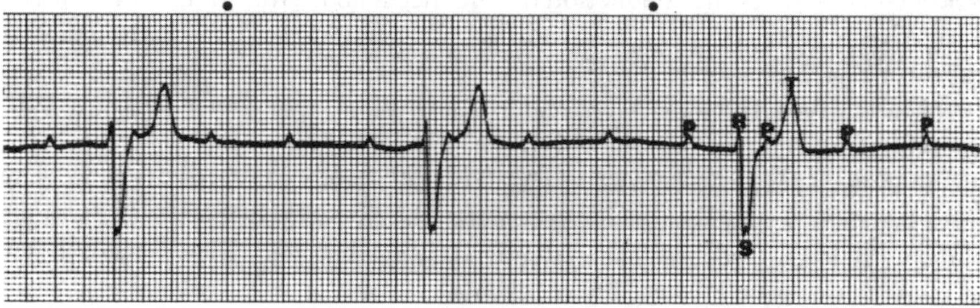

Dog

Figure 31-12
Third degree AV block. The cardiac impulse is completely blocked in the region of the AV junction and/or all bundle branches. The atrial rate (P-P interval) is normal. The idioventricular escape rhythm is slow. (From Tilley, LR and Burtnick, NL: Electrocardiography for the Small Animal Practitioner. Teton NewMedia, 1999.)

Pathogenesis. Third degree heart block tends to be associated with organic heart disease. Idiopathic myocardial fibrosis in older dogs (especially Cocker Spaniels), infiltrative cardiomyopathy (amyloidosis or neoplastic) and congenital defects (aortic stenosis or ventricular septal defects) may be predisposing factors. Complete heart block may be observed secondary to severe digitalis toxicity, β-2 adrenergic drugs (xylazine, medetomidine), endocarditis, infectious myocarditis, myocardial damage, and hyperkalemia.

Clinical Presentation. Exercise intolerance, weakness, syncope, seizures, or congestive heart failure can accompany complete AV block. The magnitude of clinical signs will depend upon the rate of the idioventricular escape rhythm. Complete AV block should always be considered an emergency due to possibility of sudden death.

ECG Findings. There is complete atrioventricular dissociation (*i.e.*, P waves have no association with the QRS complexes). The P-P interval and the R-R intervals are relatively constant; therefore a slow regular ventricular escape rhythm with a more rapid atrial rate will be present. Ventricular rate depends on the latent pacemaker location. Escape rhythms associated with the AV junction are faster and more reliable (dogs 40–60 bpm and cats 60–100 bpm) than those associated with the ventricles (heart rate less than 40 bpm). The AV pacemaker location will also influence QRS morphology; QRS complexes originating below the His bundle bifurcation will be wide and bizarre.

Diagnostic Evaluation. Diagnostic evaluation should be directed toward identifying underlying factors including systemic disease, cardiac abnormality, or medications. A complete physical examination, detailed history, CBC, biochemical profile, thoracic radiographs, and echocardiogram can help to determine the underlying cause and exclude extracardiac variables.

Treatment. Medical therapy has a limited role in third-degree heart block but it may be useful in emergent situations until cardiac pacing can be initiated. Atropine and isoproterenol are used for temporary management of medically responsive cases. Both medications can increase SA node activity and improve conduction through the AV node. Terbutaline (2.5 to 5 mg/kg P.O.) has been also suggested in refractive cases.

Permanent pacemakers are the only reliable therapy for symptomatic bradyarrhythmias. Temporary pacemakers may be required for emergent use to stabilize the patient until a permanent pacemaker may be implanted.

Prognosis. Prognosis is related to the underlying disorder. Following pacemaker implantation, dogs with idiopathic heart block tend to clinically improve with marked resolution of clinical signs. The prognosis in animals with structural heart disease is related to the underlying cause and tends to be guarded to poor.

Pulseless Electrical Activity

Pulseless electrical activity (PEA), formerly referred to as electromechanical dissociation (EMD), is characterized by organized electrical activity without effective myocardial contraction (Fig. 31-13). The term PEA was adopted to more accurately identify a heterogeneous group of arrhythmias including pseudo-EMD, ventricular escape rhythm, post-fibrillation idioventricular rhythm, and brady-asystolic rhythm.

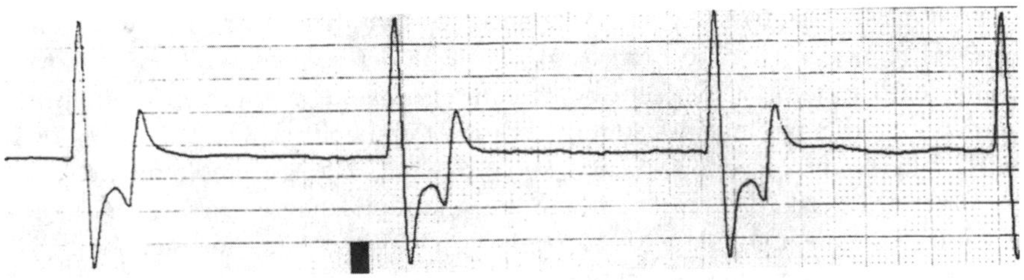

Figure 31-13
Pulseless electrical activity is characterized by sinus origin complexes that demonstrate QRS widening and S-T segmental baseline changes reflecting myocardial ischemia. Absence of mechanical activity in conjunction with electrical signalling is the hallmark of this disorder.

Pathogenesis

PEA represents failure of organized electrical depolarization to produce synchronous myocardial contraction. Loss of electromechanical coupling may be due to abnormal intracellular calcium metabolism, intracellular acidosis, or adenosine triphosphate depletion.

PEA is often associated with hypovolemia, hypoxia, metabolic acidosis, hyper/hypokalemia, hypothermia, cardiac tamponade, tension pneumothorax, coronary or pulmonary thrombosis, and drug overdoses. In humans, the most common PEA etiology is prolonged cardiac arrest or end-stage heart disease. Cardiac arrest associated PEA appears to be the more common clinical presentation in veterinary medicine.

Clinical Presentation

Clinical presentation is compatible with cardiac arrest. Apnea, cyanosis, non-palpable pulses or audible heart sounds, and pupillary dilation are noted. PEA is often noted as part of the physiologic process of dying.

ECG Findings

The presence of organized electrical activity other than VT or VF on electrocardiography with absence of a detectable pulse are the hallmark signs of PEA.

Diagnostic Evaluation

Every effort should be made to identify the initiating cause of the cardiac arrest (*i.e.*, hypovolemic shock, hypoxia, tension pneumothorax) by performing an abbreviated physical examination and quick assessment tests (PCV/TS, blood gas, and electrolyte analysis) during resuscitation.

Treatment

Aggressive therapy for cardiac arrest is warranted in those animals not expected to die. Initial therapy includes intubation, ventilation, cardiac massage, intravenous fluids, identifying the PEA pattern on ECG, and administration of resuscitation drugs (see Chapter 30). Specific PEA therapy should be targeted towards identification and correction of the underlying causes (*i.e.*, hypovolemia, cardiac tamponade, tension pneumothorax, or pulmonary embolism). Nonspecific therapy includes administration of epinephrine (1ml/ 5 kg IV or 1 ml/ 2.5 kg IT) and atropine (1 ml/5 kg IV or 1 ml/ 2.5 kg IT). Naloxone (0.02 mg/kg to 0.1 mg/kg IV), dexamethasone sodium phosphate (2 mg/kg IV), and calcium (calcium chloride 500–1000 mg/kg IV or calcium gluconate 1 ml/10 kg) are secondary rescue medications.

Prognosis

The experience to date in veterinary medicine has been that PEA is poorly responsive to resuscitation.

ARRHYTHMIAS OF FAST RATE ORIGIN (TACHYARRHYTHMIAS)

Sinus Tachycardia

Sinus tachycardia is a frequently noted rhythm in critically ill patients (Fig. 31-14). Sinus tachycardia is diagnosed when all criteria for sinus rhythm are present but the heart rate is faster than species normal (dog > 200 bpm, cats > 230 bpm). There is an overlap between sinus rhythm and sinus tachycardia; in many cases classification is determined by co-existing factors as well as heart rate.

Pathogenesis

Sinus tachycardia is generally associated with sympathetic nervous system activation. Excitement is a common underlying cause in healthy animals. Possible causes in sick or critically ill patients include fever, hypovolemia, hypotension, (shock), anaphylaxis, hypoxemia, hypercapnia, cardiac tamponade, heart failure, pain, hyperthyroidism, and anesthetic emergence.

Clinical Presentation

Animals with sinus tachycardia may be clinically asymptomatic or demonstrate symptoms associated with their primary disease. Cases of heart failure and hypoxemia will demonstrate clinical signs of their primary disease and have a persistent high heart rate. Cases that have noncardiac reasons for sinus tachycar-

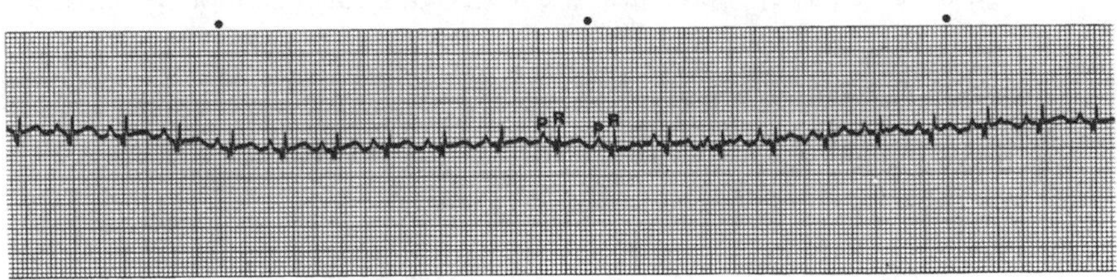

Cat

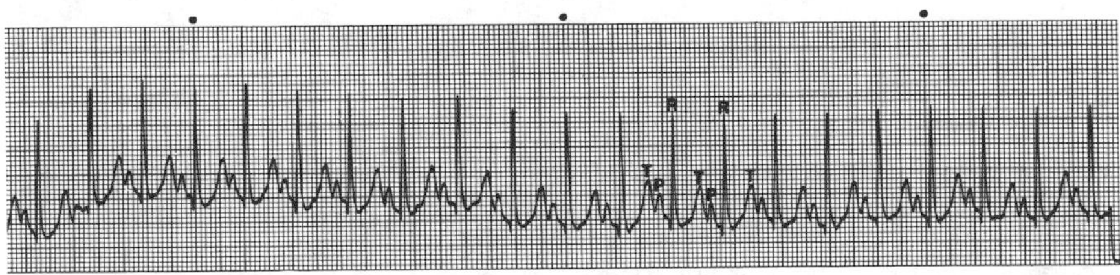

Dog

Figure 31-14
Sinus tachycardia is a regular sinus rhythm with a heart rate above normal discharge rates. Ocular pressure produces only a gradual transient slowing of the heart rate, if and change at all. (From Tilley, LR and Burtnick, NL: Electrocardiography for the Small Animal Practitioner. Teton NewMedia, 1999.)

dia have transient elevation in heart rate that normalizes with passage of the acute phase of the underlying disorder.

ECG Findings

Electrocardiographic criteria for sinus rhythm are present. Sinus tachycardia is distinguished by a rate greater than expected for the clinical situation. There is no clear cut off point between sinus rhythm and sinus tachycardia.

Diagnostic Evaluation

The major differential diagnosis for sinus tachycardia is supraventricular tachycardia. The two arrhythmias may look identical on ECG. Supraventricular tachycardia is differentiated based on a heart rate that is too fast for the clinical situation, nonresponsiveness to vagal maneuvers (carotid sinus massage, ocular pressure), and documented heart disease.

Treatment

Treatment is generally focused on the underlying reason for sinus tachycardia. Primary modification of heart rate without correction of the underlying cause is contraindicated.

Prognosis

Prognosis is generally good unless the underlying cause cannot be managed.

Supraventricular Tachycardia

Supraventricular tachycardia (SVT) is generally noted in dogs secondary to organic heart or serious systemic disease states.

Pathogenesis

SVT can originate from atrial myocardium or AV junctional tissue (Fig. 31-15). Most often, SVT is a reentry class arrhythmia, but automatic SVT has been reported in humans. A reentry pathway produces a sustained "pacemaker" producing a constant heart rate and QRS-T complex on ECG. Automatic SVT may have an irregular rate and ECG appearance.

Clinical Presentation

SVT <250 beats per minute is generally asymptomatic. SVT >250 beats per minute produces clinical signs of weakness and collapse associated with insufficient diastolic filling time. Physical findings include poor pulse quality, diminished mucous membrane color, and altered level of consciousness.

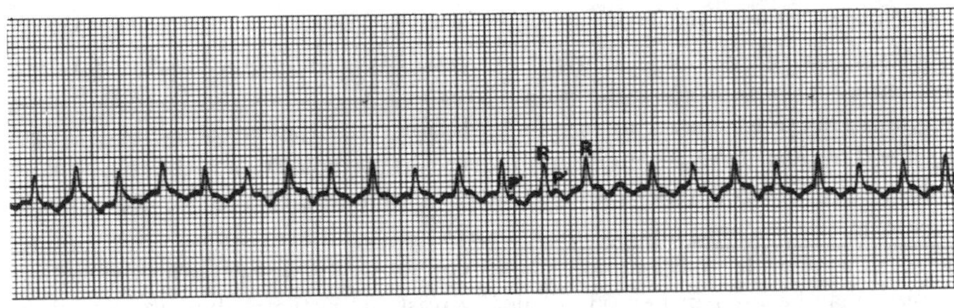

Cat

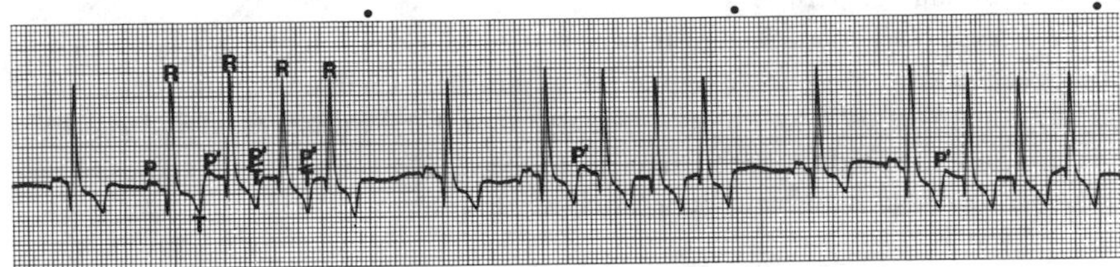

Dog

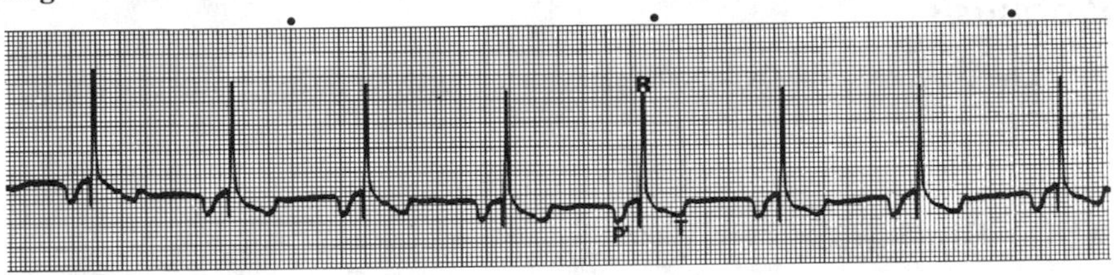

Junctional Tachycardia

Figure 31-15
Supraventricular tachycardia is a rapid regular rhythm originating from an atrial site other than the sinus node. (From Tilley, LR and Burtnick, NL: Electrocardiography for the Small Animal Practitioner. Teton NewMedia, 1999.)

ECG Findings

SVT is generally noted as normal electrical complex morphology that occurs at a higher rate than sinus rhythm. It may occur in "bursts" or may be sustained in duration. The R-R interval is constant in most cases. The QRS complexes are narrow and upright in lead II. P waves may or may not accompany each QRS complex. If present, P waves may be either positive or negative in lead II.

Echocardiographic examination reveals normal end-systolic diameter, very small end-diastolic diameter, and a decreased shortening fraction.

Treatment

SVT is a medical emergency in cases presenting with weakness and collapse. Emergency treatment includes ocular pressure (vagal reflex maneuver) and precordial thump. Precordial thump appears to be more successful in creating and sustaining cardioversion.

Several drugs have been successful in converting SVT to sinus rhythm. Calcium channel blockers including verapamil (0.05 mg/kg boluses given over 3–5 minutes up to three doses) and diltiazem (0.05–0.25 mg/kg IV over 5 minutes) are effective for acute management. β-blocking drugs propanolol (0.02 mg/kg slow bolus IV up to 0.1 mg/kg total dose) and esmolol (0.25–0.5 mg/kg slow bolus IV plus 50–200 μg/kg/min CRI) may be used for cardioversion and control except in documented myocardial failure. Class I antiarrhythmic drugs (quinidine, procainamide) may be used in automatic origin SVT. Synchronized cardioversion may be used in hemodynamically unstable patients that are refractive to medical management.

Chronic SVT management may be achieved with β-blocking drugs, calcium channel blocking drugs, or digoxin. Oral administration of propanolol or atenolol (0.5–2 mg/kg) is used for chronic management. Oral diltiazem (0.5–3 mg/kg q 8 h) may also be used for ventricular rate control. Digoxin is used in cases refractive to calcium channel and beta blocking drugs.

Prognosis

The prognosis is based on the underlying medical disorder and response to therapy.

Atrial Fibrillation

Pathogenesis

Atrial fibrillation (AF) is caused by numerous reentrant impulses creating rapid, disorganized atrial depolarization (Fig. 31-16). By definition, AF is described as >350 atrial depolarizations/minute; this may exceed 500 depolarizations per minute in some cases. The depolarization process is self-propagating due to constant regional repolarization allowing successive depolarization cycles. In AF, the AV node is under constant impulse bombardment; it conducts impulses based on its own electrophysiologic state at any instant in time. Ventricular depolarization occurs only when the AV node is physiologically capable of impulse transmission. This feature contributes to the "irregular irregularity" in cardiac rhythm associated with AF.

Constant disorganized depolarization produces poor atrial contraction. Poor atrial contraction and elevated ventricular rate render the patient at increased risk for developing congestive heart failure. Poor atrial contraction also contributes to retarded blood flow through the atrium. This predisposes to flow stagnation causing aberrant coagulation and possible thromboembolism.

Clinical Presentation

Many AF patients present with clinical signs of syncope or congestive heart failure.

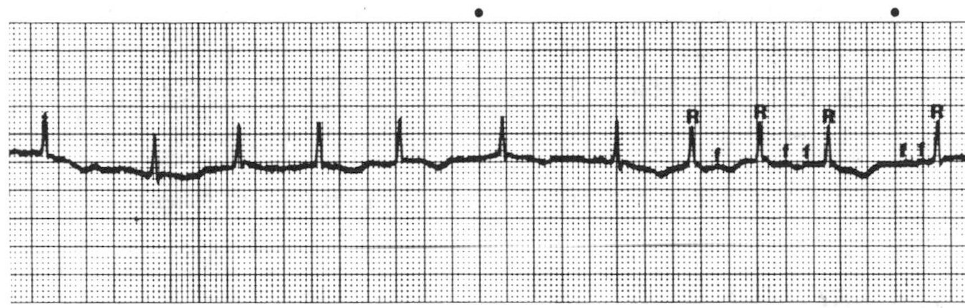

Cat

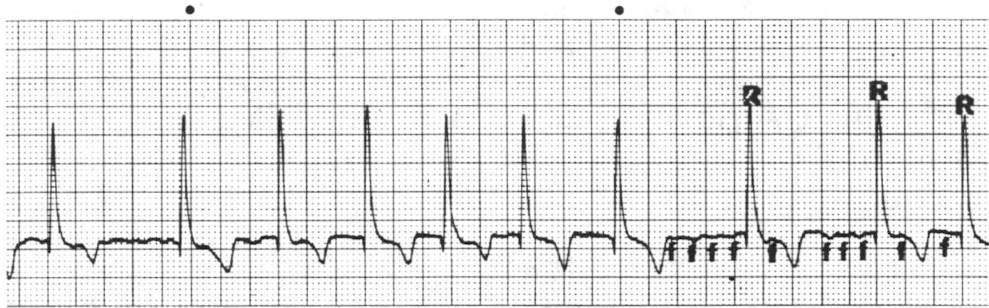

Dog

Figure 31-16
Atrial fibrillation is caused by numerous disorganized atrial impulses frequently bombarding the AV node. (From Tilley, LR and Burtnick, NL: Electrocardiography for the Small Animal Practitioner. Teton NewMedia, 1999.)

Diagnostic Evaluation

A key physical finding is an irregular heart rhythm on cardiac auscultation described as "tennis shoes in a dryer". Simultaneous pulse palpation reveals inconsistent pulse strength and character.

ECG Findings

AF has several key findings on ECG tracing. An irregular atrial and ventricular rate is evident. Normal P waves are replaced by small amplitude oscillations referred to as "f" (fibrillation) waves. QRS complexes vary in amplitude. They may be normal or wide and bizarre in configuration (due to bundle branch disease or pre-excitation). The R-R interval is inconsistent between any two complexes and does not exhibit a reproducible interval.

Treatment

Treatment is directed at managing coexisting congestive heart failure and slowing ventricular rate to increase cardiac output. Treatment goals include reducing ventricular rate to <160 beats/minute using drugs that prolong AV nodal refractory period. Digoxin, β-adrenergic blocking drugs, and diltiazem are commonly used for therapy. Digoxin is used as the initial drug in a slow digitalization protocol. If ventricular rate is not below targeted level following therapeutic doses, either propanolol (0.1–0.2 mg/kg q 8H) or diltiazem (0.5–1.5 mg/kg q8H) is supplemented for rate control. In cats with hypertrophic cardiomyopathy, diltiazem or atenolol are used for initial management. Digoxin is added if heart rate remains high. Quinidine has been used for AF cardioversion in dogs with limited success. In humans, cardioversion is successful in AF management; unfortunately it has not demonstrated long-term success in dogs and little evidence exists in cats.

Prognosis

Prognosis is guarded to poor in all cases. The origin of AF and extent of clinical signs are key factors in establishing the prognosis.

Isorhythmic Atrioventricular Dissociation (Nodal Tachycardia)

Pathogenesis

Atrioventricular (AV) dissociation occurs when the atria and ventricles are controlled by independent pacemaker sites. The term isorhythmic AV dissociation (IAVD) is used when the depolarization rate of the atrial pacemaker and ventricular pacemakers occur in approximately a 1:1 ratio (Fig. 31-17). Thus, a P wave and a QRS-T complex are present in approximately equal number but are not consistently linked in a temporal relationship. Both atrial and ventricular depolarization rate occurs at a higher rate than normal in these cases.

The pathogenesis is not completely understood. IAVD is most commonly seen in cats. Pre-existing factors include primary cardiac disease, general anesthesia, calcium-channel blocking drugs, and electrolyte or acid-base abnormalities. It has also been noted in dogs with digitalis class drug toxicity. In some cases, high AV nodal depolarization rates will decrease atrial filling to the ventricles and diminish cardiac output.

Clinical Presentation

Presentation may range from asymptomatic to overt signs of congestive heart failure. Weakness, syncope, and collapse may be noted.

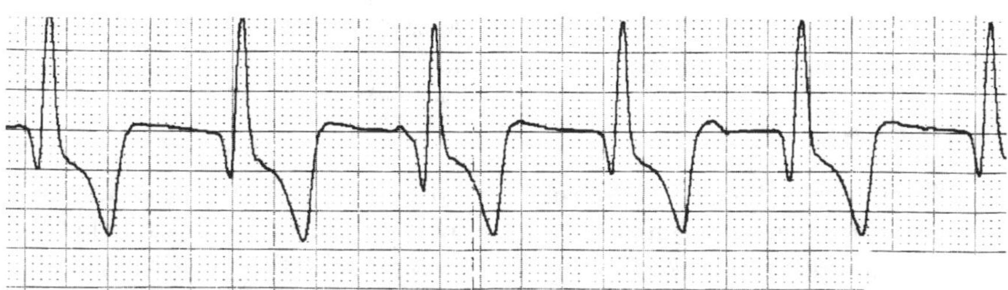

Figure 31-17
Isorhythmic atrioventricular dissociation (nodal tachycardia).

ECG Findings

Consistent P wave and QRS-T complex activity is noted. Amplitude of all waveforms may be normal or slightly widened, indicating delayed depolarization. Inconsistent relationship between the P wave and QRS-T complex is obvious on ECG rhythm analysis.

Treatment

Rate control with β-adrenergic blocking drugs is indicated if clinical signs are noted. Magnesium has been used in humans with moderate success. Management of underlying heart disease is warranted and is the likely reason for successful management.

Prognosis

Prognosis depends on the underlying reason for the arrhythmia. It varies from good in anesthesia to guarded/poor in primary myocardial disease.

Ventricular Tachycardia

Ventricular tachycardia (VT) is defined as three or more ventricular premature beats in succession (Fig. 31-18).

Pathogenesis

VT is associated with abnormal automaticity secondary to injured myocardial tissue, microreentry secondary to abnormal myocardium, or primary triggered activity. VT can be uniform or multiform. Uniform appearing complexes suggest one focus of impulse generation; multiform appearing complexes indicate several sites of impulse generation. Multiform complexes are often referred to as *multifocal*. Multifocal complexes may originate in anatomic proximity to each other and take different depolarization pathways. Differences in complex appearance are associated with site of impulse generation and the conduction pathway from site of origin. In dogs, the most common reason for VT is believed to be abnormal automaticity modulated by the autonomic nervous system.

Clinical Presentation

Clinical signs associated with VT depend on the ventricular rate, duration of the tachycardia, and underlying disease. VT in dogs without underlying myocardial disease does not produce clinical signs unless additional compromise (anesthesia, systemic disease) is present. VT greater than 250 beats/minute results in a decreased cardiac output, hypotension, and syncope.

Cardiac auscultation may reveal sudden acceleration of heart sounds that occur for short intervals. If sustained VT is present, a rapid heart rate will be evident.

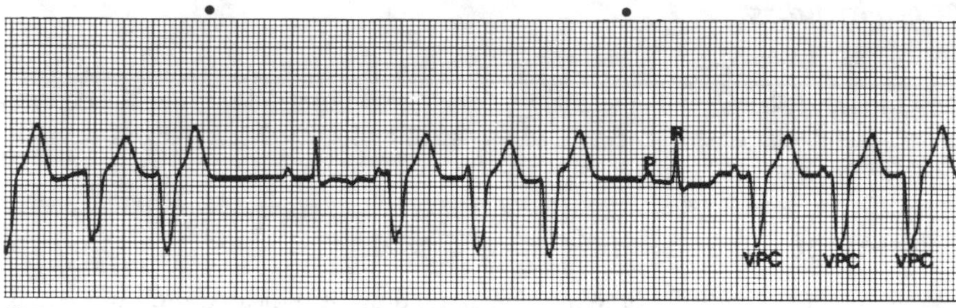

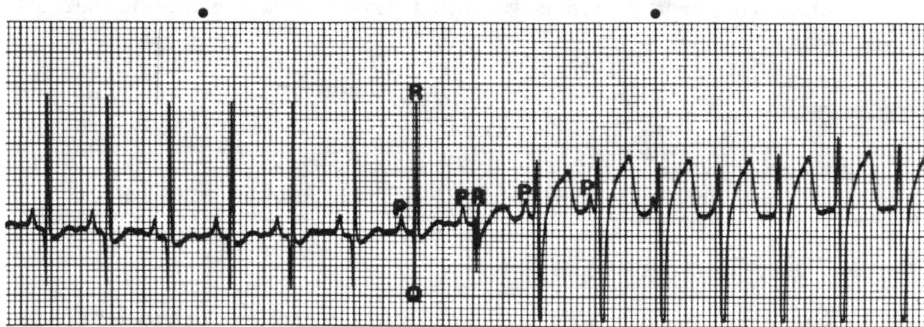

Figure 31-18
Ventricular tachycardia is three or more VPCs in succession resulting from stimulation of an ectopic focus. VT may be intermittent (paroxysmal) or sustained. Potentially life threatening, it usually signifies important myocardial disease or metabolic derangement. (From Tilley, LR and Burtnick, NL: Electrocardiography for the Small Animal Practitioner. Teton NewMedia, 1999.)

ECG Findings

VT complexes differ from regular complexes in morphology, rate, regularity, and duration on scalar ECG. Ventricular rate is highly variable ranging from 70–500 beats per minute. VT may occur for variable time periods. VT less than 30 seconds is generally classified as nonsustained VT; greater than 30 seconds is sustained VT. In general, VT is considered to be a "wide complex" arrhythmia with a QRS duration >0.12 seconds. Morphology of the ventricular complex is, in part, due to site of impulse generation. Complexes may be uniform in appearance reflecting a single site of impulse generation, or irregular in appearance indicating a multiform VT. R-R interval may be constant or irregular. Atrial depolarization may continue in a normal manner during VT periods. In many cases, P waves will be obscured on scalar ECG due to the amplitude of ventricular complexes.

"Torsades des pointes" (turning around the points) is a variant of VT characterized by phasic changes in the amplitude and polarity of the ventricular complexes. This arrhythmia is often associated with a prolonged Q-T interval. A variety of drugs including antiarrhythmic agents (quinidine, procainamide), antimicrobial agents (erythromycin, pentamidine), and psychotropic drugs (haloperidol, phenothiazines) have been associated with this rhythm. Electrolyte disturbances characterized by deficiency in calcium, magnesium, or potassium have been associated with this arrhythmia.

Treatment

Criteria for therapeutic intervention in VT are based on the underlying disease process, frequency of VT occurrence, and additional physiologic compromise that may be present (Table 31-1). Several authors note that this arrhythmia is generally "over managed" in ICU settings due to a fear that it will deteriorate into life threatening terminal arrhythmias such as ventricular fibrillation. There is no evidence to support this belief. In fact, most VT subsides as the underlying cause is corrected. Generally this occurs over a 48–72 hour period. Recommendations are consistent with published standards collated in human medicine.

Lidocaine is the primary drug used in VT management. It is generally given as an intravenous "bolus" (2–4 mg/kg) followed by a constant rate infusion (30–80 μg/kg/min). Other Class I antiarrhythmic drugs (quinidine, procainamide) have also been successfully used in management. Correction of the underlying factors (electrolytes, acid-base balance) play a key role in VT management. In cases with underlying myocardial disease, Class III antiarrhythmic drugs (amiodarone, sotalol) and β-adrenergic blocking drugs have been used to prevent VT-associated sudden death. In cases demonstrating "torsades des pointes," therapy is based on the Q-T interval. Cases with normal Q-T interval are managed with lidocaine bolus and infusion. Cases with prolonged Q-T interval will require magnesium infusion as a primary therapy (see PVC therapy section)

Hemodynamically unstable VT in the cat is acutely managed with an intra-

Table 31-1. VT Surveillance and Treatment

Criteria for Treatment	Criteria for Surveillance
At risk for developing sudden death Multifocal VT "Torsades des pointes"	Lower risk for developing sudden death Unifocal VT
>30 seconds in duration	<30 seconds in duration
VT rate greater than 250 bpm	VT rate does not exceed 250 bpm
Underlying cause is primary myocardial disease Dilated cardiomyopathy Boxer cardiomyopathy Subaortic stenosis Hypertrophic cardiomyopathy-cats	Underlying cause is not primary heart disease: Traumatic myocardial contusion Electrolyte disturbance Acid-base disturbance Anesthesia
Patient demonstrates clinical signs referable to VT episode. Syncope Hypotension Shock	Patient is asymptomatic during VT episode

venous bolus of lidocaine (0.25 to 1 mg/kg over 5 minutes up to a total of 4 mg for an average-sized cat). If the lidocaine bolus is unsuccessful, an IV bolus of esmolol (50 to 500 ug/kg) or a CRI (50 to 200 ug/kg/min) may be administered titrated to effect. Cats tend to be sensitive to the toxic side effects of lidocaine. Therefore a CRI infusion of this medication is not recommended. If both medications are ineffective, a precordial thump may be attempted. This maneuver may successfully terminate the arrhythmia by mechanically inducing a premature systole, thus interrupting the reentry circuit.

Prognosis

VT secondary to direct myocardial injury or coexisting disease carries a good to excellent prognosis if the underlying condition is successfully managed. VT associated with primary myocardial disease or valve dysfunction carries a guarded to poor prognosis.

Ventricular Fibrillation

Ventricular fibrillation (VF) is a life threatening arrhythmia that results in death if left untreated (Fig. 31-19). VF is the dominant arrhythmia associated

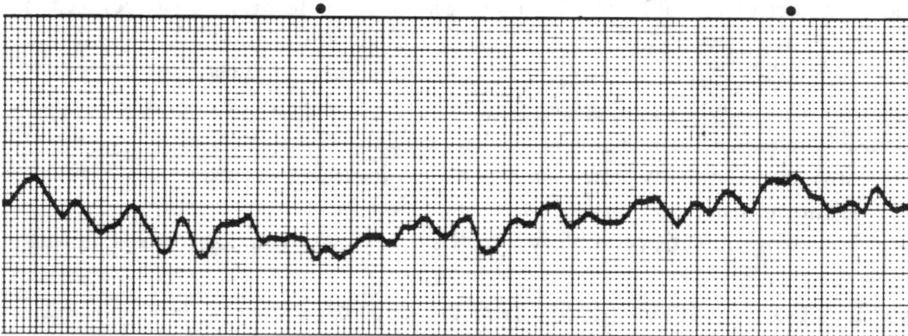

Cat

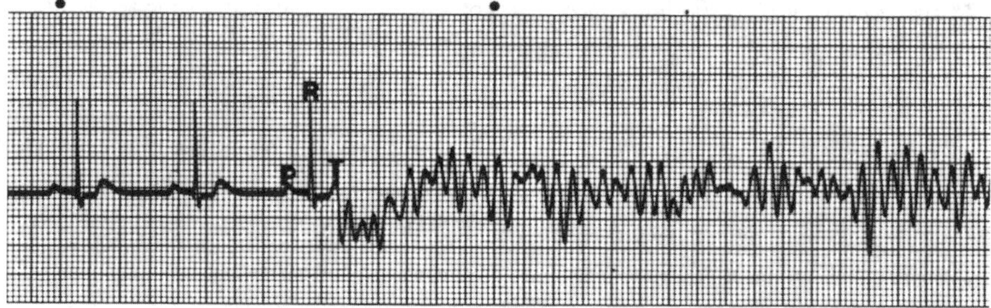

Dog

Figure 31-19
Ventricular fibrillation occurs when the cells of the ventricular myocardium depolarize in an uncoordinated menner. No pulse can be felt and cardiac output approaches zero, making this a life threatening and generally terminal rhythm.

with cardiopulmonary arrest in humans. The incidence of VF in companion animals is unknown.

Pathogenesis

VF occurs due to activation of multiple micro-reentrant circuits within the ventricular myocardium. The exact trigger mechanism varies with clinical condition and specific circumstances. It most commonly occurs as the terminal event in a patient with severe systemic or cardiac disease. It may also occur unexpectedly during various procedures including anesthesia induction, cardiac surgery, pericardiocentesis, cardiac ischemia, and endomyocardial biopsy.

Clinical Presentation

The patient is presented in acute cardiovascular collapse. Clinical signs of cardiopulmonary arrest characterized by absence of breathing, pulse, unconsciousness, and cyanosis are usually seen.

ECG Findings

No discernable P waves or QRS-T complexes are noted on scalar ECG. Low amplitude, irregular undulation of the baseline tracing is present.

Treatment

Rapid, definitive intervention is necessary to save the patient. Defibrillation (nonsynchronous cardioversion) is the treatment of choice. The initial energy level is 5–7 J/kg. Table 31-2 gives the approximate dosage.

The initial electrical dose is immediately readministered if the first attempt in restoring normal rhythm is unsuccessful. Initiation of the ABC's of CPR should occur during cardioversion efforts. Standard cardiopulmonary resuscitation measures should be performed at this point.

Prognosis

Guarded to poor depending on the underlying cause and response to initial resuscitation measures.

Table 31-2. Defibrillation and Body Size

Body Size	Electrical Dose (Total J)
Small (<10 kg)	50 J
Medium (10–20 kg)	100 J
Large (>20 kg)	200 J

SUGGESTED READINGS

Textbooks

Bistner SI, Ford RB, Raffe MR: *Handbook of Veterinary Procedures and Emergency Treatment*. Philadelphia, WB Saunders Company, 2000.

Bolton GR: *Handbook of Canine Electrocardiography*. Philadelphia, WB Saunders 1979.

Davis D: *How to Quickly and Accurately Master ECG Interpretation*, 2nd ed.. Philadelphia, JB Lippincott, 1992.

Kittleson MD, Kienle RD: *Small Animal Cardiovascular Medicine*. St. Louis, Mosby Yearbook Inc., 1998.

Marino PL: *The ICU Book*, 2nd ed. Baltimore, Williams & Wilkins, 1998

Mathews KA: *Veterinary Emergency and Critical Care Manual*. Guelph, Ont., Lifelearn Inc, 1996

Sisson D, Oyama M: *Cardiovascular Medicine of Companion Animanls*. Urbana, University of Illinois, 2001.

Tilley LP, Burtnick NL: *ECG Electrocardiography for the Small Animal Practitioner*. Jackson,Wyoming, Teton NewMedia, 1999.

Wingfield WE: *Veterinary Emergency Medicine Secrets*. Philadelphia, Hanley & Belfus, 2000.

Articles

Abbott JA: Traumatic Myocarditis. *In:* Bonagura JD, Kirk RW, eds. *Current Veterinary Therapy XII Small Animal Practice*. Philadelphia, WB Saunders Company, 1995; 846–850.

American Heart Association in Collaboration with International Liaison Committee on Resuscitation: Guidelines 2000 for Cardiopulmonary Resuscitation and Emergency Cardiovascular Care. International Consensus on Science. *Circulation (Suppl)* 2000; 102:I-1-I–380.

Balser JR: Perioperative Dysrhythmias. *In: ASA Refresher Course in Anesthesiology*. 1997; 1-13.

Dangman KH: Electrophysiologic Mechanisms for Arrhythmia. *In:* Fox PR, Sisson D, Moise NS, eds. *Textbook of Canine and Feline Cardiology Principles of Clinical Practice*. Philadelphia, WB Saunders Company, 1988; 291–305.

Fogel RI, Prystowsky EN: Management of malignant ventricular arrhythmias and cardiac arrest. *Crit Care Med*, 2001, 28:N165–N169.

Fox PR, Harpster NK: Diagnosis and Management of Feline Arrhythmias. *In:* Fox PR, Sisson D, Moise NS, eds. *Textbook of Canine and Feline Cardiology Principles of Clinical Practice*. Philadelphia, WB Saunders Company, 1988; 387–399.

Hollenberg SM, Dellinger P: Noncardiac surgery: Postoperative arrhythmias. *Crit Care Med*, 2001, 28:N145–N150.

Kaushik V, Leon AR, Forrester JS, Trochman RG: Bradyarrhythmias, temporary and permanent pacing. *Crit Care Med*, 2000, 28:N121–N128.

Keene BW: When and How to Treat Common Cardiac Arrhythmias. *In:* Proceedings IVECCS VII, Orlando, Fl, 2000; 101–105.

Moise NS. Diagnosis and Management of Canine Arrhythmias. *In:* Fox PR, Sisson D, Moise NS, eds. *Textbook of Canine and Feline Cardiology Principles of Clinical Practice*. Philadelphia, WB Saunders Company, 1988; 331–385.

Oyama MA, Sisson DD, Lehmkuhl LB: Practices and outcome of artificial cardiac pacing in 154 dogs. *J Vet Intern Med*, 2001; 15:229–239.

Rush JE, Wingfield WW: Recognition and frequency of dysrhythmias during cardiopulmonary arrest, *JAVMA*, 1992; 200:1932–1937.

Rush JE: Managment of Bradyarrhythmias. *In:* Proceedings IVECCS V, San Antonio, TX, 1996; 110–114.

Russell LC, Rush JE: Cardiac Arrhythmias in Systemic Disease. *In:* Bonagura JD, Kirk RW, eds. *Current Veterianry Therapy XII Small Animal Practice*. Philadelphia, WB Saunders Company, 1995; 161–166.

Strickland KN: Advances in antiarrhythmic therapy. *Vet Clin North Am Small Anim Pract*, 1998; 28:1515–46.

Trohman RG: Supraventricular tachycardia: Implications for the intensivist. *Crit Care Med*, 2001, 28:N129–N135.

Wood DL: Potentially lethal ventricular arrhythmias. Minimizing the danger. *Postgrad Med*, 1990; 88:65–74.

Zipes DP: Specific Arryhthmias: Diagnosis and Treatment. *In:* Braundwald E, ed. *Heart Disease: A Textbook of Cardiovascular Medicine Volume 1*. Philadelphia, WB Saunders Company, 1997; 640–704.

32
Pulmonary Hypertension

E. Christopher Orton

INTRODUCTION

The pulmonary vascular system is unique in that, unlike the vascular system of other organs, the entire cardiac output (CO) must pass through it. During passage of blood through the normal pulmonary circulation, hemoglobin is oxygenated to nearly full capacity. As a result, abnormalities of the pulmonary circulation leading to pulmonary hypertension can have dire consequences not only on the oxygenation function of the lungs, but on the entire cardiovascular system.

Definition

By definition, pulmonary hypertension is present when systolic pulmonary artery pressure (PAP) is greater than 30 mm Hg, mean PAP is greater than 20 mm Hg, or both pressure indices are elevated.

PHYSIOLOGY

The normal pulmonary circulation offers remarkably little resistance to flow. Normal pulmonary artery pressure in small animals at sea level is about 18 to 20 mm Hg systolic over 6 to 10 mm of Hg diastolic. Mean PAP normally ranges from 12 to 15 mm Hg. The arterial-venous pressure difference that drives the entire CO across the pulmonary vascular bed is generally less than 10 mm Hg, about one tenth the pressure difference necessary to drive the same amount of flow across the systemic vascular bed. Thus, resistance to flow across the normal pulmonary vascular bed is very low. Pulmonary vascular resistance (R) is defined and quantified by the pressure difference (ΔP) between PAP and the left atrial pressure (LAP) and the cardiac output (Q) according to an analogy from Ohm's law:

$$R = \Delta P/Q$$

The factors that influence R are defined by the Poiseuille relationship:

$$R = 8\eta l/\pi r^4$$

where η equals the viscosity of blood, l equals the length of the vessel, and r is the vessel radius.

From the above equations, the important role that vessel radius plays in determining vascular resistance is apparent. Two important physiologic responses

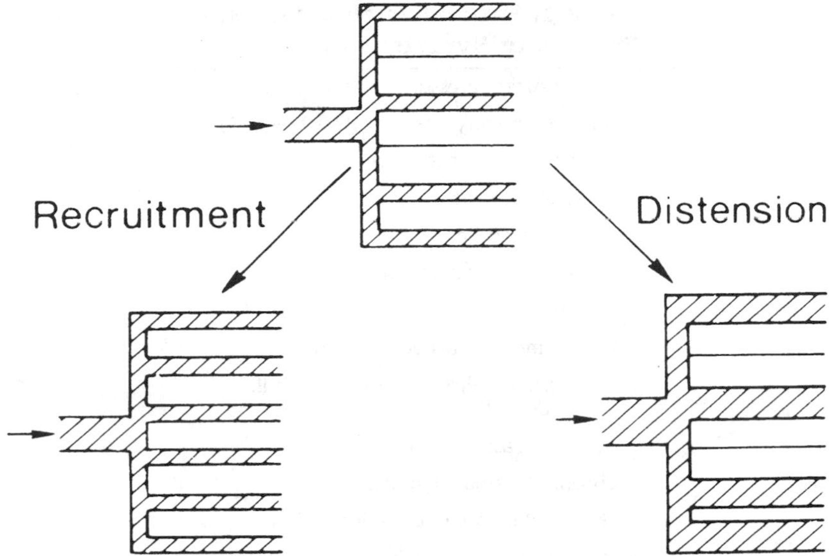

Figure 32-1
Recruitment and distention. Physiologic mechanisms in the normal pulmonary circulation that keep pulmonary vascular resistance low in the face of increasing pulmonary flow and pulmonary arterial pressure. (From West JB: Respiratory Physiology—The Essentials, 2nd ed. Baltimore, Williams & Wilkins, 1979.)

at work in the normal pulmonary circulation keep pulmonary vascular resistance and PAP low in the face of an increasing CO. These are vascular distensibility and vascular recruitment (Fig. 32-1).[1] Because normal pulmonary vessels are thin walled and elastic (*i.e.*, distensible), the radius of pulmonary vessels passively increases with increased transmural pressure and flow. Further, when pulmonary flow is low, not all available vascular channels are used. As pulmonary flow increases, additional vascular channels are recruited and this decreases vascular resistance by increasing the total cross-sectional area of the pulmonary vessels. Thus, in the normal pulmonary bed, as pulmonary flow increases pulmonary vascular resistance passively decreases. These physiologic mechanisms emphasize the importance that nature has placed on keeping vascular resistance and PAP low even during physiologic or pathologic increases in CO.

PATHOPHYSIOLOGY

Rearrangement of equation one reveals possible pathophysiologic causes of pulmonary hypertension:

$$\Delta P = R \times Q$$
$$PAP - LAP = R \times Q$$
$$PAP = R \times Q + LAP$$

Table 32-1. Pathophysiologic Causes of Pulmonary Hypertension

Pulmonary Artery Pressure = (Q R) + LAP
Increased Pulmonary Vascular Resistance (R)
Pulmonary Vasoconstriction
Alveolar Hypoxia
—Hypoventilation
—Pulmonary parenchymal disease
—Altitude
Circulating Vasoactive Substances
—norepinephrine, angiotension II, endothelin
Pulmonary Vascular Remodeling
Chronic Alveolar Hypoxia
Chronic Pulmonary Overcirculation
Pulmonary Vascular Occlusion
Pulmonary Thromboembolism
Heartworm Disease
Polycythemia
Chronic Hypoxemia
Polycythemia Vera
Increased Pulmonary Blood Flow (Q)
Left-to-Right Cardiac Shunt
Increased Left Atrial Pressure (LAP)
Mitral Valve Disease
Cardiomyopathy

A critical determinant of pulmonary vascular resistance is pulmonary vessel radius. The magnitude of this effect is illustrated by the Poiseuille relationship in which R is a function of r raised to the fourth power. Pulmonary arterial vasoconstriction increases PAP and R by decreasing vessel radius. Thus, pulmonary hypertension can result from an increase in pulmonary vascular resistance, pulmonary blood flow, or LAP (Table 32-1).

Increased Pulmonary Vascular Resistance

Pulmonary Vasoconstriction

The pulmonary vascular smooth muscle is unique compared to systemic vascular smooth muscle in that the most important stimulus for contraction is hypoxia. Although it is true that most known mediators of vasoconstriction and vasodilation active in the systemic vascular bed are active in the pulmonary vascular bed as well, alveolar hypoxia is the dominant determinant of vascular tone in pulmonary arteries. The precise cellular mechanism that mediates hypoxic pulmonary vasoconstriction has not yet been elucidated. The magnitude of hypoxic pulmonary vasoconstriction is species dependent. Dogs and cats are considered to be low to moderate responders compared to other species.[2] Nevertheless, alveolar hypoxia should be regarded as an important possible cause of pulmonary hypertension in small animals.

Pulmonary Vascular Remodeling

Pulmonary vascular remodeling is characterized by concentric thickening of the vessel and is an important pathologic cause of decreased vessel radius and increased pulmonary vascular resistance in all species (Fig. 32-2). Vascular remodeling increases both the smooth muscle cell and connective tissue matrix component of the vascular wall.[3] As a result, vascular remodeling not only causes a fixed decrease in pulmonary vessel radius, but greatly potentates the magnitude of pulmonary vasoconstriction (Fig. 32-3). Although it is true in small animals that hypoxic pulmonary vasoconstriction only causes mild pulmonary hypertension when the pulmonary vascular bed is normal, pulmonary vascular remodeling changes this in a dramatic way. In the remodeled pulmonary vascular bed, the potential for pulmonary vasoconstriction is greatly enhanced, and hypoxia can cause moderate to severe pulmonary hypertension. Known causes of pulmonary

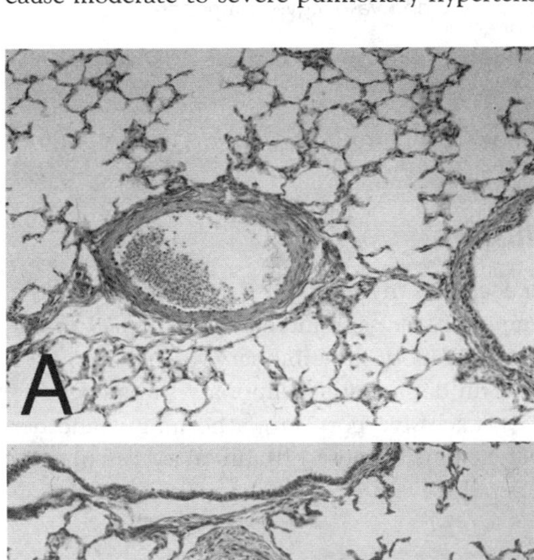

Figure 32-2
Pulmonary vascular remodeling. Photomicrograph (×100) of pulmonary artery from a normotensive (A) and pulmonary hypertensive (B) animal. Remodeling causes concentric thickening of the both the tunica adventitia and tunica media (*i.e.*, smooth muscle) layers of the vessel wall causing both a fixed increase in pulmonary arterial pressures and an increased capacity for pulmonary vascoconstriction.

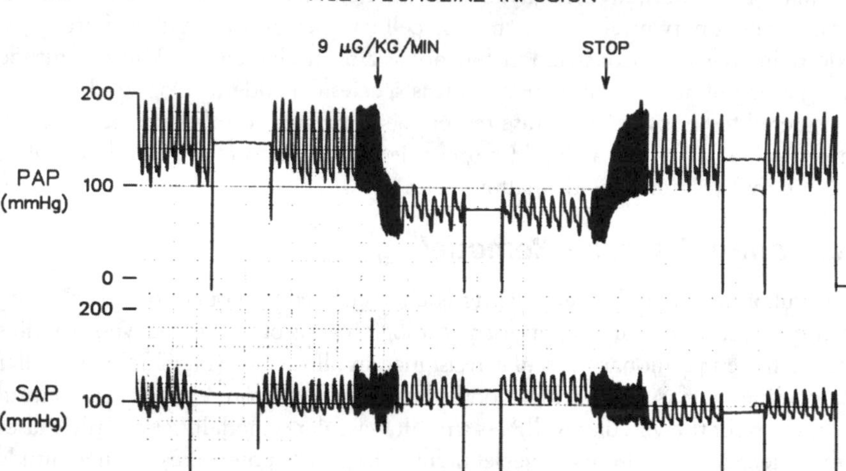

Figure 32-3
Pulmonary hypertension. Pulmonary arterial pressure (PAP) and systemic arterial pressure (SAP) during pulmonary arterial infusion of the selective vasodilator, acetylcholine, in an animal with hypoxic pulmonary hypertension. Infusion demonstrates that the pulmonary hypertension has both a fixed and vasoactive component.

vascular remodeling in small animals include chronic alveolar hypoxia or chronic pulmonary overcirculation.

Pulmonary Vascular Occlusion

Pulmonary vascular occlusion decreases the total cross-sectional area of the pulmonary vessels and is another important cause of increased pulmonary vascular resistance in small animals. The most important pulmonary vascular occlusive diseases in small animals are heartworm disease and pulmonary thromboembolism (PTE). Surgical resection of an excessive portion of the lung is another potential cause of pulmonary hypertension. Because of pulmonary vascular recruitment, vascular occlusion is generally severe before pulmonary hypertension becomes evident.

Polycythemia

According to the Poiseuille relationship, blood viscosity is a determinant of vascular resistance. Blood viscosity is primarily a function of the hematocrit. Thus polycythemia, though not a principal cause of pulmonary hypertension, does increase pulmonary vascular resistance and can exacerbate pulmonary hypertension due to other causes.

Increased Pulmonary Flow

The pulmonary circulation undergoes passive distention and recruitment of pulmonary vessels in response to an increase in pulmonary blood flow. Within limits, this allows pulmonary vascular resistance to decrease so that PAP can remain normal despite increased pulmonary blood flow. Despite these mechanisms, pulmonary overcirculation secondary to a severe left-to-right cardiac shunt can at times overwhelm these protective responses and result in pulmonary hypertension. Initially, pulmonary hypertension secondary to a left-to-right shunt is due more to an increase in pulmonary flow rather than a decrease in vascular resistance. Over time, pulmonary overcirculation becomes a potent stimulus for pulmonary vascular remodeling. As a result, pulmonary vascular resistance increases and becomes progressively more fixed over time. In the most severe cases, PAPs can actually exceed systemic arterial pressures (*i.e.*, suprasystemic pulmonary hypertension) causing flow through the cardiac shunt to become right-to-left.

Increased Left Atrial Pressure

Conditions that elevate LAP cause a proportional increase in PAP and pulmonary hypertension. This occurs without a change in pulmonary vascular resistance. The most common cause of elevated LAP in dogs is degenerative mitral valve disease, whereas hypertrophic or restrictive cardiomyopathy would be a more common cause in cats.

COR PULMONALE

Cor pulmonale is defined as right heart disease secondary to acute or chronic pulmonary hypertension. Cardiac manifestations of pulmonary hypertension include right ventricular hypertrophy, right ventricular and atrial dilation, tricuspid regurgitation, right-sided congestive heart failure (CHF), low output cardiac failure, or any combination of these.

Acute cor pulmonale is defined as right heart strain or overload due to acute-onset pulmonary hypertension, most often secondary to massive PTE. Acute cor pulmonale in dogs is characterized by rapid onset of right ventricular dilation, tricuspid regurgitation, acute systemic venous hypertension, and low CO. Low CO results from an inability of the strained right heart to push blood flow through the high resistance pulmonary vascular bed exacerbated by the presence of tricuspid regurgitation.

Chronic cor pulmonale is associated with slow-onset pulmonary hypertension most often secondary to chronic progressive hypoxic pulmonary hypertension associated with chronic respiratory disease. Right ventricular hypertrophy is an invariable finding in dogs and cats with chronic cor pulmonale. Tricuspid regurgitation may or may not be present. When tricuspid regurgitation is present, it is often accompanied by signs of right-sided CHF including hepatic congestion, ascites, or peripheral edema.

DIAGNOSIS

Physical Findings

Pulmonary hypertension, even when it is moderate to severe, can be remarkably clinically silent. Presenting complaints for animals with pulmonary hypertension include exercise intolerance, cough, dyspnea, and syncope.[4] The most consistent finding on auscultation is a loud and split second heart sound. Most small animals with significant pulmonary hypertension develop secondary tricuspid regurgitation.[4] These animals have a characteristic holosystolic murmur on the right mid-thoracic wall. This murmur may have a high intensity and be associated with a cardiac thrill due to increased right ventricular systolic pressure driving the regurgitation. Pulmonary hypertension is the most common cause of acquired tricuspid regurgitation. Animals with an acquired murmur compatible with tricuspid regurgitation should be regarded as strong candidates for pulmonary hypertension.

Other physical findings associated with pulmonary hypertension are consistent with right ventricular pressure overload. Jugular and systemic venous distention may be present. If tricuspid regurgitation is present, there may be a prominent jugular pulse. In advanced chronic cases, signs of right ventricular congestive failure (*i.e.*, chronic cor pulmonale) may be present including hepatomegaly, ascites, and peripheral edema. In animals with acute severe pulmonary hypertension (most often secondary to PTE) signs consistent with low output heart failure (*i.e.*, acute cor pulmonale) and hypoxemia may occur. If hypoxemia is secondary to PTE, it will usually be very responsive to supplemental oxygen (O_2). If hypoxemia and cyanosis are secondary to right-to-left cardiac shunt (*i.e.*, Eisenmenger syndrome), they will not be corrected by supplemental O_2.

Radiography

Thoracic radiographs of small animals with pulmonary hypertension usually show enlargement of the main pulmonary artery segment (Figs. 32-4 and 32-5). Lobar pulmonary arteries may be dilated and tortuous compared to lobar pulmonary veins, although absence of this finding does not exclude serious pulmonary hypertension (Figs. 32-5 and 32-6). Peripheral pulmonary arteries may be enlarged or show abnormal tapering. A right ventricular enlargement pattern may be evident. The later finding is more likely in animals that have developed secondary tricuspid regurgitation.

Echocardiography

Chronic pulmonary hypertension without significant tricuspid regurgitation causes thickening of the right ventricular free wall and interventricular septum (*i.e.*, concentric hypertrophy pattern) as a result of the right ventricular pressure overload. Dilation of the main pulmonary artery is another consequence of chronic pulmonary hypertension (see Fig. 25-12). Unexplained right ventricular hypertrophy and main pulmonary artery dilation on echocardiography should be regarded as strong presumptive evidence of pulmonary hypertension. If secondary

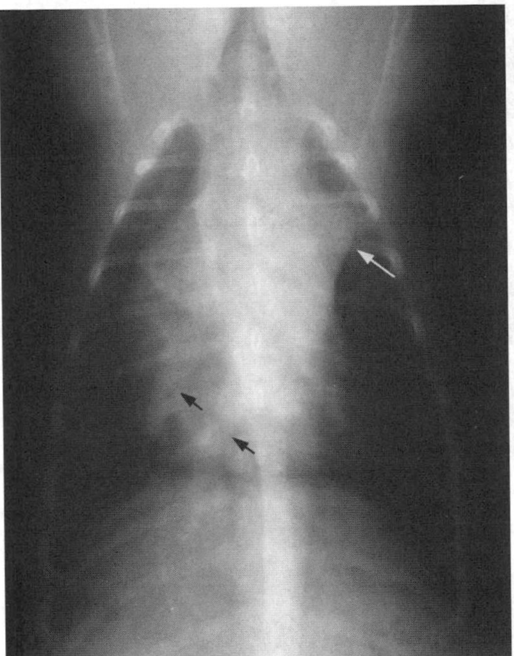

Figure 32-4
Dorsoventral radiograph from a dog with right-to-left patent ductus arteriosus (Eisenmenger syndrome) shows enlargement of main pulmonary artery segment (white arrow) and dilation of pulmonary arteries and veins (black arrows) secondary to pulmonary overcirculation.

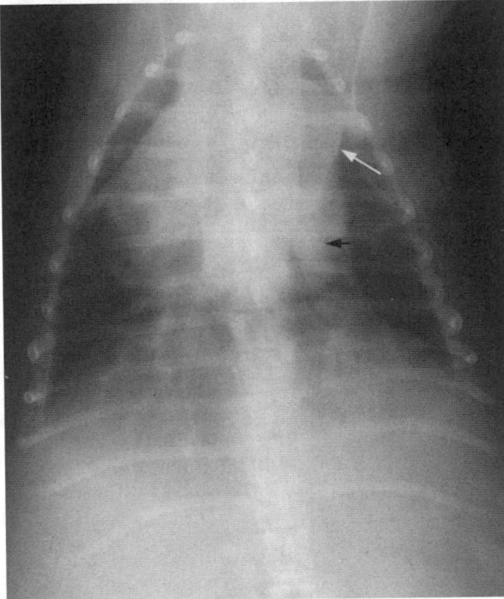

Figure 32-5
Dorsoventral radiograph from a dog with hypoxic pulmonary hypertension and cor pulmonale secondary to chronic bronchitis shows enlargement of main pulmonary artery (white arrow) and dilation of the pulmonary arteries (black arrow).

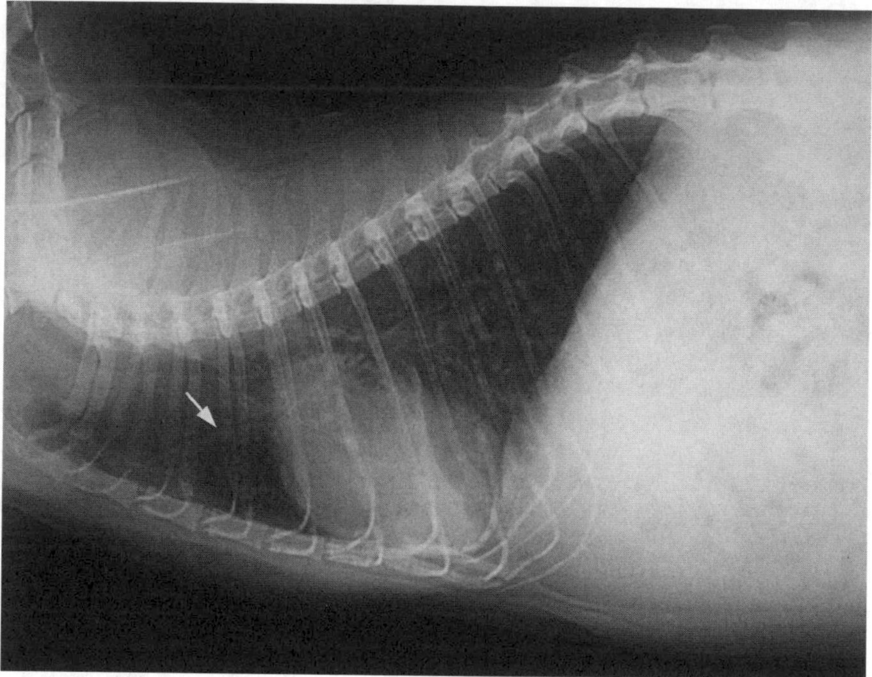

Figure 32-6
Lateral radiograph from a cat with hypoxic pulmonary hypertension and cor pulmonale secondary to feline asthma shows dilation of the pulmonary arteries (white arrow), peribronchial pattern, and ascites.

tricuspid regurgitation is prominent, then right atrial and ventricular dilation occur due to volume overload. Paradoxical motion of the interventricular septum may be present due to elevation of right-sided diastolic pressures. Left ventricular dimensions may be decreased and the left ventricular free wall may appear thickened (*i.e.*, pseudohypertrophy) because of decreased venous return to the left heart. Prolapse of the tricuspid and pulmonary valve leaflets may be evident.

Spectral Doppler evaluation of the pulmonary ejection flow profile may be abnormal in pulmonary hypertension (see Fig. 25-14). As PAPs increase, the flow profile becomes sharper, acceleration becomes more rapid, and peak velocity occurs earlier in during ejection.[4] At very high PAPs, the peak velocity may decrease and notching of the deceleration phase of the profile may be evident (*i.e.*, W-shaped profile). Direct evidence of pulmonary hypertension can be obtained from Doppler echocardiography if tricuspid regurgitation or pulmonic insufficiency are present (see Fig. 25-13).[4] Right ventricular systolic pressure can be estimated by measuring the velocity of the tricuspid regurgitant jet, calculating the systolic pressure gradient across the tricuspid valve from the modified Bernoulli equation (see Chapter 1), and adding the result to an estimated right atrial pressure or measured central venous pressure. In the absence of right ventricular outflow tract obstruction, right ventricular systolic pressure is essentially the same as systolic PAP. The same principle can be used to estimate diastolic PAP by measuring the velocity of the pulmonic insufficiency jet and calculating the resultant pressure gradient.

Right Heart Catheterization

Pulmonary artery pressure can be measured directly by passing a flow-directed Swan-Ganz balloon catheter through the right heart into the pulmonary artery (see Fig. 21-7). LAP can be estimated from the end-expiratory pulmonary wedge pressure (PWP) obtained by inflation of the balloon of a Swam-Ganz catheter positioned in the pulmonary artery. The pressure difference across the pulmonary vascular bed (ΔP) is the difference mean PAP and PWP and can be used to determine if pulmonary hypertension is the result of an increase in pulmonary vascular resistance or an elevation of LAP. Normal pulmonary ΔP is less than 10 mm Hg. Pulmonary vascular resistance is calculated by measuring pulmonary blood flow (L/min) by thermodilution, indexing the result to body surface area (m^2), and dividing it into the ΔP. A normal pulmonary vascular resistance of 21 ± 2 mm Hg/L/min/m^2 has been reported for dogs.[5] Abnormal values for pulmonary vascular resistance have not been reported for small animals.

PULMONARY HYPERTENSION SYNDROMES

There are four established syndromes of pulmonary hypertension in small animals: hypoxic pulmonary hypertension, pulmonary vascular occlusive disease, pulmonary overcirculation, and elevated LAP (Table 32-2). Two major pulmonary vascular occlusive diseases are recognized: PTE and heartworm disease. Each of these syndromes is considered a secondary cause of pulmonary hypertension. Primary pulmonary hypertension is a heritable syndrome of unknown etiology in humans. Its existence as a definable cause of pulmonary hypertension in small animals has not been established.

Hypoxic Pulmonary Hypertension

Hypoxic pulmonary hypertension is a sequela to chronic alveolar hypoxia in dogs and cats. Although these species are not considered to have an exuberant hypoxic pulmonary vasoconstriction response, they are capable of developing severe hypoxic pulmonary hypertension as a result of pulmonary vascular remodeling. Pulmonary vascular remodeling causes both a fixed increase in PAP as well as an enhanced capacity for pulmonary vasoconstriction.

Causes of hypoxic pulmonary hypertension in small animals include hypoventilation syndromes (*e.g.*, brachycephalic syndrome, obesity), restrictive pulmonary diseases (*e.g.*, pulmonary fibrosis), and obstructive airway disease (*e.g.*, chronic bronchitis, collapsing trachea, feline asthma). Although residence at altitude is not considered a common primary cause of pulmonary hypertension in small animals, it certainly accelerates its development in animals with chronic respiratory diseases.

Table 32-2. Pulmonary Hypertension Syndromes in Small Animals

Hypoxic Pulmonary Hypertension
Hypoventilation Syndromes
Restrictive Lung Disease
Obstructive Airway Disease
Altitude
Pathophysiologic mechanisms:
—Hypoxic pulmonary vasoconstriction
—Pulmonary vascular remodeling (hypoxia-induced)
—Polycythemia
Pulmonary Vascular Occlusive Disease
Pulmonary Thromboembolism
Heartworm Disease
Pathophysiologic mechanism:
—Pulmonary vascular occlusion
Pulmonary Overcirculation (Eisenmenger Syndrome)
Cardiac Shunt
Pathophysiologic mechanisms:
—Increased pulmonary blood flow
—Pulmonary vascular remodeling (flow-induced)
—Polycythemia
Elevated Left Atrial Pressure
Mitral Valve Disease
Cardiomyopathy
Congenital Heart Defects
Pathophysiologic mechanism:
—Increased left atrial pressure

Diagnosis of hypoxic pulmonary hypertension is based first on an awareness of its possibility in small animals with chronic respiratory disease. Findings on physical examination and thoracic radiographs may be subtle prior to the development of right-sided CHF compatible with chronic cor pulmonale. A strongly presumptive or definitive diagnosis of pulmonary hypertension can usually be made from Doppler echocardiography in animals with moderate or greater disease. Animals with chronic cor pulmonale will show hepatomegaly and ascites, and usually will have developed secondary tricuspid regurgitation by the time signs of congestive failure develop. In advanced cases, evidence of low output cardiac failure and severe hypoxemia may be present.

By the time clinical signs of chronic cor pulmonale occur, hypoxic pulmonary hypertension is usually severe. The cornerstone of acute therapy for hypoxic pulmonary hypertension is supplemental O_2. O_2 is the only selective pulmonary vasodilator generally available to veterinary patients. When hypoxic pulmonary hypertension has become severe, at least a portion of the increase in pulmonary vascular resistance and PAP has become fixed and unresponsive to any vasodilator therapy. Chronic therapy should be directed at the underlying respiratory disease in an attempt to improve alveolar oxygenation and minimize hypoxic pulmonary vasoconstriction. Vasodilator therapy with a direct-acting arteriodilator such as hydralazine (0.5–2.0 mg/kg q 12 h) or amlodipine (0.1–0.2 mg/kg q 24 h) may provide some benefit if systemic pressures allow systemic vascular resistance to be lowered as well. If signs of chronic cor pulmonale are present, an angiotensin-converting enzyme inhibitor such as enalapril (0.25–0.5 mg/kg q 12-24 h) or benazepril (0.25–0.5 mg/kg q 24 h) is indicated. Judicious use of diuretics may be beneficial to reduce right heart congestion although attention must be paid to the possibility of worsening CO. Combined diuretic therapy with furosemide (0.5-2 mg/kg q 12 h) and the combination of spironolactone and hydrochlorothiazide (Aldactazide, 0.5-2 mg/kg each drug q 12-24 h) is generally more effective for right heart congestion than monotherapy with furosemide.

Pulmonary Thromboembolism

Pulmonary thromboembolism is an important cause of pulmonary hypertension in dogs.[4,6,7] The condition has also been reported in cats.[8,9] Because of pulmonary vascular recruitment, pulmonary vascular occlusion must be severe (>50%) before significant pulmonary hypertension occurs. As a result, dogs with pulmonary hypertension secondary to PTE have a poor prognosis. Acute severe PTE causes diffusion impairment due to a decrease in the total area available for O_2 diffusion. The result is moderate to severe hypoxemia that is responsive to administration of supplemental O_2. The cardiac effects of acute PTE are those of acute cor pulmonale characterized by rapid onset of right ventricular dilation, tricuspid regurgitation, acute systemic venous hypertension, and low CO.

The pathogenesis and etiology of PTE is not completely understood in small animals. It is not clear whether the thrombus is generated in the systemic veins and then embolized to the lungs as it is in humans, or if it forms in situ in the pulmonary circulation. Hypercoagulable states including protein-losing nephropathy, hyperadrenocorticism, immune-mediated hemolytic anemia, and sepsis are well established predisposing factors for PTE in dogs.[6,7,10-14] Endothelial denuding injuries of the large central veins (*i.e.*, central IV catheters) and stasis of blood flow through the right heart may also be predisposing factors in dogs and cats. Pulmonary thromboembolism should be suspected in dogs that present with acute onset tachypnea and hypoxemia, especially when the hypoxemia is highly responsive to administration of supplemental O_2. Documentation of the presence of a known predisposing condition such as proteinuria or hyperadrenocorticism should increase the index of suspicion for PTE.

Thoracic radiographs can be normal or can show a patchy interstitial or

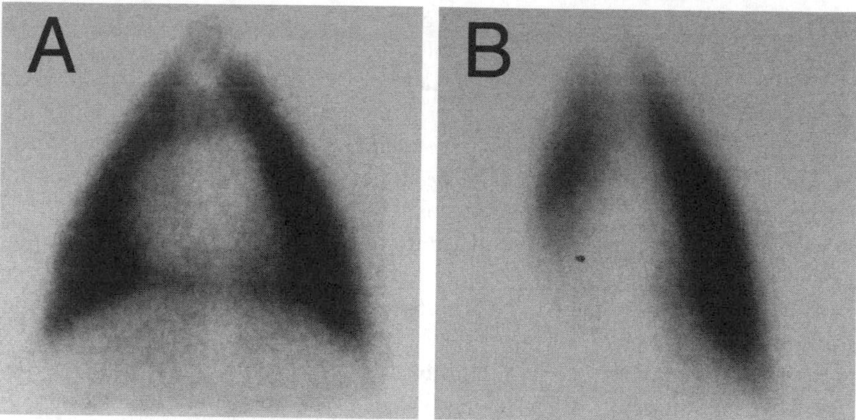

Figure 32-7
Lung perfusion scintigraphy scan from a normal dog (A) and a dog pulmonary thromboembolism of the right caudal lung lobe (B).

alveolar pattern. Echocardiographic findings are consistent with acute cor pulmonale and include right ventricular dilation, tricuspid regurgitation with a high-velocity regurgitant jet, and characteristic changes in the pulmonary flow profile. Confirmation of PTE can be obtained from a lung perfusion scintigraphy scan (Fig. 32-7) or pulmonary angiography.

Management of PTE depends on the magnitude of pulmonary vascular occlusion present. Heparin therapy (loading dose 150 IU/kg IV, maintenance dose 100 IU/kg SC q 8 h) should be instituted as soon as PTE is suspected. Therapy can be adjusted to achieve a target partial thromboplastin time (PTT) of 1.5 to 2 times the control PTT. Supportive therapy with IV fluids and supplemental O_2 are indicated during the acute phase of the disease. Jugular catheterization should be avoided in animals with hypercoagulation states. Diuretic therapy should be avoided because of the risk of worsening low CO.

Heparin constitutes only a secondary therapy for PTE because it only prevents or retards further embolization. The hope is that natural fibrinolysis will reduce the magnitude of the PTE over time. Primary therapy for PTE is indicated for patients showing evidence of acute right ventricular dilation and hypokinesis, pulmonary hypertension, and acute cor pulmonale. Primary therapies for PTE include medical fibrinolysis, catheter-based embolectomy, or surgical embolectomy. The later therapies are largely unexplored in veterinary medicine. Medical fibrinolysis can be attempted by IV infusion of streptokinase (3400 IU/kg as a loading dose over 30 minutes, followed by 1500 IU/kg/h for 6-24 hours) or recombinant tissue plasminogen activator (rt-PA; 4400 IU/kg as a loading dose over 10 minutes, followed by 4400 IU/kg/h for 6-24 hours). The efficacy of these therapies for patients with acute severe PTE have been established in human clinical trials, but not in veterinary trials.

Long-term therapy and prevention of PTE is based on chronic anticoagulation therapy with oral warfarin. Warfarin therapy can begin 3 to 5 days after initiating heparin and should be overlapped with heparin therapy until anticoagulation is established. The dose of warfarin is highly individualized and is affected by diet and numerous drug interactions. The warfarin dose should be based on measurement of the prothrombin time (PT) and calculation of the international normalized ratio (INR) based on the international sensitivity index (ISI)* of the thromboplastin reagent and the mean value of the control PT reference range[15,16]:

$$\text{INR} = (\text{patient PT}/\text{control PT})^{\text{ISI}}$$

The target INR should be between 2 and 3. Adjustments in the dose of warfarin should be based on the total weekly dose rather than the total daily dose.[15]

Pulmonary Overcirculation (Eisenmenger Syndrome)

Anatomic cardiac shunts (*e.g.*, ventricular septal defect, patent ductus arteriosus) cause overcirculation of the pulmonary vascular bed. As the physiologic mechanisms of vascular distention and recruitment work to lower vascular resistance during acute increases in pulmonary flow, chronic overcirculation causes remodeling of the pulmonary vessels eventually resulting in moderate to severe increase in pulmonary vascular resistance. Chronic hypoxia secondary to chronic respiratory conditions or residence at altitude is known to accelerate the vascular remodeling process.[17] In the most severe cases, PAP can become suprasystemic. The result is reversal of flow through the anatomic shunt (*i.e.*, right-to-left shunt), moderate to severe hypoxemia and cyanosis, and a condition known as Eisenmenger syndrome. Eisenmenger syndrome can develop within the first few weeks of life,[17] or it can occur at birth due to failure of the normal pulmonary vascular adaptation to extrauterine life.

Animals with Eisenmenger syndrome exhibit moderate to profound exercise intolerance. The dominant clinical finding is hypoxemia and cyanosis that does not respond to administration of supplemental O_2. In reverse patent ductus arteriosus, cyanosis may be restricted to the caudal half of the body. Moderate to severe polycythemia will usually be present. Diagnosis of Eisenmenger syndrome can be readily confirmed in most cases by echocardiography. A contrast bubble study can be undertaken to demonstrate the presence of right-to-left cardiac shunt. This is especially useful when the shunt is at the level of the ductus arteriosus. Tetralogy of Fallot is the most important rule out for animals with this presentation.

Limited treatment options are available for animals with Eisenmenger syndrome. Phlebotomy and replacement crystalloid fluids can be performed to reduce the magnitude of polycythemia if the hematocrit is greater than 70%. Vasodilator therapy is contraindicated because it will likely decrease systemic more than pulmonary vascular resistance and worsen the magnitude of the right-to-left shunt. The prognosis for animals with Eisenmenger syndrome is guarded but

* ISI reflects the responsiveness of the thromboplastin reagent compared to an international thromboplastin reference standard (British Comparative Thromboplastin/ human brain origin). The ISI is provided by the manufacturer of the reagent.

not hopeless and largely depends on the magnitude of polycythemia. Small animals can live for several years.

Elevated Left Atrial Pressure

Elevated LAP can cause mild to moderate pulmonary hypertension in dogs and cats. The most common cause of increased LAP in dogs is mitral regurgitation due to degenerative mitral valve disease or congenital mitral valve dysplasia.[6] Mitral valve stenosis and dilated cardiomyopathy are less common causes. In cats, possible causes include hypertrophic or restrictive cardiomyopathy or cor triatriatum sinister. The magnitude of pulmonary hypertension depends on the degree of increase in LAPs. LAP can exceed 25 mm Hg in animals with left-sided CHF and this directly increases PAP without an increase in pulmonary vascular resistance. In humans with mitral valve disease, pulmonary hypertension is exacerbated by remodeling of the pulmonary veins in response the chronically elevated pressure.[18] The importance of this mechanism in small animals is unknown.

Pulmonary hypertension resulting from elevated LAP in small animals is usually detected as an incidental finding during echocardiography. The important question is whether concurrent causes of pulmonary hypertension such as chronic hypoxic pulmonary hypertension are present. If pulmonary PAP is greater than 50 mm Hg, then concurrent causes should be suspected. Therapy is directed at lowering LAP and is essentially the same as for left-sided CHF. For chronic mitral valve disease, emphasis should be placed on decreasing the systemic systolic pressure through the use of direct-acting arteriodilator drugs such as hydralazine or amlodapine.

SUMMARY

Until recently, the incidence and importance of pulmonary hypertension has been underappreciated in small animals. With the advent of noninvasive diagnostic techniques for evaluating pulmonary hypertension, its role in several important conditions in small animals has been increasingly recognized. This increased awareness and recognition will translate into an increased understanding of the pathogenesis, diagnosis, and therapy of these conditions.

REFERENCES

1. West JB: Respiratory Physiology—The Essentials, 2nd ed. Baltimore: Williams & Wilkins, 1979, p 36.
2. Tucker A, McMurtry IF, Reeves JT, *et al.*: Lung vascular smooth muscle as a determinant of pulmonary hypertension at high altitude. *Am J Physiol* 228:762, 1975.
3. Stenmark KR, Orton EC, Crouch EC, *et al.*: Vascular remodeling in neonatal pulmonary hypertension: role of the smooth muscle cell. *Chest* 93:127S, 1988.
4. Johnson L, Boon J, Orton EC: Clinical characteristics of 53 dogs with Doppler-derived evidence of pulmonary hypertension: 1992-1996. *J Vet Intern Med* 13:440, 1999.

5. Bennett RA, Orton EC, Tucker A, *et al.*: Cardiopulmonary changes in conscious dogs with induced progressive pneumothorax. *Am J Vet Res* 50:280, 1989.
6. Johnson LR, Lappin MR, Baker DC: Pulmonary thromboembolism in 29 dogs. *J Vet Intern Med* 13:338, 1999.
7. LaRue MJ, Murtaugh RJ: Pulmonary thromboembolism in dogs: 47 cases. *J Am Vet Med Assoc* 197:1368, 1990.
8. Sottiaux J. Franck M: Pulmonary embolism and cor pulmonale in a cat. *J Small Anim Pract* 40:88, 1999.
9. Pouchelon JL, Chetboul V, Devauchelle P, *et al.*: Diagnosis of pulmonary thromboembolism in a cat using echocardiography and pulmonary scintigraphy. *J Small Anim Pract* 38:306, 1997.
10. Ritt MG, Rogers KS, Thomas JS: Nephrotic syndrome resulting in thromboembolic disease and disseminated intravascular coagulation in a dog. *J Am Anim Hosp Assoc* 33:385, 1997.
11. Bunch SE, Metcalf MR, Crane SW, *et al.*: Idiopathic pleural effusion and pulmonary thromboembolism in a dog with autoimmune hemolytic anemia. *J Am Vet Med Assoc* 195:1748, 1989.
12. Klein MK, Dow SW, Rosychuk RA: Pulmonary thromboembolism associated with immune mediated hemolytic anemia in dogs: ten cases. *J Am Vet Med Assoc* 195: 246, 1989.
13. Green RA, Kabel AL. Hypercoagulable state in three dogs with nephrotic syndrome: role of acquired antithrombin III deficiency. *J Am Vet Med Assoc* 181:914, 1982.
14. Burns MG, Kelly AB, Hornof WJ, *et al.*: Pulmonary artery thrombosis in three dogs with hyperadrenocorticism. *J Am Vet Med Assoc* 178:388, 1981.
15. Triplett DA: Current recommendations for warfarin therapy: use and monitoring. *Cardiol Clin Ann Drug Ther* 2:143, 1998.
16. Harpster NK, Baty CJ: Warfarin therapy of the cat at risk of thromboembolism. *In:* Bonagura JD, ed.: Current Veterinary Therapy XII, Philadelphia: WB Saunders, 1995, p 868.
17. Oswald GP, Orton EC: Patent ductus arteriosus and pulmonary hypertension in related Pembroke Welsh Corgi dogs. *J Am Vet Med Assoc* 202:761, 1993.
18. Hagenbottom T, Stenmark K, Simonneau G: Treatments for pulmonary hypertension. *Lancet* 343:338, 1999.

33
Pericardial Effusion

Wayne E. Wingfield

INTRODUCTION

The pericardium consists of a serous membrane and a fibrous sac. The serous membrane covers the outside of the heart (visceral pericardium) and extends a short distance beyond the atria and ventricles onto the great vessels. A serous membrane also lines the inside of the fibrous sac (parietal pericardium). The pericardial cavity, that space between the visceral and parietal pericardium, contains a small amount of clear, pale yellow fluid. This ultrafiltrate of serum has a colloidal osmotic pressure approximately 25% that of blood serum.[2] The amount of fluid generally found in the dog is 0.5 to 2.5 mL.

The fibrous pericardium is a thin, strong, flasklike sac. This sac is closed by its attachment to the great vessels and is also attached ventrally to the diaphragm. As the sternopericardial ligament, this fibrous sac is held in place in the area of the xiphoid process of the sternum.

The histology of the pericardium is flattened irregular polygonal mesothelial cells forming a smooth and glistening serous layer of the pericardium. This serous layer is attached to the fibrous layers by delicate connective tissue rich in elastic fibers.

The fibrous layer of the pericardium consists of superficial, middle, and deep layer of collagenous fibers interlaced with elastic fibers. In humans, the elastic fibers decrease in numbers from birth to adult life. The collagen fibers are practically straight in the fetus, become wavy after birth, reach the largest wave amplitude in young adults, and become straight again in old age. This change suggests that the pericardium in young adults is more elastic than that of the elderly.[3]

The pericardium functions to limit acute cardiac dilatation, maintain cardiac geometry and ventricular compliance, reduce friction, provide a barrier to inflammation from contiguous structures, and buttress the atria. Under normal conditions, a small amount of fluid is found between the epicardial (visceral pericardial) and the parietal pericardial membranes. The term pericardial effusion indicates excessive or abnormal fluid accumulation between the parietal and visceral pericardial membranes.

EPIDEMIOLOGY

Congenital hernias, acquired pericardial effusion, and constrictive (constrictive-effusive) pericardial disease represent the most clinically relevant disorders of the pericardium in small animal practice. Disease of the pericardium is generally associated with other diseases. More often than not, the effusion is chronically present. Accumulation of effusion within the pericardial space may be life-threatening. This is especially true of acute effusions. With chronic effusion the elasticity of the sac may allow compensation before the system fails and clinical signs of heart failure manifest.

Symptomatic, acquired pericardial effusion, is common in dogs and is observed sporadically in cats. In one report, the occurrence of pericardial effusion is reported at 8% in dogs and 6% of cats presented to a cardiology service.[1] Transudation into the pericardial space secondary to right-sided congestive heart failure (CHF), peritoneopericardial diaphragmatic hernia, hypoalbuminemia, or infections/toxemia (or other causes of increased vascular permeability) are findings at necropsy or with ultrasonography and do not impair heart function. There are two noteworthy clinical exceptions. Mass lesions at the heart base can obstruct lymphatic drainage leading to a large and compressive, water-like, transudative pericardial effusion. In cats with severe CHF, a large pericardial effusion may develop, which may resolve with successful therapy of heart failure.

Exudation caused by infective or noninfective pericarditis is not common in small animals. In the dog and cat, *Nocardia* infection and perforating foreign bodies are potential causes. Fungal involvement of the pericardium is recognized with *Coccidiomyocosis* in the dog or with opportunistic fungi in immunosuppressed dogs (*e.g.*, aspergillosis). Idiopathic, sterile (inflammatory) pericarditis develops occasionally in the dog and may be sequelae to some cases of recurrent, idiopathic intrapericardial hemorrhage. Pericarditis has been associated infrequently with feline cardiomyopathy but is recognized and is part of the polyserositis from infection with feline infectious peritonitis virus. Intrapericardial hemorrhage (with or without secondary pericardial reaction) is not uncommon. The most frequent cause is idiopathic pericardial hemorrhage in dogs. This is a disorder of dogs typically (but not invariably) less than 8 years of age. In some areas, male Golden retrievers and German shepherds are predisposed. Neoplasia of the heart, heart base, or pericardium frequently leads to a hemorrhagic effusion. Hemangiosarcoma of the right atrium (especially common in German shepherds, Golden retrievers, and Labrador retrievers older than 8 years), can be multicentric with splenic involvement and pulmonary metastasis. Aortic body tumors (chemodectoma) grow along the heart base (and are especially common in aged brachycephalic breed dogs). Ectopic (heart base) thyroid carcinoma can cause a large mass of the heart base, which can invade the myocardium. Mesothelioma of the pericardium also occurs but is often a controversial diagnosis in light of so-called pericardial fluids that can develop in dogs with recurrent pericardial effusion. Metastatic carcinoma to the heart is not common. Lymphosarcoma of the right atrium and ventricles is the most important cardiac neoplasm in the cat, but is considered a rare cause of pericardial effusion in dogs. Uncommon causes of pericardial hemorrhage include left atrial rupture in dogs with mitral regurgitation secondary to endocardititis or endocardiosis, blunt chest trauma (rare), puncture of the heart (knife, bullet, arrow), coagulopathies, and complicated thoracocentesis. Chyle is a rare fluid type in pericardial effusions.

PATHOPHYSIOLOGY

The function of the pericardium is variously reported. Some reports describe "no vital function"; others incriminate the pericardium as the cause of cardiac failure. The following functions of the pericardium are reported: prevention of overdilation of the heart, protection of the heart from infection and adhesions to surrounding tissues, maintenance of the heart in a fixed geometric position within the thorax, regulation of the interrelations between stroke volumes of the two ventricles, and prevention of right ventricular regurgitation when ventricular diastolic pressures are increased.[3]

Pericardectomy in the dog and cat has produced various results when its effect on heart size is studied. These reports have indicated either no apparent dilation[4] or increased size.[5,6] When large volumes of fluids, dextrans, or blood are infused, the effect of pericardectomy is more apparent. With fluid overload after pericardectomy, the venous pressure is decreased. With an intact pericardium, fluid overload produces increased venous pressures.

The intrapleural pressure and intracardiac pressures influence pericardial pressures within the sac. With inspiration the pericardial pressure increases, and expiration produces a decrease in this pressure. In the anesthetized dog, pericardial pressure fluctuates with atrial systole and during the rapid ventricular filling phase of ventricular diastole, and increases during the later part of ventricular diastole.[2]

Cardiac tamponade refers to the decompensated phase of cardiac compression resulting from an unchecked rise in the intrapericardial fluid pressure. The normally negative inspiratory pericardial pressure becomes positive. Tamponade is the mechanism by which low cardiac output and CHF develop with pericardial effusion. Development depends on the rate of fluid accumulation, not simply the volume of pericardial fluid. With few elastic fibers in the pericardium, intrapericardial pressures can rise rapidly as the elastic limits of the membrane are exceeded (Fig. 33-1). Important pathophysiologic features include increased (positive) intrapericardial pressure with diastolic collapse of the right atrium and right ventricle, compression of the vena cava, reduced right ventricular filling, decreased preload and cardiac output, and potential for arterial hypotension if compensatory mechanisms are insufficient. Coronary perfusion may be impeded by increased intrapericardial pressures. Syncope or sudden death may occur if the systemic hypotension is acute and severe. Given sufficient time, compensatory measures are activated to maintain arterial blood pressure. These include heightened sympathetic discharge, systemic vasoconstriction, renal retention of sodium and water, and elevated venous pressures. Extremely high venous pressures may develop behind the heart. CHF, with a predominately right-sided component (ascites, pleural effusion), is the consequence of chronic cardiac tamponade. Additional hemodynamic features include equilibration of diastolic pressures in the ventricles, atria, and great veins, and respiratory variation in arterial blood pressure (pulsus paradoxicus). The latter is explained by exaggeration of the normal respiratory-induced variation in right versus left-sided cardiac filling.

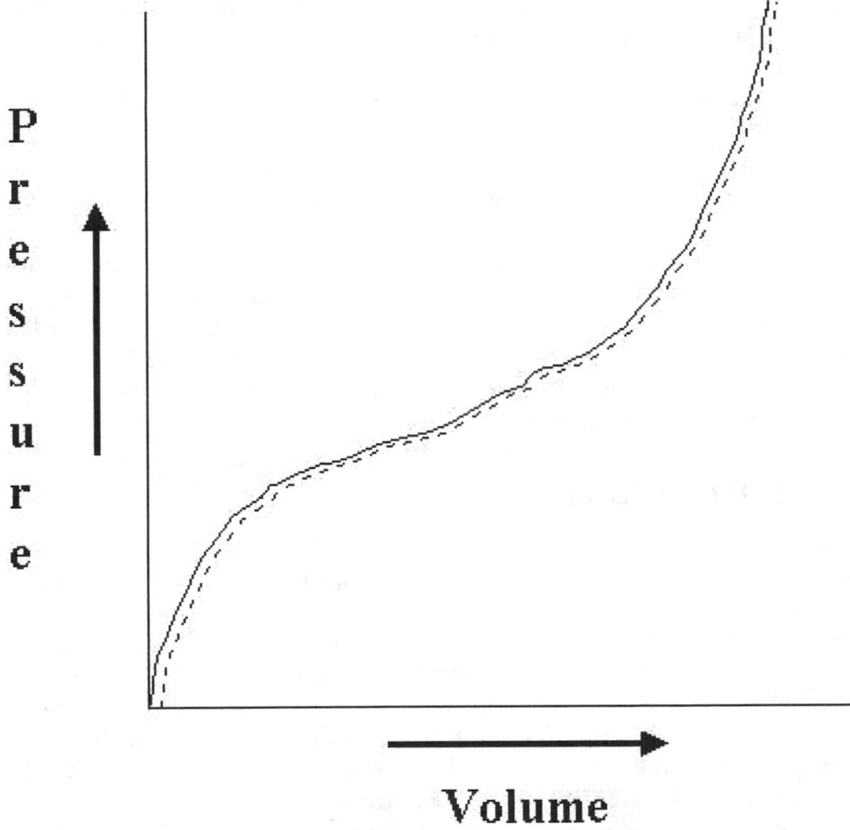

Figure 33-1
Pressure-volume curve showing that fluid accumulating in the pericardial space (solid line) results in a sigmoid curve. When fluid is removed from the pericardial space (dotted line), the curve follows the hysteresis of the volume accumulation curve. Thus, removal of a small volume of fluid results in a dramatic drop in the intrapericardial pressure.

CLINICAL FINDINGS

Species and breed predilections are noted above. The client complaint may be vague. Syncope or collapse are particularly common with acute cardiac tamponade (*e.g.*, sudden hemorrhage). Overt signs of right-sided CHF may be evident. The physical examination findings of elevated jugular venous pressure, muffled heart sounds, and ascites (with or without pleural effusion) should prompt investigation of the pericardial space. If venous distention is missed, an erroneous diagnosis of liver disease or abdominal neoplasia may be considered. If pericardial effusion is present, lying the dog on its side and observing the lateral saphenous vein as the limb is slowly elevated will show evidence of systemic venous hypertension. As the leg is raised, the vein should collapse as the vein approaches the level of the right atrium. With pericardial effusion, the lateral saphenous will be continuously distended when the leg is as much as 45° elevation above the body.

Arterial hypotension or pulsus paradoxicus may be detected. The central venous pressure (CVP) is generally quite high, often exceeding 12 cm H_20 (normal <5 cm). In acute cardiac tamponade, the major clinical signs may be low blood pressure and jugular distention but without any fluid accumulation. Fever or thoracic pain may indicate infection or inflammation within the pericardial space. Cardiac auscultation is characterized by distant heart sounds. A pericardial friction rub may indicate pericarditis, but this is rare in dogs and cats. Breath sounds are muffled and there will be tachypnea or respiratory distress if there is pleural effusion from congestive heart failure. Evidence of systemic disease, such as lymphosarcoma or hemangiosarcoma of the spleen, may be noted during a complete physical examination.

DIAGNOSTIC STUDIES

Monitoring of the CVP often leads to a diagnosis of pericardial effusion. With the tip of the venous catheter in the right atrium, an initial CVP reading greater than 15 cm H_2O is virtually diagnostic of abnormal fluid accumulation in the pericardial space. Measurement of "static" intrapericardial fluid pressure, prior to removing any pericardial effusion, can be accomplished by attaching one end of a saline-filled extension tube to the intrapericardial catheter and the other end to a CVP manometer. Cases of tamponade demonstrate a high (positive) pressure, usually greater than 15 cm H_20 above the midsternal line, with the patient resting in lateral recumbency. The pressure becomes subatmospheric following pericardiocentesis and rises and falls with ventilation. With constrictive-effusive pericardial disease, pericardial effusion without tamponade, or isolated pleural effusion, the intrapericardial pressure is essentially normal (*i.e.*, near 0 cm H_2O). Although this relatively crude method does not precisely measure intrapericardial pressure, it offers useful clinical information.

Clinical laboratory evaluation may simply reflect the consequences of heart failure or prior diuretic therapy. The complete blood count may indicate inflammation, infection, or hemorrhage. Increased numbers of circulating nucleated red blood cells, especially in susceptible breeds, are suggestive of hemangiosarcoma of the spleen (and heart). Analysis of pleural or peritoneal effusions generally indicate fluid of obstructive origin (transudate, modified transudate, or infrequently chyle). Bacterial cultures of the effusate, serum fungal titer (coccidiomycosis), or enzyme-linked immunosorbent assays for feline leukemia virus or feline infectious peritonitis may be positive when pericarditis is related to these infections.[8] Fluid can be collected by pericardiocentesis. If the pH of pericardial fluid is less than 7.0, this finding is suggestive of pericardial inflammation or idiopathic hemorrhage, although more data are needed to precisely define the predictive value of a pH greater than 7.0. Values of 7.4 or greater are more typical of neoplasia or recent hemorrhage.[6] Collected fluid can be classified as a transudate, exudate, hemorrhage, or chyle (see above). Unfortunately, except in cases of lymphosarcoma or septic inflammation, cytologic examination may not be especially helpful. It can be difficult to conclusively identify neoplastic cells within pericardial effusates. The problems include poor exfoliation or over-interpretation of reactive mesothelial cells.[9]

Radiography generally demonstrates abnormalities once there is a significant accumulation of pericardial fluid. The cardiac silhouette enlarges, loses its angles and waists, and eventually becomes globular in shape ("basketball or soccer ball heart") and sharp in outline (from diminished motion). Should a metallic foreign body be observed over the heart on two views, constrictive or constrictive-effusive disease is likely. Pulmonary vascularity is often reduced from low cardiac output (in contrast to CHF from cardiomyopathy or valvular disease). If CHF has developed, there may be increased pulmonary interstitial densities (edema), distention of the caudal vena cava, hepatomegaly, or pleural effusion. Tumors of the heart base may deviate the trachea (generally to the right and dorsad), producing a mass effect. Fluoroscopy may demonstrate reduced cardiac motion. Pneumopericardiography can identify intrapericardial mass lesions, but is rarely done because echocardiography is much less risky for the patient.

An electrocardiogram (ECG) may show any of the following: decreased amplitude (<1 mV in all leads) of the QRS complexes (most common but variable); electrical alternans (with large effusions and swinging of the heart) (Fig. 33-2); or ST-segment elevation (an epicardial injury current with pericarditis). Sinus tachycardia is typical but vagal reflexes can be invoked that promote sinus arrhythmia or bradyarrhythmias. Atrial and ventricular arrhythmias may be observed secondary to myocardial involvement, ischemia, or concurrent primary heart disease.

The echocardiogram is a highly sensitive test for detecting pericardial effusion. Abnormal fluid accumulation is evident as a sonolucent (generally black) space between the epicardium and pericardium, extending from apex to base (Fig. 33-3). Cardiac mass lesions, a mixed intrapericardial echogenic pattern (cellular exudate or recent hemorrhage), or pleural effusion are other potential echocardiographic findings. The recognition of diastolic collapse of the right atrium or right ventricular wall is supportive of increased intrapericardial pressure

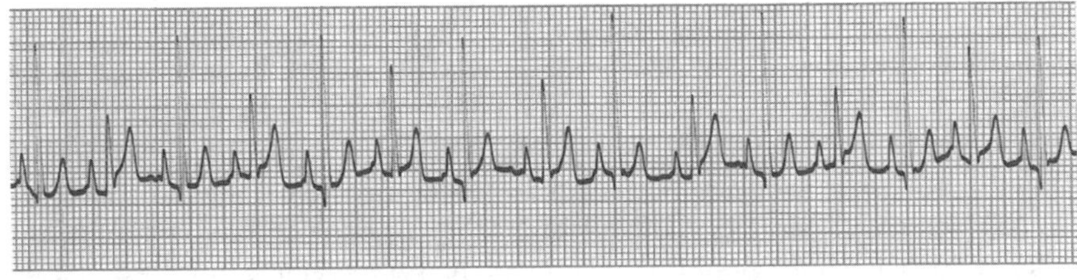

Figure 33-2
Electrical alternans results as the heart swings freely in the pericardial fluid. The alternating amplitude of the QRS complexes identifies the pattern as electrical alternans.

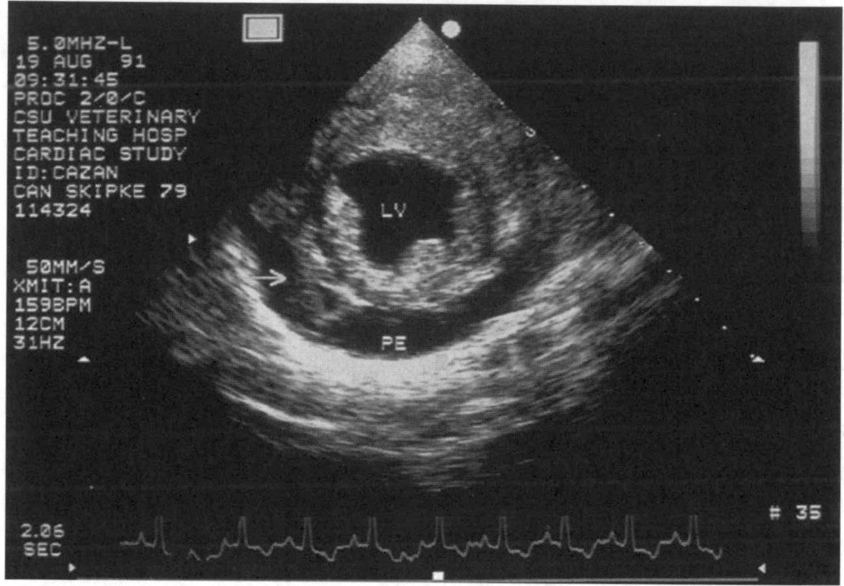

Figure 33-3
Echocardiography is the gold standard for identifying fluid in the pericardial space (PE and arrow). The left ventricle (LV) is seen in this cross-sectional view of the heart.

and corresponds to effusion with tamponade. There are both false positives (occasionally pleural effusion causes this in dogs) and false negatives (if there is concurrent right-sided CHF with elevated CVP expanding the cardiac chambers). The distinction between idiopathic hemorrhagic pericardial effusion and bleeding from a tumor may not be possible without a high-resolution, technically proficient echocardiogram recorded from each side of the thorax and use of multiple angled views. In some cases, exploratory surgery or advanced imaging (computed tomography, magnetic resonance imaging) are needed to exclude a mass lesion.

THERAPY

The treatment of choice for initial stabilization is pericardiocentesis using a needle, butterfly infusion needle (for cats or very small dogs), a through-the-needle catheter, an over-the-needle catheter, a commercial thoracocentesis trocar system, or a balloon dilation catheter (which can be used to rip the pericardium). A 14- to 16- gauge 13.2-cm, Angiocath, over-the-needle catheter is preferred. An intravenous (IV) line should be placed for emergencies or for volume loading should hypotension develop. If arterial blood pressure is stable, mild sedation is often tolerated and improves the procedure for all (buprenorphine 0.005 mg/kg mixed with acepromazine 0.025 mg/kg, both given IV). Should hypotension develop after sedation, quickly infuse a crystalloid solution IV. The dog is placed in lateral recumbency and the spine elevated slightly with a radiographic foam wedge. ECG leads are attached. The needed depth of penetration and the ideal puncture site can be guided by echocardiography (to simply identify the largest effusion space); alternatively, one can note the strongest palpable cardiac impulse (both points are usually the same). Placing the patient in a slightly oblique position, and later rotating the animal as needed, facilitates fluid withdrawal and patient restraint during the procedure. After gloving for the procedure, one additional side hole is cut into the edge of the catheter and the needle is replaced. The tap can proceed from either the right side (cardiac notch) or left hemithorax (depending on preference, the situation, radiography, and echocardiography). The right-sided intercostal approach is used to avoid the largest coronary vessels.

Following a surgical prep of the skin, a local lidocaine (2%) block of the skin, subcutaneous tissues, pleura, and superficial pericardium is made with a 25- or 23-gauge needle. Often the small-gauge needle will transiently enter the pericardial space, providing some guide to the depth needed for catheter placement. Next the catheter is advanced through the skin, subcutaneous tissue, intercostal space, and deliberately into the pericardial space. The ECG is monitored for extrasystoles in case the heart is pricked with the catheter. (Note: Dorsal approaches may cause the catheter to perforate the atrium and this will not be associated with premature ventricular beats.) Once the pericardial space is entered, fluid (usually bloody) enters the catheter lumen. If intrapericardial pressure will be measured, the line connecting the CVP manometer is immediately attached to the catheter because the intrapericardial pressure rapidly declines with aspiration of the fluid. After measuring intrapericardial pressure, fluid samples are collected for cytology (EDTA and plain tubes), culture, and pending cytology. The effusion is drained as completely as possible. Importantly, one tube of centesis fluid is placed in a red-topped tube and is continuously monitored for evidence of clotting as the pericardial space is evacuated. The presence of a clot in the tube indicates active bleeding and likely the sample was extracted from a cardiac chamber. If a clot appears, stop draining the pericardial space, remove the needle, and make another attempt. Blood in a pericardial effusion should not clot!

Owing to the relatively inelastic properties of the pericardium, the removal of even modest amounts of effusate may be very beneficial (see Fig. 33-1). The effects on the patient are often dramatic with a marked improvement in attitude, color, and peripheral pulse pressure. When complete, the aspirated fluid volume is quantified. Repeated intrapericardial pressure measurement or echocardiography can be used to verify the benefit of the procedure. A sample of the effusate is evaluated by microscopy for cellular abnormalities and bacteria and is then cultured (aerobic, anaerobic) if appropriate.

Medical therapy for pericardial effusion is not a prominent feature of this disorder. IV crystalloids, at shock doses, may be required in cases of hypotension due to severe or sudden cardiac tamponade. Thoracocentesis is a helpful adjunct in large pleural effusions. Ascitic effusions need not be tapped if pericardiocentesis is performed. Although furosemide and venodilators can decrease elevated venous pressures, they are not substitutes for pericardiocentesis in the symptomatic patient; furthermore, these drugs may reduce ventricular filling predisposing to hypotension. In general, diuretics are contraindicated except in recurrent, neoplastic-related right-sided CHF in which venous pressures can become exceptionally high.

Following successful pericardiocentesis, it is appropriate to administer 1 mg/kg furosemide subcutaneously for one or two doses to enhance renal excretion of sodium (and overcome the sodium-retaining consequences of cardiac tamponade that often persist for some time after pericardiocentesis or pericardiectomy). In patients with a negative-culture, idiopathic pericardial hemorrhage (or idiopathic pericarditis), conservative treatment with catheter drainage, may be "curative," though diligent follow-up (for at least 1 year) is needed to ensure that constrictive pericardial disease does not develop. Empirical use of antibiotics and of corticosteroids has offered no certain benefit. Drugs that prevent fibrosis might be considered, but these have not been suitably investigated in dogs and cats. Antineoplastic drugs have provided generally poor results in patients with cardiac tumors.

Surgery may be necessary for successful management of pericardial diseases. Subtotal pericardiectomy (ventral to the phrenic nerves) may be needed in recurrent idiopathic hemorrhagic effusion. The treatment for infective, suppurative pericarditis is specific antibiotic therapy based on aerobic and bacterial anaerobic culture, catheter drainage of the pericardium, and subsequent surgical removal and drainage of the pericardial space (to prevent constriction). A foreign body should be sought in these cases. Surgery is also indicated if constrictive (effusive) pericarditis is diagnosed or highly suspected, or if there is a need to explore the pericardium to rule out or to attempt removal of a tumor.

Palliative subtotal pericardiectomy (generally via pericardial window) can also be performed by thoracoscopy in some centers.[10] This approach is a reasonable palliation for neoplasia-associated pericardial effusion and it maybe a consideration for debilitated dogs with infective pericarditis (later perform pericardiectomy). Specific causes of pericardial infection (*e.g.*, coccidiomycosis) have specific adjunctive treatments.

PROGNOSIS

The prognosis of pericardial disease depends on the cause, but it is generally favorable with idiopathic hemorrhagic pericardial effusion, guarded with infective pericarditis, and unfavorable with cardiac or heart base neoplasia. Although a chemodectoma grows slowly, right atrial hemangiosarcoma has invariably metastasized by the time of diagnosis. Ectopic thyroid carcinomas can be particularly invasive.

REFERENCES

1. Smith FWK, Rush JE: Diagnosis and treatment of pericardial effusion. *In*: Bonagura JD, ed.: Current Vet Therapy XIII. Philadelphia: WB Saunders, 2000, p 772.
2. Mauer FW, Warren MF, Drinker CK: The composition of mammalian pericardial and peritoneal fluids. Studies of their protein and chloride contents, and the passage

of foreign substances from the blood stream into these fluids. *Am J Physiol* 129:635, 1940.
3. Holt JP: The normal pericardium. *Am J Cardiol* 26:326, 1970.
4. Moore TC, Schumacker HB Jr: Congenital and experimentally produced pericardial defects. *Angiology* 4:1, 1953.
5. Carlton HM: The delayed effects of pericardial removal. *Proc R Soc Lond, Series B* 105:230, 1929.
6. Spodick DH: Acute cardiac tamponade. Pathologic physiology, diagnosis and management. *Prog Cardiovasc Dis* 10:64, 1967.
7. Edwards NJ: The diagnostic value of pericardial fluid pH determination. *J Am Anim Hosp Assoc* 32:63, 1996.
8. Rush JE, Keene BW, Fox PR: Pericardial disease in the cat: a retrospective evaluation of 66 cases. *J Am Animal Hosp Assoc* 26:39, 1990.
9. Sisson D, Thomas WP, Ruehl WW, *et al.*: Diagnostic value of pericardial fluid analysis in the dog. *J Am Vet Med Assoc* 184:51, 1984.
10. Richter KP, Jackson J, Hart JR: Thoracoscopic pericardiectomy in 12 dogs. Proceedings of the 14th American College of Veterinary Internal Medicine (ACVIM) Forum, San Antonio, TX, 1996, p 746.

34
Cardiomyopathies

Julie M. Martin and Janice McIntosh Bright

INTRODUCTION

The cardiomyopathies are a heterogeneous group of myocardial diseases, all of which can result in congestive heart failure (CHF) and sudden death. A cardiomyopathy that is intrinsic to the myocardium is considered primary, whereas myocardial disease occurring from a systemic illness, infection, toxin, nutritional deficiency, or a nonmyocardial cardiac lesion is referred to as secondary cardiomyopathy. The cardiomyopathies are further classified based on structural and pathophysiologic features as dilated, hypertrophic, and restrictive cardiomyopathy. It is usually not possible to reliably distinguish primary from secondary cardiomyopathy based solely on radiographic and echocardiographic findings.

The most common form of primary myocardial disease in dogs is dilated cardiomyopathy (DCM).[1] DCM is reported to occur with a prevalence of 0.5% in the canine population.[2] In cats, hypertrophic cardiomyopathy (HCM) is the most common primary myocardial disease, occurring in 1.6% of cats presented to veterinary hospitals.[3,4]

DILATED CARDIOMYOPATHY

Dilated cardiomyopathy is a myocardial disorder characterized by reduced myocardial contractility. The cardiac chambers dilate secondarily due to volume overload and eccentric hypertrophy. Although the left ventricle (LV) and left atrium are most commonly affected, all four cardiac chambers may be involved.[1,2] An unusual form of cardiomyopathy affecting only the right ventricle and right atrium has been described in both dogs and cats.[5,6]

Feline DCM

Since discovery in the early 1980s of the causative role of taurine deficiency in feline cardiomyopathy and subsequent addition of taurine to commercial feline diets, DCM has become extremely rare in this species.[7,8] DCM is occasionally found in cats fed unusual diets and in cats with impaired nutrient absorption. Also, DCM that is unrelated to taurine deficiency is occasionally seen in feline patients. Because the cost/benefit ratio of empirical dietary taurine supplementation is favorable, cats with DCM should receive 250 mg taurine orally twice daily in addition to medications that may be needed for management of heart

Table 34-1. Canine Breeds with a High Prevalence of Primary Dilated Cardiomyopathy

Doberman pinscher
Boxer
Great Dane
Labrador retriever
American cocker spaniel
Golden retriever
Irish wolfhound
Saint Bernard
Springer spaniel
Newfoundland
English sheepdog
Afghan hound
Scottish deerhound
Dalmatian
English cocker spaniel

failure or arterial thromboembolism. However, not all cats with DCM will have taurine-responsive disease.

Canine DCM

Dilated cardiomyopathy remains an important cause of morbidity and mortality in dogs, particularly in the large and giant breeds. Impaired myocardial systolic function (reduced inotropic state) is the primary abnormality in most dogs with this disorder, and the impaired contractility typically culminates in CHF. Arrhythmias have been noted to precede the onset of mechanical dysfunction in several breeds including Doberman pinschers, boxers, and Irish wolfhounds. Primary DCM is common in a wide variety of canine breeds with the disorder being most prevalent in Doberman pinschers.[9] Table 34-1 lists the canine breeds most commonly affected.

Etiology

At this time primary cardiomyopathy is considered idiopathic in most canine patients. However, because of the high prevalence of this disorder in certain breeds, a heritable etiology is likely. The disorder is inherited as an autosomal dominant trait in the boxer dog,[10,11] and as an autosomal recessive trait in the Portuguese water dog.[12] Recently, DCM has been shown to be an autosomal dominant, heritable disorder in Newfoundlands as well.[13] Finally, a study of the pedigrees of Doberman pinschers suggests that DCM is inherited as an autosomal dominant trait with reduced penetrance in this breed.[14] Because of the high incidence of DCM in the cocker spaniel, Irish wolfhound and Great Dane, it is likely that the disease is also heritable in these breeds. Although the exact molecular and cellular mechanisms responsible for heritable forms of DCM have not been elucidated, several mechanisms have been described in people. These mechanisms include heritable abnormalities in the cytoskeletal components of the myocytes as well as abnormalities in the myocyte sarcomeric proteins.[15-17]

Secondary DCM is significantly less common than primary DCM, comprising only about 10% of the cases. Some of the recognized causes of secondary DCM in dogs include viral, parasitic, or spirochetal infection; drug toxicity; nutritional deficiencies; trauma; ischemia; chronic hemodynamic overload; sustained tachycardia; or metabolic derangements. Table 34-2 contains a list of etiologies shown to cause DCM in dogs, but only a small number of these causes are clinically important.

Nutritional deficiencies may be a contributing factor in the development

Table 34-2. Causes of Secondary Myocardial Disease in Dogs

Infectious
Parvovirus
Distemper virus
Borrelia burgdorferi
Trypanosoma cruzi
Toxoplasma gondii
Neospora canis
Drugs/Toxins
Doxorubicin
Ionophores
Nutritional
Carnitine deficiency
Taurine deficiency
Vitamin E/selenium deficiency
Ischemic
Atherosclerosis
Septic coronary embolism
Other
Chronic hemodynamic overload
Tachycardia-induced cardiomyopathy
Severe hypothyroidism
Duchenne muscular dystrophy

of DCM in the American cocker spaniel and the golden retriever.[18,19] Many American cocker spaniels are taurine deficient (plasma taurine concentration <50 μmole/mL), and taurine deficiency is believed to be at least partially responsible for the disease in this breed. Abnormally low plasma taurine concentrations have also been noted in association with DCM in several other breeds including Golden retrievers, Dalmatians, and some mixed breed dogs.[20,21] Measurement of plasma or whole blood taurine concentration should be considered in all Golden retrievers, Dalmatians, and in all dogs fed a noncommercial diet. All dogs with DCM and a measured low plasma or whole blood taurine level should receive dietary taurine supplementation (500 mg to 1 g q 12 h); unfortunately, not all dogs supplemented respond.

Some dogs with DCM may have a deficiency of myocardial carnitine. However, reduced myocardial concentration of L-carnitine has been noted in some dogs with DCM that have had no apparent response to L-carnitine supplementation. Furthermore, plasma carnitine concentration may be normal in dogs with myocardial deficiency. At this time, empirical dietary supplementation with L-carnitine (110 mg/kg L-carnitine PO q 12 h) appears to have a justifiable cost/benefit ratio in American cocker spaniels and Boxers.[18,22]

Currently, there are no data indicating that dogs with DCM are deficient in coenzyme Q_{10}. There is also no evidence that dogs with this disorder will respond to supplementation with this nutrient.[9]

Parvovirus has been associated with the development of myocarditis and secondary cardiomyopathy in dogs. Other infectious causes of cardiomyopathy in the canine include *Borrelia burgdorferi* (Lyme disease) and *Trypanosoma cruzi* (Chagas' disease). Immune-mediated events that occur secondary to these infectious agents may be responsible for the cellular damage and myocardial dysfunction.

Sustained tachycardia produced by ventricular pacing will reliably produce myocardial dysfunction and heart failure in dogs.[23] Chronic, rapid heart rates such as those that often occur with atrial fibrillation, ventricular tachycardia, or supraventricular tachycardia produce a reversible decline in myocardial contractility and a clinical syndrome identical to that of primary DCM. The extent of the dysfunction produced is related to the heart rate and duration of the tachycardia.[24] Tachycardia is often an unappreciated cause of DCM in people, and is likely to be a frequently overlooked etiology in canine patients as well.[25-27]

Pathophysiology

Although the specific mechanisms responsible for canine DCM are yet to be elucidated, it is clear that biochemical abnormalities within the myocytes of affected animals result in a progressive loss of myocardial contractility. In most dogs, the decreased contractility is initially mild but progresses with time to severe contractile dysfunction. In the intact heart, decreased myocyte shortening translates to increased ventricular end-systolic diameter and increased end-systolic volume with a subsequent drop in stroke volume. Eccentric cardiac hypertrophy (increased myocyte mass with ventricular dilation) develops as a compensatory mechanism. In addition to increased diastolic and systolic chamber size, LV geometry becomes altered with the LV becoming less elliptical and more spherical.

Reduced stroke volume that results from loss of contractility causes activation of several deleterious neurohormonal mechanisms including activation of the sympathetic nervous system, activation of the renin-angiotensin-aldosterone system, and increased secretion of arginine vasopressin (antidiuretic hormone). This neuroendocrine response initiates self-perpetuating cycles that promote antidiuresis, vasoconstriction, and sodium retention. It is also known that in patients with DCM heart failure progression will occur independently of the hemodynamic status of the patient because of an overexpression of biologically active molecules that exert toxic effects on the heart and circulation.[28] Currently, a variety of proteins including norepinephrine, angiotensin II, endothelin, aldosterone, and tumor necrosis factor (TNF) have been implicated as substances contributing to disease progression. Several of these neurohormones, such as norepinephrine, angiotensin II, and aldosterone, are actually synthesized directly within the myocardium, and, act, not as true hormones, but in an autocrine and paracrine manner. Furthermore, several of the substances implicated in myocardial remodeling and heart failure progression are synthesized by a variety of nucleated cell types within the heart, including the cardiac myocytes, and are, therefore, not necessarily of neuroendocrine origin. Nonetheless, the important concept arising from this "neurohormonal model" of CHF is that LV remodeling produces loss of myocytes (necrosis and apoptosis) as well as deleterious changes in LV shape and volume that are unrelated to preload increases, and that these changes are responsible for self-perpetuating myocardial systolic dysfunction.[28,29] Table 34-3 lists the characteristic features of LV remodeling and Figure 34-1 shows a schematic of the role of these changes in progressive CHF in dogs with DCM.

Table 34-3. Structural and Functional Features of Left Ventricular Remodeling in Patients with Myocardial Failure

Left ventricular dilation
Myocardial intersitial fibrosis
Myocyte hypertrophy
Increased expression of myocardial fetal proteins
Altered left ventricular geometry (increased sphericity)
Progressive loss of inotropic state
Increased wall stress (afterload)
Afterload mismatch
Episodic subendocardial hypoperfusion
Increased oxygen utilization
Sustained hemodynamic overloading
Worsening activation of compensatory mechanisms

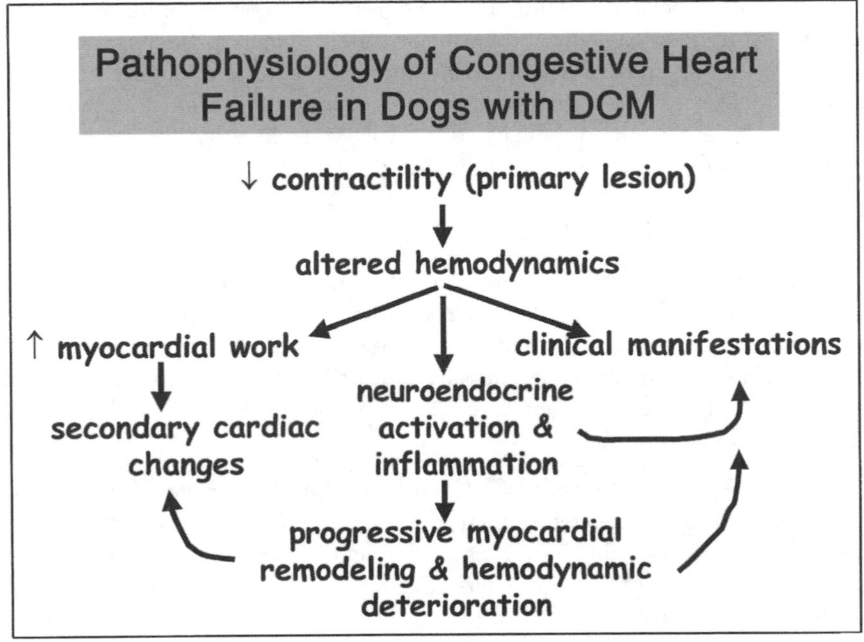

Figure 34-1
Schematic diagram of the pathophysiologic mechanisms responsible for progressive myocardial dysfunction in patients with CHF due to dilated cardiomyopathy.

As myocardial contractility progresses from mild to severe in dogs with DCM, there comes a point when the loss of inotropic state becomes severe enough that the ventricular chamber(s) cannot continue to dilate. At that point, the ventricular end-diastolic pressure begins to increase. An increase in LV filling pressure results in left atrial dilation and, ultimately, in pulmonary edema (left-sided CHF). If the right ventricular end-diastolic pressure also rises, right atrial enlargement and ascites will be noted. Increased sympathetic tone produces an increase in heart rate that helps to maintain adequate cardiac output. However, cardiac output eventually becomes inadequate despite a rapid heart rate (low output failure). Some patients may develop hypotension in terminal stages of the disorder despite an abnormally high systemic vascular resistance (cardiogenic shock).

Other pathophysiologic mechanisms may contribute to the development of CHF in dogs with DCM. Impaired ventricular filling (diastolic dysfunction) as a result of loss of ventricular compliance (increased ventricular stiffness) has been described in both people and dogs with DCM.[30, 31] Mitral regurgitation often develops because of LV dilation, and valvular incompetence adds to increased pulmonary capillary pressure and reduced forward stroke volume. Finally, arrhythmias undoubtedly play a role in the evolution of CHF in many canine patients with DCM. Atrial fibrillation is common and adversely affects cardiac function because of loss of atrioventricular synchrony. Furthermore, high heart rates typically associated with atrial fibrillation in dogs with DCM increase myocardial oxygen demand and cause further systolic dysfunction (tachycardiomyopathy). Ventricular tachyarrhythmias may also cause cardiac dysfunction in dogs with DCM. Doberman pinschers and Boxers are particularly prone to lethal ventricular tachycardia, and in these breeds ventricular tachyarrhythmias may cause syncope and sudden death prior to the onset of CHF.

Clinical Presentation

Dilated cardiomyopathy occurs in dogs of all ages, but is most commonly seen in middle-aged to older animals.[2] In contrast, cardiomyopathy seen in Portuguese water dogs develops in young dogs between the ages of 2 and 32 weeks.[12] Some studies of Doberman pinschers have described a male predisposition for the disease.[2] However, this gender bias does not seem to apply to all affected breeds.[1]

History. Typically, dogs with DCM have had a short history of problems. Most are presented for signs related to CHF. Commonly the complaint is respiratory distress as a result of pulmonary edema and pleural effusion. Other complaints include coughing, exercise intolerance, lethargy, abdominal distention, and weight loss. Some dogs with DCM present with a history of syncope, collapse, or episodic weakness. This is particularly common in boxers and in Doberman pinschers with ventricular arrhythmias, and dogs of these breeds frequently have no circulatory congestion.

Physical Examination. Dogs with early DCM or those with history of syncope may have a normal physical examination. Some dogs will have apparent arrhythmias when the thorax or arterial pulses are examined. In addition to arrhythmias, cardiac auscultation may reveal a soft (usually grade I-III) systolic regurgitant murmur over the mitral or tricuspid valve, an S_3 gallop best heard over the cardiac apex on the left hemithorax, or both a murmur and gallop. Dogs in left-sided CHF will have tachypnea and increased respiratory effort. These dogs may have a soft, moist cough producing pink-tinged pulmonary edema fluid, and auscultation of the lungs may reveal increased bronchovesicular sounds or crackles. Tachycardia due to heightened sympathetic tone is usually present. In dogs with severe myocardial failure, weak and rapid femoral arterial pulses are often palpated, and some dogs also have signs of poor perfusion such as cold extremities, cold ears, and weakness. If biventricular failure is present, ascites, hepatomegaly and jugular distention will usually be evident. A ventral fluid line may be noted on auscultation if there is significant pleural effusion. Not infrequently, a decreased body condition score will be seen due to anorexia or to cardiac cachexia.

Diagnostic Evaluation

Electrocardiography. Arrhythmias are frequent in dogs with DCM, and the main value of the electrocardiogram (ECG) in dogs with DCM is to provide a means of identifying and monitoring rhythm abnormalities. Common arrhythmias include atrial fibrillation, ventricular premature complexes, and ventricular tachycardia. Ventricular arrhythmias including ventricular premature contractions and ventricular tachycardia occur in approximately 75% of Doberman pinschers with DCM.[32,33] In this breed ventricular ectopy is often complex and frequently culminates in sudden death. A 24-hour ambulatory ECG (Holter monitor) study of Dobermans showed that the presence of more than 100 ventricular premature contractions per 24-hour period in an otherwise asymptomatic dog is usually associated with progressive cardiomyopathy.[33] Boxer dogs also commonly suffer from ventricular arrhythmias and sudden death. In this breed, ventricular ectopy typically originates from a single focus in the right ventricle producing QRS complexes that are upright in leads I, II, and III.[34]

The rhythm disturbance most commonly noted in giant breed dogs with DCM is atrial fibrillation.[1] In most breeds the atrial fibrillation is thought to be secondary to atrial enlargement, but in Irish wolfhounds atrial fibrillation has been noted to precede cardiac mechanical dysfunction by about 24 months.[35,36] It is not clear whether the atrial fibrillation in this breed is responsible for the development of mechanical dysfunction or whether atrial fibrillation is an early manifestation of a more global myocyte abnormality.

In addition to arrhythmias, other ECG abnormalities may be noted in dogs with DCM. Some affected dogs have widened or high-amplitude QRS complexes due to left-sided cardiomegaly. Although less common, low-voltage QRS complexes can also be seen. R waves are frequently notched or show sloppy R wave descent (Fig. 34-2).

Radiography. Dogs with early, subclinical DCM generally have normal survey thoracic radiographs. However, dogs with severe myocardial dysfunction consistently have radiographic cardiomegaly. The degree of enlargement of the cardiac silhouette depends on the stage (severity) of the disease and also on the breed. Giant breeds and Cocker spaniels typically have severe cardiomegaly, whereas Doberman pinschers and German shepherd dogs often appear to have only moderate radiographic cardiomegaly even when echocardiographic examination reveals severe enlargement. The cardiomegaly noted in dogs with DCM may be generalized or it may affect primarily the LV and left atrium. Pulmonary edema or pleural effusion may be apparent. If pulmonary edema is present, it is usually perihilar in distribution and is accompanied by left atrial enlargement and pulmonary venous congestion. Some Doberman pinschers, however, have pulmonary edema that is "patchy" and more generalized. In dogs with biventricular failure, enlargement of the caudal vena cava, ascites, and hepatomegaly are usually appreciable on radiographs.

Echocardiography. In normotensive dogs, echocardiography provides definitive diagnosis of dilated cardiomyopathy. The primary echocardiographic abnormality is an increase in the LV end-systolic diameter reflecting decreased myofiber shortening (see Chapter 24). In the clinical stages of the disease, this increase in LV systolic dimension is accompanied by a compensatory increase in LV end-diastolic dimension. Although reduced systolic dimension reduces fractional shortening, compensatory LV dilation increases this index. Therefore,

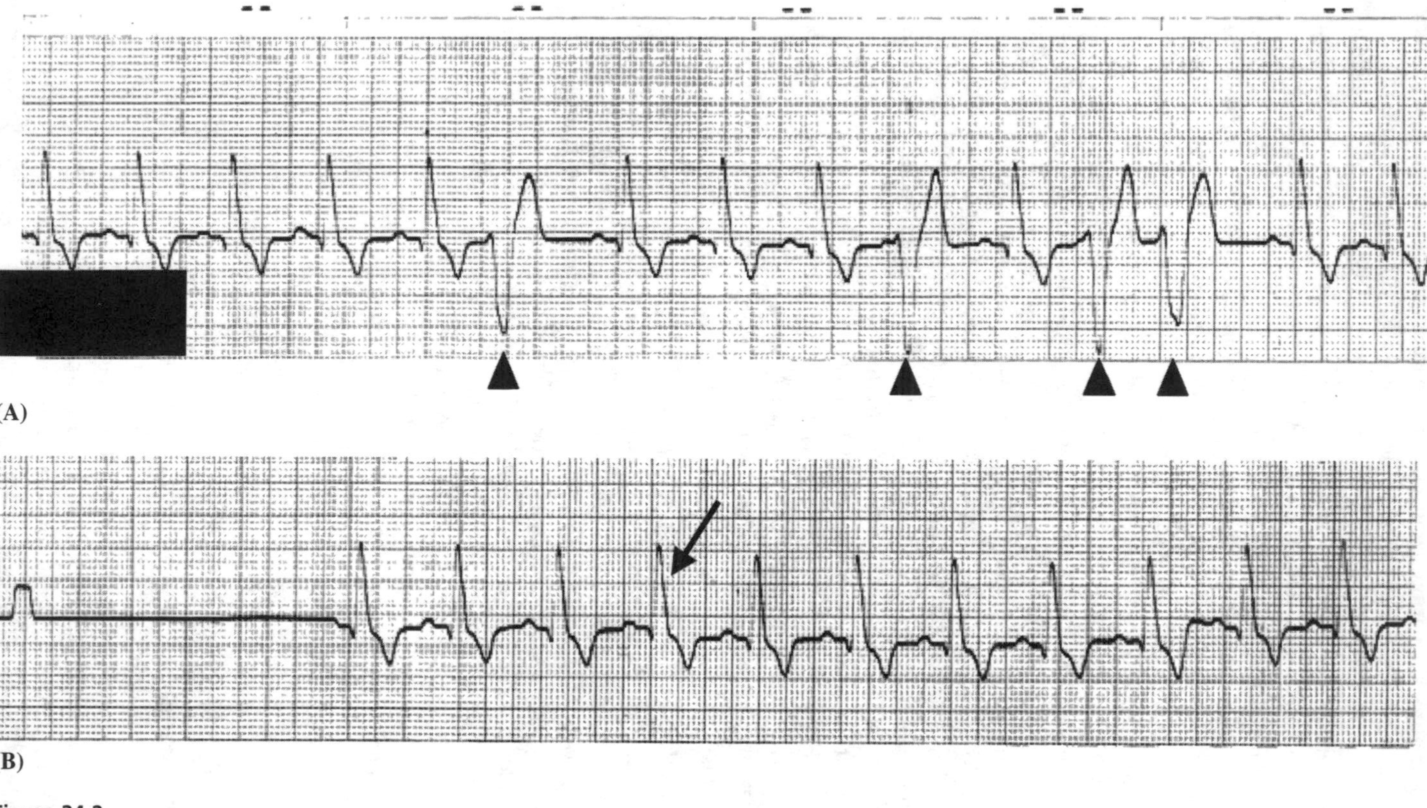

Figure 34-2
Lead II rhythm strip recorded from a 7-year-old Doberman pinscher with DCM. **(A)** The strip shows several ECG abnormalities often noted in patients with this disease including frequent premature ventricular contractions (arrowheads). **(B)** The QRS complexes are abnormally tall (R wave amplitude = 2.6 mV) consistent with LV enlargement, and there is "sloppy" R wave descent (arrow).

shortening fraction may not provide an accurate estimate of systolic function. However, dogs with left-sided CHF due to DCM generally have fractional shortening values of less than 15%. These dogs also have secondary left atrial dilation, and, unlike dogs with CHF caused by mitral regurgitation, the degree of atrial enlargement noted with DCM is comparable in degree to the LV enlargement. The LV caudal wall and interventricular septum are either normal or thinner than normal in dogs with DCM. In addition, the degree of thickening of the LV wall and septum are reduced as a result of reduced contractility.

As a result of reduced transmitral flow, excursion of the mitral valve leaflets during early diastole (rapid filling) is decreased in dogs with moderate to severe DCM. This decrease in leaflet excursion produces an increase in the distance between the tip of the anterior leaflet and the septum during early diastole (increased EPSS or E point-to-septal separation). Dogs in low output failure may have reduced aortic motion on the M-mode echocardiogram and reduced aortic flow velocity measured with spectral Doppler. When biventricular failure is present, dilation of the right atrium and right ventricle will be apparent on echocardiographic examination.

Laboratory Findings. Dogs with severe DCM usually have prerenal azotemia from decreased renal perfusion and dehydration. Alanine aminotransferase (ALT) may be increased from reduced hepatic blood flow. Dogs with severe CHF occasionally have dilutional hyponatremia caused by excessive secretion of antidiuretic hormone (ADH).[37] Hyponatremia in patients not yet receiving diuretic therapy is a poor prognostic sign.[38] Other laboratory findings commonly noted in dogs with severe DCM include lactic acidosis and reduced venous oxygen tension.

Therapy

Therapy for dogs with DCM should be determined based on the severity and the manifestations of the disease in an individual patient. Consideration should be made for seeking an underlying cause of the cardiomyopathy, particularly in young dogs or breeds not commonly affected. In this regard, transvenous endomyocardial biopsy can be done to rule out myocarditis or an infiltrative process. Serologic testing may also be helpful for identifying a cause of myocarditis leading to secondary DCM. If an underlying etiology can be identified and specifically treated, the best possible outcome can be achieved.

In most dogs DCM is primary, and often CHF is present. In these animals the goals of medical management are eliminating or reducing clinical signs, arresting or slowing progression, and preventing sudden death. Figure 34-3 shows diagrammatically the general treatment strategy that should be considered for dogs with DCM.

Because the clinical signs of CHF are caused by the hemodynamic derangements, acute intervention is aimed at reversing the hemodynamic abnormalities, in other words, at improving cardiac output and reducing increased ventricular filling pressures. These goals are achieved through combined administration of diuretics, vasodilators, and positive inotropic agents. Specific recommendations

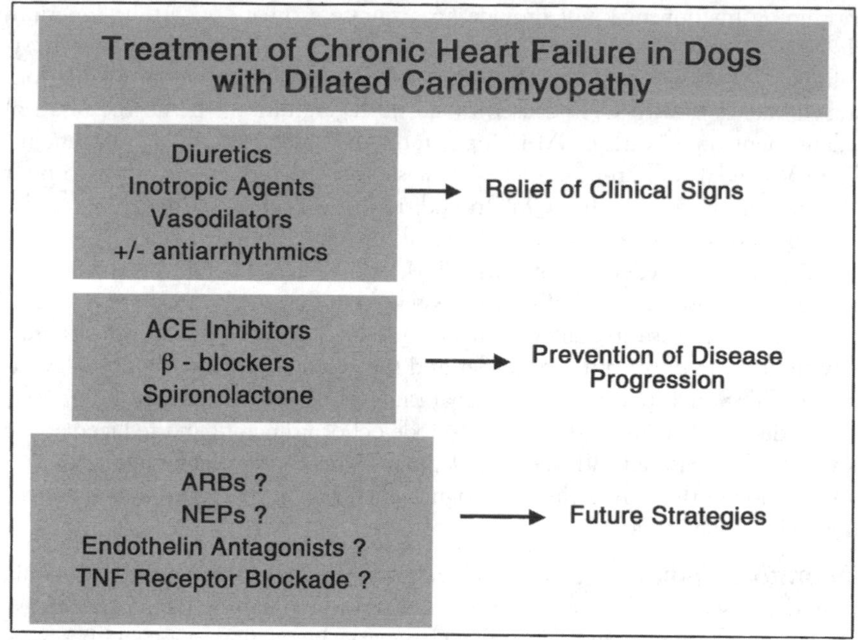

Figure 34-3
Suggested therapeutic approach for dogs with CHF due to DCM. ACE, angiotensin converting enzyme; ARBs, angiotensin receptor blockers; NEPs, neutral endopeptidases; TNF, tumor necrosis factor.

for management of acute CHF are found in Chapter 30 of this text. Dogs with hemodynamically significant arrhythmias must receive appropriate antiarrhythmic therapy as well (see Chapter 31). However, it is important to recognize that some antiarrhythmic agents, including β-adrenergic antagonists and calcium channel blockers, have significant negative inotropic effects.

Chronic treatment of CHF must be individualized. Either furosemide alone (1-3 mg/kg PO bid-tid) or combination diuretic therapy should be administered to alleviate systemic and pulmonary venous congestion. The dose of diuretic should be the least amount that will control congestion without causing excessive volume contraction. Combining diuretics that act at different sites in the nephron (sequential nephron block) is often more effective for controlling congestion than the use of extremely high doses of furosemide. Spironolactone (1 mg/kg PO bid) or Aldactazide (spironolactone/hydrochlorothiazide 1 mg/kg qd-bid) may be combined with furosemide in dogs with adequate renal function and blood pressure. Renal parameters (blood urea nitrogen and creatinine) and serum electrolytes should be monitored. Angiotensin-converting enzyme (ACE) inhibitors such as enalapril (0.5 mg/kg PO q 12 h) or benazapril (0.5 mg/kg PO q 24 h) have been shown to improve hemodynamics acutely and chronically.[39] Therapy with an ACE inhibitor has also improved survival and exercise tolerance in dogs with DCM-induced heart failure.[40] Digoxin (0.005 mg/kg PO q 12

h) is often used in patients with CHF secondary to DCM. Although digoxin has only a weak positive inotropic agent, symptomatic improvement has been noted in some DCM patients receiving this drug. However, a positive effect on long-term survival from digoxin administration has not been documented.[41] In addition to its mild positive inotropic effect, the negative dromotropic effect of digoxin is helpful in lowering the heart rate in animals with atrial fibrillation. Recent data indicates that the calcium-sensitizing inodilating agent, pimobendan (Vetmedin, Boehringer-Ingelheim), provides a superior alternative to digoxin for management of dogs with CHF caused by DCM.[42,43] Unfortunately, this agent is not yet available in North America.

Combination arteriolar dilator therapy may be needed to achieve relief of clinical signs in patients refractory to treatment with diuretics, ACE inhibition, and digoxin. If the patient is not hypotensive, the calcium channel blocking agent, amlodipine (Norvasc, Pfizer, 0.2 mg/kg PO q 24 h), or the direct-acting arteriolar dilator, hydralazine (Apresoline, CIBA, 0.5-2.0 mg/kg PO q 8-12 h) may be added to the therapeutic regimen to reduce afterload and increase cardiac output. Systemic blood pressure should be measured before and after initiating treatment with arteriolar dilating agents.

Administration of antiarrhythmic agents for suppression of ventricular ectopy is generally recommended in patients with ventricular tachycardia or other forms of complex ventricular ectopy. This is particularly important in Doberman pinschers and Boxers because sudden arrhythmic death is a recognized risk in these breeds. When antiarrhythmic agents are used, 24-hour ambulatory ECG monitoring (Holter monitoring) should be done to verify that treatment has effectively suppressed the arrhythmia. Although definitive proof that antiarrhythmic treatment reduces the incidence of sudden cardiac death is lacking at this time, treatment is generally advised.

Dogs with DCM and atrial fibrillation typically have a rapid ventricular rate, and reducing heart rate to the range of 140 to 170 beats/min becomes a therapeutic goal in these patients. If untreated, the tachycardia increases the myocardial oxygen requirement and causes progression of the systolic dysfunction. Heart rate control may be achieved in these dogs through the use of pharmacologic agents that slow conduction through the atrioventricular node or through the use of biphasic electrical cardioversion.

Long-term management of dogs with DCM should include interventions to prevent or reduce the rate of progressive myocardial dysfunction. Progressive, deleterious myocardial structural and functional changes (ventricular remodeling) result, not from the hemodynamic abnormalities associated with DCM, but from neurohormonal activation. Therefore, neurohormonal modulation has become an important component of chronic heart failure management. ACE inhibition has been shown to be an important component of the reverse-remodeling strategy.[39,44,45] It is believed that in dogs, as in people, deleterious effects of angiotensin II on the myocardium may be prevented or reduced by ACE blockade. Use of specific β-adrenergic antagonists is also an important aspect of preserving and, actually improving, LV function in humans with heart failure and in canine models of systolic dysfunction.[44-46] However, because β-blocking agents have negative inotropic properties, these agents must be used only in dogs with subclinical disease or compensated failure. Furthermore, β-adrenergic antagonists must be administered at extremely low doses initially with slow, careful upward titration (weeks to months). Finally, some β-blockers have been shown to be better tolerated and more effective reverse remodeling agents than others.[47] Specifically, the second- generation β-blocker, metoprolol (Lopressor, Geigy, 0.05-0.1 mg/kg PO q 12 h initially increasing to 0.3-0.5 mg/kg q 12 h), and the third-generation β-blocker, carvedilol (Coreg, SK Beecham, 0.05 mg/kg PO q 12 h initially increasing to 0.5 mg/kg q 12 h), have been shown to be safest and most effective.[47] Although the benefits of reverse-remodeling agents (ACE inhibition and β-blockers) have not yet been confirmed for asymptomatic DCM patients, data currently available suggest that these agents will slow progression to the symptomatic state and improve survival.[46,48]

Prognosis

In general, primary DCM has a poor prognosis. Unless an underlying etiology is found and treated, DCM is a terminal disease. In the setting of DCM with CHF, response to therapy seems to be highly variable, and it is difficult to predict an individual animal's clinical course. However, it is apparent that Doberman pinschers have a worse prognosis than other breeds. One retrospective study of 66 Dobermans with DCM and CHF of less than 2 weeks' duration, showed a mean and median survival of 9.65 and 6.5 weeks, respectively.[49] Sudden death occurred in 20% of these dogs. Biventricular failure and the presence of atrial fibrillation were negative prognostic indicators. Another study reported survival data from 37 dogs of various breeds diagnosed with DCM with or without CHF.[50] The 50% probability of survival occurred at 2.3 months, with a 1-year probability of survival of 37.5% and a 2-year survival probability of 28%. Treatment was not standardized in either of these studies. With early use of ACE inhibitors and selective β-adrenergic antagonists, prognosis may improve.

HYPERTROPHIC CARDIOMYOPATHY

Hypertrophic cardiomyopathy (HCM) is an important disease in humans and cats, but is rare in dogs.[51] HCM is a disorder of the ventricular myocardium characterized by concentric LV hypertrophy and impaired diastolic function. Not infrequently, the right ventricle is hypertrophied as well. HCM is the most common cardiac disease of cats, occurring in 81% of all feline patients with heart disease.[52] HCM is considered primary if the hypertrophy is due to an inherent defect within the myocardium itself. Secondary HCM implies that the concentric hypertrophy is due to some other primary cause. LV hypertrophy may be secondary to pressure overload, such as aortic stenosis or systemic hypertension, or it may be secondary to abnormal hormonal stimulation, such as hyperthyroidism or acromegaly.[53,54] Although secondary LV hypertrophy is often not as severe as primary HCM, primary and secondary HCM cannot be reliably distinguished based on radiographic and echocardiographic findings.

Feline HCM

Etiology and Pathophysiology

In people, HCM is often an autosomal dominant, heritable disorder. Mutations responsible for the disease have been identified in genes such as α- and β-myosin heavy-chain gene, troponin T gene, and the α-tropomyosin gene.[55,56] In most cats with HCM the disease is idiopathic. However, HCM has been shown to be heritable in several breeds including Maine Coon cats, Persians, and American short-haired cats.[57-59] HCM is inherited in Maine Coon cats as an autosomal dominant trait, with penetrance that increases to 100% in adulthood.[57] The specific genetic defects responsible for HCM in cats have not yet been identified. Hypertrophy in cats with familial HCM is often severe at a young age and may be recognized in cats as young as 12 weeks of age. However, phenotypic expression of the disease may not be apparent in some cats with heritable HCM until approximately 3 years of age.[57]

The pathophysiology of HCM involves systolic and diastolic abnormalities as well as myocardial ischemia. However, impaired diastolic function is primarily responsible for the hemodynamic and clinical manifestations of the disease. Diastolic dysfunction refers to impaired capacity of the LV to accept blood or to fill without a compensatory increase in left atrial pressure. Impaired LV filling may result in dyspnea from pulmonary edema, or it may cause lethargy, syncope, or sudden death as a result of reduced stroke volume. Also, impaired LV filling impedes normal left atrial flow predisposing to left atrial enlargement, circulatory stasis, and thromboembolism.

Impaired diastolic function in cats with HCM is the result of both reduced ventricular compliance (increased ventricular stiffness) and impaired myocardial relaxation. Reduced LV chamber compliance occurs as a result of myofiber disarray and myocardial fibrosis and also from increased ventricular mass (decreased volume/mass ratio). Impaired relaxation refers to a reduced rate of myocyte tension decline and reduced rate of LV pressure decline. Impaired relaxation attenuates early LV inflow.

Myocardial ischemia is a feature of HCM that results from reduced capillary density, narrowed intramural coronary arteries, and increased extravascular resistance. Myocardial ischemia contributes to impaired relaxation by interfering with the energy-dependent intracellular movement of Ca^{++} away from the sarcomeres into the sarcoplasmic reticulum and across the sarcolemma. In addition, myocardial ischemia predisposes to lethal arrhythmias.

Several systolic abnormalities may be present in feline patients with HCM. Occasionally, chronic ischemia and fibrosis results in impaired LV systolic performance. Some cats with HCM have mitral regurgitation from altered LV geometry or from abnormal systolic motion of the mitral valve leaflets. Finally, some feline patients develop significant intraventricular systolic pressure gradients.

Clinical Presentation

In cats with idiopathic HCM, the disease is most common in young adult, male cats. The average age of affected cats is 6.5 years, with a range of 1 to 16 years.[3]

History. Many cats with HCM show no clinical signs, and the disease is diagnosed after a murmur, arrhythmia, or gallop is detected during physical examination done for an unrelated reason. The clinical signs and history of cats with HCM are tremendously varied. Symptomatic cats are usually presented for respiratory distress due to pulmonary edema or pleural effusion. Coughing is rare. Another common complaint in affected cats is acute paresis or paralysis subsequent to thromboembolism. Posterior paresis is due to thromboembolism at the terminal aortic trifurcation. Another relatively common site for a thromboembolic event is the right forelimb, and right forelimb lameness, even intermittent, can be a sign of thromboembolism. Lethargy may be a manifestation of HCM in some cats. However, exercise intolerance often goes unnoticed in sedentary cats. Syncope may be a component of the history or the sole complaint, and syncope in cats with HCM is often secondary to cardiac arrhythmia.[60] Unfortunately, sudden cardiac death may also be the first clinical manifestation of the disease.

Physical Examination. Physical examination of cats with HCM often reveals a murmur, an arrhythmia, or a cardiac gallop rhythm. When present, murmurs are systolic and usually reflect either secondary mitral regurgitation or turbulent flow in the LV outflow tract. In many cases, systolic murmurs result from multiple sites of intraventricular and intravascular turbulence. Increased respiratory rate and effort will be present in cats with pulmonary edema or significant pleural effusion. With pulmonary edema, inspiratory crackles may be heard. When pleural effusion is present, a ventral fluid line and absence of respiratory sounds ventrally may be appreciated. Jugular venous distention with or without pulsation may accompany pleural effusion. A prominent left-sided apical beat may also be palpated. If distal aortic thromboembolism is present, the femoral pulses will be very weak or absent, and the nail beds of the affected limbs will be cyanotic. The limbs affected by the embolism will be cooler than the normal limbs, and, if the hind limbs are affected, the gastrocnemius muscle is often firmer than normal.

ECG. Numerous ECG abnormalities including ventricular and supraventricular tachycardias, premature ventricular contractions, chamber enlargement patterns, and conduction disturbances may be found. It is not unusual for affected cats to have multiple ECG abnormalities. Some, however, may have a normal ECG. Intraventricular conduction abnormalities consistent with left anterior fascicular block occur frequently. Intermittent arrhythmias causing syncope may require event recording or telemetry for diagnosis.

Radiography. Survey radiographic findings in cats with HCM may vary considerably depending on the extent of hypertrophic change, the degree of myocardial dysfunction, the presence of secondary chamber enlargement, and the severity of circulatory congestion. Thoracic radiographs are a fairly insensitive method of detecting HCM, especially in the early stages of the disease. Because cardiac hypertrophy occurs in a concentric pattern, some cats have no appreciable enlargement of the cardiac silhouette. Frequently, however, survey thoracic radiographs show mild to moderate LV enlargement with more severe left atrial enlargement (Fig. 34-4). Occasionally, more generalized enlargement of the cardiac silhouette is present

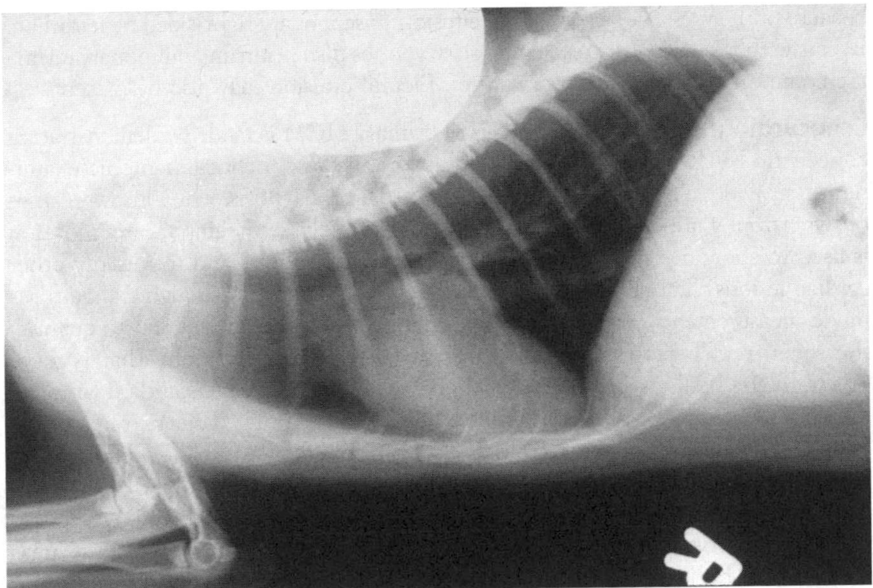

(A)

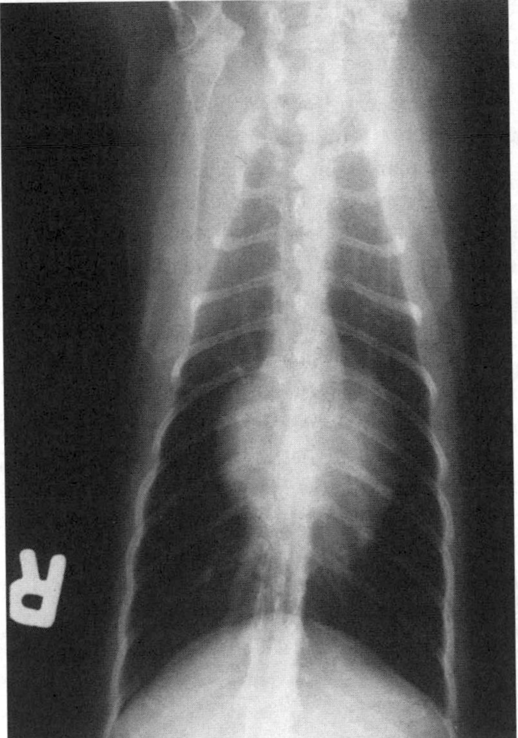

(B)

Figure 34-4
Lateral (**A**) and ventrodorsal (**B**) radiographic images from a 7-year-old cat with HCM. There is left atrial enlargement and pulmonary venous distention with minimal enlargement of the ventricles.

because of the presence of pericardial effusion or secondary right-sided heart failure. In cats with respiratory distress, pulmonary venous distention and pulmonary edema are common radiographic abnormalities. Pleural effusion may also be present.

Echocardiography. The diagnosis of primary HCM is made by demonstrating concentric LV hypertrophy without an apparent cause. Echocardigraphic examination provides a practical, noninvasive method of diagnosis, when known causes of hypertrophy are eliminated. Two-dimensional echocardiographic examination is used to show the extent and distribution of hypertrophy and to identify other cardiac lesions that may cause secondary LV hypertrophy. Although standard M-mode measurements of septal and LV caudal wall thickness are used to quantify the severity of hypertrophy, some affected cats have hypertrophy that is more severe in the basilar septal area of the ventricle. In these cats, standard M-mode measurements may be misleading if used solely for diagnosis. Four patterns of LV hypertrophy have been identified in cats with primary HCM.[61] These patterns are (1) diffuse, symmetric thickening of the interventricular septum and ventricular caudal wall; (2) hypertrophy of the ventricular caudal wall primarily; (3) hypertrophy of the interventricular septum primarily; and (4) hypertrophy of regional areas of the LV. The interventricular septum or LV caudal wall is considered thick if greater than 6 mm during diastole in adult cats.[61] Often cats with HCM have an LV chamber diameter that is decreased during both diastole and systole. In people with HCM a decrease in LV chamber size has been associated with functional limitation and history of syncope, regardless of the severity of hypertrophy.[62] Some cats have hypertrophy of the right ventricular wall in addition to LV hypertrophy.

The left atrium may or may not be dilated in cats with HCM, but left atrial enlargement is indirect evidence of significantly impaired diastolic function in cats without mitral regurgitation. With severe left atrial enlargement spontaneous echo contrast ("smoke") or thrombus may be noted on echocardiography. "Smoke" may reflect stasis of blood flow in the atria and be a precursor to thrombus formation.[63]

Spectral or color Doppler may show abnormally high blood flow velocity in the LV outflow tract and aortic root in some cats with HCM. It is unclear whether the increased velocity of blood flow reflects dynamic outflow obstruction or a hyperdynamic ventricle ejecting a small volume of blood rapidly. Systolic anterior motion (SAM) of the mitral valve, usually best appreciated on M-mode echo, may be produced as a result of this high flow velocity (Venturi effect). SAM often causes varying degrees of mitral regurgitation.[61]

Assessment of diastolic function can be accomplished with Doppler echocardiography. Pulsed-wave Doppler used to interrogate LV inflow through the mitral valve can give an estimate, noninvasively, of diastolic function and the degree of diastolic functional impairment in cats with HCM.[64]

Therapy

Commonly, the first clinical signs of heart disease cats with HCM are those associated with CHF. Respiratory distress due to pulmonary edema or pleural effusion must be treated promptly and aggressively. In this situation, parenteral administration of a loop diuretic and, possibly, therapeutic thoracocentesis are immediate therapy for relieving congestion thereby stabilizing respiratory status. Acute treatment of CHF is described in greater detail in Chapter 30 of this text.

Chronic management of HCM should include agents designed to improve diastolic function. The β-adrenergic blocking agents have been used to treat humans and cats with HCM (atenolol, 0.5-1.0 mg/kg PO q 12 h).[55,65] The beneficial effects of β-blockers arise from a reduction in heart rate which, in turn, prolongs diastole and increases the time available for passive LV filling.[55] By decreasing inotropic state, β-blockers also reduce myocardial oxygen demand and possibly prevent arrhythmias potentiated by ischemia and catecholamines. Calcium channel blockers, such as diltiazem have also been advocated for treatment of feline HCM.[66] In addition to reducing inotropic state and myocardial oxygen demand, diltiazem improves LV diastolic function by increasing the rate and extent of active relaxation. Diltiazem is a potent coronary vasodilator, an effect that may reduce myocardial ischemia in cats with HCM. At therapeutic doses, the effect of diltiazem on heart rate is less profound than the effect of β-adrenergic antagonists, and this drug should not be dosed based on heart rate reduction. Diltiazem is available in several dosage forms. Standard diltiazem may be administered using a dose of 1.75 to 2.0 mg/kg orally three times a day. The drug in this form may be mixed in a palatable liquid or formulated into a transdermal gel by a compounding pharmacy. Cardizem CD (Hoechst Marion Roussel) is administered at a dose of 10 mg/kg orally once daily. The recommended dose of Dilacor XL (Rhone-Poulenc Rorer) is 10 mg/kg orally every 12 to 24 hours.

Treatment with β-blockers versus calcium channel blockers has been compared in only a few studies of cats. In one study of 17 cats, those receiving diltiazem had greater clinical improvement than those receiving propanolol (Inderal, Wyeth-Ayerst).[66] Long-term use of diuretics in cats with CHF from HCM may not be necessary in all patients, and when used chronically, diuretics should be administered at the lowest possible dosage that will prevent recurrent edema.[67] The ACE inhibitors may be beneficial, as additional therapy, for the control of congestion in cats with refractory or biventricular failure. The results of a study of 32 cats indicates that the ACE inhibitor, benazapril (Lotensin, Novartis, 0.5 mg/kg PO q 24 h), provides some beneficial effects on clinical status and cardiac remodeling when given in addition to diltiazem.[52]

Treatment of acute arterial thromboembolism in cats should include administration of heparin to prevent extension of the thrombus. Thrombolytic therapy is an alternative strategy, but involves the risks of hemorrhage and reperfusion injury. Anticoagulation with warfarin (Coumadin, Dupont) should be considered for long-term management of cats with thromboembolism. Unfortunately, recurrence of thromboembolism occurs at a high rate (43.5%) even in cats receiving “appropriate” anticoagulation.[68]

Prognosis

The prognosis for cats with HCM is highly variable. In one study, the median survival was 732 days, with over one third of affected cats alive 5 years after diagnosis.[3] Not surprisingly, cats without clinical signs in this study survived longer than cats with heart failure or embolism. The median survival times of cats with heart failure or embolism were 92 and 61 days, respectively.[3] Some data suggest that in feline HCM patients, survival is adversely affected by the magnitude and extent of LV hypertrophy.[61]

RESTRICTIVE CARDIOMYOPATHY

Feline Restrictive Cardiomyopathy

Restrictive cardiomyopathy (RCM) is a myocardial disorder characterized by impaired ventricular filling that results from endocardial, endomyocardial, or myocardial infiltrate. Several systemic disorders, such as lymphosarcoma and amyloidosis, can produce myocardial infiltrate and secondary RCM. In cats with primary RCM, the infiltrate is fibrous and usually idiopathic.[70] Some authors have suggested that feline primary RCM be subclassified as myocardial RCM or endomyocardial RCM because of differences in echocardiographic features and possible differences in etiology.

RCM is an important disease in domestic cats. In one retrospective study looking at nearly 1500 feline necropsies, RCM represented the cause of death in more than 4%.[71]

Etiology and Pathophysiology

Some cats with RCM have inflammatory and fibrous endocardial and subendocardial infiltrate. The inflammation and fibrosis in these cats are most likely sequelae of previous viral infection or virally mediated stimulation of cellular immunity.[72,73] More commonly, cats with primary RCM have myocardial fibrous infiltrate with little inflammation. The fibrosis can be patchy, multifocal, or diffuse in distribution.[74] In these cats the fibrosis may be a long-term result of ischemia and scarring from chronic, subclinical hypertrophic disease.[75] It is probable that in cats primary RCM is, actually, an end-stage manifestation of several different etiologies. However, by the time RCM is recognized in most cats, the underlying etiology is no longer apparent.

The presence of infiltrate in the endocardium or myocardium results in a loss of normal ventricular compliance. Subsequently, there is a significant increase in diastolic ventricular pressure associated with ventricular filling (greater slope of the LV diastolic pressure volume relationship). Thus, in cats with RCM there is a greater end-diastolic pressure associated with a given end-diastolic volume. Consequently atrial pressure must increase to overcome the increased ventricular stiffness and resistance to filling. In people, RCM is associated with characteristic hemodynamic abnormalities including a rapid decline in LV pressure during early diastole (normal active relaxation), a rapid rise in early LV pressure due to a large atrial-ventricular pressure gradient immediately following mitral valve opening, an abrupt plateau in LV pressure rise associate with abrupt decline in filling during mid to late diastole, and decreased cardiac output (Fig. 34-5). Thus, the hemodynamic profile of patients with RCM is similar to that of patients

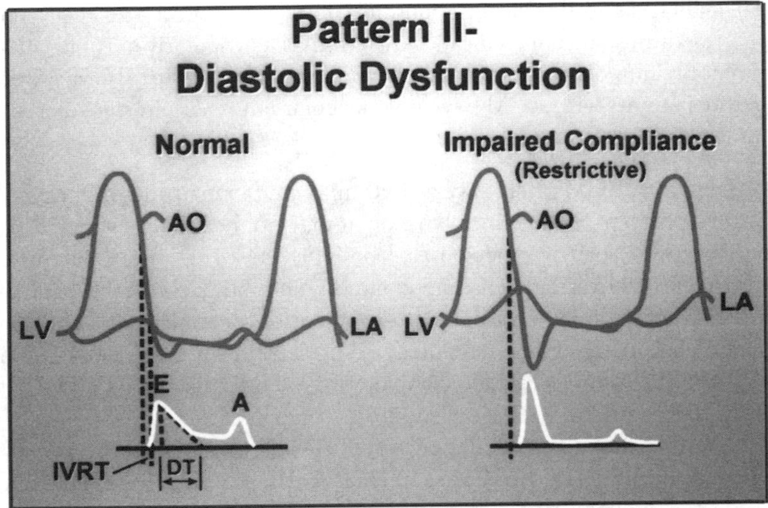

Figure 34-5
Schematic showing LV, aortic, and left atrial pressures in a normal individual and in a patient with restrictive physiology. With restriction there is a rapid, early decline in LV pressure in diastole followed by a rise and plateau in ventricular pressure during early filling. The schematic also shows typical pulsed Doppler features of RCM including reduced isovolumic relaxation time; a tall, narrow early filling peak (E wave); and attenuated atrial systolic inflow (small A wave). LV, left ventricular pressure; AO, aortic pressure; LA, left atrial pressure; IVRT, isovolumic relaxation time; DT, deceleration time of early inflow.

with constrictive pericardial disease. Pressure tracings and Doppler studies of LV filling obtained from feline patients with RCM suggest that the pathophysiology is similar in cats. Very high atrial pressures develop in cats with RCM predisposing to both left- and right-sided CHF.

Clinical Presentation

Restrictive cardiomyopathy is most common in older cats, but is occasionally found in young cats. No breed or gender predilection has been established.[53]

History. Most often, cats with RCM are brought to the veterinarian because of acute, severe respiratory distress due to CHF or because of acute paralysis from thromboembolism. Although, biventricular failure with ascites is frequently present, owners do not usually do not notice this clinical sign in cats. Some affected cats are presented for syncope, with or without other signs of cardiac disease.

Physical Examination. Physical examination findings are variable. Dyspnea or tachypnea, with or without the presence of pulmonary crackles, may be present. A ventral fluid line may be auscultated if pleural effusion is present. A soft, systolic murmur over the mitral or tricuspid valve may be heard. An S_4 gallop is often audible as well. Diastolic murmurs resulting from aortic regurgitation may be present in some affected cats. Arrhythmias, particularly atrial fibrillation, are commonly noted during physical examination of cats with RCM.[74] Because most feline patients with RCM have biventricular failure, ascites, jugular distension, and pulsation are often present.

ECG. Cats with RCM often have arrhythmias, and many times more than one arrhythmia is present. In cats with syncope, it may not be obvious which arrhythmia is responsible for the syncopal episodes (Fig. 34-6). Both supraventricular and ventricular tachyarrhythmias are common, and many cats have atrial fibrillation. Bradyarrhythmias suggestive of degeneration or infiltrate of the cardiac pacemaking and conduction system may be present in some patients. Examples of such bradyarrhythmias include complete atrioventricular block and sinus arrest with inadequate escape (see Fig. 34-6).

Left ventricular enlargement may result in widening of the QRS complexes or increased amplitude of the R wave in leads II, III, or aVF. However, the QRS amplitude may be decreased if there is significant pleural or pericardial effusion. Wide or tall P waves may be seen secondary to atrial enlargement. Intraventricular conduction disturbances resulting in splintered QRS complexes or a bundle branch block pattern can be seen. Arrhythmias such as atrial premature complexes, ventricular premature complexes, or atrial fibrillation are quite common.

Radiography. The cardiac silhouette is usually significantly enlarged often with dramatic left and right atrial enlargement. Interstitial or alveolar infiltrate in varying amounts with pulmonary venous enlargement is apparent in most cases. Pleural effusion in common. With right-sided CHF, an enlarged vena cava and hepatomegaly, usually with ascites, can be seen.

Echocardiography. Definitive diagnosis of RCM can be made using cardiac catheterization and demonstrating the classic restrictive hemodynamic pattern that indicates the abrupt, premature cessation of ventricular filling. Diagnosis of RCM is suggested noninvasively with the use of standard echocardiographic imaging and Doppler echocardiography. On the standard echocardiogram, severe left atrial enlargement is usually present, and generally the right atrium is moderately to severely dilated as well. The LV is normal in size or slightly dilated, and hypertrophy, if present is mild and often regional. Endocardial or endomyocardial fibrosis may appear as a distinct band of increased echogenicity. The LV wall can appear speckled or heterogeneous due to focal patchy infiltrate within the myocardium. Indexes of LV systolic function are normal to mildly reduced. One or more focal abnormalities are often seen on echocardiographic examination of the LV. These abnormalities include such features as focal areas of wall thinning, excessive LV moderator bands, regional hypokinesis, and areas of fibrosis.[74] In most cats the right ventricle appears slightly to moderately dilated.

Color Doppler evaluation of blood flow in cats with RCM may reveal mild mitral or tricuspid regurgitation or both, but the degree of regurgitation is disproportionate to the degree of atrial enlargement. Pulsed Doppler may be used to document the characteristic abnormalities of LV inflow associated with RCM.

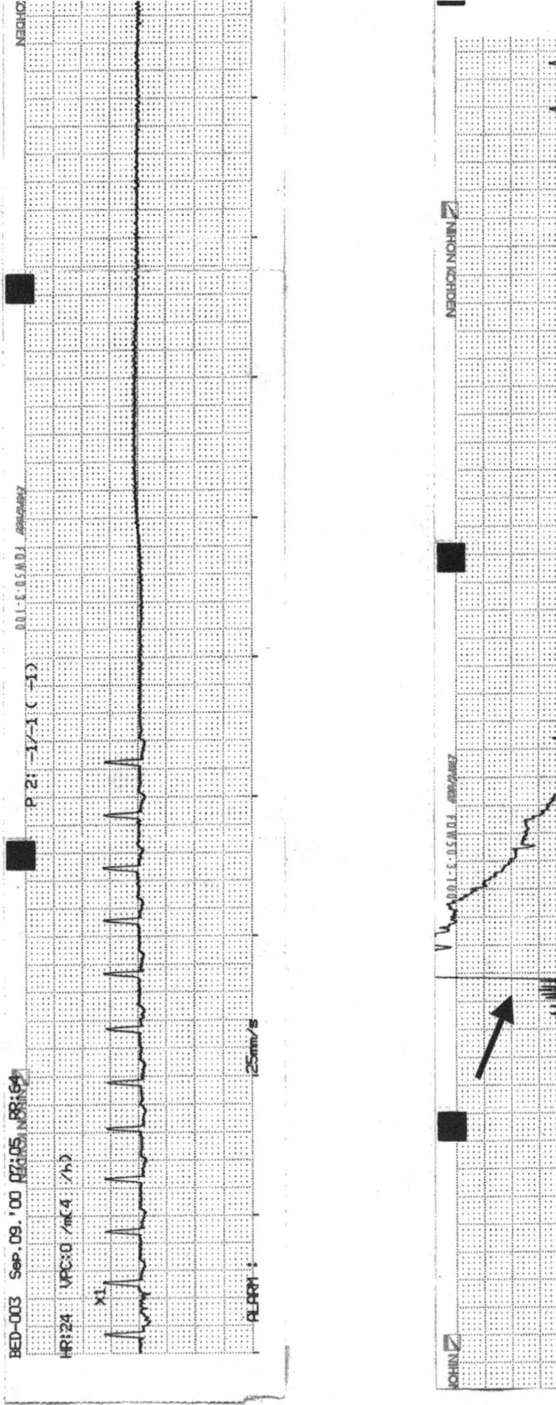

Figure 34-6
A continuous ECG rhythm obtained from a 5-year-old domestic short-haired cat with RCM. The underlying cardiac rhythm is atrial fibrillation with an average ventricular rate of 170 beats/min. There is a period of asystole lasting 11.5 seconds during which syncope occurred. The baseline deviation on the rhythm strip (arrow) resulted from delivery of a precordial thump (monitor lead, 25 mm/sec).

With restrictive physiology, the isovolumic relaxation time determined from simultaneous recording of LV inflow and outflow is reduced because of early opening of the mitral valve. There is an abnormal increase in the peak velocity of early inflow due to the very high left atrial pressure. However, the velocity of early inflow declines very quickly the atrial and ventricular pressures quickly equilibrate. Thus, the early inflow signal (E wave) is abnormally tall and narrow in affected cats. Conversely, the late diastolic inflow signal (A wave) is smaller than normal in RCM because little atrial systolic flow is achieved because of the very high intraventricular pressure in late diastole (see Fig. 34-5).[76] With rapid heart rates typically found in affected cats, the early and late diastolic filling signals often superimpose making it difficult to obtain an accurate Doppler examination of LV inflow. Nonetheless, isovolumic relaxation time can usually be measured accurately.

Therapy

Unfortunately, there are no clinically proven medical therapies for RCM in cats. Therapy is often directed at alleviating congestion or preventing thromboembolism. Diuresis to relieve pulmonary and systemic congestion must be aggressive enough to relieve edema, yet not so aggressive that cats become severely dehydrated and azotemic. Combining diuretics may be required to prevent respiratory distress caused by recurrent pulmonary edema and pleural effusion. Therapeutic thoracocentesis must be done if pleural effusion is compromising ventilation and oxygen exchange. ACE inhibitors may be helpful for relieving congestion and may also inhibit the deleterious peripheral and myocardial effects of angiotensin II. Cats with hypertrophy noted on echocardiographic examination may benefit from the lusitropic effects of diltiazem. Diltiazem may also improve coronary flow thereby reducing the ischemia that may be ongoing in some cats.[74] Stroke volume should be augmented by optimizing heart rate and rhythm. However, sinus tachycardia is usually beneficial in patients with this form of cardiomyopathy because nearly all ventricular filling occurs in early diastole. Treatment of hemodynamically significant arrhythmias should be addressed.

Prognosis

The long-term prognosis for humans and cats with RCM is poor.[70,74] Frequently, cats develop refractory CHF or fatal thromboembolism within the first several months of treatment. With medical management, cats will occasionally remain in a compensated state for 8 to 12 months following the onset of clinical signs. Sudden death is a common event.

REFERENCES

1. Sisson D, O'Grady MR, Calvert CA: Myocardial diseases of dogs. *In* Fox PR, Sisson D, Moise NS, eds.: Textbook of Canine and Feline Cardiology. Philadelphia: WB Saunders, 1999, p 581.
2. Sisson D, Thomas WP, Keene BW: Myocardial Diseases. *In* Ettinger EJ, Feldman

EC, eds.: Textbook of Veterinary Internal Medicine, 4th ed. Philadelphia: WB Saunders, 1992, p 874.

3. Atkins CE, Gallo AM, Kurzman ID, *et al.*: Risk factors, clinical signs, and survival in cats with a clinical diagnosis of idiopathic hypertrophic cardiomyopathy: 74 cases (1985–1989). *J Am Vet Med Assoc* 201:613, 1992.
4. Kittleson MD: Hypertrophic Cardiomyopathy. *In* Kittleson MD, Kienle RD, eds.: Small Animal Cardiovascular Medicine. St. Louis: Mosby, 1998, p 347.
5. Bright JM, McEntee MM: Isolated right ventricular cardiomyopathy (right ventricular dysplasia) in a bull mastiff. *J Am Vet Med Assoc* 207:64, 1995.
6. Fox PR, Maron BJ, Basso C *et al.*: Spontaneously occurring arrhythmogenic right ventricular cardiomyopathy in the domestic cat. *Circulation* 102:1863, 2000.
7. Pion PD, Kittleson MD, Rogers QR *et al.*: Myocardial failure in cats associated with low plasma taurine: a reversible cardiomyopathy. *Science* 237:764, 1987.
8. Sisson DD, Knight DH, Helinski C, *et al.*: Plasma taurine concentration and M-mode echocardiographic measures in healthy cats and in cats with dilated cardiomyopathy. *J Am Vet Med Assoc* 5:232, 1991.
9. Kittleson MD: Primary myocardial disease leading to chronic myocardial failure (dilated cardiomyopathy and related disorders). *In* Kittleson MD, Kienle RD, eds.: Small Animal Cardiovascular Medicine. St. Louis: Mosby, 1998, p 319.
10. Muers KM: Insights into the hereditability of canine cardiomyopathy. *Vet Clin North Am* 28:1449, 1998.
11. Muers KM, Spier AW, Miller NW, *et al.*: Familial dysrhythmia is inherited as an autosomal dominant trait in selected boxer families [abstract]. *J Vet Intern Med* 12: 199, 1998.
12. Dambach DM, Lannon A, Sleeper MM, *et al.*: Familial dilated cardiomyopathy of young Portuguese water dogs. *J Vet Intern Med* 13:65, 1999.
13. Dukes-McEwan J: Dilated cardiomyopathy (DCM) in Newfoundland dogs. *Proc Am Coll Vet Intern Med* 18:118, 2000.
14. Hammer TA, Venta PI, Eyster GE: The genetic basis of dilated cardiomyopathy in Doberman pinschers [abstract]. *Anim Genet* 27:109, 1999.
15. Arber S, Hunter JJ, Ross J Jr, *et al.*: MLP-deficient mice exhibit a disruption of cardiac cytoarchitectural organization, dilated cardiomyopathy, and heart failure. *Cell* 88:393, 1997.
16. Olson TM, Michels VV, Thibodeau SN, *et al.*: Actin mutations in dilated cardiomyopathy, a heritable form of heart failure. *Science* 280:750,1998.
17. Kamisogo M, Sharma SD, DePalma SR, *et al.*: Mutations in sarcomere protein genes as a cause of dilated cardiomyopathy. *N Engl J Med* 343:1688, 2000.
18. Kittleson MD, Keene B, Pion PD, *et al.*: Results of the Multicenter Spaniel Trial (MUST): taurine and carnitine responsive dilated cardiomyopathy in American cocker spaniels with decreased plasma taurine concentration. *J Vet Intern Med* 11: 204, 1997.
19. Kramer GA, Kittleson MD, Fox PR, *et al.*: Plasma taurine concentrations in normal dogs and in dog with heart disease. *J Vet Intern Med* 9:253, 1995.
20. Freeman LM, Michel KE, Brown DJ, *et al.*: Idiopathic dilated cardiomyopathy in Dalmations: nine cases (1990–1995). *J Am Vet Med Assoc* 209:1592,1996.
21. Freeman LM, Rush JE, Brown DJ, *et al.*: Relationship between circulating and dietary taurine concentrations in dogs with dilated cardiomyopathy [abstract]. *J Vet Intern Med* 14:336, 2000.
22. Keene BW, Panciera DP, Atkins CE, *et al.*: Myocardial L-carnitine deficiency in a family of dogs with dilated cardiomyopathy. *J Am Vet Med Assoc* 198:647, 1991.

23. O'Brien PJ: Rapid ventricular pacing of dogs to heart failure: biochemical and physiological studies. *Can J Physiol Pharmacol* 68:34, 1990.
24. Zupan I, Rakovec P, Budihna N, *et al.*: Tachycardia-induced cardiomyopathy in dogs; relation between chronic supraventricular and chronic ventricular tachycardia. *Int J Cardiol* 56:75, 1996.
25. Grogan M, Smith HC, Gersh BJ, *et al.*: Left ventricular dysfunction due to atrial fibrillation in patients initially believed to have idiopathic dilated cardiomyopathy. *Am J Cardiol* 69:1570, 1992.
26. Fenelon G, Wijins W, Andries E, *et al.*: Tachycardiomyopathy: mechanisms and clinical implications. *PACE* 19:95, 1996.
27. Wright KN, Mehdirad AA, Giacobbe P, *et al.*: Radiofrequency catheter ablation of atrioventricular accessory pathways in 3 dogs with subsequent resolution of tachycardia-induced cardiomyopathy. *J Vet Intern Med* 13:361, 1999.
28. Mann DL: Mechanisms and models in heart failure: a combinatorial approach. *Circulation* 100:999, 1999.
29. Cohn JN: Structural basis for heart failure: ventricular remodeling and its pharmacological inhibition. *Circulation* 91:2504, 1995.
30. Lord PF: Left ventricular diastolic stiffness in dogs with congestive cardiomyopathy and volume overload. *Am J Vet Res* 37:953, 1976.
31. Shen WF, Tribouilloy C, Rey J-L, *et al.*: Prognostic significance of Doppler-derived left ventricular diastolic filling variables in dilated cardiomyopathy. *Am Heart J* 124:1524, 1992.
32. Calvert CA, Pickus CW, Jacobs G, *et al.*: Clinical and pathologic findings in Doberman pinschers with occult cardiomyopathy that died or developed congestive heart failure: 54 cases (1984–1991). *J Am Vet Med Assoc* 210:505, 1997.
33. Calvert CA, Jacobs G, Pickus CW, *et al.*: Results of ambulatory electrocardiography in overtly healthy Doberman pinschers with echocardiographic abnormalities. *J Am Vet Med Assoc* 217:1328, 2000.
34. Harpster NK: Boxer cardiomyopathy. *In* Kirk RW, ed.: Current Veterinary Therapy XIII, Philadelphia: WB Saunders, 1999, p 329.
35. Vollmar AC: The prevalence of cardiomyopathy in the Irish wolfhound: a clinical study of 500 dogs. *J Am Anim Hosp Assoc* 36:125, 2000.
36. Brownlie SE, Cobb MA: Observations on the development of congestive heart failure in Irish wolfhounds with dilated cardiomyopathy. *J Small Anim Prac* 40:371, 1999.
37. Szatalowicz VL, Arnold PE, Chaimovitz C, *et al.*: Radioimmunoassay of plasma arginine vasopressin in hyponatremic patients with congestive heart failure. *N Engl J Med* 305:263, 1981.
38. Saxon LA, Stevenson WG, Middlekauff HR, *et al.*: Predicting death from progressive heart failure secondary to ischemic or idiopathic dilated cardiomyopathy. *Am J Cardiol* 72:62, 1993.
39. Eichhorn EJ: Medical therapy of chronic heart failure: role of ACE inhibitors and beta-blockers. *Cardiol Clin* 16:711, 1998.
40. Ettinger SJ, Benitz AM, Ericsson GF, *et al.*: Effects of enalapril maleate on survival of dogs with naturally acquired heart failure. The Long-Term Investigation of Veterinary Enalapril (LIVE) Study Group. *J Am Vet Med Assoc* 213:1573, 1998.
41. Calvert CA: Effect of medical therapy on survival of patients with dilated cardiomyopathy. *Vet Clin North Am* 21:919, 1991.
42. Luis-Fuentes V, Kleemann R, Justus C *et al.*: The effect of the novel inodilator pimobendan on heart failure status in cocker spaniels and Dobermanns with idiopathic dilated cardiomyopathy [abstract]. *Proc Ingelheimer Dialog mit Herz*, 2000.

43. Lombard CW: Therapy of congestive heart failure in dogs with pimobendan. *Proc Am Coll Vet Intern Med* 18:107, 2000.
44. Packer M, Cohn JN, eds.: Consensus recommendations for the management of chronic heart failure. *Am J Cardiol* 83 (suppl 2A):35A, 1999.
45. Sabbah HN, Shimoyama H, Kono T, *et al.*: Effects of long-term monotherapy with enalapril, metoprolol, and digoxin on the progression of left ventricular dysfunction and dilation in dogs with reduced ejection fraction. *Circulation* 89:2852, 1994.
46. MERIT-HF Study Group: Effect of metoprolol CR/XL in chronic heart failure: metoprolol CR/XL randomised intervention trial in congestive heart failure (MERIT-HF). *Lancet* 353:2001, 1999.
47. Bristow MR: What type of β-blocker should be used to treat chronic heart failure? *Circulation* 102: 484, 2000.
48. Colucci WS: Should cardio-protective therapy begin earlier? Proceedings from Challenges in Heart Failure Management: New Evidence, News Answers. November 2000, Atalnta, GA (a CME Satellite Symposium sponsored by the University of Cincinnati School of Medicine).
49. Calvert CA, Pickus CW, Jacobs G, *et al.*: Signalment, survival, and prognostic factors in Doberman pinschers with end-stage cardiomyopathy. *J Vet Intern Med* 11: 323, 1997.
50. Monnet E, Orton EC, Salman M, *et al.*: Idiopathic dilated cardiomyopathy in dogs: Survival and prognostic indicators. *J Vet Intern Med* 9:12, 1995.
51. Liu S-K, Maron BJ, Tilley LP: Canine hypertrophic cardiomyopathy. *J Am Vet Med Assoc* 174:708, 1979.
52. Amberger CN, Glardon O, Glaus T, *et al.*: Effects of benazapril in the treatment of feline hypertrophic cardiomyopathy. Results of a prospective, open label, multicenter clinical trial. *J Vet Cardiol* 1:12, 1999.
53. Fox PR: Feline cardiomyopathies. *In* Fox PR, ed.: Textbook of Canine and Feline Cardiology. Philadelphia: WB Saunders, 1999, p 621.
54. Peterson, ME, Taylor R, Greco DS, *et al.*: Acromegaly in 14 cats. *J Vet Intern Med.* 4:192, 1990.
55. Maron BJ: Hypertrophic cardiomyopathy. *In* Alexander RW, Schlant RC, Fuster V, eds.: Hurst's The Heart, 9th ed. New York: McGraw-Hill, 1998, p 2057.
56. Marian AJ, Roberts R: Molecular genetics of hypertrophic cardiomyopathy. *Annu Rev Med* 46:213, 1995.
57. Kittleson MD, Muers KM, Munro MJ, *et al.*: Familial hypertrophic cardiomyopathy in Maine Coon cats: an animal model of human disease. *Circulation* 99:3172, 1999.
58. Meurs K, Kittleson, MD, Towbin J, *et al.*: Familial systolic anterior motion of the mitral valve and/or hypertrophic cardiomyopathy is apparently inherited as an autosomal dominant trait in a family of American shorthair cats. *Proc Am Coll Vet Intern Med* 15:685, 1997.
59. Baty C: Familial hypertrophic cardiomyopathy: man, mouse, and cat. *Q J Med* 91: 791, 1998.
60. Rush JE: Therapy of feline hypertrophic cardiomyopathy. *Vet Clin North Am* 28: 1459, 1998.
61. Fox PR, Liu S-K, Maron BJ: Echocardiographic assessment of spontaneously occurring feline hypertrophic cardiomyopathy. *Circulation* 92:2645, 1995.
62. Manganelli F, Betocchi S, Losi MA, *et al.*: Influence of left ventricular cavity size on clinical presentation in hypertrophic cardiomyopathy. *Am J Cardiol* 83:547, 1999.
63. Black IW, Hopkins AP, Lee LCL, *et al.*: Left atrial spontaneous echo contrast: a clinical and echocardiographic analysis. *J Am Coll Cardiol* 18:398, 1991.

64. Bright JM, Herrtage ME, Schneider JF: Pulsed Doppler assessment of left ventricular diastolic function in normal and cardiomyopathic cats. *J Am Hosp Assoc* 35:285, 1999.
65. Fox PR: Evidence for and against beta-blockers and aspirin for management of feline cardiomyopathies. *Vet Clin North Am* 21:1011, 1977.
66. Bright JM, Golden L, Gompf R, *et al.*: Evaluation of the calcium channel-blocking agents diltiazem and verapamil for treatment of feline hypertrophic cardiomyopathy. *J Vet Intern Med* 5:272, 1991.
67. Fox PR: Feline Cardiomyopathies. *In* Fox PR, ed.: Textbook of Canine and Feline Cardiology. Philadelphia: WB Saunders, 1999, p 621.
68. Harpster NK, Baty CJ: Warfarin therapy of the cat at risk of thromboembolism. *In* Kirk RW, ed.: Current Veterinary Therapy XII. Philadelphia: WB Saunders, 1995, p 868.
69. Harpster NK, Baty CJ: Warfarin therapy of the cat at risk of thromboembolism. *In* Kirk RW, ed.: Current Veterinary Therapy XII. Philadelphia: WB Saunders, 1995, p 868.
70. Ammash NM, Seward JB, Bailey KR, *et al.*: Clinical profile and outcome of idiopathic restrictive cadiomyopathy. *Circulation* 101:2490, 2000.
71. Rush JE: Therapy of feline hypertrophic cardiomyopathy. *Vet Clin North Am* 28: 1459, 1998.
72. Stalis IH, Bossbaly MJ, Van Winkle TJ: Feline endomyocarditis and left ventricular endocardial fibrosis. *Vet Pathol* 32:122, 1995.
73. Meurs KM, Fox PR, Magnon A, *et al.*: Polymerase chain reaction (PCR) analysis for feline viruses in formalin-fixed cardiomyopathic hearts identifies panleukopenia. *J Vet Intern Med* 12:201, 1998.
74. Bonagura JD, Fox PR: Restrictive cardiomyopathy. *In* Kirk RW, ed.: Current Veterinary Therapy XII. Philadelphia: WB Saunders, 1995, p 863.
75. Kittleson MD, Kittleson JA, Mekhamer Y: Development and progression of inherited hypertrophic cardiomyopathy in Maine Coon cats [abstract]. *Proc Am Coll Vet Intern Med* 14:747, 1996.
76. Cetta F, O'Leary PW, Seward JB, *et al.*: Idiopathic restrictive cardiomyopathy in childhood: diagnostic features and clinical course. *Mayo Clin Proc* 70:634, 1995.

SECTION V
Respiratory Failure

35
Near Drowning

Sheila McCullough

Near drowning is the third most common cause of accidental death and is the second most common cause of death in humans under 44 years. Near drowning incidents in the US are estimated to be 15,000–70,000 per year.[1–3] The incidence in companion animals is unknown.

Near drowning accidents are divided into **immersion syndrome** and **submersion injuries. Immersion syndrome** results in immediate death upon cold water contact. **Submersion injury** is divided into three groups: **drowning, near drowning,** and **save.** Drowning is a submersion injury that produces death within 24 hours. Near drowning may result in either **secondary drowning** or **survival.** Secondary drowning is defined as death from complications of submersion. Patients in the survival subgroup may require medical intervention to support life during the critical post incident period. A primary save is when the victim is rescued without any adverse effects which require medical intervention.

Based on existing literature, near drowning is the patient category that requires intensive support and care. For this reason, the focus of this chapter will be based on the near drowning syndrome and associated complications.

PATHOPHYSIOLOGY OF NEAR DROWNING

The majority of submersion accidents (>85%) result in pulmonary fluid aspiration.[2–4] The saline content of the aspirated fluid (salt vs. fresh water) plays a significant role in the systemic pathology produced by the near drowning incident. Fresh or salt water aspiration may produce laryngospasm, pulmonary edema, and acute respiratory distress syndrome (ARDS). Systemic hypoxemia and hypovolemia may precipitate myocardial ischemia, acute renal failure, acute hepatic failure, and multiple organ dysfunction syndrome (MODS).[2–4] Anoxic brain damage results in cerebral edema, increased intracranial pressure and permanent ischemic damage.

Fresh Water Aspiration

Fresh water dilutes pulmonary surfactant creating an increased alveolar surface tension, alveolar collapse, and atelectasis increasing ventilation-perfusion mismatch and intrapulmonary shunt.[2–4,7–9] The physical presence of water in alveoli also interferes with normal gas exchange by creating a diffusion barrier for oxygen. Water is rapidly absorbed from the alveolus into the bloodstream expanding intravascular free water volume. This expansion does not generally cause electrolyte imbalance. Large volume aspiration may create dilutional hyponatremia and potassium shifts secondary to red cell lysis and hypoxic tissue damage.[2–4,7–9]

Salt Water Aspiration

The presence of salt water in the alveolus does not disturb surfactant production from Type II pneumocytes; thus, atelectasis is not a main feature of salt water aspiration. In contrast to fresh water, systemic hypoxemia is mainly associated with alveolar flooding.[2–4,7–9] The mechanism responsible for this effect is redistribution of intravascular fluid into the alveoli because of the increased osmolarity inherent in salt water. Intravascular fluid depletion results in hemoconcentration, hypovolemia, and hypotension.[2–9] Electrolyte disturbances (hypernatremia) are clinically significant when greater than 22 ml/kg of fluid is aspirated in adults.[2–9] Secondary electrolyte disturbances such as hypercalcemia and hypermagnesemia are seen in high mineral content water.[2–9]

A minority (less than 12%) of near drowning victims do not aspirate large water volume.[2–4] In these patients, aspirated water triggers severe laryngospasm. It is theorized that continued breathing efforts during this period will create negative pressure pulmonary edema. Intrathoracic pressure changes secondary to laryngospasm increase intrathoracic blood volume, increase pulmonary artery pressure, and decrease pulmonary interstitial pressure.[2–4,7–9] The combination of these events produces fluid movement into the interstitial space and edema formation.

Immersion in cold water will elicit the "dive reflex" that creates severe bradycardia and intense peripheral vasoconstriction. Peripheral blood is shunted to the body core and total body hypothermia occurs. Hypothermia decreases basal metabolic rate and oxygen consumption thus shielding the body from the damaging effects of prolonged hypoxemia. However, prolonged hypothermia may result in fatal arrhythmias.

CLINICAL PRESENTATION

Clinical presentation in near drowning patients is highly variable. A key diagnostic indicator is level of consciousness at time of presentation. Patients that arrive with a normal level of consciousness do not generally demonstrate vital sign changes or abnormal physical findings. Patients that arrive with a depressed level of consciousness must be carefully evaluated for systemic injury. A thorough physical exam, thoracic auscultation, and vital sign collection (ECG, BP,SaO_2, temperature) will focus the clinician on possible organ injury and secondary pathology.

If loss of consciousness is present, it must be determined if this occurred as part of or prior to submersion (concussive injuries). This point is important in that the sequence determines whether near drowning patients may have ingested large volumes of water or stomach contents.

It is imperative for the clinician to remember that prognostic indicators (mentioned below) are reliable but not absolutely predictive in every patient.

DIAGNOSTIC EVALUATION

Despite attempts to determine definitive prognostic indicators for near drowning victims, there is limited information in the literature to guide the emergency clinician. It is critical that the clinician evaluate and treat each case aggressively regardless of presentation. Near drowning victims that arrive in a conscious state without neurologic injury have an excellent chance of survival. Patients that arrive in a depressed state of consciousness should be extensively evaluated. The use of scoring systems such as the Orlowski score, Glascow Coma Scale, and Pediatric Risk of Mortality (PRISM) have been evaluated with mixed results. Evaluation of the Small Animal Coma Scale in near drowning victims has not been reported in the literature.

Initial evaluation includes a complete blood count, chemistry panel, and arterial blood gas. If possible, an arterial line should be placed and serial blood gases should be evaluated as the patient is being re-warmed. Blood gases that reveal metabolic acidosis (pH $<$ 7.1) and hypoxemia should be aggressively treated with fluid infusion and oxygen. Patients that exhibit severe hypoxemia and hypercarbia may benefit from ventilation, pulse oximetry, and capnography.

Serial monitoring of the electrolyte status is beneficial in all patients.[7–9] Patients may experience hypernatremia, hyperkalemia, and hypermagnesemia. In addition, monitoring of the patient's cardiac status is advised during re-warming due to arrhythmia potential.[3–4,8–9] Any patient that has sustained head or spine trauma should be evaluated with a CT scan. Normal CT scans within the first 24 hours are not always predictive of a positive outcome. Serial evaluation of the patient's neurological status is necessary. Unmanaged seizure activity during this period may contribute to a poor outcome.

TREATMENT

The degree of cerebral damage sustained during the immersion period is the limiting factor for survival. Resuscitation should be directed at maintaining cerebral perfusion and oxygenation and decreasing intracranial pressure.

Near drowning victims should be removed from the water and resuscitation measures immediately started. Prehospital care should include airway management, oxygen delivery, and ventilatory support. An intravascular access should be established to provide fluid support. CPR and slow re-warming should be started during transport to the nearest hospital. An electrocardiogram (EKG) should be monitored during patient re-warming.[4,7–9]

Upon arrival at a facility, vital signs (temperature, pulse, respiration), blood pressure, central venous pressure (CVP), and urine output should be continuously monitored. In fresh water aspiration cases, CVP will generally increase in the immediate post aspiration period and return to baseline values within 1 to 2 hours. Aspiration of large amounts of salt water will initially increase then decrease CVP as the onset of pulmonary edema occurs (decrease in effective circulating blood volume)[2–4,7–9] Sequential evaluation of blood gases, electrolytes, glucose, and visceral organ function is essential to determine secondary organ pathology.

Secondary survey may indicate a need for mechanical ventilation. Supplemental support using continuous positive airway pressure (CPAP) or positive end-expiratory pressure (PEEP) may be necessary to maintain lung expansion and improve gas exchange. Ventilatory therapy may required for 2–3 days until surfactant activity recovers. Fresh water injury usually requires longer ventilatory times than salt water aspiration due to surfactant dilution. The use of warm butyl alcohol in salt water aspiration victims has shown moderate success in breaking down small bubbles thought to cause small airway obstruction.

Hospital based resuscitation should also be directed at maintaining cerebral perfusion and oxygen delivery and decreasing intracranial pressure. Controversy exists regarding specific therapeutic **management of neurologic sequelae** in near drowning patients. Management of increased intracranial pressure may require use of mannitol, anti-convulsants, and controlled ventilation (see chapter 71). Administration of steroids has not been proven effective for intracranial pressure management. The treatment of secondary brain injury with free radical scavengers, prostaglandin antagonists, calcium channel blockers, dimethylsulfoxide, opiate receptor antagonists, and anesthetics is currently under investigation.[3] Antibiotic usage should be reserved for patients that have aspirated contaminated water or stomach contents.

PROGNOSIS

Numerous studies have shown that key factors in survival include the time from incident to CPR, the quality of resuscitation, and the degree of intensive care monitoring. Factors associated with a grave prognosis include submersion time greater than 5 minutes, initial pH less than 7.1 on presentation, requirement for continued CPR upon arrival at the hospital (except ice-water injuries), persistence of a coma in the emergency room, fixed and dilated pupils, elevated ICP, and young age (<3 years old).[3] The likelihood of survival increases if cold water immersion occurs.

The degree of central nervous system damage is a key prognostic indicator. Approximately 25% of near-drowning victims will die and another 6% will develop permanent neurologic sequelae.[4] Level of consciousness upon arrival at the hospital appears to be the most positive prognostic indicator. Human patients who arrive at the hospital either awake or with a blunted level of consciousness have an excellent chance for normal survival with intensive pulmonary and cardiovascular care. In one study, 40-50% of children who are comatose on admission survive normally.[3] Early prognostic evaluation of near drowning patients may be difficult. Use of scoring systems such as the Orlowski score, Glascow Coma Scale, and Pediatric Risk of Mortality (PRISM) have been evaluated for prognostic prediction with mixed results. Retrospective studies caution that in near-drowning victims normal CT scans within the first 24 hours are not always predictive of a positive outcome.[7–9] Diagnostic evaluation of human patients measuring evoked potentials is a reliable tool in predicting patient outcome.[6]

References

1. Sachdeva, RC: Near Drowning Environmental Emergencies. *Critical Care Clinics* Vol 15 No. 2, April 1999 pp 281–296
2. Gallagher TJ: Drowning. *In:* Critical Care Medicine. pp 1415–1417
3. Goodwin, SR, *et al.*: Near-Drowning: Adult and Children. *In:* Textbook of Critical Care, 3rd ed. pp 65–74.
4. Weinstein MD, Krieger BP: Near-drowning: epidemiology, pathophysiology and initial treatment. *Jrn Emerg Med,* Vol. 14, No. 4, pp 461–467, 1996.
5. Spack L, Gedeit R, Splaingard M, Havens PL: Failure of aggressive therapy to alter outcome in pediatric near-drowning. *Ped Emerg Care,* Vol. 13, No. 2, 1997.
6. Goodwin SR, Friedman WA, Bellefleur M: Is it time to use evoked potentials to predict outcome
7. Martin L: Near Drowning. Critical Care and Emergency Medicine Veterinary Secrets
8. Modell JH: Drowning. *N Eng J Med,* 328:253–6, 1993.
9. Olshaker JS: Near-drowning. *Emerg Med Clin North Am,* 10:339–50, 1992.

36
Acute Respiratory Distress Syndrome

Lesley G. King and Lori S. Waddell

INTRODUCTION AND TERMINOLOGY

Acute respiratory distress syndrome (ARDS) is a severe inflammatory disorder of the lung that is a common cause of respiratory failure in critically ill dogs and cats. Numerous synonyms exist, including "shock lung," "traumatic wet lung," "adult hyaline membrane disease," and "capillary leak syndrome." All these terms refer to the same syndrome of lung inflammation, cellular infiltration, and capillary leak, which can be classified as a form of noncardiogenic pulmonary edema. The clinical presentation of this syndrome is variable in severity, with a spectrum from subclinical to fulminating. The consensus terminology is that all degrees of this syndrome should be referred to as acute lung injury (ALI), and arbitrarily that the most severe manifestation should be termed ARDS.[1] Older terminology using the term "adult" rather than "acute" has now been discarded in human medicine in recognition of the fact that the syndrome is not found exclusively in adult humans.[1] We recommend that the term "acute" should also be used in veterinary patients for the same reason.

PATHOGENESIS AND RISK FACTORS

The response of the lung to an acute insult is fairly stereotypical and predictable. The inflammation that results in ALI and ARDS may originate in the lung itself due to a direct pulmonary insult, or it may be part of a generalized inflammatory response syndrome (Table 36-1). In the small animal CCU, ARDS is most commonly seen as a sequela of the systemic inflammatory response syndrome (SIRS) or sepsis.

In sepsis, a generalized inflammatory process (SIRS) is triggered by bacterial endotoxin, which results in activation of tumor necrosis factor and proinflammatory interleukins, thus initiating an avalanche of diverse inflammatory mediators and activation of cells such as neutrophils and macrophages. This common pathway of inflammation can affect the function of any or all organ systems in the septic patient. The progression of disease is related to a balance between proinflammatory and anti-inflammatory mediators in the lung and in the systemic circulation. Patients with SIRS that develop respiratory failure due to ARDS are simply demonstrating a local pulmonary manifestation of global SIRS.

There are a few reports of ARDS as a result of SIRS in the veterinary literature, and it is important to remember that SIRS is not always triggered by

Table 36-1. Risk Factors for Development of ALI and ARDS

Primary Pulmonary Disorders	Systemic and Nonpulmonary Disorders
• Aspiration pneumonia • Pulmonary contusion • Bacterial pneumonia • Smoke inhalation • Oxygen toxicity • Fat embolism • Near drowning • Noncardiogenic pulmonary edema ➢ Strangulation ➢ Head trauma ➢ Seizures	• Sepsis ➢ Parvoviral infection ➢ Dermatitis/cellulitis ➢ Catheter related ➢ Pyometra ➢ Endocarditis • Systemic inflammatory response syndrome ➢ Organ torsion (stomach, spleen, lung lobe) ➢ Pancreatitis ➢ Severe shock ➢ Multiple transfusions ➢ Cardiopulmonary bypass

bacterial sepsis. Organ torsion, a frequent occurrence in dogs, may trigger SIRS as a result of tissue necrosis without endotoxemia.[2,3] Sepsis due to canine parvoviral enteritis resulted in ARDS in 69% of dogs in one study of necropsy findings.[4] Necrotizing pancreatitis is another common cause of SIRS and ALI, secondary to vascular endothelial damage by activated proteases and associated inflammation.[5]

Alternatively, ARDS may be triggered by local pulmonary injury states such as severe aspiration or bacterial pneumonia, pulmonary contusions, or smoke inhalation. These insults may trigger an inflammatory response that can become generalized within the lung parenchyma. Proinflammatory cytokines may also be locally produced in the lung by inflammatory cells, lung epithelial cells, or fibroblasts. Dogs with noncardiogenic pulmonary edema after strangulation, choking, or seizures may occasionally demonstrate fulminating, rapidly progressive ARDS.[2,3] ARDS has also been reported in one dog following severe trauma and pulmonary contusions.[6] These case reports highlight another feature of ARDS; often multiple etiologies may be present and the inflammatory response may occur as a result of both direct lung injury and SIRS due to severe shock.

Occasionally, ARDS occurs for no apparent reason. In one case series of 19 dogs with histopathologically documented ARDS, predisposing factors could not be identified in 5 of the dogs.[2] Another case series of 11 related young Dalmatian dogs documented ALI similar to ARDS of unknown etiology.[7] It is unclear, however, whether this group of dogs suffered from the same syndrome commonly seen in the small animal CCU.

Because the lung has only one way to respond to inflammatory damage, the clinical and histopathologic findings are similar for all etiologies. In dogs with ARDS, the initial stages of the syndrome begin as a diffuse exudative vascular

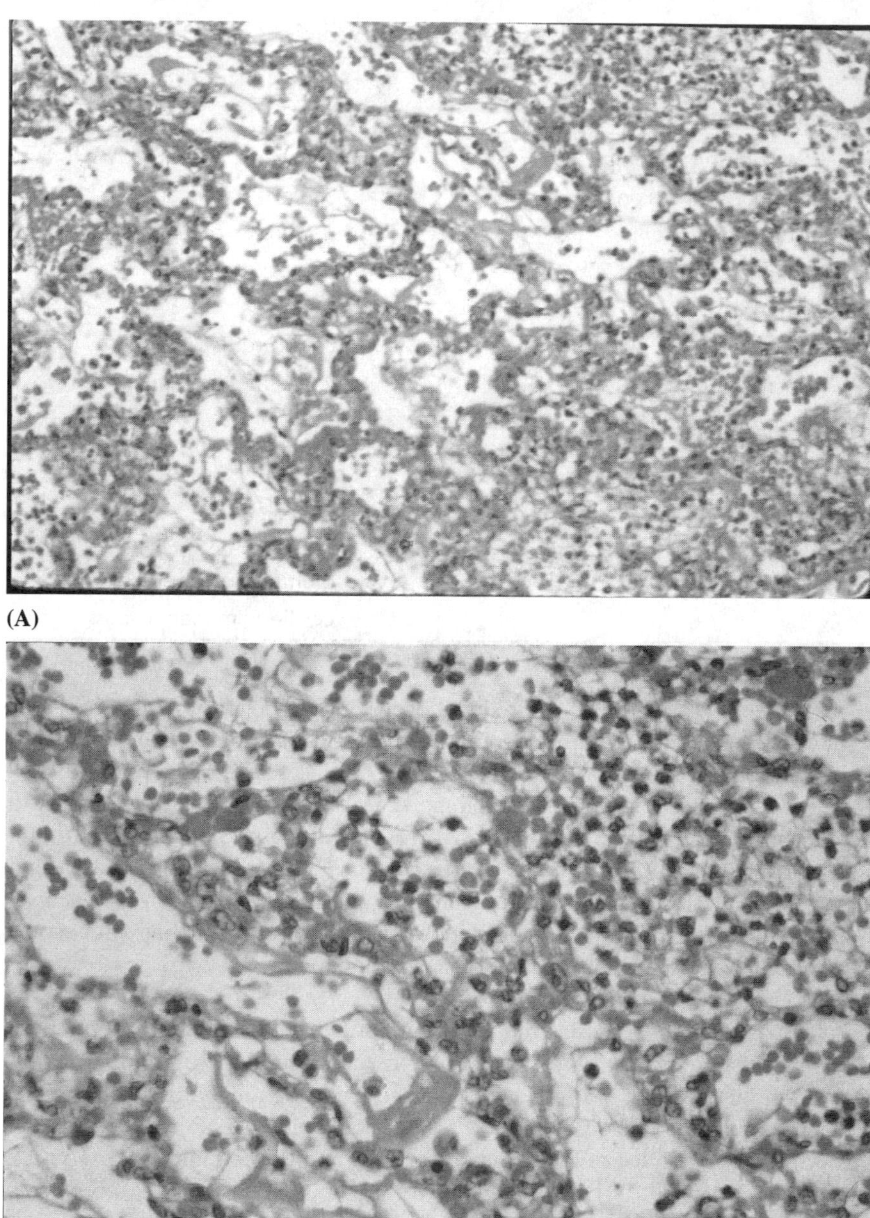

Figure 36-1
Histopathology of the lung of a dog with acute ARDS diagnosed on postmortem examination (×20 and ×40). The capillaries are dilated and filled with red blood cells. The alveoli contain a mixture of red cells, neutrophils, macrophages, and strands of fibrin. (Courtesy of Dr. Tom Van Winkle, Laboratory of Pathology, University of Pennsylvania.)

leak syndrome with infiltration of neutrophils and macrophages into the lung. This is accompanied by effusion of protein-rich fluid into the alveoli and clinical evidence of progressive pulmonary edema (Fig. 36-1) Accumulation of inflammatory cells in the lung, particularly neutrophils, occurs as a result of chemotaxis associated with the inflammation; this contributes to the severity of ongoing lung injury. As ongoing inflammation is combined with early repair attempts, there is proliferation of type II pneumocytes, formation of hyaline membranes within alveoli (organization of protein-rich fluid and cellular debris), deficiency of surfactant, and collapse and atelectasis of alveoli. This is later followed by interstitial fibrosis as the lung attempts to repair the damaged tissue. The inflammatory changes vary in severity and are often unevenly distributed in the lung. In more severely affected animals, the inflammation is profound, overwhelming, and leads to severe hypoxia.

CLINICAL PRESENTATION

Acute lung injury occurs commonly in CCU patients. The earliest signs often include progressive hypoxia and tachypnea. Low-grade productive coughing may be seen, but most of these patients do not cough. If the lung injury is severe enough to be termed ARDS, gas exchange is severely impaired and dyspnea is profound.[2] ARDS is clinically recognized by the development of pulmonary edema in an animal with a predisposing cause of an inflammatory response, and without evidence of heart failure. Animals that have ARDS are usually cyanotic when breathing room air. Auscultation reveals harsh lung sounds that rapidly progress to crackles. Dogs with ARDS may expectorate pink foam, and if intubated, sanguinous fluid may drain out of the endotracheal tube.

DIAGNOSTIC EVALUATION

Arterial blood gases usually reveal severe hypoxia.[3] Typically, hypocarbia occurs as hypoxia takes over the respiratory drive and the animal hyperventilates in an attempt to improve oxygenation. Animals with end-stage lungs or respiratory muscle fatigue may have normal or even high $PaCO_2$ values. Metabolic acidosis may be present due to poor oxygen (O_2) delivery and anaerobic tissue metabolism. Leukopenia is common, often due to sequestration of white blood cells in the periphery and in the lung. Thrombocytopenia is another frequent finding and is due to platelet sequestration or consumption. Consumptive coagulopathy may be manifested by prolonged coagulation times and elevated fibrin degradation products or D-dimers. The serum chemistry panel usually has nonspecific changes, but hypoalbuminemia occurs in many patients because of their underlying disease and exudative protein loss into the pulmonary edema fluid.

Animals with early ALI often have increased pulmonary interstitial and peribronchial markings on thoracic radiographs. As ALI progresses to ARDS, diffuse bilateral pulmonary alveolar infiltrates develop throughout all lung fields. The alveolar disease may be asymmetrical or patchy, and dependent lung lobes may be most severely affected (Fig. 36-2). A small pleural effusion may be present. For diagnosis of ARDS, it is important that the heart and blood vessels

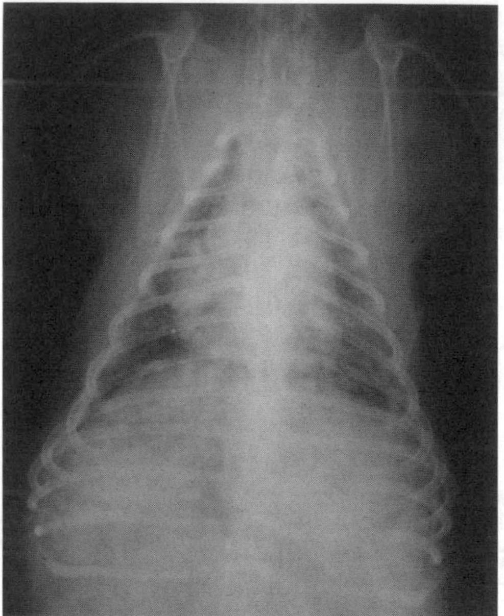

(A)

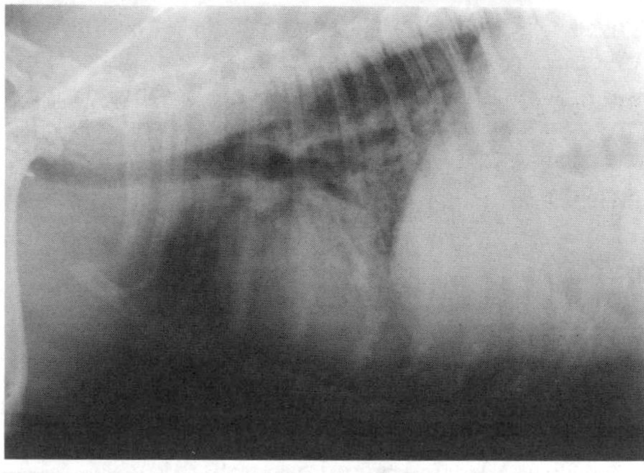

(B)

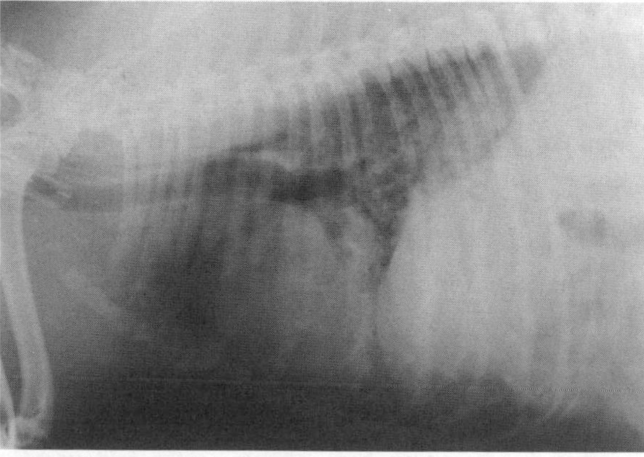

(C)

Figure 36-2
Radiographs of a 6-year-old female spayed mixed breed dog that presented with increased respiratory rate and effort. She was anesthetized for diagnostic testing, including these thoracic radiographs, which show a diffuse, patchy alveolar pattern consistent with ARDS. Her oxygenation status continued to decline despite positive pressure ventilation, and she was euthanized. On necropsy, a diagnosis of severe subacute to chronic interstitial pneumonia with ARDS was made.

are normal on the thoracic radiographs. Evidence of cardiomegaly or enlarged pulmonary vessels should prompt consideration of left-sided congestive heart failure rather than ARDS. Elevation of central venous pressure or pulmonary capillary wedge pressure (>18 mm Hg) can also help to suggest a component of congestive heart failure or fluid overload.

Oxygen tension indices are a useful way of monitoring pulmonary function in the ARDS patient. Alveolar-arterial O_2 tension gradients are usually high, routinely 500 to 600 mm Hg in one case series.[3] The ratios of PaO_2 to forced inspired O_2 (FIO_2) are also significantly low (reference range 432.4–564.6 mm Hg[8]). Typically, a PaO_2/FIO_2 ratio less than or equal to 300 is considered to be consistent with a diagnosis of ALI, whereas a PaO_2/FIO_2 ratio of less than or equal to 200 is considered to be consistent with a diagnosis of ARDS.[1] The lungs of animals with ARDS usually have poor compliance, and extremely high mean and peak airway pressures are noted when positive pressure ventilation is used. Pulmonary hypertension may occur in severely affected patients due to obliteration of the pulmonary capillary bed.

DIFFERENTIAL DIAGNOSIS

There are a number of important differential diagnoses for ALI and ARDS. Fluid overload and cardiogenic pulmonary edema are common differentials, especially in animals with documented heart disease or those that have received an aggressive volume of intravenous fluids. Atelectasis may contribute to alveolar lung disease in animals that have been recumbent or anesthetized for long periods. Atelectasis is typically associated with a mediastinal shift in the direction of the lung lobe collapse. The atelectatic alveolar pattern resolves quickly (within hours) following lung re-expansion. Pulmonary hemorrhage is another key differential diagnosis. A high index of suspicion should be noted in animals with coagulopathies or those that have developed ARDS following trauma. Pulmonary thromboembolism is a common complication of critical illness in dogs. Pulmonary thromboembolism typically causes hyperlucent lung fields, but severe thromboembolic disease can produce a diffuse alveolar pattern on thoracic radiographs. Bacterial pneumonia frequently occurs in critically ill dogs, often in addition to ALI or ARDS. However, bacterial pneumonia is typically distributed in the cranioventral lung fields on thoracic radiographs. Neoplastic infiltrates must be considered in any critically ill patient with undiagnosed disease.

MANAGEMENT OF PATIENTS WITH ALI AND ARDS

Patients with ALI or ARDS are extremely critical and require intensive management. The first priority is to address the underlying cause of SIRS or primary lung injury. For example, splenectomy would be a priority in an animal with ARDS secondary to splenic torsion. In that case, ARDS is a sequela of SIRS secondary to tissue necrosis and cytokine activation. Removal of the necrotic tissue would be a priority to arrest the inflammatory response that initiated SIRS. Most primary lung injuries such as neurogenic pulmonary edema, smoke inhalation, or traumatic pulmonary contusions occur as a single insult, rather than an ongoing process. Therefore, resolution of the underlying disease has typically already occurred by the time ARDS has become established. Aspiration pneumonia is the exception because repeated episodes often occur and should be prevented to allow resolution of the ALI.

The second priority in the patient with ALI and ARDS is to carefully evaluate fluid therapy and the possible contribution of fluid overload to pulmonary dysfunction. Administration of intravenous fluids may result in worsening lung dysfunction secondary to increased pulmonary edema formation. However, it is important to give enough fluid support to ensure adequate tissue perfusion and O_2 delivery, because inadequate tissue O_2 delivery will tend to exacerbate SIRS. Thus, the ARDS lung should be kept relatively "dry," but care should be taken not to restrict fluids so much that tissue perfusion suffers. Measurement of central venous pressure or pulmonary capillary wedge pressure can provide invaluable information about the intravascular volume status. Serial measurements of body weight interpreted in conjunction with physical examination findings can significantly aid in clinical evaluation of the patient. If volume overload is present, judicious administration of diuretics such as furosemide often improves lung function. If fluid overload is not present, furosemide may not improve lung function. Furosemide may result in a deterioration of the patient's condition by decreasing the intravascular volume, resulting in diminished tissue O_2 delivery. Colloid support should be considered in the ARDS patient, because most are hypoproteinemic. Fresh-frozen plasma is the ideal colloid, because it also supplies coagulation factors and acute phase proteins in addition to albumin. If insufficient supplies of plasma are available, especially in large patients, synthetic colloids such as hetastarch should also be administered.

Oxygen supplementation is required for any patient with impaired gas exchange that produces hypoxemia. Animals with mild ALI often respond well to O_2 supplementation alone, but hypoxia is usually so severe in ARDS that simple O_2 supplementation is insufficient to correct hypoxemia. Many animals with ARDS require positive pressure ventilation to achieve adequate gas exchange. Positive end-expiratory pressure is required to recruit alveoli and increase functional residual capacity, thereby allowing ventilation at lower FIO_2 values and prevent cyclical alveolar reopening and stretching with each breath. Ideally, FIO_2 should be kept less than 0.6 to prevent O_2 toxicity from contributing to the acute lung injury. Current recommendations suggest that tidal volumes should be kept as low as possible (ideally 6-8 mL/kg) to prevent overdistention of relatively normal alveoli and shear stress, which can result in "volutrauma" and progression of lung injury.[9,10] Excessively high airway pressures (>30 cm H_2O) can cause worsening of lung permeability and also produce pneumothorax.[11,12] Pneumothorax can rapidly progress to tension pneumothorax in the patient receiving positive pressure ventilation, resulting in life-threatening desaturation and hypotension. Immediate thoracostomy tube placement and continuous negative pressure pleural evacuation are primary therapies. Permissive hypercapnia refers to acceptance of a higher than normal $PaCO_2$ (as long as respiratory acidosis is not severe), to minimize tidal volumes and airway pressures. Concurrent administration of bias-flow O_2 is another option, flushing out carbon dioxide from the dead space, thereby improving oxygenation.[13]

Additional future options for ventilation of animals that are not responding to conventional positive pressure ventilation may include high-frequency jet ventilation or liquid ventilation with perfluorocarbons. Advances such as synthetic surfactant therapy, inhaled nitric oxide, and other new drugs, which have begun to be useful in human medicine, have not yet been evaluated in dogs with naturally occurring disease.

Because of the variety of inflammatory cascades and cells that mediate inflammatory response in ARDS, specific anti-inflammatory drugs such as corticosteroids are largely ineffective for treatment, particularly in the early exudative and proliferative stages of the disease, and may cause immunosuppression that can exacerbate sepsis.

PROGNOSIS

Human beings with ARDS have an expected survival rate of 40% to 60%, depending on the underlying cause.[14] It is not unusual to see ventilation duration of 4 to 6 weeks. In humans, recovery is associated with gradual improvement of gas exchange and lung function over 6 to 12 months. Eventually radiographic abnormalities resolve completely, and pulmonary function often returns to normal, although histopathologic resolution has not been characterized.

Dogs and cats with full-blown ARDS are difficult to ventilate, and resources to maintain them on a ventilator for several weeks are often unavailable. The prognosis for dogs and cats with ARDS remains grave at this time.

REFERENCES

1. Bernard GR, Artigas A, Brigham KL, *et al.*: Report of the American-European Consensus Conference on Acute Respiratory Distress Syndrome: definitions, mechanisms, relevant outcomes, and clinical trial coordination. *J Crit Care* 9:72, 1994.
2. Parent C, King LG, Van Winkle TJ, Walker LM: Clinical and clinicopathologic findings in dogs with acute respiratory distress syndrome: 19 cases (1985–1993). *J Am Vet Med Assoc* 208:1419, 1996.
3. Parent C, King LG, Van Winkle TJ, Walker LM: Respiratory function and treatment in dogs with acute respiratory distress syndrome: 19 cases (1985–1993). *J Am Vet Med Assoc* 208:1428, 1996.
4. Turk J, Miller M, Brown T, *et al.*: Coliform septicemia and pulmonary disease associated with canine parvoviral enteritis: 88 cases (1987–1988). *J Am Vet Med Assoc* 196:771, 1990.
5. Lopez A, Lane IF, Hanna P: Adult respiratory distress syndrome in a dog with necrotizing pancreatitis. *Can Vet J* 36:240, 1995.
6. Orsher AN, Kolata RJ: Acute respiratory distress syndrome: case report and literature review. *J Am An Hosp Assoc* 18:41, 1982.
7. Jarvinen AK, Saario E, Andresen E, *et al.*: Lung injury leading to respiratory distress syndrome in young Dalmatian dogs. *J Vet Intern Med* 9:162, 1995.
8. Beal MW, Paglia DT, Griffin GM, *et al.*: Ventilatory failure, ventilator management, and outcome in 14 dogs with cervical spinal disease (1991–1999). *J Am Vet Med Assoc*. 218:1598, 2001.

9. Amato MBP, Barbas CSV, Medeiros DM, *et al.*: Effect of a protective ventilation strategy on mortality in the acute respiratory distress syndrome. *N Engl J Med* 338: 347, 1998.
10. Acute Respiratory Distress Syndrome Network. Ventilation with lower tidal volumes as compared with traditional tidal volumes for acute lung injury and the acute respiratory distress syndrome. *N Engl J Med* 342:1301, 2000.
11. Weg JG, Anzueto A, Malk RA, *et al.*: The relation of pneumothorax and other air leaks to mortality in the acute respiratory distress syndrome. *N Engl J Med* 338:341, 1998.
12. King LG, Hendricks JC: Positive pressure ventilation in dogs and cats: 41 cases (July 1990–January 1992). *J Am Vet Med Assoc* 204:1045, 1994.
13. Nahum A, Ravenscraft SA, Adams AB, Marini JJ: Inspiratory tidal volume sparing effects of tracheal gas insufflation in dogs with oleic acid-induced lung injury. *J Crit Care* 10:115, 1995.
14. Ware LB, Matthay MA: The acute respiratory distress syndrome. *N Engl J Med* 342: 1334, 2000.

37
Aspiration Pneumonitis

Elisa M. Mazzaferro

INTRODUCTION

Pulmonary inflammation resulting from aspiration of exogenous material into the respiratory system is known as aspiration pneumonitis.[1] Healthy animals frequently aspirate small amounts of foodstuff and fluid without complications.[2,3] However, numerous conditions including debilitation, altered level of consciousness, neuromuscular disease, immobility, compromised upper airway defense mechanisms, and breakdown of immunity predispose some animals to aspiration pneumonitis and its negative sequelae (Table 37-1).[2,4,5] Following aspiration, airway defense mechanisms must be compromised for aspiration pneumonitis to progress and produce pathology.[2] Four types or classifications of aspiration pneumonitis have been defined: (1) chemical pneumonitis, (2) reflex airway closure, (3) mechanical obstruction, and (4) infection.[2]

PATHOGENESIS

The development and extent of aspiration pneumonitis depends on the frequency, amount, and character of the aspirate and the status of normal host defense mechanisms (Table 37-2). The most common material aspirated is gastric contents. Three factors are involved in the pathogenesis of aspiration pneumonitis. First, bronchoconstriction and reflex airway closure occur when gastric contents with a pH less than 2.5 are aspirated. Second, damage to the respiratory endothelial membranes occurs immediately and dilutes and denatures the surfactant necessary for normal alveolar structure and opening.[6,7] Within 3 minutes of aspiration, alveoli collapse and contribute to atelectasis.[8] Further, necrosis of the epithelial layer and separation of endothelial cells from their basement membrane allows flooding of the alveoli with hemorrhage and proteinaceous edema fluid.[9] The interstitial and alveolar edema decreases lung compliance, increases work of breathing, pulmonary vascular resistance, and diffusion distance for oxygen (O_2) and carbon dioxide (CO_2). This contributes to regions of low ventilation (V/Q mismatch), intrapulmonary shunting, and venous admixture.[1,9] The resultant hypoxemia causes pulmonary vasoconstriction. In extreme cases, pulmonary vasospasm also promotes retention of CO_2.[9] Marked increases in pulmonary vascular resistance lead to right heart failure and right-to-left shunting.[9] Finally, the patient's condition is further complicated, within several hours by

Table 37-1. Predisposing Conditions for Aspiration Pneumonitis

Gastrointestinal System
Esophageal Disorders
Reflux esophagitis
Esophageal motility disorder
Vascular ring anomalies
Esophageal foreign body
Esophageal stricture
Megaesophagus
Idiopathic
Secondary to chronic vomiting
Myasthenia gravis
Cricopharyngeal achalasia
Gastric Disorders
Chronic vomiting
Pyloric outflow obstruction (mechanical or physiologic)
Gastroesophageal instussusception
Oropharygneal Disorders
Cleft palate
Force feeding
Nasopharygeal or nasoesophageal feeding
Swallowing disorder
Laryngeal paralysis
Dentistry
Nervous System
Altered level of consciousness
Central injury or disease
Anesthesia
General
Sedation
Seizures
Coma
Immobility
Myasthenia gravis
Coonhound paralysis
Botulism

Table 37-1. Continued

Altered airway defense mechanisms
Pharyngostomy tube
Endotracheal tube
Tracheostomy tube
Misplaced feeding tubes

rapid influx of neutrophils and edema fluid into the damaged areas of lung. Depending on the extent of injury, systemic hypotension and hypovolemia occur and worsen tissue perfusion, systemic hypoxemia, and lactic acidosis.

Aspiration of inert substances such as water, barium, and saline often causes a transient, self-limiting hypoxemia. However, large volumes of these substances can become life-threatening by causing mechanical obstruction of the airways and acute asphyxiation.[2] Regardless of pH, aspiration of particulate matter causes both mechanical obstruction and damage to the lower respiratory tree.[10,11] The severity and duration of lung injury following aspiration of particulate matter are more severe than aspiration of acidic fluids with a pH less than 2.5[2] (Fig. 37-1). Within 6 hours, flooding of alveoli with red blood cells, inflammatory cells, and edema fluid occurs. Within 48 hours, a granulomatous reaction composed of giant cells and macrophages is observed.[9,10,12] The severe inflammatory exudates cause further bronchiolitis and airway obstruction. Experimental inoculation of colloidal antacid solutions results in severe parenchymal pneumonitis and chronic inflammation.[13] Exogenous administration of lipoid compounds such as mineral oil also causes profuse chronic granulomatous inflammation within the lung parenchyma.[14]

Finally, the most common complicating factor in aspiration pneumonitis is the presence of bacteria. In animals, inoculation of aerobic, facultative, and anaerobic bacteria from the oropharynx, esophagus, and stomach is common.[15-17] The aspiration of gastric acid impairs the lung's normal ability to clear bacteria, resulting in an excellent medium for bacterial colonization.[15] Infection occurs immediately or appears days after the inciting event.[1] In humans, anaerobic bacteria appear to have an important role in the pathogenesis of bacterial aspiration

Table 37-2. Host Defense Mechanisms That Prevent Aspiration Pneumonitis

Reflex airway closure during swallowing
Cough reflex
Mucociliary transport apparatus
Normal pulmonary inflammatory cell function

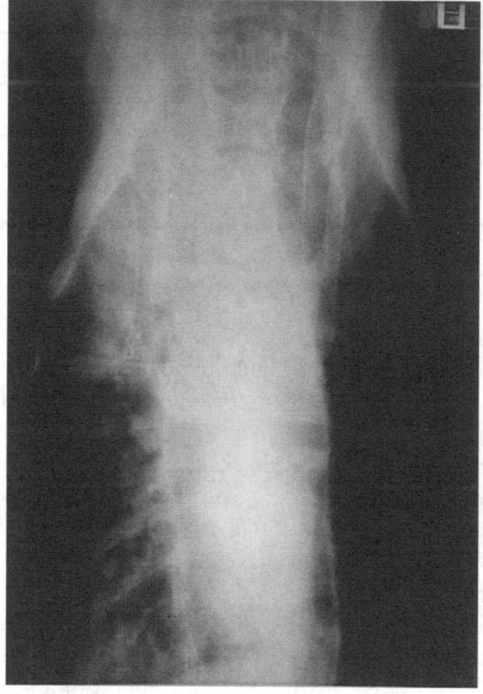

Figure 37-1
Pathophysiology of aspiration pneumonitis. Pathologic changes that occur following the aspiration event depend on the type and amount of substance aspirated. The presence or absence of particulate matter and whether the pH less than or greater than 2.5 are among the most important factors that determine if the aspiration pneumonitis will be self-limiting or become severe.

pneumonitis. Treatment against anaerobic bacteria alone, even in the presence of mixed infection, results in complete disease resolution.[18]

EPIDEMIOLOGY

The exact incidence of aspiration pneumonitis in veterinary patients is unknown. Conditions that predispose patients to aspiration pneumonitis are listed in Table 37-1. Aspiration pneumonitis occurs frequently in dogs with megaesophagus and laryngeal paralysis. Approximately 53% of human patients with dysphagia develop aspiration pneumonitis.[19] Although many acquired conditions predispose veterinary patients to aspiration, diagnostic and therapeutic procedures and treatments can also result in iatrogenic aspiration. These conditions include tube feeding,[20] general anesthesia with endotracheal intubation,[21] and tracheostomy.[22] Fifty-six percent of human tracheostomy patients develop aspiration pneumonitis.[22] The incidence of aspiration decreases with the use of high-volume low-pressure endotracheal cuffs and prescribing a period of fasting prior to general anesthesia.

CLINICAL PRESENTATION

Aspiration pneumonitis should be considered in any patient with a known predisposing condition (see Table 37-1). Aspiration under general anesthesia may go unnoticed. Clinical signs develop on anesthetic recovery or shortly thereafter. Clinical signs include respiratory difficulty (dyspnea), cough, and wheezing. Cyanosis occurs when pulmonary damage is extensive. Patients often appear depressed, weak, and are inappetant. Many times, aspiration of gastric contents with a pH less than 2.5 has an acute onset of clinical signs, whereas aspiration of more inert substances results in the development of signs 6 to 8 hours after the aspiration event.[2] In comatose or recumbent animals, a change in respiratory rate and effort can signify potential aspiration. Thoracic auscultation often reveals harsh airway sounds with crackles in the affected areas. Inflammation and the presence of bacterial infection can produce fever. In more severe cases, systemic hypotension occurs as edema fluid floods damaged alveoli, resulting in tachycardia and poor pulse quality. In some cases, a frothy, nonpurulent sputum may be present.[15] A thorough examination of the oropharynx should be performed to investigate whether vomitus, foreign material, cleft palate, or an abnormal gag reflex is present.[23] Ballooning of the esophagus at the thoracic inlet, during exhalation, is often noted with megaesophagus.[23]

DIAGNOSTIC EVALUATION

Physical Examination and Ancillary Diagnostic Tests

Diagnosis of aspiration pneumonitis is often based on a clinical history of vomiting or regurgitation followed by respiratory difficulty. Although physical examination findings are often supportive of aspiration pneumonitis, the diagnosis is based on radiographic signs of lung consolidation and arterial blood gas data. With suspected or confirmed aspiration pneumonitis, every patient should have a minimum database consisting of a complete blood count, serum biochemistry panel, arterial blood gas analysis, and urinalysis performed. Serum lactate levels, which increase with conditions causing hypoxemia and poor tissue perfusion, are elevated.[24] Other ancillary tests used to document and characterize aspiration pneumonitis include bronchoalveolar or transtracheal lavage with cytology and bacterial culture with susceptibility. Tests to rule out the presence of an underlying cause of aspiration pneumonitis should be performed as based on each patient's physical status, history, and clinical signs (*i.e.*, serum thyroid hormone levels to rule out hypothyroidism, adrenocorticotropinc hormone stimulation testing to rule out hypoadrenocorticism, serum acetylcholine receptor antibody titers to rule out myasthenia gravis, and laryngeal examination under heavy sedation to rule out laryngeal paralysis).

Arterial Blood Gases

The most characteristic feature of aspiration pneumonitis is the hypoxemia seen with an arterial blood gas sample. The causes of hypoxemia include diffusion impairment, ventilation-perfusion mismatch (V/Q mismatch), intrapulmonary shunting, and venous admixture. Hypoxemia and decreased tissue perfusion cause anaerobic metabolism and lactic acidosis. CO_2 is more readily diffusible than O_2. Therefore, hypercarbia (CO_2 retention) usually does not occur unless end-stage pulmonary parenchymal disease is present.[25]

Radiography

Severe interstitial to alveolar lung patterns are seen on radiography with aspiration pneumonitis. Radiographic signs of aspiration pneumonia may not be apparent in the first several hours after the aspiration event and may progress and worsen in the first 24 to 36 hours[1] (Figs. 37-2 and 37-3). Alveolar consolidation in dependent lung areas (right middle; left and right cranial lung lobes) is most commonly observed. However, any pulmonary region can be affected, depending on the position of the patient at the time of aspiration. Aspiration under general anesthesia often occurs with the patient in lateral or dorsal recumbancy. Cough can further scatter the aspirated debris throughout the lung field. Secondary development of acute respiratory distress syndrome results in more

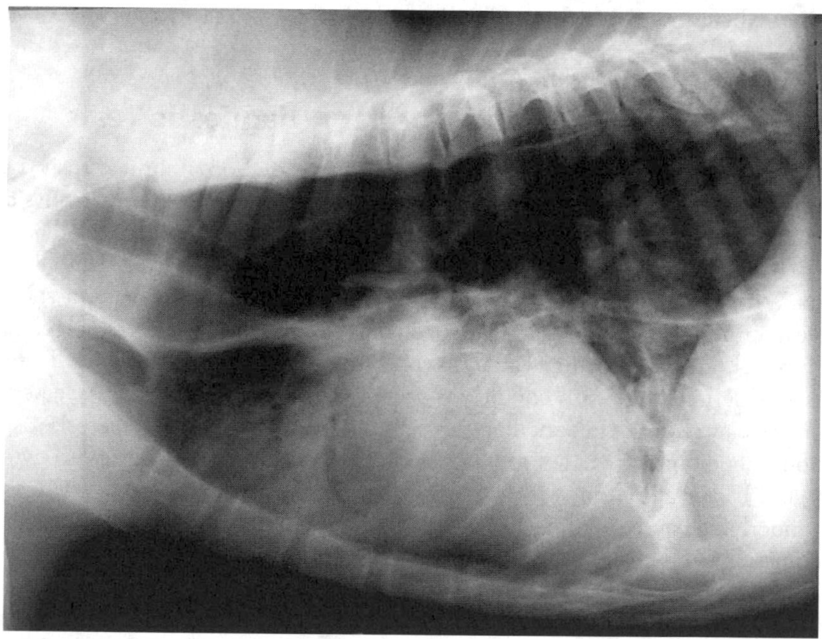

Figure 37-2
Lateral thoracic radiograph from a dog with severe megaesophagus and aspiration penumonitis. Note the air bronchograms in the crainioventral lung field, increased interstitial densities in the caudodorsal lung field, and widened air-filled esophagus throughout its length in the thorax. This patient also had a history of bilateral laryngeal paralysis. Laryngeal paralysis and megaesophagus are two conditions that predispose patients to the development of aspiration pneumonitis.

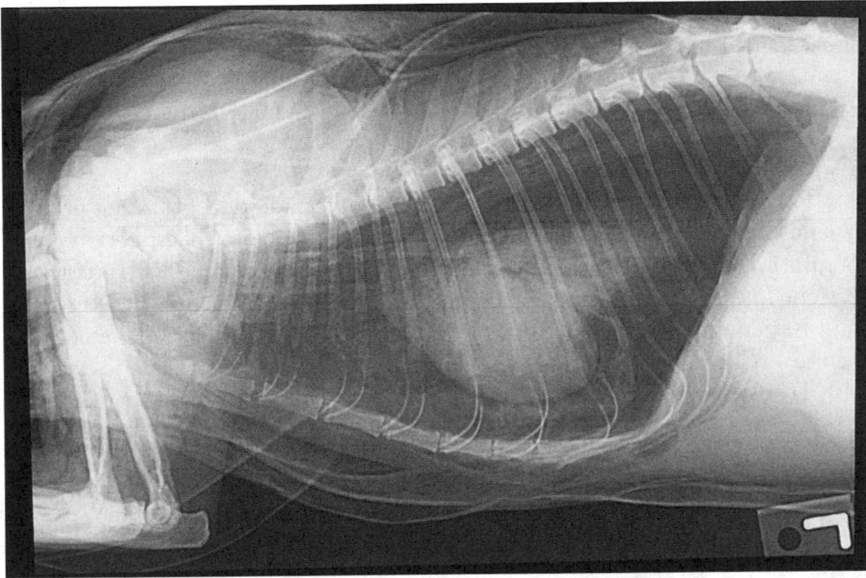

Figure 37-3
Ventrodorsal radiograph of the patient described in Figure 37-2. Note the widened air-filled esophagus and increased interstitial to alveolar densities in the right cranial, right middle, and right caudal lung fields.

diffuse and severe areas of alveolar collapse, atelectasis, and consolidation. Aspiration of material, such as mineral oil, may produce small nodular densities secondary to granuloma formation, rather than alveolar consolidation. The radiographic differential diagnoses in this case would include neoplasia or a fungal pneumonia.

Radiographic contrast studies may be performed to document the presence of megaesophagus, vascular ring anomalies, or esophageal motility disorders. However, the risk of aspirating contrast material often precludes the benefits of this type of study. Radiographs must also be carefully evaluated for the presence of cranial mediastinal masses consistent with lymphoma or thymoma. These conditions are often associated with acquired myasthenia gravis, megaesophagus, and esophageal motility disorders.[26-28] It is important to appreciate that the severity of radiographic signs at the time of diagnosis has no prognostic value in predicting morbidity and mortality.[29]

Bronchoscopy

Bronchoscopy may be performed as a therapeutic tool to remove particulate material from large airways. Bronchoalveolar lavage can also be performed for cytology and bacterial culture/susceptibility. However, due to the risk of general anesthesia, bronchoscopy is often not performed due to the patient's fragile condition. Aerobic and anaerobic bacterial cultures should be performed on all samples obtained via bronchoalveolar lavage or transtracheal wash.

PREVENTION AND TREATMENT

Prevention

Prevention of aspiration pneumonitis involves a period of fasting prior to general anesthesia. In humans there is an increased incidence of aspiration pneumonitis following anesthesia for emergency treatment compared with anesthesia for scheduled elective procedures following a period of fasting.[21] If anesthesia must be performed in an emergency situation (*i.e.*, cesarean section, hemoabdomen secondary to neoplasia), specific therapies to increase pH of gastric contents with H_2-blockers (cimetidine 5 mg/kg IV or IM or ranitidine 2.0 mg/kg IV or IM) and motility modifiers to promote gastric emptying (metoclopramide 0.2-0.4 mg/kg, maximum dose 10 mg/dog) are administered.[15] In patients with predisposing conditions, routine use of H_2-blockers is not indicated and may promote bacterial aspiration by disrupting normal gastrointestinal flora.[1] Metoclopramide may also be useful in preventing aspiration of gastric contents by tightening the lower esophageal sphincter. The use of emetic agents such as apomorphine or empirical gastric lavage prior to anesthesia does not reduce the incidence of anesthetic-related aspiration events and may cause undue stress to the already compromised patient. The administration of colloidal antacid compounds is contraindicated, because they can form large granulomas within the lungs if aspirated.[14,30] There is no documented benefit in discontinuing oral fluids prior to anesthesia.[31]

Treatment

Successful treatment of aspiration pneumonitis depends on the cause and severity of pathology. The most important features of treatment include maintaining airway patency, oxygen therapy to combat hypoxemia, fluid therapy to combat hypovolemia and subsequent shock, antibiotics, and ancillary treatments.[1,2] Treatment of any underlying illness is necessary to eliminate the potential for repeated aspiration events.

Establishing a Patent Airway

The patient's airway must be carefully evaluated for mechanical obstruction and debris immediately on presentation or discovery of aspiration/regurgitation. Immediate suctioning of the oropharyngeal area and airway should occur. If the patient cannot protect its airway due to anesthesia or loss of consciousness, an endotracheal tube should be placed to allow adequate oxygen delivery. If an endotracheal tube cannot be placed, a temporary tracheostomy is considered. The cuff on the endotracheal or tracheostomy tube should be inflated to prevent further aspiration of gastric contents. If the aspiration occurs under anesthesia, the patient's esophagus should be carefully lavaged with 1 to 2 liters of warm saline (0.9% NaCl) to prevent esophagitis and possible stricture. Bronchial lavage following aspiration is usually unnecessary. The pulmonary defense mechanisms often neutralize acid within several minutes of the aspiration event, making exogenous buffering unnecessary. Instilling large volumes of fluid into the compromised airway can spread debris further into smaller airways and contribute to pulmonary edema fluid.

Oxygen Supplementation

O_2 therapy should be initiated Immediately on establishing a clear airway. The hypoxemia associated with aspiration pneumonitis is often responsive to O_2 administration in the early stages of disease. When patients are awake and alert, supplemental humidified O_2 in the form of nasal O_2,[32] hood O_2, or O_2 cage is administered. Mechanical ventilation with positive end-expiratory pressure or continuous positive airway pressure helps expand collapsed alveoli.[3,33] Indications for mechanical ventilation include refractory hypoxemia, persistent hypercarbia ($PaCO_2$ >60 mm Hg), and persistent respiratory distress or fatigue.[15] In an experimental dog model of aspiration pneumonitis, rapid initiation of mechanical ventilation following aspiration improved survival.[3,12] Arterial blood gases and calculation of alveolar-arterial O_2 tension gradients are useful in monitoring a patient's response to therapy.[34]

Fluid Therapy

Intravenous fluid therapy is extremely important in patients with aspiration pneumonitis. Tracheobronchial secretions are normally 95% water.[2] Many patients develop hypovolemic shock secondary to alveolar flooding with edema fluid. Diuretics, therefore, are contraindicated because they will further decrease cardiac preload, decreases cardiac output, and will worsen dehydration. Dehydration will interfere with normal mucociliary clearance mechanisms, causing retention of sputum and debris within the airways. Fluid therapy requires judicious use of crystalloids and careful patient monitoring to meet each patient's fluid requirements without causing volume overload and its negative consequences. In humans, pulmonary arteriolar occlusion pressure (pulmonary capillary wedge pressure) via Swan-Ganz monitoring is the gold standard to monitor fluid resuscitation and prevent overhydration. Because this technique is invasive, and not commonly used in veterinary medicine, other parameters such as central venous pressure via jugular catheterization are used to avoid overhydration in patients with pulmonary parenchymal damage. Crystalloid fluids should be administered as partial shock bolus increments to alleviate hypovolemic shock. There is no documented benefit in using colloids over crystalloids in patients with aspiration pneumonitis.[15]

Antibiotics

The prophylactic use of antibiotics in patients with documented aspiration pneumonitis is controversial. Empirical antibiotic coverage following an aspiration event favors the development of resistant bacteria. However, several studies have documented that bacterial aspiration from the oropharynx is more common in animals than in human patients.[15] Damage to the lung epithelium favors bacterial colonization by inhibiting normal lung clearance mechanisms. Therefore, the use of broad-spectrum antibiotic therapy is warranted. Clinical signs of infection include fever and inflammation/left shift neutrophilia. Whenever possible, a transtracheal wash with cytology, bacterial culture, and susceptibility should be performed prior to starting antibiotic therapy. Coverage with a second-generation cephalosporin such as cefoxitin (22 mg/kg IV tid), or four-quadrant antibiotic approach with ampicillin (22 mg/kg IV tid) and enrofloxacin (5 mg/kg IV bid), is often the treatment of choice in veterinary patients with aspiration pneumonitis. Aminoglycosides are also effective in treating aspiration pneumonitis, but should be used only when culture and susceptibility prove them necessary. Because many patients with aspiration pneumonitis are dehydrated and hypovolemic, the use of aminoglycoside antibiotics in these patients is potentially dangerous due to the risk of nephrotoxicity. Antibiotic therapy should be continued for 10 to 14 days following complete resolution of clinical and radiographic signs of aspiration pneumonitis.[35] Often, this requires a minimum of 3 to 4 weeks of therapy.

Ancillary Therapy

Other therapies that are beneficial in treating aspiration pneumonitis include saline nebulization followed by physiotherapy and patient mobilization. Nebulization with small inhaled saline particles helps moisten and loosen airway debris. Thoracic physiotherapy assists in promoting coughing and expelling sputum from the airways. Patient mobilization helps promote alveolar expansion and prevent atelectasis. If mobilization and mild exercise cannot be tolerated, frequent turning every 2 to 4 hours, or keeping a patient in sternal recumbancy, helps prevent atelectasis and further aspiration events.

Controversial Therapies

The use of bronchodilators and corticosteroids in patients with aspiration pneumonitis is controversial. Bronchodilators enhance contractility of diaphragmatic muscle contraction, which promotes bronchodilation, as well as decrease inflammation and prevent respiratory muscle fatigue.[37] However, their use may also enhance infection and contribute to V/Q mismatch.[15] Immediately following aspiration of acid material, reflex bronchoconstriction causes severe respiratory distress. In such cases, the use of bronchodilators such as aminophylline (6-10 mg/kg IV tid-qid) or terbutaline (0.01 mg/kg IV or SQ bid) may be beneficial. Parenteral isoproterenol (0.01-0.04 ug/kg/min IV or 0.5 mL in a nebulizer) can be used for emergency bronchodilation.[15] Bronchodilators are only useful in the first 24 to 48 hours after the aspiration event.[37] Prolonged use beyond this time period likely has no advantage and is therefore unnecessary.[36]

There have been no documented benefits to corticosteroid use in patients with aspiration pneumonitis.[38,39] Although steroids may decrease inflammation and potentially stabilize cell membranes, they also interfere with normal cellular defense mechanisms and promote bacterial colonization. Therefore, the use of corticosteroids is unwarranted.

PROGNOSIS

The prognosis in patients with aspiration pneumonitis largely depends on the type and amount of substance aspirated, the degree of pulmonary infiltration and damage, whether any underlying illness is present, and the patient's response to therapy. Prognosis is always guarded with underlying conditions such as persistent megaesophagus following vascular ring anomaly, neuromuscular dysfunction, or laryngeal paralysis. Negative sequelae of aspiration pneumonitis include pulmonary abscess, persistent lung consolidation, lung lobe torsion, and persistent foreign material.

REFERENCES

1. Hawkins EC: Aspiration pneumonia. *In:* Bonagura JD, ed.: Current Veterinary Therapy XII. Philadelphia, WB Saunders, 1995, p 915.
2. Tams TR: Aspiration pneumonia and complications of inhalation of smoke and toxic gases. *Vet Clin North Am Sm Anim Pract* 15:971, 1985.
3. Cameron JL, Sebor J, Anderson RP, *et al.*: Aspiration pneumonia. *J Surg Res* 8:447, 1968.
4. Graham KL, Buss MS, Dhein CR, *et al.*: Gastroesophageal intussusception in a Labrador retriever. *Can Vet J* 39:709, 1998.
5. Hackett TB, VanPelt DR, Willard MD, *et al.*: Third degree atrioventricular block and acquired myasthenia gravis in four dogs. *J Am Vet Med Assoc* 206:1173, 1995.
6. Awe WC, Fletcher WS, Jacob SW: The pathophysiology of aspiration pneumonitis. *Surgery* 60:232, 1966.
7. Greenfield LJ, Singleton RP, McCaffree DR, *et al.*: Pulmonary effects of experimental graded aspiration of hydrochloric acid. *Ann Surg* 170:74, 1969.
8. Cohen SE: The aspiration syndrome. *Clin Obstet Gynecol* 9:235, 1982.
9. Boysen PG, Modell JH: Pulmonary aspiration. *In:* Grenvik A, ed.: Textbook of Critical Care, 4th ed. Philadelphia, WB Saunders, 2000, p 1432.
10. Teabeaut JR II: Aspiration of gastric contents: an experimental study. *Am J Pathol* 28:51, 1952.
11. Moran TJ: Experimental food-aspiration pneumonia. *Arch Pathol* 52:350, 1951.
12. Wynne JW and Modell JH: Respiratory aspiration of stomach contents. *Ann Intern Med* 87:466, 1977.
13. Gibbs CP, Schwartz DJ, Wynne JW, *et al.*: Antacid pulmonary aspiration in the dog. *Anesthesiology* 51:380, 1979.
14. Becton DL, Lowe JE, Falletta JM: Lipoid pneumonia in an adolescent girl secondary to use of lip gloss. *J Pedriatr* 105:421, 1984.
15. Tams TR: Pneumonia. *In:* Kirk RW, ed.: Current Veterinary Therapy X. Philadelphia: WB Saunders, 1989, p 376.
16. Greene CE: Gastrointestinal, intra-abdominal and hepatobiliary infections. *In:* Greene CE, ed.: Clinical Microbiology and Infectious Diseases of the Dog and Cat. Philadelphia: WB Saunders, 1990, p 125.
17. Syed SA, Svanberg M, Svanberg G: The predominant cultivatable dental plaque flora of beagle dogs with gingivitis. *J Periodont Res* 15:123, 1980.

18. Bartlett JG, Gorbach SL, Finegold SM: The bacteriology of aspiration pneumonia. *Am J Medicine* 56:202, 1974.
19. Lundy DS, Smith C, Colangelo L, *et al.*: Aspiration: causes and implications. *Otolaryngol Head Neck Surg* 120:474, 1999.
20. Kadakia SC, Sullivan HO, Starnes E: Percutaneous endoscopic gastrostomy to jejunostomy and the incidence of aspiration in 79 patients. *Am J Surg* 164:114, 1992.
21. Mellin-Olsen J, Fasting S, Gisvold SE: Routine preoperative gastric emptying is seldom indicated. A study of 85,594 anaesthetics with special focus on aspiration pneumonia. *Acta Anaesthesiol Scand* 39:1184, 1996.
22. Spray SB, Zuidema GD, and Cameron JL. Aspiration pneumonia: incidence of aspiration with endotracheal tubes. *Am J Surg* 131:701, 1976.
23. Hawkins EC: Pulmonary parenchymal disease. *In:* Ettinger SJ, Feldman EC, eds.: Textbook of Veterinary Internal Medicine. Philadelphia, WB Saunders, 2000, p 1084.
24. Lagutchik MS, Ogilvie GK, Hackett TB, *et al.*: Increased lactate concentrations in ill and injured dogs. *J Vet Emerg Crit Care* 8:117, 1998.
25. Wingfield WE, Matteson VL, Hackett TB, *et al.*: Arterial blood gases in dogs with bacterial pneumonia. *J Vet Emerg Crit Care* 7:75, 1997.
26. Atwater SW, Powers BE, Park RD, *et al.*: Thymoma in dogs: 23 cases (1980B1991). *J Am Vet Med Assoc* 205:1007, 1994.
27. Day MJ: Review of thymic pathology in 30 cats and 36 dogs. *J Sm Anim Pract* 38: 393, 1997.
28. Rusbridge C, White RN, Elwood CM, *et al.*: Treatment of acquired myasthenia gravis associated with thymoma in 2 dogs. *J Sm Anim Prac* 37:376, 1996.
29. Bynum LJ, Pierce AK: Pulmonary aspiration of gastric contents. *Am Rev Respir Disease* 114:1129, 1976.
30. Toung TJ, Rosenfeld BA, Yoshiki A, *et al.*: Sucralfate does not reduce the risk of aspiration pneumonitis. *Crit Care Med* 21:1359, 1993.
31. Phillips S, Hutchinson S, Davidson T: Preoperative drinking does not affect gastric contents. *Br J Anaesth* 70:6, 1993.
32. Marks SL: Nasal oxygen insufflation. *J Am Anim Hosp Assoc* 35:366, 1999.
33. Orton EC, Wheeler SL: Continuous positive airway pressure therapy for aspiration pneumonia in a dog. *J Am Vet Med Assoc* 188:1437, 1986.
34. VanPelt DR, Wingfield WE, Wheeler SL, *et al.*: Oxygen-tension based indices as predictors of survival in critically ill dogs: clinical observations and review. *J Vet Emerg Crit Care* 1:19, 1991.
35. Stone MS, Pook H: Lung infections and infestations: therapeutic considerations. *Probl Vet Med* 4:279, 1992.
36. Plumb DC: Veterinary Drug Handbook, 3rd ed. Ames, IA: Iowa State university Press, 1999, p 23.
37. Arms RA, Dines DE, Tinstman TC: Aspiration pneumonia. *Chest* 65:136, 1974.
38. Wilson JW: Treatment or prevention of pulmonary cellular damage with pharmacologic doses of corticosteroid. *Surg Gynecol Obstet* 134:675, 1972.
39. Chapman RL, Downs JB, Modell JH, *et al.*: The ineffectiveness of steroid therapy in treating aspiration of hydrochloric acid. *Arch Surg* 108:858, 1974.

38
Laryngeal and Tracheal Disorders

Adam J. Reiss and Brendan C. McKiernan

INTRODUCTION

Laryngeal and tracheal diseases are commonly reported in small animals. Impairment of structure or function of the upper airway may result in audible airflow changes during respiration at rest or during exercise, altered voice (bark or purr), and frequent coughing.

ETIOLOGY AND CLINICAL PRESENTATION

Laryngeal Obstruction/Disease

The larynx is the point of maximum air flow resistance within the respiratory tract; relatively small changes in diameter may therefore be associated with significant clinical signs. Brachycephalic breeds, such as Pekingese, Pugs, and English bulldogs, have anatomic distortion of their upper airways resulting in obstruction and increased airway resistance. Animals that fall into the brachycephalic category may have one or more of the following anatomic features: stenotic nares, elongated soft palate, laryngeal edema, laryngeal collapse, edematous/everted laryngeal saccules and, in some instances, hypoplastic trachea. Factors such as fever, anxiety, respiratory infection, obesity, exercise, and increased ambient temperature or humidity can precipitate an acute respiratory crisis. Heat should be considered extremely dangerous because polypnea necessary for thermolysis produces turbulent airflow that may cause edema of the upper airways and further respiratory compromise. These events lead to increased body temperature and anxiety that results in a vicious cycle of increasing body temperature and respiratory distress.[1] Although cats such as Persians and Himalayans may have similar anatomic problems, clinical symptoms are rarely encountered.

Laryngeal Paralysis

Most commonly, laryngeal paralysis presents as a slowly progressive disease in middle-aged to older (≥7 years), large and giant breed dogs (*e.g.*, Labrador retrievers, Saint Bernard's, Golden retrievers, and Siberian huskies).[5,6] The majority of acquired cases are considered idiopathic in origin. Laryngeal paralysis diagnosed in young patients, without other explainable etiologies, may be congenital in origin. Congenital laryngeal paralysis appears to be inheritable and has been proven in the Bouvier des Flandres as an autosomal dominant trait, and suspected to be inheritable in Siberian huskies, Dalmatians, Rottweilers, and Bull terriers.[3,6,7] The average age of congenital laryngeal paralysis patients at the time of diagnosis has been reported to be 14 months,[3] although many are encountered as young at 6 weeks.

Underlying causes affecting the recurrent laryngeal nerves such as trauma, lymphosarcoma, or a generalized neuromuscular disease (such as polyneuropathy or myasthenia gravis) may be identified. Although hypothyroidism has been suggested as a potential underlying cause of acquired laryngeal paralysis,[8] at least one published study has refuted this theory.[9]

Laryngeal paralysis is an uncommon cause of airway obstruction in the cat.[10] A report of 16 cases in cats found no breed or sex predilection.[10] Twelve of the 16 cats had bilateral paralysis, and 4 had unilateral paralysis (interestingly, all were left-sided). Clinical signs similar to those described in the dog were present in cats with both unilateral and bilateral disease.[10]

Laryngeal paralysis is characterized by airflow limitation, primarily during inspiration, resulting in varying degrees of respiratory distress.[2] The inability to abduct the anatomic borders of the rimma glottidis (the vocal folds and arytenoid cartilages) is due to the loss of innervation of the intrinsic dilators of the larynx.[3-5] The abductors of the vocal folds and arytenoid cartilages are the paired dorsal cricoarytenoid muscles,[3,4] which are innervated by the recurrent laryngeal nerves.[3] Increased resistance to gas flow occurs when the borders of the rimma glottidis, the anatomic opening to the larynx, are drawn into a median position by the subatmospheric, intraluminal glottic pressure created during inspiration. The decreased diameter of the rimma glottidis is the cause of clinical signs associated with laryngeal paralysis.[3,4]

Bilateral laryngeal paralysis is usually noted with clinical signs.[4,6] Clinical signs commonly reported are respiratory distress (increased effort or rate), inspiratory stridor, a change in the animal's purr or bark, stress or exercise intolerance, gagging or coughing associated with ingestion of food or water, heat intolerance, cyanosis, and syncope.[3-5] The severity of clinical signs usually correlate with the degree of abductor dysfunction (unilateral versus bilateral paralysis) and level of exertion.[6]

Laryngeal Trauma

Hemorrhage and edema secondary to laryngeal trauma may impede normal airflow and result in a life-threatening event.[6] Cervical trauma from bite wounds and the use of choke chains may cause injury to the larynx and trachea.[4] Iatrogenic trauma may be secondary to direct manipulation of the laryngeal tissues, injury of the recurrent laryngeal nerves (*e.g.*, during surgery on the neck), or traumatic intubation techniques.[6] Although foreign bodies rarely lodge in the larynx, they can irritate and injure the sensitive lining of the airway.[4] The authors have diagnosed laryngeal obstruction secondary to a pharyngeal hematoma in dogs with acquired coagulopathies.

Laryngeal Inflammation

Granulomatous and inflammatory laryngitis has been reported in both the dog and cat.[11] Granulomatous laryngitis is a chronic proliferative inflammatory disease that can be confused with neoplasia. It is usually localized to the larynx, especially to the arytenoid processes. Biopsy is necessary to differentiate granulomatous disease from neoplasia.[4] There has been no evidence of bacterial or fungal infection associated with granulomatous laryngitis.[11] Less severe inflammatory causes of laryngitis in dogs and cats, on the other hand, have been attributed to infectious causes such as *Bordatella bronchiseptica*, canine distemper, *Calici* virus, and viral rhinotracheitis.[4,11] Other causes of laryngeal inflammation and edema include snake or insect bites and caustic chemicals.[6,11]

Laryngeal Neoplasia

Laryngeal neoplasia is rare in the dog. The most common primary tumor of the larynx in the dog is squamous cell carcinoma. Other reported neoplastic diseases of the canine larynx include melanoma, osteosarcoma, mast cell tumor, oncocytoma, leiomyoma, rhabdosarcoma, and mixed cell tumor.[4,6] Lymphosarcoma and squamous cell carcinoma are the most commonly reported laryngeal neoplasms in the cat.[11] Lymphosarcoma may present as a solitary mass or as diffuse laryngeal mucosal thickening.[11] Adenocarcinoma, epidermoid carcinoma, and undifferentiated carcinoma have also been described in the cat.[11] Clinical signs associated with laryngeal neoplasia are similar to the laryngeal diseases discussed above.

Laryngeal Web Formation

Laryngeal webbing occurs when the mucosa of the larynx is disrupted and scar tissue is allowed to form.[6] Web formation in the airways secondary to surgery or trauma is an uncommon but recognized problem in both dogs and cats.[4] During the routine debarking procedure, care must be taken to preserve the ventral one fifth of each vocal fold to prevent web formation by scar tissue postoperatively.[12] Unilateral arytenoidectomy, use of a surgical laser, reapposition of mucosal borders, and the laryngeal tieback procedure are techniques that may help to prevent web formation.[3] Clinical signs associated with web formation, usually appearing 2 to 6 weeks after the inciting cause, are similar to other laryngeal disorders discussed above.[4]

Tracheal Obstruction/Disease

Tracheal Collapse

Tracheal collapse is a dynamic event that results from a combination of weakened cartilagenous support and small airway disease. Tracheal collapse is a common cause of airway obstruction in middle-aged toy and miniature breed dogs.[13-15] Yorkshire terriers, Chihuahuas, Pomeranians, toy Poodles, and Maltese are commonly affected.[13-15] Although several etiologies for tracheal collapse have been suggested, the disease is probably multifactorial in origin.[14,15] Tracheal cartilage in affected animals is hypocellular and contains less chondroitin sulfate, resulting in weakened cartilages and the tendency to collapse.[15,16] Small airway inflammation leads to increased expiratory pressures (clinically seen as an active abdominal press) that narrow and collapse intrathoracic airways. Loss of intrinsic tracheal support most commonly results in dorsoventral flattening of the cartilaginous tracheal rings, stretching of the dorsal tracheal membrane, and dynamic collapse as pressures outside the trachea exceed the ability of the cartilaginous tracheobronchial support to maintain airway patency.[13-15]

Tracheal narrowing due to other causes (*e.g.*, congenital malformations, extratracheal masses) should be differentiated from dynamic tracheal collapse. Airway collapse may involve airways of any size from the trachea or mainstem/lobar bronchi to more distal airways. The breakdown of the tracheal infrastructure results in partial or complete airway obstruction that in severe cases is heard clinically as the characteristic "goose honk" cough.[13] More frequently an "end-expiratory snap" can be heard at peak expiration (during a cough) as the walls of the trachea or mainstem bronchi snap together. Other clinical signs include exercise intolerance, respiratory distress, syncope, and cyanosis.[13,15] In contrast to intrathoracic tracheal collapse, cervical tracheal collapse occurs during inspiration and may be associated with upper airway obstruction.

Once airway collapse occurs, coughing itself may act as a perpetuating factor by initiating tracheal inflammation.[15] If the cycle of coughing, inflammation, and excess mucous production continues, pathologic changes characteristic for chronic bronchitis occur (loss of epithelium, subepithelial glandular hypertrophy, squamous metaplasia) that further exacerbate the condition.[15]

Neoplasia

Reports of tracheal neoplasia in dogs and cats are rare. A comprehensive review of reported tracheal neoplasia described 23 cases that were all presented with a complaint of airway obstruction.[17] The majority of tumors were evident radiographically as a distinct intratracheal mass, most of which appear mineralized. The most common type of canine tracheal tumor appears to be the osteochondroma, which routinely arises in dogs less than 1 year of age and may be amenable to tracheal resection.[17] Other reported canine tracheal tumors include mast cell tumor, osteosarcoma, plasmacytoma, adenocarcinoma, chondroma, chondrosarcoma, leiomyoma, and carcinoma.[17,18] Reported feline tracheal tumors include lymphosarcoma, adenocarcinoma, squamous cell carcinoma, and seromucinous carcinoma.[17] The seromucinous carcinoma was the only tumor described in the cat to appear as an annular mass.[17] The prognosis for tracheal tumors should be assumed to be poor and most likely dependent on the tumor type,[17,18] but we are unaware of any reports that describe the long-term outcome of these cases.

Trauma

Bite wounds of the neck are reported to be one of the most common sites of injury.[19] The shallow position of the larynx and trachea make them susceptible to injuries due to tears, crushing, or avulsion.[20] External trauma resulting in disruption of tracheal integrity may result in subcutaneous emphysema, pneumomediastinum, and pneumopericardium.[20] It is important to note that bite wounds may result in relatively minor injury to the epidermis; deeper structures, such as the trachea, are more severely damaged. For this reason a high index of suspicion for tracheal injury should be maintained when animals with injuries to the neck present, or in those with wounds to the cervical region, subcutaneous emphysema, and respiratory distress.

Internal trauma to the trachea, although infrequent, has been reported. The tracheal lining may be damaged by foreign bodies, parasites, smoke (heat and chemical), iatrogenic injuries, most of which occur during intubation. Two recent reports found that iatrogenic tracheal rupture was most commonly associated with dental procedures in cats.[21,22] Overinflation of the endotracheal tube cuff, to ensure that fluid and debris are not aspirated, was suggested as the cause of tracheal rupture in these reports.[21,22] Hardie and colleagues found, in a cadaver study, that as little as 6 mL of air in the endotracheal tube cuff was needed to cause tracheal rupture.[21] In clinically normal cats, the mean volume of air needed to obtain an airtight seal was only 1.6 ± 0.7 mL.[21] Iatrogenic tracheal injuries have also been reported during procedures such as jugular venipuncture and transtracheal washes.[23]

Subcutaneous emphysema is the most common clinical sign specific to tracheal rupture. Other common clinical signs included respiratory distress, coughing, gagging, stridor, anorexia, lethargy, and depression.[21,22] Conservative medical treatment consisting of supplemental oxygen, needle aspiration of subcutaneous air, cage rest, and light sedation is indicated in most cases.[22] Surgical intervention should be reserved for cats with signs of severe respiratory distress (open mouth breathing, cyanosis), worsening subcutaneous emphysema, or the development of a clinically significant pneumothorax.[22]

Inflammation

Inflammation of the tracheal epithelium, tracheitis, can be caused by either infectious or noninfectious etiologies.[23] Noninfectious tracheitis is caused by irritation from excessive barking, collapsing trachea, chronic cardiac disease, or dental disease. Most animals with tracheitis present with a cough as the only clinical sign. These patients are sensitive to palpation of the trachea; palpation initiates a harsh and often paroxysmal cough that characteristically terminates with gagging and production of a clear liquid topped with white foam.[23]

The clinical signs of infectious tracheitis (kennel cough) are similar. Nearly all cases have a recent history of exposure to other animals as might occur in a training class, groomers, kennel, hospital, or dog show.[23] *B. bronchiseptica*, the most commonly implicated agent in cases of infectious tracheitis in dogs, has a predilection for ciliated airways and is frequently cultured from dogs with tracheitis.[24] Some authors have suggested viral infections and or impaired airway defenses permit *B. bronchiseptica* to colonize in the lower airways.[23] Other agents implicated as causes of infectious tracheitis include mycoplasmas, canine parainfluenza virus, canine adenovirus, canine herpes virus, and canine distemper.[23] These infections are contagious and may be spread either by aerosol or direct contact.[23,24] Clinical signs usually develop 3 to 5 days after initial exposure.[23] Tracheitis is unusual in cats and most commonly is associated with viral agents or allergic airway disease.[23] Feline bronchopulmonary disease may also initiate tracheal inflammation.

Two clinical presentations may be seen with infectious canine tracheobronchitis. The mild form is typically found in older, vaccinated animals and is usually a self-limiting disease with few symptoms other than a nonproductive cough. The more severe form is encountered in younger dogs, often in those with little or no vaccination history. These animals are typically more systemically ill with fever, a productive cough, depression, and anorexia being noted frequently; pneumonic infiltrates are often present. Although systemic antibiotics have not been shown to reach significant concentrations in tracheobronchial secretions or to shorten the course of infection, prophylactic therapy has, nonetheless, been recommended.[23] The mild and self-limiting disease associated with *B. bronchiseptica* may preclude the need for systemic antimicrobials.[24] These infections are typically nonresponsive to systemic antibiotic administration but may benefit from the local delivery of antibiotics into the airways.[25] In the authors' practice, transtracheal injection of an aminoglycoside (2 mg/kg Gentocin, Schering), once or twice daily for 3 consecutive days, has been successful in resolving infections and symptoms that do not respond to systemic antibiotics. Systemic absorption of gentamicin appears to be negligible in dogs after aerosolization.[25] Systemic antibiotics are indicated in more severe form of the disease; their use should be based on culture and sensitivity tests.[24] In the absence of culture and sensitivity results recommended antibiotics include cephalosporins, chloramphenicol, or a fluoroquinolone.[23,25]

Intranasal *Bordetella* vaccines elicit high levels of secretory antibodies as soon as 4 days after inoculation; their use is recommended because they may reduce both clinical disease and the duration of organism shedding.[24]

Foreign Bodies

Tracheal foreign bodies are infrequently reported in dogs. Hunting dogs, due to their use and activity, are reported to be most commonly affected. In a report of 153 dogs, all extracted tracheobrochial foreign bodies were identified as plant material (*i.e.*, grass awns).[26] Coughing, which begins almost immediately after aspiration, is the most commonly reported clinical sign. If foreign bodies are not extracted in a timely manner, severe tracheobronchitis may ensue followed by more severe lung damage including bronchiectasis, pneumonia, and finally migration through the bronchi/lung parenchyma and visceral pleura. The inevitable consequence of foreign body migration includes abscess formation, pyothorax, or draining fistulas. Diagnosis is based on history, physical examination, radiographic findings, and fiberoptic endoscopy. Endoscopy may be used to remove these foreign bodies if diagnosed early; surgical intervention will be necessary in more chronic cases.[26]

Hypoplasia

Hypoplasia of the trachea is a congenital anomaly commonly affecting bulldogs and other brachycephalic breeds.[23,27,28] The condition is caused by inadequate growth of tracheal rings and often results in the overlap of tracheal rings.[23,27] Clinical signs are consistent with those described with laryngeal and tracheal diseases. Due to poor secretion clearance from the narrowed trachea, many cases are incorrectly diagnosed as having episodes of recurring pneumonia.

In contrast with tracheal collapse, tracheal hypoplasia is a static disease and tracheal diameter will not be dramatically altered by the phase of respiration when viewed radiographically.[27] Different methods have been described to radiographically diagnose hypoplastic trachea. The diagnosis of hypoplastic trachea is suggested when the lumen diameter is less than three times the width of the third rib where they cross.[29] Another proposed method for diagnosing this disorder involves the comparison of the tracheal diameter (TD) to the thoracic inlet (TI) diameter.[28] The TI diameter is determined by measuring from the ventral aspect of T1 to the manubrium at its point of minimum diameter; TD is defined as the perpendicular distance at the point where the TI line crosses the midpoint of the tracheal lumen[28] (Fig. 38-1). Reported normal values for the

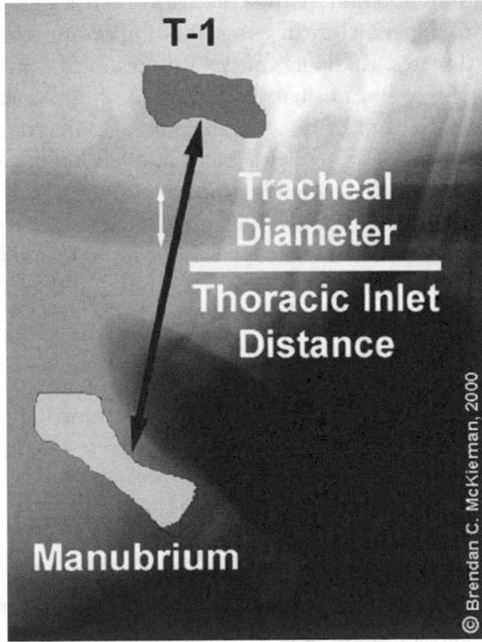

Figure 38-1
Diagram of one method used to determine whether tracheal hypoplasia is present in the dog. (Adapted from Harvey CE: Tracheal diameter: analysis of radiographic measurements in brachycephalic and nonbrachycephalic dogs. *J Am Anim Hosp Assoc* 18: 570, 1982.)

ratio of the TD to the TI diameter are 0.127 in bulldogs, 0.160 in non-bulldog brachycephalic dogs, and 0.204 in nonbrachycephalic dogs.[28] The TD/TI ratio is the preferred method of assessing tracheal diameter, because both measurements are obtained from structures in the same radiographic planes.[28] The prognosis for dogs depends on the degree of hypoplasia as well as the presence or absence of concurrent congenital defects.[23] Young dogs with this diagnosis may outgrow this condition.[23] Weight loss and treatment of concurrent airway problems as well as any inflammation/infection will improve outcome in many of these cases.

DIAGNOSIS

Physical examination and history are essential components in the diagnosis of upper airway disease. The owner should be questioned about the animal's typical environment and recent travel history, exposure to other animals, current medications, and voice changes. In addition to a routine physical examination the following are suggested: careful observation of respiration efforts at rest prior to examination, careful oropharyngeal examination, airflow evaluation from both nares, and auscultation of the thorax, trachea, and larynx while clinical signs are being exhibited and during laryngeal and tracheal manipulation.

Performing complete blood count, chemistry panel, and endocrine studies may identify concurrent and underlying conditions. Although clinical pathology is rarely diagnostic of upper airway diseases, it is important to screen for concurrent or underlying diseases. Radiographic examination of lung parenchyma and airways should be part of the evaluation of laryngeal and tracheal diseases. Be sure to stabilize the patient prior to obtaining radiographs so further respiratory compromise does not occur. Three views (right and left lateral, and ventrodorsal) are necessary to evaluate all lung fields properly. Oxygen supplementation and dorsoventral or standing lateral projections may be necessary to avoid additional stress in these patients.[1] When fluoroscopy is not available and a dynamic disease is suspected, lateral chest radiographs should be obtained on both peak inspiration and peak expiration.

Endoscopy is the gold standard for the evaluation of the respiratory tract. Direct visualization using fiberoptic endoscopes is considered essential for evaluation of pharyngeal and laryngeal anatomy and function. It not only allows for the visualization of anatomic and functional changes, but it also permits the clinician to obtain selected biopsy and culture samples. Readers are directed to recent reviews of small animal bronchoscopy for additional details on the procedure.[30,31]

Airway cytology is a useful aid in the diagnosis of these airway diseases, specifically those of infectious, allergic, inflammatory, or neoplastic etiologies. Cytologic samples may be obtained by transtracheal wash or bronchoalveolar lavage. Refer to the Chapter 42 for a more in-depth discussion regarding airway cytology.

Other diagnostic tools such as electromyograms, tidal breathing flow volume loops, and planimetric measurement of the tracheal cross-sectional area have proven useful in diagnosing abnormalities of the upper airways.[2,5,32] The equipment and expertise required for these techniques is not readily available, however, precluding their everyday use.

TREATMENT

Medical Treatment

The overall treatment goals should be aimed at relieving airway narrowing, reducing airway inflammation, and improving oxygen delivery to the lungs. Patients in severe respiratory distress should be stabilized before additional diagnostic studies are performed. Oxygen therapy is the mainstay of initial therapy. Unfortunately, some animals may not tolerate mask or hood delivery of oxygen. These methods may cause increased anxiety, an increase in oxygen demand and may precipitate decompensation. Flow-by oxygen, provided with an open oxygen line aimed directly at the nares may provide short-term support to prevent decompensation during subsequent diagnostic evaluation.

When flow-by oxygen does not provide adequate support and other methods of oxygen delivery are not tolerated, sedation may be required. Careful sedation will not only help decrease oxygen demand but also prevent further trauma to laryngeal structures (*e.g.*, mucosal edema) by decreasing the velocity and turbulence of airflow. In the authors' practice, acepromazine (PromAce, Ft. Dodge) in combination with opioids such as morphine (Elkins-Sinn), fentanyl (Baxter) and butorphanol (Torbugesic, Ft. Dodge) have been safe and effective in most cases. Rapid intubation and ventilatory support may be required in some patients and should be available at all times. Initial administration of sedatives should use the lowest recommended doses, followed by incremental increases until the desired effect (*e.g.*, relief of anxiety) is achieved. These patients must have continuous monitoring available.

If edema and swelling of laryngeal mucosa is suspected (or the results of sedation are inadequate) corticosteroids should be administered. Short-acting steroids such as dexamethasone sodium phosphate (Azium SP, Schering), at anti-inflammatory dosages, are recommended (Table 38-1). Long-term use of steroids is reserved for cases of chronic bronchitis or allergic airway disease.

Impaired laryngeal reflexes, recurrent aspiration, and compromise of local immune defense mechanisms facilitate bacterial colonization and infection of the lower airways. Antibiotic selection should be based on airway cytology and culture/sensitivity results, but this is not always possible in acute diseases. Most lower airway infections are due to gram-negative bacteria. The β-lactam antibiotics (penicillins) and first-generation cephalosporins are excellent first-choice drugs for the treatment of lower airway bacterial infections in small animals.[25] Serious, life-threatening gram-negative infections may be addressed with third-generation cephalosporins (Cefotan, Zeneca Pharmaceuticals), fluorinated quinolones (Baytril, Miles), extended-spectrum penicillins (Clavamox, Beecham), and aminoglycosides[25] (see Table 38-1). Aerosolization of aminoglycosides can enhance their efficacy, especially in treatment of *Bordetella* and *Pseudomonas* tracheobronchitis

Table 38-1. Doses of Drugs Used to Treat Respiratory Diseases

Drug	Route	Dose	Frequency
		Bronchodilators	
Albuterol	PO	20–50 μg/kg (D)	bid-tid (increase slowly)
Terbutaline	PO, SQ (C)	1.25 mg/kg up to 10kg (D) 2.5 mg/kg up to 25kg (D) 5 mg/kg over 25kg (D) 0.625 mg total (C) 0.01 mg/kg SQ (C)	bid
Sustained-release theophylline: Slo-bid Gyrocaps (Rhone-Poulenc Rorer) Theo-dur (Key Pharm)	PO	20 mg/kg (D) 25 mg/kg (D)	bid bid
		Anti-inflammatory	
Prednisone or predniso-lone (Delta-Cortef, Up-john)	PO	0.5 to 1 mg/kg	sid, bid
Dexamethasone	IV, IM	0.2–2.2 mg/kg	sid, bid
		Antimicrobial	
Amoxicillin (Amoxi, SK Beecham)	PO, SQ	10 mg/kg	bid
Amoxicillin/clavulanic acid	PO	10-20 mg/kg	bid-tid
Cefazolin (Kefzol, Lilly)	IV	20 mg/kg	tid
Cephalexin (Keflex, Dista)	PO	22 mg/kg	tid
Cefotan	IV	30 mg/kg	tid
Doxycycline (Vibramycin, Pfizer)	PO	2.5-5.0 mg/kg	bid
Enrofloxacin	PO, IM	5-10 mg/kg	sid, bid
Gentamicin	IV, IM, SQ, IT	1-2 mg/kg	sid, bid

Adapted from Boothe DM, McKiernan BC: Respiratory therapeutics. *Vet Clin North Am* 22:1231, 1992.

infections, which can colonize the mucosal surfaces of the airways.[25] Aerosol delivery of antibiotics should be used in concert with systemic therapy.[25]

Some patients with concurrent upper and lower airway disease may benefit from treatment with bronchodilators (see Table 38-1). Because of a shared mechanism of action, some of the drugs that induce bronchodilation may also reduce inflammation. Theophylline has been a cornerstone of long-term bronchodilator therapy in human and veterinary medicine.[25] In addition to its bronchodilatory effects, theophylline inhibits mast cell degranulation, increases mucociliary clearance, prevents microvascular leakage, and increases strength of respiratory muscles.[25] The effects of these drugs should benefit animals in respiratory distress secondary to airway compromise. Because of pharmacokinetic differences, only specific sustained-release theophylline products (see Table 38-1) are recommended for use in dogs and cats; generic sustained-release products and regular aminophylline (oral or injectable) are not recommended. The β-receptor agonists, terbutaline (Brethine, Geigy) and albuterol (Proventil, Schering), are also excellent bronchodilators. Injectable terbutaline is recommended in emergencies when acute bronchodilation is required (see Table 38-1).

Surgical Treatment

Airway Management

Temporary tracheostomy may be required on presentation of animals with severe airway obstruction or during postoperative recovery from laryngeal or pharyngeal procedures.[1] Permanent tracheostomy should be considered for animals with upper airway obstruction secondary to nonresectable tumors, intractable swelling and edema, or following failure of upper airway surgical intervention. Owner acceptance of and the dog's quality of life after permanent tracheostomy has been reported to be good.[13]

Laryngeal and Pharyngeal Diseases

Diseases that have progressed to the point of severe airway compromise (*e.g.*, laryngeal paralysis, elongated soft palate, everted saccules, and laryngeal collapse) often require surgical intervention. Surgical enlargement of the rimma glottidis and improved airflow can be achieved with laryngeal tieback or partial laryngectomy procedures. The potential success of a tieback procedure should be evaluated preoperatively by manually attempting to enlarge the rimma glottidis with forceps *per os*. Older patients may have calcified, fixed laryngeal cartilages that do not move easily and may not lateralize well with the standard arytenoid lateralization procedure.[3] If a failure to increase the diameter of the airway is noted, laryngectomy may be required. A unilateral tieback procedure is most commonly performed as bilateral laryngeal procedures increase the risk of aspiration.

Laryngectomy enlarges the rimma glottidis by partial resection of the vocal cords, lateral saccules, or the corniculate process of one arytenoid cartilage.[3,5] If primary mucosal closure is not obtained during laryngectomy, the rimma glottidis may become compromised as scar tissue forms a web across the ventral airway.[33] The chance of scar tissue formation may be reduced by using a carbon dioxide surgical laser for tissue resection, preserving the ventral fifth of each vocal fold, avoiding the use of electrocautery, and most importantly achieving primary closure of the mucosa.[5,12]

Silastic implants (*e.g.*, the Hood stent) have been recommended as another method of preventing (or treating) laryngeal mucosal web formation. This stent is surgically placed between the exposed raw surfaces of the ventral larynx, left in place until mucosal healing occurs, and then later removed.

Tracheal Diseases

Surgical intervention for tracheal diseases is considered only when medical therapy is deemed unsuccessful. Three surgical procedures that have been performed in dogs and cats include tracheostomy, tracheal ring prosthesis, and tracheal resection.

Tracheostomy may be temporary or permanent. Although the main purpose is to bypass obstructions of the upper airways, tracheostomy can also be used to provide ventilatory support in the awake animal. Temporary tracheostomy should be considered in patients recovering from surgery of the upper airways.[1] The tracheostomy will provide a patent airway if postoperative swelling of the pharynx and larynx occurs.[1] In addition to providing a patent airway, tracheostomy allows swollen and edematous tissues to heal and avoid further trauma caused by turbulent airflow. If the airway obstruction is not correctable, a permanent tracheostomy must be performed. Long-term complications of permanent tracheostomy may include tracheitis, pneumonia, and respiratory distress secondary to stoma occlusion.[12] Patients with permanent tracheostomies are not allowed to swim, should be kept from dusty environments, and may require intermittent long-term antibiotic therapy.[12]

Tracheal ring prosthesis has been advocated as the treatment of choice for management of cervical tracheal collapse.[14,15] Dogs should be considered candidates for this procedure if their symptoms have not responded to at least 2 weeks of medical therapy.[15] Application of an extraluminal prosthetic ring has been the surgical procedure of choice (due to the high incidence of severe complications, the spiral prosthesis should not be used in the authors' opinion). Commonly reported postoperative complications include loosening or breakage of the rings, infection, and laryngeal paralysis.[13] To date intraluminal stents have not been successfully used in clinical cases.

Tracheal resection and anastomosis is indicated for patients suffering from occlusive lesions and tracheal transection. In these patients intubation may be difficult, but endotracheal tubes should extend beyond the proposed site of resection whenever possible. Excessive tension on the surgical site is the main cause of complications such as dehiscence and stenosis. The amount of tension that causes anatomosis breakdown varies with age. Tension at the site of anastomosis can be reduced by placement of tension sutures and maintaining cervical flexion postoperatively. As with the larynx, mucosal defects may facilitate the development of scar tissue and subsequent stenosis.[34]

PROGNOSIS

The prognosis is variable for laryngeal and tracheal disorders. Signalment, etiology, concurrent diseases, and duration of the disease all play a role in therapeutic success. This prognosis is worse when chronic damage (malacia) of the cartilagenous infrastructure of the airways is present. Improved outcomes will be achieved when therapeutic intervention is initiated early in disease process.

REFERENCES

1. Hendricks JC: Brachycephalic airway syndrome. *Vet Clin North Am* 22:1145, 1992.
2. Amis TC, Smith MM, Gaber CE, *et. al.*: Upper airway obstruction in canine laryngeal paralysis. *Am J Vet Res* 47:1007, 1986.
3. Aron DN: Laryngeal paralysis. *In* Kirk RW, ed.: Current Veterinary Therapy X. Philadelphia: WB Saunders, 1989, p 343.
4. Wykes PM: Canine laryngeal diseases: Part I. Anatomy and disease syndromes. *Compend Contin Educ Pract Vet* 5:8, 1983.
5. Bjorling DE: Laryngeal paralysis. *In* Bonagura JD, ed.: Current Veterinary Therapy XII. Philadelphia: WB Saunders, 1995, p 901.
6. Venker-van Haagen AJ: Diseases of the larynx. *Vet Clin North Am* 22:1155, 1992.
7. BraundKG: Laryngeal paralysis-polyneuropathy complex in young dalmation dogs. *In* Bonagura JD, ed.: Current Veterinary Therapy XII. Philadelphia: WB Saunders, 1995, p 1136.
8. Harvey HJ, Irby NL, Watrous BJ: Laryngeal paralysis in hypothyroid dogs. *In* Kirk RW, ed.: Current Veterinary Therapy VIII. Philadelphia: WB Saunders, 1983, p 694.
9. Gaber CE, Amis TC, LeCouteur RA: Laryngeal paralysis in dogs: a review of 23 cases. *J Am Vet Med Assoc* 186:377, 1985.
10. Schachter S, Norris CR: Laryngeal paralysis in cats: 16 cases (1990–1999). *J Am Vet Med Assoc* 216:1100, 2000.
11. Griffon DJ: Upper airway obstruction in cats: pathogenesis and clinical signs. *Compend Contin Educ Pract Vet* 22:822, 2000.
12. Petersen SW, Rosin E, Bjorling DE: Surgical options for laryngeal paralysis in dogs: a consideration of partial laryngectomy. *Compend Contin Educ Pract Vet* 13:1531, 1991.
13. Buback JL, Boothe HW, Honbson HP: Surgical treatment of tracheal collapse in dogs: 90 cases (1983–1993). *J Am Vet Med Assoc* 208:380, 1996.
14. Figland RB: Tracheal collapse. *In* Kirk RW, ed.: Current Veterinary Therapy X. Philadelphia: WB Saunders, 1989, p 353.
15. Jerram RM, Fossum TW: Tracheal collapse in dogs. *Compend Contin Educ Pract Vet* 19:1049, 1997.
16. Dallman MJ, McClure RC, Brown EM: Histochemical study of normal and collapsed trachea in dogs. *Am J Vet Res* 49:2117, 1983.
17. Carlisle CH, Biery DN, Thrall DE: Tracheal and laryngeal tumors in the dog and cat: literature review and 13 additional patients. *Vet Radiol* 32:229, 1991.
18. Chaffin K, Cross AR, Allen SW, Mahaffey EA, *et al.*: Extramedullary plasmacytoma in the trachea of the dog. *J Am Vet Med Assoc* 212:1579, 1998.
19. Kolata RJ: Patterns of trauama in urban dogs and cats: a case study of 1000 cases. *J Am Vet Med Assoc* 164:499, 1974.
20. Davidson EB: Managing bite wounds in dogs and cats. Part I. *Compend Contin Educ Pract Vet* 20:811, 1998.
21. Hardie EM, Spodnick GJ, Gilson SD, *et al.*: Tracheal rupture in cats: 16 cases (1983–1998). *J Am Vet Med Assoc* 214:508, 1999.
22. Mitchell SL, McCarthy R, Rudloff E, *et al.*: Tracheal rupture associated with intubation in cats: 20 cases (1996–1998). *J Am Vet Med Assoc* 216:1592, 2000.

23. Ettinger SJ, Kantrowitz B, Brayley K: Diseases of the trachea. *In* Ettinger SJ, ed.: Textbook of Veterinary Internal Medicine. Philadelphia: WB Saunders, 2000, p 1040.
24. Bemis DA: Bordatella and mycoplasma respiratory infections in dogs and cats. *Vet Clin North Am* 22:1173, 1992.
25. Boothe DM, McKiernan BC: Respiratory therapeutics. *Vet Clin North Am* 22:1231, 1992.
26. Lotti U, Niebauer GW: Tracheobronchial foreign bodies of plant origin in 153 hunting dogs. *Compend Contin Educ Pract Vet* 14:900, 1992.
27. Coyne BE, Figland RB: Hypoplasia of the trachea in dogs: 103 cases (1974–1990). *J Am Vet* Med *Assoc* 201:768, 1992.
28. Harvey CE: Tracheal diameter: analysis of radiographic measurements in brachycephalic and nonbrachycephalic dogs. *J Am Anim Hosp Assoc* 18:570, 1982.
29. Suter PF: A text atlas of thoracic diseases of the dog and cat. Wettswil: Switzerland, 1984, p 238.
30. McKiernan, BC: Bronchoscopy in the small animal patient. *In* RW Kirk, ed.: Current Veterinary Therapy X. Philadelphia: WB Saunders, 1989, p 219.
31. Padrid PA, McKiernan BC: Endoscopy of the upper respiratory tract of the dog and cat. *In* Tams TR, ed.: Small Animal Endoscopy, 2nd ed. St. Louis: Mosby, 1999, p 357.
32. Huber ML, Henderson RL, Finn-Bodner S: Assessment of current techniques for determining tracheal luminal stenosis in dogs. *Am J Vet Res* 58:1051, 1997.
33. Payne JT, Martin RA, Rigg DL: Abductor muscle prosthesis for correction of laryngeal paralysis in 10 dogs and 1 cat. *J Am Anim Hosp Assoc* 26:599, 1990.
34. Nelson AW: Lower respiratory system. *In* Slatter D, ed.: Textbook of Small Animal Surgery. Philadelphia: WB Saunders, 1993, p 777.

39
Allergic Airway Disease

Carrie Miller and Brendan C. McKiernan

INTRODUCTION

Allergic airway disease is a broad and poorly understood disease in small animals. The disease is typically characterized by bronchial and/or alveolar inflammatory changes including submucosal wall edema, increased bronchial secretions, smooth muscle hypertrophy, and smooth muscle constriction of the bronchioles and small bronchi. Labored breathing, rapid shallow breathing, increased expiratory effort, and cough characterize the clinical signs of lower airway disease. Studies have shown that small animals with airway disease have variable degrees of hypersensitivity in the bronchiolar smooth muscle.[1,2] The disease can have an acute onset with completely reversible changes, or it can become a chronic disease (a duration of more than 2 months) and be associated with irreversible bronchial wall changes.[3] Diseases commonly included in this definition include allergic bronchitis, "feline asthma," and pulmonary infiltrates with eosinophils (PIE).

HUMAN ASTHMA

The pathogenesis of allergic asthma in humans has been more thoroughly investigated than it has in small animals.[4] One should avoid terming small animal allergic airway disease as "asthma" because the pathogenesis is much less clear than in humans.[5] Human asthma is defined as a disease of the airways that makes the airways prone to narrow too easily in response to a wide variety of provoking stimuli. The ease with which these airways narrow is termed hyperreactivity.[6] Asthmatic patients develop high concentrations of IgE antibodies in response to these various inhaled allergens. Mast cells within the lungs, located in close association with the bronchioles and small bronchi, bind to IgE antibodies. Once bound, the mast cells degranulate via complex intracellular pathways, releasing inflammatory mediators (*e.g.*, histamine, leukotriennes, eosinophilic chemotactic factor, and bradykinin). The inflammatory mediators cause immediate airway bronchoconstriction. Leukotriennes also contribute to a late phase inflammatory response that takes place several hours after mediator release[7,8] and causes mucosal edema, smooth muscle hypertrophy, the accumulation of secretions, and airway narrowing (Figure 39-1).

In humans, these pathophysiologic changes lead to an increase in lower airway resistance and a decrease in compliance as measured by pulmonary func-

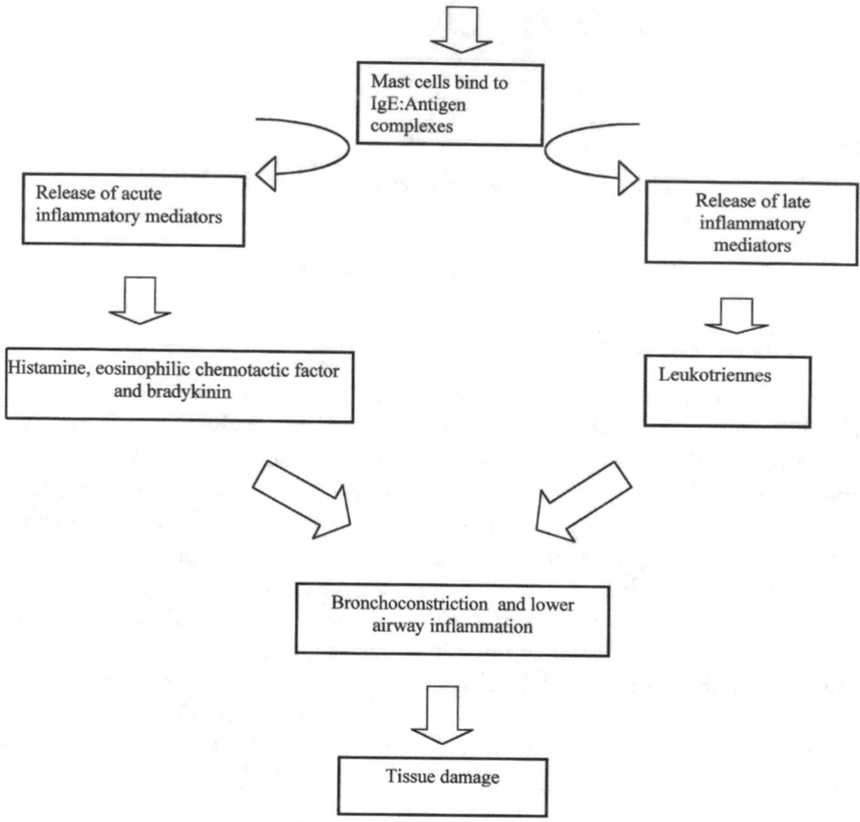

Figure 39-1
Pathophysiology of human asthma showing that both acute and late phase inflammatory mediators are involved.

tion tests. Because of pulmonary elasticity and interdependence, inspiratory measurements are affected less than expiratory measurements. This phenomena causes "air trapping" within the lungs and may lead to a radiographically apparent hyperinflation of the lungs as well as an increase in functional residual capacity (FRC). Expiratory values such as forced expiratory volume at one second (FEV1) markedly decrease.[4,8]

PATHOGENESIS OF SMALL ANIMAL ALLERGIC RESPIRATORY DISEASE

The pathophysiology of small animal allergic respiratory disease is less well understood than asthma in humans, but it is becoming clearer that allergic respiratory disease in small animals encompasses a broad spectrum of clinical findings on examination of affected animals. Diseases that should be included in small animal allergic respiratory disease include allergic bronchitis, parasitic larval migration, pulmonary infiltrates with eosinophilia, and feline asthma. Although similar in presentation and treatment, diseases such as canine and feline bronchitis have not been shown to be allergic in nature. Factors contributing to the development of allergic respiratory disease in small animals include lower airway inflammation in response to either an extrinsic noxious stimuli or intrinsic hypersensitivity to antigenic stimulation. These factors cause mucosal edema, airway smooth muscle hypertrophy and constriction, and excessive production of airway secretions.[3,9]

PARASITIC ALLERGIC AIRWAY DISEASE

Intestinal parasite migration as well as primary pulmonary parasitism can cause a parenchymal or lower airway allergic inflammatory response. *Toxocara canis*, for example, can cause pulmonary disease in young dogs when larval migration takes place as part of the normal parasite development. An inflammatory "allergic reaction" can take place in the lower airways and parenchyma because of antigenic stimulation and the eosinophilic infiltrate induced by the larvae. Usually, the inflammatory reaction is mild, and young dogs recover well with deworming alone.

Clinical signs associated with larval migration vary markedly from asymptomatic to severe coughing, wheezing, and respiratory distress. A complete blood count (CBC) may show eosinophilia or basophilia, although this finding is variable. On chest radiographs, a variety of changes may be seen including interstitial infiltrates, bronchial thickening, and even alveolar consolidation. A clinician should be suspicious of larval migration in a young dog with acute onset of cough and increased respiratory effort with or without a positive fecal. Ova may be difficult to find on fecal examination because larvae usually begin to migrate before shedding ova into the intestinal tract.[10] Other parasites known to migrate through the lungs include *Ancylostoma caninum* and *Strongyloides stercoralis*. *Ancylostoma caninum* and *T canis* ova can be seen with routine fecal floatation techniques. *Strongyloides stercoralis* is more reliably found by use of the Baermann technique.[10,11]

Primary lung parasites include *Paragonimus kellicotti*, *Aelurostrongylus abstrusus*, *Capillaria aerophilia*, and others (Table 39-1). In certain parts of the United States, primary pulmonary parasites are a common rule out with a dog or cat in respiratory distress. In cats, lung parasite infection can easily be confused with feline asthma. Diagnosis is primarily by demonstrating ova or larvae in pulmonary fluid or on fecal examination. Thoracic radiographs reveal either a diffuse interstitial, bronchial, or alveolar pattern. Frequently, no organisms are found, and a presumptive diagnosis is made by observation of airway eosinophilia in the appropriate geographical setting. History often aids in the diagnosis as well. An outdoor cat with a history of eating snails, for example, has a greater chance of infection with *Paragonimus* sp than a completely indoor cat.

PULMONARY INFILTRATES WITH EOSINOPHILS

Pulmonary infiltrates with eosinophils is thought to be a type I hypersensitivity reaction occurring in the pulmonary parenchyma in response to various stimuli,

Table 39-1. Pulmonary Parasitic Diseases

Parasite Name	Species	Location	Diagnosis	Treatment
Aelurostrongylus abstrusus	Cats	Southern US-worldwide	Larvae in tracheal wash or fecal (Baermann technique)	Fenbendazole or Ivermectin if clinical
Capillaria aerophilia	Dogs/Cats	Worldwide	Eggs in tracheal wash or fecal floatation	Fenbendazole or Levamisole (dogs)
Filaroides hirthi	Dogs	North America, Japan, Europe	Zinc sulfate floatation or Baermann; larvae in tracheal wash.	Albendazole or fenbendazole
Crenosoma vulpis	Dogs	Worldwide	Larvae in tracheal wash or fecal Baermann technique	Fenbendazole, Levamisole
Paragonimus kellicotti	Dogs/Cats	Great Lakes, Midwest, Southern, US	Eggs in tracheal wash or fecal sedimentation	Praziquantel or Fenbendazolel
Intestinal parasite migration: Toxocara canis*	Dogs	Worldwide	Ova on fecal floatation	Pyrantel pamoate; for larval migration, use either Fenbendazole or Ivermectin

The table lists parasitic diseases that may result in an inflammatory pulmonary reaction. Clinical signs may include cough, respiratory distress and, often, peripheral eosinophilia. *Other intestinal parasites to consider with allergic lung disease include *Ancylostoma caninum* and *Strongyloides stercoralis.*

including pulmonary or migrating parasites, heartworms, drugs, or inhaled allergens. It occurs mainly in adult dogs with no particular predominant age group. One study showed that 65% of PIE cases were associated with heartworm disease.[12] Although PIE appears to be allergic in origin, one should know that PIE mainly affects the pulmonary parenchyma and not the airways. Affected dogs classically have respiratory distress (characterized by rapid, shallow breathing), some coughing, and possible cyanosis. Radiographically, a diffuse interstitial, bronchial, or alveolar pattern is seen. Hilar lymphadenopathy is commonly seen as well. Eosinophils are the predominant cell type on airway cytologic examination. Basophils have been identified in some cases. Peripheral eosinophilia is common, although it is not seen in all cases of PIE.[10,12] Morbidity and mortality depend greatly on whether or not an inciting cause can be found and removed or the signs controlled with medical therapy.

FELINE BRONCHOPULMONARY DISEASE

Feline bronchopulmonary disease is a broad term that encompasses several different disease processes. Although some affected cats may truly be allergic and asthmatic, others may have chronic changes (chronic bronchitis) due to prolonged and persistent irritation and inflammation to the lower airways related to nonallergic stimuli.

Pathogenesis

The most predominant cell type found in bronchial washings of cats affected by bronchopulmonary disease are neutrophils and eosinophils. Dye et al.[2] reported that moderately and severely affected cats had statistically significantly higher percentages of eosinophils, neutrophils, and combined neutrophils and eosinophils when compared with healthy cats. Mast cells, however, were infrequently found and at most represented 8% of all the cell types.[2] Moise et al. found the predominant cell type in affected cats to be eosinophils (24% of cats), neutrophils (33% of cats), macrophages (22% of cats), or a mixed cell population (21% of cats).[3] Out of 65 cats, 58 had bronchial washings consistent with an exudate. Clearly, the pathogenesis of the feline bronchopulmonary inflammatory response is variable. Defining the feline pulmonary inflammatory response is complicated further by some reports that up to 30% eosinophils may be seen in the bronchoalveolar lavage fluid of healthy cats.[13] The cellular inflammatory response is only partially responsible for feline bronchopulmonary disease. Another important factor is lower airway hyperreactivity, which may be defined as the ease with which airways narrow in response to a nonspecific (nonallergic or nonsensitizing) stimulus.[14] While some small animal patients may have inherently reactive airways to allergic stimuli, studies also suggest that many animals have a degree of airway responsiveness to extrinsic noxious stimuli. Patients have had exacerbations of clinical signs apparently associated with exposure to scented hair sprays or changing the brand of litter to a clay-based product.[2] Other suggested factors included changing to a dustier type of litter, use of a scented air freshener near the litter box, and smokers in the household. It is suggested but not clearly substantiated that clinical improvement may be seen in a cat with feline bronchopulmonary disease by simply removing the patient from these noxious stimuli.

Clinical Signs in Feline Allergic Airway Disease

Clinical signs vary in cats with allergic airway disease. Respiratory distress (with increased expiratory effort and rapid, shallow breathing) is a common clinical sign. Cats often display open-mouth breathing on examination; excessive coughing is typical. The onset of distress may be acute with marked tachypnea, although this does not necessarily indicate an acute disease. More severe respiratory distress in cats with allergic airway disease is characterized by increased expiratory effort. Wheezes and forced abdominal expiration are common and are the result of airway narrowing caused by the inflammation and bronchoconstriction in the lower airways. One can often see (and even feel) a marked abdominal push as the animal attempts to force trapped air out of its lungs.[1,15] Seventy-five percent of cats in one retrospective study had signs of coughing on examination. Of these, 50% also showed other respiratory signs including obstruction (*i.e.*, wheezing, sneezing and a noisy or abnormal breathing pattern). Signs of lower airway obstruction with no history of cough were seen in 16% of the cats.[2] Evidence supports that the Siamese breed is over-represented in cats with lower airway disease.[2,3] While one study suggests that feline bronchopulmonary disease is more common in female cats, other studies find that there is no sex predilection. No age group seems to be predominant.

DIAGNOSTIC EVALUATION IN FELINE ALLERGIC AIRWAY DISEASE

In any cat with respiratory distress, a routine CBC, biochemical analysis, and urinalysis should be performed to rule out other systemic diseases. Typically with allergic airway disease, these test results are within normal limits. Less than 40% of cats with allergic airway disease are found to have peripheral eosinophilia, yet this remains a common misconception.[2,3] In one study of 312 cats with peripheral eosinophilia, only 28/312 (9%) were diagnosed with feline allergic airway disease.[16] In the study by Moise, only 14% of bronchial lavage specimens from cats with bronchial disease contained eosinophils as the predominant inflammatory cell. These findings strongly suggest that a diagnosis of allergic airway disease in a cat with peripheral eosinophilia should not be made without cytologic evidence demonstrating concurrent *airway* eosinophilia.

Fecal examination and heartworm testing should be included in order to rule out parasitism. A heartworm test is an important diagnostic test in any cat with labored breathing and signs of interstitial disease. Most cats experimentally infected with *Dirofilaria immitis* showed radiographic signs of bronchointerstitial lung disease, lobar arterial enlargement, and pulmonary hyperinflation. In many of these cats, radiographic signs of lobar arterial enlargement resolved by 270 days postinfection, while the pulmonary hyperinflation and bronchointerstitial patterns persisted and even worsened in some cats.[17] Feline heartworm disease should be diagnosed by an antibody rather than an antigen test since the amount of antigen can be extremely low in some cats.[18]

Radioallergosorbent (RAST) Testing

Recent work has explored the use of hyposensitization in treating feline allergic disease. Some evidence exists to support that feline allergic airway disease may be linked to an atopic process.[19] Halliwell reported that hyposensitization led to a 86% improvement in clinical signs in four cats with presumed allergic asthma. He suggests in this study that the RAST test be performed in cats with allergic airway disease in which no specific cause can be found for the disease. It is hypothesized that by determining which IgE allergen-specific antibodies are in the patient, one can desensitize the patient by giving small amounts of this antigen on a frequent basis.[19,20] The study unfortunately does not prove that the clinical response seen was directly the result of hyposensitization therapy since many of the patients were given anti-inflammatory doses of steroids before or during the time of desensitization as well.

Radiology and Bronchoscopy

Thoracic radiographs should be part of the workup for any respiratory distress case. Patients in severe respiratory distress should be stabilized before risking the stress of the positioning required for routine chest radiography. Changes on thoracic radiographs are variable; an increased interstitial and/or alveloar pattern and, most typically, increased bronchial densities are reported. Common terms used to describe the bronchial pattern include "doughnuts" and "tramlines," representing the thickened bronchial walls viewed end-on or from the side, respectively.[10] The severity of radiographic changes has been shown to vary. Dye et al.[2] demonstrated that radiograph findings did not correlate well with pulmonary function testing. Moise et al.[3] also demonstrated that allergic cats can have radiographic changes ranging from very mild to severe, and that these changes do not correlate with the severity of other diagnostic tests. Alveolar infiltration and consolidation of the right middle lung lobe has been reported in 11% of cats with bronchopulmonary disease.[3] It is hypothesized that this consolidation is the result of decreased mucus clearance, bronchial obstruction, and subsequent atelectasis.

Bronchoscopy is an extremely valuable tool that can be used to obtain diagnostic information from the pulmonary system. Bronchoscopy allows direct visualization of the internal aspect of the trachea and bronchial tree. Animals with allergic airway disease commonly have excessive, thick mucus secretions in their lower airways. The mucosa of the airways is typically hyperemic and edematous.[2,3] Bronchoscopy also aids in ruling out common differentials including neoplasia, foreign body, and granulomatous processes. During bronchoscopy, a bronchoalveolar lavage should be performed. This procedure allows the clinician to evaluate cytopathologic changes in the lower airways. Bronchoalveolar lavage is generally preferred over transtracheal wash since the former yields a cell population that is more representative of the distal airways and interstitium. Particularly in large-breed dogs, transtracheal wash does not yield the cell population of the distal airways but rather exfoliated cells within the larger central airways. Fluid obtained from the lower airways by either procedure should be cultured to exclude bacteria as a potential cause of the inflammatory response. Quantitated culture is recommended, although a clinically significant bacterial colony count is not commonly obtained in a dog or cat with chronic bronchial disease.[2,21] Finally, bronchoalveolar lavage has been shown to be more accurate than transtracheal wash in the diagnosis of bacterial and mycotic infection of the lower airways.[21] Bronchoscopy also allows for the clinician to obtain bronchial mucosal specimens for histologic examination, if indicated. Biopsy can be extremely helpful in patients in which fungal or neoplastic growths are involved. The benefit of mucosal biopsy over cytologic examination (by bronchoalveolar or transtracheal wash) in a cat with suspected allergic airway disease is questionable.

Lung Function Testing

Pulmonary function testing is the gold standard for diagnosing and treating asthma in humans. Characteristic changes include an increase in resistance, decrease in compliance and FEV1, and an increase in FRC.[4] Unfortunately, in small animals, current limitations of equipment and training make these techniques of limited availability. An additional drawback in small animal pulmonary function testing is that our patients are unable to cooperate by voluntarily and forcefully exhaling on command. This makes it essentially impossible to measure variables such as FEV1 and FRC. Work is being done, however, to make pulmonary function testing more accessible and to determine other variables that may be used to evaluate lung function in small animals. In an anesthetized patient, one can indirectly measure transpulmonary pressure by placing an esophageal balloon catheter. Flow can also be indirectly measured by means of a pneumotachograph attached to the endotracheal tube. With these measurements, one can calculate compliance, resistance, and other measures of lung mechanics. Unfortunately, studies to date have demonstrated marked variation in the lung mechanics in small animals with lower airway disease.[2,22,23] Dye et al.[2] showed that while some cats have hyperreactive airways in response to metacholine challenge, variability exists as to the extent of hyperreactivity in each patient. Hoffman et al.[22] demonstrated that even in healthy cats, airway reactivity is highly variable and not predictable from baseline pulmonary measurements. Hyperreactivity of the small airways to bronchoconstricting agents appears variable in both healthy animals as well as in those displaying signs of lower airway disease.[2,22,23] This makes it difficult to define the degree that airway hyperreactivity contributes to small animal allergic airway disease.

TREATMENT OF FELINE ALLERGIC AIRWAY DISEASE

Once a diagnosis of allergic airway is confirmed, both intrinsic and extrinsic factors should be addressed when considering therapy. The veterinarian should advise clients to remove possible inhalant irritants from the animal's environment, including such things as dusty litter, perfumes, aerosols, and cigarette smoke. Owners have also reported that their pets condition seems to worsen when heaters or air conditioners are turned on for the first time during the season, perhaps reflecting recirculation of debris trapped in air filters and suggesting that routine filter changing and cleaning be done.[3]

In most animals, medical management in addition to irritant avoidance is necessary. Several options exist for medical management of these patients. Steroids, bronchodilators, and oxygen therapy are the mainstay of emergency therapy[24] (Table 39-2). Steroids are used in emergency situations and also on a long-term basis to decrease inflammation and airway resistance in the lower airways. Steroids inhibit inflammation by several different mechanisms. These mechanisms include stabilization of lysosomal membranes, decreased migration of white blood cells, decreased production of interleukin 1, and decreased reproduction of lymphocytes.[4] Steroids also inhibit phospholipase A2, blocking the arachidonic pathway and leading to a decrease in inflammatory mediators such as prostaglandins and leukotriennes.[25]

Table 39-2. Recommended Emergency Medical Therapy for Allergic Airway Disease.

Drug	Mechanism	Dosage
Steroids	Immunosuppressive: stabilize membranes, decrease WBC migration, decrease IL-1 and lymphocytes	1 mg/lb divided q12h SQ/IV/PO; taper dose to q24h use if possible; may try to discontinue seasonally
β-agonists	Bronchodilation via Beta receptor sympathetic pathway	
Albuterol		Start at 20 ug/kg q12h PO; can go up to 50 ug/kg q8h PO depending on side effects
Terbutaline		0.01 mg/kg SQ/IV
Time Release Theophylline	Phosphodiesterase inhibitor—increases intracellular cAMP	
Theo-Dur tablets		25 mg/kg q24h PO (evening) for cats, 20 mg/kg q12h PO BID for dogs
Slo-bid Gyrocaps		25 mg/kg q24h PO (evening) for cat, 25 mg/kg q12h PO for dogs
Oxygen	Increases diffusion gradient	

These are mainstay drugs used for emergency allergic airway disease. Terbutaline and theophylline should only be used once cardiac disease has been ruled out.

Two primary classes of bronchodilators are available that can be used to treat respiratory distress. These classes include methylxanthines (theophylline, aminophylline) and selective β–2 receptor agonists (terbutaline or albuterol). In a distressed animal, injectable terbutaline should be administered for the quickest effect. The clinician should rule out cardiac disease before administering these medications since tachyarrhythmia is a possible side effect of the beta agonists.[26] If the animal shows a clear response to bronchodilator administration, there is support for continuing oral administration of medication for long-term therapy. Response can be measured by noticing changes in such things as airway resistance, respiratory rate, expiratory effort and even the degree of hyperinflation on thoracic radiographs. The authors prefer using either of two sustained-release theophylline products (Theo-Dur tablets or Slo-bid Gyrocaps) on the basis of studies demonstrating acceptable pharmacokinetics with these two products.[27] Dosing in cats is once daily *at night* because less variability and higher peak concentrations were observed compared with morning dosing.[28]

Antihelminthics are routinely recommended for animals with allergic airway disease. Although bronchoscopy and bronchial washings offer the best chance of diagnosing parasitic allergic lung disease, there are times when either these resources are not available to the clinician or treatment is started on a prophylactic basis. In these situations, various antihelminthics are available (Table 39-1).[11] Response to treatment should be monitored by clinical response, thoracic radiography, and periodic fecal examination.

It has been suggested that antihistamines and hyposensitization may be of benefit in the treatment of the inflammatory response associated with allergic airway disease.[19,20] This line of reasoning assumes that small animal allergic airway disease mimics the pathophysiology of human asthma, and that mediator release (histamine, bradykinin, leukotriennes) is the underlying cause of bronchoconstriction. Many studies, however, have shown that mast cells are not a predominant cell type in bronchial washings in small animals with allergic airway disease.[3,2] Furthermore, recent studies have shown that cats challenged with histamine aerosolization have variable responses of pulmonary resistance and compliance. Some cats demonstrate bronchodilation in response to histamine challenge.[1,2] This would argue that antihistamines would not be an efficacious drug in the treatment of allergic airway disease in cats. Padrid[29] has also suggested that cyproheptadine (a serotonin receptor antagonist) may have potential in treating allergic airway disease in cats. *In vitro*, serotonin has been shown to cause contraction of tracheal and bronchial strips of feline smooth muscle. It is presumed that the serotonin originates from mast cell degranulation, although this has not been directly proven. Serotonin does not appear to have similar effects on human or equine pulmonary smooth muscle.[29] It has yet to be determined whether cyproheptadine will work *in vivo* as well in cats with airway disease.

Many human asthmatics are now treated with new drug therapies such as leukotrienne receptor blockers or inhibitors of the enzyme 5-lipoxygenase, which is responsible for the formation of leukotriennes themselves. These drugs include Zileuton (Zyflo), an inhibitor of 5-lipoxygenase, and montelukast (Singulair) and zfirlukast (Accolate), both leukotrienne receptor blockers. Clinical efficacy in humans has been demonstrated in a number of large clinical trials.[30] Patients treated with both β-agonists and either zileuton, zafirlukast, or montelukast showed significant improvement in FEV1 over a period of 4 to 6 weeks, and their use of rescue β-agonist therapy decreased as well.[31] Padrid[29] was unable to show efficacy using a lipoxygenase blocker in his model of experimentally-induced, allergic airway disease in cats. Although the human literature is encouraging, to date no clinical studies have been performed on animals with allergic airway disease to evaluate the efficacy of these drugs.

PROGNOSIS

The prognosis for small animals with allergic airway disease is variable depending on the cause, chronicity, and continuing exposure to irritants. The overall clinical picture can be exacerbated by concurrent underlying cardiac or other respiratory disease. The disease in cats is often a chronic disorder, one that will exhibit either persistent signs or episodic flare-ups. While mortality is not greatly affected, morbidity is high in affected cats because of the chronicity of the disease.

REFERENCES

1. Padrid PA: CVT update: feline asthma. *In* Bonagura JD, ed.: Kirk's Current Veterinary Therapy XIII. Philadelphia: WB Saunders, 2000, p 805.
2. Dye JA, McKiernan BC, Rozanski EA, et al.: Bronchopulmonary disease in the cat: historical, physical, radiographic, clinicopathologic, and pulmonary functional evaluation of 24 affected and 15 healthy cats. *J Vet Int Med* 10:385, 1996.
3. Moise NS, Weidenkeller D, Yeager AE, et al.: Clinical, radiographic, and bronchial cytologic features of cats with bronchial disease: 65 cases (1980–1986). *J Am Vet Med Assoc* 194:1467, 1989.
4. Guyton AC and Hall JE: Textbook of Medical Physiology, 9th ed. Philadelphia: WB Saunders, 1996.
5. Johnson L: Diseases of the bronchus. *In* Ettinger SJ, Feldman EC, eds.: Textbook of Veterinary Internal Medicine. Philadelphia: WB Saunders, 2000, p 1055.
6. Woolcock AJ: Asthma *In* Murray JF, Nadel JA, eds.: Textbook of Respiratory Medicine, 2nd ed. Philadelphia: WB Saunders, 1994, p 1289.
7. Felsburg PJ: Respiratory Immunology. *In* Kirk RW, ed.: Current Veterinary Therapy IX. Philadelphia: WB.Saunders, 1986, p 228.
8. West JB: Respiratory Physiology, 4th ed. Baltimore: Williams and Wilkins, 1990.
9. Bauer T: Pulmonary Hypersensitivity Disorders. *In* Kirk RW, ed.: Current Veterinary Therapy X . Philadelphia: WB Saunders, 1989.
10. Hawkins E: Pulmonary Parenchymal Diseases. *In* Ettinger S, Feldman E, eds.: Textbook of Veterinary Internal Medicine. Philadelphia: WB Saunders, 2000.
11. Urquhart GM, Armour J, Duncan JL et al.: Veterinary Parasitology. New York: Churchhill Livingstone, 1987.
12. Calvert CA, et al.: Pulmonary and disseminated eosinophilic granulomatosis in dogs. *J Am Anim Hosp Assoc* 24:311, 1988.
13. Padrid PA, Feldman BF, Funk K, et al.: Cytologic, microbiologic, and biochemical analysis of bronchoalveolar lavage fluid obtained from 24 healthy cats. *Am J of Vet Res* 52:1300, 1991.

14. Boushey HA, Holtzman MJ, Sheller JR, et al.: State of the art-bronchial hyperreactivity. *Am Rev Respir Dis* 121:389, 1980.
15. Corcoran BM, Foster DJ, Fuentes VL: Feline asthma syndrome: a retrospective study of the clinical presentation in 29 cats. *J Small Anim Pract* 36:481, 1995.
16. Center SA, Randolph JF, Erb HN, et al.: Eosinophilia in the cat: a retrospective study of 312 cases (1975 to 1986). *J Am Anim Hosp Assoc* 26:349, 1990.
17. Selcer BA, Newell SM, Mansour AE, et al.: Radiographic and 2-D echocardiographic findings in eighteen cats experimentally exposed to D. Immitis via mosquito bites. *Vet Radiol* 37:37, 1996.
18. Dillon R: Dirofilariasis in dogs and cats: *In* Ettinger SJ, Feldman EC, eds.: Textbook of Veterinary Internal Medicine. Philadelphia: WB Saunders, 2000, p 956.
19. Halliwell RW: Efficacy of hyposensitization in feline allergic disease based upon results of in vitro testing for allergen-specific immunoglobulin E. *J Am Anim Hosp Assoc* 33:282, 1997.
20. Prost C: Immunotherapy treatment in nine cats with feline asthma syndrome. *Veterinary Dermatology, Scientific Abstracts* 11(Suppl1):15.
21. Peeters DE, McKiernan BC, Weisiger RM: Quantitative bacterial cultures and cytological examination of bronchoalveolar lavage specimens in dogs. *J Vet Intern Med* 14:534, 2000.
22. Hoffman AM, Dhupa N, Cimetti L: Airway reactivity measured by barometric whole body plethysmography in healthy cats. *Am J Vet Res* 60:1487, 1999.
23. McKiernan BC, Dye JA, Rozanski EA, et. al.: Tidal breathing flow-volume loops in healthy and bronchitic cats. *J Vet Intern Med* 7:388, 1993.
24. Diehl KJ: Repiratory Emergencies. *In* Wingfield WE, ed.: Veterinary Emergency Medicine Secrets. Philadelphia: Hanley and Belfus, 1997, p 149.
25. Schimmer B, Parker K: Adrenocorticotropic Hormone; Adrenocortical Steroids and Their Synthetic Analogs. *In* Goodman A, ed.: The Pharmacological Basis of Therapeutics, 9th ed. New York: McGraw-Hill, 1996.
26. Plumb DC: Veterinary Drug Handbook. White Bear Lake: Pharma Vet Publishing, 1999, p 29.
27. Koritz GD, McKiernan BC, Neff-Davis CA, et al.: Bioavailability of four slow release theophylline formulations in the Beagle dog. *J Vet Pharmacol Ther* 9:293, 1986.
28. Dye JA, McKiernan BC, Jones SD, et al.: Sustained release theophylline pharmacokinetics in the cat. *J Vet Pharmacol Ther*12:133, 1989.
29. Padrid PA, Mitchell RW, Ndukwu IM, et al.: Cyproheptadine induced attenuation of type I immediate hypersensitivity reactions of airway smooth muscle from immune sensitized cats. *Am J Vet Res* 56:109, 1995.
30. Villaran C, O'Neill SJ, Helbling A, et al.: Montelukast versus salmeteraol in patients with asthma and exercise induced bronchoconstriction. *J Allergy Clin Immunol* 104:547, 1999.
31. Edelman JM, Turpin JA, Bronsky EA, et al.: Oral montelukast compared with inhaled salmeterol to prevent exercise induced bronchoconstriction. A randomized, double-blind trial. *Ann Intern Med.* 132:197, 2000.

40
Pulmonary Edema

Dez Hughes

INTRODUCTION

Pulmonary edema is one of the most life-threatening and challenging conditions faced by the critical care specialist. The term *pulmonary edema* is often used synonymously, but incorrectly, with cardiogenic pulmonary edema; however, the strict definition refers to any condition that results in an increase in the extravascular water content of the lung. Pulmonary edema can be classified into two major forms on the basis of the underlying pathogenesis. *High-pressure edema* refers to increased lung water due to an elevated pulmonary capillary hydrostatic pressure and transudative losses of low-protein fluid through an intact pulmonary microvasculature.[1] In most cases this is due to increased left atrial pressure from heart failure or fluid overload. *Increased permeability edema* results from damage to the microvascular endothelium and/or alveolar epithelium thereby providing a direct conduit for leakage of high-protein fluid and even blood cells into the pulmonary interstitium and alveolar air spaces.[1] Most, if not all, causes of high-permeability edema have an inflammatory component and are conditions that can progress to the acute respiratory distress syndrome (ARDS) in severe cases.

Basic concepts of body fluid compartments and the fluid fluxes between compartments are often greatly oversimplified. To manage the patient with pulmonary edema to the level befitting critical care medicine, a more complex understanding is required. Appreciation of the normal water, solute, and protein fluxes in the lung, the processes involved in the generation of edema, the defense mechanisms that protect against fluid accumulation, and the ways in which excess fluid is cleared from the pulmonary interstitium and alveolar spaces should allow a more informed, rational, and hopefully successful approach to the management of the patient with pulmonary edema.

BODY FLUID COMPARTMENTS AND TRANSVASCULAR FLUID EXCHANGE

There are three major fluid compartments in body tissues: the intracellular space within cells, the interstitial space between cells, and the intravascular space within blood vessels. Together the intravascular space and interstitial space comprise the extracellular space. Movement of fluid between compartments depends on the permeability of the relevant barrier and the concentration of molecules contained within each compartment. The cell membrane is only freely permeable to water. Movement of water across the cell membrane depends on the relative concentration of molecules within cells compared to the concentration around the cell. Osmotic movement of water will occur into an area with a higher concentration of molecules. The microvascular barrier in most tissues is freely permeable to water, small solutes, and relatively (but not completely) impermeable to macromolecules.[2] This means that a protein concentration gradient exists from the vasculature to the interstitium. The higher concentration of impermeant solutes within the capillaries exerts an osmotic pressure, termed the intravascular colloid osmotic pressure (COP) that acts to retain fluid. Fluid exchange between the vasculature and the interstitium is governed by the balance between hydrostatic and osmotic pressure gradients between the intravascular compartment and the interstitium.[3]

$$\text{Flow} = K_{fc}\left(\left(\begin{matrix}\text{capillary}\\ \text{hydrostatic}\\ \text{pressure}\end{matrix} - \begin{matrix}\text{interstitial}\\ \text{hydrostatic}\\ \text{pressure}\end{matrix}\right) + \sigma\left(\begin{matrix}\text{capillary}\\ \text{COP}\end{matrix} - \begin{matrix}\text{Interstitial}\\ \text{1COP}\end{matrix}\right)\right.$$

The filtration coefficient, K_{fc}, is basically a measure of how well a specific tissue allows fluid efflux from the vasculature. It depends on the capillary surface area and hydraulic conductivity; that is, the greater the surface area available and higher the hydraulic conductivity of a membrane system, the greater the transvascular fluid flow will be in that tissue. The reflection coefficient, σ, indicates the relative permeability of the membrane to protein. A value of 1.0 corresponds to complete impermeability, 100% of the possible colloid osmotic gradient can be maintained across that membrane and exert its full effect to retain fluid within the intravascular space.

A hydrostatic pressure gradient in excess of the COP gradient at the arterial end of the capillary bed results in a net transudation of fluid into the interstitium. At the venous end of the capillary bed, plasma proteins exert an osmotic force in excess of the hydrostatic gradient resulting in a net fluid flux into vessels. The hydrostatic and COP gradients governing transvascular fluid flux and the permeability of the microvascular barrier can vary between different tissues and at different levels of the capillary bed within the same tissue.

PHYSIOLOGY AND PATHOPHYSIOLOGY OF PULMONARY FLUID BALANCE

The pulmonary ultrastructure is highly specialized to facilitate and protect gaseous diffusion (Fig. 40-1). The alveolar epithelial cells and capillary endothelial cells are extremely thin and have a fused basement membrane to minimize the width of the diffusion barrier. In normal lung there is a constant extravasation of fluid from the pulmonary microvasculature into the interstitium that is cleared via the lymphatic system. Because the endothelial and epithelial cells on the gas exchange side of the capillary are fused, normal interstitial fluid flow occurs on the opposite side of the capillary to gas exchange. Furthermore, the distensibility of the pulmonary interstitium increases toward the peribronchovascular

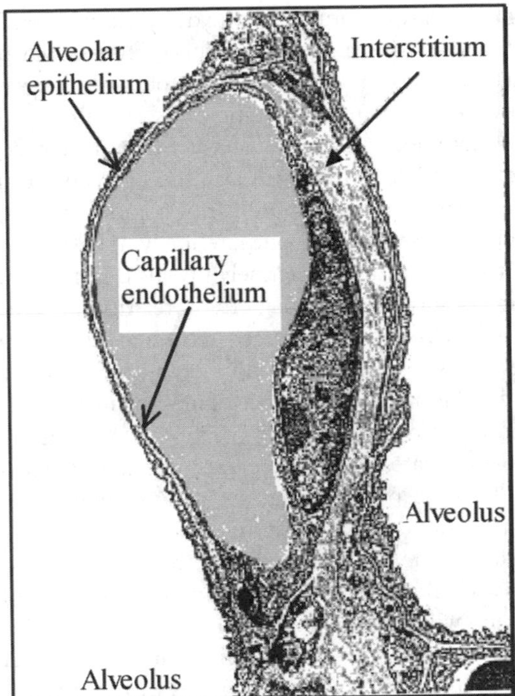

Figure 40-1
Schematic of electron photomicrograph of normal lung.

regions, thereby ensuring that excess fluid not cleared by pulmonary lymphatics will tend to accumulate where gas exchange will be least affected.[4]

In small arterioles, capillaries, and small venules, the pulmonary microvascular endothelium is permeable to water and electrolytes, but restricts the movement of protein. In contrast, the alveolar epithelium is essentially impermeable to all blood solutes and is only freely permeable to water. As in all tissues, extravasation of fluid from the pulmonary microcirculation depends on the balance of hydrostatic pressure and COP between the pulmonary capillaries and the interstitium.

It is important to realize that *hydrostatic pressure is the **only*** major force that results in extravasation of fluid from pulmonary microvessels in normal lungs and in both types of pulmonary edema.[1] In the treatment of pulmonary edema there has been a tendency to focus on hydrostatic pressure modification (diuretics and vasodilators) in high-pressure edema and not in increased permeability edema. In severe permeability edema where protein can freely cross into the interstitium reducing hydrostatic pressure reduction may be the only means by which to reduce fluid extravasation.

Pulmonary edema will occur when the rate of interstitial fluid formation overwhelms the clearance mechanisms. The mechanisms by which tissues protect themselves against edema are collectively named the tissue safety factors[5] and comprise (1) increases in interstitial hydrostatic pressure, (2) decreases in interstitial COP, and (3) increased lymph flow. The normal perimicrovascular pulmonary interstitium has a relatively low compliance; therefore, as fluid passes into the interstitium the tissue hydrostatic pressure will rise, thereby opposing filtration. Furthermore, extravasated fluid with low protein concentration will reduce the interstitial COP, which will also limit further filtration. Lastly, because the perimicrovascular interstitium is not compliant, increased interstitial fluid results in an increased driving pressure for lymphatic drainage.

The interstitial matrix may be actively involved in the modulation of small and especially large solute fluxes through the interstitium.[6] The complex, coiled structure of the huge, negatively charged molecules in the interstitial matrix hinders movement of water and solute and thereby contributes to the permeability of the microvascular barrier. This maze of meshed macromolecules also serves to resist expansion and collapse during conditions of edema and dehydration. In mild edematogenic states, small increases in volume result in large increases in interstitial hydrostatic pressure that act to limit extravasation of fluid and increase lymphatic drainage. In most tissues, the interstitium remains noncompliant until a threshold is reached and the interstitial structure abruptly breaks down. This is called stress relaxation and it is important because it means that the interstitium will become distensible and edema can rapidly progress. In the lung, the critical point may be when alveolar or airway cell separation and alveolar flooding occur. Fluid then accumulates in the interstitium and alveoli without a corresponding protective rise in interstitial pressure and lymph flow. Furthermore, during conditions of increased interstitial fluid flow, the components of the interstitial matrix can actually be washed out via the lymphatic system, further reducing interstitial resistance to fluid flow. From a clinical standpoint, this means that as gradual expansion of the interstitium occurs with overhydration from fluid therapy, edema can abruptly worsen.

High-Pressure Edema

As pulmonary capillary pressures gradually increase over the intravascular COP (usually due to left-sided heart failure or fluid overload), fluid extravasation increases and ultimately overwhelms the capacity for removal by pulmonary lymphatics. Although the lung is extremely resistant to edema formation from hypoproteinemia alone,[7] lower intravascular COP reduces the hydrostatic pressure at which edema occurs.[8] Fluid then begins to accumulate in the interstitium and flows toward the peribronchovascular interstitium. Eventually edema fluid will distend all parts of the pulmonary interstitium and fluid will begin to fill the alveoli. It appears that, because the alveolar membrane is so impermeable to solutes, alveolar filling does not occur by fluid flow through the epithelium, but rather it spills into the airspaces at the junction of the alveolar and airway epithelia. Blood vessel rupture can also occur with hydrostatic edema as evidenced clinically by the serosanguineous nature of edema fluid seen in some cases of cardiogenic pulmonary edema. Because many forms of left heart failure are gradual, rises in hydrostatic pressure often occur over a relatively long time period.

In contrast, fluid therapy can cause more precipitous increases in hydrostatic pressure especially if cardiac insufficiency is present.

Increased Permeability Edema

Injury to the microvascular barrier by direct chemical injury or inflammatory cells and mediators results in a reduction of the selective permeability of the capillary endothelium to protein. This significantly reduces or abolishes the ability of colloid osmotic pressure to retain intravascular fluid. Similarly, the protective fall in interstitial COP that occurs with extravasation through an intact barrier is diminished or negated. Consequently, capillary hydrostatic pressure becomes the major determinant of edema formation.[1] Edema formation then occurs at normal or even low pulmonary pressures and even small increases in capillary hydrostatic pressure result in much greater edema formation than when the microvascular barrier remains intact. If the alveolar epithelial cells are also damaged, then interstitial edema rapidly progresses to alveolar flooding, which explains the increased clinical severity and fulminant course seen in increased permeability edema compared to hydrostatic edema.

Resolution of Pulmonary Edema

Resolution of pulmonary edema involves clearance of interstitial and alveolar fluid. Although lymphatic drainage is one of the most important mechanisms limiting interstitial fluid accumulation, it plays a minor role in edema resolution in high-pressure edema.[9] Most interstitial edema fluid is cleared via the bronchial circulation[10] likely because of the peribronchovascular pooling of edema fluid. Absorption of water, solutes, and protein from alveoli occurs via different mechanisms and at vastly different rates. When the alveolar epithelium remains intact, alveolar free water, such as is seen in fresh water drowning, can be absorbed from the alveoli over the course of minutes. This is because the alveolar epithelium is virtually impermeable to solutes and, consequently, transepithelial osmotic gradients of up to 5000 mm Hg can exist! Resorption of sodium-containing alveolar fluid occurs in a period of hours mainly via active transport by the alveolar epithelium, most likely via a sodium–potassium pump with glucose cotransport.[11] Fluid absorption occurs against a colloid osmotic gradient, which increases as fluid is resorbed and protein remains behind. The mechanism of macromolecule clearance is less well understood but occurs at a very slow rate over a period of days.[12,13] Slow macromolecule clearance, the presence of inflammatory cells, and alveolar epithelial cell damage or death likely explain the protracted resolution or progression to ARDS often seen with increased permeability edemas.

EPIDEMIOLOGY/ETIOLOGY

Causes of pulmonary edema potentially relevant to veterinary medicine are listed in Table 40-1.

Any animal that develops systemic inflammatory response syndrome or diseases associated with systemic vasculitis is at risk for developing increased perme-

Table 40-1. Causes of Pulmonary Edema in Dogs and Cats

Increased Permeability Edema	High-Pressure Edema
Infectious pneumonia	Left-sided heart failure
Pulmonary contusions/hemorrhage	Fluid overload
SIRS	
Sepsis	Uncertain or mixed etiology
Pancreatitis	Neurogenic edema
Metastatic neoplasia	Re-expansion edema
Severe tissue trauma	High altitude edema
Immune mediated disease	Feline endomyocarditis
Systemic vasculitis	
ARDS	Other
Pulmonary thromboembolism	Near drowning
Toxic lung injury	
Smoke inhalation	

SIRS, systemic inflammatory response syndrome; ARDS, acute respiratory distress syndrome.

ability edema. Animals with bacterial, fungal, or protozoal pneumonia have pulmonary edema due to parenchymal inflammation.[14] Many causes included under increased permeability and uncertain or mixed etiology edemas could also be antecedents of ARDS. As such, ARDS is the end result of an underlying disease process. Notwithstanding, ARDS represents one of the most refractory and challenging forms of increased permeability pulmonary edema. Because ARDS carries such a poor prognosis, severe cases of pulmonary alveolar disease and impending respiratory failure should be vigorously pursued and aggressively treated to avoid the often irreversible condition of ARDS. Only two necropsy-based case series have been published related to ARDS in dogs,[14,15] so survival rate cannot be determined from the literature; however, clinical experience suggests that it is very low.

Left-sided heart failure is covered in detail in Chapter 31. When managing cardiac disease in dogs and cats it can be helpful to remember that there are only a small number of common conditions in both species. Most middle-aged to older dogs will have either mitral valve disease or dilated cardiomyopathy, whereas most cats will have hypertrophic, thyrotoxic, or restrictive cardiomyopathy or endomyocarditis. Fluid overload has been largely ignored in the veterinary literature, ostensibly because many stable animals are able to deal with a wide variety of fluid types and infusion rates.[16] With the development of veterinary critical care, increasing numbers of cases are encountered where the resilience of the cardiovascular, respiratory, neurologic, and renal systems cannot be relied on. Furthermore, subsequent to the aggressive fluid therapy of the late 1980s and early 1990s, it has become apparent that, although aggressive fluid therapy is certainly indicated in many cases, it can be detrimental in others, especially those with respiratory parenchymal disease. To cause severe fluid overload in normal dogs requires large volumes of intravenous fluids (up to 360 mL/kg/h) and even these rates did not result in death.[16] Cats are more sensitive to fluid overload especially those with renal insufficiency. A common mistake is to underestimate the relative intravascular volume-expanding effects of colloids versus crystalloids, again especially in cats. Because approximately five times the volume of colloid is retained within the intravascular space compared to crystalloid, the colloid infusion rate can be multiplied by 5 to obtain an equivalent rate of crystalloid. If a rate of 50 mL/h of crystalloid is too much for a feline patient, 10 mL/h of colloid may also be a relative overdose. All comments regarding colloid infusion apply equally to artificial hemoglobin solutions, which have a colloid action.

Toxins that can cause pulmonary edema include volatile hydrocarbons, paraquat, and *cis*-platinum in cats. Re-expansion edema is a poorly understood phenomenon reported in dogs and cats after chronically collapsed lung lobes are acutely re-expanded.[17,18,19] Suggested mechanisms include decreased surfactant concentrations, negative interstitial pressures, and oxygen (O_2) free radical formation.

Neurogenic edema is an incompletely understood condition that results in both increased hydrostatic pressure and increased microvascular permeability. It occurs much more commonly in dogs and is usually due to head trauma or seizures, upper airway obstruction, or electric cord bite. The majority of affected dogs are under 1 year of age. In young dogs, the nature of the head trauma or upper airway obstruction can be trivial, such as a slap on the nose or a pull on a leash. Older dogs usually have more serious underlying causes such as seizures or laryngeal paralysis. Signs of dyspnea occur immediately after the incident. The prognosis is usually extremely good in young dogs and depends on the underlying cause in older animals.

Feline endomyocarditis is an intriguing and frustrating condition of unknown etiology seen in cats often following a stressful episode such as a veterinary visit.[20] Cats are often young and present with an acute onset of severe dyspnea. Endocardial inflammation and interstitial pneumonia are seen in the majority of cases. The author's clinical experience of this condition suggests that prognosis is very poor; however, given the extreme difficulty of establishing a definitive diagnosis prior to death, this may reflect severe cases only.

CLINICAL PRESENTATION AND DIAGNOSTIC EVALUATION

The most serious consequence of pulmonary edema is reduced arterial oxygenation from ventilation-perfusion mismatching. Affected areas also have decreased compliance that can result in reduced lung volume and also overdistention of nonedematous regions with the potential for barotrauma in artificially ventilated patients.

Dogs and cats usually present for respiratory distress or become dyspneic during hospitalization. Successful management of the animal with difficulty breathing demands that the clinician remain acutely aware of the fragility of the dyspneic patient. Even a brief major body system evaluation can prove fatal, especially in cats. Consequently, the risks of any manipulation must be carefully weighed against the potential benefits. Once an animal has suffered a respiratory arrest the odds are hugely stacked against a successful outcome. Apart from the most severe upper airway obstructions, most animals will benefit from a period in 100% O_2 in an O_2 cage prior to a complete evaluation of major body systems.

The management goals for the patient with respiratory distress are to identify the severity of the disease process and to identify the underlying cause. The instability of the patient may preclude any diagnostic testing before empirical stabilization. Clinical severity is determined by physical examination and pulse oximetry or arterial blood gas evaluation. In a critical patient, the possibility of more than one cause is not uncommon.

Initial diagnostic evaluation should be directed at identifying the presence of respiratory versus nonrespiratory causes of dyspnea (such as pain, stress, excitement, metabolic acidosis, or brain disease). Respiratory causes may be due to upper airway obstruction, small airway disease, pulmonary parenchymal disease, pleural space disease, or defects or dysfunction of the chest wall and diaphragm. Once parenchymal disease is confirmed, the diagnostic evaluation then proceeds to identify its cause or causes.

Historical Information

Some causes of pulmonary edema have obvious historical indicators such as smoke inhalation, pulmonary contusions, re-expansion pulmonary edema, or previously diagnosed cases of congestive heart disease. In dogs with dyspnea, vomiting or regurgitation should raise suspicion of aspiration pneumonia. An older large breed dog with historical findings suggestive of laryngeal paralysis (such as changes in bark and exercise intolerance) may also have aspiration pneumonia or neurogenic pulmonary edema.[21] Upper airway obstruction, seizures or head trauma, and electric shock account for almost all of the cases of neurogenic pulmonary edema. Quite minor upper airway obstruction or head trauma can cause severe neurogenic edema. Any suspicion of rodenticide exposure should prompt coagulation testing because pulmonary hemorrhage is common with anticoagulant rodenticide toxicity.[22–24] A recent stressful episode such as a veterinary visit is noted in many cats with endomyocarditis.[20]

Physical Examination

The majority of pulmonary edema cases will have moderate to severe tachypnea and dyspnea, the severity of which can be inversely proportional to the chronicity of disease. Some dogs with slowly progressive mitral valve disease can tolerate quite severe edema surprisingly well. Animals with neurologic disease, severe hypoperfusion, or respiratory muscle paralysis may not manifest appropriately severe respiratory distress. Paradoxically, some of the most severe pulmonary edema cases can clinically appear less dyspneic, potentially due to decreased lung compliance or respiratory muscle fatigue. Not all animals with pulmonary edema have crackles on pulmonary auscultation, but most will have either harsh lung sounds or crackles. With careful auscultation the abnormal area can be localized to a specific region. For example, a perihilar distribution with cardiogenic edema in dogs or a predominantly dorsocaudal distribution with neurogenic edema, or with aspiration pneumonia will have cranioventral harsh lung sounds or crackles.

Diagnostic Testing

Ultimately, chest radiographs are the initial test to identify the underlying cause of dyspnea because they provide information about the anatomy of the whole chest cavity and its organs. They can only be used to discriminate cardiogenic versus noncardiogenic caused pulmonary edema. Unfortunately, chest radiographs are also arguably the most stressful part of the initial diagnostic evaluation and empirical therapy such as O_2 and diuretics may have to be instituted first. With severe dyspnea, dogs will often tolerate a quick lateral radiograph, often the most useful view. In contrast, cats will sit in sternal recumbency for a dorsoventral view with minimal restraint. When taking radiographs of dyspneic patients, the equipment should be fully set up before beginning the procedure and O_2 supplementation should always be available. Even short periods without O_2 can be life-threatening, especially if the animal struggles during restraint. A cranioventral alveolar pattern is most compatible with aspiration pneumonia, whereas as dorsocaudal alveolar or interstitial pattern suggests neurogenic pulmonary edema. Alveolar disease, worse in the perihilar region, is often seen with cardiogenic edema in dogs. Notably, cats sometimes show perihilar edema but can also have patchy alveolar patterns that can sometimes appear almost nodular. Distended pulmonary veins relative to the corresponding pulmonary artery can be supportive of increased venous pressures in some cases. Not all animals with these diseases will have classic radiographic patterns and almost all causes of pulmonary edema can cause a diffuse pattern.

With a skilled echocardiographer, cardiac ultrasound can be a relatively quick and easy way to provide useful information on a possible cardiac component to pulmonary parenchymal disease. Most dogs will have mitral valve disease or dilated cardiomyopathy and cats usually have hypertrophic or restrictive cardiomyopathy, or endomyocarditis. Difficulty in appropriately positioning a dyspneic animal can limit the ability to perform a meaningful study and adequately assess chamber sizes or wall thickness.

Although chest radiographs provide anatomic information, blood gas analysis and pulse oximetry can provide objective physiologic documentation of the severity of the underlying disease. Blood gas analysis or pulse oximetry, though useful, are not absolutely essential if they pose a serious risk. Obtaining a metatarsal arterial blood sample is usually much less stressful than using the femoral artery. Arterial blood gas analysis allows calculation of the alveolar-arterial O_2 tension difference (A-a gradient). The majority of patients with pulmonary edema will have an increased gradient and it is hard to consider a diagnosis of pulmonary edema without one. Pulse oximetry is useful providing a meaningful waveform is obtained. An accurate reading may be difficult in cats, in patients with poor peripheral perfusion, fast heart rates, or pigmented skin, or in moving patients. If the accuracy of the reading is uncertain it should be viewed with appropriate skepticism especially if it is at odds with the clinical picture.

Arterial blood pressure measurement is rarely of diagnostic value. However, because almost all conditions resulting in pulmonary edema can be associated with hypovolemic, cardiogenic, or septic shock, it is wise to monitor arterial blood pressure. Metatarsal arterial lines can be placed quickly by surgical cut-down under local anesthesia providing the criticalist or surgeon is familiar and proficient with the technique.[25] Central venous pressure (CVP) can be helpful in managing the patient with pulmonary edema. In the absence of fluid overload an elevated CVP can occur with right-sided heart failure, pericardial effusion, and right-sided cardiac obstruction such as masses or heartworm disease. Its main use, however, is in guiding fluid therapy in these patients. In advanced practices, a flow-guided pulmonary arterial catheter can be used to measure pulmonary capillary wedge pressures (an indicator of left atrial pressure) and with special thermistor-tipped catheters cardiac output can also be determined. Furthermore, systemic vascular resistance and O_2 transport and consumption variables can then be calculated allowing intense scrutiny of cardiopulmonary status. In research facilities, these catheters can be used to calculate extravascular lung water (EVLW), a direct measure that can detect fluid accumulation in the lungs prior to oxygenation defects and guide fluid therapy.[26]

In cases where infectious pneumonia or neoplasia are suspected, specimens should be obtained for cytology and microbiologic analysis via transtracheal lavage, endotracheal lavage, or endobronchial lavage. Edema fluid protein concentration is lower on average in patients with high-pressure versus increased permeability edema.[27] Importantly, the amount of overlap between groups limits its diagnostic utility in specific cases. A negative result does not rule out the presence of either disease. Positive bacterial cultures should be viewed in light of clinical findings and the possibility of contamination should always be considered.

Several ancillary tests may be considered depending on the potential disease processes present. Pulmonary thromboembolism is notoriously difficult to confirm in vivo and is often a diagnosis based on clinical features with documentation of another disease known to be associated with hypercoagulability such as hyperadrenocorticism or protein-losing nephropathy. Pulmonary angiography and more recently computered tomographic digital subtraction angiography can sometimes be helpful but require advanced expertise and equipment. Coagulation screening is often indicated with increased permeability due to the high incidence of coagulopathy with these diseases. Abdominal ultrasound can detect pancreatitis, intra-abdominal neoplasia, or potential septic foci. Blood cultures and fungal, protozoal, or rickettsial titers may be indicated in certain cases. In extremely challenging cases, especially in ventilated animals, lung biopsy may be necessary.

TREATMENT

Treatment of pulmonary edema depends largely on the underlying cause; however, in all cases O_2 supplementation must be supplied to allow adequate tissue oxygenation. When PaO_2 falls below 60 mm Hg there is a more rapid decline in hemoglobin saturation (which is the main determinant of arterial O_2 content) and serious tissue hypoxia becomes more likely. Hypoxemic animals that are not moving often have sufficient tissue O_2 delivery to support their major organ systems; however, increased skeletal muscle O_2 demand due to agitation or restraint can be sufficient to precipitate cardiopulmonary arrest. Hence, it is important to restrict movement in patients with pulmonary edema especially those with concurrent heart disease.

An O_2 cage provides a quiet, less stressful environment and allows an inspired O_2 concentration up to 100%. Nasal cannulation can be used with moderate hypoxemia when animals will tolerate nasal cannulae or prongs; however, placement can be extremely stressful for some patients. When placing a nasal cannula with local anesthetics it is important to realize that full desensitization can take up to 10 minutes to occur. Artificial positive pressure ventilation is necessary in patients in which O_2 saturation cannot be maintained above 90% with noninvasive methods of O_2 supplementation, in animals with concurrent hypoventilation and an $PaCO_2$ above 50 mm Hg, and in cases where respiratory fatigue is a concern. Some evidence suggests that positive end-inspiratory pressure can facilitate edema resolution but this remains controversial. Body position can significantly affect arterial O_2 concentration. In general, gas exchange is best in a sternal position; however, in cases with disease that is worse on one side it may be necessary to position the animal with that side down. Placing an affected animal with the diseased side up can precipitate life-threatening hypoxemia.

Diuretics, initially administered as furosemide, are the mainstay of treatment in high-pressure edema. Furosemide decreases pulmonary capillary pressure and also increases COP.[28,29] Some evidence also suggests that furosemide also increases perfusion to ventilated regions of the lung. In view of the fact that hydrostatic edema is the force causing fluid extravasation in permeability edema, diuretic administration may well be indicated in these cases when hypoxemia is life-threatening. Concerns regarding slowing clearance via the mucociliary escalator are not really applicable when dealing with a life-threatening situation. In humans with heart failure constant rate infusions have been shown to be more effective in increasing diuresis than bolus administration.

Vasodilators such as nitroglycerin or nitroprusside are the other main strategy of reducing pulmonary capillary hydrostatic pressure. The main concern with administration of vasodilators is their potential to cause arterial hypotension and to worsen ventilation-perfusion mismatching by decreasing hypoxic pulmonary vasoconstriction. Nitroglycerin is primarily a venodilator with minimal effects on arterial blood pressure at recommended doses and is usually safe; however, some authorities have questioned its efficacy. Nitroglycerin is available as a transcutaneous paste and is used somewhat empirically at 1/4 to 2 inches per dog (1 inch contains 15 mg nitroglycerin). Nitroprusside is a balanced vasodilator that, because of its short half-life, must be given via a constant rate infusion. Because of its potential to cause severe hypotension, it should be used with constant monitoring, ideally of direct arterial pressures. Recent experimental evidence indicates that phosphodiesterase inhibitors and β_2-agonists, especially terbutaline, facilitate reabsorption of fluid from the alveolar space.[30,31]

Fluid Therapy in the Management of Pulmonary Edema

Restriction of fluid therapy in the patient with pulmonary edema must be weighed against the potential risks such as compromised renal function and multiple organ failure. Experimental and clinical studies of fluid therapy with pulmonary edema lean toward the conclusion that prudent fluid restriction is beneficial in high-pressure and increased permeability edema. The relative importance of the hydrostatic pressure gradient in both forms of pulmonary edema cannot be overemphasized. Moreover, when permeability is increased, the hydrostatic pressure gradient may be the main determinant of transvascular fluid flow. Because the protective effects of the intravascular colloid osmotic pressure are reduced, relatively small rises in pulmonary capillary pressure will result in large increases in fluid loss into the lung. Even in normal lungs, the pulmonary endothelium is relatively permeable to protein compared to other tissues,[32] and albumin[33] and hetastarch[34] equilibrate more rapidly with the interstitial space. If an increase in endothelial permeability is sufficient that the majority of colloid molecules can pass through the pulmonary capillary endothelium, then colloid therapy may worsen pulmonary edema.[35,36] Because of the extremely slow clearance of macromolecules from the alveolar space, this increase in edema is even more dangerous. Because the increase in permeability cannot be reliably estimated in a clinical setting, assessing the response to a test infusion of colloid may be useful. An increase in COP should be titrated against changes in clinical signs and arterial O_2 concentration. If respiratory parameters worsen following colloid administration this raises the possibility that extravascular leakage of colloid could be contributing to the deterioration.

Cautiously increasing intravascular COP by colloid administration can protect against cardiogenic pulmonary edema[37] providing this is accomplished without increasing pulmonary capillary hydrostatic pressure. Monitoring the gradient between pulmonary artery occlusion pressure and COP has been suggested to be useful in the management of pulmonary edema.[38,39] Because conventional therapy with O_2, cage rest, diuretics, and vasodilators is successful in many cases, colloid therapy should only be considered for left heart failure when close supervision and invasive hemodynamic monitoring is possible.

PROGNOSIS

General statements regarding prognosis with pulmonary edema are meaningless. For hydrostatic edema, the prognosis in animals without serious underlying disease is excellent. In contrast, prognosis in the animal with multisystem disease is guarded to poor. Prognosis with cardiogenic edema depends on the severity of underlying cardiac disease. Some dogs with mitral insufficiency survive for years, whereas patients with severe dilated cardiomyopathy fail to survive to hospital discharge despite intensive care. Severe cases of increased permeability edema can be challenging and carry a poor prognosis; however, treatment of mild to moderate disease is often successful. Outcome in animals that require positive pressure ventilation is poor for two reasons. First, many owners elect euthanasia without ventilation and second, even when advanced intensive care is provided survival is only of the order of 20%.[40]

REFERENCES

1. Demling RH, LaLonde C, Ikegami K: Pulmonary edema: pathophysiology, methods of measurement, and clinical importance in acute respiratory failure. *New Horiz* 1:371, 1993.
2. Rippe B, Haraldsson B: Transport of macromolecules across microvascular walls: the two pore theory. *Physiol Rev* 74:163, 1994.
3. Starling EH: On the absorption of fluid from the connective tissue spaces. *J Physiol (Lond)* 19:312, 1896.
4. Conhaim RL, Lai-Fook SJ, Staub NC: Sequence of perivascular liquid accumulation in liquid-inflated dog lung lobes. *J Appl Physiol* 60:513, 1986.
5. Guyton AC, Granger HJ, Taylor AE: Interstitial fluid pressure. *Physiol Rev* 51:527, 1971.
6. Aukland K, Reed RK: Interstitial-lymphatic mechanisms in the control of extracellular fluid volume. *Physiol Rev* 73:1, 1993.
7. Zarins CK, Rice CL, Peters RM, *et al.*: Lymph and pulmonary response to isobaric reduction in plasma oncotic pressure in baboons. *Circ Res* 43:925, 1978.
8. da Luz P, Shubin H, Weil MH, *et al.*: Pulmonary edema related to changes in colloid osmotic and pulmonary artery wedge pressure in patients after acute myocardial infarction. *Circulation* 51:350, 1975.
9. Mackersie RC, Christensen J, Lewis FR: The role of pulmonary lymphatics in the clearance of hydrostatic pulmonary edema. *J Surg Res* 43:495, 1987.
10. Fukue M, Serikov VB, Jerome EH: Bronchial vascular reabsorption of low-protein interstitial edema liquid in perfused sleep lungs. *J Appl Physiol* 81:810, 1996.
11. Sakuma T, Okaniwa G, Nakada T, *et al.*: Alveolar fluid clearance in the resected human lung. *Am J Respir Crit Care Med* 150:305, 1994.
12. Folkesson HG, Matthay MA, Westrom BR, *et al.*: Alveolar epithelial clearance of protein. *J Appl Physiol* 80:1431, 1996.
13. Matthay MA, Berthiaume Y, Staub NC: Long-term clearance of liquid and protein from the lungs of unanesthetized sheep. *J Appl Physiol* 59:928, 1985.
14. Parent C, King LG, Walker LM, *et al.*: Clinical and clinicopathologic findings in dogs with acute respiratory distress syndrome: 19 cases (1985–1993). *J Am Vet Med Assoc* 208:1428, 1996.
15. Turk J, Miller M, Brown T, *et al.*: Coliform septicemia and pulmonary disease associated with canine parvoviral enteritis: 88 cases (1987–1988). *J Am Vet Med Assoc* 196:771, 1990.
16. Cornelius LM, Finco DR, Culver DH: Physiological effects of rapid infusion of Ringer's lactate solution into dogs. *Am J Vet Res* 39:1185, 1978.
17. Stampley AR, Waldron DR: Reexpansion pulmonary edema after surgery to repair a diaphragmatic hernia in a cat. *J Am Vet Med Assoc* 203:1699, 1993.
18. Raptopoulos D, Papazoglou LG, Patsikas MN: Re-expansion pulmonary oedema after pneumothorax in a dog. *Vet Rec* 136:395, 1995.

19. Fossum TW, Evering WN, Miller MW, *et al.*: Severe bilateral fibrosing pleuritis associated with chronic chylothorax in five cats and two dogs. *J Am Vet Med Assoc* 201:317, 1992.
20. Stalis IH, Bossbaly MJ, Winkle TJ: Feline endomyocarditis and left ventricular endocardial fibrosis. *Vet Pathol* 32:122, 1995.
21. Drobatz KJ, Saunders HM, Pugh CR, *et al.*: Non-cardiogenic pulmonary edema in dogs and cats: 26 cases (1987–1993). *J Am Vet Med Assoc* 206:1732, 1995.
22. Sheafor SE, Couto CG: Anticoagulant rodenticide toxicity in 21 dogs. *J Am Anim Hosp Assoc* 35:38, 1999.
23. Berry CR, Gallaway A, Thrall DE, *et al.*: Thoracic radiographic features of anticoagulant rodenticide toxicity in fourteen dogs. *Vet Radiol Ultrasound* 34:391, 1993.
24. Hess RS, Kass PH, Shofer FS, *et al.*: Evaluation of risk factors for fatal acute pancreatitis in dogs. *J Am Vet Med Assoc* 214:46, 1999.
25. Hughes D, Beal MW: Emergency vascular access. *Vet Clin North Am Small Anim Pract* 30:491, 2000.
26. Mitchell JP, Schuller D, Calandrino FS, *et al.*: Improved outcome based on fluid management in critically ill patients requiring pulmonary artery catheterization. *Am Rev Respir Dis* 145:990, 1992.
27. Rozanski EA, Dhupa N, Rush JE, *et al.*: Differentiation of the etiology of pulmonary edema by measurement of the protein content. *J Vet Emerg Critl Care* 8:256, 1998.
28. da Luz P, Shubin H, Weil MH, *et al.*: Pulmonary edema related to changes in colloid osmotic and pulmonary artery wedge pressure in patients after acute myocardial infarction. *Circulation* 51:350, 1975.
29. Schuster CJ, Weil MH, Besso J, *et al.*: Blood volume following diuresis induced by furosemide. *Am J Med* 76:585, 1984.
30. Seibert DG, Thomson WJ, Taylor A, *et al.*: Reversal of increased microvascular permeability associated with ischemia-reperfusion: role of cAMP. *J Appl Physiol* 72:389, 1992.
31. Sakuma T, Okaniwa G, Nakada T, *et al.*: Alveolar fluid clearance in the resected human lung. *Am J Respir Crit Care Med* 150:305, 1994.
32. Parker JC, Perry MA, Taylor AE: Permeability of the microvascular barrier. *In* Staub NC, Taylor AE, eds.: Edema. New York: Raven Press, 1984, p 143.
33. Vaughan TRJ, Erdmann AJ, Brigham KL, *et al.*: Equilibrium of intravascular albumin with lung lymph in unanesthetized sheep. *Lymphology* 12:217, 1979.
34. Korent VA, Conhaim RL, McGrath AM, *et al.*: Molecular distribution of hetastarch in plasma and lung lymph of unanesthetized sheep. *Am J Respir Crit Care Med* 155:1302, 1997.
35. Holcroft JW, Trunkey DD, Carpenter MA: Extravasation of albumin in tissues of normal and septic baboons and sheep. *J Surg Res* 26:341, 1979.
36. Rutili G, Parker JC, Taylor AE: Fluid balance in ANTU-injured lungs during crystalloid and colloid infusions. *J Appl Physiol* 56:993, 1984.
37. Guyton AC, Lindsay NW: Effect of elevated left atrial pressure and decreased plasma protein concentration on the development of pulmonary edema. *Circ Res* 7:649, 1959.
38. Rackow EC, Fein IA, Leppo J: Colloid osmotic pressure as a prognostic indicator of pulmonary edema and mortality in the critically ill. *Chest* 72:709, 1977.
39. Rackow EC, Fein IA, Siegel J: The relationship of the colloid osmotic-pulmonary artery wedge pressure gradient to pulmonary edema and mortality in critically ill patients. *Chest* 82:433, 1982.
40. King LG, Hendricks JC: Use of positive-pressure ventilation in dogs and cats: 41 cases (1990–1992). *J Am Vet Med Assoc* 204:1045, 1994.

41
Pneumonia

Adam J. Reiss and Brendan C. McKiernan

INTRODUCTION

Pneumonia may be defined as any inflammation of the lung parenchyma resulting in alveolar air spaces filling with exudate.[1] The presence of exudate in the alveolar spaces and smaller airways leads to regional hypoventilation and, clinically, to hypoxemia. Most cases of pneumonia in small animals are caused by bacterial infection. Other causes of pneumonia include fungal, viral, parasitic, aspiration of gastric contents, and chemical and smoke inhalation.

PATHOGENESIS

Infectious

Bacterial

Bacterial infection of the lower respiratory tract is one of the most commonly recognized causes of pneumonia in small animals. Pneumonia attributed to bacterial infection is reported more often in dogs than cats.[2] Bacterial pneumonia may, on occasion, be a primary disease but most often is secondary to other types of lung injury.[3] The most common organisms identified in dogs with bacterial pneumonia are gram negative bacteria such as *Escherichia coli, Pseudomonas* sp, *Klebsiella* sp, and *Bordetella* sp.[4-8]

Although *Mycoplasma* spp have been cultured from many dogs with bacterial pneumonia, its role as a primary pathogen is debatable.[9] In a retrospective study of 93 dogs with bacterial pneumonia, 58 dogs cultured positive for both *Mycoplasma* and another organism, while 7 dogs were positive for *Mycoplasma* only, and the remaining 28 dogs were negative for *Mycoplasma*. The authors observed that favorable clinical response was achieved when antibiotic selection was based on susceptibility of bacterial isolates other than *Mycoplasma*, therefore suggesting that *Mycoplasma* is not likely a primary invader.[9]

The chances of resolving bacterial pneumonia are significantly improved when the selection of antibiotics is based on culture and sensitivity results.[3,5,7,10] Antibiotic selection before culture and sensitivity results should be based on Gram stain and cytologic findings (*e.g.*, the finding of intracellular organisms).[5]

Viral

Viral pneumonia is not commonly confirmed in small animals. Cost and technical expertise make viral isolation procedures difficult to perform. In addition, viral pneumonia is commonly complicated by secondary bacterial invasion, making its diagnosis even more difficult.[2] Viral species commonly associated with pneumonia in small animals include canine distemper virus, canine adenovirus, canine parainfluenza, and feline calici virus.[2,3]

Fungal

Fungal pneumonia is common in certain geographic areas of the country (*e.g.*, histoplasmosis and blastomycosis are common in the midwest and southeastern river valleys; coccidioidomycosis is common in the southwest). Travel history is an essential part of the diagnosis of fungal pneumonia; usually, clinical infection develops within 4 to 8 weeks of exposure. These are systemic fungal infections, which start following inhalation of infective spores into the lungs. The inhaled spores of dimorphic fungi convert to a yeast at body temperature and disseminate to other organs throughout the body (sites of distribution varies with the agent involved).[3]

Aspiration

Aspiration of liquid or particulate matter into the lower respiratory tract may lead to pneumonia. A history of vomiting or regurgitation followed by respiratory distress shortly afterwards is typical of aspiration into the lower airways.[11] Animals with megaesophagus and laryngeal disease are at increased risk for aspiration pneumonia.[3,11] Aspiration may not be observed in these patients, but it is wise to have a high index of suspicion. Infection may develop immediately as the result of contaminated material within the airway or later because of impaired pulmonary defense mechanisms.[11] The full extent of radiographic changes usually lags behind the aspiration incident by 24 to 36 hours. Radiographic abnormalities due to aspiration pneumonia classically involve dependent (*i.e.*, right middle, left and right cranial) lung lobes.[11]

Hypoxemia is a common finding in animals with aspiration pneumonia and can be caused by airway obstruction by particulate matter or secondary derangement of normal gas exchange mechanisms as outlined in this section.[3,11] Aspiration of gastric contents with pH <2.5 causes alveolar collapse, bronchoconstriction, edema, hypotension, and ventilation/perfusion mismatch, all of which can result in clinical hypoxemia[11,12]; aspiration of moderate amounts of gastric acid (>3 ml/kg) is usually fatal.[12] Epithelial necrosis caused by aspirated gastric acid leads to capillary leakage and edema, both of which further impair oxygen exchange.[11] Acids are diluted by airway secretions, alleviating the need for neutralization by solutions with a basic pH.[3] Bronchoalveolar lavage is contraindicated unless performed immediately after aspiration because it may lead to alveolar collapse secondary to surfactant dilution and result in worsening of respiratory signs.[3,10,11] In the few cases in which bronchoalveolar lavage is indicated, sterile saline is recommended as the lavage solution.[3,10,11] Bronchoscopy is useful in animals in which removal of particulate matter is needed to resolve airway obstruction.[10]

Smoke

Mechanisms by which smoke inhalation can cause pneumonia include heat and chemical injuries to the respiratory tract.

Heat

Inhalation of soot and superheated particles results in upper airway damage.[10] Thermal injuries are usually confined to the larynx and supralaryngeal airways because of the efficient heat dissipation of the upper airways.[3,13] Indicators of airway injury due to heat include the presence of facial and oral burns, wheezing, voice change, and carbon containing sputum.[3,10] The inhalation of vaporized liquids in the form of steam, containing particles small enough to bypass the upper airways, is required to injure the lower airways.[3,13] Retrospective studies of smoke inhalation in dogs and cats show survival rates between 70% and 90%.[13,14] Animals with smoke inhalation that had no respiratory abnormalities on initial examination were not likely to develop any during the subsequent hospital stay.[13,14] In the same study, all dogs (7/7) with respiratory signs that progressed after examination died or were euthanized.[13]

Chemical

Carbon monoxide poisoning results in hypoxia due to carbon monoxide's potent affinity for hemoglobin. A cherry red appearance to the mucous membranes and skin is a common clinical sign of COHb poisoning. A definitive diagnosis of COHb poisoning cannot be made by blood gas analysis or oxygen saturation measurement; specific measurement of the COHb concentration must be made to diagnose this poisoning. Clinical signs of COHb intoxication can be seen with blood concentrations as low as 10% to 20%. Treatment of COHb poisoning consists of administration of 100% oxygen, which improves blood oxygen content and decreases half-life of COHb to approximately 30 minutes.[10]

Smoke poisoning results from the release of toxic byproducts of burned materials.[10] Irritation and inflammation of respiratory epithelium can result from inhalation of smoke containing such chemicals as aldehydes, ammonia, oxides of sulfur, acrolein, and nitrogen.[10,13] Some burned plastics produce large amounts of benzene, which has anesthetic action and may facilitate the passage of acids and alkali deeper into the respiratory tract.[10] Smoke can also poison alveolar macrophages, impairing their function and potentially contributing to the onset of bacterial infection in some patients.[10]

Allergic

Pulmonary infiltrates with eosinophils and allergic or hypersensitivity pneumonia are discussed in the chapter entitled "Allergic Airway Disease" (Chapter 39).

EPIDEMIOLOGY

Animals with Altered Protective Airway Reflexes

Numerous clinical syndromes put animals at risk for pneumonic diseases. The proximity of the upper airway to the proximal aspect of the gastrointestinal tract make pneumonia an important concern in animals with diseases such as megaesophagus, laryngeal paralysis, any pharyngeal dysfunction, and severe dental disease. In addition, animals undergoing corrective procedures such as laryngeal tieback and tracheostomy are at increased risk for aspiration pneumonia. Brachycephalic airway syndrome dogs often have difficulty eating (because of airway obstruction and marked inspiratory pressure while breathing) and frequently are dysphagic; these dogs have an increased risk of developing chronic airway disease and subsequent pneumonia.

Postoperative and heavily sedated patients often have an impaired gag reflex making them susceptible to aspiration and subsequent pneumonia. In addition to anesthetized patients, those suffering from neuromuscular blockade or paralysis (*e.g.*, those with botulism, tick paralysis, or Coonhound paralysis) may develop an impaired gag reflex and require ventilatory assistance. Providing ventilatory assistance increases the chance that oropharyngeal flora will be transported to the lower airways and result in airway colonization. Invasive devices such as intravenous catheters and urinary catheters that bypass normal protective mechanisms also increase the risk of systemic infection and subsequent pneumonia.[15]

Immunocompromised Animals

Because of their potential for suppressing host defenses, systemic metabolic conditions (*e.g.*, diabetes mellitus, hyperadrenocorticism, and uremia), viral infection (*e.g.*, feline leukemia virus and feline immunodeficiency virus infections), trauma (*e.g.*, pulmonary contusions), and parasitic infestation may also be considered predisposing causes of pneumonia.

Very young and very old animals as well as those suffering from malnutrition are commonly considered populations at risk for development of pneumonia.[2] Malnutrition has profound adverse effects on systemic and pulmonary defense mechanisms. Protein-calorie malnutrition specifically impairs macrophage recruitment to the lungs in response to organisms whose clearance requires normal cell mediated immunity.[16]

Diseases including ciliary dyskinesia and IgA deficiency, which impair the removal of airway pathogens, also put animals in this at-risk group for the development of pneumonia.[2] Immunosuppressed animals (*e.g.*, those on corticosteroids or chemotherapy) have impaired pulmonary defense mechanisms and are more susceptible to respiratory tract infection.[2]

Chronic Airway Disease

Animals with chronic airway disease frequently have excessive respiratory tract secretions and some degree of airway obstruction, both of which alter local defense mechanisms and increase the risk of bacterial colonization and infection.[17]

CLINICAL PRESENTATION

A review of 42 dogs with confirmed bronchopneumonia found that no single clinical finding was pathognomonic for the diagnosis of bacterial pneumonia.[7] Less than 50% of dogs with confirmed bacterial pneumonia had fever on initial examination.[7] Common clinical findings in animals with bacterial pneumonia include dehydration, anorexia, lethargy, exercise intolerance, cough, and nasal discharge.[7] More severely affected animals may have respiratory distress and a restrictive breathing pattern (rapid and shallow respirations) on examination. Orthopnea and cyanosis may be seen in severely affected animals.[3,7,10]

DIAGNOSTIC EVALUATION

History

A complete history can be helpful in diagnosing pneumonia. Pertinent historical information includes any exposure to other animals, recent travel, current medications, smoke or chemical exposure, as well as any history of vomiting or procedures requiring anesthesia. It is also important to quiz owners on subtle changes in their pet's attitude, voice, appetite, or history of coughing.[3]

Physical Examination

Oral and Pharyngeal Examination

The following abnormalities may be associated with pneumonia: excess secretions, severe dental or tonsillar disease, masses, an abnormal gag reflex, or the finding of foreign material or gastric contents.

Tracheal Palpation

Tracheal palpation can be used to elicit a cough and confirm epithelial irritation. Pneumonia is most often associated with excessive secretions and a moist or productive cough.[3]

Auscultation and Percussion

Abnormal lungs sounds have been reported to be the most consistent physical examination finding in dogs with confirmed bronchopnuemonia.[7] Classically, these patients have increased bronchovesicular sounds as well as crackles and wheezing.[3] The lack of normal or abnormal sounds may indicate complete consolidation of that area of lung.[3] Percussion of consolidated areas of lung elicits a low-pitched or dull sound.[3]

Thoracic Radiography

Thoracic radiographs are key in diagnosing pneumonia. Caution should be used when taking radiographs of patients in respiratory distress. Acute respiratory distress can occur when these animals are positioned for thoracic radiographs. Supplemental oxygen and used of standing lateral or dorsoventral views may prevent respiratory decompensation. Three views (L and R latent and ventrodorsal/dorsoventral) of the thorax are recommended in order to examine all lung fields and improve the recognition of small lesions. Radiographic findings vary in animals with pneumonia and can change depending on the etiologic agent. In animals with acute pneumonia, the appearance of radiographic abnormalities may be delayed, and radiographs should be repeated every 24 to 48 hours to monitor disease progression.[3,11] Typical radiographic findings based on the type of pneumonia are given in Table 41-1.

Clinical Pathology

Blood culture and evaluation of the clotting cascade should be performed in patients in which severe sepsis is a concern.

Blood Gas Analysis

Arterial blood gases can be used to monitor disease progression and the response to therapeutics.[3] In a comparison of blood gas samples from 62 dogs with culture-confirmed bacterial pneumonia with samples from 46 clinically normal dogs, significantly low partial pressure of oxygen (PaO_2) and low oxygen saturation (SaO_2) values with high alveolar-arterial gradients were found in pneumonic dogs.[8] Although respiratory acidosis (hypoventilation, high $PaCO_2$ value) was not diagnosed in any of these patients, it has been suggested that this is a grave prognostic indicator.[3]

Table 41-1. Typical Radiographic Findings in Small Animal According to Type of Pneumonia

Bacterial pneumonia[3]

Mixed patterns may be seen
Air bronchograms
Alveolar infiltrates, from patchy to lobar consolidation
Pleural effusion uncommon

Fungal pneumonia[3]

Generalized miliary, nodular, or interstitial pattern
Hilar lymphadenopathy
Solitary granuloma or lobar consolidation less common

Aspiration[11]

Classically located in dependent lung lobes, *i.e.,* right middle and left and right cranial
Patterns similar to those of bacterial pneumonia

Smoke Inhalation[13,14]

Patterns commonly seen include alveolar, interstitial, and bronchial patterns

Airway Cytology

Bronchoalveolar Lavage and Transtracheal Wash

Bronchoalveolar lavage (BAL) is currently considered the best method of obtaining samples from the deep lung.[17,18,19] Cytologic differences have been reported in BAL and transtracheal wash (TTW) samples simultaneously obtained from the same patients.[20] In general, TTW samples contain fewer cells than BAL samples.[20] There is also a difference in the normal cell distribution between samples obtained by the two techniques: normal TTW samples have few alveolar macrophages, many polymorphonuclear cells, and some epithelial cells, whereas normal BAL samples contain predominantly macrophages and fewer numbers of the other cells. The differing cytologic content of these two methods is thought to be a function of different sites of collection: TTW collects cells from the large airways and BAL from the small airways, alveoli, and interstitium.[20]

Cytologic examination of BAL samples from clinically normal animals should reveal primarily undifferentiated alveolar macrophages (80%–90%) and a mixed population of other nucleated cells (10%–20%).[19] It has been reported that >2 intracellular bacteria observed in any of 50 high power (100×) microscopic fields during examination of BAL samples is considered the threshold for airway *infection*.[18] In addition to bacteria, high numbers of degenerate neutrophils are commonly encountered in samples from animals with bacterial pneumonia.[19]

Organisms may be identified in samples obtained from animals with mycotic pneumonia, and cellular responses induced by different organisms may vary. Samples from animals with blastomycosis and coccidiomycosis are generally characterized by a purulent to pyogranulomatous response containing equal numbers of neutrophils and macrophages. Cytologic findings of a granulomatous reaction with a predominate macrophage/epithelial cell population is considered consistent with histoplasmosis.[19] Since normal BAL samples contain large numbers of macrophages, care must be taken to not over-interpret cytologic findings as indicating a pyogranulomatous response. Eosinophils are the predominant cell type seen in animals with parasitic or allergic pneumonia.[19]

Gram Stain

Gram staining is an essential cytologic evaluation component of samples obtained from the respiratory tract. Gram stain results are useful in selecting an antibiotic before culture and sensitivity test results are completed. On the basis of data from multiple studies, assumptions of pathogenic bacterial organisms can be made. In general, Gram-positive cocci should be considered to be *Staphylococcus* spp or *Streptococcus* spp.[5] Gram-negative rods (most commonly, *E coli*) have been reported to be the most common bacterial isolates cultured from dogs with bacterial pneumonia.[2,4,5,6,7,8,18]

Culture and Sensitivity

Lower airway culture of healthy dogs is reported to be positive 40% to 50% of the time.[2] *Quantitative* culture appears to be necessary to differentiate normal airway flora (bacterial colonization) from true airway infection.[18] Quantitative culture containing $>1.7 \times 10^3$ colony-forming units has been shown to be consistent with respiratory tract infection in dogs.[18] Contamination of lung samples with oral flora must be avoided when cultures are being performed. Techniques that bypass the oral cavity and its flora include TTW, BAL, lung aspirate, and use of guarded culture swabs. Transthoracic needle aspiration has been reported to be associated with high rates of complication and mortality, and the method only samples a localized area of lung. Thus, this procedure should be considered only as a last resort.[21]

Fungal Serologic Testing

The deep fungal pneumonias (*e.g.*, histoplasmosis, blastomycosis, and coccidiomycosis) often elicit a systemic response and may produce positive serologic findings. Unfortunately, serologic testing is not reliable and should be used as a "piece" of the diagnostic puzzle and not as a definitive test for establishing a diagnosis.[3]

TREATMENT

Supportive Management

Fluid and Nutritional Therapy

Tracheobronchial secretions are approximately 95% water. Dehydration increases the viscosity of secretions and their retention in the lower airways and often promotes ventilation perfusion abnormalities.[3,10] Systemic hydration is an important part of treating bacterial pneumonia in small animals. Selection of fluid type and rate depends on individual case characteristics.

Malnutrition has been shown to alter pulmonary defense mechanisms, resulting in impaired pulmonary macrophage activity and diminished clearance of organisms and foreign material.[2] Proper nutrition should not be overlooked but is addressed in Chapter 15.

Oxygen

As might be expected, dogs with bacterial pneumonia have been shown to have significantly low PaO_2 and SaO_2 values and a significantly high alveolar arterial gradient.[8] These findings indicate that hypoxemia is an important clinical problem in pneumonic dogs, most likely because of ventilation-perfusion mismatching.[8]

Supplemental oxygen is indicated in patients with $PaO_2 < 60$ mmHg or $SaO_2 < 90\%$.[2] Oxygen supplementation should also be considered in tachypneic patients and those in respiratory distress.[2] Methods of oxygen supplementation are discussed in Chapter 12.

Medical

Antibiotics

Pending results of culture and sensitivity testing, bacteriocidal antibiotics, particularly those with a good Gram-negative spectrum, should be administered. Thayer et al. found that treatment based on sensitivity test results achieved clinical resolution in 69% of canine patients versus 54% in patients treated empirically.[7] Orally administered antibiotics may need to be continued for extended periods of time (4-6 weeks after discharge).[2,10,22] The decision to discontinue antibiotic therapy should be based on resolution of radiographic and clinical signs.[10]

Nebulization

Aerosol therapy has been used in pneumonic dogs to decrease the viscosity of secretions and improve mucociliary clearance. Sterile saline is the only recommended fluid for use in patients being nebulized.[2,3,10] Ultrasonic nebulizers producing particles that range between 0.5 and 3.0 um in size (mass median diameter) are necessary to ensure that fluid particles bypass the upper airways and are deposited distal to the larynx.[2,3] Nebulization is performed by placing the patient in a sealed cage for 30 to 45 minutes 3 to 4 times daily.[2,3] Potential complications associated with cage nebulization include overhydration and overheating in very small patients as well as bacterial contamination secondary to equipment contamination.[3] Nebulization of antibiotics, mucolytics, or other drugs into these cages is not recommended. Studies show that nebulized antibiotics have not improved efficacy over systemically administered antibiotics.[3,23]

Physiotherapy

Coupage (firm hand clapping on the lateral aspects of the thoracic cage) is a form of chest wall percussion that serves to induce coughing and improve clearance of secretions. Physiotherapy should always be used following aerosol therapy. Coupage should be performed for 5 to 10 minutes, three to four times daily. Mild to moderate exercise (within limits of pulmonary reserve) also facilitates clearance of secretions from the lower airways and is an important part of physiotherapy in these patients.[3,10]

Intermittent Positive Pressure Breathing

Intermittent positive pressure breathing (IPPB) has been used in the authors' practice in attempt to open collapsed and plugged airways and further improve secretion clearance. In addition to opening blocked airways, IPPB improves pulmonary compliance by re-establishing ventilation to atelectatic areas and begins to address ventilation-perfusion abnormalities and hypoxemia.[23] Intermittent positive pressure breathing can be performed in awake, medium- and large-breed dogs with a ventilator (*e.g.*, Bird 7 or 8) in the pressure support mode and a tight-fitting face mask such as a Hall's anesthesia mask (Jorgensen Laboratories, 1450 Van Buren Ave, Loveland, CO 80538). Intermittent positive pressure breathing should be performed for 5 to 10 minutes, three to four times daily with inspiratory pressure set to approximately 15 cm H_2O. Performing IPPB in conjunction with nebulization and coupage improves efficacy of these treatment modalities.

Antifungal Therapy

While Amphotericin B remains the "gold standard" antifungal drug, newer formulations of amphotericin (*e.g.*, liposome associated, Abelcet) have proven safe (less nephrotoxic) and effective in the treatment of systemic fungal disease in dogs.[24]

The treatment of systemic fungal infection has been improved by two new imidazole drugs: itraconazole and fluconazole. The imidazoles are not only efficacious against many mycotic infections, but they have few serious side effects and can be given orally. The most common side effects of the imidazoles include anorexia and hepatoxicosis. The introduction of imidazoles has made the indication for use of regular Amphotericin B extremely rare.

Itraconizole appears to be the treatment of choice for blastomycosis and histoplasmosis. Dogs with severe lung involvement should be treated for at least 90 days. Relapse occurs in about 25% of patients regardless of treatment. While antibody titers appear to be helpful in monitoring response of coccidiomycosis to treatment, they do not provide such information in animals with histoplasmosis or blastomycosis.[24]

Surgical

Lung lobectomy has been suggested as a treatment for pneumonia in patients that are unresponsive to medical therapy. Murphy et al. reported on 59 dogs and 5 cats over a 22-year period. This study showed a resolution rate of 54% in dogs and 100% in cats. Localized pneumonia caused by foreign body was more likely to resolve after surgery compared with fungal or bacterial pneumonia.[6] Twenty-five percent of the surgical lobectomy in dogs survived lobectomy but failed to resolve their pneumonia; 20% of the patients died in the immediate postoperative period. Dogs with multiple lobes resected had a higher risk of complication and death. Dogs undergoing lobectomy during the first 10 years of the study had a significantly higher risk of postoperative death and failure to resolve pneumonia. Improved survival rates in the second 10 years of the study can be attributed to evolving critical care techniques and development of new antibiotics.

PROGNOSIS

A favorable prognosis can be given to those patients that show improvement in respiratory function within 24 to 72 hours of beginning appropriate antibiotic therapy and those who have evidence of improvement on thoracic radiographs and arterial bloodgases.[22] A poor prognosis is given in those animals that have antibiotic resistant organisms cultured, underlying disease that can not be resolved (*e.g.*, laryngeal paralysis, megaesophagus), the presence of concurrent disease (*e.g.*, fungal and viral infection, neoplasia), and hypercarbia on initial examination.[3,22]

REFERENCES

1. West JB: Pulmonary pathophysiology: the essentials. Baltimore: Williams and Wilkins, 1995, p 126.
2. Roudebush P: Infectious pneumonia. *In* Kirk RW, Bonagura JD, eds.: Current Veterinary Therapy XI. WB Saunders: Philadelphia, 1992, p 228.
3. McKiernan BC: Canine and feline pneumonia. *In* Kirk RW, ed.: Current Veterinary Therapy VII. Philadelphia: WB Saunders, 1980, p 235.
4. Angus JC, Jang SS, Hirsh DC: Microbiological study of tracheal aspirates from dogs with suspected lower respiratory tract disease: 264 cases (1989–1995). *J Am Vet Med Assoc* 210:55, 1997.
5. Hirsh DC: Bacteriology of the lower respiratory tract. *In* Kirk RW, ed.: Current Veterinary Therapy IX. Philadelphia: WB Saunders, 1986, p 247.
6. Murphy ST, Ellison GW, McKiernan BC, *et al.*: Pulmonary lobectomy in management of pneumonia in dogs: 59 cases (1972–1994). *J Am Vet Med Assoc* 210:235, 1997.
7. Thayer GW, Robinson SK: Bacterial bronchopneumonia in the dog: a review of 42 cases. *J Am Anim Hosp Assoc* 20:731, 1984.
8. Wingfield WE, Matteson VL, Hackett T, *et al.*: Arterial blood gases in dogs with bacterial pneumonia. *J Vet Emer Crit Care* 7:75, 1997.
9. Jameson PH, King LA, Lappin MR, *et al.*: Comparison of clinical signs, diagnostic findings, organisms isolated, and clinical outcome in dogs with bacterial pneumonia: 93 cases (1986–1991). *J Am Vet Med Assoc* 206:206, 1995.
10. Tams TR: Pneumonia. In Kirk RW, Bonagura JD, ed.: Current Veterinary Therapy X. Philadelphia: WB Saunders, 1989, p 376.
11. Hawkins EC: Aspiration pneumonia. In Bonagura, JD, ed.: Current Veterinary Therapy XII. Philadelphia: WB Saunders, 1995, p 915.
12. Exarhos ND, Logan WD, Abbott OA, *et al.*: The importance of pH and volume in tracheobronchial aspiration. *Dis of the Chest*, 47:167, 1965.
13. Drobatz KJ, Walker LM, Hendricks JC: Smoke exposure in dogs: 27 cases (1988–1997). *J Am Vet Med Assoc* 215:1306, 1999.
14. Drobatz KJ, Walker LM, Hendricks JC: Smoke exposure in cats: 22 cases (1986–1997). *J Am Vet Med Assoc* 215:1312, 1999.
15. Johnson JA, Murtaugh RJ: Preventing and treating nosocomial infection. Part 1. Urinary tract infections and pneumonia. *Compend Contin Educ Pract Vet* 19:581, 1997.
16. Martin TR, Altman LC, Alvares OF: The effects of severe protein-calorie malnutrition on antibacterial defense mechanisms in the rat lung. *Am Rev Respir Dis* 128: 1013, 1983.
17. McKiernan, BC: Diagnosis and treatment of canine chronic bronchitis: twenty years of experience. *Vet Clin North Am Small Anim Pract* 30:1267, 2000.
18. Peeters DE, McKiernan BC, Weisiger RM, *et al.*: Quantitative bacterial cultures and cytological examination of bronchoalveolar lavage specimens in dogs. *J Vet Intern Med* 14:534, 2000.
19. Rebar AH, DeNicola DB: The cytologic examination of the respiratory tract. *Sem Vet Med Surg (Small Anim)* 3:109, 1988.

20. Hawkins EC, DeNicola DB, Plier ML: Cytological analysis of bronchoalveolar lavage fluid in the diagnosis of spontaneous respiratory tract disease in dogs: A retrospective study. *J Vet Intern Med* 9:386, 1995.
21. Teske E, Stokhof AA, van den Ingh TS, *et al.*: Transthoracic needle aspiration biopsy of the lung in dogs with pulmonic diseases. *J Am Anim Hosp Assoc* 27:289, 1991.
22. King LG: Bacterial pneumonia in dogs. Compendium's standards of care. *Emer Crit Care* 1:1, 1999.
23. McKiernan BC: Principles of respiratory therapy. *In* Kirk RW, ed.: Current Veterinary Therapy VIII. Philadelphia: WB Saunders, 1983, p 216.
24. Krawiec DR, McKiernan BC, Twardock AR, *et al.*: Use of an amphotericin B lipid complex for treatment of blastomycosis in dogs. *J Am Vet Med Assoc* 209:2073–5, 1996.
25. Legendre AM: Antimycotic drug therapy. *In* Bonagura JD, ed.: Current Veterinary Therapy XII. Philadelphia: WB Saunders, 1995, p 327.

42
Thoracic Injuries

Catriona M. MacPhail

Thoracic injury in dogs and cats is a common cause of death after trauma. Among dogs involved in motor vehicle accidents, 31% to 39% sustain thoracic injuries, whereas thoracic trauma occurs in 39% of cats.[1-3] Other types of trauma commonly associated with thoracic injuries include gunshot wounds, bite wounds, and falling from heights. A large percentage of injured animals do not demonstrate clinical signs connected with thoracic injury. The thoracic wall is an inherently resistant structure and it is often spared from significant injury even if there are significant injuries to internal thoracic structures. Of animals with radiographic evidence of thoracic trauma, 43% to 62% have more than one type of thoracic injury. There is no correlation between the pattern of appendicular injury and the existence of thoracic trauma.[1,4]

As with all forms of injury, the extent of injury is based on the type of impact (blunt or penetrating), rate of impact, and the properties of the affected tissues. When a force strikes the thorax, kinetic energy is transmitted to the thoracic wall and underlying structures. Blunt trauma causes damage through compression, shearing, and stretching of tissue, whereas penetrating injuries create crush and stretch injuries. The velocity of impact and the viscoelastic properties of tissue also determine the extent of damage. High-velocity injuries such as gunshot wounds can be extremely destructive because shock waves are propagated through surrounding tissues. Low-velocity injuries allow displacement determined by the viscoelastic properties of the involved tissue, and injury occurs due to the extent of displacement and shearing forces.

Common thoracic injuries include pleural space lesions (pneumothorax, hemothorax), chest wall injuries (rib fractures, flail chest), diaphragmatic hernia, mediastinal injuries, cardiac injury, and pulmonary injury. It is not uncommon for an animal to sustain more than one type of thoracic injury. Respiratory compromise may result from direct pulmonary injury, pulmonary compression, loss of intrathoracic negative pressure, and pain. Early recognition of thoracic trauma through clinical signs, radiography, and blood gas analysis will help these animals receive appropriate therapy. Specifics regarding pulmonary injury and penetrating trauma are addressed elsewhere in this section.

PNEUMOTHORAX

Epidemiology

Pneumothorax occurs in approximately 13% to 50% of all traumatic thoracic injuries.[1-4] Traumatic pneumothorax primarily occurs from blunt force injury that suddenly increases intrathoracic pressure and ruptures pulmonary parenchyma. Less commonly, penetrating injury or fractured ribs will lacerate the lung, trachea, or bronchi.

Pathogenesis

Pneumothorax can be classified as open, closed, or tension. Open pneumothorax has a communication between the pleural space and the external environment. Closed pneumothorax occurs from leakage through the pulmonary tissues. Tension pneumothorax results from injured soft tissues of the thoracic wall or lung creating a one-way valve that traps air in the pleural space. This is a true emergency because the increasing intrathoracic pressure severely compromises ventilation and venous return, quickly resulting in shock then death.

Clinical Presentation

The degree of respiratory compromise depends on the amount of lung collapse and concurrent pulmonary injury. Pneumothorax is usually tolerated if there is less than 50% collapse and no other underlying injury or pulmonary pathology. However, pulmonary contusions often occur in concert with pneumothorax and may cause significant respiratory compromise.[7] The typical breathing pattern associated with pneumothorax is rapid and shallow; however, some animals may have no apparent symptoms. Open pneumothorax should be obvious from initial examination because "sucking chest wounds" create an audible flow sound during inspiration. Physical examination of closed pneumothorax reveals dorsally decreased respiratory sounds and muted heart sounds. Hyperresonance may be detected through percussion of the thoracic wall. Although the mediastinum of the dog and cat is incomplete, traumatic pneumothorax is usually more severe on one side than the other. Auscultation of all lung fields will help to localize the insult and differentiate between air and fluid occupying the pleural space.

Diagnostic Evaluation

Emergency treatment of pneumothorax is initiated on animals in respiratory distress without radiographic confirmation. Radiographs are performed once the animal is stable to assess the degree of pneumothorax and the presence of concurrent injuries. A full radiographic examination is performed if conditions allow. This includes right and left lateral views and a ventrodorsal or dorsoventral view. If the animal becomes stressed during the procedure or respiratory signs worsen, the study should be aborted or priority is given to the lateral views because this positioning is usually well tolerated and pneumothorax is best diagnosed from

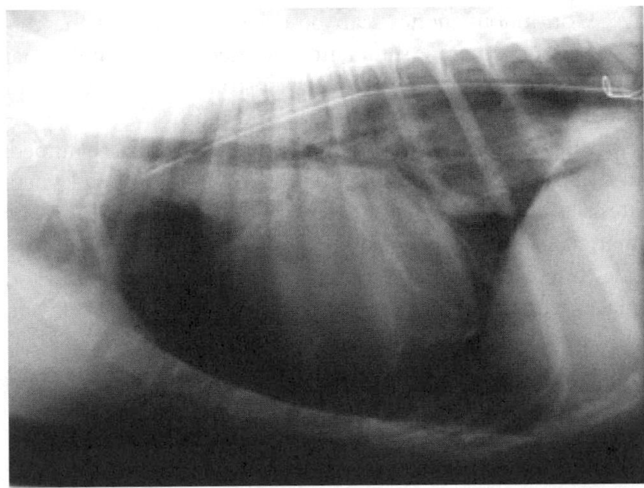

Figure 42-1
Lateral radiograph of pneumothorax.

these images. Limit unnecessary manipulation or handling of the animal during radiographic examination and have oxygen supplementation readily available.

Typical radiographic signs of pneumothorax on lateral views include elevation of the cardiac silhouette away from the sternum, visualization and retraction of visceral pleural margins away from the thoracic wall, and increased lung lobe opacity due to atelectasis (Fig. 42-1).[5] The use of horizontal beam is usually not necessary to identify pneumothorax because small volumes of air seen only on this view would be unlikely to cause significant clinical signs.

Emergency Treatment

The goal of treatment for traumatic pneumothorax is to remove the extrapulmonary, intrapleural air to allow reexpansion of the lungs. If the animal shows respiratory distress and tachypnea to any degree, or if a tension pneumothorax has been identified, thoracocentesis is indicated. This is performed by using a 20- to 22-gauge needle that is connected to an extension set, three-way stopcock, and 60-mL syringe. The needle is inserted cranial to the 8th to 10th rib at a 45° angle with the bevel facing the thoracic wall. The needle is inserted slowly and an assistant aspirates with 5 to 10 mL of pressure. Always aspirate both sides of the thorax. If air retrieval is continuous or if the animal requires multiple aspirations to alleviate clinical signs, a thoracostomy tube is indicated.

Position of the thoracostomy is critical is ensure removal of air. The tube is placed in the dorsal third of the thorax and then connected to a continuous evacuation system. Frequent intermittent evacuation may be effective; however, continuous evacuation is preferred to permit complete lung expansion and to achieve contact between the visceral and parietal pleural surfaces.[5] Also observing the underwater seal in the closed system more accurately assesses the rate of air leakage. Continuous suction can be discontinued and the thoracostomy tube removed as soon as there is sufficient evidence that the pulmonary leak has sealed. Complications associated with thoracostomy tubes include lung laceration, pleural irritation, ascending infection, and pain.

Thoracic wall wounds creating an open pneumothorax are immediately covered with an occlusive sterile dressing converting it to a closed pneumothorax. Thoracocentesis is then immediately indicated to remove the pleural air and prevent formation of a tension pneumothorax. If tension pneumothorax is suspected, needle thoracocentesis is required without delay to stabilize the patient and allow placement of a thoracostomy tube under more controlled circumstances.

If the pneumothorax persists longer that 5 to 7 days, if the animal cannot be stabilized even with continuous evacuation, or if a large airway laceration is suspected from the volume of air retrieved, thoracotomy may be indicated to definitely correct the leak. If location of the leak is not known, a median sternotomy is preferred to allow complete exploration of the thoracic cavity. However, the hilus and large airways are more accessible through an intercostal approach.

Prognosis

If tension pneumothorax is not readily identified, the animal will suffer from ventilatory and circulatory compromise and often die. However, if managed appropriately, treatment of pneumothorax is straightforward and carries a reasonable prognosis.

HEMOTHORAX

Epidemiology

Hemorrhagic pleural effusion occurs in approximately 10% of animals sustaining thoracic trauma and can occur with both blunt and penetrating trauma.[1,4] Hemothorax is a result of lung laceration or injury to major vascular structures. Considerable hemorrhage into the thoracic cavity usually results in death because the animal will bleed out before receiving emergency care.

Clinical Presentation

Lung laceration bleeding is usually clinically insignificant because the hemorrhage is self-limiting. Damage to large arteries or veins, particularly the intercostal vessels, causes significant hemorrhage. These animals will present in hypovolemic shock with tachycardia, pale mucous membranes, and decreased capillary refill time. Circulatory compromise precedes respiratory compromise as ventilation impairment will not occur until 30 mL blood per kilogram has accumulated in the pleural space.[6] Hypovolemic shock will have occurred by this point.

Diagnostic Evaluation

Auscultation of patients with hemothorax reveals muffled heart and lung sounds. A fluid–gas interface may be identified if concurrent pneumothorax is also present. Thoracocentesis is the diagnostic tool of choice because these animals are often too unstable to allow radiographic examination. Blood in the thoracic cavity is quickly defibrinated by the constant motion of the lungs and therefore will not clot after aspiration, although subacute massive hemorrhage may clot because the blood is accumulating too rapidly. The packed cell volume of the aspirated fluid is typically equal to or above the animal's peripheral packed cell volume.

Emergency Treatment

Small amounts of thoracic hemorrhage are clinically insignificant. However, more significant hemorrhage requires aggressive treatment. Drainage of the pleural cavity is performed through thoracostomy tube placement because needle aspiration will not drain the pleural space fast enough and the blood may clot within the needle if there is peracute hemorrhage. Volume replacement must be instituted to address hypovolemic shock. Transfusion is indicated if greater than 20 to 30 mL blood per kilogram is retrieved from the chest and if the packed cell drops acutely below 20%.[1] If hemothorax is a result of trauma, autotransfusion is a reasonable treatment option, especially if blood products are in short supply or not readily available. Although there are several methods of autotransfusion, direct aspiration and reinfusion is most appropriate in an emergency situation (Chapter 14).[7]

Exploratory thoracotomy is rarely indicated for hemothorax because the source of hemorrhage is rarely found or the animal is too unstable to survive the procedure. However, if the animal is not responsive to replacement therapy or if intrathoracic blood loss is continuous, surgery may be the only treatment option.

DIAPHRAGMATIC HERNIA

Pathogenesis

The pressure gradient across the diaphragm at the time of trauma dictates the nature of thoracic injury. If abdominal pressure is greater than thoracic, a diaphragmatic tear results. It has been classically thought that herniation occurs if the glottis is open at impact. A more balanced gradient across the diaphragm with a closed glottis places stress on the lung parenchyma resulting in a pneumothorax.[8] However, both pneumothorax and diaphragmatic herniation can occur simultaneously.

Diaphragmatic tears typically occur through the muscular portion, which is the weakest part of the diaphragm. The location of the diaphragmatic tear depends on the location of the viscera at the time of injury; the area least protected by abdominal organs is typically the area that ruptures. Abdominal organ displacement into the thoracic cavity depends on the location and size of the tear. Almost any organ can herniate, although the liver is the most frequent followed by the small intestine, stomach, and spleen.[9]

Clinical Presentation

Diaphragmatic hernias may go undetected after trauma and may not be diagnosed until days to weeks after injury. Animals with respiratory compromise may display respiratory distress, tachypnea, tachycardia, and cyanosis. Cardiac dysrhythmias are common due to the irritation of the heart by abdominal viscera.

Diagnostic Evaluation

Thoracic radiography may demonstrate obvious organ herniation in the thoracic cavity. Radiographic signs include loss of diaphragmatic outline and cardiac silhouette, displacement of lung fields, presence of gas-filled viscera, and pleural effusion (Fig. 42-2).[10] Effusion is usually associated with liver entrapment and venous occlusion. Abdominal radiographs may demonstrate cranial displacement of abdominal organs. Identification of stomach or intestines within the thoracic cavity makes the diagnosis of diaphragmatic hernia uncomplicated. However, if there is a large amount of pleural fluid or if the soft-tissue parenchymal organs are herniated, the diagnosis of diaphragmatic hernia may be less obvious. Repeating radiographs following thoracocentesis may identify an underlying cause that was not apparent before. Performing all radiographic views (right lateral, left lateral, ventrodorsal, and dorsoventral) may shift herniated viscera and allow better visualization.

Additional imaging procedures can be used to aid confirmation of a diaphragmatic hernia. Additional radiograph views including horizontal beam projection and standing ventrodorsal projections may confirm diaphragmatic hernia diagnosis (Fig. 42-3). Upper gastrointestinal positive contrast studies using orally administered barium sulfate will show the location of the stomach and intestines.

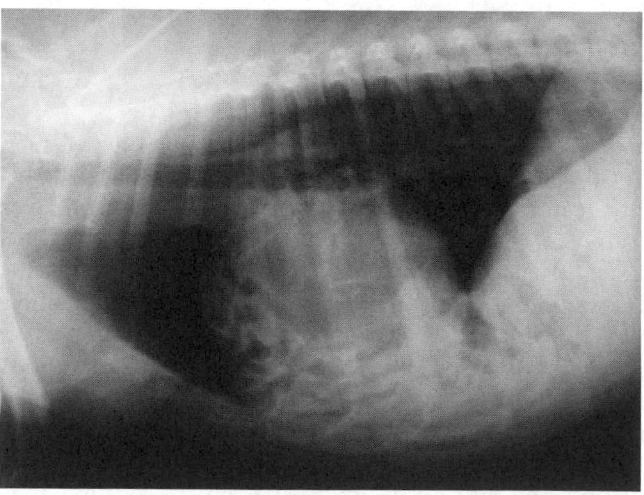

Figure 42-2
Lateral radiograph of diaphragmatic hernia.

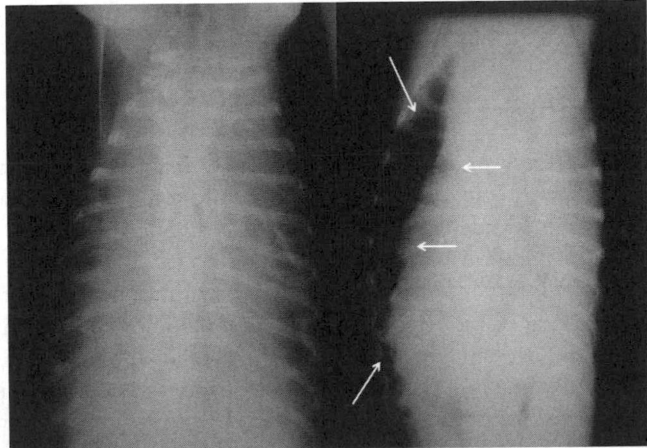

Figure 42-3
The left image is a ventrodorsal radiograph of a dog following thoracic trauma demonstrating moderate to severe pleural effusion. The right image is a ventrodorsal radiograph of the same dog in left lateral recumbancy taken with a horizontal beam; arrows show multiple loops of small intestine in the right hemithorax.

However if a large amount of pleural fluid is present, water-soluble iodinated contrast media is suggested to potentially avoid barium contamination of the pleural or peritoneal cavity due to possible gastrointestinal perforation.

Ultrasonography can also be used to diagnose diaphragmatic hernia. The diaphragm itself is not readily visualized even in normal animals. Rather, the interface between air-filled lung and hyperechoic liver identifies the location of the diaphragm.[9] A straightforward diagnosis occurs when there is identification of abdominal viscera next to the cardiac silhouette. Disruption of the lung–liver interface may contribute to information gathered from survey radiography to help diagnose a subtle diaphragmatic hernia. A common ultrasonographic artifact when imaging the diaphragm through the liver is the appearance of liver on both sides of the diaphragmatic interface. This mirror image occurs due to the extremely reflective nature of the lung–liver interface.

Positive contrast peritoneography can also be used if suspicion of diaphragmatic herniation is high but cannot be confirmed from the previously described studies. Water-soluble iodinated contrast media is injected into the peritoneal cavity. Translocation of the contrast into the thoracic cavity confirms disruption of the diaphragm.

Emergency Treatment

Mortality associated with diaphragmatic hernia is higher when surgery is performed less than 24 hours or more than 1 year after injury.[8] Anesthesia and surgery should be delayed until the animal can be stabilized. Stabilization includes shock therapy, oxygen supplementation, and antibiotic administration.

Gastric herniation is a surgical emergency because these animals are at risk for acute gastric distention and severe respiratory compromise.

Surgical Treatment

The goals of surgery are to reduce the herniated organs back into the abdominal cavity, examine the organs for any vascular compromise or perforation, and repair the diaphragmatic defect. Occasionally the diaphragmatic tear needs to be enlarged or the incision extended cranially through the sternum to allow reduction of abdominal contents and improve visualization. Tears are sutured from dorsal to ventral using a nonabsorbable monofilament suture in a simple continuous pattern. Use care when suturing near the caval, esophageal, or aortic foramina. If the diaphragm has been avulsed from its thoracic wall insertions, incorporate the ribs into the closure. Defects too large to close are rarely encountered; however, if faced with this situation autogenous flaps or synthetic implants may be used.[11] Autogenous flaps include a sliding transverse abdominus flap or an omental pedicle flap. Examples of synthetic materials include polypropylene mesh and Silastic sheeting. Following repair of the diaphragm, air is removed from the thoracic cavity by needle thoracocentesis or placement of a thoracostomy tube. Thoracic drainage is indicated if concurrent pneumothorax or pleural effusion was present.

Complications

The most serious complication associated with surgical repair of diaphragmatic hernias is re-expansion pulmonary edema, which follows rapid reinflation of atelectatic lungs. Pulmonary edema occurs as capillary integrity has been altered due to an anoxic environment in the atelectatic lung. Reperfusion of damaged vessels directs fluid into the interstitium. This is most commonly associated with chronic herniation or cats. One possible way to prevent this situation is to avoid positive pressure lung expansion during anesthesia and allow gradual reinflation of the lungs. Other less common complications include pneumothorax, hemothorax, liver lobe necrosis, gastrointestinal vascular compromise, and reherniation.[11]

Prognosis

If the animal survives for the first 12 to 24 hours postoperatively, the prognosis is very good. Reported survival rates range from 80% to 90% following surgical correction.[8,12] Deaths are usually due to concurrent injury or pulmonary edema.

RIB AND STERNAL FRACTURES

Epidemiology

Rib fractures occur in 25% of veterinary trauma patients.[1] Considerable force is required to fracture the ribs or sternum due to the inherent resiliency of the thoracic cage. Although stabilization of rib and sternal fractures is seldom necessary, identification of such injuries is crucial because underlying thoracic injury is likely. Sternal injuries require a ventrodorsally directed impact and are very uncommon in small animals. When sternal fracture does occur, it is often in association with high-rise syndrome. Rib fractures are an indicator of concurrent thoracic trauma in humans and can lead to potentially fatal cardiopulmonary complications.[13] Recognition of rib fractures is also important so that the animal's pain and discomfort from trauma are appropriately managed. Pain associated with even minor rib injury can affect respiration by impairing thoracic wall expansion, decreasing chest excursions, and exacerbating hypoxemia due to hypoventilation.

Clinical Presentation and Diagnostic Evaluation

Most rib fractures go unnoticed unless there is an open thoracic wound or flail chest. Typically fractures are not palpable, but pain is easily elicited on physical examination. Nondisplaced rib fractures can also easily go unrecognized from thoracic radiographs. Each rib should be examined closely and compared to the opposite side for symmetry (Fig. 42-4). Multiple rib fractures are more common than isolated rib injury.

Treatment

The primary goal of treatment for rib fractures is pain management. In addition to systemic administration of pain medication, local intercostal nerve blocks are effective in decreasing discomfort. In severely compromised animals, the use of local anesthesia alone can avoid the cardiovascular and respiratory depression associated with systemic narcotic administration. Intrapleural or intercostal administration of bupivacaine (0.25%-0.5%) appears to provide sufficient analgesia in dogs following rib fractures.[14] For treatment of thoracic wall pain, 0.25% bupivacaine can be injected near the proximal intercostal nerves along the caudal border of each rib. Several intercostal nerves on either side of an incision or fracture should be blocked. Use caution to avoid entering the pleural cavity and aspirate before injecting to avoid inadvertent arterial administration. Alternatively, undiluted bupivacaine (0.25% or 0.5%; up to a maximum of 1-2 mg/kg q 6 h) can be administered through a thoracostomy tube on the affected side.[14] Lidocaine may be used as an alternative to bupivacaine, however the duration of action of lidocaine is relatively short.

For open thoracic wounds with damaged ribs, the ribs may be repaired using cross-pins or wire. Sharp or splintered ends of ribs can be removed to avoid lacerating soft tissues or pulmonary parenchyma. Severely injured or contaminated ribs can be resected; however, care must be taken to preserve viable soft tissues in the area. Removal of multiple rib segments may require thoracic wall reconstruction using latissimus dorsi muscle flap, diaphragmantic advancement, or synthetic mesh implants.[15]

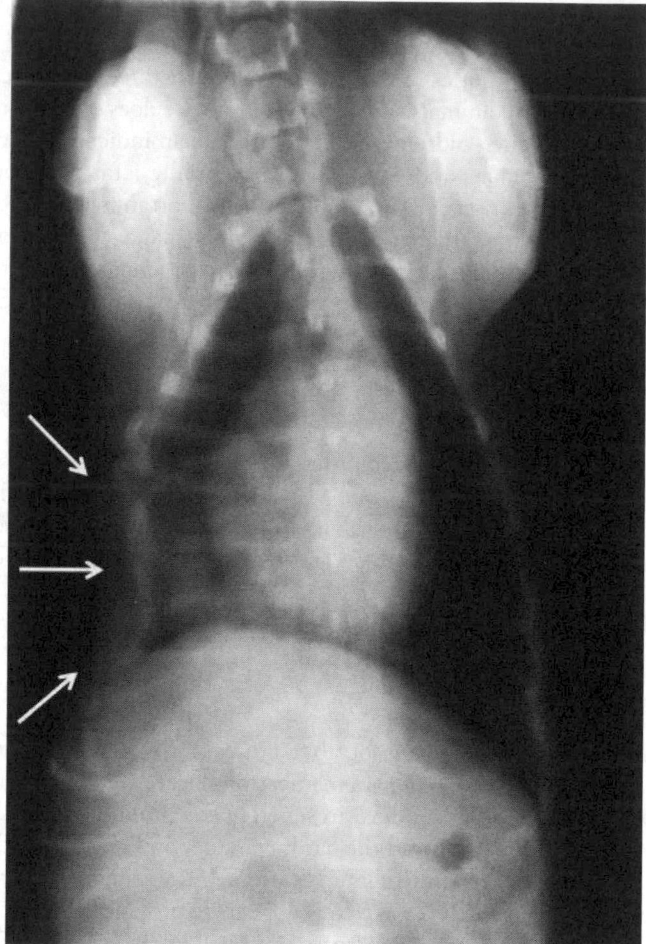

Figure 42-4
Ventrodorsal thoracic radiograph. Note fractures of the left 8th, 9th, and 10th ribs (arrows).

FLAIL CHEST

Pathogenesis

Flail chest is the fracture of several adjoining ribs resulting in a segment of thoracic wall that has lost continuity with the rest of the hemithorax. The isolated segment moves independently and paradoxically during the respiratory cycle. During inspiration, the flail segment collapses inward as pressure is reduced in the pleural cavity. The segment moves outward during expiration when pleural cavity pressure increases.

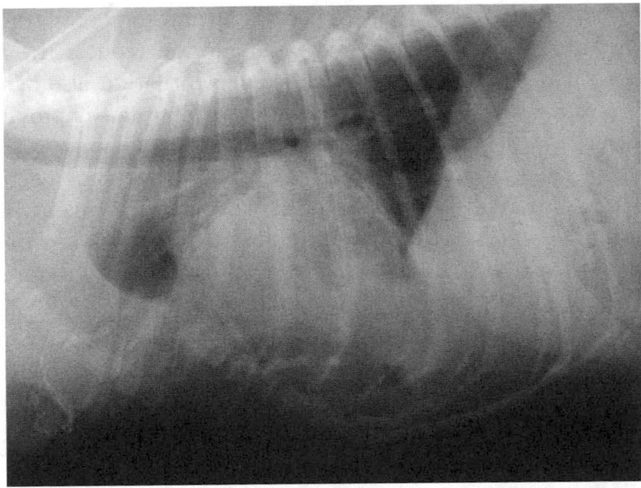

Figure 42-5
Lateral radiograph of flail chest.

Clinical Presentation

Pneumothorax, hemothorax, and pulmonary contusions may accompany flail chest and respiratory difficulty may be severe. Respiratory abnormalities are due to hypoventilation from pain and accumulation of air or fluid in the pleural cavity as well as concurrent thoracic injuries.

Diagnostic Evaluation

Flail chest is apparent on presentation. However, once the animal is stable, thoracic radiographs must be performed to determine the extent of damage and the presence of injuries (Fig. 42-5). Blood gas analysis may be helpful to characterize the severity of hypoxemia associated with hypoventilation.

Treatment

On initial presentation the animal should be placed on the side of the flail segment. This reduces the motion of the free-floating chest wall, which minimizes pain and avoids further damage to underlying structures. Stabilization of the flail segment is controversial. Some feel that the flail segment contributes little to the animal's respiratory difficulties and that stabilization of the segment is unnecessary. Instead, treatment should be focused on stabilization of the entire patient through oxygen administration, fluid therapy, pain management, and thoracocentesis if necessary. Others believe that stabilization of the free segment significantly reduces pain, thereby improving thoracic wall excursion and ventilation. The treatment of choice in human medicine for patients with pulmonary contusion and flail chest is mechanical ventilation.[16] Assisted ventilation results in decreased motion of the flail segment because intrapleural pressures are maintained above atmospheric pressure. Decreased motion reduces the amount of pain associated with rib instability. Mechanical ventilation also decreases the degree of hypoxemia by ventilating noncontused lung and improving gas exchange in damaged lung.[16]

Multiple methods of surgical stabilization of flail chest have been described in the literature. Internal fixation has been described; however, this requires general anesthesia, which may be contraindicated depending on the status of the patient. Most methods involve securing the flail segment externally using aluminum rods or plastic splints. Sutures are placed percutaneously around the ribs in multiple places to prevent pivoting of the free-floating segment. Splints may remain for up to 4 weeks after adequate immobilization of the ribs or until the animal can be taken to surgery for internal fixation. Thoracic wall bandages are not recommended because although motion of the flail segment can be reduced, expansion of the lungs is often impaired.

Prognosis

There is little information regarding the outcome of small animals with flail chest. However, a multicenter retrospective study examined 24 cases of flail chest in dogs and cats.[17] Although the majority of cases the fractured ribs were not stabilized, there was no statistical difference between stabilized and nonstabilized animals with regard to outcome.

TRAUMATIC MYOCARDITIS

Epidemiology

Myocardial contusions can result from blunt trauma to the thorax and can predispose the animal to cardiac dysrrhythmias. The term myocarditis is misleading because no true inflammatory process of the myocardium occurs. Myocardial contusion and necrosis typically are more typical lesions following blunt trauma. In fact, dysrrhythmias can occur following trauma without any evidence of damage to the cardiac muscle. The heart can be damaged by any of the following forces: unidirectional, bidirectional, indirect, decelerative, or concussive.[18] The type of dysrrhythmia depends on the type of force and location of injury; however, premature ventricular contraction is the most common dysrrhythmia associated with trauma (Fig. 42-6). Ventricular tachycardia, sinus tachycardia, and atrial fibrillation also occur. Dysrrhythmias may be exacerbated by hypovolemic shock, hypoxia, and electrolyte and acid–base disturbances. Other types of cardiac injury include myocardial laceration, tearing of major vessels, and cardiac tamponade secondary to pericardial hemorrhage, all of which are usually rapidly fatal.

Clinical Presentation and Diagnostic Evaluation

Signs of concurrent respiratory injury often mask clinical signs associated with myocardial contusions. However, traumatic myocarditis should be suspected

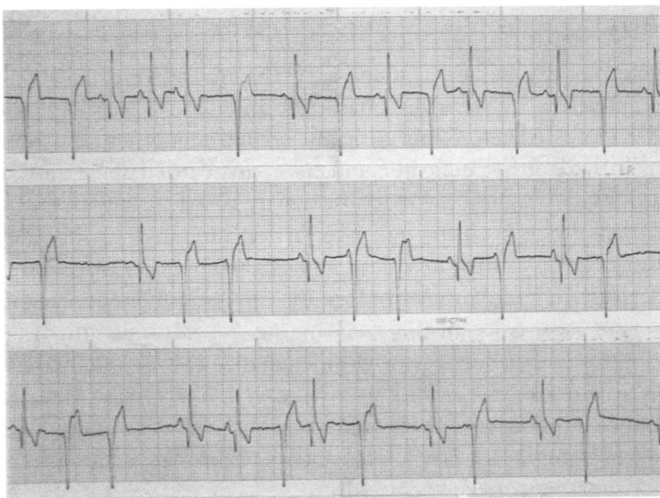

Figure 42-6
ECG obtained after blunt thoracic trauma demonstrates ventricular premature contractions.

in any animal after blunt trauma or if evidence of thoracic injury is apparent. Appropriate monitoring of trauma patients through electrocardiography (ECG) and blood pressure measurement will aid in diagnosing cardiac trauma. Ventricular dysrrhythmias commonly do not occur until 12 to 48 hours after injury; therefore, continuous ECG monitoring is ideal. If continuous monitoring is not available, the ECG should be intermittently checked every few hours while the animal is in the hospital. Direct ECG evidence of myocardial injury includes ST-segment alteration and T-wave changes.

Sinus tachycardia is common in dogs and cats following injury; it is an appropriate response to stress, pain, and hypovolemic shock. Differentiating sinus tachycardia from supraventricular tachycardia can be difficult. Although uncommon after trauma, supraventricular tachycardia results from atrial contusion, hypoxemia, or anemia. Sinus tachycardia usually resolves after appropriate shock therapy is given. Although hemodynamic alterations are uncommon with supraventricular tachycardia, antiarrhythmic therapy is often required. Vagal maneuvers may be performed before antiarrhythmic therapy is instituted although this is not commonly successful. Such maneuvers include ocular pressure and carotid sinus massage.

Ventricular dysrhythmias are by far the most common dysrhythmias associated with trauma. These ventricular disturbances are often relatively benign and rarely require treatment. However, ventricular fibrillation and cardiac arrest are possible consequences of trauma-induced ventricular dysrhythmias and therefore careful monitoring is indicated in all patients with evidence of cardiac injury.

Treatment

Correction of hypovolemia, anemia, hypoxemia, and electrolyte abnormalities often causes cardiac dysrrhythmias to spontaneously resolve. These issues should all be addressed before initiating antiarrhythmic treatment. Some antiarrhythmic agents are arrhythmogenic and cause myocardial depression; therefore, treatment should be begun only when necessary based on the ECG, blood pressure, and clinical status of the patient. Antiarrhythmic therapy should be considered in animals with supraventricular tachycardia that do not respond to vagal maneuvers. Intravenous administration of calcium channel blockers or β-blockers can be used. Esmolol (0.05-0.1 mg/kg q 5 min; maximum dose of 0.5 mg/kg) is an extremely short-acting β-blocker that can determine the response of the dysrrhythmia to β-blockers in general.[19] If conversion does not occur, diltiazem can be administered in IV boluses every 15 minutes (0.25 mg/kg; maximum dose of 0.75 mg/kg).[19] Propanolol and verapamil are other alternatives for treatment of supraventricular tachycardia.

Ventricular disturbances seldom require antiarrhythmic therapy and resolve spontaneously within a few days. However, treatment is usually recommended when clinical signs are apparent or there is significant hemodynamic alteration. Other indications include sustained ventricular tachycardia greater than 20 seconds and presence of multifocal or R-on-T complexes. Treatment is begun with an IV bolus of lidocaine (2 mg/kg). This can be repeated; however, if this is necessary a continuous rate infusion of lidocaine is indicated (40 μg/kg/min to 80 μg/kg/min).[18] If lidocaine is ineffective, procainamide can be administered intravenously or intramuscularly and can be continued orally if necessary when the animal leaves the hospital.[18]

REFERENCES

1. Spackman CJA, Caywood DD, Feeney DA, *et al.*: Thoracic wall and pulmonary trauma in dogs sustaining fractures as a result of motor vehicle accidents. *J Am Vet Med Assoc* 185:975, 1984.
2. Griffon DJ, Walter PA, Wallace LJ: Thoracic injuries in cats with traumatic fractures. *Vet Comp Orthop Traumat* 7:98, 1994.
3. Tamas PM, Paddleford RR, Krahwinkel DJ: Thoracic trauma in dogs and cats presented for limb fractures. *J Am Anim Hosp Assoc* 21:161, 1985.
4. Houlton JEF, Dyce J: Does fracture pattern influence thoracic trauma? A study of 300 canine cases. *Vet Comp Orthop Traumat* 5:90, 1992.
5. Aron DN, Roberts RE: Pneumothorax. *In* Bojrab MJ, ed.: Disease Mechanisms in Small Animal Surgery. Philadelphia: Lea & Febiger, 1993, p 396.
6. Cockshutt JR: Management of fracture-associated thoracic trauma. *Vet Clin North Am Small Anim Pract* 25:1031, 1995.
7. Purvis D: Autotransfusion in the emergency patient. *Vet Clin North Am Small Anim Pract* 25:1291, 1995.
8. Boudrieau RJ, Muir WW: Pathophysiology of traumatic diaphragmatic hernia in dogs. *Compend Contin Educ Pract Vet* 9:379, 1987.
9. Wilson GP, Hayes HM: Diaphragmatic hernia in the dog and cat: a 25-year overview. *Semin Vet Med Surg Small Anim* 1:318, 1986.

10. Williams J, Leveille R, Myer CW: Imaging modalities used to confirm diaphragmatic hernia in small animals. *Compend Contin Educ Pract Vet* 20:1199, 1998.
11. Levine SH: Diaphragmatic hernia. *Vet Clin North Am Small Anim Pract* 17:411, 1987.
12. Sullivan M, Reid J: Management of 60 cases of diaphragmatic rupture. *J Small Anim Pract* 31:425, 1990.
13. Mayberry JC, Trunkey DD: The fractured rib in chest wall trauma. *Chest Surg Clin North Am* 7:239, 1997.
14. Ludwig LL. Surgical emergencies of the respiratory system. *Vet Clin North Am Small Anim Pract* 30:553, 2000.
15. Spackman CJA, Caywood DD: Management of thoracic trauma and chest wall reconstruction. *Vet Clin North Am Small Anim Pract* 17:431, 1987.
16. Anderson M, Payne JT, Mann FA, *et al.*: Flail chest: pathophysiology, treatment, and prognosis. *Compend Contin Educ Pract Vet* 15:65, 1993.
17. Olson DA: Clinical management of flail chest in dogs and cats: a retrospective review of 24 cases (1989–1999). *Vet Surg* 29:472, 2000.
18. Abbott JA: Traumatic myocarditis. *In* Bonagura JD, Kirk RW, eds.: Current Veterinary Therapy XII. Philadelphia: WB Saunders, 1995, p 846.
19. Russell LC, Rush JE: Cardiac arrhythmias in systemic disease. *In* Bonagura JD, Kirk RW, eds.: Current Veterinary Therapy XII. Philadelphia: WB Saunders, 1995, p 161.

SECTION VI
Infection and Inflammation

43
Fever in the ICU Patient

Michael S. Lagutchik

For the intensivist, a patient's inability to maintain thermoregulation is a valuable marker of an often potentially life-threatening condition.
Michael L. Ault[1]

INTRODUCTION

Development of fever in a CCU patient often signals a serious adverse change in that patient's condition. Clinicians often launch extensive (and expensive) diagnostic procedures to define the source of a fever, and sometimes begin empirical therapeutic measures to correct the cause of the fever—actions that may carry additional risk to the patient.

An elevated body temperature is fundamentally a clinical sign reflecting the presence of either fever or hyperthermia. Fever may signal development or progression of an underlying patient problem. Hyperthermia usually reflects external environmental factors that affect the patient. Both conditions require prompt attention. The job of the intensivist is to differentiate between hyperthermia and fever, identify the cause of the elevated temperature, and manage the patient with appropriate intervention, if any, directed to the cause of the temperature change. This chapter discusses the common causes of a new fever in a CCU patient (one that develops >48 hours after a patient has been admitted to a hospital),[2] and presents an approach for evaluating a patient with a new fever.

THERMOREGULATION

Several excellent reviews of thermoregulation are available.[3-5] Briefly, body temperature is closely controlled in the hypothalamic thermoregulatory center, wherein a "set point" exists that regulates body temperature at a relatively fixed level—for dogs and cats, at about 38.3°C (101°F). Body temperature normally fluctuates less than 2°F during the day. Most clinicians define an elevated body temperature in the dog and cat as any measured temperature of 39.1°C (102.5°F) or above. Core body temperature is the temperature measured in the pulmonary artery, which requires specialized catheters, and is considered most accurate. More common measurement sites in dogs and cats are the rectum and aural tympanic membrane. Some debate exists over the accuracy of rectal and ear tympanic temperature measurements compared to core temperature. However,

Table 43-1. Temperature Conversion Calculations

°F = (9/5 × °C) + 32 *or* (1.8 × °C) + 32
°F = 5/9 × (°F − 32) *or* 0.555 × (°F − 32)

it is more important in the CCU to standardize what is considered an abnormally increased temperature, rather than debate accuracy of measurement sites. All of these methods are considered clinically accurate if properly performed, although core and rectal measurements are considered better measures of true internal temperature. Every CCU staff member must know what constitutes an abnormal temperature for optimal patient management (Table 43-1).

Pathophysiology of Increased Temperature

Hyperthermia is an elevated body temperature secondary to an imbalance between heat production (resulting from impaired heat loss, increased metabolic rate, or increased muscular activity) and heat loss. In hyperthermia, the patient produces a heat load that it is unable to handle with inherent physiologic cooling mechanisms, thus, the "set point" remains normal; the ability to regulate body temperature is lost. The most common causes of hyperthermia in CCU patients include enclosure in humid, poorly ventilated, heated oxygen cages; prolonged use of external warming devices; seizures and intense muscular activity, clinical brachycephalic syndrome or laryngeal paralysis; and select metabolic disorders (*e.g.*, hyperthyroidism, malignant hyperthermia-like syndrome).

True fever results when endogenous or exogenous pyrogens act to "reset" the hypothalamic set point to a higher level. Internal processes then act to intentionally increase core body temperature, resulting in fever. The balance between heat production and heat loss is conserved during fever; the ability to regulate body temperature is retained. Although the mechanisms by which fever is induced vary, all result from internal production of or exposure to pyrogens.

Clinical Significance of Fever

Fever represents a hallmark sign of the body's response to inflammation—fever does not conclusively prove the presence of infection! Extensive research in the last decade has markedly advanced our understanding of the underlying pathophysiology of the systemic inflammatory response system (SIRS) in people[6-8] and animals,[9,10] of which fever is a defining criteria. In SIRS, tissue injury or inflammation induced by infection and many other causes results in generation of numerous pyrogens that bind to vascular endothelial receptors in the hypothalamus and increase production of specific prostaglandins (*e.g.*, prostaglandins E_1 and E_2), which elicit a febrile response.[7] Fever does not develop in every patient with SIRS, and the degree of febrile response is not related to the severity of the underlying cause.[4]

Effects of Elevated Body Temperature

Generally, hyperthermia is considered a true emergency because extremely high body temperatures can develop—often 41.7°C (106°F) or higher—and specific measures are recommended to reduce the core temperature. Even with proper therapy, rapid irreversible tissue injury and patient death may result. Severe complications such as coma, disseminated intravascular coagulation, multiple organ failure, and decompensatory shock are common in patients with severe hyperthermia. In contrast, febrile patients seldom die or develop severe complications as a direct result of their fever. However, fever markedly reduces appetite and activity and can make management of critically ill or injured patients even more difficult because of its potent effects on nutritional intake and patient mobility and morbidity. Though not conclusively proven, it is generally believed that fever is a beneficial or protective host adaptation to inflammation. Proposed positive benefits of fever include increased neutrophil and lymphocyte activation and migration, enhanced release of proteolytic enzymes from lysosomes, enhanced interferon production, direct inhibition of some viral and bacterial agents, and decreased availability of serum iron used by some bacteria to proliferate.[4] Some studies have shown that febrile critically ill patients with systemic infections had better survival than afebrile patients, suggesting a positive role of fever against some infectious disease processes. Conversely, negative factors attributed to fever include increased metabolism, increased endotoxin activity at higher body temperatures, and clinical deterioration in patients with fever and infections caused by certain clostridial, streptococcal, and pneumococcal organisms compared to afebrile patients with similar infections.

COMMON CAUSES OF FEVER IN CCU PATIENTS

New fever in CCU patients has many possible causes, the most common of which include infection, neoplasia and paraneoplastic syndromes, tissue inflammation and injury, drugs, and immune-mediated diseases (Table 43-2).

Noninfectious Causes

"The prevalence of infection in critically ill patients means that an infection must always be sought, but complex critically ill patients are prone to many illnesses and complications that can cause fever in the absence of infection."[11] Fever is due to noninfectious causes in 26% to 31% of people in CCUs.[12-14] The incidence of noninfectious fever in veterinary patients is likely similar. Tissue ischemia and inflammation as part of the SIRS phenomenon, hemorrhage into confined spaces, transfusion and drug reactions, lung atelectasis, aspiration pneumonitis, and certain endocrinopathies are common noninfectious causes of a new fever in CCU patients. Tissue ischemia (*e.g.*, pulmonary or aortic thromboembolism, bowel infarct, crush injury), generalized inflammation (*e.g.*, vasculitis), hemorrhage into confined spaces (*e.g.*, retroperitoneal space, brain

Table 43-2. Common Causs of New Fever in CCU Patients

Infections*

- Systemic
    - Primary concern is bacterial, viral, and fungal infection.
    - Secondary considerations include parasitic, rickettsial, and protozoal infection.
    - Most common organ systems involved are the respiratory (abscess, pneumonia), cardiac (endocarditis), genitourinary (pyometra, prostatitis, urinary tract infection), and gastrointestinal tract (infectious diarrhea), and bacteremia and body cavity (pleural and peritoneal spaces) infections
- Localized
    - Catheter-induced thrombophlebitis, traumatic and surgical wounds, abscesses

Neoplasia and paraneoplastic syndromes

Tissue injury, inflammation, and necrosis

- Surgical incisions and postoperative inflammation
- Traumatic tissue injury, pancreatitis
- Head trauma, cerebrovascular occlusion, cerebral ischemia

Immune-medicated disorders

- Immune-mediated hemolytic anemia and thrombocytopenia

Drug-induced

- Tetracyclines, penicillins, sulfonamides, quinidine, amphotericin B, levamisole

Nonspecific inflammatory conditions

- Liver disease, pulmonary thromboembolism

* Nosocomial infection is the most important cause of new fever to consider initially in CCU patients.

parenchyma), and organ inflammation in the absence of infection (*e.g.*, pancreatitis) are the most common causes of noninfectious fever in veterinary patients. Fever is well documented in veterinary patients during and after intravascular transfusions of blood and blood products and is one of the hallmark signs of a transfusion reaction. Theoretically, any pharmaceutical can induce a "drug fever," and the most commonly implicated are listed in Table 43-2. Atelectasis of the lung postoperatively is presumed to be one of the most common causes of fever after surgery in people and is believed due to release of interleukin-1 from atelectatic lung tissue.[11] The incidence of atelectasis-induced fever in veterinary patients is not reported. Aspiration pneumonitis is another frequent postoperative cause of fever in people, but animal data are not available. Presumably, the incidence is similar. Although little is reported in the veterinary literature, certain endocrinopathies in people are known to be associated with noninfectious febrile episodes, to include thyroid storm, pheochromocytoma, and hypoadrenocorticism.

Infectious Causes

Fever is due to infectious causes in approximately 75% of people in CCUs.[12-14] Again, the incidence is probably similar for veterinary patients. Virtually every infective organism known can incite a febrile response. The most common agents implicated in causing new fever in ICU patients are bacterial, viral, and fungal agents from exogenous or, more commonly endogenous sources. The most frequent exogenous source of infection is transfer from contaminated hospital staff or devices. Endogenous infections develop when the patient's own bacterial flora is altered by disease or intervention, resulting in bacterial overgrowth or colonization of normally sterile areas of the body (commonly the upper respiratory tract, gastrointestinal tract, urogenital tract, and skin).[15]

Persistent, Unexplained Fever in CCU Patients

Although beyond the scope of this chapter, patients with persistent, unexplained fever (fever of unknown origin, FUO) warrant brief mention for perhaps less obvious reasons. These patients may frequently be admitted to CCUs for therapy and monitoring. CCU staff may tend to become complacent about the presence of fever when dealing with patients with FUO. Patient care and management essentially remain unchanged, but staff need to monitor body temperature more frequently, use caution with the use of invasive devices and monitoring that may induce infection, remain cognizant about complacency, and guard against ignoring or missing other problems or higher temperatures that may signal a nosocomial infection, noninfectious cause of fever, or decline in the patient's status.

NOSOCOMIAL DISEASE IN THE CCU

Nosocomial infection is a major cause of new fever and increased morbidity and mortality in CCU patients. Hospital-acquired infection *must* be the initial consideration in a critically ill or injured patient that develops a new fever. Few clinical veterinary studies have documented nosocomial infection rates,[16-18] although the topic has recently been reviewed.[15,19-21] Selected data from studies involving people in CCUs are summarized from recent literature[20] to shed light on this significant but probably overlooked clinical entity in veterinary CCUs.

- Nosocomial infection rates in people are up to five times higher in CCU patients than in non-CCU patients (infection rates range up to 25%).
- Nosocomial infection is one of the most common causes of death in critically ill people, directly by causing septic shock and indirectly by causing multiple organ dysfunction syndrome.
- Forty percent of nosocomial infections in people are catheter-related urinary tract infections, 25% are pneumonias, and 35% are postoperative wound and surgical infections, intra-abdominal infections, bacteremias, and gastrointestinal infections.

- It is estimated that 2 million people develop nosocomial infections each year; of these, 80,000 die.
- More than 50% of nosocomial epidemics occur among the 10% of the total hospitalized population who are cared for in CCUs.

Sources of Nosocomial Infection

Sources of nosocomial infection are either exogenous or endogenous. Hospital employees are the most common exogenous source and mode of transfer of nosocomial infections. Contact with fecal matter, body secretions, and urine are typically implicated in nosocomial disease. Reservoirs, fomites, and vectors are less frequently identified as sources of nosocomial infection. Contagious patients hospitalized in close proximity to critically ill patients are another common exogenous source of transmission. However, the most common source of nosocomial infection in a patient is the patient itself! For example, 60% of human urinary tract infections are caused by the patient's own bacterial flora.[22] Nosocomial infection rates are increasing and are directly related to an increased number of immunocompromised patients, more frequent use of invasive procedures and devices, greater availability of lifesaving and life-sustaining techniques, increased number of infections caused by antibiotic-resistant organisms, and an increased number of patients at extremes of life. Presumably, with recent advances in veterinary emergency and critical care medicine, the risk of increased nosocomial disease is just as real, although conclusive data are lacking.

Risk Factors for Nosocomial Disease

Common factors that increase the risks of nosocomial infection have been identified and include patient factors and external factors. Patient factors include disease- or therapy-related immunosuppression, thrombocytopenia, hypotension, dysfunctional urinary bladder with urine retention, burns and skin wounds, trauma, and increased age. External factors include admission to a CCU, patient care in a large hospital, prolonged hospitalization, presence of arterial, venous, or urinary catheters or devices or an endotracheal tube, previous antibiotic therapy, use of broad-spectrum antibiotics, and unscheduled surgery. Bypassing or weakening the patient's normal defense mechanisms significantly increases a patient's likelihood of developing a nosocomial infection.

Nosocomial infection surveillance programs and disease prevention procedures clearly reduce the incidence of hospital-acquired infection.[15-17,19,21,23-26] Every CCU should develop and use standard disease prevention and control measures.

Common Nosocomial Infections in Veterinary CCUs

Data concerning the incidence of nosocomial infection in veterinary patients is scarce. The most common hospital-acquired infections include urinary tract infections, pneumonia, catheter-related infections, bacteremia, gastrointestinal infections, and wound infections.

Nosocomial urinary tract infections occur in up to 32% to 52% of veterinary patients in which urogenital catheters are used,[15-17] and parallels the incidence in people as the most common cause of hospital-acquired infection. Open urine collection systems, prolonged duration of use of urinary catheters, contaminated closed urine collection systems, and trauma to the urogenital tract are risk factors for nosocomial urogenital infection.

Although pneumonia is reported as the second most common nosocomial infection and a leading cause of death in people in CCUs, the incidence in veterinary patients is not reported. This likely represents the less frequent use of mechanical ventilation in dogs and cats. However, as the use of such therapy increases in veterinary medicine, one can expect the incidence of hospital-acquired infection to do so as well. Infection occurs from inhalation, hematogenous, or oropharyngeal sources of organisms. Pneumonia developing in the first few days is typically from the patient's normal respiratory flora, whereas infection developing after the first few days usually is due to gram-negative bacilli that colonize the oropharyngeal area.

Catheter-related infection rates have been reported to occur in 11% to 26% of veterinary patients with indwelling intravenous catheters.[16,18] However, numerous factors affect these reported infection rates including catheter type, catheter location, duration of catheterization, underlying patient status and severity of underlying disease, hospital staff catheter-handling procedures, and use of catheters. What is clear from recent studies is that nosocomial infection is uncommon if catheters are placed using aseptic technique, staff follow rigid but simple catheter-handling procedures, catheter sites are evaluated daily, and suspected infected catheters or catheters in sites that appear infected are promptly removed. Catheter tip cultures, culture of purulent material at catheter insertion sites, and blood cultures should be considered in any CCU patient that develops a new fever and a catheter is strongly suspected of being a source of infection.

Sources of bacteremia include direct access (intravascular devices) or translocation from any heavily colonized mucous membrane surface or inflamed or infected site, such as skin wounds, urinary tract infections, gastrointestinal tract, and abscesses.[27,28] In a recent study,[28] 49% of critically ill dogs and cats had positive blood cultures for bacteria, and fever was a consistent marker of bacteremia. Additionally, mortality was 10 times greater in bacteremic animals than in animals with negative blood cultures. These results dictate that blood cultures be considered in the diagnostic evaluation of any critically ill patient with new fever and no obvious source or cause of inflammation or infection. Blood culture collection, handling, and interpretation are thoroughly discussed in available references.[27,28]

Nosocomial gastrointestinal infections, principally diarrhea, in veterinary CCUs tend to be epidemic in nature, with a reported incidence of approximately 2%.[19] Most sources of infection are either the patient's own altered flora or a common external source (contaminated thermometer, unwashed hands). Standard hospital infectious disease prevention and control procedures minimize development of nosocomial diarrhea.

Surgical wound infection rates vary markedly based on the type of surgery performed (*e.g.*, clean versus dirty), antibiotic use, postoperative care, and other factors. Nosocomial infection rates in surgical wounds are not definitively reported in veterinary patients, but the overall surgical wound infection rate is reported to range from 3% to 25%.[19] In CCU patients, proper wound care and wound evaluation are critical to reduce the likelihood of hospital-acquired infection.

APPROACH TO A CCU PATIENT WITH NEW FEVER

Because fever can have many infectious and noninfectious etiologies, a new fever in a patient in the ICU should trigger a careful clinical assessment rather than automatic orders for laboratory and radiologic tests. The goal of such an approach is to determine, in a directed manner, whether or not infection is present, so additional testing can be avoided and therapeutic options can be made.[29]

Figure 43-1 outlines an initial approach to a febrile patient in the ICU. A discussion of this approach follows to clarify key points.

Step 1: Never ignore an elevated body temperature measurement! Ensure staff has an agreed definition for fever, and "call back" orders are clear. Define that an elevated body temperature exists by taking several measurements over time with a reliable thermometer. Rule out technical errors (faulty thermometer).

Step 2: Eliminate hyperthermia as a cause. Inspect the patient's environment and check for hot cages with poor ventilation and high humidity, excessively warm heating devices, and excessive cage bedding. Iatrogenic hyperthermia is most common in patients that are recumbent, immobilized, sedated, or obtunded and unable to move away from heat sources.

Step 3: Thoroughly review the patient's history for recent changes (past 48-72 hours) that suggest nosocomial infection may have developed or that may suggest noninfectious causes of fever. Consider especially the use of new invasive devices, drug therapy, and transfusions. Consider the presence of associated clinical signs that have also recently developed that may suggest a source of the fever (*e.g.*, deep, moist productive cough suggesting pneumonia; bloody diarrhea suggesting clostridial enterocolitis). Investigate contact with other ill patients,

Figure 43-1
Approach to the febrile CCU patient. This algorithm suggests the initial approach to evaluating a CCU patient with a new fever. R/O, rule out; UTI, urinary tract infection; XR, radiographs; TTW, transtracheal wash; BAL, bronchoalveolar lavage; GIT, gastrointestinal tract. (Modified from Shatz DV, Norwood S: An approach to the febrile ICU patient. *In* Civetta JM, Taylor RW, eds.: Critical Care. Philadelphia: Lippincott-Raven, 1997, p 1590.)

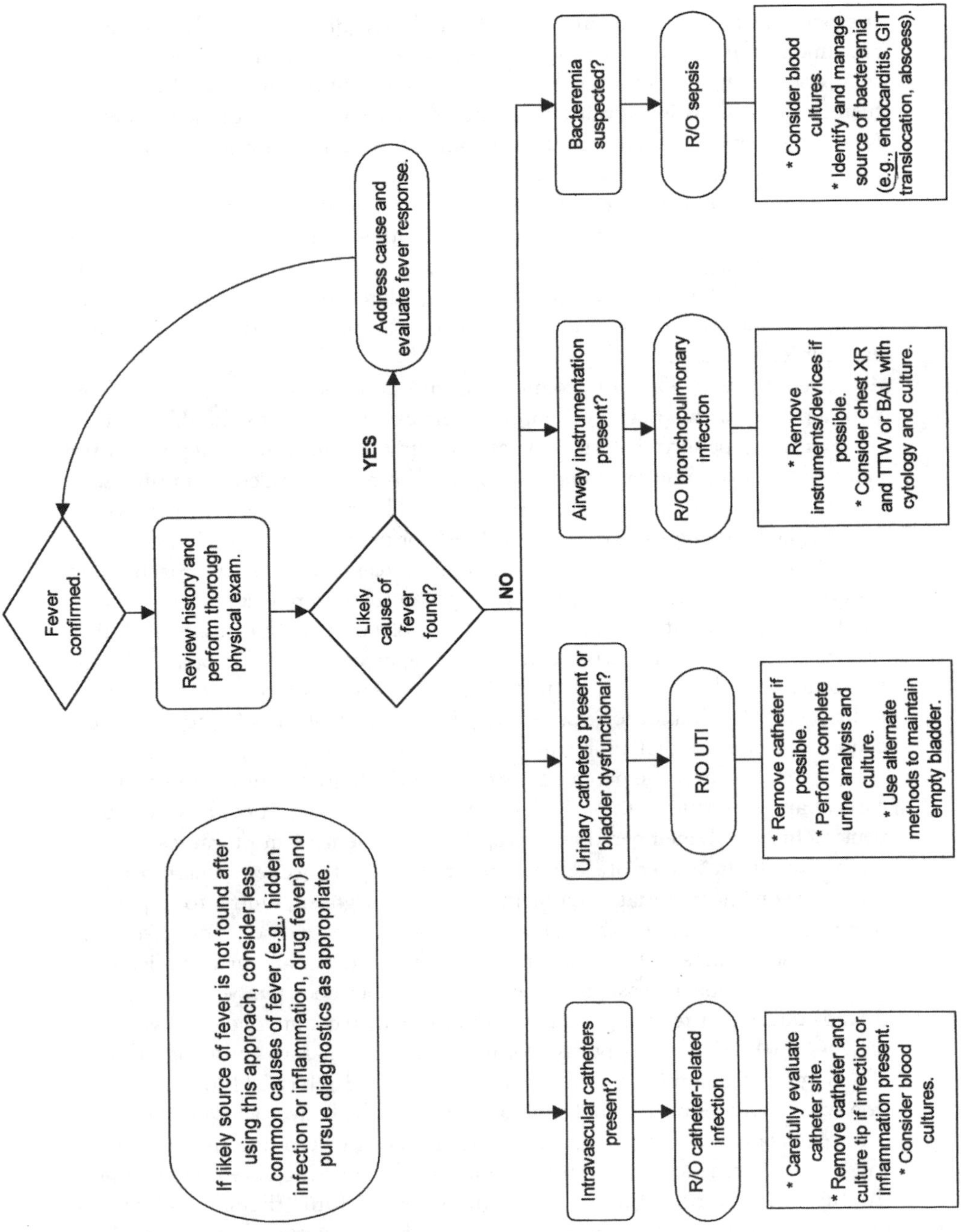

Fever confirmed.

Review history and perform thorough physical exam.

Likely cause of fever found?

YES → Address cause and evaluate fever response.

NO

Intravascular catheters present?

R/O catheter-related infection

* Carefully evaluate catheter site.
* Remove catheter and culture tip if infection or inflammation present.
* Consider blood cultures.

Urinary catheters present or bladder dysfunctional?

R/O UTI

* Remove catheter if possible.
* Perform complete urine analysis and culture.
* Use alternate methods to maintain empty bladder.

Airway instrumentation present?

R/O bronchopulmonary infection

* Remove instruments/devices if possible.
* Consider chest XR and TTW or BAL with cytology and culture.

Bacteremia suspected?

R/O sepsis

* Consider blood cultures.
* Identify and manage source of bacteremia (e.g., endocarditis, GIT translocation, abscess).

If likely source of fever is not found after using this approach, consider less common causes of fever (e.g., hidden infection or inflammation, drug fever) and pursue diagnostics as appropriate.

the patient's immunocompetence, and concurrent diseases. Review timings of placement of invasive devices such as intravascular or urinary catheters, or nasoenteric feeding tubes for any link with development of new fever. Review the history since admission for any change in or development of clinical problems (*e.g.*, development of diarrhea, postoperative wound infection) that will direct preliminary investigations for the cause of the fever.

Step 4: Thoroughly examine the patient to identify any obvious underlying cause for the fever. Concentrate especially on catheter sites (induration, swelling, pain, erythema, pus) and skin (decubital ulcers, suture site infections). If an obvious cause is found that could cause fever, address that cause first. If no obvious cause is found, consider additional diagnostic tests, based on clinical signs and clinical suspicion.

Step 5: Table 43-3 lists common diagnostic tests to consider when faced with a patient with a new fever and no overt cause. Clinicians should avoid the temptation to perform batteries of tests, hoping to gain some insight into the cause of the fever. Rather, a stepwise approach is recommended, beginning with those tests that will give the most information about global patient status (level 1 tests), and moving to more advanced tests or procedures (level 2 and 3 tests) only if initial findings are equivocal. The main reasons for this approach are to minimize costs to the client and, more importantly to minimize further invasive insults to the patient that may increase risk of nosocomial disease or clinical deterioration. Use a step-wise, conservative approach, consider financial costs to clients, consider possible risks to patients, and interpret results of tests sequentially before deciding other tests are required. If a problem is found that could cause fever, address that problem.

Step 6: Monitor the patient to assess response to intervention and to detect early changes in patient status. Reduction in fever may suggest evidence of therapeutic efficacy. Remember that appropriate treatment of most causes of fever seldom results in immediate temperature reduction. However, persistence of a fever suggests inappropriate treatment, incorrect diagnosis, failure to respond to therapy, or progression (deterioration) of disease. In these cases, a full re-evaluation of the patient's history and thorough physical exam are again indicated.

Step 7: Decide if measures are necessary to reduce body temperature. Specific therapy directed at reducing the fever is not usually recommended unless a fever of 40°C (104°F) or higher persists for more than 2 to 3 days and is significantly affecting patient morbidity, or the temperature exceeds 41.1°C (106°F). Use caution when considering external cooling measures. The body is actively increasing core temperature, and peripheral cooling may actually be counterproductive because the inherent response will be to increase (return) the core temperature to the higher set point. Also, fever-reducing measures (drug therapy and cooling measures) may be effective at reducing the body temperature, but may mask an underlying problem and delay diagnostics and therapeutic measures that a change in temperature may have prompted. External cooling measures for fever are less aggressive than measures used to reduce temperature in hyperthermic patients. Obviously, remove all external sources of heat, such as heating pads or blankets,

Table 43-3. Diagnostics Tests to Consider for New Fever in CCU Patients

Level 1—Minimum database

- Complete blood count: serial, with differential count and careful evaluation of cell morphology
- Biochemistry panel
- Urine analysis with sediment exam and culture/sensitivity testing if sediment positive
- Ancillary tests that may not have been performed as part of initial diagnostic evaluation: heartworm tests, fecal exams, infectious disease serology (feline leukemia virus, feline immunodeficiency tests), etc.
- Culture with sensitivity testing and cytology of any catheter site, wound, body cavity, or other discharges
- Consider empiric antibiotic therapy if infection strongly suspected

Level 2—Based on clinical signs and clinical suspicion

- Blood cultures if bacteremia or sepsis suspected
- Culture and sensitivity testing and cytology of samples from specific sites, based on clinical suspicion: prostatic fluid/semen, cerebrospinal fluid, joint fluid, bone marrow, pleural or peritoneal fluid, bronchoalveolar lavage fluid, transtracheal wash fluid, fecal smears, lymph node aspirates, masses, etc. May require advanced diagnostics (bronchoscopy, endoscopy, etc.).
- Radiography, ultrasonography, echocardiography, computed tomography, magnetic resonance imaging, based on clinical suspicion
- Biopsies of masses, lymph nodes, muscle, joints, etc.
- Serology (feline infectious peritonitis, protozoal titers, fungal titers, rickettsial titers, etc.)
- Immune function tests (antinuclear antibody, Coomb's test, rheumatoid factor, serum protein electrophoresis, etc.)

Level 3—Consider if patient's condition is worsening; may be diagnostic and therapeutic

- Exploratory surgery or laparoscopy
- Therapeutic trials (change antibiotics, consider antifungal therapy, antipyretics, immunosuppressive drugs)

and turn off any cage heating devices. Fans may also be helpful in improving patient comfort and reducing fever. More aggressive measures to reduce fever are not recommended. Drugs that are useful in reducing fever in veterinary patients are listed in Table 43-4. The most effective and safest of these drugs inhibit prostaglandin synthesis (acetaminophen, nonsteroidal anti-inflammatory agents), and thereby prevent the resetting of the hypothalamic set point. Glucocorticoids, although potent antipyretics, are not recommended as fever-reducing agents due to the possibility of worsening the patient's status. However, glucocorticoids may be indicated as a therapeutic course of action for some diseases that cause fever (*e.g.*, immune-mediated diseases), in which case the added benefit of fever reduc-

Table 43-4. Management Concerns for Febrile CCU Patients

- Maintain and carefully monitor fluid balance.
- Focus on patient comfort, nutritional intake, and concurrent diseases.
- Surface cooling techniques (cautious use of fans, remove external heat sources—may actually increase patient discomfort and temperature fluctuations as body attempts to return temperature to higher level).
- Antipyretic drugs*—Advised for fever ≥41.1°C (106°F); use clinical judgment for persistent symptomatic fevers ≥40°C (104°F):

  Aspirin—10 mg/kg q 8-12 h PO for dogs; 10 mg/kg q 48 h PO for cats

  Acetaminophen—10-15 mg/kg q 8-12 h PO for dogs; NOT for cats

  Ketoprofen—2 mg/kg SQ, IM, IV, PO initially, then 1 mg/kg q 24 h PO for dogs and cats for subsequent doses

  Carprofen—2.2 mg/kg q 12 h PO for dogs

  Etodolac—10-15 mg/kg q 24 h PO for dogs
- Continue thorough monitoring for response to therapy and identification of cause of fever and development of complications.

PO, orally, *per os*; SQ, subcutaneously; IM, intramuscularly; IV, intravenously.
* Clinicians must understand potential side effects and complications of these drugs before clinical use, especially in critically ill patients with concurrent diseases, and consider extralabel use implications of these drugs.

tion is welcomed. Glucocorticoids may mask a new or persistent fever and may increase the immunoincompetence of the patient, so judicious use is strongly advised. Use of drugs to reduce fever is controversial, and careful patient assessment is required. Although most clinicians probably permit a mild-to-moderate fever to persist rather than use drugs to reduce the fever, some merit is evident in improving overall patient comfort, nutritional intake, and, presumably improved outcome with such drugs, especially in patients with chronic febrile illness. A recent study, for example, demonstrated that febrile cats with various infections that received both antibiotic therapy and the nonsteroidal anti-inflammatory agent, ketoprofen, had rapid reductions in body temperature to normal, and had improved appetite and attitude than febrile cats not receiving ketoprofen. No adverse side effects of ketoprofen were noted.[30]

Step 8: Address overall patient status, especially nutrition, fluid balance, and concurrent disease management. Table 43-4 lists general management concerns for febrile CCU patients.

Nutritional Intake

It is generally assumed that fever increases the metabolic rate, and animals with fever may require an increased caloric intake of 7 kcal/kg/d.[31] This may become problematic because febrile animals typically are anorectic, and a variety of feeding techniques and inventive strategies to encourage intake may be required. It is seldom necessary to consider enteral or parenteral nutritional support for fever alone, but a persistent fever may be an additional consideration when contemplating instituting such therapy for other reasons.

Fluid Balance

Adequate fluid balance in patients in the CCU is a continuous objective and is especially important in febrile animals. Although difficult to quantitate, insensible fluid losses are considered to be substantial in febrile patients, in addition to ongoing fluid losses related to underlying disease. Coupled with the increased metabolic rate in febrile patients, it is obvious that fluid imbalances can develop covertly that may worsen the patient's status and possibly outcome. Fluid therapy is important as well because many febrile animals do not drink enough water to maintain adequate fluid balance. Careful attention to fluid requirements is essential for all patients, but especially for febrile patients in the CCU.

Concurrent Disease

Patients are seldom in the CCU simply because they are febrile. More commonly, they are hospitalized for intensive care because of major illness or injury, of which fever is a part. It is important for all staff to focus on total patient management and not restrict their attention to a single problem, such as fever. Often, the easiest parameters to measure frequently receive the most attention, including body temperature. It must be remembered that fever is a sign implicating an underlying cause, and the cause is much more important for patient management than the sign.

REFERENCES

1. Ault ML: Opioids, febrile responsiveness, and thinking outside the box. *Crit Care Med* 28:1654, 2000.
2. Marino PL: The febrile patient. *In* Marino PL, ed.: The ICU Book, 2nd ed. Baltimore: Williams & Wilkins, 1998, p 485.
3. Haskins SC: Thermoregulation, hypothermia, hyperthermia. *In* Ettinger SJ, Feldman EC, eds.: Textbook of Veterinary Internal Medicine, 4th ed. Philadelphia: WB Saunders, 1995, p 26.
4. Dunn JK, Greene CE: Fever. *In* Greene CE, ed.: Infectious Diseases of the Dog and Cat, 2nd ed. Philadelphia: WB Saunders, 1998, p 693.
5. Mackowiak PA: Concepts of fever. *Arch Int Med* 158:1870, 1998.
6. Bone RC: Systemic inflammatory response syndrome: a unifying concept of systemic inflammation. *In* Fein AM, Abraham EM, Balk RA, *et al.*, eds.: Sepsis and Multiorgan Failure. Baltimore: Williams & Wilkins, 1997, p 3.
7. Luster AD: Chemokines—chemotactic cytokines that mediate inflammation. *N Engl J Med* 338:436, 1998.
8. Members of the American College of Chest Physicians/Society of Critical Care Medicine Consensus Conference Committee. American College of Chest Physicians/Society of Critical Care Medicine Consensus Conference: Definitions for sepsis and organ failure and guidelines for the use of innovative therapies in sepsis. *Crit Care Med* 20:864, 1992.
9. Hardie EM: Life-threatening bacterial infection. *Compend Contin Educ Pract Vet* 17:763, 1995.
10. Purvis D, Kirby R: Systemic inflammatory response syndrome: septic shock. *Vet Clin North Am Small Anim Pract* 24:1225, 1994.

11. Barie PS: Fever in the ICU: noninfectious causes of fever. *Proceedings of the Society of Critical Care Medicine*, 27th Educational and Scientific Symposium. San Antonio, TX, February 4, 1998, p 275.
12. Filice GA, Weiler MD, Hughes RA, *et al.*: Nosocomial febrile illnesses in patients on an internal medicine service. *Arch Int Med* 149:319, 1989.
13. Arbo Manuel J, Fine MJ, Hanusa BH, *et al.*: Fever of nosocomial origin: etiology, risk factors, and outcomes. *Am J Med* 95:505, 1993.
14. McGowan JE, Rose RC, Jacobs NF, *et al.*: Fever in hospitalized patients with special reference to the Medical Service. *Am J Med* 82:580, 1987.
15. Johnson JA, Murtaugh RJ: Preventing and treating nosocomial infection. Part 1. Urinary tract infections and pneumonia. *Compend Contin Educ Pract Vet* 19:581, 1997.
16. Lippert AC, Fulton RB, Parr AM: Nosocomial infection surveillance in a small animal intensive care unit. *J Am Anim Hosp Assoc* 24:627, 1988.
17. Wise LA, Jones RL, Reif JS: Nosocomial canine urinary tract infections in a veterinary teaching hospital (1983 to 1988). *J Am Anim Hosp Assoc* 26:148, 1990.
18. Mathews KA, Brooks MJ, Valliant AE: A prospective study of intravenous catheter contamination. *J Vet Emerg Crit Care* 6:33, 1996.
19. Johnson JA, Murtaugh RJ: Preventing and treating nosocomial infection. Part II. Wound, blood, and gastrointestinal infections. *Compend Contin Educ Pract Vet* 19: 693, 1997.
20. Maki DG. Nosocomial infection in the intensive care unit. *In* Parrillo JE, Bone RC, eds.: Critical Care Medicine: Principles of Diagnosis and Management. St. Louis: Mosby-Year Book, 1995, p 893.
21. Murtaugh RJ, Mason GD. Antibiotic pressure and nosocomial disease. *Vet Clin North Am Small Anim Pract* 19:1259, 1989.
22. Rangel-Frausto MS, Wenzel RP: The epidemiology and natural history of bacterial sepsis. *In* Fein AM, Abraham EM, Balk RA, *et al*, eds.: Sepsis and Multiorgan Failure. Baltimore: Williams & Wilkins, 1997, p 27.
23. Civetta JM, Hudson-Civetta J, Ball S: Decreasing catheter-related infection and hospital costs by continuous quality improvement. *Crit Care Med* 24:1660, 1996.
24. Bjornson HS: Pathogenesis, prevention, and management of catheter-associated infections. *New Horizons* 1:271, 1993.
25. Price J, Ekleberry A, Grover A, *et al.*: Evaluation of clinical practice guidelines on outcome of infection in patients in the surgical intensive care unit. *Crit Care Med* 27:2118, 2000.
26. Edgeworth JD, Treacher DF, Eykyn SJ: A 25-year study of nosocomial bacteremia in an adult intensive care unit. *Crit Care Med* 27:1421, 2000.
27. Dow SW, Jones RL: Bacteremia: pathogenesis and diagnosis. *Compend Contin Educ Pract Vet* 11:432, 1989.
28. Dow SW, Curtis CR, Jones RL, *et al.*: Bacterial culture of blood from critically ill dogs and cats: 100 cases (1985–1987). *J Am Vet Med Assoc* 195:113, 1989.
29. O'Grady NP, Barie PS, Bartlett J, *et al.*: Practice parameters for evaluating new fever in critically ill adult patients. *Crit Care Med* 26:392, 1998.
30. Glew A, Keister DM, Meo NJ: Use of ketoprofen as an antipyretic in cats. *Can Vet J* 37:222, 1996.
31. Burney DP. Fever. *In:* Wingfield WE, ed.: Veterinary Emergency Medicine Secrets, 2nd ed. Philadelphia: Hanley & Belfus, 2000, p 124.

44
Multiorgan Failure

Tim Hackett

INTRODUCTION

Multiorgan failure is an important concept in the management of critical illness. As newer technologies have improved monitoring and patient care, more critically ill patients survive the initial illness only to succumb to a combination of complications involving other organ systems. The major threat to survival is often not the primary illness but rather a process of progressive failure of vital, interdependent organ systems.

Applying clinical criteria to define organ failure, sepsis, septic shock, and the systemic inflammatory response syndrome (SIRS) permits the early detection and intervention before these changes lead to irreversible organ failure. In 1991, the American College of Chest Physicians and the Society of Critical Care Medicine met in a consensus conference to provide a conceptual and practical framework to define SIRS and resulting organ dysfunctions.[1] These recommendations have been modified for use in veterinary patients[2] (Table 44-1).

Defining organ failure has been at times arbitrary with many dissimilar criteria listed from the many studies. The term "organ failure" implies a dichotomous event either present or absent. The same 1991 consensus conference settled on the term "multiple organ dysfunction syndrome" or "MODS" which better describes the inability of specific organ systems to maintain homeostasis. This process, which may be relative or absolute, describes a continuum over time and not necessarily an irreversible process. By developing clinical definitions and monitoring these variables, the intensivist strives to identify organ dysfunction before the process becomes irreversible.

Multiple organ dysfunction syndrome is a clinical constellation of severe physiologic changes occurring sequentially or concomitantly in multiple organs, most commonly in the setting of sepsis, severe inflammatory disorder, trauma, burns, or generalized perfusion deficits associated with hypovolemic shock of diverse cause.[3] The immunophysiologic response to systemic inflammation is central to an understanding of MODS. Although often thought to indicate sepsis, 15% of patients meeting the criteria for SIRS were found to have no evidence of infection.[4]

While azotemia and oliguria indicate renal dysfunction and coma scores objectively define neurologic impairment, certain organ systems have multiple immunoregulatory functions that are not subject to objective clinical measurement. While a universal classification system is lacking, the Acute Physiology

Table 44-1. Definitions and Terminology Used to Describe Multiple Organ Failure, Sepsis, SIRS, and Related Complications

Infection: Microbial invasion characterized by an inflammatory response to the presence of microorganisms or to the invasion of normally sterile host tissue by those organisms.

Systemic Inflammatory Response (SIR): The systemic response to infection characterized by two or more of the following criteria:

1. T > 103.5°F or < 100°F
2. Heart rate > 160 bpm (dogs) and > 250 bpm (cats)
3. Respiratory rate > 20 bpm or $PaCO_2 < 32$ mmHg
4. WBC > 12,000 cells/µl, < 4,000 cells/µl or > 10% bands

Sepsis: The systemic response to confirmed infection characterized by two or more of the criteria above.

Septic shock: Sepsis with refractive hypotension and the presence of perfusion abnormalities that may include, but are not limited to, lactic acidosis, oliguria, or acute changes in mental status.

Multiple Organ Dysfunction Syndrome (MODS): The presence of altered organ function in the acutely ill patient such that homeostasis cannot be maintained without intervention. Examples include hepatic, renal and cardiac failure, stupor and coma, acute respiratory distress syndrome (ARDS), cardiac arrhythmias, and disseminated intravascular coagulation (DIC).

From: Kirby R: Septic Shock. *In* Bonagura JD, ed.: Current Veterinary Therapy XII. Philadelphia: W.B. Saunders Company, 1995, p 139.

and Chronic Health Evaluation II (APACHE II) scoring system is used to objectively assess organ function.[5] A similar scoring system has been evaluated and validated in veterinary medicine (see Chapter 27). Useful to objectively compare the degree of physiologic derangements, these scoring systems do not address the pathogenic significance of specific organ dysfunction.

PATHOGENESIS

The cumulative effect of impaired host defenses and inappropriate host regulation of immune and inflammatory responses result in SIRS and MODS. Infectious and noninfectious processes resulting in tissue ischemia or trauma lead through multiple pathways to cell injury and organ damage.[6] Although noninfectious systemic disorders can activate the cascade of events resulting in organ dysfunction, gram-negative endotoxemia has been the most widely studied.[5] Gram-negative endotoxin is a lipopolysaccharide in the outer cell wall. Lipopolysaccharide interacts with vascular endothelial cells, neutrophils, platelets, lymphocytes, macrophages and other cells to release the inflammatory cytokines required to initiate the host's inflammatory response.[7] Tumor necrosis factor-alpha (TNF-α) and isoforms of interleukin (IL)-1 are pivotal early proinflammatory mediators of the host response to injury and have multiple effects which contribute to MODS. Other products of inflammation including eicosanoid metabolites of the arachidonic acid cascade, platelet activating factor, and nitric oxide mediate the actions of TNF-α and both IL-1α and IL-1β.[3] Progression from an initial, local response to injury to MODS depends on the balance (or lack thereof) between the pro-inflammatory cytokines and their anti-inflammatory counterparts (IL-4, IL-6, IL-10, granulocyte colony-stimulating factor).[8] When these mediators reach systemic concentrations, what normally functions to contain infection may culminate in progressive cardiovascular dysfunction, vasomotor collapse, increased vascular permeability, impaired tissue perfusion, organ failure, and death.

When bacterial or fungal organisms start this cascade, the associated hypotension is referred to as septic shock. In patients with noninfectious disease such as trauma and severe pancreatitis, the same cascade can occur. Septic shock and SIRS are characterized by low systemic vascular resistance, a maldistribution of blood flow, and cardiac output inadequate to maintain normal metabolic function.

EPIDEMIOLOGY

Multiple organ dysfunction syndrome has been defined as severe acquired dysfunction in at least two organ systems after critical illness, injury, or a major operation that lasts at least 24 to 48 hours.[3] Information concerning the incidence of MODS in human critical care patients comes from prospective and retrospective surveys in medical, surgical, and mixed intensive care unit populations. These surveys include data from clinical sepsis trials. Studies used to validate the various severity-of-illness scoring systems have also provided information on large numbers of critically ill patients. Large numbers from veterinary medicine are not yet available. However, with the validation and use of similar scoring systems in veterinary medicine, this information will also be collected. Using this definition, critical care researchers have found that MODS complicates 15% of all ICU admissions, is the principal cause of death in such patients, and that the mortality rate increases with the number of acquired dysfunctions of the cardiovascular, respiratory, renal, gastrointestinal, hepatic, hematologic, or central nervous systems.[3]

DIAGNOSTIC EVALUATION

Serial monitoring of the major organ systems is necessary to detect early derangements in function. Monitoring to evaluate the function of multiple organ systems should include objective blood tests such as a complete blood count (CBC), arterial blood gas analysis, serum biochemical profile, and tests of coagulation function. In addition to biochemical analysis of blood urea nitrogen and creatinine, urine should be checked for inflammatory cells, casts, and protein. Urine production should be closely monitored and values <1 ml/kg/day should signal the need for aggressive therapy. Tissue perfusion can be assessed subjectively by examining mucous membranes. Color and capillary refill times provide information about the adequacy of cardiac output and the state of peripheral vascular resistance. More objective assessment of perfusion includes measurement of serum creatinine and blood lactate.

Suspicion of sepsis or septic shock demands that diagnostic material be collected immediately and appropriate monitoring and therapeutic procedures instituted. A diagnosis of SIRS is one of exclusion, and every effort must be made to identify and treat potential sources of sepsis. Areas of particular concern include the urinary tract, reproductive tract, abdominal cavity, respiratory tract, gingiva, and the heart valves. The clinician must begin an "infection hunt." Historic questions are asked concerning gastrointestinal signs, reproductive status (neutered, recent estrus), abnormal urination, recurrent infections, travel, or a recent dentistry. A thorough physical examination is performed with attention to oral examination, cardiac and thoracic auscultation, and abdominal palpation. Blood samples are drawn for CBC, serum biochemical profile, coagulation testing, rickettsial, fungal, and immune testing if indicated. Urine is collected for analysis and culture. Blood for culture should be taken from the jugular vein. Because blood cultures can have a relatively low yield, multiple samples should be taken 15 minutes to 1 hour apart, ideally during peak rises in body temperature. Antibiotic administration should be withheld until samples are collected, but there should be minimal delay in starting treatment.

Radiographs and ultrasound of the abdomen may reveal masses, organomegaly, or fluid-filled lesions. Loss of abdominal detail suggests abdominal fluid. Radiographs of the chest and echocardiography help to evaluate the lungs and heart (radiographs for lungs, echo for heart). When decreased detail or fluid is seen in the chest or abdomen, sterile collection (either by abdominocentesis or diagnostic peritoneal lavage) for cytologic examination and fluid analysis should be performed. If interstitial changes in the lung fields and clinical findings support possible pulmonary disease, bronchoscopy or a transtracheal wash may provide samples for a diagnosis.

TREATMENT

Initial treatment of MODS should focus on restoring normal oxygen delivery to vital organs.

CARDIOVASCULAR DYSFUNCTION

Myocardial failure in SIRS manifests as decreased contractile function and decreased left ventricular compliance.[3] Cardiac arrhythmias are also a common feature. Supraventricular and ventricular tachycardias can impair ventricular filling and lead to reduced cardiac output. Ventricular tachycardia with R on T phenomenon can lead to sudden death from ventricular fibrillation, and such patients should receive antiarrhythmic therapy immediately (Figure 44-1). Third-degree atrioventricular block (Figure 44-2) can lead to functional bradycardia and reduced cardiac output. Treatment may be complicated by lack of conduction through the atrioventricular node. Usually unresponsive to atropine, a beta-agonist (isoproterenol) may be necessary to increase ventricular escape and pulse rate. Because a patient with SIRS is at risk for any number of potentially harmful arrhythmias, constant monitoring is important.

Increasing either heart rate or stroke volume increases cardiac output and

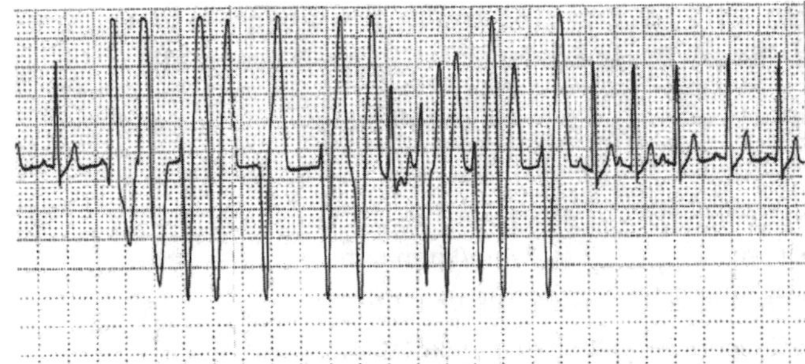

Figure 44-1
Multiform ventricular tachycardia. The high rate and close (R on T phenomenon) complexes contribute to poor cardiac output and place the patient at risk for ventricular fibrillation and sudden death.

oxygen delivery. Increasing heart rate will only work when enough time exists for normal diastolic filling. When the heart rate is too high, stroke volume decreases and prevents further rise in cardiac output. Stroke volume is optimized with intravenous fluid therapy. Fluid type will depend on the patient and may need to include both crystalloids and colloids.

Serum albumin should be monitored and kept above 2.0 g/dl with plasma or whole blood transfusions. Persistent hypoalbuminemia is associated with increased mortality in critically ill animals. When patient size and albumin deficit makes plasma transfusion alone impractical, any one of the synthetic colloid solutions can bridge the gap and help maintain plasma oncotic pressure. Another variable in determining arterial oxygen content (and oxygen delivery) is the red blood cell mass. The use of crystalloid, plasma, and synthetic colloids during resuscitation and rehydration can dilute red blood cells (RBCs) and blood proteins. Although the improvement in cardiac output is important, whole blood or packed red blood cell transfusions should be used to maintain a packed cell volume of between 27% and 33%.

Tachycardia is also the result of pain. Often, patient comfort takes a back seat to convenience in a 24-hour critical setting. The appropriate use of analgesics, padding, clean dressings, and personal contact will reduce the anxiety level allowing the patient to rest and recover.[2]

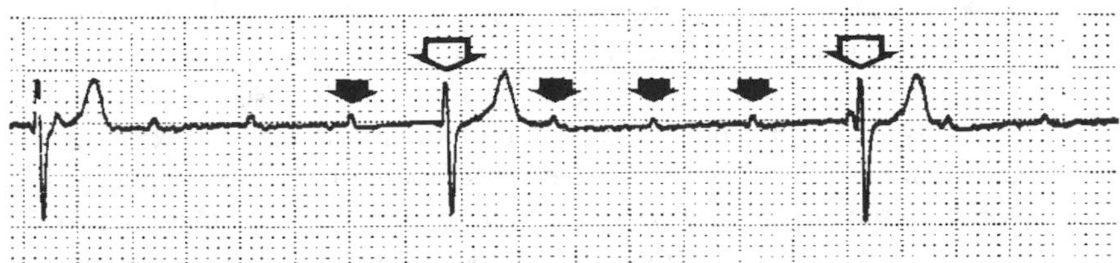

Figure 44-2
Third-degree atrioventricular block. There is no relationship between the ventricular complexes (open arrows) and the p-waves (closed arrows). Pulse rate and cardiac output are determined by the rate of ventricular contraction.

Table 44-2. Strategies for Optimizing Fluid Volume and Blood Pressure in Critically Ill Animals

Crystalloid fluids	Up to 90 ml/kg/hour (dogs), 45 ml/kg/hour (cats)
Hypertonic saline	4 ml/kg one time over 5–10 minutes
Synthetic colloids	20 ml/kg/day
Dopamine	2 to 20 μg/kg/minute
Dobutamine	5–20 μg/kg/minute
Norepinephrine	0.01–0.4 μg/kg/minute

Optimal blood volume is vital; however, vasomotor tone is also important in MODS patients. Inflammatory mediators in circulation can cause profound vasomotor collapse leading to relative hypovolemia and shunting of blood from vital organs to peripheral tissues. Treatment options for the cardiovascular system are summarized in Table 44-2.

PULMONARY DYSFUNCTION

Respiratory failure can be a failure of gas exchange, hypoventilation, or a combined failure of both. Factors contributing to respiratory dysfunction include pneumonia, atelectasis, muscle weakness, and impaired immune function. The response to hypoperfusion in the lungs is a progressive increase in vascular permeability and decrease in pulmonary compliance resulting in the acute respiratory distress syndrome (ARDS).[9] (See chapter 36.)

Arterial blood gas analysis is the most objective assessment. Hypoxemia with a high alveolar to arterial (A-a) oxygen gradient is seen with impaired gas exchange. Daily calculation of the A-a gradient allows the clinician to objectively assess gas exchange over time.

Providing supplemental oxygen is one of the simplest ways to optimize oxygen saturation. Raising SaO_2 will in turn improve CaO_2. Oxygen can be administered by oxygen cage or nasal cannula. Nasal cannulation is often easier to manage with intensively monitored patients because it avoids the drop in FiO_2 that occurs every time the oxygen cage door is opened for patient assessment or treatment. By use of oxygen flow rate of 3 to 5 liters per minute, an FIO_2 of approximately 40% to 50% can be attained and maintained comfortably. Patients remaining hypoxic despite supplementation and an increased inspired oxygen concentration may benefit from pressure ventilation. Atelectasis from prolonged recumbency, aspiration pneumonitis, and pulmonary edema are examples of postsurgical complications resulting in decreased pulmonary compliance. With the decreased compliance, energy required for normal ventilation increases. Positive pressure ventilation can reduce the work of breathing, improve gas exchange, and assure adequate alveolar ventilation.

Hypoventilation is defined as an increase in PCO_2. With inadequate ventilatory efforts, the CO_2 concentration will rise and the patient will develop respiratory acidosis. Supplemental oxygen corrects the hypoxia in these patients;

however, these patients will require positive pressure ventilation to improve CO_2 elimination.

ACUTE RENAL FAILURE

Acute renal failure is a common complication of critical illness. In humans, 10–20% in intensive care units appear to develop clinically important renal dysfunction.[3] Reduced renal blood flow, tubular obstruction, tubular back leak, and altered glomerular permeability affect glomerular filtration rate (GFR) and may lead to oliguria.[10] Renal hypoperfusion results in a renal medullary ischemia. Most countercurrent and energy-dependent solute transport takes place in the outer medulla, an area of high oxygen consumption that is uniquely sensitive to ischemia. Acute renal injury may manifest as polyuria in normotensive, normovolemic patients. Other clinical indications of ARF include hyperkalemia, azotemia, metabolic acidosis, and abnormal urine sediment.

Urine output is an objective, easily measured variable. Urine production should be frequently quantitated, even to the point of placing an indwelling urinary catheter in a critically ill patient for continuous assessment. Renal function is most commonly estimated by following serum creatinine. Since creatinine production is relatively stable and its elimination dependent on glomerular filtration, serum creatinine provides an estimate of the glomerular filtration rate in the steady state. It may take several days to reach a new steady state following a single insult.

Prevention of acute renal failure caused by prerenal factors is one of the important therapeutic goals in critical care. A balanced electrolyte fluid is chosen on the basis of the patients' electrolyte status. If indicated, blood products or synthetic colloids may be necessary to maintain intravascular volume and adequate oxygen delivery. Recognition of acute renal failure during the initiation of tubular injury provides the best opportunity to reverse the damage. The foremost goal is restoration of adequate circulatory blood volume. Volume is continually assessed by arterial blood pressure, pulse quality, and central venous pressure. Only after blood volume has been optimized should any pharmacologic treatments be considered.

LIVER AND GASTROINTESTINAL DYSFUNCTION

The liver and gastrointestinal systems are important in the host immune response. With circulatory shock and splanchnic ischemia, the gastrointestinal tract can become the source of pathogenic bacteria access to the systemic circulation. The resulting bacteremia and secondary septicemia contribute to the failure of other organ systems.[11]

Neither the liver nor the gastrointestinal tract is as accessible for study as the cardiovascular system, lungs, or kidneys. Acute dysfunction is not as immediately evident as circulatory shock, acute lung injury, or renal failure. Liver function tests are sensitive to parenchymal injury but provide little information about protein biosynthesis or immunologic function. Likewise, assessment of gastrointestinal dysfunction by monitoring fecal character or the frequency and character of vomiting are nonspecific and may tell little about intestinal permeability or splanchnic oxygenation. Signs of gastrointestinal dysfunction can be as subtle as anorexia or a serious as acute hemorrhagic diarrhea.

Malnutrition results in compromised host defenses. Short-term use of a nasogastric feeding tube can provide important nutrients to animals that will not eat on their own. Enteral feeding with a gastrostomy or jejunostomy tube may be necessary. Lack of enteral nutrition can cause a loss of bowel integrity, leading to bacterial translocation.

OTHER THERAPIES

In addition to volume support, septic patients must receive antibiotics that are effective against the inciting organism.[12] Since definitive culture results may take days, it is imperative to start parenteral administration of four-quadrant (effective against gram positive, gram negative, aerobic, and anaerobic bacteria) antibiotics when sepsis is a possibility. When culture data are available, the spectrum of coverage can be changed accordingly. The specific choice varies with every patient, and one should consider the underlying disease, the presence of localized sites of infection, and renal function (Table 44-3).

Calcium, sodium, chloride, and potassium should be maintained within normal limits. Potassium should be added to maintenance fluids to avoid iatrogenic hypokalemia. Blood glucose should be maintained between 100 and 200 gm/d. Low blood glucose or a concentration that is not above normal in the face of added dextrose can be seen in patients with acute sepsis.

Table 44-3. Monitoring Goals for Patients Suffering Systemic Inflammatory Response Syndrome at Risk of Multiple Organ Dysfunction Syndrome

Core temperature	98–104°F
Core/toe-web	<7°F
Heart rate	70–120 (dogs) 100–140 (cats)
Capillary refill	<2 seconds
Arterial blood pressure	>120/80/90 systolic/diastolic/mean
Central venous pressure	5–10 cm H20
Urine output	1–2 ml/kg/hr
Packed cell volume	30–35%
Total solids	3.5–5.0
PaO2	85–120
PaCO2	<35, >28
Blood glucose	70–150 mg/dl

Disseminated intravascular coagulation (DIC) is a common component of systemic illness. Daily screening in at-risk patients can help the clinician intervene before fulminant DIC develops. Examination of a blood smear for low platelets and fragmented RBCs is inexpensive and easy. Activated clotting time is another excellent screening test for acute defects in the intrinsic and common pathways of coagulation. More specific tests for fibrin degradation products (FDP) and antithrombin III (AT III) concentration may help guide therapy. Treatment is directed toward decreasing microthrombi (heparin and AT III), providing missing factors (fresh frozen plasma), and improving perfusion.

Mentation is a subjective but important way to gauge neurologic dysfunction. Support of blood glucose, oncotic pressure, and serum osmolality reduces the risk of neurologic injury. Hepatic encephalopathy develops in patients with liver failure and can be treated supportively with gastrointestinal decontamination and ammonia trapping.

Based on new information about cytokine biology, there have been many attempts to mitigate the biological activity of cytokines on target cells (see Chapter 45).[12] The management of patients with life-threatening infection and systemic inflammation still largely consists of hemodynamic and pulmonary support, administration of appropriate antibiotics, and timely surgical intervention. Despite the exponential growth in our understanding of the basic biology of inflammation, our arsenal does not yet include a magic bullet to normalize the mediators of the pro-inflammatory and anti-inflammatory response.

PROGNOSIS

Mortality associated with MODS is directly related to the number of organ systems that fail. As more organ systems fail, the chances for survival diminish. In one human study, any single organ system failure lasting more than 1 day resulted in an in-hospital mortality risk of approximately 40%, failure of two systems in the same interval led to 60% mortality, while failure of any three systems for >72 hours brought the mortality rate close to 100%.[5] While similar information is lacking in veterinary medicine, these numbers reflect the grave prognosis with even the most intensive monitoring and therapies. Efforts to validate disease severity scoring systems in veterinary medicine will be useful to monitor our progress and gauge the benefit of new therapies that are developed to ameliorate MODS in our most critical patients.

REFERENCES

1. Bone RC, Balk RA, Cerra FB, *et al.*: American College of Chest Physicians/Society of Critical Care Medicine Consensus Conference: Definitions for sepsis and organ failure and guidelines for the use of innovative therapies in sepsis. *Crit Care Med* 20:864, 1992.
2. Kirby R: Septic shock. *In* Bonagura JD, ed.: Current Veterinary Therapy XII. Philadelphia: WB Saunders Company, 1995, p 139.
3. Matuschak GM: Multiple organ system failure: clinical expression, pathogenesis, and therapy. *In* Hall JB, Schmidt GA, Wood LDH, eds.: Principles of Critical Care. New York: McGraw-Hill, 1998, p 221.

4. Bone RC: Toward an epidemiology and natural history of SIRS (the systemic inflammatory response syndrome). *J Am Med Assoc* 25:270, 1993.
5. Knaus WA, Wagner DP: Multiple systems organ failure: epidemiology and prognosis. *Crit Care Clin* 5:221, 1989.
6. Ahmed AJ, Kruse JA, Haupt MT, *et al.*: Hemodynamic responses to gram-positive versus gram-negative sepsis in critically ill patients with and without circulatory shock. *Crit Care Med* 19:1520, 1991.
7. Bone RC: The pathogenesis of sepsis. *Ann Intern Med* 115:457, 1991.
8. Bone RC: Immunologic dissonance: a continuing evolution in our understanding of the systemic inflammatory response syndrome (SIRS) and the multiple organ dysfunction syndrome (MODS). *Ann Intern Med* 125:680, 1996.
9. Donnelly TJ, Meade P, Jagels M, *et al.*: Cytokine, complement, and endotoxin profiles associated with the development of the adult respiratory distress syndrome after severe injury. *Crit Care Med* 22:768, 1994.
10. Kirby R: Acute renal failure as a complication in the critically ill animal. *Vet Clin of North Am* 19:1189, 1989.
11. Biffl WL, Moore EE: Role of the Gut in Multiple Organ Failure. *In* Grenvik A, ed.: Textbook of Critical Care. Philadelphia: WB Saunders Company, 2000, p 1627.
12. Bone RC, Balk RA, Cerra FB, *et al.*: Definitions for sepsis and organ failure and guidelines for the use of innovative therapies in sepsis. *Chest* 101:1644, 1992.

45
Sepsis

Cynthia M. Otto

INTRODUCTION

The definitions used throughout this chapter are taken from the American College of Chest Physicians/Society of Critical Care Medicine Consensus Conference and are presented in Table 45-1.[1]

Inflammation is the body's response to limit host damage. Controlled inflammation is essential to contain and eliminate pathogens and remove damaged tissue. Macrophages recognize foreign pathogens or damaged host tissues. In response, cellular signals (cytokines, eicosanoids, and free radicals) are synthesized and released.[7] These factors act on white blood cells (monocytes, neutrophils, and lymphocytes) and endothelial cells to coordinate an inflammatory response. This response is fully equipped with amplification signals and negative feedback controls.[5] The clinical picture of inflammation results from the cardinal signs of pain, heat, redness, swelling, and loss of function.

The inflammatory response can be initiated by a spectrum of factors. In general, an appropriate response is initiated to control and reduce the inciting factors. It has long been recognized that there is an increased potential for aberrant inflammation in certain clinical situations. Patients with a higher than average risk for triggering abnormal inflammation include those presented with infectious pathogens, tissue trauma (including burns, crush injury, and major surgery), pancreatitis, neoplasia, hypoxia, and hypoperfusion. In addition, patients with a controlled inflammatory response ("one hit," *e.g.*, trauma or localized infection) are at risk for developing an exaggerated inflammatory response when exposed to a second "hit" (*e.g.*, hypoxia, hypoperfusion, infection, or surgery)[3] (Fig. 45-1). Immunosuppressive drug therapy may also contribute to the exaggerated response by unbalancing the inflammatory response. This unbalanced response renders the patient more susceptible to pathogens and interferes with endogenous regulatory mechanisms. The serious morbidity and mortality associated with sepsis and systemic inflammatory response results from extensive and generalized activation of the host immune system.[4-6]

The clinical picture of systemic inflammation results from either excess amplification, loss of negative feedback, or immune paralysis.[4,8] Failure to contain the systemic inflammatory response may lead to organ dysfunction, organ failure, and death.

Table 45-1. Definitions Pertinent to Sepsis

Bacteremia: the presence of live bacteria in the bloodstream

Systemic inflammatory response syndrome (SIRS): the clinical manifestation of systemic inflammation in response to a variety of severe insults. This is a clinical diagnosis and as such there is no gold standard for diagnosis. The criteria for the systemic inflammatory response include tachypnea, tachycardia (or in cats bradycardia), leukocytosis or leukopenia, and fever or hypothermia. The suggested criteria for diagnosis of the systemic inflammatory response in dogs and cats are listed in Table 45-2. The Consensus conference on Sepsis in Humans states that only two of the four criteria are required for the diagnosis of SIRS. This lack of specificity may contribute to heterogeneity of cases and confuse our understanding of the clinical picture of SIRS. The sensitivity of the proposed SIRS criteria for dogs was only 64%.[2]

Sepsis: systemic inflammatory response to infection, which can be caused by gram-negative, gram-positive, fungal, or viral organisms.

Severe sepsis: sepsis associated with organ dysfunction, hypoperfusion, or hypotension. Clinical manifestations of hypoperfusion may include lactic acidosis, oliguria, hypoxemia, or altered mental status.

Septic shock: sepsis with hypotension (systolic blood pressure <90 mm Hg) despite fluid resuscitation. This term is defined for humans and there is no consensus definition for animals. Patients may require vasopressors for maintenance of blood pressure.

Multiple organ dysfunction syndrome (MODS): Derangements of cardiovascular, pulmonary, renal, neurologic, coagulation, gastrointestinal, and hepatic function in patients with sepsis or SIRS that require intervention to maintain homeostasis.

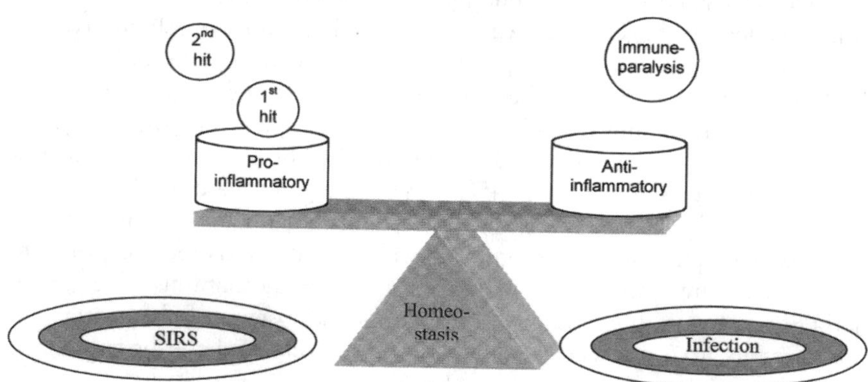

Figure 45-1
The balance between proinflammatory and anti-inflammatory mediators. A second inflammatory insult (second hit) can result in the development of SIRS in a previously compensated patient. Immune paralysis will lead to overwhelming infection.

PATHOGENESIS

Sepsis

The study of gram-negative sepsis and endotoxemia have substantially contributed to our understanding of the pathophysiology of both sepsis and systemic inflammatory response syndrome (SIRS).[11,12] One of the key observations is the relationship between presence of bacterial endotoxin (lipopolysaccharide [LPS]) and inflammation. The inflammatory response to LPS provides the framework for our understanding of both sepsis and SIRS.

The most common sepsis source in small animals is gram-negative enteric bacteria (Table 45-2).[13-17] Studies have demonstrated that LPS can also trigger clinical signs of sepsis in the absence of live bacteria. LPS binds with an acute phase protein (LPS binding protein [LBP]) and is delivered to a cell surface receptor (CD14) on the macrophage. The activated receptor then interacts with a second cell surface receptor (the toll-like receptor [TLR]) and initiates a series of reactions that initiate inflammatory mediator production.[18] Inflammatory mediators activate the inflammatory response and are essential in the development of clinical signs. Despite our understanding of SIRS activation in response to LPS, clinical trials with agents that neutralize or prevent LPS binding and activation have failed to show a therapeutic benefit.[10] Common infections that carry an increased sepsis risk include peritonitis, pneumonia, and traumatic bite wounds/infected wounds. Animals that do not have a primary infection site may develop bacteremia or endotoxemia via translocation across the gastrointestinal tract.[44] The mechanisms for translocation include primary damage to the intestinal barrier (*e.g.*, dogs with parvoviral enteritis[45]) or injury secondary to intestinal ischemia and reperfusion.

Gram-positive sepsis is not typically associated with a fulminant inflamma-

Table 45-2. Summary of Reports of Bacterial Isolates Obtained from Small Animals According to Frequency and Origin of Culture[13-17]

	Lung (dog)	Peritoneum (dog and cat)	Blood Cultures (dog and cat)	Bacteremia (dog)
Enterics	26.1%	73%	33% (dogs) 36% (cats)	51%
Anaerobes	18.7%	16%	24% (dogs) 14% (cats)	not reported
Pasteurella	12.8%	—	—	—
Streptococcus	6.9%	26%	18% (dogs) 0% (cats)	8%
Staphylococcus	5.4%	—	11% (dogs) 0% (cats)	34%

(Reprinted with permission from Otto CM: *Suppl Compend Contin Educ Pract Vet* 22:47, 2000.)

tory response as seen with gram-negative sepsis; however, recent reports describe an acute inflammatory response associated with streptococcus fasciitis in the dog.[19,20] The most common pathogen in gram-positive sepsis is *Streptococcus canis*. The mechanism is thought to be a massive cytokine response to a soluble toxin (superantigen) released from the bacteria.[21]

SIRS

It is critical to recognize that patients with signs of the SIRS may not have any infectious component. Risk factors for development of SIRS are listed in Table 45-3. As noted above, the common theory to explain SIRS and sepsis development is that the host immune response produces an excess of proinflammatory mediators.[5, 29] This may result from increased mediator production or failure to modulate the inflammatory response. Basic research has helped to identify a cohort of SIRS mediators.[30] Clinical research has provided evidence to support the role of these mediators in clinical disease.[31] There are several reports associating cytokine levels with disease severity and prognosis.[32-34] Mediators associated with initiation and amplification of the inflammatory response include tumor necrosis factor (TNF) and interleukin (IL) 1.[35, 36] Experimental infusion of these mediators induces sepsis.[37, 38] These mediators have been the focus of several experimental therapies which failed to demonstrate benefit.[10] IL-8 is also an important chemokine produced as part of the inflammatory response.[39] IL-8 is chemoattractant for neutrophils. Inhibiting neutrophil activation may be beneficial in SIRS[40]; however, clinical trials have not been performed. Vasoactive agents (*e.g.*, endothelin and nitric oxide), stress hormones, and complement and coagulation cascades contribute to the clinical and pathologic manifestations of SIRS.[35]

An alternative hypothesis to explain the exaggerated proinflammatory response in SIRS is an inadequate anti-inflammatory response. Several mediators down-regulate the inflammatory response (*e.g.*, IL-4, IL-10, and soluble receptors to TNF and IL-1).[8] Inadequate production of these mediators allows the inflammatory response to go unchecked. A recent theory suggests that excess production of anti-inflammatory mediators may contribute to SIRS by paralyzing the immune system.[4] Studies in human trauma and sepsis patients demonstrate immune dysfunction.[23,41] People who develop compensatory anti-inflammatory re-

Table 45-3. Risk Factors for SIRS

Trauma
Extensive surgery
Hypoxia
Hypotension
Pancreatitis
Burns
Immunosuppressive drugs

sponse syndrome (CARS) are more susceptible to infections and associated complications. In summary, either amplified inflammation or excessive activation of the anti-inflammatory response can lead to MODS and death. The difficulty in treating individuals lies in identifying where their inflammatory response is functioning. This is particularly difficult in dogs and cats because of limited tests and reagents to identify the mediators and characterize the immune status.

EPIDEMIOLOGY

Sepsis

The incidence of sepsis and septic shock in humans has increased over the past 15 years (Fig. 45-2).[9] There is no nationwide tracking system to monitor sepsis and SIRS in companion animals. Diagnosis codes entered by clinicians at the Veterinary Hospital of the University of Pennsylvania between 1987 and 1997 suggest that sepsis in animals has increased over the past decade (Fig. 45-3). The information available is based on microbiology studies and postmortem reports.[13-17,42] One of the biggest challenges in diagnosing sepsis and SIRS in dogs and cats is that there are no consensus guidelines. The diagnosis of sepsis/SIRS is based on clinical criteria; recent studies suggest that adopting criteria established for humans is inappropriate for dogs[2] and inaccurate for cats.[42] Despite these limitations, the research and veterinary clinical and human literature can provide some case profiles in dogs and cats that have increased risk of sepsis and SIRS. It is unknown what percentage of animals that develop sepsis or SIRS will progress to MODS and death; however, prevention is the best therapy. All patients with sepsis or SIRS should be considered at risk for MODS and death.

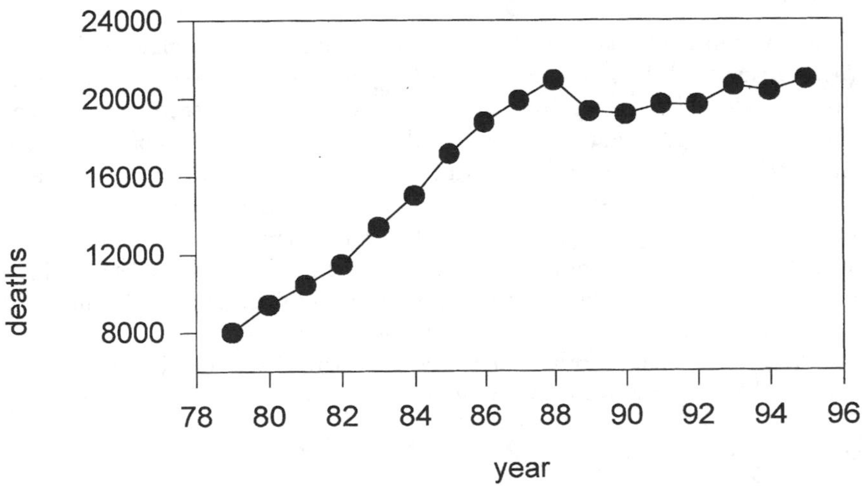

Figure 45-2
The annual number of human deaths due to sepsis in the United States between 1979 and 1995. (From Anderson RN, Kochanek KD, Murphy SL: Report of final mortality statistics 1995. *Monthly Vital Statistics Report* 45:suppl 2, 1997.)

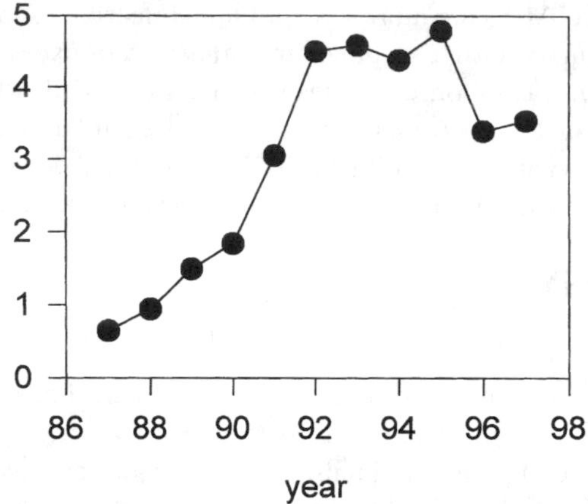

Figure 45-3
The annual incidence of sepsis in dogs, reported as number of septic cases per 1000 hospital cases, at the University of Pennsylvania Veterinary Teaching Hospital between 1987 and 1997.

In children, the definition of sepsis has been modified to include cases with clinical suspicion of infection.[43] This modification may blur the lines between sepsis and SIRS, but it recognizes that blood cultures may be negative despite bacteremia and previous treatment may prevent the culture of organisms.

Sirs

Trauma

In humans, 50% of deaths from traumatic injuries occur immediately, 30% within hours, and the remaining 20% occur within days to weeks.[48] Major surgery, periods of hypoxemia, or hypotension may provide a second insult that activates a primed immune system into the destructive cascade of SIRS. Late deaths from trauma are associated with the development of sepsis, SIRS, and MODS.[22,49] It is also possible for sepsis to occur secondary to SIRS as result of bacterial translocation or nosocomial infection.[3,22] Trauma patients have also been shown to have alterations in their immune system that predispose them to secondary infection.[23] Burn injury triggers rapid activation of the inflammatory cascade, metabolic and immune derangements, and a high incidence of secondary infections similar to other trauma class patients. The incidence of sepsis, SIRS, and MODS following extensive trauma in dogs and cats is unknown.

Hypoxia/Hypotension

Tissue hypoxia can result from inadequate oxygen delivery or defects in oxygen utilization (typically associated with toxins and endotoxemia).[24] It has been recently recognized that hypoxia can alter gene expression, including expression of inflammatory mediators.[25,26] Although hypoxia alone may not be sufficient to induce SIRS in patients that have experienced one insult, multiple episodes of hypoxia may be sufficient to amplify the inflammatory response and trigger SIRS. Tissue hypoxia can result from inadequate perfusion. Hypotension has been identified as a risk factor for the development of sepsis following trauma.[22]

Inflammation

Excess inflammatory response in the absence of infectious agents is probably best recognized in pancreatitis.[27,28] Acute fatal pancreatitis is reported in dogs and cats. Clinical signs in dogs with acute pancreatitis are consistent with SIRS.[47] Clinical signs in cats are frequently insidious and may be difficult to diagnose.[46]

CLINICAL PRESENTATION

The clinical picture of sepsis depends on the stage of the disease. In general, animals with early sepsis show the signs described in Table 45-5. In early sepsis, the animal mounts a compensatory response to maintain perfusion to the heart and brain.[50] Cardiac output is maintained at normal or elevated levels. As sepsis progresses, cardiac output is decreased; however, normal systemic vascular resistance is maintained. Ultimately, vasodilation and vascular leak result in decreased venous return, decreased cardiac output, and development of decompensated sepsis.[52] Cardiac function is impaired in all stages of septic shock, but becomes clinically apparent in decompensated and hypovolemic sepsis.[50,51] Signs of late sepsis are listed in Table 45-4.

All organ systems are affected by SIRS. Dogs appear to develop intestinal failure as an early manifestation of SIRS. This is clinically noted as diarrhea, melena, and ileus associated with enterocyte injury and bacterial translocation. Vascular endothelial dysfunction leads to coagulopathy characterized by early hypercoagulability and disseminated intravascular coagulation in the later disease phases.[54,55] Endothelial failure contributes to increased vascular permeability leading to edema. Maldistribution of blood flow is clinically and physiologically noted as peripheral vasodilation, venous pooling, and nonresponsive hypoten-

Table 45-4. Physical Parameters Associated with Sepsis

Early Sepsis	Late Sepsis
Tachypnea	Tachypnea
Bounding pulses	Thready pulses
Capillary refill time <1 sec	Capillary refill time >2 sec
Red mucous membranes	Pale mucous membranes
Mental depression	Stupor, coma
Hyperthermia	Hypothermia
	Organ failure

(Adapted with permission from Otto CM: *Suppl Compend Contin Educ Pract Vet* 22:47, 2000.)

Table 45-5. Proposed Criteria for SIRS in Dogs and Cats

Criteria for SIRS (≥2 of the following)	Dogs[2]	Cats[42]
Tachypnea	>20 breaths/min	>40 breaths/min
Tachycardia (or in cats bradycardia)	>120 beats/min	<140, >225 beats/min
Increased or decreased rectal temperature	<38° or >39°C (<100.4° or >104°F)	<37.8° or >39°C (<100° or >104°F)
Increased or decreased white blood cell count (cells/mm^3)	>18,000, <5000	>19,000, <5000

sion.[52] Myocardial function is severely compromised secondary to circulating mediators, local thrombosis, and tissue hypoxia. This is clinically noted as systolic dysfunction and arrhythmias. Severe sepsis in cats results in cardiovascular failure, hypotension, and bradycardia.[42] Tissue oxygenation can be impaired as a result of maldistribution of flow, shunting of blood, and mitochondrial failure.[24]

In humans, the lung is one of the first affected organs. Patients with SIRS develop acute respiratory distress syndrome (ARDS). ARDS has also been reported in dogs.[53] Progressive organ dysfunction leading to acute tubular necrosis and renal failure, hepatic dysfunction and bilirubinemia, neurologic dysfunction, and mentation abnormalities has also been reported.

DIAGNOSTIC EVALUATION

The diagnosis of sepsis is confirmed if there is a known infection source in an animal exhibiting the signs of sepsis (see Table 45-4) and systemic inflammatory response (see Table 45-5). A complete physical examination is critical to identify subtle signs of SIRS prior to progression of sepsis, septic shock, and MODS. Typical physical examination findings are listed in Tables 45-4 and 45-5. Systemic inflammation results in both hematologic and biochemical changes. The source of inflammation and the severity of illness will influence these changes. Common findings are listed in Table 45-6.

The diagnosis of sepsis relies on positive identification of an infectious organism, most commonly a positive bacterial culture.[1] Aerobic and anaerobic cultures should be obtained from patients with suspected sepsis prior to initiation of antibiotic therapy. In animals with an unknown infection source, blood and urine cultures should be obtained.

TREATMENT

The inflammatory response has been the target of multiple studies and clinical trials, but the complex and interrelated nature of the response has eluded all attempts to control it.[10] The most critical goal in treating a sepsis patient is preventing disease progression to severe sepsis, septic shock, or MODS. Controlling the infection source and inflammation is paramount. The early and appro-

Table 45-6. Hematologic and Biochemical Parameters Associated with Sepsis

Early Sepsis	Late Sepsis
Increased (early) or decreased blood glucose	Hypoglycemia
Leukocytosis (or leukopenia)	Leukopenia (or leukocytosis)
Mild to moderate thrombocytopenia	Thrombocytopenia
Hypercoagulability (diagnosis difficult, ±increased FSP, d-dimer, thromboelastographic changes)	Hypocoagulability (increased PT/APTT/FSP/d-dimers, decreased ATIII)
Hypoalbuminemia	Severe hypoalbuminemia
	Evidence of organ dysfunction: Increased bilirubin, ± liver enzymes Increased BUN/creatinine Decreased PaO_2, Increased $PaCO_2$

APTT, activated partial thromboplastin time; ATIII, antithrombin III; BUN, blood urea nitrogen; FSP, fibrin split products; PT, prothrombin time.

priate use of antibiotics is essential. It has been reported that antibiotic administration may stimulate inflammation through the release of LPS from dying bacteria.[56] Although this phenomenon can occur, evidence of negative clinical impact is minimal.[56] In addition, delay in providing antibiotics will allow bacteria to multiply, presenting the host with a larger bacterial burden thus producing more LPS. In septic patients, empirical administration of antibiotics is warranted; however, cultures of blood, urine, or sites of infection are important to ensure appropriate therapy. Although antibiotics are necessary, they are not the only treatment necessary. Surgical drainage or debridement may be necessary to remove sources of infection and inflammation.

In addition to controlling ongoing infection and inflammation, the septic patient has systemic abnormalities that need supportive care. All systems must be supported to optimize recovery. Key organ systems include cardiovascular, pulmonary, coagulation, renal, gastrointestinal, and central nervous system. The mainstay of cardiovascular support is fluid therapy. Both crystalloids and colloids are used in treatment of patient with sepsis/SIRS, although there is no proven advantage of one fluid type.[6,52] Fluid selection and administration should be tailored to the individual patient's needs. Guidelines are provided in Table 45-7. Altered vascular reactivity in sepsis, frequently leads to the use of vasopressors for blood pressure support (Table 45-8). Potential sequelae to vasopressor use include blood flow maldistribution (especially to the intestinal tract) and increased the cardiac workload. This added workload in the presence of myocardial depression secondary to cytokines frequently necessitates use of positive inotropic agents. In humans, a series of studies promoted "supranormal" resuscitation. The goal of this therapy was to increase oxygen delivery beyond normal values. This required the aggressive use of inotropes, fluids, and blood products.[57] In

Table 45-7. Overview of Treatment of the Septic Patient

Clinical Finding	Evaluation	Intervention	Monitor
Tachycardia Dogs >160 beats/min Cats >220 beats/min	Check ECG and auscultation to rule out primary heart disease	**Fluid therapy** *Crystalloids* Dogs: 90 mL/kg to effect Cats: 60 mL/kg to effect *Colloids* Dogs: 20 mL/kg to effect Cats: 10-15 mL/kg to effect	CVP, auscultate lungs, PCV, TS
Hypotension Systolic BP <90 mm Hg	Check if volume replaced (CVP >8 cm H_2O or increased by 3 from baseline)	**Vasopressor** Phenylephrine 1-3 µg/kg/min in saline **Combined inotrope and vasopressor** Epinephrine Dogs: 0.05–1.0 µg/kg/min Cats: 0.01–1.0 µg/kg/min	Monitor cardiac function; likely to require inotropes
Hypoglycemia Blood glucose <60 g/dL	Samples with very high PCV or those that were in contact with red cells for a prolonged period may be falsely low.	**IV Dextrose** Bolus 0.5 g/kg (dilute to <10% for peripheral administration) Supplement fluids with 2.5%, if persistent hypoglycemia supplement with 5% dextrose	Recheck glucose q 4-6 h
Fever T >39.7°C (103.5°F)	Check for excessive muscle activity, laryngeal dysfunction that could contribute to hyperthermia	Provide cold fluids, start antibiotics. Cool with ice, fans if T >40.3°C (104.5°F)	Stop external cooling at 39.4°C (103°F), monitor T q 2-4 h.
Hypothermia T <37.2°C (99°F)	Most commonly associated with hypoperfusion.	Fluid therapy with warm fluids. Prevent external heat loss (blankets, warm environment). DO NOT *surface* warm until volume replaced.	Monitor T q 2-4 h.

BP, blood pressure; CVP, central venous pressure; ECG, electrocardiogram; PCV, packed cell volume; TS, total solids. (Adapted with permission from Otto CM: *Suppl Compend Contin Educ Pract Vet* 22:47, 2000.)

Table 45-8. Inotropes and Vasopressors for Support in Sepsis

Inotropes	Dobutamine	Dogs: 5-20 μg/kg/min in D_5W or saline
	Dopamine	Dogs and cats: 2-10 μg/kg/min in D_5W
	Epinephrine	Dogs: 0.005–0.05 μg/kg/min in D_5W or saline
		Cats: 0.01–1.0 μg/kg/min in D_5W or saline
	Norepinephrine	0.1–1.0 μg/kg/min in D_5W
Vasopressors	Phenylephrine	1-3 μg/kg/min in saline
	Epinephrine	0.05–1.0 μg/kg/min in D_5W or saline
	Norepinephrine	0.5–2.0 μg/kg/min in D_5W

some patients, this strategy appeared to be beneficial; however in large clinical trials no benefit was demonstrated.[58]

Coagulation and fibrinolytic abnormalities are common in sepsis.[55] Early hypercoagulable changes are difficult to identify clinically and thus most treatment is directed at disseminated intravascular coagulation. The use of anticoagulants (low molecular weight heparins) and replacement therapy (plasma, antithrombin III) is under investigation.

Specific Care

Over the last 25 years, there have been a series of promising treatments for sepsis. These therapies, listed in Table 45-9, have all failed to improve survival in human studies.[10] New treatments continue to be investigated; however, it has been suggested that specific treatments will need to be tailored to the individual. Until specific therapies are developed, the key component of therapy is prevention. This includes prevention of ongoing inflammation by appropriate antimicrobials and surgery and prevention of secondary insults (hypotension, hypoperfusion, hypoxemia, secondary infections).[59]

Table 45-9. Specific Anti-inflammatory Therapies for Sepsis

Therapy	Outcome of Human Clinical Trials[10]
High-dose glucocorticoids	No improvement
Anti-LPS	No improvement
Anti-prostaglandins (ibuprofen)	No improvement
Anti-TNF	No improvement
TNF receptor antagonists	Worse outcome (p80)
Inhibitors of IL-1	No improvement
Nitric oxide antagonists	Increased mortality in phase III[62]
Bradykinin antagonists	No improvement
Platelet activating factor antagonists	No improvement

IL-1, interleukin 1; LPS, lipopolysaccharide; TNF, tumor necrosis factor.

PROGNOSIS

There have been no prospective studies in veterinary medicine to evaluate the incidence of SIRS or sepsis, nor the progression to septic shock or MODS or death. In a prospective study in people admitted to a tertiary care center, 68% met at least two of the four SIRS criteria. In that study, the mortality rate with SIRS was reported as 7%. The mortality has been reported to be 16% with sepsis that did not progress to septic shock or MODS.[60] In this study, the greater number of SIRS criteria that were met, the greater the probability of developing evidence of infection or sepsis.[61] Mortality of humans with septic shock is between 40% and 70% and is the leading cause of CCU deaths.[60] Risk factors for human mortality associated with sepsis include elderly patients, septic shock, the infection source, and inappropriate antibiotic selection.[61] In humans, the prognosis rapidly deteriorates as sepsis progresses to severe sepsis and septic shock. The development of MODS is also a poor prognostic indicator. Both the number of organs affected and the severity of the dysfunction affect prognosis. Veterinary patients are likely to have an even poorer prognosis with development of MODS due to the restricted availability of long-term positive pressure ventilation and hemodialysis.

REFERENCES

1. American College of Chest Physicians/Society of Critical Care Medicine Consensus Conference: Definitions for sepsis and organ failure and guidelines for the use of innovative therapies in sepsis. *Crit Care Med* 20:864, 1992.
2. Hauptman JG, Walshaw R, Olivier NB: Evaluation of the sensitivity and specificity of diagnostic criteria for sepsis in dogs. *Vet Surg* 26:393, 1997.
3. Moore FA, Moore EE: Evolving concepts in the pathogenesis of postinjury multiple organ failure. *Surg Clin North Am* 75:257, 1995.
4. Bone RC, Grodzin CJ, Balk RA: Sepsis: a new hypothesis for pathogenesis of the disease process. *Chest* 112:235, 1997.
5. Davies MG, Hagen PO: Systemic inflammatory response syndrome. *Br J Surg* 84:920, 1997.
6. Wheeler AP, Bernard GR: Treating patients with severe sepsis. *N Engl J Med* 340:207, 1999.
7. Evans T: The role of macrophages in septic shock. *Immunobiology* 195:655, 1996.
8. van der Poll T, van Deventer S: Cytokines and anticytokines in the pathogenesis of sepsis. *Infect Dis Clin North Am* 13:413, 1999.
9. Anderson RN, Kochanek KD, Murphy SL: Report of final mortality statistics 1995. *Monthly Vital Statistics Report* 45:suppl 2, 1997.
10. Zeni F, Freeman B, Natanson C: Anti-inflammatory therapies to treat sepsis and septic shock: A reassessment. *Crit Care Med* 25:1095, 1997.
11. Hinshaw LB, Tekamp-Olson P, Chang AC, *et al.*: Survival of primates in LD100 septic shock following therapy with antibody to tumor necrosis factor (TNF alpha). *Circ Shock* 30:279, 1990.
12. Feuerstein G, Hallenbeck JM, Vanatta B, *et al.*: Effect of gram-negative endotoxin on levels of serum corticosterone, TNF alpha, circulating blood cells, and the survival of rats. *Circ Shock* 30:265, 1990.

13. King LG: Postoperative complications and prognostic indicators in dogs and cats with septic peritonitis: 23 cases (1989–1992). *J Am Vet Med Assoc* 204:407, 1994.
14. Dow S, Curtis C, Jones R, *et al.*: Bacterial culture of blood from critically ill dogs and cats: 100 cases (1985–1987). *J Am Vet Med Assoc* 195:113, 1989.
15. Angus J, Jang S, Hirsh D: Microbiological study of transtracheal aspirates from dogs with suspected lower respiratory tract disease: 264 cases (1989–1995). *J Am Vet Med Assoc* 210:55, 1997.
16. Greenfield C, Walshaw R: Open peritoneal drainage for treatment of contaminated peritoneal cavity and septic peritonitis in dogs and cats: 24 cases (1980–1986). *J Am Vet Med Assoc* 191:100, 1987.
17. Calvert C, Greene C: Bacteremia in dogs: diagnosis, treatment, and prognosis. *Compend Contin Educ Pract Vet* 8:179, 1986.
18. Ingalls RR, Heine H, Lien E, *et al.*: Lipopolysaccharide recognition, CD14, and lipopolysaccharide receptors. *Infect Dis Clin North Am* 13:341, 1999.
19. Prescott J, Miller C, Mathews K, *et al.*: Update on canine streptococcal toxic shock syndrome and necrotizing fasciitis. *Can Vet J* 38:241, 1997.
20. Miller C, Prescott J, Mathews K, *et al.*: Streptococcal toxic shock syndrome in dogs. *J Am Vet Med Assoc* 209:1421, 1996.
21. Sriskandan S, Cohen J: Gram-positive sepsis. Mechanisms and differences from gram-negative sepsis. *Infect Dis Clin North Am* 13:397, 1999.
22. Morgan AS: Risk factors for infection in the trauma patient. *J Natl Med Assoc* 84: 1019, 1992.
23. Guillou PJ: Biological variation in the development of sepsis after surgery or trauma. *Lancet* 342:217, 1993.
24. Ince C, Sinaasappel M: Microcirculatory oxygenation and shunting in sepsis and shock. *Crit Care Med* 27:1369, 1999.
25. Fandrey J: Hypoxia-inducible gene expression. *Respir Physiol* 101:1, 1995.
26. Ghezzi P, Dinarello CA, Bianchi M, *et al.*: Hypoxia increases production of interleukin-1 and tumor necrosis factor by human mononuclear cells. *Cytokine* 3:189, 1991.
27. Giroir B: Pancreatitis, cytokines, and sirs: Deja vu all over again? *Crit Care Med* 27:680, 1999.
28. Brivet FG, Emilie D, Galanaud P: Pro- and anti-inflammatory cytokines during acute severe pancreatitis: an early and sustained response, although unpredictable of death. Parisian study group on acute pancreatitis. *Crit Care Med* 27:749, 1999.
29. Nystrom PO: The systemic inflammatory response syndrome: definitions and aetiology. *J Antimicrob Chemother* 41:1, 1998.
30. Creasey AA, Stevens P, Kenney J, *et al.*: Endotoxin and cytokine profile in plasma of baboons challenged with lethal and sublethal *Escherichia coli*. *Circ Shock* 33:84, 1991.
31. Suter PM, Suter S, Girardin E, *et al.*: High bronchoalveolar levels of tumor necrosis factor and its inhibitors, interleukin-1, interferon, and elastase, in patients with adult respiratory distress syndrome after trauma, shock, or sepsis. *Am Rev Respir Dis* 145:1016, 1992.
32. Calandra T, Baumgartner JD, Grau GE, *et al.*: Prognostic values of tumor necrosis factor/cachectin, interleukin-1, interferon-alpha, and interferon-gamma in the serum of patients with septic shock. Swiss-Dutch J5 immunoglobulin study group. *J Infect Dis* 161:982, 1990.
33. Kern P, Hemmer CJ, Van-Damme J, *et al.*: Elevated tumor necrosis factor alpha and interleukin-6 serum levels as markers for complicated *Plasmodium falciparum* malaria. *Am J Med* 87:139, 1989.

34. Waage A, Halstensen A, Espevik T: Association between tumour necrosis factor in serum and fatal outcome in patients with meningococcal disease. *Lancet* 1:355, 1987.
35. Beishuizen A, Vermes I, Haanen C: Endogenous mediators in sepsis and septic shock. *Adv Clin Chem* 33:55, 1998.
36. Brouckaert P, Fiers W: Tumor necrosis factor and the systemic inflammatory response syndrome. *Curr Top Microbiol Immunol* 216:167, 1996.
37. Tracey KJ, Lowry SF, Fahey Td, *et al.*: Cachectin/tumor necrosis factor induces lethal shock and stress hormone responses in the dog. *Surg Gynecol Obstet* 164:415, 1987.
38. Butler LD, Layman NK, Cain RL, *et al.*: Interleukin 1-induced pathophysiology: induction of cytokines, development of histopathologic changes, and immunopharmacologic intervention. *Clin Immunol Immunopathol* 53:400, 1989.
39. Takala A, Jousela I, Jansson SE, *et al.*: Markers of systemic inflammation predicting organ failure in community-acquired septic shock. *Clin Sci* 97:529, 1999.
40. Carvalho GL, Wakabayashi G, Shimazu M, *et al.*: Antiinterleukin-8 monoclonal antibody reduces free radical production and improves hemodynamics and survival rate in endotoxic shock in rabbits. *Surgery* 122:60, 1997.
41. Heidecke CD, Hensler T, Weighardt H, *et al.*: Selective defects of T lymphocyte function in patients with lethal intraabdominal infection. *Am J Surg* 178:288, 1999.
42. Brady C, Otto C, Van Winkle T, *et al.*: Severe sepsis in cats: a retrospective study of 29 cases (1986–1998). *J Am Vet Med Assoc* 217:531, 2000.
43. Anderson MR, Blumer JL: Advances in the therapy for sepsis in children. *Pediatr Clin North Am* 44:179, 1997.
44. Van Leeuwen PA, Boermeester MA, Houdijk AP, *et al.*: Clinical significance of translocation. *Gut* 35:S28, 1994.
45. Otto CM, Drobatz K, Soter C: Endotoxemia and TNF activity in canine parvoviral enteritis [abstract]. *Shock* 5:36, 1996.
46. Steiner J, Williams D: Feline pancreatitis. *Compend Contin Educ Pract Vet* 19:590, 1997.
47. Hess R, Saunders H, van Winkle T, *et al.*: Clinical, clinicopathologic, radiographic, and ultrasonographic abnormalities in dogs with fatal acute pancreatitis: 70 cases (1986–1995). *J Am Vet Med Assoc* 213:665, 1998.
48. Trunkey D: Initial treatment of patients with extensive trauma. *N Engl J Med* 324:1259, 1991.
49. Abraham E: Physiologic stress and cellular ischemia: relationship to immunosuppression and susceptibility to sepsis. *Crit Care Med* 19:613, 1991.
50. Parillo JE, Parker MM, Natanson C, *et al.*: Septic shock in humans. Advances in the understanding of pathogenesis, cardiovascular dysfunction, and therapy. *Ann Intern Med* 113:227, 1990.
51. Natanson C, Fink MP, Ballantyne HK, *et al.*: Gram-negative bacteremia produces both severe systolic and diastolic cardiac dysfunction in a canine model that simulates human septic shock. *J Clin Invest* 78:259, 1986.
52. Astiz ME, Galera-Santiago A, Rackow EC: Intravascular volume and fluid therapy for severe sepsis. *New Horizons* 1:127, 1993.
53. Parent C, King LG, Walker LM, *et al.*: Clinical and clinicopathologic findings in dogs with acute respiratory distress syndrome: 19 cases (1985–1993). *J Am Vet Med Assoc* 208:1419, 1996.
54. Otto C, Rieser T, Brooks M, *et al.*: Evidence of hypercoagulability in dogs with parvoviral enteritis. *J Am Vet Med Assoc* 217:1500. 2000.

55. Vervloet MG, Thijs LG, Hack CE: Derangements of coagulation and fibrinolysis in critically ill patients with sepsis and septic shock. *Semin Thromb Hemost* 24:33, 1998.
56. Hurley JC: Antibiotic-induced release of endotoxin. A therapeutic paradox. *Drug Safety* 12:183, 1995.
57. Shoemaker WC, Appel PL, Kram HB, *et al.*: Hemodynamic and oxygen transport monitoring to titrate therapy in septic shock. *New Horizons* 1:145, 1993.
58. Heyland DK, Cook DJ, King D, *et al.*: Maximizing oxygen delivery in critically ill patients: A methodologic appraisal of the evidence. *Crit Care Med* 24:517, 1996.
59. Quezado ZM, Natanson C: Systemic hemodynamic abnormalities and vasopressor therapy in sepsis and septic shock. *Am J Kidney Dis* 20:214, 1992.
60. Rangel-Frausto MS, Pittet D, Costigan M, *et al.*: The natural history of the systemic inflammatory response syndrome (SIRS). A prospective study. *JAMA* 273:117, 1995.
61. Rangel-Frausto MS: The epidemiology of bacterial sepsis. *Infect Dis Clin North Am* 13:299, 1999.
62. Cobb JP: Use of nitric oxide synthase inhibitors to treat septic shock: The light has changed from yellow to red. *Crit Care Med* 27:855, 1999.

46
Immune-Medicated Hemolytic Anemia

Leah S. Faudskar

INTRODUCTION

Immune-mediated hemolytic anemia (IMHA) is the most common form of hemolytic anemia in dogs. In this disease process, red blood cells (RBCs) are coated with antibody, which leads to an accelerated rate of RBC destruction. Clinical signs vary widely depending on the severity and the rate of onset of the anemia. Several life-threatening complications are associated with this disease and its treatment, making these patients some of the more challenging intensive care unit patients.

PATHOGENESIS

Red blood cell destruction occurs as the result of an immune reaction involving immunoglobulin, complement, or both. Antibodies are produced against RBC membrane antigens. The trigger for antibody production may be unknown, as in animals with primary (idiopathic) IMHA, or it may be secondary to infection by a virus, bacteria, or RBC parasite, other immune-mediated disease, exposure to a drug or vaccine, or neoplasia. There may be a change in the RBC membrane antigens or exposure of hidden antigens causing the production of antibodies against the RBC by a normal immune system. Alternately, there may be an abnormality in the immune system allowing antibody production against self antigens.[1]

After antibody production and RBC coating, destruction occurs by one of three mechanisms: intravascular agglutination, intravascular hemolysis, or extravascular hemolysis. Intravascular agglutination with subsequent phagocytosis and extravascular hemolysis reaction is known as class I IMHA and results in a positive slide agglutination. Intravascular hemolysis class II IMHA, usually involves immunoglobulin M (IgM) antibodies, which fix complement in sufficient quantities to produce hemolysis. Red blood cells heavily coated with immunoglobulin G (IgG) may also fix so much complement that intravascular lysis occurs. Class I and class II IMHA are acute in onset and rapidly progressive. In animals with class III IMHA, RBCs coated with antibody in insufficient quantity to cause hemolysis or agglutination are destroyed by phagocytosis in the reticuloendothelial system. Slide agglutination does not occur. Class III IMHA is more chronic in nature.

Phagocytosis may be IgM or IgG mediated with or without complement. Macrophages recognize the constant fragment (Fc) portion of the IgG molecule.

Immunoglobulin binding by Fc receptors on the macrophage can result in complete erythrophagocytosis. Alternately, only a portion of the membrane may be removed by the phagocyte leaving the RBC with reduced surface, thus forming a spherocyte. These are small, dense, rigid RBCs that have lost the typical biconcave shape of canine RBCs. The deformability of spherocytes is impaired. These cells are trapped in the spleen and subsequently destroyed. Macrophages also have receptors for complement components. Complement together with IgG enhances the phagocytic process, particularly for hepatic macrophages. Macrophages do not have receptors for the Fc component of IgM. Destruction of IgM coated RBCs is mediated by complement.

Affected dogs are typically middle aged. Some studies suggest older females are more frequently affected, whereas males predominate in animals <1 year of age. Other studies have shown no sex predilection. A higher incidence of IMHA is reported in the Old English Sheepdog, Poodle, American Cocker Spaniel, English Springer Spaniel, Lhasa Apso, Shih Tzu, and Irish Setter, but a familial tendency has not been established. A seasonal tendency was suggested in one study, in which 40% of the cases developed in May and June.[2] Sixty to 75 percent of IMHA in dogs is primary or idiopathic.

CLINICAL AND LABORATORY FINDINGS

History and physical examination findings vary widely with and depend on the severity of the anemia, the rate of onset of the anemia, and the presence of underlying disease. Common findings include lethargy, weakness, exercise intolerance, pale mucous membranes, tachycardia, tachypnea, bounding pulses, systolic heart murmur, icterus, pigmenturia (bilirubinuria or hemoglobinuria), splenomegaly, hepatomegaly, fever, petechia, vomiting, anorexia, syncope, collapse, peripheral lymphadenopathy, polydipsia, and dermatitis.

A list of differential diagnoses for hemolytic anemia is provided in Table 46-1. The diagnostic approach for IMHA may include a complete blood count, slide agglutination test, cytologic examination of RBCs, biochemical analysis, urinalysis, serologic testing for tick disease, antinuclear antibody testing, direct antiglobulin test (DAT), thoracic and abdominal radiographs, abdominal ultrasound, bone marrow biopsy, and coagulation testing. It is important to assess for underlying disease and determine the impact of the anemia on multiple organ systems.

Key laboratory findings are spherocytosis with a positive slide agglutination or direct antibody test. Table 46-2 lists other common laboratory abnormalities in patients with IMHA. Demonstration of antibodies directed against RBCs by a positive slide agglutination or DAT is definitive for IMHA.

Autoagglutination is represented by grape-like clusters of cells seen microscopically or clumps of cells grossly visible in anticoagulated blood or on a slide. It must be differentiated from rouleau, which may be caused by high serum proteins. Rouleau appears as cells stacked like coins and tends to disperse when one drop of blood is diluted by several drops of saline.

Two thirds of patients with IMHA are DAT positive. The DAT detects antibody or complement on the surface of the RBCs when the antibody strength

Table 46-1. Causes of Hemolytic Anemia

Immune-mediated	RBC Defects	Microangiopathy	Bacterial	Parasites	Chemical	
Autoimmune hemolytic anemia	Chondrodysplasia (malmutes)	Babesia	*C. perfringens* *C. haemolyticum*	*Anaplasma*	Acetominophen	Onion
Feline leukemia	Congenital feline porphyria	Dirofilarisis	Endotoxemia	*Babesia*	Bee venom	Penicillin
Glomerulonephritis	Elliptocytosis	DIC	Leptospirosis	*Cytauxzoon*	Benzocaine	Phenazopyridine HCl
Histoplasmosis	Heinz body anemia	Hemangiosarcoma		*Ehrlichia*	Castor bean	Prenothiazines
Idiopathic	Methemoglobin reductase deficiency	Heat stroke		*Hemobartonella*	Cephalosporin	Propothiouracil
Incompatible transfusions	Phosphofructokinase deficiency	Splenic torsion		Piroplasmosis organism	Chronic hepatitis (Bedlington terriers)	Quinidine
Lymphocytic leukemia	Pyruvate kinase deficiency	Vasculitis			Copper	Sulfonamide
Lymphosarcoma	Spur cell anemia				Dipyrone	Zinc
Neonatal isoerythrolysis	Stomatocytosis				Heparin	
Reticulum cell sarcoma					Hypophosphatemia	
Endocarditis					Methimazole	
Systemic lupus erythematosis					Methylene blue	

(Modified from Stewart et al.: Immune-mediated hemolytic anemia part II: Clinical entity, diagnosis and treatment theory. Comp Cont Educ Pract Vet 15:479, 1993)

Table 46-2. Laboratory Finding in Animals with Immune-Mediated Hemolytic Anemia

Definitive
Positive slide agglutination
Positive direct antiglobulin test
Strongly suggestive
Spherocytosis
Frequently observed
Profound anemia
Polychromasia
Anisocytosis
Reticulocytosis, >60,000/μl
Leukocytosis, neutrophilia ± left shift
Thrombocytopenia
Erythroid hyperplasia, bone marrow
Hemoglobinemia
Hemoglobinuria
Bilirubinemia
Bilirubinuria
Coagulation abnormalities
Elevated ALT
Elevated ALP
Azotemia

or concentration is too low to cause spontaneous agglutination. IgG, IgM, and complement (C3b) reagent is added at various concentrations to the patient's washed RBCs. Agglutination is reported from 1+ to 4+. Identification of complement alone suggests an underlying disease process. The strength of the DAT does not predict the severity of the anemia. False-positive results may be seen with hyperglobulinemia, rouleau, and inadequate washing of RBCs, and in previously transfused patients.[4] False-negative test results can be caused by insufficient quantity of antibody, low affinity of antibody, drug reaction, corticosteroid therapy, or technical problems.[4]

Spherocytosis is mild to marked depending on the type of RBC destruction, and spherocytes are found in approximately 80% of patients with IMHA. Spherocytosis is suggested by a low mean corpuscular volume (MCV) and a high mean corpuscular hemoglobin concentration (MCHC).

Reticulocytosis is found in 60% to 70% of IMHA patients and suggests a regenerative response. Number of reticulocytes should be evaluated relative to the degree of anemia.[5]

The corrected reticulocyte count (CRC) = % reticulocytes × PCV/normal PCV (45% in dogs, 37% in cats). Normal CRC < 0.4%. Regenerative response >1%.

THERAPY

The therapeutic plan for IMHA patients must encompass three goals. First, deficits in oxygen delivery resulting from severe reduction in red cell mass must

Table 46-3. Therapeutic and Monitoring Plan for Animals with Immune-Mediated Hemolytic Anemia

Specific Care		
Provide adequate oxygen carrying ability. Remove/treat underlying cause. Begin immunosuppressive therapy with glucocorticosteroids.	PRBCs 10 ml/kg Oxyglobin 5–30 ml/kg—dog 5–10 ml/kg—cat Prednisolone 2–4 mg/kg divided q 12 h PO, IM, IV	PCV or plasma hemoglobin q 4–24 h Note mm color, CRT, pulse quality, heart rate and rhythm, respiratory rate, mentation, strength, body temperature.
Immediate Care		
Correct dehydration and electrolyte imbalances. Correct coagulation abnormalities. Provide gastrointestinal protection, antiemetics. Consider other immunosuppressive agents in the face of refractory anemia. Consider anticoagulants in the face of thromboembolic disease.	Balanced electrolyte solutions supplemented as needed. FFP 10 ml/kg H_2 blockers, synthetic prostaglandins, coating agents. Cyclophosphamide,[1] azathioprine,[6] danazol, IVGG,[7,8] cyclosporine Heparin, streptokinase	BUN, glucose, electrolytes q 12–24 h Note: body weight, ins and outs, CVP Platelets, coagulation profile q 12–24 h Note: petechia, hematuria, emesis, ochezia, hyphema, epistaxis Gastrointestinal mucosal integrity q 6 h Note: appetite, presence of vomiting, diarrhea, hematemesis, hematochezia, melena.
General Care		
Monitor for infection, organ failure. Provide nutritional support. Provide nursing care/patient hygiene.	Serial CBC, biochemical, coagulation profiles Enteral and parenteral support, antiemetics as needed Catheter, bandage care	Bilirubin, ALT q 24–48 h Note: mm and scleral color, urine bilirubin. CBC q 24h-weekly Note: temperature change, hypo- or hyperglycemia, pyuria, dyspnea, inflammation at catheter sites, as part of monitoring with bone marrow suppressive agents such as cyclophosphamide or azathioprine

be alleviated. Second, modulation of the immune process and removal of the underlying cause (antigen), is imperative. Third, supportive care is needed to minimize the complications of RBC destruction, tissue hypoxia and to ameliorate the side effects of immunosuppressive drugs (Table 46-3).

Patients whose RBC mass is severely reduced, *i.e.*, hemoglobin <7 mg/dl or who show signs of oxygen debt (tachycardia, tachypnea, syncope, arrhythmia) should receive hemoglobin in the form of packed RBCs or a hemoglobin based, oxygen carrying solution such as Oxyglobin (Biopure). Packed RBCs are administered intravenously (IV) as rapidly as needed and at a dose required to alleviate clinical signs of severe anemia. Typically, patients receive 10 ml/kg over a 4-hour period. Autoagglutination may prevent accurate blood typing and cross-matching. Donors selected for packed RBC transfusion should be DEA 1.1 negative. Transfused RBCs are expected to be lysed at the same rate as the patient's RBCs until immune suppression occurs, and multiple transfusions may be needed. Oxyglobin may be administered in dogs at 10 to 30 ml/kg IV over a 4- to 6-hour period. This represents an increase in plasma hemoglobin of 2 to 4 g/dl or an equivalent increase in the packed cell volume (PCV) of 6% to 12%. Oxyglobin may be the hemoglobin source of choice because it eliminates the need for cross matching or blood typing, it is immediately available, and has no storage lesions to reduce the oxygen carrying ability of the hemoglobin. Oxyglobin may discolor the mucous membranes and the sclera. It will render further tests of plasma bilirubin inaccurate. The half-life of Oxyglobin is dependent on the dose administered. Plasma hemoglobin concentration may be monitored, and Oxyglobin redosed as needed to maintain an acceptable concentration or resolution of the clinical signs of anemia. Volume overload is a potential consequence of packed RBC or Oxyglobin administration in the IMHA patient. Careful observation for pulmonary edema is required.

Glucocorticosteroids are the primary drug for immunosuppressive therapy in IMHA patients. Glucocorticosteroids inhibit amplification of the complement cascade, T cell activation and can inhibit prostaglandin and leukotriene production. These drugs also inhibit the clearance of antibody coated RBCs reticuloendothelial system by blocking Fc and complement (C3b) receptors on the macrophage. Over weeks, antibody production decreases because of a diminished number of lymphocytes in the circulating T helper cell pool and a reduction in lymphocyte cell division.[1] Glucocorticosteroids are most effective in reducing the clearance of IgG-coated cells and less effective in preventing the clearance of IgG-complement or IgM-coated cells. Drug dosage varies with the immunosuppressive potency of the glucocorticosteroid used. Response to therapy is reflected by increasing PCV, appropriate reticulocytosis, reduced spherocytosis, and reduced autoagglutination. Complications from glucocorticosteroid use are increased vulnerability to infection, gastrointestinal ulceration, increased risk of thromboembolism, increased water consumption, and increased urination.

Reports vary regarding the efficacy of other immunosuppressive agents for patients who fail to respond to glucocorticosteroid therapy. Other drugs may be added to or used in place of glucocorticosteroids, but there are no conclusive studies to support their use in standard acute therapeutic protocols (Table 46-4). Plasmapharesis and splenectomy are alternate therapies that have been proposed; however, plasmapharesis is not readily available and the response to splenectomy is transient.

Table 46-4. Commonly Used Therapeutic Agents in Animals with Immune-Medicated Hemolytic Anemia

Red Cell Fluid Support

Crystalloids to correct deficit, provide for ongoing losses, and meet maintenance fluid needs IV; electrolyte supplementation is needed.

Oxyglobin (Biopure) 15–30 ml/kg over 4–12 hours IV

Packed red blood cells 10 ml/kg over 4 hours IV

Fresh frozen plasma 10 ml/kg over 4 hours IV

Immunosuppression

Prednisolone 2–4 mg/kg/day divided q 12 h PO, IM until PCV is stable or rising then taper by 25% per week to 4 weeks until 0.5 mg/kg/day then alternate-day therapy

Dexamethasone 0.1–0.3 mg/kg/day IV, IM, PO

Cyclophosphamide (Cytoxan, Meade-Johnson Oncology) 50 mg/m^2 × 4 days, 3 days off or 200 mg/m^2 IV or PO as a component of initial therapy

Azathioprine (Imuran, Glaxo Wellcome) 2 mg/kg q 24 h PO

Danazol (Danocrine, Sanofi-Winthrop) 5–10 mg/kg q 12 h PO

Cyclosporine A (Sandimune, Sandoz Pharmaceuticals) 10 mg/kg q 24 h IV then adjust to achieve blood concentration of 200–400 ng/ml

Human intravenous gamma globulin 5% (Gamimune 0.5%, Bayer Corporation-Biologics) 0.5 gm/kg over 4 hours or 1.0 gm/kg IV over 6–12 hours

Gastrointestinal Protection

Misoprostol (Cytotec-Searle) 2–5 mcg/kg PO q 8 h

Cimetidine (Tagamet-SK Beecham) 10 mg/kg q 6–8 h IV, IM, PO

Famotidine (Pepcid-Merck) 0.5 mg/kg q 12–24 h IV, PO

Sucralfate (Carafate-Hoechst Marion Roussel) 0.5–1.0 gm q 8 h PO

Support Therapy

Metoclopramide (Reglan-Robins) 2 mg/kg/day constant rate infusion IV

Heparin 250 IU/kg q 6 h SQ

Streptokinase 150,000 IU over 30 min then 75,000 IU/h for 24 hours IV

Aspirin 1–5 mg/kg q 24 h PO

Doxycycline (Vibramycin, Pfizer) 5 mg/kg q 24 h PO

COMPLICATIONS

Complications often encountered in IMHA patients include thrombocytopenia, disseminated intravascular coagulation (DIC), thromboembolism, gastrointestinal ulceration and bleeding, infection, renal failure, and refractory anemia.

Thrombocytopenia has been reported in approximately 70% of patients with IMHA. Two theories for concurrent thrombocytopenia have been examined. Thrombocytopenia can develop as a result of concurrent, immune-mediated destruction of platelets (Evans syndrome) or as a result of platelet consumption. Patients with thrombocytopenia, petechia, or schistocytes may have RBC fragmentation and platelet consumption associated with DIC. A coagulation profile should be done in these patients to evaluate for coagulation abnormalities. Patients with IMHA may be more vulnerable to DIC and thromboembolism because of thromboplastic substances released from RBC membranes, tissue ischemic injury secondary to anemia, and the coagulopathic or bone marrow suppressive effects of immunosuppressive drugs. Evidence of prolonged clotting times in combination with thrombocytopenia should be treated by transfusion of fresh frozen plasma at 10 ml/kg IV over 4 hours or as tolerated or until prothrombin time (PT) and activated partial thromboplastin time (aPTT) are normal. The use of anticoagulants such as heparin or fractionated heparin remains controversial. Difficulty in monitoring heparin therapy and increased risk of bleeding must be weighed against any beneficial effects in prevention of coagulation factor consumption or thromboembolism.

The incidence of thromboembolism in animals with IMHA is not known. Pulmonary thromboembolism (PTE) is a potentially fatal complication of IMHA. One study demonstrated a 30% incidence of PTE in patients with IMHA.[9] Thromboembolism has been suggested to develop as the result of the release of thromboplastic substances from the RBC membrane or because of an endothelial-cell dependent pathway triggered by the presence of immune complexes.[10] Patients with a high bilirubin (>10 mg/dl), multiple IV catheters, and frequent blood transfusions are at high risk for thromboembolism.[9] Signs of PTE include acute onset of dyspnea and pain, hypoxemia with normo- or hypocapnia on arterial blood gas analysis, increased alveolar to arterial oxygen gradient, high central venous pressure secondary to pulmonary hypertension, interstitial pattern, pleural effusion, abruptly terminating pulmonary vessels on thoracic radiography, or ventilation-perfusion abnormality on pulmonary scintigraphy.[10] Therapy includes oxygen administration and heparin for control of thrombus growth or streptokinase for thrombus dissolution.

Gastrointestinal blood loss may occur secondary to coagulopathy or injury to gastrointestinal mucosa and may represent clinically important blood loss for the anemic patient. Gastrointestinal ulceration can develop secondary to use of glucocorticosteroid through the inhibition of prostaglandins and the loss of the protective gastrointestinal mucous production. Patients with IMHA in a severely anemic state are also prone to ischemic injury of gastrointestinal mucosa. Anorexia leads to atrophy and increased vulnerability to injury of the gastrointestinal mucosa. Thrombocytopenia and coagulation abnormalities can cause gastrointestinal bleeding. Gastrointestinal protectants are indicated throughout the entire course of immunosuppressive therapy. Enteral nutritional support helps to maintain gastrointestinal mucosal viability.

Patients with IMHA are particularly vulnerable to infection. Careful evaluation of the patient is needed because leukocytosis and left shift may develop because of infection or as part of the leukemoid response to severe anemia and bone marrow stimulation from inflammatory cytokines. Monitoring of catheter sites, leukogram, urine sediment, blood glucose levels, chest radiographs, body temperature and pressure points will help identify occurrence of new infection.

Prophylactic antibiotics are not recommended because antibiotics are implicated in drug reactions that stimulate antibody production against erythrocytes.

Renal injury associated with IMHA is thought to be caused by vasoconstriction and hypoperfusion.[11] Some heme pigments may precipitate and form casts in the distal renal tubule. However, tubular necrosis and acute renal failure are rarely seen in animals with severe and chronic hemoglobinuria.[5] Results of renal function tests may be high because of prerenal azotemia secondary to dehydration from anorexia, vomiting, or diarrhea. Renal azotemia may be caused by underlying renal disease. Crystalloid fluid therapy is used to protect renal perfusion and replace fluid deficits.

Approximately 10% of IMHA patients are refractory to glucocorticosteroids. Other patients may fail to show a regenerative response in spite of aggressive, multimodal therapy. Refractory anemia may be the result of failure to suppress the immune response, direct immune injury to erythroid precursors, blood loss through gastrointestinal bleeding, microangiopathic injury to RBCs, or suppressed erythropoiesis by immunosuppressive agents.[12] A bone marrow biopsy is indicated in patients with nonregenerative anemia that persists longer than 5 to 7 days. The bone marrow response in patients with IMHA typically shows increasing erythropoiesis and concurrent granulopoiesis with a decreasing M:E ratio. Diminished or absent erythropoiesis may represent a type of IMHA in which antibodies are directed against RBC precursors.[1]

PROGNOSIS

In patients that achieve remission, medications are tapered individually over weeks to months, and the hemogram is monitored closely. Prognosis remains guarded. Mortality rates have been reported from 20% to 79%. Most deaths occur within 90 days of diagnosis.[12] Higher mortality rates have been associated with intravascular hemolysis, low initial PCV, persistent reticulocytosis of $<3\%$, multiple blood transfusions, and high bilirubin concentration.[12]

CATS

Immune-mediated hemolytic anemia is rare in cats. Antibodies may be directed against self antigens, as in patients with true autoimmune disease, or against foreign antigens adsorbed onto or incorporated into cell membranes. The disease may be idiopathic or associated with feline leukemia infection (FeLV), hemobartonellosis, lymphoid or myeloid neoplasia, or systemic lupus erythematosis or it may be drug induced.[13] A diagnosis of IMHA in a cat should prompt the clinician to look carefully for underlying disease.

Clinical signs are similar to those in dogs. IgM antibody is more common in cats, whereas IgG is the more prevalent antibody in dogs.[13] Autoagglutination occurs when IgM antibody is present. Extravascular hemolysis results in RBC destruction. Spherocytes are not readily identified because of the morphology of feline RBCs. Partial phagocytosis is manifested by increased osmotic fragility.

A diagnosis of IMHA is made by demonstrating evidence of hemolysis, such as increased osmotic fragility, increased agglutination, or a positive DAT. Other diagnostic tests commonly performed are direct fluorescent antibody test for FeLV on peripheral blood or bone marrow, antinuclear antibody test, and cytologic examination of bone marrow and lymph node aspirates. Erythrophagocytosis may be observed in smears of blood or bone marrow or lymph node aspirates.

Anemia is typically regenerative, with >50,000 reticulocytes/µl. Reticulocytes in cats are of two types, punctate and aggregate. Aggregate reticulocytes correspond to the reticulocytes seen in dogs and indicate an active regenerative response. Aggregate reticulocytes mature to punctate reticulocytes in less than one day. Punctate reticulocytes circulate for one to two weeks.[4] Nonregenerative anemia may result from dysplastic or hypoplastic bone marrow secondary to myeloproliferative disease.

Direct agglutination test-positive anemia may precede the development of feline leukemia viremia. Cats should be retested for FeLV 4 to 6 weeks after diagnosis of IMHA if the initial FeLV test is negative. It is important to know that not all cats with IMHA have FeLV infection.

Blood smears are evaluated for *Hemobartonella* sp. Organisms take two forms: a signet ring shape superimposed on the cell or a rod shape at the periphery of the cell.

Therapy is similar to that for dogs with IMHA. Prednisolone (2–4 mg/kg/day divided) or dexamethasone (0.2 mg/kg/day) are the initial drugs for immunosuppression.[11] Packed RBCs or Oxyglobin may be used as needed. Oxyglobin is not labeled for use in cats and must be used with caution. Cats are extremely sensitive to volume overload. Initial doses are 5 to 10 ml/kg IV over 4 to 6 hours. Feline patients are often started on tetracycline (Panmycin, Upjohn; 20 mg/kg q 8 hours PO) or doxycycline (Vibramycin, Pfizer; 5 mg/kg q 24 hours PO). Other immunosuppressive agents have been use such as chlorambucil (Leukeran, Burroughs Wellcome). Cyclophosphamide is not well tolerated in cats. Azathioprine is not recommended because of bone marrow toxicity.

REFERENCES

1. Aird B: Immune-mediated hemolytic anemia. Proceedings, 13th Forum Am Col Vet Int Med, 1995, p 41.
2. Klag AR, Giger U, Shofer FS: Idiopathic immune-mediated hemolytic anemia in dogs: 42 cases (1986–1990). *J Am Vet Med Assoc* 202:783, 1993.
3. Stewart AF, Feldman BF: Immune-mediated hemolytic anemia part II. Clinical entity, diagnosis and treatment theory. *Comp Contin Educ Pract Vet* 15:1479, 1993.
4. Honeckman AL, Knapp DW, Reagan, WJ: Diagnosis of canine immune-mediated hematologic disease. *Comp Contin Educ Pract Vet* 18:113, 1996.
5. Giger U: Regenerative anemia caused by blood loss or hemolysis. *In* Ettinger SK, ed.: Textbook of Veterinary Internal Medicine, 4th ed. Philadelphia: WB Saunders: p 1784.
6. Beale KM: Azathioprine for treatment of immune-mediated diseases of dogs and cats. *J Am Vet Med Assoc* 192:1316, 1988.
7. Kellerman DL, Bruyette DS: Intravenous human immunoglobulin for the treatment of immune-mediated hemolytic anemia in 13 dogs. *J Vet Int Med* 11:329, 1997.
8. Scott-Moncrieff JCR, Reagan WJ, Snyder PW, *et al.*: Intravenous administration

of human immune globulin in dogs with immune-mediated hemolytic anemia. *J Am Vet Med Assoc* 210:1623, 1997.

9. Klein MK, Dow SW, Rosychuk AW: Pulmonary thromboembolism associated with immune-mediated hemolytic anemia in dogs: ten cases (1982–1987). *J Am Vet Med Assoc* 195:246, 1989.
10. Lifton SJ: Managing immune-mediated hemolytic anemia in dogs. Vet Med p. 532 6/1999.
11. Miller E: CVT update: Diagnosis and treatment of immune-mediated hemolytic anemia. *In* Bonagura JD, ed.: Current Veterinary Therapy XIII, Philadelphia: WB Saunders, 2000, p 427.
12. Reimer ME, Troy GC, Warnick, LD: Immune-mediated hemolytic anemia: 70 cases (1988–1996). *J Am Anim Hosp Assoc* 35:384, 1999.
13. Werner LL, Gorman, NT: Immune-mediated diseases of cats. *Vet Clin North Am Small Anim Pract* 14:1039, 1974.

47
Acute Tumor Lysis Syndrome

Gregory K. Ogilvie

INTRODUCTION

Dogs and cats with a large tumor burden or rapidly proliferating tumors may experience treatment-related acute tumor lysis syndrome (ATLS). This under-recognized clinical condition results from the destruction of tumor cells and subsequent rapid discharge of intracellular electrolytes and nucleic acids resulting in acute illness that can lead to death.[1-8]

The hyperkalemia associated with ATLS may be accentuated by associated renal insufficiency or renal failure and may cause electrocardiographic (EGC) alterations and a potentially fatal cardiac arrhythmia. The major manifestation of hyperphosphatemia is secondary to hypocalcemia caused by precipitation of calcium phosphate in the soft tissues and the kidney. The clinical consequences are due to resultant renal failure and metabolic effects secondary to the hyperkalemia and hypocalcemia.

PATHOGENESIS

ATLS is most common in lymphoma or leukemia patients, partly because the intracellular concentration of phosphorus in human lymphoma and leukemic cells is four to six times higher than in normal cells.[3-8] Canine and feline patients at highest risk are volume-contracted dogs and cats with stage IV or V lymphoma that are treated with chemotherapy and that undergo very rapid remission; therefore, this condition may be identified within 48 hours after the first treatment.

The actual pathogenesis of ATLS in dogs and dogs and cats is unstudied; however, it is hypothesized that the pathogenesis is similar to that seen in people.[1,2] A large tumor burden, a high growth fraction, and pre-existing renal insufficiency increase the risk of ATLS. Reduced renal perfusion or glomerular filtration including acute renal insufficiency or failure further aggravate the metabolic abnormality. The syndrome usually occurs within 6 to 72 hours after the initiation of therapy. In humans, and presumably in dogs and cats, rapid tumor lysis may cause an acute release of intracellular phosphate and potassium. This release of electrolytes causes hypocalcemia, hyperkalemia, and hyperphosphatemia. In human patients, hyperuricemia is also seen. The hyperkalemia associated with ATLS may cause ECG alterations and potentially fatal cardiac arrhythmias. The major manifestation of hyperphosphatemia is secondary hypocalcemia caused by precipitation of calcium phosphate in the soft tissues and the kidney. The clinical consequences are due to resultant renal failure and metabolic effects secondary to hyperkalemia and hyopcalcemia.

CLINICAL PRESENTATION

Dogs and cats with suspected ATLS are often diagnosed after acute collapse and decompensation following chemotherapy administration and, less commonly, radiation therapy.[2-8] Some cases are evaluated in the hospital after electrolyte changes have partially or completely normalized yet demonstrate severe clinical signs. Hypocalcemia may lead to alterations in mental status, neuromuscular irritability, involuntary twitching of the extremities, and seizures. Hyperkalemia can result in weakness and abnormalities in gastrointestinal and cardiac function. Clinically affected patients may have relatively mild symptoms or they may rapidly go into renal failure and shock, leading to multiple organ failure and death if untreated.

DIAGNOSTIC EVALUATION

A rapid diagnosis is essential to reduce morbidity and mortality.[1,2] The history of recent chemotherapy or radiation therapy coupled with a rapid decline in health and a reduction in the size of tumor should increase the suspicion of ATLS. The initial work-up should include a rapid assessment of the patient and concurrent placement of vascular access devices while obtaining blood and urine. A diagnosis can be made by assessing results from a hemogram, biochemical profile, urinalysis, and a blood gas analysis. Because of the common concurrent cardiac arrhythmias, an ECG should be obtained. Whenever possible, a urinary catheter, central venous catheter, and blood pressure monitoring should be secured for sequential monitoring for overhydration, urinary output, and blood pressure. Sequential biochemical analyses may confirm the presence of serum hypocalcemia, hyperkalemia, and hyperphosphatemia. Hyperuricemia (seen in humans with ATLS) has not been identified in dogs and cats. In the presence of elevated serum phosphate levels, hypocalcemia develops as a result of calcium and phosphate precipitation. Without effective treatment, cardiovascular collapse, shock, or renal failure may occur in this syndrome; therefore, urinary output, blood urea nitrogen (BUN), and creatinine concentrations should be monitored closely. The hyperkalemia may result in bradycardia, diminished P-wave amplitude, and spiked T waves on an ECG.

TREATMENT

Anticipation and controlled management of tumor lysis are the keys to preventing the syndrome. Patients who are at risk should be hospitalized and fully hydrated, before, during, and after treatment. These patients should receive frequent electrolyte monitoring. Because the kidneys are the main source of electrolyte excretion, metabolic abnormalities may be exacerbated in dogs and cats with renal dysfunction. Identification of at risk dogs and cats and correction of any volume depletion or azotemia may reduce the risk of ATLS, and chemotherapy should be delayed until metabolic disturbances, such as azotemia, are corrected.

If ATLS is identified, the condition should be treated with aggressive crystalloid fluid therapy and careful monitoring of electrolytes and renal parameters. Treat for shock, provide daily fluid needs, correct dehydration, correct electrolyte abnormalities, and compensate for external fluid losses. In ATLS, 0.9% NaCl may be ideal until hyperkalemia and hyperphosphatemia are corrected. Fluids can be administered during acute shock or shocklike states at a rate of 40 to 60 mL/kg for the first hour, followed by 10 mL/kg/h with very close monitoring to adjust fluid rate as needed. Patients who have either symptomatic hypocalcemia or the ECG changes associated with hypocalcemia should be treated with an infusion of calcium gluconate. The hypocalcemia may persist beyond the period of observed hyperphosphatemia. Life-threatening hyperkalemia should be treated aggressively. Further chemotherapy should be withheld until the patient is clinically normal and all biochemical parameters are within normal limits.

PROGNOSIS

Untreated patients have a high fatality rate. Patients diagnosed and treated shortly after clinical signs begin have a good prognosis.

REFERENCES

1. Marcus SL, Einzig AI: Acute tumor lysis syndrome: prevention and management. *In* Dutcher JP, Wiernik PH, eds.: Handbook of Hematologic and Oncologic Emergencies. New York: Plenum Press, 1987, p 9.
2. Woodlock TJ: Oncologic emergencies. *In* Rosenthal S, Carignan JR, Smith BD, eds.: Medical Care of the Cancer Patient, 2nd ed. Philadelphia: WB Saunders, 1993, p 236.
3. Ogilvie GK, Moore AS: Acute tumor lysis syndrome. *In* Managing the Veterinary Cancer Patient: A Practice Manual. Trenton, NJ: Veterinary Learning Systems, 1995, p 157.
4. Rostom AY, El-Hussainy G, Kandil A, Allam A: Tumor lysis syndrome following hemi-body irradiation for metastatic breast cancer. *Ann Oncol* 11:1349, 2000.
5. Calia CM, Hohenhaus AE, Fox PR, Meleo KA: Acute tumor lysis syndrome in a cat with lymphoma. *J Vet Intern Med* 10:409, 1996.
6. Piek CJ, Teske E: Tumor lysis syndroom bij een hond. *Tijdschr Diergeneeskd* 121:64, 1996.
7. Laing EJ, Carter RF: Acute tumor lysis syndrome following treatment of canine lymphoma. *J Am Anim Hosp Assoc* 24:691, 1988.
8. Brooks DG: Acute tumor lysis syndrome in dogs. *Compend Contin Educ Pract Vet* 17: 1103, 1995.

48
Peritonitis

Andrew J. Staatz

INTRODUCTION

The peritoneal cavity has a large surface area covered with a serosal membrane. This membrane is semipermeable, allowing passive diffusion of small molecules such as electrolytes, urea, and water. Similarly, certain drugs and toxins can rapidly cross the serosal membrane to the systemic circulation. Normally there is a small amount of clear fluid in the peritoneal space. This fluid is a transudate with a cell count ranging from 200 to 2500 cells. A typical distribution of the cells in the peritoneal fluid is 50% macrophages and 50% lymphocytes.[1]

The omentum is an important component of normal peritoneal physiology. The omentum has a large surface area and is relatively mobile within the peritoneal cavity. This mobility is manifested by the adherence and clumping of the omentum to areas of inflammation virtually anywhere in the peritoneal cavity. The omentum can induce local vascularization and increase delivery of immune and phagocytic function via the secretion of an angiogenic factor.[2]

Peritonitis is defined as inflammation of the peritoneal lining; it may affect the omentum as well as visceral and parietal peritoneal surfaces. Peritonitis is a common cause of admission of dogs and cats to the CCU. Prompt diagnosis and treatment will reduce mortality. An understanding of the normal physiology of the peritoneum and omentum is essential to diagnosis and treatment.

PATHOGENESIS AND EPIDEMIOLOGY

Peritonitis has many etiologies. Etiology can be grouped into chemical, septic, and combined chemical/septic peritonitis. Chemical peritonitis is due to the presence of sterile irritating substances on the peritoneal lining including urine, bile, and pancreatic enzymes. Urine causes a diffuse, mildly inflammatory reaction, whereas bile is irritating but remains localized. Pancreatic enzymes tend to create regional inflammation. Trauma, infection, and neoplasia are known inciting causes of chemical peritonitis. The initiating event in chemical peritonitis, particularly pancreatitis, remains unknown.

Septic peritonitis is due to free bacteria in the abdominal cavity. Most cases are due to break down of the gastrointestinal wall including perforating foreign bodies, erosive neoplasia, and necrosis of the gastrointestinal wall following obstruction, gastric dilatation/volvulus, or intussusception. Inoculation of bacteria from outside the body is a less common cause of septic peritonitis. Liver, kidney, prostate, and uterine infection can occasionally serve as a source of bacteria to initiate septic peritonitis. Inflammation produced by chemical peritonitis can lead to secondary septic peritonitis. The direct connection of the biliary tree to the duodenum and the highly inflammatory nature of bile result in sterile bile peritonitis progressing to septic peritonitis. Bile peritonitis uncomplicated by the presence of bacteria has an improved survival over septic bile peritonitis.[3]

Bacteria or chemical irritants cause increased permeability of serosal capillaries resulting in leakage of protein, solutes, and water into the peritoneal cavity. Exudation of protein-rich fluid can result in hypoproteinemia and bacteria proliferation. At the same time, endotoxins are absorbed across the more permeable serosal capillaries. Bacteria 0.5 to 2 μm in size can pass directly into the lymphatics.[4] This can happen rapidly; bacteria have been detected in the blood within minutes of inoculation in the peritoneal cavity.[5] The combined effect of fluid loss to the peritoneal cavity and the vasodilatory effects of absorbed toxins can produce profound hypotension and hypovolemia.

Endotoxins absorbed from the peritoneum have systemic effects leading to hypotension, shock, systemic inflammatory reaction syndrome (SIRS) and disseminated intravascular coagulation (DIC). Endotoxins, myocardial depressant factor, acid–base and electrolyte disturbances directly affect cardiac function leading to further reduced cardiac output. Renal hypoperfusion and insufficiency exacerbates electrolyte abnormalities and azotemia. Direct renal damage from endotoxins and bacteremia can lead to acute renal failure.

CLINICAL PRESENTATION

Animals with peritonitis typically present with a nonspecific history. Owners report anorexia and lethargy that can be acute or gradual in onset. Occasionally vomiting, diarrhea, or a hunched posture will be noted. Animals may be ambulatory or recumbent, reflecting the gravity of systemic involvement. Standing patients will often exhibit a wide-based posture with an arched back and may have a lowered front posture. This has been referred to as a "praying position." Clinical signs are primarily those of shock with weak peripheral pulses and tachycardia. Dull mentation and fever may be present. The abdomen is typically tense to overtly painful and may have positive ballotment sign indicating effusion.

DIAGNOSIS AND TREATMENT

Diagnosis

Diagnosis and treatment proceed simultaneously because these animals are often moribund on presentation. Diagnosis can be divided into identifying the abdominal pathology present and assessing the patient's systemic condition. Initially, a complete blood count (CBC) and complete serum chemistry panel including lipase and amylase are required. This gives the clinician baseline information regarding the presence and degree of dehydration, anemia, thrombocytemia, electrolyte disturbances, azotemia, and specific organ involvement. If available, a coagulation profile including one-stage prothrombin time

Table 48-1. Normal Peritoneal Fluid

1. Clear fluid with a total protein <3 g/dL
2. Volume <1 mL/kg
3. Cytology
4. Cell number ≤2500 cells/mm^3
5. 50% monocytes and 40% lymphocytes

(OSPT), activated partial thromboplastin time (aPTT), and fibrin/fibrinogen degradation products (FDP) is helpful in guiding the selection of blood products. The presence of abdominal discomfort or peritoneal effusion are indications for abdominocentesis. Cytology and peritoneal fluid chemistries including albumin, creatinine, bilirubin, and amylase are performed to classify the effusion (Table 48-1). Fluid should be submitted for culture and susceptibility. Abdominocentesis, although a rapid technique, sometimes does not yield an adequate sample. The clinician can use diagnostic peritoneal lavage to enhance sampling (Table 48-2).

The presence of degenerative neutrophils and bacteria in peritoneal fluid indicate septic peritonitis. Total white cell count does not correlate with severity. Creatinine levels in the peritoneal fluid greater than serum creatinine levels are suggestive of a uroabdomen. Any bilirubin or amylase is abnormal in the peritoneal fluid. In cases of septic peritonitis the clinician will have to weigh the value of additional information against the value of rapid surgical intervention. Chemical peritonitis patients benefit from fluid and electrolyte management in the critical care unit with surgery performed later, if necessary. Further diagnostics can be performed pending the patient's response to initial treatment.

Abdominal radiographs may help define the abdominal pathology. The presence of gas free in the abdominal cavity is strong evidence of septic peritonitis. Foreign objects, gastrointestinal displacement (intussusceptions, mesenteric torsion, gastric dilatation volvulus) and gastrointestinal obstructions can be discerned from radiographs. More commonly, abdominal fluid in peritonitis leads to loss of detail. This can be regionally noted as in pancreatitis. Thoracic

Table 48-2. Diagnostic Peritoneal Lavage Technique

1. Lidocaine is infused in the skin and linea alba around the umbilicus.
2. A small stab incision is made with a no. 11 blade.
3. A sterile 8 or 10 Fr red rubber feeding tube is inserted 6–10 cm into the abdominal cavity. Cutting extra side holes into the feeding tube will help with the recovery of fluid.
4. Isotonic sterile saline is flushed into the abdomen (5 mL/kg).
5. The patient is gently turned and the abdomen is agitated.
6. The fluid is aspirated. Typical fluid recovery is 80% of the volume instilled.
7. Fluid analysis is the same performed for standard abdominal centesis.

radiographs can be also taken at this time to investigate possible heart disease and look for evidence of metastasis. The simultaneous presence of abdominal and thoracic effusion (dual infusion) may suggest pancreatitis.

Abdominal ultrasound is an excellent tool to refine location and dissemination of abdominal pathology as in the case of bile peritonitis or suspected gastrointestinal neoplasia. Caution must be exercised in establishing prognosis based on ultrasound findings.

A cystourethrogram and/or an excretory urogram should be performed on animals with suspected or documented uroabdomen. These contrast procedures can often be performed after initial stabilization in the CCU.

Treatment

The treatment of peritonitis involves removal of the inflammation source followed by drainage and supportive care. Due to the rapid systemic effects of peritoneal inflammation, virtually all patients with peritonitis will have derangements in hydration, electrolyte, acid–base, or clotting status. Consequently, immediate fluid and electrolyte support is required. Large fluid volumes need to be rapidly administered because these patients are at risk for developing hypovolumic, distributive, and septic shock. Repeated assessment of the packed cell volume (PCV), total solids, platelets and activated clotting times (ACT), OSPT, aPTT, and FDP will guide blood, plasma, or other colloid administration. Colloids have a more sustained effect than crystalloids in maintaining vascular volume. In a study of 42 dogs and cats with septic peritonitis, survival was improved in animals given plasma or blood over those that did not receive blood or plasma.[6]

Cytologic evidence of septic peritonitis is an indication for broad-spectrum intravenous antibiotics. Frequently, multiple bacterial isolates are identified on culture including gram-negative rods, gram-positive cocci, and anaerobes. The clinician must initiate antibiotic therapy before culture and susceptibility results are available. Individual antibiotics (cefoxitin) or combination antibiotics (enrofloxacin and ampicillin) can be used.

Peritonitis is almost always painful and can be misinterpreted by the clinician as "dullness." Opioids including fentanyl, morphine, oxymorphone, butorphanol and bupranorphine offer therapeutic analgesia. However, the clinician must be attentive to mentation changes secondary to these analgesics. Specific drug preference is clinician based and probably reflects the emergency environment. Intravenous fentanyl is the author's preference for pain management in peritonitis cases because dosage can be changed quickly. However, it requires an infusion pump and 24-hour monitoring (see Chapter 7).

Surgery is usually indicated to eliminate the contamination source. The urgency of surgical intervention is high for cases of septic peritonitis because the benefit of eliminating further contamination and removing mediators of inflammation from the peritoneal cavity is higher than the risks of anesthesia. Surgical technique will not be reviewed here. The surgeon must perform a thorough abdominal exploration and be prepared to operate on any organ in the abdomen. Meticulous attention to detail must be balanced with expediency because prolonged anesthesia is poorly tolerated. Following identification and surgical correction of the septic source, large volumes of warm sterile isotonic fluid are used to lavage the peritoneal cavity. In those patients where peritoneal contamination and inflammation are not adequately resolved, the surgeon can elect to leave the abdomen open. This technique is a delayed closure; the abdomen is loosely closed with suture to leave a 2-cm gap the length of the incision in the linea alba. Sterile laparotomy pads and towels are layered over the gaping incision and secured with bandage materials around the patient's abdomen. Under sedation or general anesthesia these patients can be repeatedly lavaged, on a daily basis, until contamination and inflammation are adequately resolved to permit complete closure of the abdomen.

Open abdomen patients present special challenges to the critical care clinician. These patients are vulnerable to ascending nosocomial infection and rapid onset of hypoproteinemia due to protein loss in draining peritoneal fluid.[7,8] Managing an abdomen in an open manner is even more time and labor intensive than a managing a primary closure peritonitis and the expense correspondingly greater. In a series of 42 septic peritonitis cases, survival has been shown to be similar for patients managed with primary closure and patients managed with open peritoneal lavage.[6] However, assignment of an animal to the open abdominal management group was based on the appreciation of especially severe abdominal contamination by the attending clinician.

Surgical treatment of chemical peritonitis follows the same strategy used for septic peritonitis. Bile peritonitis and uroabdomen require closure of the source of contamination and generous lavage. The value of surgery for pancreatitis is still unresolved. Potential benefits include the ability to perform lavage to remove pancreatic enzymes from the peritoneal cavity and allow placement of a jejunostomy permits alimentation aboral from the pancreas.

The hemodynamically fragile status of peritonitis patients requires continuous electrocardiogram (ECG) and blood pressure monitoring. Ideally monitoring includes central venous pressure. A urinary catheter is needed to monitor urine output. Evaluation of PCV, total solids, glucose, electrolytes, platelets, white blood cell counts, and temperature are made frequently (q 4–12 h initially). These parameters combined with the continuous blood pressure and ECG monitoring give the clinician the necessary information to assess fluid balance, adequacy of sepsis control, and the presence of arrhythmias. Decreased platelet number, bleeding from venipuncture sites, or presence of petecchiae suggests the possibility of DIC. Early detection of changes in hemostasis is essential to prevent DIC associated mortality. This can be done with repeated assessment of ACT, platelet numbers, OSPT, APTT, FDP, or antithrombin III. Serial evaluation of urea nitrogen, creatinine, amylase, lipase, total bilirubin, and albumin may be performed depending on the specific type of peritoneal pathology. In septic peritonitis, serial abdominal fluid cytology is a valuable tool to follow the progression of disease. Declining counts of bacteria and degenerative neutrophils are expected. Although no bacteria are expected in chemical peritonitis, serial analysis of abdominal fluid is useful in assessing resolution of abdominal pathology.

Nutritional support should be anticipated because many peritonitis patients will not eat. Although oral alimentation is ideal, vomiting or anorexia may force the clinician to seek alternate avenues. The placement of a feeding tube prior to surgical closure is ideal.[9] Esophagostomy, gastrostomy, or jejunostomy tubes can be placed. Gastrostomy or esophagostomy tubes allow feeding of a complete diet. Elemental diets must be used with jejunostomy tubes. Jejunostomy tubes can be used in vomiting patients and alimentation can be started immediately on placement. Feeding directly into the gastrointestinal tract promotes the health of the intestinal mucosa and reduces translocation of bacteria from the gastrointestinal tract.[10] Total parenteral nutrition (TPN) refers to feeding through an intravenous catheter. This method does not require surgery but also does not play a role in maintaining the health of the intestinal mucosa. Sepsis may be a complication of TPN.[10]

Other drugs that can be used to symptomatically manage peritonitis patients include antiemetics, gastric acid release blockers, motility modifiers, and cytoprotective drugs. The use of flunixine meglumine and glucocorticoids is controversial. Although both drugs are anti-inflammatory, they have significant side effects. Flunixine meglumine reduces normal gastric cytoprotection and decreases renal and gastrointestinal blood flow. Glucocorticoids reduce immune response and lend to gastrointestinal ulceration. Peritonitis patients are challenged by sepsis and shock and consequently are more vulnerable to the negative side effects of flunixine meglumine and glucocorticoids.

PROGNOSIS

Survival depends on multiple factors including the etiology of peritonitis, promptness of presentation and recognition, and skill of treatment. A guarded to grave prognosis must be given to these patients. Chemical peritonitis generally carries a better prognosis to septic peritonitis. In our institution overall survival of septic peritonitis cases treated with both open and closed peritonitis was 23%.[6] Owners must be made aware that even with intensive care and considerable expense that mortality still remains significant.

REFERENCES

1. Crowe DT, Bjorling DE: Textbook of Small Animal Surgery. Philadelphia: WB Saunders, 1993, p 407.
2. Hosgood G: The omentum—the forgotten organ: physiology and potential surgical applications in dogs and cats. *Compend Contin Educ Pract Vet* 12:45, 1990.
3. Ludwig LL, McLoughlin MA, Graves TK, *et al.*: Surgical treatment of bile peritonitis in 24 dogs and 2 cats: a retrospective study (1987–1994). *Vet Surg* 26:90, 1997.
4. Allen L, Weatherford T: Role of fenestrated basement membrane in lymphatic absorption from the peritoneal cavity. *Am J Physiol* 1997:551, 1959.
5. Steinberg B: Infection of the Peritoneum. New York: Hoever, 1944.
6. Staatz AJ, Monnet E: Open peritoneal drainage versus primary closure for the treatment of septic peritonitis in dogs and cats: 42 cases (1992–1999). Poster presentation ACVS 35th Annual Scientific Conference, Arlington, VA, September, 2000.
7. Greenfield CL, Walshaw R: Open peritoneal drainage for the treatment of contam-

inated peritoneal cavity and septic peritonitis in dogs and cats: 24 cases (1980–1986). *J Am Vet Med Assoc* 191:100, 1987.

8. Woolfson JM, Dulish ML: Open abdominal drainage in the treatment of generalized peritonitis in 25 dogs and cats. *Vet Surg* 15:27, 1986.
9. Thatcher CD: Nutritional needs of critically ill patients. *Compend Contin Educ Pract Vet* 18:1303, 1996.
10. Deitch EA: Role of the gut in the pathogenesis of sepsis and multiple organ failure. *Proceedings IVECCS*, San Antonio, TX, 1996.

49
Disorders of Hemostasis

Michael S. Henson and Stephanie A. Smith

INTRODUCTION

The hemostatic system involves a complex interplay between the blood vessel wall, platelets, and multiple procoagulant and anticoagulant factors in the peripheral blood. This complex defense mechanism prevents excessive hemorrhage and helps localize repair to the site of injury without prolonged obstruction of blood flow (thrombosis). For the most common disorders of hemostasis in dogs and cats, a presumptive diagnosis sufficient for initial management can be made from the signalment, history, and clinical signs along with a blood smear and a rapid cage-side assessment of the coagulation cascade. Treatment usually consists of supportive care, treatment of any underlying disease, and replacement of the deficient hemostatic factors.

REVIEW OF NORMAL HEMOSTASIS

Normal hemostasis consists of four major components: vascular integrity, primary hemostasis (platelet-vessel wall interaction resulting in a platelet plug), secondary hemostasis (coagulation cascade resulting in a fibrin clot), and fibrinolysis (clot lysis). Vascular integrity can be disrupted by trauma, neoplasia, inflammation, or necrosis. Disruption in arteries and large veins may require ligation to control hemorrhage, but the normal hemostatic mechanism is sufficient to control bleeding in most other vessels. Shortly after vessel damage, local vasoconstriction occurs. This minimizes blood loss and decreases the rate of blood flow resulting in less shear forces on the forming platelet plug.

Platelets adhere to the damaged endothelium and subendothelial collagen via circulating von Willebrand factor (vWF). Platelet adhesion stimulates a conformational change in the platelet (spreading) and release of granule contents that promote further platelet aggregation and activation of the coagulation cascade. The result is a platelet plug that stops hemorrhage (primary hemostasis) and localizes the coagulation cascade to the site of injury (Fig. 49-1). The platelet plug is unstable and can dissociate within minutes unless a fibrin clot is formed (so-called rebleeding).

Secondary hemostasis consists of a chain reaction in coagulation proteins, enzymes, and cofactors that circulate in an inactive form. When activated, these enzymes activate other enzymes in the cascade. This amplification system allows

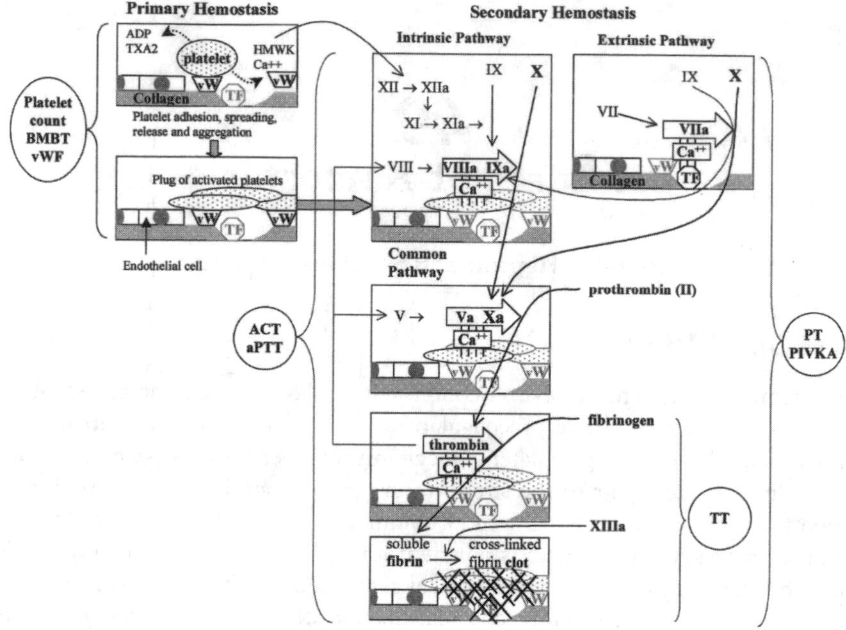

Figure 49-1
Pathways of normal hemostasis. Abbreviations: ADP = adenosine diphosphate; TXA_2 = thromboxane A_2; HMWK = high-molecular-weight kininogen; Ca^{++} = calcium; vW = von Willebrand factor; TF = tissue factor; BMBT = buccal mucosal bleed time; ACT = activated clot time; APTT = activated partial thromboplastin time; TT = thrombin time; PT, prothrombin time; PIVKA = proteins induced by vitamin K absence.

relatively few initiator molecules to induce sequential activation proteins ending in fibrin production at the site of injury. Factors II, VII, IX, and X require vitamin K to become functional. Vitamin K_1 is a cofactor required for post-translational modifications that allows these coagulation proteins to bind via calcium ion bridges to tissue factor or activated platelet membranes. This binding is a rate-limiting step in the formation of enzymatically active complexes in the cascade. The coagulation cascade is usually initiated by exposure of tissue factor when the vessel wall is damaged (extrinsic cascade), but can also be initiated through activation of factors within the circulating blood (intrinsic cascade). The two pathways are distinct regarding testing in vitro, but are closely interrelated in vivo. Both pathways result in activation of factor X, the beginning of the common pathway. Factor X converts prothrombin to thrombin. Thrombin cleaves fibrinogen to form soluble fibrin monomers. These polymerize and are covalently cross-linked by factor XIII to form a stable fibrin clot.[1,2]

Clot formation is localized to the site of injury by activated platelet membranes and tissue factor. Clot formation downstream from the injury is inhibited in normal individuals by quiescent endothelium, dilution of activated clotting factors in flowing blood, and circulating anticoagulant factors. Antithrombin III (AT III) and heparin cofactor II inactivate thrombin, especially when catalyzed by heparin. Protein C and protein S, in conjunction with thrombomodulin, inactivate factors V and VIII, preventing further participation in the cascade.[3]

The process of clot dissolution (fibrinolysis) is initiated at the same time that the clot is forming. Fibrinolysis is mediated by plasmin, which circulates as the inactive proenzyme plasminogen. Plasminogen binds to both fibrinogen and fibrin and is trapped in the fibrin meshwork as the clot is formed. Tissue plasminogen activator (tPA), released from damaged endothelial cells, converts plasminogen to plasmin inside the clot. Plasmin then digests fibrin into fragments called fibrin degradation products (FDPs). FDPs are released into the circulation and then cleared by the liver. The plasmin released from the clot is rapidly inhibited by circulating α_2-antiplasmin, so that fibrinolysis is limited to the healing site of injury (Fig. 49-2).[3] The relatively slow pace of lysis allows healing of the wound to occur before blood flow is re-established.

Excessive fibrinolysis (*e.g.*, in disseminated intravascular coagulation [DIC]) may cause a bleeding tendency. Clots are destroyed before the area has

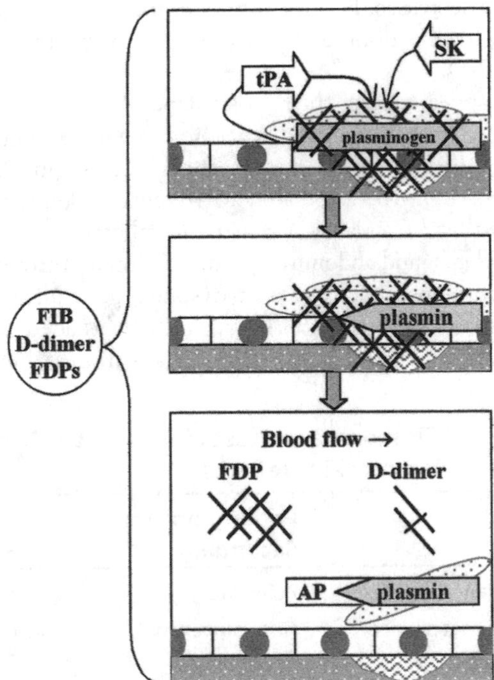

Figure 49-2
Fibrinolysis. Abbreviations: tPA = tissue plasminogen activator; SK = streptokinase; FIB = fibrinogen; FDPs = fibrin(ogen) degradation products; AP = α_2 anti-plasmin.

healed causing rebleeding. In addition, FDPs decrease platelet function and inhibit thrombin, resulting in anticoagulant activity. Defective fibrinolysis can also lead to inappropriate formation of thrombi.[1]

CLINICAL PRESENTATION

Abnormalities in primary hemostasis are usually characterized by superficial bleeding: petechiae, ecchymoses, and mucosal hemorrhage. Common manifestations include cutaneous and gingival petechiae, epistaxis, hyphema, scleral and vitreal hemorrhage, hematemesis and melena, and hematuria. If platelet function is normal, bleeding from thrombocytopenia never occurs with counts greater than 50,000 cells/μL and is rare with counts above 20,000 cells/μL.[2] Even with profound thrombocytopenia, cats are less likely than dogs to bleed spontaneously.[4] The sites of hemorrhage are not helpful in distinguishing platelet disorders from vascular disease.

Secondary hemostatic defects are associated with deep bleeding.[5] Coagulation factor deficiencies are usually manifested by bruising, hematomas, hemarthroses, muscular hemorrhage, or body cavity hemorrhage.[2] Anticoagulant rodenticide toxicity sometimes also presents as pulmonary, mediastinal, or retrobulbar hemorrhage.[6] Clinical bleeding generally does not occur unless factor levels are markedly decreased. Because of the multiple hemostatic defects present in DIC, patients with this disorder may experience hemorrhage of any type and location (Table 49-1).

The clinical appearance of thrombosis depends on the site. Appendicular venous thrombosis may be associated with limb edema and erythema distal to the thrombus, pain, and a palpable cord in the affected vein. Portal and mesenteric vein thrombosis may be associated with acute abdominal pain, anorexia, vomiting, and diarrhea.[7] Caudal vena cava thrombosis may be associated with ascites, rear limb edema, and abdominal pain. Pulmonary thromboembolism usually presents as acute-onset tachypnea or dyspnea, generally with hypoxemia.[8] Appendicular arterial thromboembolism will present as acute loss of limb function, with cold, cyanotic, pulseless limbs. Arterial thromboembolism of visceral

Table 49-1. Site of Hemorrhage Associated with Primary versus Secondary Hemostasis Defects

Primary	Primary and/or Secondary	Secondary
Cutaneous petechiae/ecchymoses	Pulmonary	Mediastinal
Mucous membrane petechiae/ ecchymoses	Gastrointestinal	Pleural cavity
Ocular (hyphema, scleral, vitreal)	Central nervous system	Abdominal cavity
Epistaxis	Venipuncture	Joint
	Surgical site	Muscle

organs presents as acute loss of function of that organ. Patients with cerebral or cardiac thrombosis may present with sudden death.

SIGNALMENT AND HISTORY

Patient signalment may help prioritize differential diagnoses for the underlying cause of the hemostatic defect. Anticoagulant rodenticide toxicity is more common in young dogs. Severe inherited bleeding tendencies usually present at a young age.[2] A variety of breeds are predisposed for vWD, with Doberman Pinscher, Scottish Terrier, German Shepherd, Shetland Sheep Dog, and German Short-haired Pointer well described.[9] Although most hereditary coagulopathies are inherited as autosomal traits, hemophilia primarily affects males due to sex-linked inheritance. Immune-mediated thrombocytopenia most commonly affects middle-aged, female dogs, with Cocker Spaniels, Poodles, and Old English Sheepdogs predisposed.[10]

In addition to routine historical questions, specific information regarding the bleeding may help determine the most likely cause. Questions should relate to the affected sites, duration of bleeding, previous episodes of bleeding (especially that associated with previous trauma or surgery), possible exposure to an anticoagulant rodenticide, the potential for unobserved trauma, and recent drug or vaccine exposure. A history of potential tick exposure may increase clinical suspicion for infectious disease such as Rocky Mountain spotted fever or ehrlichiosis.

Clients with pets presenting with evidence of arterial, venous, or pulmonary thromboembolism should be questioned regarding previous diagnosis of, or history suggestive of, an underlying prothrombotic disorder. Polyuria/polydipsia may suggest underlying glomerulonephropathy or hyperadrenocorticism. Coughing, dyspnea, or syncope may suggest underlying cardiac disease.

PHYSICAL EXAMINATION

A detailed examination of all body systems should be performed to identify all sites of hemorrhage. Common sites of hemorrhage due to bleeding disorders include eyes, skin, mucous membranes, joints, urinary tract, lungs, and pleural and peritoneal cavity. The distribution of the hemorrhage may help distinguish local hemorrhage (*e.g.*, from trauma or necrosis) from a systemic hemostatic defect (see Clinical Presentation).

DIAGNOSTIC EVALUATION

Cage Side Hemostasis Evaluation

For a bleeding patient, several rapid cage-side tests usually can provide sufficient information for initial management and allow for rapid elimination of some possible causes of hemorrhage from the list of differential diagnoses. All bleeding patients should have packed cell volume (PCV), total protein (TP), fresh blood smear (see platelet estimate below) and activated clotting time

Table 49-2. In-house Rapid Screening Tests to Differentiate the Most Common Bleeding Disorders

	Type of Bleeding	Platelet Estimate	RBC Morphology	ACT	BMBT
IMT	Superficial	⇓⇓⇓	N or spherocytes with IMHA	N to ⇑	*⇑⇑⇑
Rodenticide	Deep	N to ⇓⇓	N	⇑⇑⇑	*N
DIC	Variable	⇓ to ⇓⇓⇓	RBC fragments	⇑ to ⇑⇑⇑	N to ⇑⇑⇑
vWF deficiency	Superficial Deep if severe	N	N	N	⇑ to ⇑⇑⇑
Vasculitis	Superficial	⇓ to ⇓⇓	N	N	⇑ to ⇑⇑⇑
NSAID toxicity	Superficial	N to ⇓	N	N	⇑ to ⇑⇑
Liver failure	Deep	N	N	⇑ to ⇑⇑⇑	N

* BMBT not clinically indicated in these circumstances as it fails to provide any additional information regarding the cause of hemorrhage.
IMT, immune-mediated thrombocytopenia; DIC, disseminated intravascular coagulation; VWF, von Willebrand factor; NSAID, nonsteroidal anti-inflammatory drug; N, normal; IMHA, immune-mediated hemolytic anemia; RBC, red blood cell; ACT, activated clot time; BMBT, buccal mucosal bleed time.

(ACT) (Table 49-2). Buccal mucosal bleeding time (BMBT) may be measured for breeds at high risk for vWD.

Disorders of hemostasis are frequently secondary to other primary diseases (*e.g.*, neoplasia, infection, liver failure) and may themselves cause organ dysfunction. Therefore, in addition to assessing various aspects of hemostasis, appropriate diagnostic testing may include a complete blood count (CBC), biochemistry profile, urinalysis, serology, imaging, or biopsies. Ideally, most samples should be collected before treatment (see below for proper handling of samples).

Suspected primary hemostatic deficits need to be evaluated for adequate platelet numbers, proper platelet and vascular function, and in some cases, vWF levels. Platelet numbers can be rapidly estimated from a fresh blood smear, counted by a hemocytometer or hematology analyzer, or measured as part of a reference laboratory analysis. If hemorrhage suggests a primary hemostatic defect but platelet numbers are adequate, perform a BMBT and vWF antigen level.

Secondary hemostatic defects can be rapidly screened with the use of an immediate ACT or cage-side coagulation monitor that can perform prothrombin time (PT) and activated partial thromboplastin time (aPTT). Reference laboratories are then used to further characterize the hemostatic defect. DIC should be suspected when hemorrhage is associated with neoplasia, inflammation, or trauma. Because this is a defect of multiple hemostatic mechanisms as well as activated fibrinolysis, all portions of the hemostatic process should be evaluated.

Platelet Morphology, Estimates, and Counts

Because of activation during sample collection, platelets frequently clump causing inaccurate counts and estimates. Examination of a fresh blood smear is necessary to identify clumping, usually most notable at the feathered edge, as well as platelet morphology. Numerous large platelets suggest active thrombopoiesis. If clumping is noted, redraw the sample. If not, the sample can be analyzed to determine the platelet count or the blood smear can be used to estimate platelet number. To estimate the platelet count, examine the slide in the monolayer area where erythrocytes infrequently touch each other (erythrocytes will be farther apart in anemic animals). Count the number of platelets in 10 oil immersion fields (100×) and determine the average. A normal smear should include more than 10 platelets per oil immersion field. Each platelet in the field represents approximately 15,000 platelets/μL, but the numerical estimate is a rough approximation. It is better to categorize the estimate as very low, low, normal, and so forth. A manual count of platelets can be performed in-house using a hemocytometer and the Unopette system. Automated in-house hematology analyzers that measure the thickness of the platelet layer of the buffy coat (QBC) will not provide an accurate count when platelet size is abnormal (*e.g.*, thrombocytopenia with large regenerative platelets). When using an impedance type automated cell counter (*e.g.*, Coulter type), large canine platelets and normal feline platelets will appear falsely decreased.[2]

Buccal Mucosal Bleed Time

The BMBT is a cage-side test to evaluate platelet function. It is indicated in animals whose platelet numbers are normal but have a clinical presentation suggestive of a primary hemostatic defect. A lancet instrument is used to make a standardized shallow cut in the buccal mucosa. Filter paper is then used to blot away each drop of blood, without contact with the cut so that the platelet plug is not disturbed. Bleeding will stop within 1.7 to 4.2 minutes in normal dogs, and 1.4 to 2.4 minutes in normal cats.[2] This test is difficult to perform in the nonsedated cat, but can be accomplished in most dogs without sedation.

Activated Clot Time

The ACT is performed using a special gray-topped tube containing diatomaceous earth, a contact activator. Tubes need to be warmed to body temperature before use. This can be done in a specialized heated block or water bath at 37°C (98.6°F). Whole blood (2 mL) is drawn via atraumatic venipuncture and added to the tube. The time is noted and the tube is rapidly inverted 5 times. The tube is then kept warm for 60 seconds, after which the tube is inverted every 5 seconds. When a hard clot forms, the time is noted. Automated analyzers are also available to measure ACT. Normal ACT is 60 to 110 seconds for dogs and 50 to 75 seconds for cats. The ACT is primarily dependent on the intrinsic and common portions of the coagulation cascade. Because platelets provide the phospholipid required for clot formation, profound thrombocytopenia can prolong the ACT despite normal factor levels. Mild to moderate thrombocytopenia does not affect the ACT.[2] The ACT is a rough indicator of secondary hemostasis. If an ACT is within normal range, marked deficiencies in secondary hemostasis can be ruled out.

Reference Laboratory Hemostasis Evaluation

Additional coagulation tests are evaluated using citrated plasma and require special handling for reliable results. Whole blood should be collected by atraumatic venipuncture and immediately mixed with the citrate to minimize sample contamination with tissue thromboplastins and consumption of coagulation factors. A new needle is used for sample transfer, or the needle is removed and the tube filled after removing the stopper. Blue-topped tubes contain an appropriate amount of citrate to achieve a ratio of 1 part sodium citrate to 9 parts blood. Proper filling is required for accurate results. If the tests cannot be performed in-house, the whole blood should be centrifuged and the plasma separated and frozen within 1 hour of collection. The plasma needs to be shipped to the laboratory with cold packs or dry ice so that it will arrive frozen. Citrate is currently available in two concentrations (3.2% and 3.8%). Check with the reference laboratory as to which type was used to establish normal ranges. If the laboratory used does not have an established species-specific reference range, citrated control plasma from a normal individual should also be submitted.

Prothrombin Time

The PT is the test used primarily to evaluate the extrinsic pathway, but it also indicates deficiencies in the common pathway. Prolongation of PT is indicative of deficiencies primarily of factors VII and X. It may also be prolonged with lack of hepatic synthesis of factors, vitamin K deficiency due to vitamin K antagonists, and with consumptive coagulopathies.

Proteins Induced by Vitamin K Absence

Thrombotest is a specialized form of PT that is sensitive to the presence of unactivated vitamin K-dependent factors II, VII, IX, and X ("proteins induced by vitamin K absence" or PIVKA). It will be abnormal prior to the PT and be more markedly prolonged than the PT in patients with anticoagulant rodenticide exposure. The PIVKA test may also be prolonged with hepatic synthesis failure or dietary vitamin K deficiency.[11]

Activated Partial Thromboplastin Time

The aPTT evaluates the intrinsic and common portions of the coagulation cascade. It is more sensitive than ACT in identifying factor deficiencies and will not be affected by thrombocytopenia. The aPTT will be prolonged with use of heparin, so it is the primary test used to evaluate degree of anticoagulation when a patient is receiving this drug. The aPTT can be prolonged in animals with hemophilia A (factor VIII deficiency), hemophilia B (factor IX deficiency), vitamin K deficiency, and DIC. Inherited factor XII deficiency will also prolong the aPTT, but this is not associated with a bleeding tendency.

Thrombin Time

The thrombin time (TT) measures the time required for excess exogenous thrombin to catalyze the conversion of fibrinogen to fibrin. TT will be prolonged with decreased or abnormal fibrinogen and in the presence of thrombin inhibitors like heparin and FDPs. The most common cause for prolonged TT is a consumptive coagulopathy.

Fibrinogen

Fibrinogen levels (FIB) can be semiquantitatively measured with heat precipitation, although the test is subjective and not highly reliable. Decreased fibrinogen concentration may be indicative of consumptive coagulopathy. Increased concentrations may be associated with nephrotic syndrome and marked inflammation.

Antithrombin III

Antithrombin III is measured through a chromogenic assay available through reference laboratories. Because AT III is a small protein, excessive losses occur with protein losing enteropathy and glomerulonephropathy. AT III is excessively consumed in DIC, so decreased concentration may be a marker for this complication.

Fibrin Degradation Products

Fibrin(ogen) degradation products, derived from the breakdown of both cross-linked fibrin and fibrinogen, can be estimated using a latex particle agglutination test kit. Elevated FDPs indicate increased fibrinolysis or fibrinogenolysis. Increased fibrinolysis is present in DIC, thrombosis, and anticoagulant rodenticide toxicity. FDPs may also be elevated with hepatic failure due to decreased hepatic clearance of these proteins.[2]

D-dimer

D-dimer is the neoantigen formed as a result of plasmin digestion of cross-linked fibrin. The D-dimer test specifically measures fibrinolysis as opposed to fibrinogenolysis. Therefore, it is a better indicator of excessive clot formation and dissolution. A variety of kit methods have recently become commercially available for measuring D-dimer in dogs, but have not been validated for use in cats. D-dimers have been documented as a useful indicator of active thrombosis in humans and are currently being investigated for clinical usefulness in supporting this diagnosis in veterinary patients. Elevated D-dimers may support a diagnosis of DIC.[12]

von Willebrand Factor

Both the quantity and the quality of vWF antigen can be measured through a reference laboratory. This test is the only reliable means of diagnosis of vWD and will allow identification of both the type of and severity of vWF deficiency.

THERAPY FOR DISORDERS OF HEMOSTASIS

In general, therapy for bleeding disorders involves correcting deficiencies (replacement of fluid volume, blood cells, coagulation factors, vitamin K), improving the function of existing hemostatic components, treating any underlying disease, and minimizing the consequences of the coagulopathy for the patient during therapy.

Emergency Management

Patients presenting with bleeding and signs of hypovolemia should be given colloids and/or crystalloids while diagnostic testing is started and other necessary therapies are determined and prepared (*e.g.*, blood products). Emergency transfusion is rarely needed. However, rapid transfusion with fresh whole blood (FWB) or packed red blood cells (PRBCs) mixed with fresh-frozen plasma (FFP) may be appropriate and lifesaving in certain situations.

Correct Deficiencies

Correct fluid, electrolyte, and acid–base abnormalities to improve organ function. Vitamin K may be necessary in animals with chronic hepatic disease or anticoagulant rodenticide toxicity (see below) to allow production of functional factors II, VII, IX, and X. In emergency situations, transfusion of FFP can supply functional coagulation factors to control hemorrhage. Transfusion of cellular blood components (PRBCs or FWB) are indicated: (1) for anemias severe enough to cause tachypnea, tachycardia, and weakness at rest regardless of PCV (assuming thoracic causes for these signs have been ruled out), (2) anemia with large expected losses (*e.g.*, before splenectomy), or (3) PCV less than 25% in the dog or less than 20% in the cat.[13] Transfusion of platelet-containing products (FWB or platelet-rich plasma) may be appropriate when thrombocytopenic animals need emergency surgery or if there is life-threatening hemorrhage (*e.g.*, hemorrhage in the brain or lungs). However, the benefit for animals with immune-mediated thrombocytopenia (IMT) and DIC is expected to be very small and transient due to the rapid rate of destruction of platelets in these patients. Platelet transfusions may be most helpful in bleeding thrombocytopenic patients with bone marrow production defects.

Improve the Function of Existing Hemostatic Components

Hypothermia impairs the function of both platelets and the coagulation cascade. Ideally, use warmed fluids to improve patient comfort and to prevent exacerbation of the coagulopathy even if normothermic. Fluid therapy may also reduce uremic toxins and dilute platelet inhibitors (*e.g.*, FDPs). Avoid medications that impair platelet function (Table 49-3). Because hetastarch, dextrans, and hemoglobin-based oxygen-carrying solutions (Oxyglobin) can prolong in vitro clotting times, monitor animals with coagulopathies carefully when using these products.

Minimize the Clinical Consequences of the Coagulopathy

Continued bleeding can exacerbate anemia, cause organ dysfunction, and result in further consumption of limited coagulation factors. Minimize trauma with cage rest, gentle restraint (avoid neck leads), and soft foods. If possible, give drugs orally or intravenously through an indwelling catheter. Avoid intramuscular injections, use small-gauge needles, and keep gentle pressure on injection sites for several minutes. Bandage or suture wounds, even small ones, if bleeding.

Primary Hemostatic Defects

Thrombocytopenia

Thrombocytopenia may result from decreased platelet production, increased destruction, increased utilization, and sequestration. A complete blood count and blood smear can give many clues to the etiology. Platelet sequestration due to hepatomegaly or splenomegaly rarely decreases platelet count below 100,000/µL.[14] Through loss and increased utilization, severe hemorrhage can cause thrombocytopenia, particularly when the bleeding occurs into the gastrointestinal tract or body cavities. However, it is rare for this to decrease the platelet count below 50,000/µL. Severe thrombocytopenia (<20,000 platelets/µL) is most often associated with IMT, DIC, or bone marrow production defects. Large platelets suggest platelet regeneration, whereas microthrombocytes (decreased mean platelet volume) may be seen with IMT, particularly in the early stages before bone marrow response. Later stage IMT may have both small and large platelets with an increase in platelet distribution width (a parameter provided by some laboratories). Concurrent neutropenia is usually associated with production problems (*e.g.*, aplastic anemia, myelophthisis, chronic ehrlichiosis), whereas inflammatory leukograms are more commonly seen with sepsis, IMT, and Rocky Mountain spotted fever. In rare cases, *Ehrlichia morulae* may be noted on the blood count. Red blood cell fragments (keratocytes, schizocytes) are commonly seen with DIC. If the animal is receiving medication and lacking signs of other causes of

Table 49-3. Selected Drugs that Adversely Affect Platelet Function

Nonsteroidal Anti-inflammatories	Antibiotics	Sedatives/ Anesthetics	Calcium Agonists	Cardioactive Drugs	Other Drugs
Aspirin	Ampicillin	Halothane	Diltiazem	Lidocaine	Antihistamines
Ibuprofen	Penicillin G	Phenothiazines	Nifedipine	Nitroprusside	Chondroitin sulfate
Indomethacin	Carbenicillin	Nitrous oxide	Verapamil	Nitroglycerin	Estrogens
Phenylbutazone	Gentamicin			Propranolol	Heparin
	Sulfonamides				

thrombocytopenia, it should be presumed that the thrombocytopenia is due to the drug until proven otherwise. The diagnosis is confirmed by return of the platelet count to normal within 5 days of discontinuing the drug.

Assessment of the coagulation cascade is indicated for animals with thrombocytopenia, particularly if there is evidence of secondary hemorrhage or clinical signs other than superficial bleeding. Depending on the clinical signs and initial laboratory findings, additional testing may be indicated for animals with thrombocytopenia including bone marrow examination or serology (*Ehrlichia* spp., Rocky Mountain spotted fever, *Babesia*, feline leukemia virus, feline immunodeficiency virus). Platelets can be evaluated for evidence of immune attack with a test for the presence of platelet surface associated immunoglobulin, although a positive test will not differentiate primary from secondary immune disorders.[15] Animals with DIC, sepsis, or tick-borne disease almost always show significant clinical abnormalities in addition to bleeding, whereas IMT and drug-related thrombocytopenia may show only superficial bleeding.

Bone marrow examination is indicated in thrombocytopenic animals with neutropenia or nonregenerative anemia or when the cause of the thrombocytopenia is uncertain. Excessive bleeding from bone marrow biopsies is extremely rare even in severe thrombocytopenia. Bone marrow examination may provide a definitive diagnosis in some cases (*e.g.*, myelophthisis) and it is helpful in most others. For instance, megakaryocytic hypoplasia or aplastic anemia can be associated with drug toxicity. Hypoplastic marrow with increased plasma cells is frequently seen with chronic *Ehrlichia canis* infection. Megakaryocytic hyperplasia suggests peripheral destruction or increased use. Direct immunofluorescence on bone marrow slides can identify antimegakaryocyte antibodies, which supports a diagnosis of IMT. Because IMT is a diagnosis of exclusion, serologic tests for tick-borne diseases are appropriate for dogs with thrombocytopenia in endemic areas. The definitive diagnosis of IMT is often based on eliminating other potential causes and a response to therapy. The lowest platelet counts (*i.e.*, $<10{,}000/\mu L$) are seen with IMT.[10]

While titers are pending, therapy can be instituted for both IMT and rickettsial diseases (doxycycline 5–10 mg/kg bid) without significant harm to the patient. The primary therapy for IMT is prednisone starting at 1 to 2 mg/kg PO q 12 h. Any nonessential drugs should be discontinued. Transfuse as needed to manage anemia. Transfusion of platelet-containing products (FWB or platelet-rich plasma) may be appropriate if the patient needs emergency surgery or if there is life-threatening hemorrhage (*e.g.*, in the brain or lungs). However, the benefit is expected to be very small and transient due to the rapid rate of destruction of platelets in this disease and the very low platelet yield in these products.[16]

The initial dose of prednisone is typically given for 2 to 3 weeks. If recheck platelet counts are greater than $75{,}000/\mu L$, the dose can be tapered by 25% every 2 weeks. When the daily dose is approximately 0.25 mg/kg, the interval can be increased to every other day. If the platelet count returns to normal within 10 days of starting prednisone therapy, and there are no relapses during tapering, it is likely that therapy can be safely discontinued after several months of every-other-day therapy. If the platelet count increases more slowly, ranges between

75,000/μL and 150,000/μL, drops during tapering, or requires additional drug therapy, it is likely that long-term (perhaps lifetime) every-other-day therapy will be necessary.[14]

Although efficacy is not well documented in dogs, other medications used to treat IMT include azathioprine (starting dose 2 mg/kg PO q 24 h), cyclophosphamide (starting dose 200 mg/m^2 PO or IV weekly), cyclosporine (starting dose 10 mg/kg PO q 12 h), vincristine (0.01-0.025 mg/kg slowly IV weekly), or danazol (5 mg/kg PO q 12 h for induction dose). These medications are most commonly used in cases refractory to corticosteroids, when recrudescence occurs as the corticosteroid dose is tapered, or when the side effects of corticosteroids are severe.[16]

Platelet Function Defects

Platelet function defects can be either inherited or acquired. Unique inherited defects have been noted in specific breeds (basset hounds, otterhounds, foxhounds, spitz),[17] but by far the most common inherited platelet function disorder is vWD, which affects many breeds. Acquired disorders include those secondary to drugs (particularly nonsteroidal anti-inflammatory drugs [NSAIDs]), renal failure, pancreatitis, liver disease, malignancies, IMT, and DIC.[10] The inhibitory effects of aspirin and other NSAIDs on platelet function are irreversible. Normal function does not return until new platelets are released. Therefore, aspirin should not be used in animals with thrombocytopenia or inherited platelet functional defects.

von Willebrand Disease

A diagnosis of vWD is based on measurement of vWF levels. As stated above, animals with vWD rarely present for bleeding, rather the bleeding tendency is noted after trauma or surgery. In addition to controlling platelet adherence, vWF is a carrier protein for factor VIII. With severe vWF deficiency, there may be a deficiency of factor VIII resulting in a moderately prolonged APTT.

Transfusion of functional vWF may be appropriate for animals with active hemorrhage or those requiring surgery. Blood components containing functional vWF include FWB, FFP, and cryoprecipitate. Cryoprecipitate is a concentrated source of vWF, factor VIII, and fibrinogen. Each unit is produced from 1 unit FFP. Because of the smaller volume, cryoprecipitate is preferred over FFP because there is less risk of volume overload when multiple units are needed. Start with 1 U/10 kg body weight for cryoprecipitate and 10 mL/kg for FFP. Repeat as needed to control hemorrhage.

Desamino-8-arginine vasopressin (DDAVP) is a synthetic analog of vasopressin with fewer pressor effects. It temporarily increases circulating vWF in normal dogs and may help dogs with some forms of vWD (particularly type I). The intranasal preparation may be given subcutaneously (1 μg/kg) either to help control ongoing hemorrhage or 15 to 30 minutes before surgery. Repeated doses would not be expected to be beneficial. Avoid drugs known to adversely affect platelet function (see Table 49-3).[5] Although some reports suggest that thyroxine therapy may be of benefit for dogs with vWD, supplementation should be reserved for those patients with documented hypothyroidism, confirmed through testing in addition to total T_4 values.[18]

Secondary Hemostatic Defects

As with platelet problems, coagulation factor dysfunction and deficiencies can be either inherited or acquired. Inherited factor deficiencies are rare, the most common being the X-linked hemophilias: factor VIII deficiency (hemophilia A) and factor IX deficiency (hemophilia B). The most common acquired deficiencies include vitamin K deficiency (activation defect), liver failure (production defect), and DIC (consumption and localization defect).[1]

Vitamin K Deficiency

Although vitamin K deficiency may result from chronic malabsorption, oral antibiotic use, or cholestasis, the most common cause is ingestion of anticoagulant rodenticides. Most intoxications today are due to second-generation anticoagulant rodenticides (*e.g.*, brodifacoum, bromodiolone) with much longer half-lives than warfarin. The first clinical signs are typically seen several days after ingestion. Although some patients present for overt bleeding, more commonly the clinical signs are vague (anorexia, depression, weakness) or relate to a site of internal hemorrhage (*e.g.*, neurologic signs with nervous system hemorrhage, dyspnea with bleeding into the chest or lungs). Diagnosis is often based on history, evidence of a coagulopathy (prolonged aPTT, ACT, PT), and rapid response to vitamin K_1 therapy. Some laboratories can determine the specific anticoagulant via chromatographic analysis of samples of blood or vomitus. This can be helpful in determining the duration of vitamin K_1 therapy necessary. By the time an animal presents with hemorrhage, there is a deficiency of multiple factors and both the intrinsic and extrinsic pathways are prolonged. If animals are presented for potential exposure to an anticoagulant rodenticide before clinical signs occur (*i.e.*, ingestion is uncertain), the PT and PIVKA tests will be prolonged first because of the shorter life span of factor VII.

When ingestion is witnessed, induce vomiting within 12 hours. Removal of stomach contents is not recommended for patients with bleeding tendencies because of potential hemorrhage and because anticoagulant rodenticide exposure precedes clinical signs by several days. At this point, you can either assume toxicity and treat with vitamin K_1 or confirm/refute toxicity by measuring PT or PIVKA at 24 and 48 hours. For animals presenting with hemorrhage, it is appropriate to treat with phytonadione (vitamin K_1, not K_3) while diagnostic tests are pending. However, vitamin K alone will not stop hemorrhage until the liver synthesizes new clotting factors (12–24 hours). Transfusion of active clotting factors may be necessary to control hemorrhage. Depending on the degree of anemia, start with either 6 to 12 mL/kg FFP or 12 to 20 mL/kg FWB. Repeat until bleeding is controlled. Rapid whole blood transfusion (12–20 mL/kg) may be lifesaving for animals presenting in shock. Give 50% rapidly, then reassess. Vitamin K_1 therapy should be started with a dose of 2 to 5 mg/kg/d subcutaneously. Note that vitamin K should not be given intramuscularly due to possible hemorrhage and cannot be given intravenously due to the potential for anaphylaxis. Oral therapy can begin at similar doses once the patient is eating. The length of oral therapy needed may be as long as 4 to 6 weeks depending on the toxin and the degree of exposure.[19]

Liver Disease

Animals with coagulopathies secondary to liver disease usually present with clinical signs related to liver disease. Coagulopathies may be suspected after excess hemorrhage from minor procedures or noted on a coagulation panel. The coagulopathy may be due to inadequate production of coagulation factors, vitamin K deficiency, or inadequate clearance of plasminogen activators and FDPs. For animals with severe liver disease, if their condition will not be compromised by delay, it may be advisable to treat with vitamin K_1 for several days before proceeding with invasive diagnostic tests. Therapy involves treatment of the underlying disease and supportive care. Plasma transfusion may be necessary to control hemorrhage in some cases.

Disseminated Intravascular Coagulation

Any disorder causing widespread activation of the coagulation cascade can cause DIC. Because DIC is always a secondary event, most animals with DIC present with clinical signs associated with the primary illness rather than overt hemorrhage. The most common causes are those that cause systemic inflammation such as intravascular hemolysis, malignancies, gastric dilatation-volvulus, sepsis, pancreatitis, heatstroke, massive tissue trauma, toxins, and snakebites. A diagnosis of DIC is supported by identification of a primary disease, thrombocytopenia, red cell fragmentation, prolonged coagulation times (APTT, PT, TT), increased FDPs, and decreased fibrinogen or AT III.[20] Confirmation of the diagnosis is not critical because the therapy is always tailored to the patient's current clinical signs. The most important factors in managing DIC are treatment of the primary disease and supportive care. Administer fluid therapy to improve tissue perfusion, inhibit vascular stasis, and dilute activated coagulation and fibrinolytic factors. In addition, correct acid–base and electrolyte abnormalities, warm if hypothermic, and provide nutritional support. Transfusion may be appropriate to manage anemia and replace deficient coagulation factors and inhibitors. Heparin has been advocated at a wide range of doses (*e.g.*, 5–500 U/kg q 8 h to q 6 h) with little evidence showing efficacy. The clearest indications for use are when signs of thrombosis predominate (see below) or after transfusion of products containing AT III (FFP or FWB). If heparin therapy is started, theoretically it is best to decrease the dose over several days to prevent a hypercoagulable state following discontinuation.

Inappropriate Thrombosis and Thromboembolism

Thrombosis and thromboembolism have been described as complications in a variety of clinical disorders in veterinary patients, including cardiac disease, infectious diseases, neoplasia, endocrinopathies, and immune-mediated disorders. The site of thrombosis may be venous, pulmonary, or arterial. Newer diagnostic techniques, including ultrasonography, Doppler flow evaluation, and nuclear scintigraphy have improved the veterinary clinician's ability to diagnose thrombosis in small animal patients.

Anticoagulant Therapy

Heparin. Subcutaneous heparin therapy is indicated in the acute phase of clinical thrombosis because it rapidly inhibits coagulation. It catalyzes the binding of AT III and heparin cofactor II to various coagulation factors, preventing their participation in the coagulation cascade. Heparin may also promote clot dissolution through increased release of tissue plasminogen activator.

Heparin is rapidly absorbed from subcutaneous injection sites. It should not be administered intramuscularly due to injection site hemorrhage. The appropriate dose for use in thrombosis has not been determined for veterinary patients. Clinical trials in humans have suggested that plasma heparin concentrations of 0.35 to 0.70 U/mL (as measured by chromogenic factor Xa assay) are associated with highest clinical efficacy and minimal hemorrhagic complications. In normal experimental animals, doses of 250 U/kg SQ q 6 h (dogs)[26] or 200 U/kg SQ q 8 h (cats)[27] were most consistently associated with this target plasma concentration. Heparin plasma concentration monitoring in canine clinical patients with immune-mediated hemolytic anemia and feline patients with aortic or pulmonary thromboembolism has suggested that appropriate doses to achieve this heparin concentration are highly variable. Clinical patients have tended to require higher doses of heparin than normal individuals.[28]

Monitoring of heparin therapy is most commonly accomplished by measuring the aPTT or ACT. The suggested target range is a prolongation over normal plasma control aPTT by a factor of 1.5 to 2.5, or prolongation of the ACT by 15 to 20 seconds. Wide variation in the sensitivity of aPTT reagents and in individual patients' aPTT response to a given heparin concentration results in inconsistencies in degree of anticoagulation measured with this approach. The ACT is even less predictive of plasma heparin concentration.

Because heparin requires frequent administration to achieve consistent anticoagulation, it is generally not suitable for long-term outpatient therapy. Because heparin therapy may cause decreased levels of AT III, which may result in hypercoagulability, heparin therapy should be gradually discontinued if the hypercoagulable state no longer exists or overlapped with oral anticoagulant in patients requiring long-term anticoagulation.

Aspirin. Acetylsalicylic acid irreversibly prevents the production of thromboxane A_2 (TXA_2) in platelets. Because TXA_2 is a potent platelet aggregator, aspirin decreases platelet aggregability. Published recommendations for aspirin therapy in feline patients at risk for thromboembolism range from 10 to 25 mg/kg PO q 3 d.[29] Aspirin has been widely used at these doses for decades, but clinical evidence suggests that it is ineffective at preventing thromboembolism in cats at risk. In humans, low doses of aspirin (1 mg/kg q 24 h) are effective in preventing recurrence of thrombosis in a variety of disorders. This lower dose may be effective in part because it is sufficient to irreversibly inhibit platelet cyclooxygenase (thereby limiting platelet aggregation) without significantly inhibiting prostaglandin I_2 (PGI_2) synthesis in endothelial cells. Endothelial PGI_2 is important in inhibiting platelet aggregation outside the area of injury, which is vital for limiting thrombus growth. Whether or not lower doses of aspirin may be of benefit in veterinary patients with hypercoagulability remains to be seen.

Warfarin. Warfarin (a 4-hydroxycoumarin compound) exerts its anticoagulant effect by blocking the recycling of vitamin K, thus reducing body stores.

Pharmacokinetic/pharmacodynamic study of warfarin suggested an initial oral dose of 0.22 mg/kg q 12 h in normal dogs[30] and 0.06 to 0.09 mg/kg/d in cats.[31] Warfarin (Coumadin) is supplied as a 1-mg tablet. Analysis of crushed tablets suggested unequal distribution of the drug in different portions of the tablet. The author consequently does not recommend that tablets be broken for administration because this may result in variation in dose administered. When the tablets were crushed into a powder and mixed well, analysis suggested even distribution of the drug. The powder can be weighed out by a compounding pharmacist and used to fill gelatin capsules.[32]

The PT is the most commonly performed laboratory test for monitoring of warfarin therapy. Monitoring of PT after initiation of warfarin therapy is usually performed with the patient hospitalized for the first few days because most patients are still currently receiving heparin as described previously. The potential for hypercoagulability early in warfarin therapy due to decreased protein C levels suggests that warfarin should only be initiated once anticoagulation is achieved with heparin. Most patients will require that warfarin be overlapped with heparin for at least 4 to 5 days. The patient PT should be monitored daily for the first 4 to 5 days of therapy, until the PT stabilizes. The timing of sample collection in relation to the administration of the warfarin dose for the day is unimportant, because PT is dependent on coagulation factor levels at the time of sampling rather than plasma warfarin concentration. Monitoring of anticoagulant therapy with the PT must be adjusted for variations in thromboplastin reagent and laboratory technique. The laboratory should provide an index of specificity of the thromboplastin reagent called an international sensitivity index (ISI). The ISI may be different depending on whether the PT was performed by manual or automated methodology. The international normalization ratio (INR) is calculated as follows: $INR = (\text{Patient PT}/\text{Control PT})^{ISI}$. The ideal INR for anticoagulation to prevent thrombosis in dogs and cats has not been determined. In humans, the recommended therapeutic range depends on the condition predisposing to thrombosis. No prospective studies evaluating the effectiveness of any warfarin regimen have as yet been reported for veterinary patients. Until such information is available, an INR of 2.0 to 3.0 is recommended because this lower intensity approach is associated with less hemorrhage and reasonable efficacy in humans. Experience to date with use of warfarin in cats and dogs would suggest that although an INR of 2.0 to 3.0 is an ideal goal, a wider range for INR might have to be acceptable to the veterinary clinician. Future experience may allow for better dose adjustments in response to an inadequate INR and result in better control.[33]

Once the INR indicates appropriate anticoagulation, heparin therapy (if used concurrently) is discontinued. Because the INR may decrease once heparin is discontinued, the PT should be repeated 6 to 8 hours following the last heparin dose. If the INR is within therapeutic range, the patient is discharged with instructions to return twice weekly for PT measurements until consistent anticoagulation is achieved. Monitoring is then reduced to once weekly for several weeks to several months, then every 2 months assuming an appropriate and consistent response. Because of the high rate of drug interactions with warfarin, an adjustment in any other concurrent drug therapy is an indication to reevaluate patient anticoagulation status.[33]

Thrombolysis

Streptokinase (SK) is a bacterial protein that binds to plasminogen. This results in exposure of a plasminogen enzyme center that activates other plasminogen molecules, resulting in their conversion to plasmin. When administered systemically, it accelerates activation of fibrin-bound plasminogen. It has been successfully used to lyse experimentally created thrombi in cats and naturally occurring thrombi in dogs. Dogs have been successfully treated with 90,000 U IV as a loading dose over 30 minutes, followed by a 45,000 U/h IV continuous infusion for 7 to 12 hours.[21] Cats with aortic thromboembolism treated similarly had mortality rates of 70% to 100%.[22,23] The main side effect of SK in dogs is inappropriate hemorrhage because of the systemic thrombolytic state. SK is potentially allergenic and costly to administer.

Tissue plasminogen activator is a naturally occurring glycoprotein that catalyzes the conversion of plasminogen to plasmin in the presence of fibrin. It has been produced for clinical use through recombinant gene technology. Anecdotal reports detail its successful use for aortic thromboembolism in both cats and dogs. The reported dog dose was 1 mg/kg IV q 1 h for 10 doses. Advantages of tPA over SK include more rapid thrombolysis, less antigenicity, and potentially less hemorrhage. This agent is cost prohibitive for many clients.[24,25]

REFERENCES

1. Brooks M: Coagulopathies and thrombosis. *In:* Ettinger SJ, Feldman EC, eds.: Textbook of Veterinary Internal Medicine. 5th ed. Philadelphia: WB Saunders, 2000, p 1829.
2. Hackner SG: Approach to diagnosis of bleeding disorders. *Comp Contin Ed* 17:331, 1995.
3. Welles EG: Antithrombotic and fibrinolytic factors. A review. *Vet Clin North Am Small Anim Pract* 26:1111, 1996.
4. Jordan HL, Grindem CB, Breitschwerdt EB: Thrombocytopenia in cats: a retrospective study of 41 cases. *J Vet Intern Med* 7:261, 1993.
5. Thomas JS: von Willebrand's disease in the dog and cat. *Vet Clin North Am Small Anim Pract* 26:1089, 1996.

6. Berry CR, Gallaway A, Thrall DE, *et al.*: Thoracic radiographic features of anticoagulant rodenticide toxicity in fourteen dogs. *Vet Radiol Ultrasound* 34:391, 1993.
7. Van Winkle TJ, Bruce E: Thrombosis of the portal vein in eleven dogs. *Vet Pathol* 30:28, 1993.
8. Dennis JS: Clinical features of canine pulmonary thromboembolism. *Comp Contin Ed Pract Vet* 15:1595, 1993.
9. Meyers KM, Wardrop KJ, Meinkoth J: Canine von Willebrand's disease: pathobiology, diagnosis, and short-term treatment. *Comp Contin Ed Pract Vet* 14:13, 1992.
10. Mackin A: Canine immune-mediated thrombocytopenia. Part I. *Comp Contin Ed* 17:353, 1995.
11. Center SA, Warner K, Corbett J, *et al.*: Proteins invoked by vitamin K absence and clotting times in clinically ill cats. *J Vet Intern Med* 14:292, 2000.
12. Stokol T, Brooks MB, Erb HN, *et al.*: D-dimer concentrations in healthy dogs and dogs with disseminated intravascular coagulation. *Am J Vet Res* 61:393, 2000.
13. Kristensen AT, Feldman BF: General principles of small animal blood component administration. *Vet Clin North Am Small Anim Pract* 25:1277, 1995.
14. Ruiz de Gopegui R, Feldman BF: Hemostatic diseases. *In:* Leib MS, Monroe WE, eds.: Practical Small Animal Internal Medicine. Philadelphia: WB Saunders, 1997, p 973.
15. Lewis DC, Meyers KM, Callan MB, *et al.*: Detection of platelet-bound and serum platelet-bindable antibodies for diagnosis of idiopathic thrombocytopenic purpura in dogs. *J Am Vet Med Assoc* 206:47, 1995.
16. Mackin A: Canine immune-mediated thrombocytopenia Part II. *Comp Contin Ed Pract Vet* 17:515, 1995.
17. Boudreaux MK: Platelets and coagulation. An update. *Vet Clin North Am Small Anim Pract* 26:1065, 1996.
18. Panciera DL, Johnson GS: Plasma von Willebrand factor antigen concentration in dogs with hypothyroidism. *J Am Vet Med Assoc* 205:1550, 1994.
19. Murphy MJ: CVT Update: rodenticide toxicosis. *In:* Bonagura JD, ed.: Kirk's Current Veterinary Therapy XIII. Philadelphia: WB Saunders, 2000, p 211.
20. Bateman SW, Mathews KA, Abrams-Ogg AC, *et al.*: Diagnosis of disseminated intravascular coagulation in dogs admitted to an intensive care unit. *J Am Vet Med Assoc* 215:798, 1999.
21. Ramsey CC, Burney DP, Macintire DK, *et al.*: Use of streptokinase in four dogs with thrombosis. *J Am Vet Med Assoc* 209:780, 1996.
22. Ramsey CC, Riepe RD, Macintire, DK, Burney DP: Streptokinase: a practical clotbuster? *Proc ACVIM Vet Med Forum* 225, 1996.
23. Moore K, Dhupa N, Rush JE *et al.*: Clinical experience with streptokinase administration in 27 cats [abstract]. *J Vet Emerg Crit Care Soc* 8:262, 1998.
24. Clare AC, Kraje BJ: Use of recombinant tissue-plasminogen activator for aortic thrombolysis in a hypoproteinemic dog. *J Am Vet Med Assoc* 212:539, 1998.
25. Pion PD: Feline aortic thromboemboli and the potential utility of thrombolytic therapy with tissue plasminogen activator. *Vet Clin North Am Small Anim Pract* 18:79, 1988.
26. Kellerman DL, Lewis DC, Bruyette DS: Determining and monitoring of a therapeutic heparin dosage in the dog [abstract]. *J Vet Intern Med* 9:187, 1995.
27. Kellerman DL, Lewis DC, Myers NC, Bruyette DS: Determination of a therapeutic heparin dose in the cat [abstract]. *J Vet Intern Med* 10:231, 1996.
28. Smith SA, Lewis DC, Kellerman DL: Adjustment of intermittent subcutaneous hep-

arin therapy based on chromogenic heparin assay in 9 cats with thromboembolism [abstract]. *J Vet Intern Med* 12:200, 1998.

29. Fox PR: Evidence for or against efficacy of beta-blockers and aspirin for management of feline cardiomyopathies. *Vet Clin North Am Small Anim Pract* 21:1011, 1991.
30. Neff Davis CA, Davis LE, Gillette EL: Warfarin in the dog: pharmacokinetics as related to clinical response. *J Vet Pharmacol Ther* 4:135, 1981.
31. Smith SA, Kraft SL, Lewis DC, *et al.*: Pharmacodynamics of warfarin in cats. *J Vet Pharmacol Ther* 23:339, 2000.
32. Smith SA, Kraft SL, Lewis DC, *et al.*: Plasma pharmacodynamics of warfarin enantiomers in cats. *J Vet Pharmacol Ther* 23:329, 2000.
33. Harpster NK, Baty CJ: Warfarin therapy of the cat at risk of thromboembolism. *In:* Bonagura JD, ed.: Kirk's Current Veterinary Therapy XII. Philadelphia, PA: WB Saunders, 1995, p 868.

SECTION VII
Digestive Disorders

50 Gastric Dilatation-Volvulus

Wayne E. Wingfield

INTRODUCTION

Gastric dilatation-volvulus (GDV) is an acute, polysystemic, life-threatening disease predominantly affecting large or giant, purebred, deep-chested dogs. Untreated this disease will rapidly progress to death.

This disease is variously termed bloat, canine bloat, torsion, gastric torsion, gastric dilatation, and now, appropriately, gastric dilatation-volvulus or GDV. First reported in 1906 in the dog, GDV has become one of the more feared diseases by owners due to its sudden, unexpected onset and relatively high mortality rate. Most disturbing is the failure of researchers and clinical investigators to identify an etiology for the condition.

PATHOGENESIS

Risk Factors

Gastric dilatation-volvulus is a syndrome primarily affecting dogs although it is also reported in cats and primates. The syndrome is characterized by rapid accumulation of air in the stomach, malposition of the stomach, increased gastric pressure, and shock. Although the etiology and pathogenesis are unknown, specific risk factors have been identified in case reports and retrospective studies.[1]

Large and giant breed dogs are the most common breeds affected by GDV. The likelihood of these breeds developing GDV during their lifetime is 21.6% for giant and 24% for large breed dogs, assuming the normal life spans for giant and large breed dogs are 8 and 10 years, respectively. The Great Dane has the highest incidence and is at greatest risk of developing GDV (42.4%).[1]

The incidence of GDV increases with age in giant breed dogs. In dogs, body size is inversely related to longevity.[2] This implies the aging process is somehow accelerated in larger dogs, and diseases such as GDV develop earlier in life in larger dogs, compared to smaller dogs. The incidence of GDV in the Great Dane and Irish wolfhound (giant breeds) continuously increases with increasing age, whereas in the other giant and large breed dogs, the incidence of GDV does not increase until dogs are older (>4.9 years).[1]

Genetically linked breed characteristics, such as conformation and temperament may be related to incidence of GDV. Dogs with a narrow and deep conformation of the thoracic cavity have a higher incidence of GDV. Using thoracic radiographs, measurements for thoracic depth are taken as the distance from the ventral border of the eighth thoracic vertebrae to the cranial dorsal limit of the xyphoid sternebra. Thoracic width is measured from the lateral aspect of the left ninth rib to the lateral aspect of the right ninth rib. The depth/width ratios are calculated, and studies reported that dogs with reduced thoracic depth/width ratios are at greater risk of GDV.[2,4] More recently a study noted depth/width ratios ($P < 0.20$), depth of the abdomen, and in female dogs, height are all positively correlated with incidence of GDV. When these breed conformational characteristics are included in a multiple linear regression analysis, none are associated with incidence of GDV.[1]

Owner-perceived personality and temperament traits among dogs that are positively ($P < 0.20$) associated with GDV include fearfulness ($r = 0.61$; $P = 0.05$) or agitation in response to strangers or environmental changes ($r = 0.55$; $P = 0.08$), whereas the only trait negatively associated with the incidence of GDV is happiness ($r = -0.79$; $P = 0.004$). When these three breed-related personality and temperament traits are included in a multiple linear regression analysis, happiness is associated with a decreased incidence of GDV among male ($P = 0.01$) and female ($P = 0.02$) dogs.[1] This does not necessarily mean that within a given breed, the happier the dog, the lower the incidence of GDV. However, in a recent case-controlled study,[5] the risk of GDV in dogs characterized by their owners as happy is reduced by 78%, compared to dogs not characterized as happy. Moreover, risk of GDV is increased by 257% in fearful versus nonfearful dogs. These authors postulated that the differences between happy and fearful dogs might affect function and motility of the gastrointestinal tract, especially under conditions of stress.

Proposed etiologic mechanisms in GDV include the role of gastrin, myoelectric dysfunction, esophageal dysfunction, and dietary factors. Gastrin has a trophic effect on gastric mucosa resulting in delayed emptying, increased gastroesophageal sphincter pressure, thus inducing esophageal spasm, initiating aerophagia, and decreasing the likelihood of vomiting with gastric distention. Dogs with GDV have significantly higher gastrin concentrations than seen in normal dogs during acute GDV and during the postoperative period.[6] In a study of six postoperative dogs with GDV, gastroesophageal sphincter function and plasma gastrin concentrations are not significantly different than normal dogs.[7] Whether gastrin is important in the pathogenesis of GDV is yet unresolved.

It is frequently speculated that delayed gastric emptying may predispose to GDV. The rate of gastric emptying of a solid, radionucleotide-labeled test meal in 10 dogs with a previous GDV was not significantly different than 10 clinically normal dogs.[8] In another study, gastric emptying following circumcostal gastropexy was delayed when compared to normal dogs with the same surgery. Thus, it was assumed that the delay in gastric emptying was due to GDV.[9] Whether gastric emptying is important in the pathogenesis of GDV is as yet unresolved.

Abnormal esophageal motility in dogs with recurrent GDV is reported.* It is unknown whether these animals had previous gastric surgery. Aerophagia is

* van Sluijs FJ, Wolvekamp WTC: Abnormal esophageal motility in dogs with recurrent gastric dilatatation-volvulus [abstract]. *Vet Surg* 22:250, 1993.

seen mainly when primary esophageal peristalsis failed to transport a food bolus to the stomach. The ingestion of air elicited secondary peristaltic waves strong enough to transport the food to the stomach. Whether abnormal esophageal motility is important in the pathogenesis of GDV is unresolved.

Because most people associate the stomach with food, many attempts to relate food or feeding practices to GDV are available in existing literature.[10] Unfortunately no study can implicate any dietary foodstuff or specific feeding practice with the development of GDV.[11] It is highly unlikely that food is associated with this syndrome. Dogs that eat rapidly and feeding dogs with a raised feeding bowl results in a 20% increase in large, and 50% increase in giant, breeds in occurrence of GDV.[11a]

Mechanism of Gastric Dilatation

A source of fluid or gas and an obstruction to emptying that prevents relief of gastric distention are required for the development of GDV. In young dogs (<6 months), there is usually no abnormal quantity of gas or fluid. Instead there is usually overconsumption of food. In the mature animal the stomach is most commonly filled with gas in GDV. The source of this gas is consistent with aerophagia.[12]

Why the stomach is unable to relieve itself of this accumulation of gas is unknown. Normally, swallowed air leaves rapidly from the stomach. Eructation, emesis, absorption, or passage of the gas into the small bowel usually accounts for the rapid movement of swallowed air. As air is swallowed, some is refluxed from the stomach back into the esophagus. This air is then either belched or returned to the stomach via peristaltic contractions. A tightening of the distal esophageal sphincter in humans is known to elicit a feeling of fullness. When one feels full, aerophagia is more pronounced. Whether this happens in dogs is still controversial. Interestingly, with the extreme distensibility of the dog's stomach, instillation of 1000 cc gas results in only slight intragastric pressure changes.

Negative intrathoracic pressure can also suck air into the esophagus. This occurs if the cranial esophageal sphincter is relaxed. Normally this sphincter is contracted and prevents atmospheric air from entering the esophagus. The cause for this relaxation is unknown but has been noted in human patients with debility or disease, stimulation of the vagus nerve below the diaphragm, or in the presence of hypoxia.

Anatomic Changes

As the stomach dilates, a torsion of the distal esophagus and gastroesophageal junction of the stomach develops. This rotation is continued onto the greater curvature of the stomach towards the antrum. With increased dilatation, the pylorus shifts from its normal position to a dorsal, cranial, and leftward location. Experimentally this requires laxity of the gastrohepatic ligament. The continued dilatation results in a ventral displacement of the stomach in the abdomen resulting in an acute angle being formed at the gastroesophageal junction effectively creating a one-way valve. With further aerophagia the air is effectively prevented from escaping.

As the stomach dilates, the spleen is passively dragged rightward within the abdomen. Eventually the splenic vessels come to lie ventrally across the esophagus and become partially obstructed leading to venous congestion and a secondary splenomegaly.

Also, as the stomach dilates it exerts pressure on the caudal vena cava.[13] The blood in the vena cava is shunted via the ventral vertebral sinuses to the azygos vein and back to the cranial vena cava. Failure of some to realize venous occlusion is not complete has led to the false belief that intravenous fluids should not be administered via the lateral saphenous vein. This vein is an excellent place for an intravenous catheter and there is not an impediment to fluid administration. Additionally, the rotation of the stomach also actively occludes the portal vein leading to venous congestion of abdominal splanchnic viscera. This occlusion promotes the onset and severity of shock.

Physiologic Responses

With the mechanical enlargement of the stomach, the intraluminal pressures increase and the arterial pressure to the stomach is maintained, but venous drainage is compromised and intraluminal vascular stasis results. Peristaltic activity decreases with the onset of ischemic hypoxia. Severe damage to the ganglion cells of Auerbach's plexus is produced. If the hypoxia is corrected within 3.5 to 4 hours, the neurologic damage is reversible. With the increasing intragastric luminal pressures, injury to the gastric mucosa develops. The local hypoxia leads to the development of subepithelial hemorrhage and edema. Ulcers may develop, resulting in large areas of necrotic mucosa.

The spleen is passively dragged with the dilating stomach. Stretch is applied to the splenic vessels and eventually venous congestion results from the stretching and occlusion of the vessels by the dilating stomach. The portal vein is also obstructed by the rotating stomach, thus retarding the venous return from the spleen and other abdominal viscera. With occlusion of the vasa brevi to the gastroepiploic and left gastric veins, gastric ulceration is augmented.[14] During splenic ischemia the production of coagulation factors VIII and IX is decreased.[15] This is of theoretical importance in the development of disseminated intravascular coagulation. Torsion of the splenic pedicle can occur independently or in association with GDV.

The respiratory system is also affected by gastric dilatation. In the clinical patient there will be an increased respiratory rate. The enlarged stomach encroaches on the thoracic space leading to a decrease in tidal volume with an increased respiratory rate. This increased rate allows the minute volume to be maintained. As diaphragmatic excursions are further impaired by the enlarging stomach, inspiratory and expiratory resistance increases and pulmonary compliance is decreased.

With a decrease in venous return to the heart via the caudal vena cava and portal circulation, the right ventricle is hampered in its ability to provide blood for oxygenation and thus leads to inadequate alveolar ventilation and a ventilation-perfusion mismatch.

As the stomach dilates it impinges on the caudal vena cava. Blood in the vena cava begins to shunt to the ventral vertebral sinuses and returns blood to the cranial vena cava via the azygos vein and to the cranial vena cava.[13] Continued distention of the stomach results in a progressive fall in arterial blood pressure while the pressure in the caudal vena cava progressively rises. Blood becomes sequestered in the skeletal muscles, portal system, splanchnic organs, and caudal vena cava. Sequestration results in oxyhemoglobin desaturation in blood collected from the caudal vena cava and right atrium.[13]

Sequestration of blood also promotes a fall in cardiac output. The predominant cause of this decreased output is a decrease in venous return. Neurogenic factors may also be important in this fall in cardiac output. Gastric distention will result in stimulation of the splanchnic sympathetics, resulting in hypotension. The consequences of the hypotension are manifest as a low velocity flow. At low velocity, blood tends to increase in viscosity.

When the portal system is occluded, endotoxemia likely results. Acutely occluding the portal vein leads to a high mortality in the dog. The mechanism of this high mortality is either hypovolemia, a neurogenic enhancement of shock, or a failure of the reticuloendothelial system's capacity to neutralize endotoxins. As gram-negative bacteria within the gut release their endotoxins, they contribute to the shock associated with portal venous occlusion. This endotoxin apparently enters to the circulation either via the peritoneal surface or lymphatic channels.

CLINICAL PRESENTATION

Clinical signs of GDV usually present soon after the dog has eaten. Owners see their dog with severe cranial abdominal distention with tympany, retching with the inability to vomit, restlessness, excessive salivation, and often panting or making grunting signs indicative of the animal's pain and discomfort. Depending on the duration of the GDV, the animal may also be found in its pen recumbent, moribund, or even dead. It is not unusual to elicit a history of excitement, stress, or chronic gastrointestinal symptoms such as vomiting, loose stools, belching, or flatulence.

Physical examination findings include a rapid, weak pulse, labored breathing, pale mucous membranes, prolonged capillary refill times, cranial abdominal distention with tympany, an irregular heart rhythm with, or without, pulse deficits. Again, the findings are extremely variable and extend from mild signs in the bright, alert, ambulatory dog, to the moribund signs in the seriously ill dog.

Not all dogs presented as GDV have a rotated stomach. In fact, there appears to be at least three commonly diagnosed conditions: GDV, acute gastric dilatation (GD), and chronic GDV. In GD dogs, simple gluttony is the usual cause. Young dogs are most commonly presented with simple GD. These dogs seem to be unable to relieve themselves effectively by vomiting, probably because of the tremendous volume of food ingested. Occasionally it is not food causing this distention. Rather, it may be straw or hay used in the dog's bedding or the bedding cover itself! Young dogs too are prone to ingest garbage materials and will proceed to gastric outflow obstruction.

Some GDV dogs will spontaneously untwist their stomachs and present without the classical picture of shock seen in acute GDV. These are the chronic GDV dogs. Their histories usually include chronic vomiting, loss of weight, eructation, flatulence, and intermittent episodes of gastric distention that spontaneously resolve.[16] Regardless, these dogs should be taken to surgery and a gastropexy performed.

DIAGNOSTIC EVALUATION

Most dogs with GDV have their diagnosis made on the basis of the patient's profile (large breed, deep-chested, usually purebred), history, and the physical findings of cranial abdominal distention with tympany, restlessness, abdominal pain, labored breathing, and shock signs. In some cases, abdominal radiography is helpful. This is especially true when distinguishing the GD from the GDV dog. No dog should be taken to radiography until the stomach is decompressed via orogastric tube or gastrocentesis and intravenous fluids have been started to combat the dog's state of shock. Radiography can usually confirm the diagnosis with plain radiographs and no radiographic contrast material.

The radiographic view of choice is a right lateral recumbency.[17] With gastric volvulus, the pylorus is positioned dorsally, cranially, and to the left of the abdominal midline and the pylorus will appear filled with gas. The stomach will be distended and filled with gas, and will appear compartmentalized with a tissue-dense soft-tissue line representing a fold in the stomach. Splenomegaly is often noted and the spleen is displaced to the right of the midline. Presence of gas within the walls of the stomach is indicative of gastric necrosis. Free gas within the peritoneal cavity arises from two sources: gastric perforation or gastrocentesis prior to radiography. Evidence of free peritoneal gas requires an exploratory surgical procedure. In most dogs with GD and GDV, the intestine is also noted to be gas filled most likely from the aerophagia inducing the gastric distention.

Electrocardiographic monitoring is essential in dogs with GDV. In most cases there will only be a sinus tachycardia on presentation. This is undoubtedly due to shock and the catecholamines associated with the excitement and handling in the emergency room. Ventricular tachycardia represents the most common abnormal rhythm but almost any arrhythmia may be seen.[18]

A strong association between plasma lactate concentration and outcome of dogs with GDV is reported.[19-21] A dog with a plasma lactate concentration of less than 6.0 mmol/L is likely to survive, whereas a dog with GDV and a plasma lactate concentration greater than 6.0 mmol/L has an almost equal chance of either surviving or dying. The prognostic value of plasma lactate is attributable not only to its association with gastric necrosis, but also to its association with severity of systemic hypoperfusion. Hyperlactatemia develops when the rate of lactate production in ischemic tissue exceeds the rate of lactate metabolism in the body. Thus, the increase in plasma lactate concentration is proportional to the severity of circulatory compromise. Using plasma lactate concentrations seems logical as a means to potentially identify those dogs with gastric necrosis and are thus more likely to die.[19]

In experimentally induced GDV, consistently researchers have reported dogs in shock with cardiac output values 50% that of typical values for clinically normal dogs. Additionally, the experimental studies report mean arterial pressures (MAP) significantly less than reference range.[22,23] Recently a study of naturally occurring GDV reported that cardiac index (CI) and MAP are slightly lower than, but not statistically different from, normal or anesthetized dogs.[24] This study only involved six dogs and 67% of these dogs had received intravenous fluids prior to anesthesia. Following derotation of the stomach, CI increased significantly. This increase is a result of an increased stroke volume, presumably by restoration of venous return. Systemic vascular resistance decreased at the same time, most likely because of removal of external compressive forces from the vasculature of stomach and cranial part of the gastrointestinal tract, or perhaps from release of endogenous vasoactive mediators from the compromised bowel and stomach. Interestingly, the MAP did not significantly change with derotation of the stomach. This reminds us that pressure does not necessarily correspond with flow. Many clinicians tend to rely on MAP values to indicate hemodynamic status, because MAP is easy to measure.

The importance of reperfusion injury in the pathogenesis of naturally occurring GDV is not determined. Experimentally, the role of xanthine oxidase and iron-dependent lipid peroxidation (purported mechanisms of reperfusion injury) are reported.[26,27]

TREATMENT

Preoperative treatment for a dog with GDV involves the decompression of the stomach and treatment for shock. Decompression of the stomach is important because it results in an increase in CI presumably through increasing venous return. One should minimize stress on the animal as the orogastric tube is passed. Sedation is unlikely required. The most efficient and successful means for passing the tube is to allow the animal to assume any position most comfortable. Ideally, the dog is in a sternal recumbancy. The tube is premeasured from the tip of the nose to the thirteenth rib. Place a roll of 2-inch adhesive tape or a mouth speculum behind the canine teeth, have an assistant hold the mouth closed around the tape, and gently pass a well-lubricated orogastric tube. (A foal-sized stomach tube works best.)

If resistance is encountered or the animal struggles, it is best to use gastrocentesis. Using a 14- to 16-gauge needle, percuss the *right* paracostal region until tympanic sounds are resonated. The hair is clipped and prepped with routine methods, and the needle inserted. Gas will escape and one should place gentle pressure on the cranial abdomen to evacuate as much gas as possible. It is very important to remember that if gastrocentesis is used, later radiographs of the abdomen may show free gas. At that point it will be impossible to distinguish between a ruptured stomach and iatrogenic free air. Either way, the dog is going to surgery and thus it may be more academic than clinically relevant. After gastrocentesis, an orogastric tube is passed and the stomach lavaged with warmed tap water. If gastric bleeding is encountered, cold or even ice water is used for the lavage to slow bleeding. Lavage removes any food and also provides a means to investigate mucosal injury (bleeding, coffee grounds-colored digested blood, or even gastric mucosa). Temporary gastrostomy has been reported but cannot be recommended at this time. It is more important to prepare the animal for immediate surgery.

Surgery decreases the likelihood of gastric perforation, gastric or splenic infarction, and an increasing prevalence of serious cardiac dysrhythmias. The belt-loop gastropexy is the preferred technique for preventing reoccurrence of GDV. It is an easy and efficient surgical procedure. During surgery, careful inspection of the stomach is required to identify areas of gastric necrosis or questionably viable stomach. If in doubt, resect this area. Most commonly the area of the greater curvature where the short gastric arteries from the spleen anastomose to the left gastroepiploic artery will be the affected area of the stomach. If the spleen does not return to normal size or there is evidence of infarction, a splenectomy (partial or total) is recommended.

Postoperative Management

Complications expected in the postoperative period following GDV surgery include cardiac arrhythmias, shock, gastroparesis, vomiting, hypokalemia, and gastric distention. Less commonly, vomiting, pancreatitis, disseminated intravascular coagulopathy, incisional dehiscence, peritonitis, and gastric ulcers, ischemia, or necrosis, are seen.

The ideal monitoring during the first 48 hours of the postoperative period will include the following: electrocardiograms measured continuously; electrolytes monitored every 8 hours; acid–base status measured every 12 hours; packed cell volume, total solids, and activated clotting time monitored every 8 hours; and appropriate parameters monitored to identify other complications likely to result.

The major electrolyte disturbance in GDV is hypokalemia. It potentiates cardiac arrhythmias, gastroparesis, and ileus. Potassium chloride should be added to the intravenous fluids. If the serum potassium remains low despite supplementation, the problem is often one of hypomagnesemia. Supplementing the intravenous fluids with magnesium chloride will help alleviate the hypokalemia.

PROGNOSIS

The lifetime risk of dying from GDV in large and giant breed dogs, given a case mortality rate of 30%, is approximately 7%.[1] The Great Dane's likelihood of death is higher (12.6%).

Mortality for dilatation in the absence of confirmed gastric displacement is only 0.9%.[19] Postoperative mortality for dogs is reported at 15%[5] to 18%.[21] When gastric necrosis is so severe as to require resection (13.5%), mortality increased to 30% to 35%.[5,27] In dogs with gastric necrosis, the morbidity likely increases as a result of associated disease processes including splenectomy and preoperative cardiac dysrhythmias.[6] Importantly, the age of the dog does not adversely affect survival following surgery.[6]

REFERENCES

1. Glickman LT, Glickman NW, Schellenberg DB, *et al.*: Incidence of and breed-related risk factors for gastric dilatation-volvulus in dogs. *J Am Vet Med Assoc* 216: 40, 2000.
2. Patronek GJ, Waters DJ, Glickman LT: Comparative longevity of pet dogs and humans: implications for longevity research. *J Gerontol Biol Sci* 52:B171, 1997.
3. Glickman LT, Glickman NW, Pérez C, *et al.*: Epidemiologic studies of bloat in dogs. *Vet Previews* 2:10, 1995.
4. Glickman L, Emerick T, Glickman N, *et al.*: Radiological assessment of the relationship between thoracic conformation and the risk of gastric dilatation-volvulus in dogs. *Vet Radiol Ultrasound* 37:174, 1996.
5. Glickman LT, Glickman NW, Schellenberg DB, *et al.*: Multiple risk factors for the gastric dilatation-volvulus syndrome in dogs: a practicioner/owner case-control study. *J Am Anim Hosp Assoc* 33:197, 1997.
6. Leib MS, Wingfield WE, Twedt DC, *et al.*: Plasma gastrin immunoreactivity in dogs with gastric dilatation-volvulus. *J Am Vet Med Assoc* 185:205, 1984.
7. Hall JA, Twedt DC, Curtis CR: Relationship of plasma gastrin immunoreactivity and gastroesophageal sphincter pressure in clinically normal dogs and dogs with previous gastric dilatation-volvulus. *Am J Vet Res* 50:1228, 1989.
8. van Sluijs FJ, van den Brom DE: Gastric emptying of a radionucleotide-labeled test meal after surgical correction of gastric dilatation-volvulus in dogs. *Am J Vet Res* 50:433, 1989.
9. Hall JA, Willer RL, Seim HB, *et al.*: Gastric emptying of nondigestible radiopaque markers after circumcostal gastropexy in clinically normal dogs and dogs with gastric dilatation-volvulus. *Am J Vet Res* 53:1961, 1992.
10. Van Kruiningen HG, Gregoirie K, Meuten DJ: Acute gastric dilatation: a review of comparative aspects by species, and a study in dogs and monkeys. *J Am Anim Hosp Assoc* 10:294, 1974.
11. Van Kruiningen HJ, Wojan LD, Stake PE, *et al.*: The influence of diet and feeding frequency on gastric function in the dog. *J Am Anim Hosp Assoc* 23:145, 1987.

11a. Glickman LT, Glickman NW, Schellenberg DB, *et al.*: Non-dietary risk factors for gastric dilatation-volvulus in large and giant breed dogs. *J Am Vet Med Assoc* 217, 1492, 2000.

12. Caywood D, Teague HD, Jackson DA, *et al.*: Gastric gas analysis in the canine gastric dilatation-volvulus syndrome. *J Am Anim Hosp Assoc* 13:459, 1977.
13. Wingfield WE, Cornelius LM, Ackerman, N, *et al.*: Experimental acute gastric dilation and torsion in the dog. 2. Venous angiographic alterations seen in gastric dilation. *J Small Anim Pract* 16:55, 1975.
14. Baronofsky I, Wangensteen OH: Obstruction of splenic vein increases weight of the stomach and predisposes to erosion of ulcer. *Proc Soc Exp Biol Med* 59:234, 1945.
15. Tsapagas MJ, Peabody RA, Karmody AM, *et al.*: Pathophysiological changes following ischemia of the spleen. *Ann Surg* 178:179, 1973.
16. Leib MS, Blass CE: Acute gastric dilatation in the dog: various clinical presentations. *Compend Contin Educ Pract Vet* 6:707, 1984.

17. Hathcock JR: Radiographic view of choice for the diagnosis of gastric-volvulus: the right lateral recumbent view. *J Am Anim Hosp Assoc* 20:967, 1984.
18. Muir WW: Gastric dilatation-volvulus in the dog, with emphasis on cardiac arrhythmias. *J Am Vet Med Assoc* 180:739, 1982.
19. de Papp E, Drobatz KJ, Hughes D: Plasma lactate concentration as a predictor of gastric necrosis and survival among dogs with gastric dilatation-volvulus: 102 cases (1995–1998). *J Am Vet Med Assoc* 215:49, 1999.
20. Brockman DJ, Washabau RJ, Drobatz KJ: Canine gastric dilatation/volvulus syndrome in a veterinary critical care unit: 295 cases (1986–1992). *J Am Vet Med Assoc* 207:460, 1995.
21. Brourman JD, Schertel ER, Allen DA, *et al.*: Factors associated with perioperative mortality in dogs with surgically managed gastric dilatation-volvulus: 137 cases (1988–1993). *J Am Vet Med Assoc* 208:1855, 1996.
22. Merkley DF, Howard DR, Eyster GE, *et al.*: Experimentally induced acute gastric dilatation in the dog: cardiopulmonary effects. *J Am Anim Hosp Assoc* 12:143, 1976.
23. Orton EC, Muir WW: Hemodynamics during experimental gastric dilatation-volvulus in dogs. *Am J Vet Res* 44:1512, 1983.
24. Wagner AE, Dunlop CI, Chapman PL: Cardiopulmonary measurements in dogs undergoing gastropexy without gastrectomy for correction of gastric dilatation-volvulus. *J Am Vet Med Assoc* 215:484, 1999.
25. Badylak SF, Lantz GC, Jefferies M: Prevention of reperfusion injury in surgically induced gastric dilatation-volvulus in dogs. *Am J Vet Res* 51:294, 1990.
26. Lantz GC, Badylak SF, Hiles MC, *et al.*: Treatment of reperfusion injury in dogs with experimentally induced gastric dilatation-volvulus. *Am J Vet Res* 53:1594, 1992.
27. Clark G, Pavletic M: Partial gastrectomy with an automatic stapling instrument for treatment of gastric necrosis secondary to gastric dilatation-volvulus. *Vet Surg* 20: 61, 1991.

51

Acute Hemorrhagic Diarrhea

Tim Hackett

INTRODUCTION

Gastrointestinal problems are a common presenting complaint in veterinary medicine. Not only are problems like anorexia, vomiting, and diarrhea frequent reasons for pet owners to seek veterinary care, animals may develop gastrointestinal dysfunction as a complication of systemic illness. The gastrointestinal tract and liver are considered the shock organs of dogs[1] and are therefore subject to damage with a variety of other systemic problems. These problems tend to occur following states of poor perfusion and impaired oxygen delivery because the splanchnic circulation is particularly vulnerable to hypoperfusion. This vulnerability is evident in hemorrhagic models of shock where splanchnic perfusion decreases rapidly and out of proportion to other major organ systems.[2] Splanchnic hypoperfusion and gastrointestinal dysfunction can be clinically seen as mild changes in appetite, anorexia, to loss of intestinal mucosal integrity, hemorrhagic diarrhea, enteric bacterial translocation, septicemia, and death.

While azotemia and oliguria clearly indicate renal dysfunction and coma scores objectively define neurologic impairment, the gastrointestinal tract has many functions that are not subject to objective clinical measurements. The gut is not just for digestion and nutrient absorption. It is a metabolically active, immunologically unique reservoir of potential pathogens.[3] However clinically difficult it may be to monitor splanchnic perfusion; the intensivist must remain diligent and attempt to diminish the risk of complications associated with gastrointestinal dysfunction.

Of all the clinical manifestation of gastrointestinal failure, acute, hemorrhagic diarrhea is one of the most serious.[4] Uncontrolled diarrhea causes massive fluid, electrolyte, and protein loss. Hemorrhagic diarrhea, regardless of cause, signals a loss of normal mucosal integrity. With loss of this barrier, normal enteric flora can cross into the bloodstream leading to septicemia. The combination of dehydration, anemia, hypoproteinemia, and septicemia reduce systemic perfusion and oxygen delivery putting the patient at risk of multiple organ dysfunction.[3] The intensivist needs to address the life threatening complications of hemorrhagic diarrhea while determining the cause.

PATHOGENESIS

The small intestine functions to propel, mix, and digest food, secrete enzymes and fluids, and selectively absorb water, electrolytes, and nutrients. Enormous quantities of fluid and electrolytes are cycled through the intestine each day. Almost half of the total volume of extracellular fluid is secreted into the upper gastrointestinal tract each day, an amount that greatly exceeds normal intake. Normal fecal water and electrolyte loss is less than 0.1% of the fluid cycled through the gastrointestinal tract.[1] With abnormal secretion and/or impaired absorption, the potential exists for massive fluid and electrolyte loss.

Diarrhea results from accumulation of osmotically active particles in the intestinal tract, excess solute secretion, impaired absorption, or alterations of intestinal motility. It is important to review all these mechanisms as one or all may occur together in the individual patient with diarrhea.[1,4]

Osmotic diarrhea results when unabsorbable solutes increase fecal water content. Osmotic diarrhea can result from overeating, sudden dietary changes, maldigestion, or malabsorption. Bacterial enterotoxins will enhance secretion. Bacterial pathogens that are known to cause secretory diarrhea include *Escherichia coli*, *Staphylococcus aureus*, *Klebsiella pneumoniae*, *Yersinia enterocolitica*, *Salmonella typhimurium*, *Campylobacter* spp., and *Clostridium perfringens*.[1,4,5]

Enteric hormones, fatty acids, and bile acids also stimulate intestinal secretion. Malabsorption is caused by anything affecting the mucosal or submucosal layers of the intestine. With damage to the mucosa, normal sodium reabsorption is impaired, fecal water increases, and diarrhea results. Motility changes that speed intestinal transit cause diarrhea. By decreasing transit time, insufficient water is resorbed and diarrhea results. Hookworm infection, canine and feline dysautonomia, and colitis have been associated with deranged intestinal motility.[1]

Of all the causes of diarrhea, the mechanism most frequently associated with hemorrhagic diarrhea is an increase in intestinal permeability. The normal mucosa of the large and small intestine forms a semipermeable barrier to control and movement of fluid and electrolytes while preventing the loss of larger molecules and is made up of a glycocalyx and epithelial cells. The epithelial cells are connected with tight junctions on their apical borders that are important in maintaining the integrity of the mucosal barrier. The morphology and number of tight junctions in various regions of the intestinal tract alters permeability and absorption. While the tight junctions high in the small intestine are permeable to fluid, electrolytes, and other small solutes, the barrier in the colon is impermeable to fluid and electrolytes. Fluid moves in a passive manner into and out of the small intestine, while active transport systems move electrolytes in the colon. Finally, the capillaries and lymphatics of the mucosa help maintain normal integrity by conserving plasma protein and removing absorbed fluid to prevent an increase in interstitial hydrostatic pressure. In addition to fluid and electrolyte homeostasis, the integrity of the mucosal barrier is closely guarded by cellular and humoral components of the immune system and the mononuclear/phagocyte system of the liver. Even bile salts play a role in defense by binding endotoxin into detergent-like complexes within the intestinal lumen. With normal intestinal integrity, a functioning local immune system and liver, fluid, and protein balance is achieved and the plethora of potential pathogens kept in their place.

Mild changes in intestinal permeability will permit electrolytes to flow back into the lumen of the bowel. Normally the enterocytes and their tight junctions retain electrolytes creating a gradient for the conservation of water. With the loss of the normal osmotic gradient, fecal water concentration increases and when it exceeds the absorptive capacity of the remaining bowel, diarrhea results. With further damage to the mucosal barrier, interstitial proteins are lost into the bowel. If the process extends into the lamina propria and blood vessels, more plasma proteins and even blood will be lost. The loss of red blood cells requires over a 10,000-fold increase in intestinal pore size.[1]

Increased intestinal permeability can result from epithelial erosion and ulceration, inflammation, cellular infiltration with inflammatory or neoplastic cells, lymphatic and interstitial hypertension, and ischemia. Erosions and ulceration can be seen with severe inflammation (inflammatory bowel disease), neoplasia (lymphoma), and infectious diseases (parvovirus enteritis).[6] Anti-inflammatory drugs, toxins, and excess gastrin (renal insufficiency or gastrin producing tumors), and mast cell tumors have also been implicated.[1,4,6]

Parvovirus enteritis is a common clinical problem in young (10–16 week old) dogs. Starting with anorexia and vomiting, the disease can quickly progress to severe diarrhea, dehydration, and even death.[7,8] Lesions begin in the distal duodenum, which becomes thickened and discolored. As the disease progresses, the jejunum becomes more severely affected. Intestinal lesions are characterized by necrosis of the crypt epithelium. The villi become shortened or completely obliterated as the virus impairs normal epithelial replacement.[9] Therapy is supportive as described for all causes of hemorrhagic diarrhea. Because of the immaturity of the parvovirus patient's immune system, plasma replacement should be considered in addition to crystalloid fluid therapy and broad-spectrum antibiotics.

Hemorrhagic gastroenteritis syndrome of dogs (HGE) is a unique clinical entity of unknown etiology that seems to be separate from other causes. The syndrome usually occurs in young adult dogs with a median age of 5 years. Signs begin with acute vomiting and rapidly progress to severe hemorrhagic diarrhea. Profound hypovolemia results in signs of circulatory shock and hemoconcentration. Treatment is as previously described with antibiotics to prevent bacterial translocation, aggressive crystalloid fluid therapy, and colloid fluids, if indicated.[10]

DIAGNOSTIC EVALUATION

Obtunded, dehydrated, febrile animals with diarrhea should be evaluated for systemic disease. A complete physical examination should identify life-threatening complications associated with blood and fluid loss. Priority is given to stabilizing the cardiopulmonary system with intravenous fluids, supplemental oxygen, electrolyte replacement, and parenteral antimicrobials while a definitive diagnosis is pursued. Increased intestinal permeability is clinically characterized by hypoproteinemia, melena, and hematochezia.[1,4] A complete blood count should always be evaluated. Animals with idiopathic hemorrhagic gastroenteritis may have packed cell volumes as high as 75%. Severe intestinal blood loss can lead to anemia and panhypoproteinemia. Infection with either *Salmonella* spp. or canine parvovirus is associated with neutropenia. Leukocytosis with lymphopenia and eosinopenia (stress leukogram) is a common finding in any debilitated animal with gastroenteritis. A normal leukogram in a sick animal with gastrointestinal disease should prompt an ACTH stimulation test to evaluate possible adrenocortical insufficiency.

A complete serum biochemical profile is necessary to evaluate other organ systems. Glucose should be checked on admission and at least once a day thereafter to detect hypoglycemia associated with sepsis. Electrolytes including sodium, chloride, potassium, and magnesium can drop precipitously in anorectic animals with diarrhea. Hyperkalemia with hyponatremia is another indication of adrenocortical insufficiency, but these changes can also be seen with whipworm (*Trichuris vulpis*) infections. Hypocholesterolemia is another common finding with hypoadrenocorticism. Samples for baseline renal function including BUN, creatinine, phosphorous, calcium, and urine specific gravity should be collected before intravenous fluid therapy begins.

Examination of feces is indicated in any diarrheic state. In one study, infectious agents were identified in over 25% of dogs presenting to a veterinary teaching hospital with diarrhea.[11] Direct fecal examination should be performed, as should zinc sulfate flotation. Some parasites, *Giardia* spp. and *Trichuris*, may be difficult to find so multiple examinations should be performed. Using a saline-moistened swab, a thin smear of feces is rolled onto a glass slide. The slide is air dried and stained with a Romanowsky-type stain. The smear is examined for abnormal numbers of inflammatory cells, abnormal populations of bacteria or *Clostridium perfringens* spores. Acid fast staining is useful to pick out *Campylobacter jejuni*. Enzyme linked immunosorbent assays (ELISA) are available to detect canine parvovirus, *Giardia* spp., and *Cryptosporidium parvum* antigens. The canine parvovirus ELISA test will detect the feline panleukopenia parvovirus. Electron microscopy can be used to identify other viral pathogens in the stool.

Fecal culture is indicated in animals with inflammatory changes on the fecal smear. Pathogenic and zoonotic bacteria causing enterocolitis include *Salmonella* spp., *Campylobacter jejuni*, *Shigella* spp., and *Yersinia enterocolitica*. These species are of particular concern for hospitalized patients, in multi-animal households, kennels, and homes of immunocompromised individuals.[11] At least 3 grams of fresh stool should be collected for culture.

TREATMENT

Nutrition

There are enough serious, predictable, systemic complications of acute hemorrhagic diarrhea to warrant immediate supportive care. Animals with acute gastroenteritis have often been fasted for 12 to 48 hours and then fed small amounts of a low-fat diet for several more days.[1] The absence of nutrients in the gastrointestinal tract reduces secretions and decreases the concentration of osmotically active particles. For this reason, fasting seems a logical step for secretory and osmotic diarrhea. When fasting animals with acute gastrointestinal disease it is important to remember that the gastrointestinal tract receives much of its nourishment from food passing through the bowel. Early feeding of patients with diarrhea may make more sense in those cases with increased mucosal permeability. Enteral feeding maintains greater mucosal barrier integrity and helps minimize malnutrition.[12] Experimental studies have shown that antibacterial host defenses, such as lymphocyte, neutrophil, and gut-associated immune functions are better preserved in enterally fed humans and animals.[13] A study with human volunteers demonstrated impaired neutrophil function, an exaggerated catabolic hormone response and increased cytokine production after endotoxin challenge in subjects receiving total parenteral nutrition and complete bowel rest for 7 days when compared to subjects receiving an enteral diet.[14] Glutamine is the main metabolic substrate exerting trophic effects on enterocytes supporting their normal function. Primarily extracted via luminal absorption, enough glutamine is also synthesized in the normal gut to be considered a non-essential amino acid. However, during states of illness, this synthetic ability is inadequate to meet these metabolic needs of the enterocytes. Mucosal integrity may require glutamine supplementation to form and repair intracellular tight junctions. Glutamine is also important in the synthesis of the protective mucus gel layer and is an essential nutrient for proper cellular immune functions.[15] Dosages for glutamine supplementation have been extrapolated from the human literature. The recommended dose for dogs with hemorrhagic diarrhea secondary to parvovirus enteritis is 0.5 g/kg/day divided BID in the drinking water.[8]

Fluid Therapy

Parenteral fluid therapy is aimed at restoring lost fluids (dehydration), provided normal requirements (maintenance) and, importantly, keeping up with ongoing losses. While oral fluid therapy may be adequate for simple diarrhea in a hydrated animal, animals with marked dehydration or hemorrhagic diarrhea should have an intravenous catheter to receive parenteral fluids and antibiotics. Fluid therapy must be individualized for each patient based on acid base status, electrolyte concentrations, plasma protein concentrations, and packed cell volume, as these can be highly variable in patients with diarrhea. Choices of which crystalloid fluid to use, the use of whole blood, packed red blood cells, plasma, or synthetic colloids should be based on serial physical examination, monitoring of packed cell volume, serum total solids, and electrolyte concentrations.

In severely dehydrated patients, fluid therapy is started with an isotonic crystalloid fluid at rates up to 90 mL/kg/hour in the dog and 45 mL/kg/hour in the cat. Rapid administration of crystalloid fluids will expand the intravascular space. However, within an hour, 75% to 85% of the infused crystalloid will have moved out of the vascular space and into the interstitial fluid compartment.[16] Patients with gastrointestinal protein loss will already have low plasma oncotic pressures. With crystalloid fluid resuscitation, plasma oncotic pressure is further reduced. Colloids are indicated to expand and maintain intravascular volume in hypovolemic patients with reduced plasma oncotic pressures. The choice of colloid depends on the source of protein loss and the need for other blood pro-

Table 51-1. Common Antibiotic Protocols for the Treatment of Hemorrhagic Diarrhea.

Cephoxitin (22 mg/kg IV TID)
Enrofloxacin (5–10 mg/kg IV BID) *and* ampicillin (22 mg/kg IV BID to TID)
Amikacin (20 mg/kg IV once daily) *and* ampicillin (22 mg/kg IV BID to TID)
Gentamicin 6.6 mg/kg IV once daily *and* ampicillin (22 mg/kg IV BID to TID)
Trimethoprim-sulfadiazine (30 mg/kg SQ BID)

teins. In addition to oncotic support, fresh frozen plasma transfusion can provide albumin, amino acids, coagulation precursors, and anticoagulants (protein C and antithrombin III).[17] Synthetic colloids, such as hydroxyethyl starch, are less expensive, easier to store, and provide more cardiovascular support than albumin.[18] When the goal is improved plasma oncotic pressure, hetastarch and Dextrans 70 provide more predictable oncotic support than plasma in patients with ongoing protein loss.[16]

Antibiotics

Resident microbial flora in the intestinal tract include anaerobic bacteria which outnumber the aerobic gram-negative organisms 100 to 1000 times.[3] Because the anaerobic flora occupy the mucous layer adjacent to the epithelial cells their presence can prevent the adherence of other potential pathogens. Antibiotic therapy should not simply target the anaerobes. Instead, the clinician should employ a balanced approach toward both gram-negative and anaerobic pathogens (Table 51-1). The use of antibiotics is controversial with simple diarrhea. However, with severe hemorrhagic diarrhea, the clinician must assume the patient has a serious loss of intestinal mucosal integrity and parenteral bactericidal antibiotic therapy is indicated. The goal of antibiotic therapy is aimed at eliminating enteric bacteria that have passed through the mucosa, entered the bloodstream, and possibly taken up residence in distant organs like the liver. Care is taken to provide coverage for both gram-negative pathogens and anaerobic bacteria. Gentamicin should be used with extreme caution in dehydrated or hypokalemic animals. Trimethoprim-sulfadiazine is only bacteriostatic and therefore is only recommended for mild cases without signs of systemic disease. Animals with fecal cultures positive for bacterial pathogens may be treated according to the sensitivity pattern of the culture. Animals with positive blood cultures should have an antibiotic plan chosen based on the organisms identified.

Other Therapies

Analgesia should be considered in patients showing signs of abdominal pain. Objective serial monitoring of critically ill patients is necessary when pain is appropriately treated. Nonsteroidal and steroidal anti-inflammatory drugs may complicate gastrointestinal hemorrhage by inhibiting the production of normal protective prostaglandins. Narcotic analgesics can be used as long as respiratory and pulmonary function is monitored.

Animals with acute inflammation of the gastrointestinal tract may be extremely nauseous. Nausea may manifest clinically as anorexia, hypersalivation, or emesis. Anti-emetic drugs can provide a degree of relief not offered by fluids or analgesics. Metclopramide by continuous infusion at 1 to 2 mg/kg/day is the preferred agent at our hospital. Other anti-emetics include chlorpromazine (0.2 to 0.4 mg/kg IM or SQ TID to QID) and ondansetron (0.1 mg/kg IV or PO TID). Chlorpromazine is an alpha-blocker and should be used in caution with hypovolemic patients.

PROGNOSIS

The prognosis for patients with acute gastrointestinal hemorrhage is dependent on etiology and the presence of concurrent organ dysfunction. Young dogs with HGE syndrome generally respond quickly to volume replacement and have an excellent prognosis.[10] Parvoviral enteritis can produce severe dehydration, shock, and multiple organ failure. With aggressive supportive care, survival rates of 5% to 12% have been reported.[8,19] Morbidity and mortality for other causes of acute gastrointestinal hemorrhage depend on the primary cause, the presence of bacterial translocation and sepsis, and concurrent organ failure. The challenge to the intensivist is to replace lost fluids, electrolytes, and proteins while preventing septic complications. It is vital to monitor major organ function, and treat the primary disease and secondary organ dysfunction in a timely manner.

REFERENCES

1. Guilford WG, Strombeck DR: Classification, Pathophysiology, and Symptomatic Treatment of Diarrheal Diseases. *In* Guilford WG, ed., *Strombeck's Small Animal Gastroenterology*. Philadelphia: W.B. Saunders Company, 1996, p 351.
2. McNeill JR, Srark RD, Greenway CV: Intestinal vasoconstriction after hemorrhage: Roles of vasopressin and angiotensin. *Am J Physiol* 219:1342, 1970.
3. Biffl WL, Moore EE: Role of the Gut in Multiple Organ Failure. *In* Grenvik A, ed., *Textbook of Critical Care*. Philadelphia: W.B. Saunders Company, 2000, p 1627.
4. Dow SW: Acute medical diseases of the small intestine. *In* Tams TR ed., *Handbook of Small Animal Gastroenterology*. Philadelphia: W.B. Saunders Company, 1996, 246–266.
5. Sasaki J, Goryo M, Asahina M, *et al.*: Hemorrhagic enteritis associated with *Clostridium perfringens* type A in a dog. *J Vet Med Sci* 61:175, 1999.
6. Moreland KJ: Ulcer disease of the upper gastrointestinal tract in small animals: Pathophysiology, diagnosis, and management. *Comp Contin Ed Pract Vet* 10:1265–1280, 1988.
7. Smith-Carr S, Macintire DK, Swango LJ: Canine parvovirus part I: Pathogenesis and vaccination. *Compend Contin Educ Pract Vet* 19:125–133, 1997.
8. Macintire DK, Smith-Carr S: Canine parvovirus part II: Clinical signs, diagnosis and treatment. *Compend Contin Educ Pract Vet* 19:291–302, 1997.
9. Hoskins JD: Canine viral enteritis. *In* Green CE, Ed. *Infectious Diseases of the Dog and Cat*. Philadelphia: W.B. Saunders Co. Philadelphia, pp 40–49, 1990.
10. Spielman BL, Garvey MS: Hemorrhagic gastroenteritis in dogs. *J Amer Anim Hosp Assoc* 29:341–344, 1993.

11. Hackett TB, Lappin MR: Prevalence of enteric pathogens in dogs. *Journal of Veterinary Internal Medicine* 14:382, 2000.
12. Deitch EA: Role of the gut in the pathogenesis of sepsis and multiple organ failure. *Proceedings, Fifth International Veterinary Emergency and Critical Care Symposium*. San Antonio, TX, pp 1–4, 1996.
13. Mainhous MR, Block EF, Deitch EA: Nutritional support of the gut: How and why. *New Horizons* 2:193, 1994.
14. Fong Y, Marano M, Barber A, *et al.*: Total parenteral nutrition and bowel rest modify the response to endotoxin in humans. *Ann Surg* 210:449, 1989.
15. Mazzaferro EM, Hackett TB, *et al.*: Role of glutamine in health and disease. *Comp Contin Ed Pract Vet* 22:1094–1103, 2000.
16. Concannon KT: Colloid oncotic pressure and the clinical use of colloidal solutions. *J Vet Emerg Crit Care* 3:49–62, 1993.
17. Haskins SC: Management of septic shock. *J Am Vet Med Assoc* 200:1915–1924, 1992.
18. Haupt MT, Rackow EC: Colloid osmotic pressure and fluid resuscitation with hetastarch, albumin, and saline solutions. *Crit Care Med* 10:159–162, 1981.
19. Houston DM, Ribble CS, Head LL: Risk factors associated with parvovirus enteritis in dogs: 283 cases (1982–1991). *J Am Vet Med Assoc* 208:542–546, 1996.

52
Acute Pancreatitis in the Dog

Donald S. Westfall

INTRODUCTION

Canine pancreatitis is subdivided into chronic and acute forms.[1,2] Chronically recurring mild pancreatitis results in intermittent vomiting and anorexia; this syndrome can lead to progressive pancreatic glandular damage and eventual fulminant acute pancreatitis.[1,2] Because this text is focused on critically ill patients, the remainder of this section will be directed toward the acute form of pancreatitis.

Pancreatitis is a diagnostic challenge. A combination of history, clinical signs, laboratory abnormalities, and diagnostic imaging studies is necessary to arrive at a correct diagnosis. Pancreatitis is also a therapeutic challenge. The high incidence of secondary complications can lead to high mortality rates if one is not careful in monitoring and aggressively anticipating and treating complications.

PATHOGENESIS

The most widely accepted theory in the development of acute pancreatitis is that pancreatic digestive enzyme activation occurs within the gland, resulting in autodigestion. Normally, autodigestion is prevented by pancreatic storage of digestive enzymes as inactive zymogens, which are activated once enzymatic cleavage of a peptide bond occurs.[1-4] Activation occurs within the small intestinal lumen as a series of events. The mucosal enzyme enterokinase, which is produced by duodenal enterocytes, cleaves trypsinogens to make trypsins.[1-4] The physical separation of enterokinase (within the duodenum) from the zymogen, trypsinogen (within the pancreas), is one protective mechanism against autodigestion.[3] Trypsins, in turn, activate other zymogens, including chymotrypsinogen, proelastase, procarboxypeptidases A and B, procolipase, and prophospholipase A.[1-3] Protection against autodigestion is also achieved by sequestration and separation of digestive enzymes and lysosomal enzymes within the lumen of the pancreatic rough endoplasmic reticulum.[1-4] The two remain separated as lysosomal enzymes are incorporated into lysosomes and pancreatic enzymes into zymogens, which prevents intrapancreatic activation of zymogens by lysosomal proteases.[1-4]

If intrapancreatic activation of trypsinogen occurs, defense mechanisms limit autodigestion. The first defense is the ability of trypsin to self-hydrolyze.[1,2]

The second is trypsin inhibition by low- molecular-weight pancreatic secretory trypsin inhibitor, a substance released by pancreatic acinar cells.[1-4] Finally, the plasma protease inhibitors α_2-macroglobulin (α_2-M) and α_1-protease inhibitor (α_1-antitrypsin) bind with any digestive enzymes that are released into circulation to prevent widespread systemic damage.[1-6]

With pancreatitis, there is activation of pancreatic enzymes with lysosomes and zymogen granules fusing in the acinar cells, resulting in autodigestion.[1-4,6] It is thought that abnormal segregation of lysosomes and zymogens may be responsible for this process.[1,2] Autodigestion results from the action of proteases and activated trypsin on pancreatic tissue. Trypsin activates other zymogens, which furthers pancreatic inflammation.[1-4,6] Once autodigestion begins, inflammatory mediators, free radicals, and other vasoactive substances perpetuate the progression of disease.[1-4,6] Inflammatory mediators are directly injurious to pancreatic tissue, resulting in more damage, and increased enzyme activation and release.[1-4,6] Free radical damage is primarily mediated by peroxidation of lipid membranes.[1,2] Peroxidative damage to endothelial cells and vascular injury by phospholipase A_2 and elastase results in increased capillary permeability and pancreatic edema.[1-4] As pancreatic digestive enzymes are activated, edema progresses to hemorrhagic

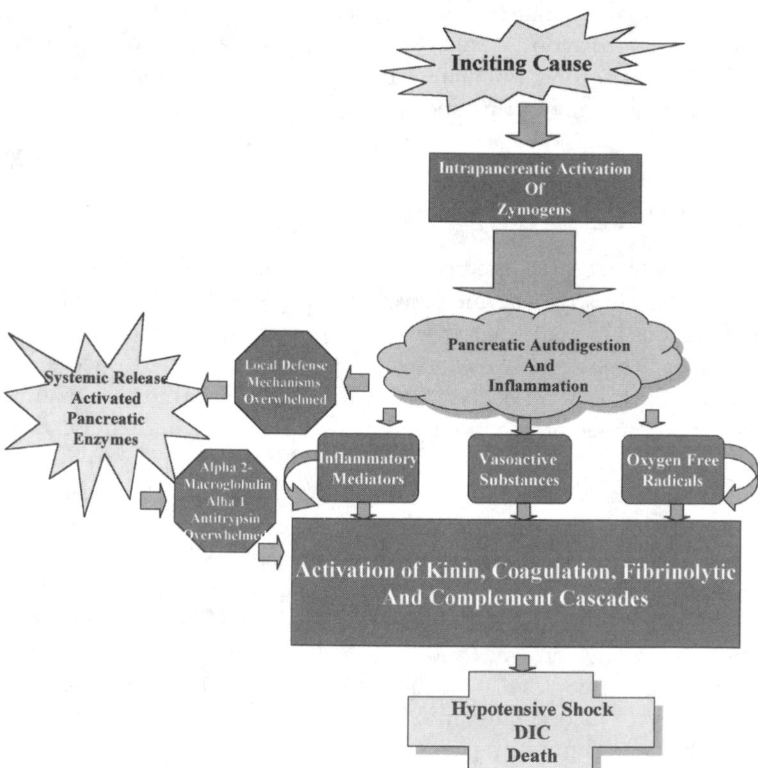

Figure 52-1
Pathogenesis of acute pancreatitis in the dog.

or necrotic pancreatitis.[1,2,6] Pancreatic digestive enzymes are released systemically as additional damage occurs.[1-4,6] Plasma protease inhibitors are overwhelmed, resulting in venous pooling, vascular compromise, hypotension, hypovolemia, and multisystemic organ damage as the inflammation spreads.[6] Activation of the kinin, coagulation, fibrinolytic, and complement cascade systems may lead to shock and disseminated intravascular coagulation (DIC)[1-4] (Fig. 52-1).

ETIOLOGY

Many etiologies have been proposed for the pathogenesis of pancreatitis; however, the underlying cause remains largely unknown.[1-5] Potential etiologies include nutritional factors, drugs and toxins, biliary duct obstruction, abdominal or surgical trauma, pancreatic ischemia, and infectious causes.[1-6] Classically, pancreatitis is associated with the ingestion of a high-fat meal or dietary indiscretion.[1-7] Concurrent endocrinopathies such as diabetes mellitus, hyperadrenocorticism, and hypothyroidism are risk factors for the development of fatal acute pancreatitis.[7] A prior history of gastrointestinal disease is also a risk factor for the development of fatal acute pancreatitis.[7]

Nutritional Factors

Obesity has been recognized as a predisposing condition leading to pancreatitis.[1-6,8] The presence of appropriate clinical signs in an obese patient raises the index of suspicion for pancreatitis. Because the pancreas responds to dietary influences, certain types of nutrients are more highly associated with the development of pancreatitis than are others. Classically, high-fat, low-protein diets are associated with the development of pancreatitis.[1-7] This is probably due to the action of lipase on high levels of triglyceride in pancreatic capillaries resulting in the production of toxic fatty acids.[1-3] Hyperlipidemia syndromes are also associated with pancreatitis.[1-8] Idiopathic hyperlipidemias occur in miniature Schnauzer dogs.[1,8,9] It is possible that underlying endocrinopathies that result in hypertriglyceridemia may predispose to the development of pancreatitis through this mechanism.[7] Hyperlipidemia, however, may also be the end result of pancreatitis, due to peripancreatic mesenteric fat necrosis, rather than an inciting cause.[1-3]

Drugs and Toxins

Drugs that have been associated with pancreatitis in veterinary medicine include the thiazide diuretics, furosemide, estrogens, azathioprine, L-asparaginase, sulfonamides, tetracyclines, metronidazole, cimetidine, ranitidine, acetaminophen, procainamide, and nitrofurantoin.[1-6] However, reports are only anecdotal and no cause-and-effect relationship has been proven.[1-3] Corticosteroids and H_2-receptor antagonists also have been associated with pancreatitis.[1,2] Cholinesterase inhibitor insecticides and anticholinergic or cholinergic drugs may overstimulate the pancreas and result in pancreatitis.[1,2,4] Overstimulation may also occur with hypercalcemia and scorpion stings.[1-3]

Pancreatic Duct Disease

Any cause of pancreatic duct obstruction may lead to pancreatic inflammation and edema.[1,2] Reflux of duodenal contents through the pancreatic duct leads to severe acute pancreatitis.[1,2,4,6] This is a result of the direct action of enterokinase, activated pancreatic enzymes, bacteria, and bile on the pancreatic tissue.[1,2] Associated conditions include protracted vomiting, duodenal trauma, or any disease process resulting in abnormally high duodenal pressures sufficient to overwhelm the sphincter of the pancreatic duct's opening.[1,2,4]

Trauma and Ischemia

Surgical manipulation or biopsy of the pancreas may result in clinical pancreatitis. However, the risk of inducing pancreatitis when properly handling pancreatic tissue or biopsying the pancreas is minimal.[1,2,4] Direct trauma to the pancreas resulting from abdominal injury is a rare cause of pancreatitis in veterinary medicine.[1,2] Pancreatic ischemia secondary to hypovolemic shock or anesthesia may result in pancreatitis, and failure to maintain adequate volume in cases of clinical pancreatitis may worsen clinical signs and delay recovery.[1-6]

Infection

Bacterial infection is not usually a primary cause of pancreatitis; however, concurrent sepsis may worsen the severity of the disease.[1,2] This may occur as a consequence of pancreatitis and loss of intestinal mucosal integrity, resulting in bacterial translocation.[1,2,8] Inflamed, necrotic pancreatic tissue may be a suitable media for bacterial growth.[3,4] Viral and protozoal causes of pancreatitis have been reported.[1,2]

CLINICAL PRESENTATION

Historical Findings

Historical findings in cases of canine pancreatitis include lethargy, depression, anorexia, vomiting, weakness, diarrhea, dehydration, abdominal pain, and fever.[1-6,8] Ingestion of a dietary indiscretion or fatty meal supports a diagnosis of pancreatitis; however, many cases have no such history.[1,2,4,6] Most dogs that develop pancreatitis are over 5 years old.[1,2,6,7]

Clinical Signs

Polyuria, polydipsia, and weight loss may accompany the clinical signs of pancreatitis due to concurrent diseases such as diabetes mellitus.[8] The dog may assume a praying position due to abdominal pain.[1,2,4,6]

Physical Examination

The dog is likely to be obese on physical examination.[6,8] Dehydration is a result of anorexia and protracted vomiting, and, in severe cases, hypovolemic

Table 52-1. Historical and Physical Examination Findings in Dogs with Fatal Acute Pancreatitis

Historical Findings		Physical Examination Findings	
Anorexia	91%	Dehydration	97%
Vomiting	90%	Abdominal pain	58%
Weakness	79%	Obesity	43%
Painful abdomen	59%	Fever	32%
Polyuria/polydipsia	50%	Icterus	26%
Diarrhea	33%	Heart murmur	20%
Neurologic signs	20%	Coagulation abnormalities	
Melena	16%	Petechiation Ecchymoses Epistaxis Bruising	11%
Seizures	11%		
Weight loss	11%	Hematoma	
Hematemesis	10%	Harsh lung sounds	11%
Hematachezia	4%	Hypothermia	7%

Adapted from Hess RS, Saunders HM, Van Winkle TJ, *et al.*: Clinical, clinicopathologic, radiographic, and ultrasonographic abnormalities in dogs with fatal acute pancreatitis: 70 cases (1986–1995). *J Am Vet Med Assoc* 213:665, 1998.

shock. These result in clinical signs such as tachycardia, weak and thready pulses, cardiac dysrhythmias, and collapse. If significant bile duct compression is a consequence of pancreatic inflammation, icterus may be noted.[1-3,6,8,9] Abdominal effusion and a palpable mass or mass effect within the right cranial quadrant of the abdomen may be present[1,2,6] (Table 52-1).

DIAGNOSTIC EVALUATION

Complete Blood Count

A complete blood count usually reveals an inflammatory leukogram characterized by leukocytosis and neutrophilia with a left shift.[1-4,6,8,9] Severe cases with overwhelming infection, endotoxemia, or shock may have a degenerative left shift.[3,7,9] Hemoconcentration is usually present with dehydration.[1-4] Thrombocytopenia is present with DIC.[2-4,8,9]

Serum Chemistry Panel

Azotemia (increased serum urea nitrogen, creatinine, and phosphorous) results from dehydration or from acute renal failure due to hypovolemia, sepsis, lipid thrombi, or microthrombi associated with DIC.[1-4,6,8,9] Liver enzymes and total bilirubin are increased due to direct hepatotoxicity of systemically released activated pancreatic enzymes, hypovolemia resulting in hepatic ischemia, or secondary to cholestasis associated with biliary duct compression due to pancreatic inflammation.[1-4,6,8,9] Hyperglycemia develops in cases of acute necrotizing pancreatitis due to hyperglucagonemia and release of cortisol and catecholamines, or from the development of diabetes mellitus.[1-4,6,8,9] Hypoglycemia may also occur as a result of insulin therapy or sepsis.[8] Hypoalbuminemia results from third-space losses.[4,8] Hypocalcemia (once corrected for hypoalbuminemia) may result from fat breakdown by pancreatic lipase and calcium soap deposition,[1,2,6] by shifting of calcium into soft tissues such as muscle due to alterations in cell membranes,[4] or by altered levels of thyrocalcitonin and parathyroid hormone.[4] Hypercalcemia may occur more commonly than hypocalcemia.[8] Hyperlipidemia, hypertriglyceridemia, and hypercholesterolemia are common.[1-4,6,8,9]

Urinalysis

Hypersenthuria may be noted due to dehydration; isosthenuria or hyposthenuria and the presence of tubular casts in the urine sediment may be noted secondary to the development of renal failure.[3,4,8] Glucosuria and bilirubinuria may be present.[3,4] Ketonuria indicates the presence of concurrent diabetic ketoacidosis.[8]

Radiographs

The reported radiographic findings are seldom seen clinically, and a diagnosis made solely on radiographic signs should be approached with caution. The use of abdominal radiographs in the patient with pancreatitis enables the clinician to rule out other etiologies leading to acute vomiting, such as gastrointestinal obstruction.

Radiographic findings may include a mass effect in the right cranial quadrant of the abdomen, displacing the stomach to the left and cranially, the duodenum to the right, the transverse colon caudally, and increasing the distance between the proximal duodenum and pylorus.[1-4,6,8,11] Generalized ileus is often seen; a gas-distended proximal duodenum may also be noted.[1-4,6,8,11] Loss of abdominal detail due to presence of fluid within the peritoneal cavity may be seen.[1-4,6,11] A ground-glass appearance or presence of gas pockets in the peripancreatic area is also suggestive of pancreatitis.[1-4,6,11] Dual effusions in the abdomen and thoracic cavity may be noted.[8,9,12]

Because diagnosis based on radiographs is difficult, the use of abdominal ultrasound is recommended. A recent retrospective of necropsy-verified acute pancreatitis found that radiographs are consistent with pancreatitis 24% of the time, whereas ultrasound is consistent 68% of the time.[8]

Ultrasound

Ultrasound can be used to document pancreatitis and may help to differentiate pancreatitis, pancreatic neoplasia, pancreatic pseudocysts, and pancreatic abscesses.[1-2,4,6,11] Ultrasonographic findings suggestive of pancreatitis include a mixed echogenicity or a mass effect in the area of the pancreas, fluid-filled areas within the pancreas, a fluid- and gas-filled descending duodenum, a thick-walled

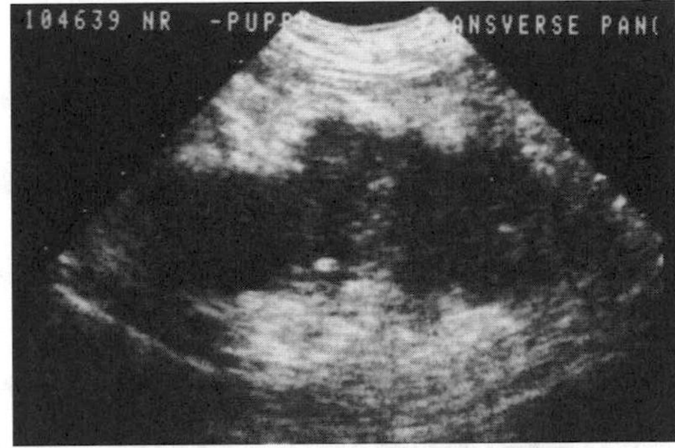

Figure 52-2
Ultrasonographic appearance of acute pancreatitis in the dog. Note the mixed echogenicity of the pancreas, and the fluid accumulation within the tissues surrounding the pancreas.

descending duodenum, an atonic duodenum, and abdominal effusion.[1-2,4,6,8,11] Dilation of the biliary system may occur with biliary obstruction[4,8,11] (Figs. 52-2, 52-3, and 52-4). Ultrasound can also be used to perform abdominocentesis on small pockets of effusion to aid in the diagnosis (see below).

Adjunct Laboratory Tests

Serum amylase and lipase activities can be used to support a diagnosis of pancreatitis; however, levels of these enzymes do not always correlate well with disease.[1-4,6,8,9,13-17] There is no correlation between severity of disease and magnitude of amylase and lipase elevation.[1,2,9] Organ-specific isoamylase determination may be helpful; however, this test is not widely available.[4,6] Enzyme levels may be elevated due to nonpancreatic diseases or may not be elevated in true cases of pancreatitis. Renal insufficiency, dehydration leading to prerenal azotemia, hepatic dysfunction, neoplasia, small intestinal disease, gastric disease, and other

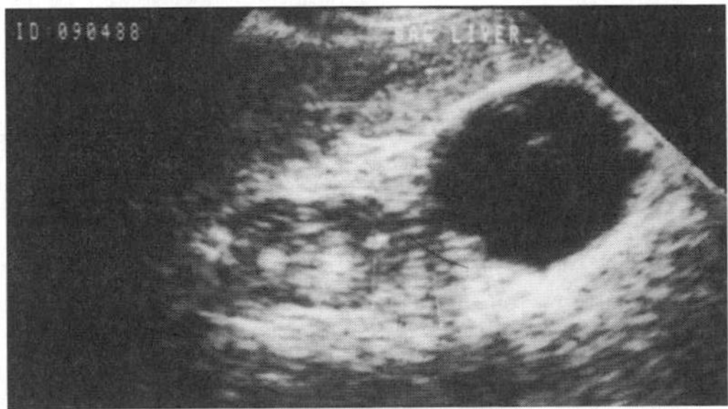

Figure 52-3
Ultrasonographic appearance of a pancreatic pseudocyst. There is a mixed echogenicity within the pancreas suggesting chronic inflammation. Note the peripancreatic walled-off fluid-filled structure (pancreatic pseudocyst). The appearance of a pancreatic pseudocyst is ultrasonographically indistinguishable from a pancreatic abscess.

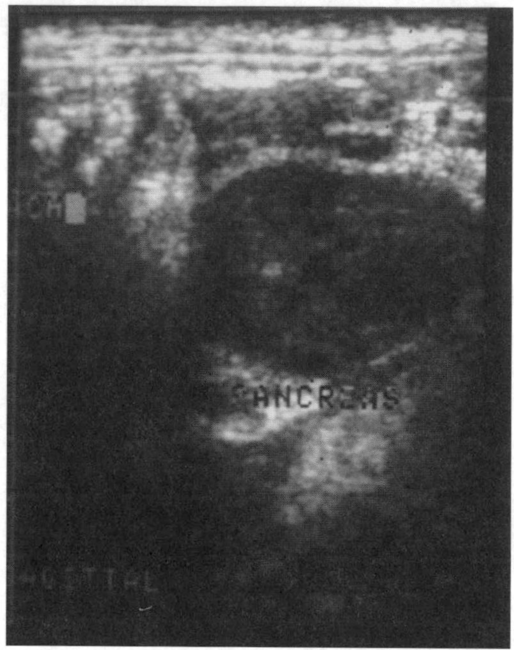

Figure 52-4
Ultrasonographic appearance of pancreatic adenocarcinoma.

pancreatic diseases (neoplasia) may lead to extrapancreatic sources of enzyme production or decreased excretion.[1-4,6,8,9,15,16] Amylase and lipase may also be falsely elevated due to glucocorticoid administration[1-3,6,9,14] and after abdominal surgery.[12] Amylase and lipase can be measured from recovered abdominal fluid to aid in the diagnosis of pancreatitis.[3,4,9] In pancreatitis, the activities of these enzymes in recovered abdominal fluid are dramatically higher than serum.

Serum phospholipase A_2 levels are high in cases of pancreatitis due to systemic release of activated pancreatic enzymes. Phospholipase A_2 assay has similar drawbacks to amylase and lipase determination, including lack of sensitivity and specificity.[1,2]

Trypsin-like immunoreactivity (TLI) is pancreas specific enzyme which originates from pancreatic and extrapancreatic tissues.[1,2,6,9,17,18] TLI measurement in canine pancreatitis is helpful because it rises sooner and to a greater degree than amylase and lipase activities.[1,2,6,17] The magnitude of TLI elevation may correlate with severity of disease.[18] TLI may also be increased due to decreased excretion with renal failure or dehydration.[3,4,9] Reduced levels of α_2-M and α_1-antitrypsin have been documented in cases of pancreatitis, although testing for these is not widely available.[4,6]

Clotting times should be performed in all suspected cases, especially if thrombocytopenia is present. Prothrombin time, activated partial thromboplastin time, activated clotting time, and fibrin degradation products may all be prolonged or elevated in pancreatitis cases.[8,9] It is important to serially monitor these tests to monitor for DIC development. In a recent study of fatal acute pancreatitis, 61% of the dogs had abnormal coagulation function tests.[8]

Cytologic examination of abdominal fluid is nonspecific; a nonseptic, suppurative exudate is characteristic of pancreatitis and other types of peritonitis.[3,4]

Summary of Diagnosis

Pancreatitis remains a diagnostic challenge. No single test can definitively obtain a diagnosis. The author prefers to use a combination of clinical signs, physical examination findings, laboratory abnormalities, and diagnostic imaging studies to arrive at a diagnosis. Additional diagnostic support can be obtained by abdominocentesis. Serum amylase and lipase activities are compared to the amylase and lipase activities within recovered abdominal effusion. If abdominal values are higher than the serum values, active pancreatitis is likely present.

TREATMENT

The foundation of treatment for pancreatitis is fluid and electrolyte support, plasma transfusion, maintenance of nutrition while suppressing pancreatic secretion, antiemetic therapy, pain management, prevention of bacterial translocation, and monitoring to prevent and quickly treat complications.[1-6] Severe cases may also require surgery for peritoneal lavage to alleviate clinical signs, to relieve biliary obstruction, for placement of an enteral nutrition feeding tube, and for biopsy of the pancreas.[1-6]

Fluid and Electrolyte Support

A balanced electrolyte crystalloid solution is the initial maintenance fluid of choice.[1-4,6] Potassium supplementation should be sufficient for maintenance (20 mEq/L) unless a potassium deficiency warrants additional supplementation.[1-3,5,6] If shock is present, a shock fluid rate is indicated while vital signs and packed cell volume and total solids are monitored.[3] Further volume resuscitation is achieved with the use of synthetic colloids. Once signs of hypovolemic shock have subsided, a maintenance fluid rate should be based on correction of preexisting dehydration and maintenance needs.[5] Estimations of fluid losses in vomitus and diarrhea should be appropriately replaced.[1,2,4-6]

Fluid resuscitation and maintenance of normovolemia may be sufficient to ensure adequate blood flow to the kidneys and pancreas. Additional perfusion is achieved by the use of dopamine hydrochloride at a dose that stimulates both dopaminergic and β-adrenergic receptors (2.0–5.0 μg/kg/min constant rate infusion [CRI] IV).[2]

Plasma Transfusion

Plasma is valuable in the treatment of pancreatitis.[1,2,4-6] α_2-M and α_1-antitrypsin are present in fresh-frozen, fresh plasma and whole blood. These constituents bind with and inactivate systemically circulating and locally activated pancreatic enzymes.[1-6] Albumin also binds detergents such as free fatty acids and lysolecithin, which are produced by the actions of phospholipase A_2 and lipase, that may disrupt cell membranes.[1,2,6]

Additionally, clotting factors and antithrombin III present in plasma help to prevent and treat DIC.[3] Prevention of DIC and thromboembolic sequelae can be achieved by the addition of heparin (Elkins-Sinn, Cherry Hill, NJ), 100 U/kg q 8 h SC. Heparin therapy is continued (see Section VI).

Nutrition

Historically, pancreatitis patients are held off of food and water for the duration of illness.[3-6] This prevents gastrin and cholecystokinin release, thereby decreasing pancreatic secretion.[3] Inhibitors of pancreatic secretion (anticholinergic drugs, somatostatin, acetazolamide, glucagon, and calcitonin) have not been proven effective in canine patients.[1-3,5,6] Nasogastric suction has been attempted to indirectly decrease pancreatic secretion; however, this is also ineffective in canine patients.[1,2,5,6]

Enteral nutrition, rather than parenteral nutrition has been advocated in canine pancreatitis,[1,2,19] and is preferred over parenteral nutrition in cases of human pancreatitis.[20-22] Enteral nutrition reduces intestinal villous atrophy and bacterial translocation, which decreases the incidence of sepsis and morbidity, and speeds recovery.[20-22] A weighted nasojejunal feeding tube (Pedi-Tube, Sherwood Medical, St. Louis, MO) can be used. The tube is placed via the ventral middle meatus through the esophagus and into the stomach. The weighted distal portion is carried by gastrointestinal peristalsis through the pylorus, duodenum, and into the jejunum. Radiographic or fluoroscopic examination verifies proper placement. Other options for parenteral nutrition include surgical or laparoscopic placement of a jejunal feeding tube, partial parenteral nutrition, or total parenteral nutrition. Advantages of surgical placement of a feeding device include the ability to perform exploratory laparotomy, debridement or resection of the pancreas, biopsy of the pancreas, and peritoneal lavage.[1-6]

Antiemetic Therapy

Currently, the most often used antiemetics are metoclopramide (1.0 to 2.0 mg/kg/24 h CRI IV) and the newer serotonin antagonists dolasetron mesylate (0.6 to 3.0 mg/kg q 24 h IV) and ondansetron hydrochloride. The recommended dosages are (0.1to 0.2 mg/kg q 8 to 12 h IV). Metoclopramide is typically used for routine cases, whereas serotonin antagonists are chosen in cases of intractable vomiting. The use of H_2-receptor antagonists such as famotidine (0.5 to 1.0 mg/kg q 24 h IV), or the proton pump inhibitor omeprazole (0.7 mg/kg/24 h PO), and sucralfate (0.5 to 1.0 g mixed with water in a slurry q 8 h PO) is indicated for suspected gastric ulceration or esophagitis associated with vomiting.

Pain Management

There are several alternatives used for pain management in dogs with pancreatitis (see Chapter 7). Fentanyl citrate (1.0 to 4.0 μg/kg/hr CRI IV) is a commonly used method of pain control. Fentanyl transdermal patches (2.5 mg for dogs 10 to 40 lb, 5.0 mg for dogs 40 to 80 lb, and 10 mg dogs over 80 lb) are also available. These take approximately 12 to 24 hours to begin taking effect; thus, additional pain management is warranted in the interim. Other pain management protocols include subcutaneous morphine (0.5 to 2.0 mg/kg q 4 to 6 h IM or SC), oxymorphone (0.11 to 0.22 mg/kg q 4 to 6 h IM, SC, or IV), or butorphanol tartrate (0.1 to 0.4 mg/kg q 6 to 12 h IM or SC). Intrapleural bupivacaine (1.5 to 3.0 mg/kg q 4 to 6 h) with or without lidocaine (2.0 mg/kg q 4 to 6 h) is also used successfully to treat abdominal pain. Lidocaine has an immediate effect, lasting for approximately 1 hour; bupivacaine has a slower onset of action, but lasts for up to 12 hours. These drugs are administered via a catheter inserted into the pleural space.[23,24] These drugs are warmed to room temperature and mixed with 1 part sodium bicarbonate to 3 parts local analgesic agent to reduce pain on administration.

Prevention of Bacterial Translocation

The routine use of antibiotics is controversial.[1-5] Although antibiotic therapy is not aimed at treating the underlying cause, it may be of benefit in the prevention of bacterial translocation due to loss of intestinal mucosal integrity or secondary pancreatic infection.[1-7] Antibiotic therapy should be effective against both anaerobes and gram-negative bacteria. Cefoxitin (22 mg/kg q 8 h IV) or other broad-spectrum antibiotic combinations such as enrofloxacin (2.5 to 10.0 mg/kg q 12 h IV) and ampicillin (22 mg/kg q 8 h IV) are suitable choices.

Exploratory Laparotomy

Indications for surgery include intractable or progressive clinical signs, suspicion of pancreatic neoplasia, sepsis or septic peritonitis, pancreatic abscess, biliary duct obstruction, and enteral feeding tube placement.[1-5] Lavage of the abdomen helps to lessen severity of disease by removing and diluting activated pancreatic enzymes from the abdominal cavity.[1-6] Peritoneal dialysis is another option to remove activated pancreatic enzymes and fluid from the peritoneal cavity.[1-4,6] If one lobe of the pancreas is affected and the remainder normal, pancreatic debridement and resection are performed.[6]

Miscellaneous Treatments

Treatment with a protease inhibitor, such as intraperitoneal aprotinin, is currently experimental.[5] There is a report that selenium (0.1 mg/kg q 24 h IV) is beneficial.[5] Future prospective studies are necessary to determine if this is an effective treatment strategy.

Monitoring

The pancreatitis patient should be monitored routinely to evaluate for development of electrolyte and acid–base disturbances, acute renal failure, hepatocellular necrosis, DIC, cardiac dysrhythmias, multiorgan failure, and respiratory distress (thromboembolic disease, pulmonary edema, or pleural effusion).[1-6]

Recovery

Following cessation of vomiting and return to normal clinical parameters, small amounts of water or oral glucose-electrolyte solutions are initially offered for the first 6 to 12 hours. If vomiting does not develop, small amounts of food are offered. Appropriate diets are low in fat and protein with a high-carbohydrate content. Fat and protein stimulate pancreatic secretion to a greater degree than carbohydrates.[1,2,6] Once the animal returns to eating and drinking normal amounts, the owners should be counseled on weight loss if the animal is obese. A lifelong low-fat diet is recommended for severe cases of pancreatitis or in cases of repeat offenders. Hyperlipidemic dogs should be placed on fat-restricted diets (Hills Science Diet R/D, Pet Nutrition, Topeka, KS or Eukanuba Veterinary Diets Restricted Calorie Formula, Iams, Dayton, OH).

PROGNOSIS

Pancreatitis is an extremely variable disease. Severe cases developing life-threatening consequences (DIC, renal failure, thromboembolic disease) have a poor prognosis. The prognosis for pancreatic abscess is likewise poor. Mild cases that are responsive to dietary adjustments may have a better prognosis, although the owner should be warned that an acute episode might be only a dietary indiscretion away.

REFERENCES

1. Williams DA: Exocrine pancreatic disease. *In* Ettinger SJ, Feldman EC, eds.: Textbook of Veterinary Internal Medicine, 5th ed, vol 2. Philadelphia: WB Saunders, 2000, p 1345.
2. Williams DA: The pancreas. *In* Guilford WG, Center SA, Strombeck DR, Williams DA, Meyer DJ, eds.: Strombeck's Small Animal Gastroenterology, 3rd ed. Philadelphia: WB Saunders, 1996, p 381.
3. Hall JA, Macy DW: Acute canine pancreatitis. *Compend Contin Educ Vet Pract* 10: 403, 1988.
4. Bunch SE: The exocrine pancreas. *In* Nelson RW, Couto CG, eds.: Small Animal Internal Medicine, 2nd ed. St. Louis: Mosby, 1998, p 555.

5. Williams DA, Steiner JM. Canine pancreatitis. *In* Bonagura JD, ed.: Kirk's Current Veterinary Therapy XIII Small Animal Practice. Philadelphia: WB Saunders, 2000, p 607.
6. Williams DA: Diagnosis and management on pancreatitis. *J Small Anim Pract* 35: 445, 1994.
7. Hess RS, Kass PH, Shofer FS, *et al.*: Evaluation of the risk factors for fatal acute pancreatitis in dogs. *J Am Vet Med Assoc* 214:46, 1999.
8. Hess RS, Saunders HM, Van Winkle TJ, *et al.*: Clinical, clinicopathologic, radiographic, and ultrasonographic abnormalities in dogs with fatal acute pancreatitis: 70 cases (1986–1995). *J Am Vet Med Assoc* 213:665, 1998.
9. Whitney MS: The laboratory assessment of canine and feline pancreatitis. *Vet Med* 88:1045, 1993.
10. Whitney MS, Boon GD, Rebar AH, *et al.*: Ultracentrifugal and electrophoretic characteristics of the plasma lipoproteins of Miniature Schnauzer dogs with idiopathic hyperlipoproteinemia. *J Vet Intern Med* 7:253, 1993.
11. Saunders HM: Ultrasonography of the pancreas. *In* Kaplan PM, Kay WJ, Brown NO, eds.: Problems in Veterinary Medicine, Ultrasound. Philadelphia: JB Lippincott, 1991, p 583.
12. Steyn PF, Wittum TE: Radiographic, epidemiologic, and clinical aspects of simultaneous pleural and peritoneal effusions in dogs and cats: 48 cases (1982–1991). *J Am Vet Med Assoc* 202:307, 1993.
13. Bellah JR, Bell G: Serum amylase and lipase activities after exploratory laparotomy in dogs. *Am J Vet Res* 50:1638, 1989.
14. Parent J: Effects of dexamethasone on pancreatic tissue and on serum amylase and lipase activities in dogs. *J Am Vet Med Assoc* 180:743, 1982.
15. Polzin DJ, Osborne CA, Stevens JB, *et al.*: Serum amylase and lipase activities in dogs with chronic primary renal failure. *Am J Vet Res* 44:404, 1983.
16. Strombeck DR, Farver T, Kaneko JJ: Serum amylase and lipase activities in the diagnosis of pancreatitis in dogs. *Am J Vet Res* 42:1966, 1981.
17. Simpson KW, Batt RM, McLean L, *et al.*: Circulating concentrations of trypsin-like immunoreactivity and activities of lipase and amylase after pancreatic duct ligation in dogs. *Am J Vet Res* 50:629, 1989.
18. Ruaux CG, Atwell RB: Levels of total alpha-macroglobulin and trypsin-like immunoreactivity are poor indicators of clinical severity in spontaneous canine acute pancreatitis. *Res Vet Sci* 67:83, 1999.
19. Wingfield WE: Acute pancreatitis. *In* Wingfield WE, ed.: Veterinary Emergency Medicine Secrets, 2nd ed. Philadelphia: Hanley & Belfus, 2000, p 295.
20. Kalfarentzos F, Kehagias J, Kokkinis K, *et al.*: Enteral nutrition is superior to parenteral nutrition in severe acute pancreatitis: results of a randomized prospective trial. *Br J Surg* 84:1665, 1997.
21. Windsor ACJ, Kanwar S, Li AGK, *et al.*: Compared with parenteral nutrition, enteral feeding attenuates the acute phase response and improves disease severity in acute pancreatitis. *Gut* 42:431, 1998.
22. Kotani J, Makoto U, Nomura H, *et al.*: Enteral nutrition prevents bacterial translocation but does not improve survival during pancreatitis. *Arch Surg* 134:287, 1999.
23. Skarda RT: Local and regional anesthetic and analgesic techniques: dogs. *In* Thur-

mon JC, Tranquilli WJ, Benson GJ, eds.: Lumb and Jones' Veterinary Anesthesia, 3rd ed. Baltimore: Williams & Wilkins, 1996, p 440.

24. Quandt JE, Rawlings CR: Reducing post-operative pain for dogs: local anesthetics and analgesic techniques. *Compend Contin Educ Small An Pract* 18:101, 1996.

53
Severe Liver Disease

Ronald S. Walton

INTRODUCTION

The liver is a complex organ that is essential to vital metabolic functions of every animal. The functions of the liver include pivotal roles in protein, carbohydrate, and fat metabolism; detoxification and excretion of toxins, toxicants, and drugs; formation and elimination of bile; and a central role in the formation of most coagulation factors. The liver has a tremendous reserve capacity (70%–80% functional mass) and a remarkable capacity for regeneration. Because of this large reserve capacity, the clinical signs of liver disease tend to become apparent only when the reserve capacity becomes exhausted. With the vast number of possible diseases of the liver and secondary involvement from systemic disease, it is impossible to fully discuss hepatic pathophysiology in the space allowed. Instead this chapter focuses on the pathophysiology and treatment of acute and chronic hepatic failure as an emergency and intensive care condition.

The approach and management of severe hepatic disease is often determined by the onset of the disease. Classifying a patient with severe liver disease as having acute or chronic disease carries many diagnostic, therapeutic, and prognostic implications. The clinical syndrome of acute liver failure (ALF) occurs when the liver rapidly becomes functionally impaired and is unable to perform its synthetic and excretory homeostatic roles without prior evidence or history of liver disease. Acute hepatic failure is a true medical emergency because of the rapid onset and clinical progression as well as the high mortality rate associated with the disease. The clinical outcome of ALF and the subsequent ability of liver to regain its functional roles depends on rapid and aggressive supportive care.

ETIOLOGY

The most frequent etiologies of severe liver disease are listed in Table 53-1.

Infectious Agents

Infectious agents are a well known but uncommon cause of severe liver disease and liver failure in the veterinary patient. Viral hepatitis has largely been eliminated with routine vaccination programs for canine type I adenovirus. Cats may present in severe hepatic failure due to pyogranulomatous inflammatory

Table 53-1. Common Causes of Severe Liver Disease in the Dog and Cat

Infectious Agents	Drugs	Chemical Agents, Toxins, and Toxicants	Infiltrative and Metabolic Disease	Traumatic, Hypoxic, or Thermal
Viral Infectious canine hepatitis (CAV1) Canine herpes virus Feline infectious peritonitis (FIP) Canine acidophil hepatitis **Bacterial** Clostridiosis Leptospirosis *Bacillus piliformis* (Tyzzer's) Liver abscess *Salmonella* sp. *Francisella tularensis* (Tularemia) **Fungal** Histoplasmosis Coccidiomycosis Blastomycosis **Protozoal** Toxoplasmosis Babesia *Cytauxzoon felis* **Metazoan** *Dirofilaria immits* **Rickettsial** *Ehrlichia canis* *Rickettsia rickettsii*	Acetaminophen Aprindine Aspirin Carprofen Diazepam Griseofulvin Halothane Itraconazole Ketoconazole Mebendazole Methotrexate Methoxyflurane Mithramycin Phenytoin Primidone Phenobarbital Sulfadiazine Tetracycline Thiacetarsemide Tolbutamide Trimethoprim	**Toxin** Aflatoxin Amanita mushrooms Blue-green algae Cycad seeds (*Zamia floridana*) Hornet sting Pennyroyal oil Sago palm **Major Toxicants** Carbon tetrachloride Dimethylnitrosamine Galactosamine metals (Cu, Fe, P) Organochloride pesticides Zinc phosphide	Hepatic lipidosis Inflammatory bowel disease Pancreatitis Septicemia/endotoxemia Hemolytic anemia Copper storage disease Neoplasia Lymphoma Myeloproliferative Primary hepatic neoplasia Metastasis	Blunt or penetrating abdominal trauma Diaphragmatic hernia Shock Liver lobe torsion Massive ischemia Heat stroke

Listings are grouped by type of pathologic insult.

cell infiltrate associated with feline infectious peritonitis (FIP). Severe bacterial-related liver disease is seen most commonly with leptospirosis, Tyzzer disease (*Bacillus piliformis*), or clostridial infections. The incidence of fungal hepatic infections is variable by geographic location (see Table 53-1). *Dirofilaria immitis* can lead to acute hepatic necrosis by causing severe hepatic congestion and obstruction of blood flow in a case with caval syndrome. Disseminated toxoplasmosis, babesiosis, and cytauxzoonosis are the protozoal diseases most often associated with liver failure. Rickettsial organisms have infrequently been associated with liver failure in the dog.

Chemical and Pharmaceutical Agents

Organic chemicals/biotoxins/toxicants, anesthetic agents, and even antibiotics can and have caused hepatic necrosis and failure (see Table 53-1). Idiosyncratic drug reactions and direct toxicity have resulted in ALF in both dogs and cats; although drug reactions account for 25% of the cases of ALF in humans, incidences in the dog and cat are unknown. Agents that have been implicated in producing ALF include acetaminophen and diazepam in the cat and carprofen and thiacetarsemide in the dog.

Infiltrative Disease

Acute liver failure can result from hepatic infiltration with neoplastic cells, inflammatory cells, or lipid. Indeed, the most common cause of ALF is extensive infiltration of neoplastic cells such as lymphoma. Hepatic lipidosis is both an infiltrative and a metabolic disease. This disease is commonly seen and undoubtedly is the most common cause of potentially reversible ALF in the cat.

Ischemia and Hypoxic Injury

Reduced blood flow can lead to massive hepatic ischemia, cellular necrosis, and organ failure. Severe shock, right-sided heart failure, thrombosis, neoplasia, and vascular anomalies are the most common reasons for arterial or venous occlusion or restricted blood flow.

Metabolic

Acute copper-associated liver disease is seen frequently in Bedlington Terriers and has been associated with acute hepatic failure. Copper accumulation occurs over a long period and the dogs are usually asymptomatic until hepatic copper levels reach high levels (>2000 ppm).

Hepatic lipidosis occurs in both dogs and cats; the incidence is higher in cats. The condition results from intracellular accumulation of lipid when an imbalance exists between the rates of deposition and mobilization of hepatic fat. The end result is a progressive hepatic dysfunction leading to severe intrahepatic cholestasis and generalized hepatic failure.

Anatomic Variants

Portosystemic shunting of blood via either congenital or acquired vascular connections between the portal and systemic circulations is an important cause of severe liver disease and may produce signs of hepatoencephalopathy in the dog and cat. The reader is referred to chapter 54 for further information.

PATHOGENESIS

Hepatic Response to Injury

Hepatocellular degeneration is a common response to inflammatory, toxic, metabolic, and ischemic insult. The mechanisms that lead to cell necrosis and cell death are not completely understood. Postulated mechanisms include hypoxia, free radical exposure or generation, membrane lipid peroxidation, depletion of essential intracellular compounds, intracellular toxin production, toxin binding to DNA and RNA, cholestatic injury, as well as direct effects of endotoxin or viral, parasitic, and immune complexes on the hepatobiliary system. These factors all play a role in possible liver diseases that produce cellular dysfunction, cell death, and ultimately organ dysfunction.

The liver does have a unique capability of rapid regeneration following injury. The liver has the capability to regenerate large sections that may become damaged if the reticular framework is not destroyed in the disease process. Although the healing mechanisms and compensatory regrowth of injured tissue is poorly understood, it is known that the regenerative process involves the complex and interlinked functions of hypertrophy and hyperplasia. This connective tissue stroma acts as a foundation to support the regeneration of hepatic parenchyma.

Hepatic Dysfunction

The following categories reflect the functional parameters the liver regulates under normal conditions and changes associated with severe liver disease.

Carbohydrate Metabolism

The liver has a central role in carbohydrate metabolism, acting to maintain normal blood glucose concentrations in the fasting state. Hepatic gluconeogenesis and glycogenolysis are key metabolic steps to achieve glucose homeostasis. Gluconeogenesis and glycogenolysis are stimulated via glucagon, epinephrine, and corticosteroid release and are inhibited by insulin. Depleted glycogen reserves lead to protein catabolism for gluconeogenesis.

Hypoglycemia is frequently a complication of acute hepatic failure. Signs of hypoglycemia will only appear when 70% or more of the functional hepatic mass is lost.

Lipid and Cholesterol Metabolism

The liver has a lipogenic role in the conversion of fatty acids to triglycerides. The liver can regulate the metabolic fate of lipids and can also determine storage needs, synthesis of lipoproteins, or oxidization depending on the energy needs of the body. Cholesterol enters the liver via hepatic extraction of chylomicron remnants and low-density lipoproteins from plasma, but the liver is also capable of independent cholesterol synthesis. Posthepatic obstruction can lead to increased plasma cholesterol levels. Hypocholesterolemia is seen in more than 60% of dogs and cats with PSS. Hypocholesterolemia is less common, however, in hepatic parenchymal disease and dysfunction.

Nitrogen and Protein Metabolism

The liver is responsible for approximately 20% of the total protein turnover of the body. The liver is also the primary site of synthesis of albumin, numerous transport proteins, most coagulation factors, and many anticoagulant proteins, as well as many of the activators and inhibitors of the coagulation cascade. The liver is the source of most α-globulins, half of the β-globulins, and a small percentage of the γ-globulin production. Many of the key serum enzymes are also derived within the liver. When the functional capacity of the liver fails, clinical signs manifest as bleeding tendencies, encephalopathic signs due to ammonia and toxin retention, hypoalbuminemia leading to edema and ascites, and cellular and immune dysfunction that increase susceptibility to infection.

Microsomal Enzyme System

More than 200 compounds have been associated with the hepatic microsomal enzyme system. The activity of the cytochrome P-450 system can dramatically affect drug metabolism and enzyme production. The influence of severe liver disease on the cytochrome P-450 system is unpredictable. As a rule, histologic lesions do not correlate with the degree of cytochrome P-450 enzyme dysfunction between patients. The elimination of drugs may be markedly delayed, resulting in overdosage using routine therapeutic dosages. Careful attention must therefore be paid to drug effects and dosages adjusted accordingly in any patient with hepatic compromise.

Hepatic Encephalopathy

Metabolic abnormalities associated with advanced hepatic disease/dysfunction may include abnormal function of the central nervous system (CNS) known as hepatic encephalopathy (HE). Many hypotheses have been suggested as to the pathogenesis of HE including hyperammonemia, accumulation of false neurotransmitters, and increased aromatic amino acids concentration. Ammonia, mercaptans, γ-aminobutyric acid (GABA), endogenous benzodiazepines, and short-chain fatty acids are all potential encephalopathic toxins. They are typically produced in the colon where they are absorbed and transported to the liver via the portal circulation. The liver normally detoxifies these substances, which prevents them from reaching the systemic circulation and CNS. As the liver fails, these toxins reach the CNS in higher than normal concentrations and result in the typical clinical signs of HE.

Cerebral Edema

Cerebral edema and increased intracranial pressure are seen in cases of uncontrolled HE. The mechanisms are not fully known; current hypotheses range from the development of cerebral hyperemia and vasogenic edema due to excess transfer of extracellular fluid across the blood–brain barrier to the accumulation of cytotoxic intracellular substances that osmotically attract water into the brain tissue. The signs of cerebral edema are often a primary result of increased intracranial pressure (ICP). Severe increase in ICP can result in displacement of brain structures which produce clinical signs including pupillary abnormalities and decerebrate and decorticate posturing.

Coagulopathy

The liver is the site of synthesis of all coagulation factors except factor VIII, von Willebrand factor, calcium, and local tissue thromboplastin. The liver is also responsible for activation of the vitamin K-dependent factors II, VII, IX, and X. The liver synthesizes or regulates anticoagulant and fibrinolytic factors including plasminogen, antithrombin III, α_2-macroglobulin, α_2-antiplasmin, and plasminogen activators. Dogs and cats with severe hepatic dysfunction can develop a tendency to bleed from one or combination of factor deficiencies. These tendencies typically manifest as upper GI hemorrhage (hematemesis and melena), oozing and hematoma formation at venipuncture sites, petechiae, ecchymoses, and severe cases of disseminated intravascular coagulation (DIC).

Bilirubin Metabolism and Jaundice

Bilirubin is a product of hemoprotein catabolism and is the major pigment in bile. Bilirubin is normally conjugated with glucouronic acid in the liver. Conjugated bilirubin is transported to the biliary system and released as a bile component into the small intestine. Hyperbilirubinemia is caused by excessive production of bilirubin, impaired processing by hepatocytes, or interference with excretion into the small intestine. Jaundice is a condition of hyperbilirubinemia in which the patient becomes visibly discolored with a yellow tone that is typically observed in the mucous membranes and sclera. In severe cases the skin will have a yellow tone in hairless areas. Jaundice is classified as prehepatic (excessive production due to hemolysis), hepatic (abnormal uptake and conjugation by hepatocytes), and posthepatic (obstruction of bile flow). Jaundice can develop early or late in the disease timeline depending on the degree of injury focused on the periportal triad. If jaundice is present, acholic feces are diagnostic for bile duct obstruction.

Portal Hypertension and Ascites

Portal hypertension (PH) is a result of blood flow impedance from the splanchnic circulation, portal vein, liver, or caudal vena cava to the right side of the heart. PH is classified as prehepatic (constriction or obstruction of the portal vein), hepatic (hepatic parenchymal lesion decreasing sinusoidal flow), or posthepatic (resistance in major hepatic veins, vena cava, or heart). In patients with acute failure, massive sinusoidal collapse can create a blockade against intrahepatic flow and cause a significant portal pressures elevation. Rapid onset of PH leads to systemic collapse due to endotoxin absorption into the systemic circulation. Acute PH can lead to ascites and profound splenomegaly; it is considered a grave prognostic sign. The patient with chronic liver failure is more likely to develop PH due to cirrhosis that alters the sinusoidal circulation and increases vascular resistance. PH can lead to the development of severe congestion of the splanchnic vasculature and cause or exacerbate gastrointestinal tract hemorrhage.

Hepatorenal Syndrome

The association of unexplained oliguric renal failure with severe liver disease is known as hepatorenal syndrome. Although the cause of the disease in unknown, the condition is recognized in humans in decompensated hepatic insufficiency from both acute and chronic origins. A similar syndrome exists in dogs, especially in Doberman Pinschers with decompensated hepatic failure. The reported pathologic lesions are minimal and are not consistent between patients. Cases of hepatorenal syndrome in dogs have had poor clinical outcomes.

DIAGNOSTIC EVALUATION PLAN

History

The historical findings and client concerns are typically vague and share a commonality with many disease processes. Due to the great functional reserve of the liver, much of the reserve capacity must be lost before the owner may even notice signs or symptoms in their pet. A patient will often present with acute signs of hepatic dysfunction that represent the final decompensation period of a long-term but unrecognized disease process. A history of exposure to known hepatotoxins (*e.g.*, acetaminophen or amanita mushrooms), administration of a known hepatotoxic drug (*e.g.*, itraconazole or phenobarbital), infectious organisms (*e.g.*, leptospirosis), physiologic extremes (*e.g.*, thermal or traumatic injury), vascular compromise of the liver, liver lobe entrapment or torsion, or severe systemic disease leading to multiorgan involvement help the clinician to determine rapid, directed therapies. More often the patient with severe liver disease will present without a defined causative history.

Clinical Signs

Clinical signs are often not specific for hepatic disease. General clinical signs of hepatic disease include anorexia, depression, polyuria/polydipsia (PU/PD), vomiting, diarrhea, weight loss, variable cranial abdominal compartment pain, abdominal effusion, melena, and dehydration. Defining clinical signs as ALF or acute decompensation of chronic disease can be difficult. Massive hepatic necrosis is the classic disease that produces signs of ALF. Typical clinical signs include depression, vomiting, HE, hepatomegaly, hepatodynia, abnormal bleeding tendency, jaundice, fever, and ascites. Signs of HE often predominate and are demonstrated as depressed menace reflex, mentation changes, visual deficits, circling, pacing, ptyalism, anxiety, seizures, head pressing, stupor, or coma. The signs of HE may be interspersed with periods of normal behavior and mentation. Findings of weight loss, ascites, jaundice, anorexia, and microhepatica are more typical findings of chronic liver failure.

CLINICOPATHOLOGIC FINDINGS

Hematology

Mild to moderate anemia is common and often due to hemorrhage or erythropoiesis failure. When the patient is anemic and icteric, icterus must be separated from hemolysis. An icteric patient with regenerative anemia and normal plasma proteins is likely in a hemolytic crisis rather than hepatic failure. Poikilocytosis is a common finding in dogs and cats with hepatic disease. Microcytosis is a common finding with PSS. Cats frequently display acanthocytes and dogs display target cells on peripheral blood smears. The white blood cell count can vary from high in an acute or active inflammatory process to low in sepsis. Platelet count can also vary from normal to low if the platelets are consumed in excessive hemorrhage or DIC.

Biochemical Testing

Liver Enzymes

Liver enzyme levels are used as a primary screening test to detect liver disease. Due to its many integral functions, the clinical and laboratory abnormalities associated with liver disease are diverse and no single diagnostic test has 100% sensitivity and specificity for hepatic disease. Abnormal values for liver enzymes are a key feature in linking the liver to clinical signs, although increases in liver enzyme activity are often not specific for the underlying hepatic disorder. Commonly measured enzymes are alanine aminotransferase (ALT), aspartate aminotransferase (AST), alkaline phosphatase (ALP), and γ-glutamyltransferase (GGT). An important note to remember is that liver enzyme levels do not evaluate liver function. The level of enzyme increase may be proportional to the number of cells involved, but severe chronic hepatic dysfunction can exist with normal liver enzyme activity. Conversely, high liver enzyme levels can be seen in patients without appreciable hepatic dysfunction. An increase in serum ALT levels is associated with hepatocyte injury and leakage of the enzyme from the cytoplasm; the magnitude of the increase correlates with the number of hepatocytes injured. For example, large increases in ALT are often associated with hepatocellular necrosis and inflammation; moderate increases are associated with hepatocellular leakage induced by hypoxia, secondary to cholestasis, anticonvulsant therapy steroid hepatopathy. In hepatic injury, both ALT and AST are concurrently increased; elevation in both enzyme levels serves as a more sensitive index of hepatocyte injury than either value alone. ALP and GGT are membrane-bound enzymes in the biliary epithelium; the activity of each of these enzymes is stimulated by cholestasis and drug induction. Increases in ALP are not specific to liver injury; activity can arise from bone and drug-induced isoenzymes. Although dogs exhibit corticosteroid- or drug-induced isoenzyme elevations in ALP, cats do not. Cats typically have smaller increases in ALP than dogs and the enzyme has a very short half-life in cats. Because of this, small increases in ALP are significant in cats and generally imply significant cholestasis. Increased serum GGT reflects cholestasis and increased production by hepatocytes. Cats tend to demonstrate a greater GGT than ALP response in most hepatobiliary diseases except in hepatic lipidosis. In hepatic lipidosis, the GGT levels may be normal or minimally elevated in the presence of significant ALP elevations.

Hepatic Function Testing

Liver enzymes can reflect damage but not function of the hepatobiliary system. Specific function testing is required to determine the degree of functional hepatic impairment. The use of serum bile acid (SBA) testing has largely replaced the use of organic dyes (bromsulphalein and indocyanine green). SBA concentrations tend to increase with most types of liver disease. Increased SBA occurs in hepatocellular and cholestatic disorders that affect hepatic uptake and secretion of bile acids and PSS, which diverts bile acids directly into the systemic circulation. Decreases in SBA are almost never seen due to a large hepatic synthetic reserve. The measurement of postprandial SBA is an endogenous challenge test of liver function and may be used with great efficacy to test all hepatic disorders in cats. In dogs, a major difference in postprandial SBA value is noted only with PSS or cirrhosis (dogs can have near normal resting bile acids with PSS and cirrhosis). The ammonia tolerance test (ATT) is another function test to document portosystemic shunting and hepatic dysfunction. This test should never be administered when baseline ammonia levels are elevated. The use of SBA testing has largely replaced ammonia tolerance test in most clinics.

Other Biochemical Testing

Many tests can be used to support the diagnosis of hepatobiliary disease. These tests include bilirubin, albumin, globulin, blood urea nitrogen (BUN), glucose, electrolytes, and cholesterol. Elevation in serum bilirubin concentration can occur secondary to cholestasis or hemolysis. Jaundice is not clinically detectable until bilirubin concentrations reach more than 2.5 to 3.5 g/dL. Low serum albumin levels are typically seen only in chronic hepatic disease. The synthesis of albumin exclusively occurs in the liver; hypoalbuminemia does not occur until 70% to 80% of the functional mass is reduced. Remember, hypoalbuminemia is not diagnostic for liver disease because significant albumin loss can occur from the urinary and gastrointestinal systems. Globulin levels may be elevated in acute and chronic hepatic disease due to antigenic stimulation. Hypoglobulinemia is rarely seen. BUN levels may be decreased in advanced liver disease. Because the liver is responsible for metabolism of ammonia to urea, functional impairment may manifest as a decrease in BUN with or without concomitant elevations in blood ammonia levels. Glucose measurement is an important but insensitive index of hepatic function. The liver can adequately maintain euglycemia until over 70% to 80% of the functional mass becomes impaired. Many nonhepatic causes of hypoglycemia are possible and should be ruled out before diagnosing hepatic failure based on this measurement alone. Although not specific for hepatic disease, elevation in cholesterol is associated with acute cholestatic disorders. Hypocholesterolemia is rarely seen even in chronic disease. Serum electrolyte levels are variable and dependent on the type and stage of the disease process. In patients with ALF, the values of commonly measured electrolytes (Na^+, K^+, Cl^-) are frequently normal. In chronic liver disease, sodium levels tend to increase; potassium levels are low due to sodium and water retention and altered adrenal steroid metabolism.

Urinalysis

Urine bilirubin is a sensitive indicator of abnormal bilirubin metabolism, especially in dilute urine. Trace amounts of bilirubin are a normal finding in concentrated urine samples in the dog, but bilirubinuria is always an abnormal finding in the cat. High bilirubin concentrations impart an orange color to the urine and very high bilirubin concentrations can result in the formation of bilirubin crystals in urine. Elevations in urinary bilirubin will be seen in advance of clinical evidence of hyperbilirubinemia and icterus. Urobilinogen is a colorless product of bacterial degradation of bilirubin in the gut and is routinely measured on a urinalysis. Normally, a small portion of the total urobilinogen escapes the enterohepatic circulation to be excreted in the urine. Urobilinogenuria is only found with an intact enterohepatic circulation. A urinalysis with negative urobilinogen and jaundice suggests common bile duct obstruction.

Coagulation Abnormalities

Laboratory evaluation of coagulation function includes measures of prothrombin time (PT), activated partial thromboplastin time (APTT), and activated clotting time (ACT). Moderate prolongation of PT, APTT, and ACT times are more commonly seen than overt signs of bleeding as acute liver disease. Specific coagulation factor analysis will often demonstrate specific or multiple factor deficiency. Vitamin K deficiency is commonly caused by malabsorption due to cholestasis. The PIVKA (proteins induced by vitamin K antagonism) test is a very sensitive clotting diagnostic test routinely used to diagnose rodenticide toxicity; it can also be used to predict bleeding tendencies in dogs and cats with liver disease. The PIVKA test is more sensitive than PT or APTT in patients with liver disease. The test may normalize with parenteral vitamin K administration alone.

Imaging

Radiography

Routine survey radiographs can be useful to evaluate liver size and to detect abdominal effusion. Liver size in hepatic failure can be enlarged (hepatomegaly), normal, or small (microhepatica). Normal to large liver size is more commonly associated with acute processes, whereas microhepatica tends to occur with chronic hepatic disease and cirrhotic changes.

Ultrasound

Ultrasound examination may be used to noninvasively assess parenchymal abnormalities, mass lesions, evaluate the status of the gallbladder and biliary tract, and assist in the diagnosis of vascular lesions. Information gained from abdominal ultrasound may allow the determination of hepatic and extrahepatic involvement in the disease process. Ultrasound also is a useful tool to improve safety for hepatic biopsy.

Ancillary Testing

Abdominal Paracentesis

Abdominal fluid obtained from an animal with hepatic disease can be helpful in determining a diagnosis. The sample is usually evaluated for total protein content, nucleated cell count, and cytologic evaluation. The typical ascitic fluid associated with liver disease is a transudate (protein ≥2.5 g/dL and <2500 cells/µL). The fluid may become a modified transudate (protein ≥.5 g/dL) if the disease process involves severe hepatic venous congestion or obstruction of the vena cava. The fluid may have an exudative character in cases of biliary tract rupture, hepatic abscess, parenchymal trauma, FIP, or neoplasia. Cytologic evaluation and biochemical testing for bilirubin may help diagnosis. In contrast to dogs, cats with severe liver disease rarely form ascites.

Serology

A suspected infectious agent may be identified via serologic testing. The test results often can take several days and may be falsely negative depending on the diagnostic accuracy of the test and stage of the disease.

Biopsy

Histopathologic elevation can establish a cause, determine if the disease process is acute or chronic, and provide the clinician with valuable prognostic information.

Evaluation of coagulation parameters and platelet counts should be performed on every patient before to attempting a liver biopsy. Biopsy samples should be handled carefully and prepared for cytology, histopathology, culture, and copper analysis as indicated. Samples should be packaged and shipped according to supporting pathology department instructions.

Fine-Needle Aspirate (FNA). This technique is the easiest to accomplish. Generally, FNA is performed blind but can be performed with ultrasound guidance to yield a more representative sample. FNA can provide information about diffuse infiltrative disease such as hepatic lipidosis, neoplasia, and inflammation.

However, it does have the potential to seed tumor cells into the abdominal cavity or along needle tracks.

Percutaneous Needle Biopsy. This technique is successful when the liver is large and the pathologic process is diffuse. The technique can be performed blind or with the aid of ultrasound guidance. Ultrasound guidance is preferred if available to improve diagnostic yield and safely avoid damage to adjacent organs and vessels. Needle biopsy techniques are generally contraindicated in cases of suspected cyst, bile duct obstruction, peritonitis, cystic lesion or abscess, microhepatica, severe uncorrectable coagulation abnormalities, or with lesions adjacent to bile ducts or major vessels. Obese patients are difficult to biopsy without ultrasound guidance. The primary disadvantage is the small sample size (usually 4-5 portal triads without complete hepatic lobules or acini).

Laparoscopy. The advantage to laparoscopy is direct visualization of the liver, biliary system, and adjacent organs. Laparoscopy allows the clinician to obtain directed large biopsy specimens with a minimally invasive technique. Laparoscopy can often be accomplished with heavy sedation. The technique does require some specialized training and a modest amount of equipment.

Exploratory Laparotomy. The best evaluation of the hepatobiliary system and abdominal organs is achieved via exploratory laparotomy. A laparotomy allows the clinician tactile as well as visual evaluation and enhanced ability to control hemorrhage not available by other means. Generally, this technique is selected in cases of biliary obstruction or hepatic resection due to mass lesions. General anesthesia and delayed wound healing are disadvantages in a decompensated patient with hepatic disease.

TREATMENT

The overall objective is to provide supportive care and management of many of the complications associated with liver failure. Potential complications include hepatic encephalopathy, gastrointestinal ulceration, coagulopathy, ascites, edema, anemia, infection, and endotoxemia. By controlling these signs and providing supportive care, the clinical problems associated with hepatic failure can be eliminated or minimized while diagnostics continue. Every effort should be made to determine the cause of the liver disease. Therapy and prognosis can be better determined if the etiology is known (see Table 53-1). Basic therapy guidelines for a patient with suspected liver failure patient are listed in Table 53-2. Administration of directed therapies (Table 53-3) when etiology is known (*i.e.*, antimicrobials for infectious agents, discontinuation of suspect medication, antidotal and antioxidant therapy for known toxicity and drug reactions, and immunosuppression for immune-mediated disease) should be initiated as soon as possible. When functional impairment is evident, the large reserve capacity of the liver has been exhausted and therapy is directed at supportive measures to allow the remaining hepatic tissue to regenerate if possible.

Table 53-2. Therapy Guideline for the Treatment of Hepatic Failure

Goal	Therapy
Prevent formation and absorption of enteric toxins	For *Critical Patient/Hepatic Coma:* Cleansing enema with warm H_2O until clear effluent obtained. Retention enemas Povidone iodine solution (1:10 dilution with H_2O) leave in 10 min then flush with H_2O or a 30% lactulose solution (5-10 mL/kg) mixed with neomycin at 22 mg/kg leave for 20-30 min. For *Maintenance Therapy:* Metronidazole (7.5 mg/kg q 12 h PO), or amoxicillin (22 mg/kg q 12 h PO), or neomycin (22 mg/kg q 8-12 h PO) and lactulose (0.25-0.5 mL/kg q 8-12 h PO)
Control GI hemorrhage	*Treat GI Ulceration:* Famotidine (0.5-1.0 mg/kg q 12-24 h PO) Carafate (1 g/25 kg q 8 h PO) *Correct Coagulopathy:* Vitamin K_1 (1.5-2 mg/kg q 12 h SC or IM, *fresh* plasma transfusion, Treat GI parasites if present Discontinue drugs that exacerbate GI hemorrhage (glucocorticoids, aspirin, NSAIDs)
Control seizures	Avoid benzodiazepines. Consider IV phenobarbital (7 mg/kg IV), oral loading of sodium bromide (600-100 mg/kg q 6 h for 24 h then decease to 20-40 mg/kg or potassium bromide per 24 h PO. *Stable long-term seizure management:* Potassium bromide 20-40 mg/kg q 24 h. *Refractory seizures/status epilepticus.* General anesthesia with propofol or pentobarbital with intubation and mechanical ventilation to maintain normal PaO_2 and $PaCO_2$.
Decrease cerebral edema	Mannitol (0.5-1.0 g/kg IV) followed by furosemide (1-2 mg/kg q 12 h)
Nutritional support	Initial NPO. Long-term management; provide easily digested high-carbohydrate diet. Moderate protein restriction on a dry matter basis to 18%–22% for dogs and 30%–35% for cats. Protein source should be dairy or vegetable source. Provide 60-100 kcal/kg/d. Multivitamin supplement, high in B vitamins. Include soluble dietary fiber (psyllium mucolloid 1-3 tsp/d)
Prevent and control hypoglycemia	*Severe hypoglycemia:* Administer 50% dextrose IV (0.5-1.0 mL/kg diluted in sterile H_2O to 20%–25% solution. Add dextrose to IV fluids as needed (2%–5%) to maintain adequate blood glucose levels

Table 53-3. Directed Therapies For Selected Acute Hepatic Injury

Disease Process	Therapy
Ischemic hepatic injury	Ensure adequate volume support Ensure adequate O_2 delivery Fresh transfusion with whole blood or packed red cells and supplemental O_2 as needed Ensure euglycemia (see Table 55-2) Glucocorticoids (hydrocortisone sodium succinate 30-100 mg/kg)
Oxidative hepatic injury (general or suspected toxin nonspecific injury)	Cimetidine 5 mg/kg IV (only if blocking P-450 enzyme system indicated S-Adenosyl-methionine 700-1200 mg/d Silymarin/Silbinin 50-150 mg/kg IV in Ringer's solution administered over 1 h Vitamin E 100-400 IU PO/d Ursodeoxycholic acid (10-15 mg/kg q 24 h PO)
Oxidative hepatic injury (specific toxin) Acetaminophen toxicity	N-Acetylcystine (140 mg/kg IV loading dose and 7-17 subsequent doses of 70-140 mg/kg IV or PO q 6 h) Cimetidine 5 mg/kg IV or PO for duration of N-acetylcystine therapy
Amanita mushroom intoxication	Gastric decontamination if acute ingestion Dexamethasone (0.3-0.5 mg/kg q 1h IV) Penicillin G 250 mg/kg/d Silymarin/Silbinin 50-150 mg/kg IV in Ringer's solution administered over 1 h
Hepatitis infectious/suppurative (CAV-1) Leptospirosis Hepatic abscess Cholagiohepatitis (acute suppurative)	General supportive care (see Table 55-2) Broad-spectrum antibiotics Penicillin G 40,0000-80,000 IU/kg IM 24 h Surgical excision/drainage Broad-spectrum antibiotic Vitamin K_1 (1.5-2 mg/kg SQ or PO 3-4 doses) Amoxicillin (20-40 mg/kg PO, SQ q 8 h) or Metronidazole (7.5 mg /kg PO q 12 h)
Neoplastic Hepatic neoplasia solitary/discrete Hepatic neoplasia infiltrative	Resect affected lobes. Can resect up to 75 % and regain function Chemotherapy largely ineffective, palliative therapy
Metabolic Hepatic lipidosis (feline) Acute crisis Hepatic copper accumulation Acute crisis	General supportive symptomatic (all) Nutritional Esophagostomy tube or PEG tube Blenderized canned commercial cat food, gradual increase to full calorie requirement increase over 3-4 days. Total daily caloric requirement divided over 6-8 feedings. Protein restriction only if encephalopathic signs. Thiamine supplementation 50-100 mg/cat q 12 h × 3

Table 53-3. Continued

Disease Process	Therapy
	Metaclioprimide (0.4 mg/kg SC q 8 hr, 30 min prior to feeding) Multivitamin supplements Supportive care Chelator therapy D-Penicillamine (10-15 mg/kg PO q 12 h for months) Zinc (100 mg PO q 12 h) Vitamin E 400 IU/d Ursodeoxycholic acid (10-15 mg/kg q 24 h PO)

Specific therapies would be directed to the conditions above. General therapeutic guidelines would be indicated for all patients as needed (see Table 53-2). For detailed therapeutic information and chronic therapies, refer to alternate texts.

General Support

Major Organ Systems

When caring for any critical patient, the basic principles of care are the same regardless of the disease process (see Table 53-2). Basic therapeutic priorities are established for the cardiovascular, respiratory, renal, and neurologic systems. Aggressive therapeutic support must be provided to each patient to prevent complications in secondary organ systems leading to the development of multiorgan failure.

Fluid, Electrolyte, and Acid—Base Balance

Patients with liver disease typically need aggressive fluid support, traditionally provided by administration of balanced crystalloid fluids. Early aggressive fluid therapy is required to support the hepatic microcirculation and decrease the possibility of adverse complications such as shock, renal failure, DIC, and HE. However, sodium retention, portal hypertension, hypoalbuminemia, and hypoglycemia are common complicating factors. The use of 0.45% NaCl in 2.5% dextrose with potassium and dextrose supplementation as needed is recommended in suspected hepatic disease. The addition of either natural (plasma) or synthetic (hetastarch or dextrans) colloids may be required to restore oncotic pressure in cases of severe hypoalbuminemia. Avoid routine use of alkalizing agents such as lactate and $NaHCO_3$, because alkalosis can exacerbate the signs of hepatic encephalopathy. Choosing an alkalizing agent that does not require hepatic metabolism to function (*i.e.*, acetate and gluconate in Normosol or Plasmalyte or judicious amounts of $NaHCO_3$) is more reliable. If acidosis is a feature of the disease process, avoid lactated Ringer's solution.

Hepatoencephalopathy

The goals for treating HE are to: (1) minimize or eliminate symptoms by diet modification; (2) prevent the formation and absorption of enteric toxins;

(3) control gastrointestinal hemorrhage; (4) correct metabolic imbalances; (5) avoid drugs that can exacerbate or perpetuate HE signs; and, (6) control seizures. Table 53-2 lists steps in treating the patient with HE.

Cerebral Edema

Life-threatening cerebral edema can be a serious complication of liver disease. Rapid institution of therapy with an osmotic and loop diuretic (mannitol and furosemide) has been the standard of therapy (see Table 53-2). Corticosteroids are not effective in treating this condition in humans, but early use in animal models has demonstrated some beneficial effects.

Hemorrhage and Anemia

Treat coagulopathy with fresh plasma and whole blood as needed. Stored blood progressively develops increasing ammonia concentrations that may exacerbate signs of HE. Early use of GI protective agents such as famotidine (0.5–1.0 mg/kg q 12-24 h PO or IV) and carafate (1 g/25 kg q 8 h PO) are indicated if ulceration is expected. Cimetidine (5 mg/kg q 8 h IV, PO) and ranitidine (2-3 mg/kg q 8-12 h IV, PO) cause variable action on the hepatic microsomal enzyme systems and are usually avoided unless enzyme blocking action is desired, as in acetaminophen toxicity.

Ascites

The primary treatment for ascites is restriction of dietary sodium intake and diuretic use to promote sodium and water excretion. Commonly used diuretics include furosemide (1-2 mg/kg q 12 h IV or PO) and spironolactone/hydrochlorothiazide (2 mg/kg q 12 h PO). Abdominal paracentesis is not performed routinely as a treatment for ascites except when severe abdominal distention leads to respiratory distress. Rapidly removing large amounts of abdominal fluid can lead to rapid fluid shifts and severe hypotension. Ascites and edema can be temporarily managed with natural (plasma) or synthetic colloids (hetastarch or dextrans) (at a dose range of 10-20 mL/kg/d IV).

Infection and Endotoxemia

An increased incidence of infection may be seen in cases of hepatic disease. Impaired phagocytic system clearance allows enteric bacteria and endotoxin to gain access to the systemic circulation and may lead to septicemia and endotoxemia. Although prophylactic use of systemic antibiotics is controversial, antibiotics should always be used when clinical signs of a fever, infection, or endotoxemia exist. If possible, avoid antimicrobial drugs that require significant hepatic biotransformation or elimination. Amoxicillin, ampicillin, penicillin, and second-generation cephalosporins are good first-choice drugs, because most hepatic bacterial infections tend to be anaerobic and are eliminated by renal mechanisms.

Modification of antibiotic therapy may be necessary based on culture and serology results or on response to therapy.

Nutritional

Although NPO may be part of the initial therapy plan in cases of acute encephalopathic crisis, hepatic disease does not benefit from starvation. Nutritional support is critical to the regeneration process and also allows the animal to gain and or maintain body weight. It is important to avoid high-protein diets that may exacerbate HE signs, but adequate protein levels are critical to normal hepatic regeneration. Excess protein restriction leads to a negative nitrogen balance and increased blood ammonia, with a concomitant increase in the potential to develop HE. When protein restriction is required, dogs require a minimum of 2.1 g protein/kg/d, whereas cats require a minimum of 4 g/kg/d. Soy and milk proteins are well tolerated in both species. The use of branched-chain amino acids (BCAA) has been advocated, but this nutritional alteration has not yielded consistent results. Supply the bulk of the caloric needs with easily digestible carbohydrates. Feeding frequent small meals is also indicated to improve the nutritional status and decrease catabolism, particularly in cirrhotic patients.

Placement of feeding tubes may be required in anorectic patients, especially cats with hepatic lipidosis. Successful treatment of feline hepatic lipidosis hinges on providing adequate nutritional support. The addition of soluble fiber may help acidify the colonic contents and minimize ammonia absorption. With the exception of vitamin K, few vitamin and mineral deficiencies have been documented in veterinary medicine. Nevertheless, home-prepared diets should always be mixed with a complete multivitamin supplement. Zinc supplementation (2 mg/kg/d) may reduce lipid peroxidation and have antifibrotic properties, and vitamin E (400 IU/d) is recommended for its antioxidant properties. Potassium supplementation may also help stem fluctuations due to glucose intolerance, vomiting, diarrhea, and excessive diuretic use.

Oxidative Injury

S-Adenosyl-L-methionine (SAMe) acts as a donor of methyl groups in transmethylation reactions that help maintain cellular structure and function. Studies have shown SAMe helps maintain cell membrane fluidity, helps prevent collagen accumulation and fibrosis, and has significant anticholestatic activity. In humans, SAMe helps decrease clinical signs and enzyme elevations when used to treat intrahepatic cholestasis secondary to chronic liver disease. In the canine liver, SAMe can modify some of the deleterious effects of high dose glucocorticoid administration. SAMe, through the transsulfuration pathway, also serves as a precursor for hepatic synthesis of glutathione (a critical cellular antioxidant). In humans, liver cirrhosis is associated with decreased SAMe formation. Additionally, SAMe synthetase (the enzyme responsible for conversion of methionine to SAMe) is inhibited by hypoxia, oxygen free radicals, and various cytokines. Cats are particularly sensitive to oxidative stress. They have a decreased capacity for the hepatic glucuronidation and sulfation reactions necessary in xenobiotic conjugation. Therefore, dogs and cats with liver disease may benefit from administration of SAMe.

PROGNOSIS

The prognosis for animals with severe hepatic disease depends on rapid recognition, aggressive therapeutic support, and the degree of damage and remaining regenerative ability of the liver. ALF has a good prognosis if it is recognized early and the causative agent is suppressed or eliminated before damage beyond the regenerative capacity of the liver occurs. Infectious and parasitic disease carries a variable prognosis that often depends on the degree of secondary organ involvement and the organism involved. Acute necrotic cholestasis or bile duct rupture can lead to septic bile peritonitis, which many animals do not survive. Chronic hepatitis has a variable prognosis because it represents a heterogeneous group of diseases. Chronic copper-associated hepatitis with moderate failure responds favorably to supportive care, but prognosis is poor for end-stage cirrhotic failure of any cause. Doberman Pinchers have a breed-associated form of chronic hepatitis that carries a very poor prognosis. Most die within weeks to months when presenting in failure, regardless of the therapy instituted. Feline hepatic lipidosis usually responds well to aggressive nutritional support in 50% to 60% of cases. The origin of hepatocutaneous syndrome is unknown (probably immune mediated) and the prognosis is poor. Hepatic neoplasia may be cured if it is isolated to an individual lobe (or lobes) that can be surgically resected; chemotherapy is not an effective means of control. Evidence of multilobe involvement and metastasis is a grave prognostic sign.

SUGGESTED READINGS

Bunch SE: Acute hepatic disorders and systemic disorders that involve the liver. *In* Ettinger SJ, Feldman EC, eds.: Textbook of Veterinary Internal Medicine, 5th ed. Philadelphia: WB Saunders, 2000, p 1326.

Center SA: Pathophysiology of liver disease. *In* Guilford G, Center SA, Williams D, Stombeck D, eds.: Strombeck's Small Animal Gastroenterology. Philadelphia: WB Saunders, 1996, p 553.

Center SA: Acute hepatic injury: hepatic necrosis and fulminant hepatic failure. *In* Guilford G, Center SA, Williams D, Stombeck D, eds.: Stombeck's Small Animal Gastroenterology. Philadelphia: WB Saunders, 1996, p 654.

Center SA: Nutritional support for dogs and cats with hepatobiliary disease. *J Nutr* 128(12 suppl):2733S, 1998.

Center SA: Chronic liver disease: current concepts of disease mechanisms. *J Sm Anim Pract* 40:106, 1999.

Center SA: S-Adenosyl-methionine (SAMe) an antioxidant and anti-inflammatory nutraceutical. Proceedings of the 18th annual meeting, ACVIM, Seattle, WA, 2000, p 550.

Gange JM, Armstrong PJ, Weiss DJ, *et al.*: Clinical features of inflammatory liver disease in cats: 41 cases (1983—1993). *J Am Vet Med Assoc* 214:513, 1999.

Hughes D, King LG: The diagnosis and management of acute liver failure in dogs and cats. *Vet Clin North Am Small Anim Pract* 25:437, 1995.

Johnson SE, Sheriding RG: Diseases of the liver and biliary tract. *In* S. Birchard, R. Sherding, eds.: Saunders Manual of Small Animal Practice, 2nd ed. Philadelphia: WB Saunders, 2000, p 824.

Lieber CS: Role of S-adenosyl-L-methionine in the treatment of liver diseases. *J Hepatol* 30:1155, 1999.

Rothuizen J, Myer HP: History, physical examination and signs of liver disease. *In* Ettinger SJ, Feldman EC, eds.: Textbook of Veterinary Internal Medicine, 5th ed. Philadelphia: WB Saunders, 2000, p. 1272.

Twedt DC: Diagnosis of liver disease in companion animals. *Vet Q* 20(suppl):S44, 1998.

54
Portosystemic Shunts

Sheldon Padgett

INTRODUCTION

Portosystemic shunt (PSS) is a vascular anomaly that bridges the portal and systemic circulation. This allows portal blood draining the stomach, intestines, pancreas, and spleen to bypass the liver. The abnormal physiology created leads to important clinical and biochemical abnormalities, which can have life-threatening consequences.

EPIDEMIOLOGY AND PATHOPHYSIOLOGY

Single vessels located between the portal and systemic vasculature are a congenital anomaly. Single portosystemic shunts can be divided into intrahepatic and extrahepatic based on their location relative to the liver. The majority of single shunts (60%–80%) are extrahepatic in location (portocaval, gastrocaval, and portoazygous). These types of shunts are most common in small-breed dogs such as the schnauzer, Yorkshire terrier, poodle, and dachshund. Single extrahepatic shunts are the most common type of shunt found in cats.

Single intrahepatic shunts are most common in large-breed dogs. German shepherd dogs, Golden retrievers, Labrador retrievers, Old English sheepdogs, and Irish setters are reported to be the most commonly affected breeds. Often an intrahepatic shunt is found to be a persistent patent fetal ductus venosus, although many other abnormalities have been reported. Multiple extrahepatic shunts are usually acquired lesions that form because of high portal pressure. This type of shunt is seen more commonly in older animals with chronic liver disease.

Reports of microvascular portal shunting (hepatic microvascular dysplasia) have been published.[1,2] This is a syndrome characterized by blood shunting at the level of the hepatic lobule without demonstrable vascular anomaly. Canine breeds such as the Maltese, Yorkshire terrier, and cairn terrier have been reported to be predisposed. The clinicopathologic changes associated with this syndrome are similar to those in animals with gross vascular shunts. Other less reported causes for portosystemic shunt include portal atresia and intrahepatic arteriovenous fistula.

Hepatoencephalopathy (HE) refers to the neurologic abnormalities caused by hepatic insufficiency. The pathogenesis of this disorder relates to systemic release of neurotransmitter-like substance produced in the gastrointestinal tract.

These substances normally detoxified in the liver include ammonia, endogenous benzodiazapenes, aromatic amino acids, and mercaptans. Presence of these substances in the systemic circulation have been implicated as causative factors in animals with hepatoencephalopathy.[3] These substances are produced by protein metabolism, or by bacterial production, primarily in the colon. Precipitating factors for hepatoencephalopathy include excess dietary protein, gastrointestinal bleeding, infection, catabolism, and constipation. Administration of methionine-containing medications (such as urinary acidifiers) can lead to HE due to a high concentration of mercaptans.

Animals with a portosystemic shunt are predisposed to ammonium biurate crystalluria. Presumably, decreased clearance of ammonia and decreased uric acid conversion leads to an increase in the excretion of both these substances into the urine, allowing crystal precipitation. Some of these patients form either ammonium or urate stones in either the kidneys or bladder.

CLINICAL PRESENTATION

Portosystemic shunt patients can have a spectrum of historical findings. These usually include: failure to grow, intermittent anorexia, vomiting, diarrhea, polyphagia, polyuria, polydipsia, and prolonged anesthetic recovery.

Animals with a portosystemic shunt commonly have a small body size and may be have poor body condition. Other congenital abnormalities may be seen, such as cryptorchidism (up to 50% incidence) and heart murmurs (especially in cats). Ptyalism is the most common clinical abnormality in cats with a portosystemic shunt. Additionally, cats commonly have copper-colored irises. Liver margins may not be palpable on abdominal examination. Animals that have multiple extrahepatic (acquired) shunts usually have signs consistent with hepatic disease and cirrhosis or fibrosis.

Hepatoencephalopathy develops in most patients with a portosystemic shunt. Dementia, cortical blindness, head pressing, stupor and, sometimes, aggression (especially in cats) can be seen. Approximately 25% to 50% of patients experience seizures.

DIAGNOSTIC EVALUATION

Serum biochemical analysis may reveal mild elevations of liver enzymes including in serum alanine aminotransferase (ALT), aspartate aminotransferase (AST), and alkaline phosphatase (ALP). In young animals, an increase in ALP may actually be caused by bone turnover (increase in bone isoenzyme) instead of hepatic changes. A low albumin concentration is commonly encountered, presumably because of the impaired ability of hepatocytes to produce albumin. Blood urea nitrogen (BUN), normally produced as an end-product of ammonia detoxification in the liver, is commonly low in portosystemic shunt patients. Hematologic abnormalities may include microcytic, normochromic anemia and formation of target cells. In patients with multiple extrahepatic shunts, blood abnormalities may be more profound because of the chronicity of liver disease.

Urinalysis may reveal a low urine specific gravity and crystalluria. Low specific gravity is usually a reflection of polydipsia and resultant polyuria and not primary renal disease. Ammonium biurate crystalluria in dogs (other than the dalmatian) should support suspicion of liver disease.

Liver function tests are more reliable for assessing the PSS diagnosis. Serum bile acid measurement, taken after a 12-hour fast and 2-hour postprandial, is the most popular test because of availability and ease of sample collection. An increase in the postprandial serum bile acid concentration indicates a failure of the liver to recycle bile acid from the portal circulation. While this is not pathognomonic for a portosystemic shunt, it does provide evidence of severely compromised liver function.

Ammonia metabolism is abnormal in patients with a portosystemic shunt, commonly leading to a high blood ammonia concentration. Resting ammonia concentration alone can be unreliable. Over 20% of dogs with a portosystemic shunt have a normal fasting blood ammonia concentration. As an alternative to measuring the resting ammonia, ammonia tolerance testing can be performed by measuring the blood ammonia concentration before and 30 minutes after administering a known dose of ammonia. This is more reliable in demonstrating hepatic insufficiency and is similar in sensitivity to measuring serum bile acid. However, many clinicians prefer measuring serum bile acid as a means of liver function testing because intolerance to an ammonia challenge can be profound (exacerbating hepatoencephalopathy), and concerns with sample lability make handling more difficult.

A wide range of diagnostic imaging is available to support the diagnosis of portosystemic shunt. Abdominal radiographs may indicate microhepatica caused by absence of hepatatrophic factors. Ammonium biurate uroliths may be seen on radiographs, although they may be subtle because they are less radiopaque than most uroliths. Abdominal ultrasonography can be a sensitive method of demonstrating a shunt, especially in the hands of an experienced ultrasonographer. This modality offers a noninvasive method of assessing presence and location (intrahepatic or extrahepatic) of a shunt, assessing portal vein blood flow, and documenting urinary tract abnormalities.

When available, transcolonic sodium pertechnetate scintigraphy offers a noninvasive method of diagnosis with good reliability. If radiation activity is seen in the heart before being seen in the liver, the scan is consistent with a PSS diagnosis.

The definitive test for a portosystemic shunt is contrast angiography, which documents portal blood flow anomalies (portogram). This is usually accomplished by catheterizing a jejunal vein during laparotomy and radiographically recording the flow of contrast media injected into the jejunal vein, either by intraoperative standard radiography or by fluoroscopy. This method of diagnosis is more complex and time consuming, requires the patient to be stable enough to undergo anesthesia, and is usually not performed until definitive surgical treatment of the shunt is planned. Many surgeons elect to explore the abdomen in search of a shunt and, if none is found, proceed with a portogram.

Animals with hepatic microvascular dysplasia have abnormal serum bile acid concentration, but scintigraphic studies and ultrasounds are normal. A diagnosis of hepatic microvascular dysplasia should be suspected in the patient who has clinical signs consistent with portosystemic shunting and an abnormal serum bile acid concentration but has no demonstrable shunt and a normal-appearing scintigraphy or portogram. The diagnosis is confirmed by liver biopsy, usually at the time of portography or exploratory laparotomy.

TREATMENT

Medical Therapy

Mild hepatoencephalopathy, metabolic derangements, and urinary tract abnormalities may require hospitalization but are not emergencies. Seizures and severe metabolic derangements warrant immediate and urgent care.

The primary goal of medical therapy is to minimize clinical signs of hepatoencephalopathy by decreasing the number of false neurotransmitters in the bloodstream. Hepatoencephalopathy can manifest as lethargy, stupor, listlessness, dementia, aggressive behavior, or seizures. Predisposing factors include dehydration, constipation, infection, catabolism, alkalosis, hypokalemia, high-protein meals, and gastrointestinal bleeding.

If an animal has active seizure activity or is comatose because of encephalopathy, immediate treatment is needed. Because endogenous benzodiazapenes have been implicated as causing hepatoencephalopathy, conventional treatment with exogenous benzodiazepine (intravenous diazepam administration) for seizure control is not indicated. A bolus of dextrose should be administered after collecting pretreatment blood samples to empirically treat hypoglycemic seizures. If there is no response, general anesthesia is indicated. A propofol constant rate infusion is generally favored over barbiturate agents because of propofol's decreased reliance on hepatic metabolism for clearance. Anesthesia is maintained with propofol for 6 hours and then is discontinued. If seizures start again, the animal is re-anesthetized for another 4 to 6 hours. Careful monitoring of vital signs, blood glucose, and appropriate respiration is necessary during anesthesia. Patients exhibiting signs of high intracranial pressure (*e.g.*, cranial nerve abnormalities, hyperventilation, abnormal pupil responses, decerebrate posture) should be treated for cerebral edema.

While the animal is anesthetized, or if the animal is comatose on examination, a cleansing enema is performed to reduce the amount of feces available for bacterial breakdown. Additionally, a lactulose retention enema is performed to reduce the pH of the colon. A solution of one part 50% lactulose and two parts warm water is used at a dose of 5 to 10 ml/kg. A Foley catheter with balloon inflated at the rectum is used to instill and retain the lactulose solution in the colon for 20 to 30 minutes. Orally administered lactulose and antibiotics are initiated after the swallowing reflex is regained.

Management of hepatoencephalopathy consists of preventing or removing factors that may initiate or exacerbate pathologic changes. Lactulose is a mainstay of treatment for hepatoencephalopathy. In the colon, lactulose is hydrolyzed to organic acids, thus creating osmotic diarrhea and decreasing the pH of the colon. In a more acidic environment, the ammonium ion is trapped in the bowel, and less of the ammonia molecule, which is more absorbable, is formed. Lactulose is administered orally (0.25 ml–0.5 ml) two to three times daily. The dose is titrated until two to three soft stools are produced per day. If an animal is constipated on initial examination, a cleansing enema (10–20 ml/kg of warm water) should be performed.

Orally administered antibiotics are used to reduce the number of ammonia-producing bacteria in the colon. Typically, an aminoglycoside such as neomycin (12–22 mg/kg PO q 18 h to q 12 h) is used. Because aminoglycosides are not normally absorbed in the intestines, systemic toxicity is usually not a concern. Care should be exercised in patients with inflammation of the gastrointestinal system, however, because enough drug could be absorbed to cause concern for nephrotoxicity. Care should be exercised in an animal with any signs of renal insufficiency. Alternatively, ampicillin can be used in the azotemic patient. Metronidazole (7.5 mg/kg PO, IV, IM, or SC q8h) is also effective, although drug-associated neurotoxicity is a potential complication, which can be difficult to distinguish from hepatoencephalopathy.

Metabolic derangements such as dehydration, hypokalemia, and catabolism exacerbate hepatoencephalopathy. Adequate hydration is attained with intravenous administration of 0.9% sodium chloride fluids, with supplementation if the animal has hypokalemia or hypoglycemia. Sodium chloride promotes renal correction of metabolic alkalosis. Fluids containing lactate should be avoided because they can lead to alkalosis in an animal with impaired liver function.

For long-term medical therapy, dietary manipulation is recommended to reduce nitrogenous waste products. A highly digestible, high-quality diet should be used to minimize the amount of fecal material available in the colon for bacterial breakdown. On a dry matter basis, the diet should contain 14% to 17% protein for dogs, and 30% to 35% for cats. This is roughly equivalent to 1.75 to 2.5 g/kg/day for dogs and 3 to 3.5 g/kg/day for cats. Prescriptions diets u/d and k/d (Hill's Pet Products, Topeka, KS) are commonly used, with supplementation of protein as needed to meet recommendations.

Medical treatment of urate urolithiasis has been suggested. With appropriate dietary therapy, urinary bladder stones have been reported to resolve without surgical removal, although renal uroliths have not. While alkalization of the urine has been suggested to help prevent the formation of urate uroliths, the potential for exacerbation of hepatic encephalopathy is a concern.

Surgical Therapy

Traditionally, single extrahepatic shunts have been treated by ligation at the time of surgery. Portal pressure and central venous pressure are measured with a water manometer, while the shunt is gradually attenuated with a silk ligature. To avoid portal hypertension, portal pressure should not increase more than 10 cm of water over baseline measurement. Central venous pressure should not decrease more than 1 cm of water. Additionally, the intestines are observed for 5 to 10 minutes for gross signs of hypertension such as cyanosis, hypermotility, or bounding vasculature. It is not always possible to fully ligate the shunting vessel; therefore, partial occlusion is performed. It has been reported that long-term prognosis diminishes with partial occlusion; therefore a second surgery is recommended approximately 3 months after partial ligation to fully ligate the shunting vessel. This delayed complete ligation increases the prognosis for a more normal life after surgery.

If attenuation of the vessel is too acute, portal hypertension may occur. This is a severe and possibly life-threatening condition, leading to cardiovascular collapse, sepsis, and loss of integrity of the gastrointestinal barrier.

To prevent acute portal hypertension, multiple methods of slow occlusion have been described. The most common method of slow occlusion is placement of an amaroid constrictor, which is a ring of casein with a steel casing.[5] The constrictor is placed at the time of surgery, and medical therapy is continued for a number of weeks while the constrictor slowly decreases the lumen of the vessel. Most patients improve clinically and have a more normal serum bile acid concentration within 3 months. Medical therapy is slowly weaned after bile acids normalize. The use of this technique precludes the need for portal pressure measurement, reduces the risk of portal hypertension, and eliminates the possible need for a second surgery to completely ligate a partial shunt ligation.

Intrahepatic vessels can also be attenuated, although the morbidity and mortality associated with surgical therapy tends to be significantly higher. Multiple surgical methods have been described to treat intrahepatic shunts, and advanced equipment such as an ultrasonic aspirator is helpful to dissect through hepatic parenchyma.[6]

After surgical therapy of a single portosystemic shunt, monitoring for portal hypertension is necessary in the immediate postoperative period. As noted above, clinical signs of portal hypertension include severe abdominal pain, vomiting, diarrhea, tachycardia, cardiovascular collapse, and signs of sepsis.[7] Portal hypertension must be treated as soon as it is recognized because it can be rapidly fatal. Treatment consists of emergency surgery to alleviate the ligature on the shunting vessel. Animals exhibiting portal hypertension that has progressed to bloody diarrhea have a poor prognosis.

Surgical therapy of multiple extrahepatic portosystemic shunts has been described. The goal of the procedure is to increase pressure in the vena cava, by using a procedure known as caval banding. While the procedure has been reported to improve quality of life in some patients, it has also been reported to be no more efficacious than medical therapy.[8]

Postoperative prolonged generalized motor seizures have been reported in many dogs after ligation of a portosystemic shunt. These seizures can start 1 to 3 days after surgery and commonly lead to death if not treated aggressively. General anesthesia is often necessary because benzodiazepines are contraindicated, and treatment for hepatic encephalopathy should be instituted as described above. A propofol constant rate infusion is recommended for anesthesia because barbiturate metabolism is erratic because of diminished liver function. Anesthesia should be maintained for 6 hours, as described above.

PROGNOSIS

Surgical therapy of a congenital shunt is considered high risk. The reported mortality rate ranges from 14% to 21% for a single extrahepatic shunts and 11% to 25% for a single intrahepatic shunts.

Prognosis for normal function after surgery for a congenital shunt is associated with the ability to fully ligate the shunt. Animals with partial shunt ligation have a much greater incidence of recurrence of clinical signs and patient morbidity than those with complete ligation.[9] For this reason, a portosystemic shunt that is not completely ligated should undergo additional ligation after the portal vasculature has had the opportunity to accommodate to the change in blood flow. The rate of complete ligation in nonencephalopathic dogs is much higher than that in dogs showing signs of encephalopathy.[10] Animals that undergo only partial occlusion of the shunt may need continued medical therapy and dietary modification. Alternatively, ameroid constrictor placement slowly occludes the vessel and obligates the need for a second surgery.

Animals that have seizures before treatment do not carry a poor prognosis, except if prolonged seizures lead to cerebral edema and neurologic damage. Seizures after ligation of a shunt are ominous and carry a guarded prognosis.[11]

REFERENCES

1. Schermerhorn T, Center SA, Dykes NL, *et al.*: Characterization of hepatoportal microvascular dysplasia in a kindred of cairn terriers. *J Vet Intern Med* 10: 219, 1996.
2. Tisdall PL, Hunt GB, Malik R: Post-prandial bile acid concentrations and ammonia tolerance in Maltese dogs with and without hepatic vascular anomalies. *Aust Vet J* 72:121, 1995.
3. Maddison JE: Hepatic encephalopathy, current concepts of the pathogenesis. *J Vet Int Med* 6:341, 1992.
4. Center SA: Evaluation of twelve-hour preprandial and two-hour postprandial serum bile acids concentrations for diagnosis of heptobilitary disease in dogs. *J Am Vet Med Assoc* 199:217, 1991.
5. Vogt JC, Krahwinkel DJ, Bright RM, *et al.*: Gradual occlusion of extrahepatic portosystemic shunts in dogs and cats using the ameroid constrictor. *Vet Surg* 25:495, 1996.
6. Tobias KMS, Rawlings CA: Surgical techniques for extravascular occlusion of intrahepatic shunts. *Compend Contin Educ Small Animal Pract* 18:745, 1996.
7. Holt D: Critical care management of the portosystemic shunt patient. *Compend Contin Educ Small Animal Pract* 16:879, 1994.
8. Boothe HW, Howe LM, Edwards JF, *et al.*: Multiple extrahepatic portosystemic shunts in dogs: 30 cases (1981–1993). *J Am Vet Med Assoc* 208:1849, 1996.
9. Hottinger HA, Walshaw R, Hauptman JG: Long-term results of complete and partial ligation of congenital portosystemic shunts in dogs. *Vet Surg* 24:331, 1995.

10. Harvey J, Erb HN: Complete ligation of extrahepatic congenital portosystemic shunts in nonencephalopathic dogs. *Vet Surg* 27:413, 1998.
11. Hardie EM, Kornegay JN, Cullen JM: Status epilepticus after ligation of portosystemic shunts. *Vet Surg* 19:412, 1990.

55
Esophageal Disorders

Sheldon Padgett

INTRODUCTION

Normally, the esophagus propels a food bolus from the pharynx to the stomach. Dogs have skeletal muscle throughout the length of the esophagus; cats have a large quantity of smooth muscle in the distal one-third of the esophagus. Disorders of the esophagus usually result in clinical signs of regurgitation and weight loss. Disorders can be separated into mechanical and functional abnormalities.

PATHOGENESIS

Mechanical Abnormalities

Mechanical obstruction is not uncommon in dogs and cats. Foreign body obstruction represents the most common mechanical abnormality. Objects with an irregular shape or an ability to penetrate tissue have a tendency to remain in the esophagus after swallowing. The foreign body location often correlates with areas of physiologic narrowing. These areas include the pharyngeal esophagus, the thoracic inlet, the base of the heart, and the distal esophageal sphincter (at the level of the diaphragmatic esophageal hiatus). The area of the gastroesophageal junction is the most common location.[1] Depending on the chronicity and type of the foreign body, pathologic changes can range from mucosal irritation to perforation of the esophagus. Perforation can lead to mediastinitis and pneumomediastinum.[2]

Stricture of the esophagus can develop secondary to foreign body, gastroesophageal reflux, ingestion of caustic agents, thermal burns, or trauma. Stricture usually develops 2 to 8 weeks after the inciting cause. Stricture arises from extension of severe local inflammation to the esophageal lamina propria and muscularis. General anesthesia has been implicated in relaxing the lower esophageal sphincter and allowing gastric acid reflux. One study showed that abdominal surgery increases the incidence of gastric acid reflux, but body positioning does not.[3]

Esophageal neoplasia can also produce mechanical obstruction. Squamous cell carcinoma, leiomyosarcoma, fibrosarcoma, and osteosarcoma have been described as primary tumors of the esophagus. Less commonly, an extraesophageal mass can produce clinical abnormalities due to transmural compression. Secondary megaesophagus may occur proximal to the compression site. In one report, 11 of 25 dogs with thymoma also had megaesophagus.[4]

Esophageal diverticula are focal wall dilatations producing a functional pouching effect of the esophagus. Pulsion diverticula are created by supranormal esophageal wall pressure, usually caused by exaggerated local peristalsis or obstruction interfering with normal peristalsis. Traction diverticula develop secondarily to adhesion of the esophagus to other thoracic structures and leads to bulges or distortion in the esophagus wall.[5] Diverticula can develop congenitally and are believed to be the result of congenital weakness of the esophageal wall, abnormal separation of tracheal and esophageal embryonic buds, or eccentric vacuole formation.[5] Traction diverticula occur as fibrous extraesophageal tissue contracts away from the esophagus, and pulls the esophagus with it.

Functional Obstruction

Regional or diffuse dilation of the esophagus with diminished or absent motor activity is known as megaesophagus. Many causes of this condition have been described (Table 55-1).

Acquired megaesophagus is most common form. Any chronic obstructive esophageal lesion can result in megaesophagus orad to the lesion site; this is commonly described as secondary megaesophagus. The most common obstructive lesion in young animals is a vascular ring anomaly, most frequently a persistent right aortic arch. Obstruction induced by neoplasia or stricture can also lead to chronic, progressive megaesophagus.

Table 55-1. Diseases Reported to Be Associated with Megaesophagus[7,14]

Central Nervous System	Distemper	Brain Stem Lesions
	Neoplasia	Trauma
Peripheral Neuropathies	Toxicity (lead, thallium, acrylamide)	Polyneuritis
	Spinal muscular atrophy	Polyradiculoneuritis
	Dysautonomia	Ganglioradiculitis
	Giant cell axonal neuropathy	Mediastinitis
	Bronchoesophageal fistula	Bilateral vagal damage
Neuromuscular Junction	Myasthenia gravis	Botulism
	Tetanus	Anticholinesterase toxicity
Esophageal Musculature	Systemic lupus erythematosus	Glycogen storage disease
	Polymyositis	Dermatomyositis
	Hypoadrenocorticism	±Hypothyroidism
Obstructive Lesion	Neoplasia (esophageal or mediastinal)	Vascular ring anomaly
	Foreign body	Stricture
	Granuloma	

A number of diseases that feature neurologic or muscle abnormalities also increase risk for development of secondary megaesophagus. Of this category, myasthenia gravis is the most common. One form of myasthenia is localized only to the esophagus.

Endocrinopathies such as hyperadrenocorticism, hypoadrenocorticism, and hypothyroidism are also implicated in causing megaesophagus. The absolute cause of the megaesophagus with these disorders is controversial. Hypoadrenocorticism is thought to alter muscle carbohydrate metabolism and deplete muscle glycogen stores, leading to megaesophagus.[6,7]

Congenital megaesophagus is much less common than acquired. A congenital abnormality can accompany any abnormality of the esophageal afferent nervous system and many congenital polyneuropathies or myopathies.

EPIDEMIOLOGY

A large, esophageal foreign body is more common in young dogs, which tend to indulge in indiscriminate eating. Small dogs are reported to be more likely than large dogs to have an esophageal foreign body, and the foreign body is more likely to result in perforation in small dogs. Bone esophageal foreign body is the most common type in dogs.[8] Cats, having a tendency to hunt and play, have a higher prevalence of needles than large objects such as bones.

Esophageal neoplasia is seen in older animals. In cats, squamous cell carcinoma is more commonly seen in females in the middle third of the esophagus.

The German shepherd, Irish setter, Boston terrier dogs, and Siamese and Persian cats are most commonly diagnosed with vascular ring anomaly. There is no breed, sex, or age predilection for diverticula.

Congenital megaesophagus is an inherited condition in dogs, reported in the wirehair fox terrier and miniature schnauzer. Additionally, a predisposition may exist in the great Danes, German shepherd, Irish setter, Labrador retriever, Newfoundland, and Chinese shar-pei. Predisposed cat breeds are the Siamese and Siamese-related breeds.[7] The signalment for animals with acquired megaesophagus varies with the underlying cause. In a report of 136 dogs with acquired megaesophagus, the mean age was 8.1 years with a range of 0.75 to 18 years of age.[9]

CLINICAL PRESENTATION

Client complaints often include regurgitation, dysphagia, dyspnea, gagging, ptyalism, weight loss, and distress. It is important to discern regurgitation from vomiting, as many owners report vomiting with esophageal disease when regurgitation is actually seen. Occasionally, both vomiting and regurgitation are seen in an animal with esophageal disease.

Animals with a congenital vascular ring anomaly such as a persistent right aortic arch are usually examined at the time of weaning because solid food does not pass as easily as milk. Acquired stricture caused by gastroesophageal reflux or ingestion of a caustic substance usually leads to clinical signs in 2 to 8 weeks, depending on the exuberance of the fibroplasia.

Megaesophagus leads to recurrent regurgitation and can cause aspiration pneumonia. Some patients are initially examined with a primary history of respiratory disease and will have fever and harsh respiratory sounds. Suspicion of megaesophagus or other esophageal disease should be high if the owner reports that recurrent regurgitation or vomiting took place before respiratory signs developed.

Clinical signs that increase the suspicion of an underlying systemic disorder usually accompany megaesophagus secondary to polyneuropathy or metabolic disease. The exception would be focal esophageal myasthenia gravis, which is seen in approximately 25% of myasthenic animals.

DIAGNOSTIC EVALUATION

A complete blood count and serum biochemical analysis should be performed, although no specific abnormalities are associated with esophageal disease. Neutrophilia can be found in animals with aspiration pneumonia secondary to megaesophagus and mediastinitis secondary to esophageal perforation. Chemistry profile abnormalities may support an endocrinopathy as the cause of megaesophagus. Additional testing for causative diseases such as adrenocortical disease, thyroid disease, immune-mediated disease, and toxicity should be pursued as clinical suspicion indicates.

Thoracic radiography is helpful in any animal suspected of having esophageal disease. Most esophageal foreign bodies are radiopaque (*i.e.*, bones, fish hooks, and needles). Radiographic signs of an esophageal foreign body include abnormal esophageal gas patterns, dilation of the esophagus orad to the foreign body, and presence of an obvious foreign body.

Megaesophagus is seen on survey radiographs as a dilated esophagus (Figure 55-1). Generalized megaesophagus involves the entire esophagus, and strictures (including vascular ring abnormalities) lead to dilation orad to the lesion. It is important to know that aerophagia can sometimes lead to a local, transient megaesophagus that can be seen on radiographs.

Perforation of the esophagus secondary to foreign body or trauma can produce radiographic signs of mediastinitis. Loss of mediastinal detail including obliteration of the caudal vena cava shadow has been shown to be significantly associated with esophageal perforation. Pneumomediastinum was not seen in 10 cases of esophageal perforation in dogs.[8]

Positive contrast esophagography can be used to delineate a foreign body, mass, stricture, or diverticula of the esophagus. Contrast studies can be useful in delineating an esophageal irregularity, stricture, mass, and esophagitis (Figure 55-2). Liquid contrast is usually used first but may pass through more mild strictures in a relatively normal fashion. Food mixed with barium can be used if a stricture is strongly suspected because it will more likely become lodged orad to a stricture, although regurgitation is an important concern. Esophageal endoscopic evaluation is preferred over food mixed with barium to avoid aspiration of the food and barium mixture. Leakage of contrast material into the mediastinum is diagnostic for esophageal perforation, although a high rate of false negatives

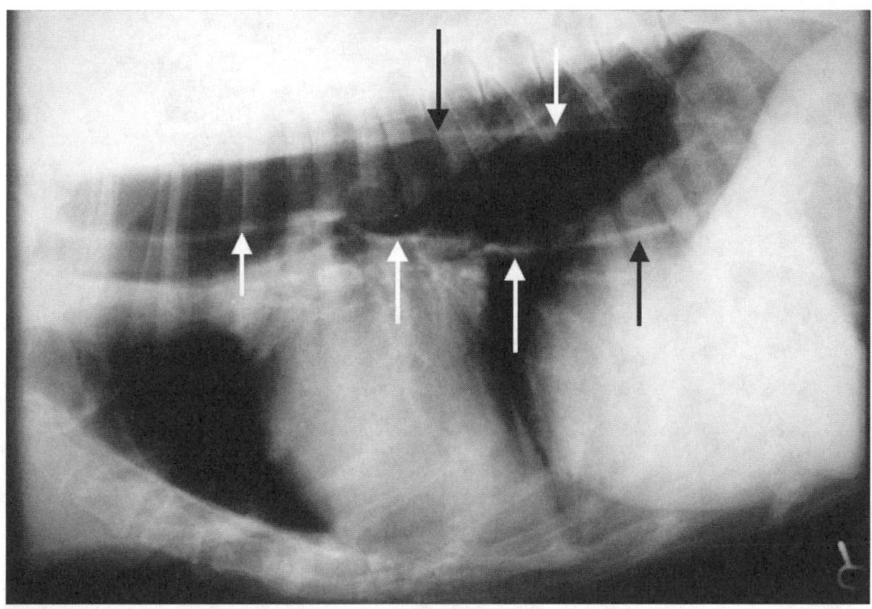

(A)

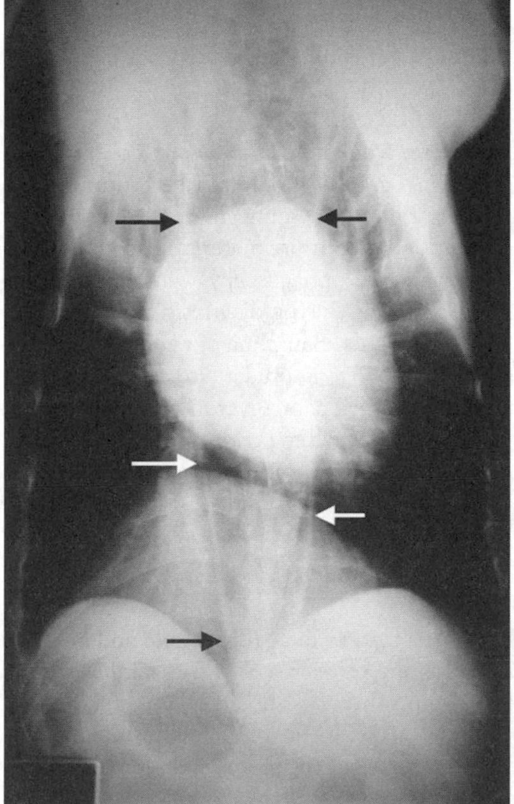

(B)

Figure 55-1
Lateral (**A**) and ventrodorsal (**B**) thoracic radiographs of a patient with megaesophagus. The megaesophagus is outlined by arrows in each view.

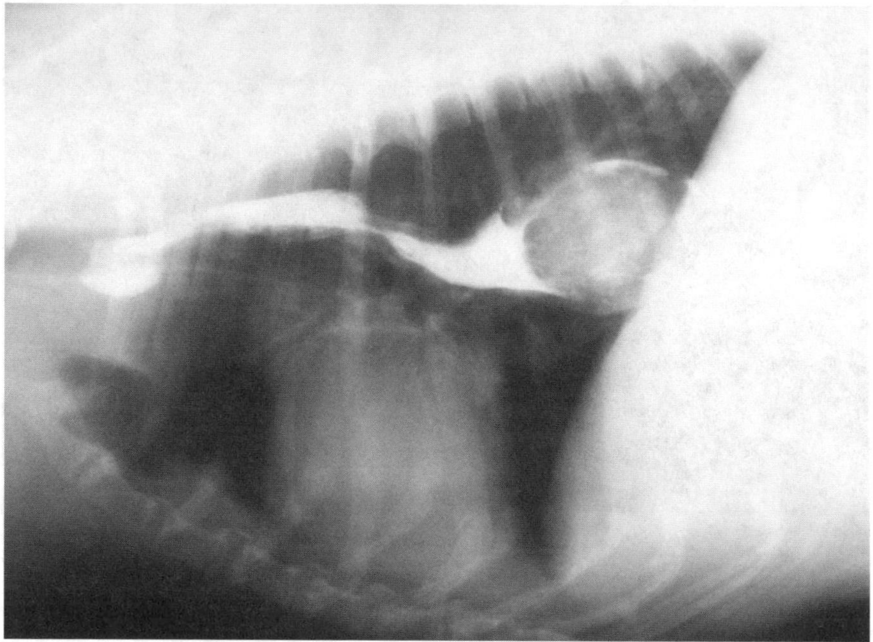

Figure 55-2
Lateral positive contrast esophagram of a patient with a caudal esophageal mass.

(25%–50%) have been reported; therefore, a negative esophagram does not rule out the possibility of perforation.[8] Esophagography should not be routinely performed in an animal with known, generalized megaesophagus because regurgitation is common and can lead to aspiration of contrast material into the lungs.

Endoscopic evaluation of the esophagus (esophagoscopy) can be a valuable diagnostic tool. Visualization by endoscopy aids in the diagnosis of esophagitis, foreign body, neoplasia, stricture, and diverticula. Sampling of neoplastic lesions is also possible at the time of esophagoscopy. It is prudent to be prepared to perform surgery after esophagoscopy if perforation or severe necrosis is found. Caution must be exercised during esophagoscopy when perforation is a possibility because as life-threatening tension pneumothorax can result from aggressive insufflation.

TREATMENT

Since most abnormalities of the esophagus lead to diminished tone and possible gastroesophageal reflux, prophylactic therapy to decrease gastric acidity is indicated. Histamine blockers or proton pump inhibitors should be used for 7 to 10 days after the inciting cause has been removed. The use of sucralfate as a mucosal protective drug is controversial because of the need for an acidic environment for maximal effect. Sucralfate slurries may lead to mild improvement of esophagitis but do not prevent esophagitis from developing in humans.[10]

While it may be assumed that antibiotics are indicated in cases of esophagitis, no benefit has been found in human studies of esophagitis. Human patients do not receive antibiotics while being treated for esophagitis unless fever or infection develops.[10]

Removal of an esophageal foreign body varies depending on the location and composition. If possible, endoscopic removal with grasping forceps is ideal. Large objects distal in the esophagus can be pushed into the stomach to dissolved or be removed via gastrotomy. A surgical approach to the esophagus may be necessary if the patient has marked necrosis or perforation of the esophagus. As suggested, it is important to be judicious in the use of insufflation, because esophageal perforation may allow air to escape, leading to a pneumothorax. Fishhooks were found to be more difficult to remove via endoscopy if they were treble-barb as opposed to single barb. Orientation or location in the esophagus was not indicative of ability to remove the fishhook.[11] A foreign body that is not lodged in the esophageal wall can sometimes be removed blindly by passing a deflated Foley catheter distal to the foreign body, then inflating the balloon and retracting the catheter.

Vascular ring anomaly is treated by ligation and transection of the anomalous vessel. Treatment should be initiated as soon as possible after diagnosis because the degree of esophageal dilation is thought to progress with time.

Strictures other than vascular ring anomaly should be managed conservatively before surgery is attempted. Progressive dilation by bougienage or balloon dilation can be attempted. Sequentially larger bougies or balloons are used to break down fibrous constricting bands. Medical treatment of gastric acid reduction should be continued during this time. Multiple dilations may be needed.

Animals with stricture of the esophagus should be fed a soft food gruel in an upright position to allow gravitational flow of food past the stricture. Ideally, the animal should be held so that the forelimbs are higher than the hindlimbs for 10 to 20 minutes after feeding.

Surgery of the esophagus commonly necessitates thoracotomy. Esophagostomy is performed if a foreign body cannot be removed by advancing into the stomach or endoscopy. Patients with marked esophageal necrosis or esophageal neoplasia can be candidates for partial esophageal resection. While 20% to 50% of the esophagus can be resected without a tension relieving technique, the surgeon should be prepared to perform a reconstructive procedure if necessary. Small diverticula can often be managed by feeding the animal a soft diet and elevating the food. Larger diverticula require surgical excision. The reader is referred to a surgical text for complete description of these procedures.

Treatment of megaesophagus is directed at the underlying cause in addition to conservative treatment such as pharmacologic manipulation and positional feeding as described. Antibiotic administration is indicated if the patient has aspiration pneumonia. Prokinetic agents are controversial because they have not been shown conclusively to increase peristalsis in the esophagus. Prokinetic drugs may, however, be beneficial due to their ability to increase the tone of the lower esophageal sphincter, thereby decreasing acid reflux.[7]

PROGNOSIS

Conditions without perforation or necrosis of the esophagus generally have a favorable prognosis. Perforation of the esophagus warrants a more guarded prognosis.

Diverticula of the esophagus can be managed conservatively with success. If surgery is necessary, the prognosis is good as long as esophageal reconstruction is possible.

Prognosis for megaesophagus varies with the cause. If the underlying cause can be treated, as in a patient with a vascular ring anomaly, the prognosis can be good. Commonly, treatment for primary or idiopathic megaesophagus is supportive with a poor, long-term prognosis. In patients with megaesophagus secondary to myasthenia gravis, multiple forms of the disease complicate prognostication, although it is known that aspiration pneumonia is commonly the cause of death in these animals.[13] Thymoma-associated megaesophagus has a poor prognosis; in one study, six of nine animals undergoing surgery for thymoma died within 1 week.[4]

Masses of the esophagus are commonly large by the time of diagnosis. For this reason, surgery may be difficult, and prognosis is guarded. Palliation of clinical signs may be achieved if esophageal reapposition or reconstruction is possible.

REFERENCES

1. Spielman BL, Shaker EH, Garvey MS: Esophageal foreign body in dogs: a retrospective study of 23 cases. *J Am Anim Hosp Assoc* 28:570, 1992.
2. Rogers KS, Walker MA: Disorders of the mediastinum. *Compend Contin Educ Pract* Vet 19:69, 1997.
3. Galatos AD, Raptopoulos D: Gastro-esophageal reflux during anaesthesia in the dog: the effect of age, positioning and type of surgical procedure. *Vet Record* 137: 513, 1995.
4. Atwater SW, Powers BE, Park RD, *et al.*: Thymoma in dogs: 23 cases (1980–1991). *J Am Vet Med Assoc* 205:1007, 1994.
5. Hedlund CS: Surgery of the esophagus. *In* Fossum TW, ed.: Small Animal Surgery. St. Louis: Mosby-Year Book, 1997, p 232.
6. Shelton GD: Pathogenesis of canine megaesophagus: neuromuscular disorders. *In* Proceedings, 14th Forum Am Col Vet Int Med, 1996, p 581.
7. Mears EA, Jenkins CC: Canine and feline megaesophagus. *Compend Contin Educ Pract* Vet 19:313, 1997.
8. Parker NR, Walter PA, Gay J: Diagnosis and surgical management of esophageal perforation. *J Am Anim Hosp Assoc* 25:587, 1989.
9. Gaynor AR, Shofer FS, Washabau RJ: Risk factors for acquired megaesophagus in dogs. *J Am Vet Med Assoc* 211:1406, 1997.
10. Weyrauch EA, Willard MD: Esophagitis and benign esophageal strictures. *Compend Contin Educ Pract* Vet 20:203, 1998.
11. Michels GM, Jones BD, Huss BT, *et al.*: Endoscopic and surgical retrieval of fish-

hooks from the stomach and esophagus in dogs and cats: 75 cases (1977–1993). *J Am Vet Med Assoc* 207:1194, 1995.

12. Muldoon MM, Birchard SJ, Ellison GW: Long-term results of surgical correction of persistent right aortic arch in dogs: 25 cases (1980–1995). *J Am Vet Med Assoc* 210:1761, 1997.
13. Dewey CW, Bailey CS, Shelton GD, *et al.*: Clinical forms of acquired myasthenia gravis in dogs: 25 cases (1988–1995). *J Vet Int Med* 11:50, 1997.
14. Moses L, Harpster NK, Beck KA, *et al.*: Esophageal motility dysfunction in cats: a study of 44 cases. *J Am Anim Hosp Assoc* 36:309, 2000.

56
Gastric Outflow Obstruction

Sheldon Padgett

INTRODUCTION

Inability to pass stomach contents into the duodenum is known as gastric outflow obstruction. Normally, smooth muscle of the stomach contracts in peristaltic waves, which vary with the amount of ingesta in the stomach and neural influences. The canine stomach contracts with an aboral peristalsis four to five times per minute during feeding.[1,2] Inability to appropriately empty the stomach due to outflow obstruction can lead to clinical signs such as vomiting and weight loss. Disorders of gastric motility, pyloric abnormalities, neoplasia (extrinsic or intrinsic), and foreign bodies have been reported to lead to gastric outflow obstruction.

PATHOGENESIS

Mechanical Gastric Outflow Obstruction

Obstructions can be classified as either functional or mechanical (Table 56-1). A foreign body at the level of the pylorus is the most common type of mechanical obstruction. Pyloric foreign bodies tend to be either ball-shaped, acting as a valve at the pylorus, or a mass of foreign material (often cloth) that is entangled with a linear foreign body. The linear foreign body extends into the small intestine, pulling the mass of foreign material into the pylorus and acting as an anchor.

Mechanical obstruction due to changes in pyloric anatomy is also encountered. The most common pathologies are hypertrophy of the circular muscles at the level of the pylorus and hypertrophy of the pyloric mucosa or a combination thereof. Inflammation of the pyloric area can lead to exacerbation of the obstruction. Two syndromes involving hypertrophy of the pyloric area have been named. Congenital pyloric stenosis is caused by hypertrophy of the pyloric circular smooth muscle layer in young dogs.[1] The pathogenesis is unclear, but gastrin excess has been implicated since gastrin has trophic effects on gastric smooth muscle. The second syndrome is chronic hypertrophic pyloric gastropathy, which can be associated with circular muscle hypertrophy (type I), both muscle hypertrophy and mucosal hypertrophy (type II), or only mucosal hypertrophy (type III).[1] Many causes have been proposed for this syndrome. Chronic gastric distention due to long-term sympathetic stimulation, chronic gastritis, or neurogenic abnormality can lead to gastrin release. This hypothesis appears to be a plausible

Table 56-1. Type and Cause of Common Gastric Outflow Obstruction with Associated Signalments and Histories

Type of pyloric obstruction	Cause	History/Signalment
Mechanical obstruction	Foreign body	Young patient most commonly; history of ingesting foreign body
	Neoplasia	Middle-aged to older patient
	Congenital pyloric stenosis	Young, brachycephalic dog
	Chronic hypertrophic pyloric gastropathy	Middle-aged, small-breed dogs (male more often than female)
Functional obstruction	Idiopathic delayed gastric emptying	No predisposed breed or age
	Secondary delayed gastric emptying	Varies with primary cause (hypokalemia, hypoadrenocorticisim, diabetes mellitus, uremia, drug therapy, stress, abdominal inflammation, pancreatitis)

explanation for hypertrophic pyloric changes, mucosal and muscular hypertrophy, as well as an increase in the amount of gastric hydrochloric acid released.

Pyloric stenosis is uncommon in cats. Siamese cats are most commonly affected, and many have concurrent megaesophagus, suggesting an underlying neuropathologic cause.[1,2]

Gastric neoplasia can also lead to mechanical outflow obstruction. Malignant neoplasia is more common in dogs, with adenocarcinoma being the most prevalent.[3,4] Other gastric malignancies include leiomyosarcoma, lymphoma, plasmacytoma, and fibrosarcoma.[3,5] Benign tumors of the canine stomach include leiomyoma and adenoma. The most commonly diagnosed gastric tumor in cats is lymphoma, with adenocarcinoma diagnosed rarely.[3] Extrinsic neoplasia originating from the pancreas and liver can also lead to extramural compression and outflow tract obstruction in both species.

Functional Gastric Outflow Obstruction

Functional disorders of gastric emptying (also known as delayed gastric emptying or gastroparesis) can be either transient or chronic in nature. The disorder can be a primary pathologic condition, such as an underlying motor abnormality resulting from dysfunction of the myenteric plexus or smooth muscle. Secondary pathologic change leading to altered gastric emptying (functional) is common. Systemic conditions such as hypokalemia, hypoadrenocorticisim, diabetes mellitus, uremia, drug therapy (*e.g.*, anticholinergics, β-adrenergic agonists, opiates), acute stress, acute abdominal inflammation, and pancreatitis can result in delayed gastric emptying. It is most common, however, to find no underlying pathologic cause, and this condition is referred to as idiopathic delayed gastric emptying.[2]

Secondary gastric ulceration may result from delayed gastric emptying caused by a high gastrin concentration. Inflammatory gastritis and ulcerative disease can also be primary inciting causes of diminished gastric motility and, therefore, functional outflow obstruction.

Pathophysiology of Metabolic Alkalosis

Metabolic alkalosis is a disorder characterized by a primary increase in plasma bicarbonate concentration or a loss of hydrogen ion that tends to increase the blood pH. This alkalosis results from frequent and profuse vomiting of gastric contents, with two exceptions (*i.e.*, marked potassium depletion and primary aldosteronism). Metabolic alkalosis requires a chloride deficiency for its genesis and chloride repletion for its correction. The fact that metabolic alkalosis may persist even when no new bicarbonate is added to the extracellular fluid is *a priori* evidence that the kidney is reabsorbing more bicarbonate than under normal circumstances.

The kidneys attempt to maintain electroneutrality of extracellular fluid by reabsorbing appropriate amounts of cations and anions. Since the major inorganic anions are chloride and bicarbonate, the reabsorption of these anions in the kidneys is inversely proportional to each other. Thus, with excess loss of chloride in vomitus, the kidneys compensate for the resulting hypochloridemia by increasing bicarbonate reabsorption.

Hypokalemia and alkalosis are often directly related because of the renal response to either. Hypokalemia due to a true body deficit of potassium causes the intracellular concentration of this ion to fall. This intracellular deficit of cation is replaced partially by hydrogen ion, and this can produce extracellular alkalosis or potentiate it if it has already developed. Because sodium reabsorption in the distal tubule is linked to an exchange for other cations, chiefly potassium and excess hydrogen, it will cause excess hydrogen secretion into the urine when distal sodium reabsorption is required. This situation is found in patients with metabolic alkalosis in which sodium bicarbonate reabsorption in the proximal nephron is decreased because of the excess of plasma bicarbonate. Distal nephron avidity for sodium is increased to protect extracellular fluid volume, and the increased distal sodium reabsorption is at the expense of hydrogen ion secretion.

The treatment of hypochloremic, hypokalemic metabolic alkalosis usually requires only correction of extracellular fluid volume and sodium and chloride deficits by saline infusion. Providing adequate chloride ion allows the sodium to be reabsorbed without bicarbonate. Increased proximal reabsorption of sodium decreases distal acid secretion because less sodium is presented to the distal nephron. As less bicarbonate is reabsorbed and less acid is secreted, plasma pH returns to normal. Concurrently, some intracellular potassium ions are replaced by hydrogen ions, and this pH-mediated cation shift also aids the return to normokalemia.

EPIDEMIOLOGY

Mechanical Gastric Outflow Obstruction

Foreign body patients tend to be young because young animals are more likely to ingest objects that are too large to pass through the pylorus. Trichobezoars in cats may be related to underlying motility disorders.

Congenital pyloric stenosis is seen particularly in young, brachycephalic dogs.[1,6] The most common time of occurrence is at the point of weaning: liquid passes through the stenosed pylorus but solid food is retained. Chronic hypertrophic pyloric gastropathy is a disease in middle-aged, small-breed dogs, more commonly seen in males.[1,6] Rarely, mechanical outflow obstruction has been reported as a sequela of percutaneous gastrostomy and gastric surgery.[7,8]

Functional Gastric Outflow Obstruction

Primary motility disorders are found in animals with neurologic disorders, those who have undergone gastric surgery, and those with gastritis (commonly infectious or inflammatory).[2] Secondary functional abnormalities are seen in animals with signalments common for the underlying disease.

CLINICAL PRESENTATION

Clinical signs are secondary to obstruction of gastric outflow. Duration of vomiting, frequency of vomiting, and length of time after eating vary widely. Some animals do well with liquid or soft foods but vomit solid foods.

Physical examination findings are nonspecific and vary with the severity and frequency of vomiting. Weight loss, anorexia, lethargy, and dehydration may be observed. Results of abdominal palpation are often normal, except in a patient with an obvious, extramural neoplastic lesion or with pain due to peritonitis or pancreatitis.

DIAGNOSTIC EVALUATION

Results of blood work may reflect an underlying disease state responsible for a secondary functional outflow abnormality such as azotemia, hypokalemia, or hypoadrenocorticism. Prerenal azotemia may be found depending on the frequency of vomiting and ability of the animal to maintain hydration. Complete gastric outflow obstruction, most commonly caused by a pyloric foreign body, classically causes hypokalemic, hypochloremic, metabolic alkalosis due to loss of gastric secretions. This metabolic derangement is not always found, especially with incomplete obstruction due to pyloric stenosis or chronic hypertrophic pyloric gastropathy. Peritonitis leading to gastric paresis may be associated with neutrophilia.

Survey abdominal radiographs may show gastric distention with any type of gastric outflow disease. Abdominal ultrasonographic examination may show pyloric hypertrophy. Extramural masses may be revealed by radiography or, more typically, ultrasound. Positive contrast radiography can be useful to delineate outflow tract obstruction. Unfortunately, false-negative studies are possible, and one cannot differentiate between hypertrophy, benign neoplasia, and malignant neoplastic disease by this diagnostic modality. For these reasons, gastroduodenoscopy is usually more appropriate than contrast radiography as a diagnostic tool when outflow obstruction is suspected. This allows the clinician to both see the outflow tract and obtain biopsy specimens. Biopsy of a thickened pylorus revealed by endoscopy is imperative because it is not possible to visually differentiate between hypertrophy, benign neoplasia, and malignant neoplasia. Foreign bodies can often be removed by endoscopy, thereby avoiding a more invasive procedure such as gastrotomy.

TREATMENT

Dehydration and electrolyte abnormalities should be corrected before anesthesia for either endoscopy or surgery. Treatment of any underlying metabolic or systemic abnormality should be initiated to achieve a metabolically stable condition.

Mechanical obstruction secondary to a pyloric foreign body can be removed either by endoscopy or gastrotomy. Treatment of these patients is usually straightforward, and supportive care is needed in the perianesthetic and postanesthetic periods.

When mechanical obstruction is caused by hypertrophy of the pyloric musculature, pyloric mucosa, or both, surgery is indicated. Several surgical procedures have been described in detail to treat benign hypertrophic outflow obstruction. If the patient has hypertrophy of the muscular layer without mucosal hypertrophy, the Heineke-Mikulicz pyloroplasty is easy to perform and effective in relieving outflow obstruction. If the patient has mucosal hypertrophy, however, this procedure can be ineffective, and a Y-U pyloroplasty is indicated. A more advanced technique such as gastroduodenal resection (Bilroth I or Bilroth II) may be necessary in a patient with an intrinsic or extrinsic mass in the area of the pylorus. The Bilroth procedures carry more risk of surgical and postoperative functional complications and therefore should not be used if a less aggressive procedure would be effective. The reader is referred to surgical texts for a complete description of the surgical procedures mentioned here.[6] A full-thickness biopsy of the pyloric area should always be done to confirm lack of neoplasia.

If ulcerative disease is suspected or confirmed caused by hypergastrinemia, a primary inflammatory disease, or underlying metabolic disease, treatment should be initiated. An antisecretory agent such as an H2-receptor antagonist (ranitidine [Zantac, Glaxo Wellcome] 1–2 mg/kg q 12 h PO) or proton pump inhibitor (omeprazole [Prilosec, Astra-Zeneca] 0.7–2.0 mg/kg q 24 h PO) should be used.[2] As discussed below, ranitidine can also be prokinetic.

The following therapies are *contraindicated* for an animal with mechanical obstruction. For patients with a functional pyloric obstruction such as primary idiopathic or secondary gastroparesis, gastric promotility agents are used to promote emptying. Cisapride (Propulsid, Janssen), a serotonergic drug, is currently the drug of choice for use in stimulating gastric emptying. Although a dosage of 0.1–0.5 mg/kg q 8h to q12 h PO increases gastric motility in normal dogs, a higher dosage (0.5–1.0 mg/kg q 8h–12 h PO) may be needed in dogs with a functional abnormality of gastric emptying.[2] Metoclopramide (Reglan, Robins), while a classic drug to promote gastrointestinal motility, may not be as effective for solids as it is for liquids. Studies have shown that metoclopramide administration can lead to accelerated gastric emptying in normal dogs, but does not change gastric myoelectric and motor activities in a way that would promote emptying in dogs with delayed gastric emptying.[2]

Erythromycin (Erythro-100, Rhone Merieux) may be selected if cisapride is not effective. Erythromycin is used to promote motor activity during nonfed states and probably does not change the gastric emptying of a fed animal. The suggested prokinetic dosage for erythromycin (0.5–1.0 mg/kg q 8 h PO) is much lower than the antimicrobial dosage (10–20 mg/kg q 8 h PO).[2] Ranitidine has been found to be prokinetic at antisecretory dosages; therefore, it can have a dual benefit when used in patients with ulcerative gastritis.

PROGNOSIS

Patients with a mechanical obstruction secondary to foreign body have an excellent prognosis in the absence of co-existing pathology. Patients with mucosal or muscular hypertrophy also have a good to excellent outcome with appropriate surgical therapy. The most common cause of poor outcome is poor surgical technique or inappropriate choice of surgical procedure.

The prognosis for malignant neoplasia of the stomach is poor. Patients with gastric adenocarcinoma do not usually live longer than 6 months, even with surgery and chemotherapy.[3] Those with leiomyosarcoma that survive the perioperative time have a mean survival time of 1 year.[3] Complete excision of benign neoplasia is curative.

The prognosis for patients with a functional abnormality depends on the ability to resolve the underlying cause and the patient's response to appropriate, prokinetic medication.

REFERENCES

1. Stanton ML: Gastric outlet obstruction. *In* Bojrab MJ, Smeak DD, eds.: Disease mechanisms in small animal surgery, 2nd ed. Malvern, PA: Lea & Febiger, 1993, p 235.
2. Hall JA, Washabau RJ: Diagnosis and treatment of gastric motility disorders. *Vet Clin North Am Small Anim Pract* 29:377, 1999.
3. Withrow SJ: Gastric cancer. *In* Withrow SJ, MacEwen EG, eds.: Small Animal Clinical Oncology, 2nd ed. Philadelphia: WB Saunders, 1996, p 244.
4. Gualtieri M, Monzeglio MG, Scanziani E: Gastric neoplasia. *Vet Clin North Am Small Anim Pract* 29:415, 1999.

5. Kapatkin AS, Mullen HS, Matthiesen DT, *et al.*: Leiomyosarcoma in dogs: 44 cases (1983–1988). *J Am Vet Med Assoc* 201:1077, 1992.
6. Fossum TW: Surgery of the stomach. *In* Fossum TW, ed.: Small Animal Surgery. St. Louis: Mosby-Year Book, 1997, p 261.
7. Glaus TM, Cornelius LM, Reusch C, *et al.*: Complications with non-endoscopic percutaneous gastrotomy in 31 cats and 10 dogs: a retrospective study. *J Small Anim Pract* 39:218, 1998.
8. Fossum TW, Rohn DA, Willard MD: Presumptive, iatrogenic gastric outflow obstruction associated with prior gastric surgery. *J Am Anim Hosp Assoc* 31:391, 1995.

57
Intestinal Obstruction

Joseph Harari

INTRODUCTION

Partial or complete bowel obstruction is a common indicator for intestinal surgery in small animals. Most frequently, single or multiple foreign bodies cause the obstruction.[1-6] Intussusception and neoplastic conditions can also occur. Less often, intestinal volvulus, intramural hematoma, extramural adhesions, herniations, strangulations, cecal inversion, rupture of duodenocolic ligament, and pelvic malunions have been identified as causes of obstruction. Clinical signs, surgical treatments, and prognosis vary with the location, etiology, and severity of the lesion(s) (Table 57-1).

PATHOGENESIS

A partial or complete small intestine obstruction may be in a "high" (duodenum, proximal jejunum) or "low" (distal jejunum, ileum) location.[2-5] A high obstruction causes vomiting and loss of gastrointestinal fluids including acidic gastric secretions and alkaline secretions from the gallbladder, pancreas, and duodenum. Electrolyte abnormalities (hypokalemia, hypochloremia) and an acid–base disturbance (metabolic alkalosis or acidosis) may occur. Obstruction of the distal jejunum or ileum produces intestinal distention with fluid and gas accumulation proximal to the lesion. The latter is due to aerophagia, decomposition of intesti-

Table 57-1. Causes of Intestinal Obstruction

Lesion	Location	Comment
Linear foreign bodies	Jejunum	Cats (tethered under tongue)
Mass objects	Pylorus, duodenum, ileocolic valve	Dogs
Intussusception	Jejunum, ileum	Young dogs
Volvulus	Jejunum	Large dogs
Neoplasia	Small intestine, rectal strictures	Lymphosarcoma, adenocarcinoma
Herniations, strangulations	Small intestine	Traumatic, congenital lesions
Adhesions	Small intestine	Trauma, surgery patients

nal contents, and diffusion from blood.[2] The collection of fluid is due to increased production, decreased absorption, alteration of vascular supply, and increased intestinal bacterial population. Bacterial overgrowth and intestinal stasis (ileus) leads to endotoxemia and septicemia.

Vascular compromise secondary to strangulation, herniation, torsion, or invagination of the bowel will deleteriously affect mucosal integrity. In chronic cases, intraluminal objects produce pressure-related wall necrosis and, thus, contribute to increased bacterial absorption.

Linear foreign bodies in cats can be attached proximally at the base of tongue and erode through the mesenteric side of a peristaltic small intestine. In dogs with linear foreign objects, conversely, lodgment at the pylorus along with perforations and peritonitis have been described.[7]

Colonic obstructions are characterized by persistent distention leading to abnormal motility and loss of smooth muscle function. Continued water absorption from colonic contents produces dry feces that are unable to be evacuated.

EPIDEMIOLOGY

Linear foreign bodies are most frequently identified in cats, whereas dogs have a propensity to ingest masslike objects. Intussusception occurs commonly at the ileocecal junction in young dogs with hypermotile intestines secondary to parasitism, stress, surgery, dietary changes, or unknown causes. The ileum (*intussusceptum*) telescopes into the large colon (*intussuscipiens*). Herniations, strangulations, extramural adhesions, and pelvis-associated obstructions are identified in patients after trauma (including surgery). Intestinal volvulus has most often been diagnosed in large (German shepherd) dogs.[8] Intra- or extraluminal neoplasia would be suspect in older animals.

CLINICAL PRESENTATION

Signs of obstruction are variable and include vomiting, depression, anorexia, and dehydration. Weight loss and bloody diarrhea or obstipation (colonic obstruction) are also clinical findings. Abdominal palpation can reveal pain/discomfort and abnormal intestinal contents, bowel loops, or bowel masses. Rectal palpation will reveal pelvic strictures (neoplasia) or compromised canal (malunion). Peracute signs of abdominal distention, circulatory collapse, and death are unique features of intestinal volvulus.[8]

DIAGNOSTIC EVALUATIONS

A review of the clinical history and signs, along with physical examination, laboratory, and imaging evaluations are helpful in identifying the lesion(s). Inconclusive findings in a worsening patient warrant an abdominal exploratory or laparoscopic procedure.

Survey radiographic changes in patients with obstruction include abnormal size, shape, density, and location of bowel loops.[9] Accumulation of gas, fluid, and ingesta occurs proximal to the obstruction. The diameter of the small bowel

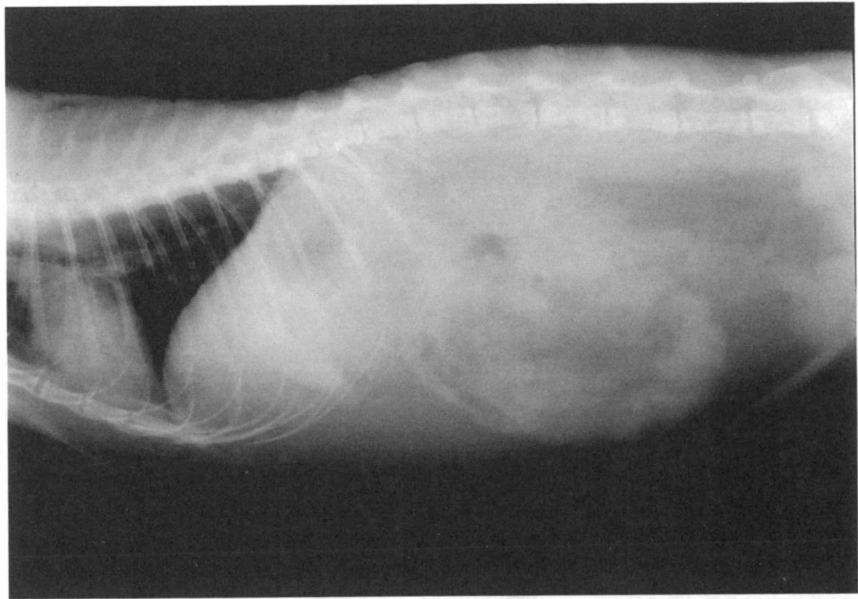

Figure 57-1
Plication of the small bowel secondary to linear foreign body (string) in a cat.

should not exceed the width of a lumbar vertebra (ventrodorsal projection) or the diameter of the colon. Radiography of animals with rectal strictures or pelvic malunions reveals a dilated, feces-impacted colon (megacolon). Plication of the small bowel, especially on the right side of the abdomen, is a feature of linear foreign body ingestion[9] (Fig. 57-1). Opaque foreign bodies are easily discerned. Persistent abnormal findings on serial examinations in an ill patient suggest a clinically significant lesion. Contrast radiography or a gastrointestinal series may reveal abnormal transit of contrast medium or mass outlines (Fig. 57-2) in some cases. Barium enemas can delineate lesions of the large bowel but compromise colonoscopy. Ultrasonography is most helpful in delineating mass lesions and intussusception (alternating layers of hyper- and hypoechoic tissues).[6,9] Peristalsis, or the lack thereof (ileus), can be recognized during ultrasound examination. Advanced imaging techniques (computed tomography, magnetic resonance imaging) may prove useful, although they are today mostly limited to specialty centers and university teaching hospitals.

Laboratory findings are unremarkable in mild, early, or incomplete obstructions.[4] Chronic or severe lesions can produce a neutrophilia, anemia, hypokalemia, variable sodium and chloride values, metabolic acidosis, and prerenal azotemia.

Abdominocentesis may be inconclusive unless bowel rupture has occurred. Laparoscopy is useful for diagnostic purposes, especially in a morbid patient. Endoscopy (gastroduodenal lesions) and colonoscopy are helpful for diagnostic purposes, as well as biopsy procedures.

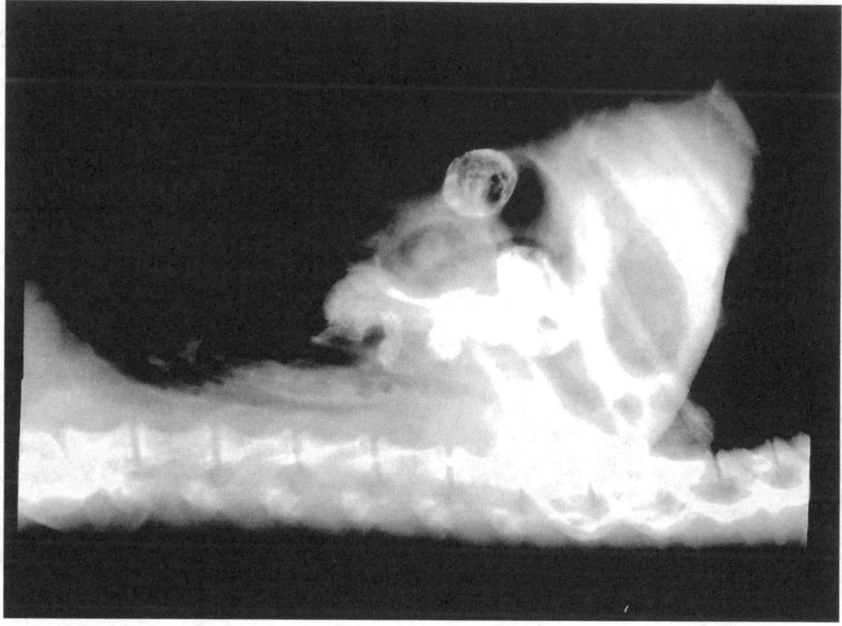

Figure 57-2
Foreign body (corncob) outlined by contrast medium in a young dog. Note proximal dilated, gas-filled bowel loops and contrast medium in the transverse colon (*i.e.,* incomplete obstruction).

TREATMENT

Surgical relief of the obstruction, including intestinal resection and anastomosis, is required for most patients. Unattached linear and small objects (needles, coins) may pass uneventfully through the gastrointestinal tract. Serial radiography and absence of clinical signs are helpful in identifying these nonsurgical patients. Minimally invasive surgical procedures using laparoscopy may gain widespread support in the future as veterinarians become familiar with the equipment and techniques.[10]

General guidelines for obstructive small intestinal surgery include use of prophylactic intravenous antibiotic (cefazolin, 20 mg/kg; enrofloxacin, 10 mg/kg) medication, approximating sutures (monofilament synthetic absorbable or nonabsorbable) placed through the submucosa, replacement of contaminated instruments before closure, and abdominal lavage with warm physiologic solutions.[2,3,5,6] Volume-depleted animals should be resuscitated with fluids perioperatively. Postoperative adhesion formation can be avoided by gentle tissue handling, prevention of dehydration and infection, careful hemostasis, use of nonstrangulating sutures, and irrigation/suction to remove debris.[11] Anesthesia with nitrous oxide should be avoided in surgical patients to avoid diffusion into dilated gas-filled, bowel loops, which increases pressure and volume in a closed system.[12] Epidural morphine given preoperatively or intraoperative infusion of lidocaine will reduce anesthetic requirements, provide postoperative analgesia, and hasten return of bowel function.[13,14]

For surgery, a generous ventral midline celiotomy is performed and the entire gastrointestinal tract is isolated and examined. Removal of a foreign body obstruction requires single or multiple enterotomy(ies) performed in viable tissue. Closure of the incision(s) is by a single layer interrupted or continuous pattern of monofilament synthetic absorbable or nonabsorbable suture.[15] Incisional dehiscence is minimized by use of a serosal or omental patch sutured over the enterotomy.[2,3,5] Dilated, flaccid, discolored, avascular, necrotic bowel loops secondary to chronic obstructions, strangulations, or irreducible intussusception require resection and anastomosis at viable, vascularized regions. End-to-end or side-to-side anastomosis can be performed manually or with stapling devices.[2,5] Enteropexy or bowel plication is recommended to prevent recurrence of intussusception.[2,3,5,6] Typhlectomy is recommended for cecal inversion; constrictive adhesions or ligaments are resected. In cases of uncertain or recurrent pathology, histologic examination of removed tissues is beneficial.

For colonic surgery, similar principles apply as indicated for small intestinal surgery. Additionally, the high bacterial content may be reduced by dietary manipulations (elemental/low residue diets, withholding food), laxatives, enemas, or oral antibiotics (neomycin, kanamycin, metronidazole, trimethoprim-sulfadiazine), although these attempts may not be realistic in morbid animals requiring immediate surgery.[2,5] Second- and third-generation cephalosporins (cefoxitin, cefmetazole, cefotetan, cefotaxime, ceftizoxime) provide enhanced coverage against anaerobes and gram-negative organisms.[16] Colectomy can be performed using manual or stapling procedures. Malunions of pelvic fractures will require corrective osteotomies or ostectomy to relieve obstruction in the pelvic canal.[2,5] Preservation of the ileocecocolic valve during resection and anastomosis is technically difficult due to tension at the surgery site; in cats, removal of the valve may not cause a small intestine bacterial overgrowth problem as it does in dogs, although this is debatable.[2,5,17]

PROGNOSIS

Short- and long-term recoveries are based on the underlying cause of the obstruction. Resection of up to 70% of the small bowel is tolerated by most patients.[2,3,5] Adherence to proper surgical and medical principles reduces complications such as dehiscence, infection (abscess or peritonitis) septic or hypovolemic shock, lesional recurrence, and malnutrition. Volvulus of the bowel is frequently fatal despite therapy.

REFERENCES

1. Wylie KB, Hosgood G: Mortality and morbidity of small and large intestinal surgery in dogs and cats. *J Am Anim Hosp Assoc* 30:469, 1994.
2. Orsher RJ, Rosin, E: Small intestine. *In* Slatter D, ed.: Textbook of Small Animal Surgery, 2nd ed. Philadelphia: WB Saunders, 1993, p 594.

3. Tobias KS: Alimentary system. *In* Harari J, ed.: NVMS Small Animal Surgery. Baltimore: Williams & Wilkins, 1996, p 133.
4. Williams DA: Diseases of the Small Intestines. *In* Morgan RV, ed.: Handbook of Small Animal Practice, 3rd ed. Philadelphia: WB Saunders, 1997, p 367.
5. Fossum TW: Small Animal Surgery. St. Louis: Mosby, 1997, p 299.
6. Aronson LR, Brockman DJ: Gastrointestinal emergencies. *Vet Clin North Am Small Anim Pract* 30:555, 2000.
7. Evans KL, Smeak DD: Gastrointestinal foreign bodies in 32 dogs. *J Am Anim Hosp Assoc* 30:445, 1994.
8. Harari J: Intestinal volvulus. *In* Harari J, ed.: Small Animal Surgery Secrets. Philadelphia: Hanley & Belfus, 2000, p 142.
9. Burk RL, Ackerman N: Small Animal Radiology and Ultrasonography. Philadelphia: WB Saunders, 1996, p 296.
10. Freeman LJ: Veterinary Endosurgery. St. Louis: Mosby, 1999, p 121.
11. Henderson RA: Controlling peritoneal adhesions. *Vet Surg* 11:30, 1982.
12. Muir WW, Hubbell JAE: Handbook of Veterinary Anesthesia. St. Louis: Mosby, 2000, 168.
13. Tranquilli WJ, Benson JG: Essentials of Small Animal Anesthesia and Analgesia. Baltimore: Lippincott, Williams & Wilkins, 1999, p 52.
14. Groudine SB, Fisher HA: Intravenous lidocaine speeds the return of bowel function and decreases postoperative pain and hospital stay in prostatectomy patients. *Anesth Analg* 86:235, 1998.
15. Weisman D, Smeak DD: Comparison of a continuous suture pattern with a simple interrupted pattern for enteric closure in dogs and cats. *J Am Anim Hosp Assoc* 214:1507, 1999.
16. Papich MG: Antibacterial drug therapy. *Vet Clin North Am Small Anim Pract* 28:215, 1998.
17. Sweet DC, Hardie EM: Preservation versus excision of the cecocolic junction during colectomy for megacolon in cats. *J Small Anim Pract* 35:358, 1994.

SECTION VIII
Endocrine Disorders

58
Adrenal Dysfunction

Douglass K. MacIntire

INTRODUCTION

Four types of adrenal dysfunction can occur in CCU patients: hypoadrenocorticism, hyperadrenocorticism, pheochromocytoma, and postoperative adrenalectomy complications.

PATHOGENESIS

The normal hypothalamic-pituitary-adrenal axis is important in the adaptive response to stress. Corticotropin-releasing hormone (CRH) is released by cells in the paraventricular nucleus of the hypothalamus. In response to CRH, adrenocorticotropic hormone (ACTH) is released from the pituitary gland to stimulate the adrenal gland. The adrenal cortex has three layers. The outermost layer is the zona glomerulosa and produces aldosterone in response to stimulation by angiotensin II and hyperkalemia. The effect of ACTH on this layer is minimal. The zona fasciculata (middle layer) produces cortisol, and the zona reticularis (inner layer) produces androgens in response to ACTH secretion. The adrenal medulla produces catecholamines (epinephrine and norepinephrine) in response to stress. Under normal conditions glucocorticoids stimulate appetite, promote a sense of well-being, maintain glucose homeostasis, promote renal free water loss, maintain blood pressure, and protect against shock. Mineralocorticoids promote renal retention of sodium and water and renal excretion of potassium and hydrogen ion. Lack or excess of adrenal hormones can have profound systemic consequences.

Hypoadrenocorticism can be primary or secondary. Primary hypoadrenocorticism (Addison's disease) results from atrophy or destruction of all layers of the adrenal cortex, resulting in inadequate production of both mineralocorticoids and glucocorticoids. Causes include immune-mediated destruction, iatrogenic (mitotane administration), infectious disease (fungal, viral), neoplasia, trauma, hemorrhage, or infarction. Secondary hypoadrenocorticism is characterized by insufficient glucocorticoid production but normal mineralocorticoid production in response to inadequate ACTH secretion. It is most commonly caused by abrupt cessation of long-term or high-dose exogenous corticosteroid therapy. Rarely, secondary hypoadrenocorticism can be caused by destructive lesions of the hypothalamus or pituitary gland.

Lack of mineralocorticoid secretion can cause-life threatening hyperkalemia, hyponatremia, and severe hypovolemia resulting in weakness and collapse. Lack of glucocorticoids may cause depressed mentation, lethargy, anorexia, and inability to respond to stress.

Hyperadrenocorticism results from the excessive production of cortisol from the adrenal cortex. The most common form in dogs is pituitary-dependent hyperadrenocorticism, accounting for 80% to 85% of cases. Bilateral adrenocortical hyperplasia and overproduction of cortisol most commonly are the result of a functional pituitary microaderoma. If accompanying neurologic signs are present, a pituitary macroadenoma should be suspected. Adrenal tumors are responsible for 15% to 20% of spontaneous hyperadrenocorticism in dogs. Iatrogenic hyperadrenocorticism is clinically indistinguishable from spontaneous hyperadrenocorticism and results from excessive or prolonged administration of exogenous glucocorticoids. Chronic suppression of ACTH resulting from negative feedback causes bilateral adrenal atrophy.

Pheochromocytoma is a tumor arising from the chromaffin cells of the adrenal medulla. Metastasis is rare, but local invasion of the caudal vena cava may occur. Excessive catecholamine release can result in systemic hypertension and cardiac arrythmias.

Adrenalectomy is the treatment of choice for adrenal tumors. Postoperative complications may occur because the contralateral adrenal gland is atrophied. Exogenous glucocorticoid supplementation is needed to overcome the stress of surgery and must be continued until the adrenal gland regains normal function (2–3 months).

EPIDEMIOLOGY

Hypoadrenocorticism may occur in any breed, but breeds at higher risk include standard Poodles, Portuguese water dogs, Great Danes, Labrador retrievers, Rottweilers, West Highland white terriers and Wheaten terriers. Most dogs are less than 7 years old; females are more commonly affected. Hypoadrenocorticism is rare in cats.

Hyperadrenocorticism occurs primarily in middle-aged to older dogs, usually small breeds of either sex. Poodles, Dachshunds, Boston terriers, Beagles, terriers, German shepherds, and Boxers are predisposed, although any breed can be affected. Spontaneous hyperadrenocorticism is rare in cats and is most commonly diagnosed in middle-aged to older cats with insulin-resistant diabetes mellitus.

Pheochromocytomas are rarely diagnosed antemortem. There appears to be no sex predilection. Affected dogs are usually older animals.

Adrenal tumors can occur in both large and small breed dogs. Breeds at risk for adrenal tumors include poodle, dachshunds, German shepherds, Labrador retrievers, and terriers. Adrenal tumors may be slightly more common in female dogs.

CLINICAL PRESENTATION

Hypoadrenocorticism has been called "the great pretender" because clinical signs associated with this syndrome can mimic renal disease, gastrointestinal disease, and other causes of episodic weakness and acute collapse (cardiovascular, metabolic, neurologic or muscular). Clinical signs are listed in Table 58-1.

Hyperadrenocorticism can complicate treatment and predispose to infection in affected CCU patients. Clinical signs associated with hyperadrenocorticism are listed in Table 58-2. CCU patients with hyperadrenocorticism are at risk for developing diabetes mellitus, systemic infections, delayed wound healing, glomerulonephritis, impaired hepatic metabolism of drugs, pulmonary thromboembolism, pancreatitis, hypertension, and impaired ability to handle stress. Strict asepsis should be used in these immunocompromised patients when intravenous, arterial, or urinary catheters are required for patient care.

Pheochromocytoma causes vague, nonspecific signs making antemortem diagnosis difficult. Signs are listed in Table 58-3.

Adrenalectomy results in the signs associated with hypoadrenocorticism (see Table 58-1) if glucocorticoid replacement is not provided during surgery and the postoperative period until normal adrenal function is restored. Inadequate glucocorticoid replacement during adrenalectomy can result in anesthetic death, prolonged recovery, refractory hypotension, hypoglycemia, and signs consistent with multiple organ dysfunction. Unilateral adrenalectomy generally does not require mineralocorticoid supplementation.

Table 58-1. Clinical Signs Associated with Hypoadrenocorticism

Chronic Presentation

- Weight loss
- Trembling, shivering, hypothermia
- Episodic weakness or collapse
- Anorexia, lethargy, depression
- Intermittent melena, hematochezia, diarrhea
- Polyuria and polydipsia
- History of improvement following glucocorticoid or fluid therapy

Acute Presentation

- Severe dehydration
- Hypovolemic shock—weak pulses, prolonged capillary refill time, pale mucous membranes, collapse
- Bradycardia in a clinical shock state

Table 58-2. Clinical Signs Associated with Hyperadrenocorticism

- Polyuria and polydipsia
  - Pollakiuria, hematuria, pyuria, or stranguria may indicate a urinary tract infection
- Polyphagia, weight loss, polyuria, and polydipsia
- Severe respiratory distress may occur because animals with hyperadreocorticism are at risk for pulmonary thromboembolism
  - Panting occurs with pulmonary mineralization and abdominal distention
  - Cyanosis may be present with hypoxemia

May indicate secondary diabetes mellitus

- Central nervous system signs ranging from lethargy and disorientation to stupor, aimless wandering, ataxia, or tetraparesis

May indicate pituitary macroadenoma

- Catabolic muscle wasting and atrophy
- Hepatomegaly, pendulous abdominal distention
- Neuropathies, myopathies, weakness
- Bilaterally symmetrical alopecia
- Thin skin, easily bruises
- Hyperpigmentation
- Testicular atrophy

Table 58-3. Clinical Signs Associated with Pheochromocytoma

- Tachypnea, restlessness
- Dilated pupils
- Pulse deficits, arrhythmias, tachycardia
- Epistaxis
- Hyperemia of skin and mucous membranes
- Retinal hemorrhage, hyperemia, bounding pulses, and cardiac abnormalities may occur secondary to hypertension
- Shock, collapse, syncope
- Peripheral edema of one or both rear legs may occur if the mass invades the vena cava
- Palpable abdominal mass?
- Signs may be intermittent or sustained

DIAGNOSTIC EVALUATION

Hypoadrenocorticism can often be tentatively diagnosed on the basis of history, clinical signs, and routine laboratory findings. "Classic" abnormalities include increased hematocrit from dehydration or mild nonregenerative anemia, lymphocytosis, eosinophilia, hyponatremia, hyperkalemia, sodium/potassium ratio less than 27:1, azotemia, hypercalcemia, low to normal blood glucose, metabolic acidosis, and urine specific gravity less than 1.030. Thoracic radiographs may reveal microcardia and decreased pulmonary vascularization secondary to hypovolemia. In rare cases, megaesophagus may be present. Electrocardiographic (ECG) abnormalities depend on the degree of hyperkalemia present. Mild hyperkalemia causes increased T-wave amplitude. Moderate hyperkalemia is associated with flattening of the P wave (atrial standstill) and slowing of the heart rate. Severe hyperkalemia causes a widening of the QRS complexes and bradycardia characterized by a sinoventricular rhythm.

Definitive diagnosis of hypoadrenocorticism requires the ACTH stimulation test (Table 58-4). Most glucocorticoids, except for dexamethasone, cross-react with the test and should not be administered for 24 to 48 hours prior to testing.

Hyperadrenocorticism can be suspected when the hemogram exhibits lymphopenia, eosinopenia, erythrocytosis, and lipemia. Serum chemistry abnormalities include elevated serum alkaline phosphatase, hyperglycemia, hypercholesterolemia and urine specific gravity less than 1.020. A urine culture should be performed when hyperadrenocorticism is suspected, because approximately 50% of dogs with hyperadrenocorticism have urinary tract infections.

Critically ill animals are most likely stressed, and screening tests may be too sensitive in these animals to be of any use. The best tests for critically ill animals are the ACTH stimulation test (performed as described in Table 58-4) and endogenous ACTH levels. The ACTH stimulation test will be exaggerated in 85% to 90% of dogs with pituitary-dependent hyperadrenocorticism and in

Table 58-4. Protocol for ACTH Stimulation Test

- Obtain plasma or serum sample for baseline cortisol measurement.
- Administer 0.25 mg synthetic ACTH IV (Cortrosyn; Organon Pharmaceuticals, West Orange, NJ).
- Obtain plasma or serum sample for cortisol measurement 1 h later
- In cats, administer 0.125 mg ACTH and obtain three samples: before and 1 and 2 h after injection.
- If ACTH gel is used instead of synthetic ACTH, 2.2 U/kg is administered IM and the samples are obtained before and 2 h after injection.
- Animals with primary hypoadrenocorticism will have a "flat" response with before and after cortisol concentrations usually <1 μg/dL or <30 nmol/L.
- Animals with secondary hypoadrenocorticism will have a "blunted" or decreased response to ACTH. Before and after values are usually <2.5 μg/dL or <70 nmol/L.

60% of dogs with adrenal tumors. Endogenous ACTH levels are elevated in dogs with pituitary tumors and decreased in dogs with adrenal tumors. A urine cortisol/creatinine ratio rules out hyperadrenocorticism if it is normal, but an elevated ratio occurs with either stress or hyperadrenocorticism. In a stressed animal, the low-dose dexamethasone screening test may not suppress enough to differentiate stress from hyperadrenocorticism.

Ultrasonography can also be helpful in diagnosis. Bilateral adrenal enlargement is consistent with pituitary-dependent hyperadrenocorticism, whereas unilateral adrenomegaly with distortion of normal architecture is consistent with adrenal tumor.

Pheochromocytoma is difficult to diagnose antemortem because signs are nonspecific (weight loss, lethargy, tachypnea). An abdominal mass may be palpable in approximately 10% of affected dogs. Abdominal ultrasound may reveal an adrenal mass. Arterial blood pressure is often elevated, but hypertension may be missed because of the episodic nature of catecholamine secretion. Urine or plasma catecholamines can be measured but the tests are expensive and not widely available.

Adrenalectomy can result in postoperative complications because of reduced adrenal function. The ACTH stimulation test (see Table 58-4) can be performed to initially diagnose adrenal suppression and monitor the recovery of adrenal function postoperatively while glucocorticoid supplementation is gradually tapered off.

TREATMENT

Treatment of hypoadrenocorticism involves correcting hypotension and hypovolemia, providing glucocorticoid replacement, and restoring electrolyte and acid–base balance. Treatment recommendations are listed in Table 58-5. Electrolytes, blood urea nitrogen, and creatinine should be initially monitored weekly, then every 3 to 4 months once values have stabilized.

Hyperadrenocorticism is usually medically treated with mitotane if the cause is pituitary dependent and with adrenalectomy if the cause is adrenal tumor. Mitotane causes necrosis of the zona fasciulata and zona recticularis. The most common medical treatment protocol is listed in Table 58-6. Mitotane should not be used in cats. Hyperadrenocorticism is rare in cats. Metyrapone and adrenalectomy have been successful in treating feline patients with hyperadrenocorticism.

Pheochromocytoma is treated by adrenalectomy. The animal must be medically stabilized before surgery to reduce excessive sympathetic stimulation. Phenoxybenzamine (0.2-1.5 mg/kg PO q 12 h) is started at a low dose and gradually increased until hypertension is controlled for 7 to 10 days before surgery. Cardiac arrhythmias are controlled with propranolol (0.15-0.5 mg/kg PO q 8 h) or atenolol (0.2-1.0 mg/kg PO q 12-24 h). The α- and β-blockers should be given concurrently.

For anesthesia, phenothiazines should be avoided because of the potential for hypotension. Thiobarbiturates and halothane should not be used because of

Table 58-5. Treatment Recommendations for Hypoadrenocorticism

I. Fluid therapy—IV 0.9% NaCl

- Correct dehydration over 2-6 h (Percent dehydration × Body weight [kg] = No. liters fluid).
- Continue IV fluids at a rate of 4-6 mL/kg/h until azotemia and electrolyte imbalances are resolved.

II. Glucocorticoid replacement

- Dexamethasone $NaPO_4$: 0.2-0.4 mg/kg IV q 8-12 h

III. Correct severe hyperkalemia (life-threatening bradyarrhythmias, atrial standstill). Three options include:

(1) Regular insulin 0.1 U/kg IV followed by 1-2 g 25% dextrose/U insulin. Add 100 mL 50% dextrose to 1 liter IV fluids to make a 5% concentration.

(2) Calcium gluconate 10%: 50-100 mg/kg IV slowly over 2-5 min while monitoring ECG.

(3) Sodium bicarbonate: 1-2 mEq/kg IV slowly

IV. Correct hypoglycemia

- 25% dextrose: 0.5 g/kg IV bolus followed by 5% solution IV

V. Correct metabolic acidosis

- No. mEq $NaHCO_3$ = 0.3 × Body weight (kg) × Base deficit
- For severe cases, give 1-2 mEq/kg slowly IV and add the remainder to IV fluids to be administered over 12 h.

VI. Mineralocorticoid replacement—two options:

(1) Fludrocortisone acetate (Florinef; Squibb): 0.02 mg/kg/d PO

(2) Desoxycorticosterone pivalate (DOCP; CIBA-Geigy): 2.2 mg/kg IM or SQ q 25-30 d

VII. Maintenance glucocorticoid supplementation

- Prednisone: 0.2 mg/kg/d PO
- May not be required in dogs receiving fludrocortisone
- Prednisone dosage can be increased (0.4-2.0 mg/kg) in times of stress (surgery, travel, boarding, etc.).

the potential for catecholamine-induced arrhythmias. Preferred preanesthetics are narcotics and glycopyrrolate followed by isoflurane anesthesia. Animals should be monitored with direct arterial blood pressure and ECG. Hypertensive crises caused by tumor manipulation can be managed with phentolamine (0.02-0.1 mg/kg IV). Animals should be monitored for hypotension following tumor removal and treated with aggressive fluid therapy if it occurs.

Adrenalectomy usually results in hypoadrenocorticism when the adrenal tumor is removed because the normal adrenal gland is atrophied. Preoperative treatment for 2 to 6 weeks with ketoconazole (10 mg/kg PO q 12 h) may minimize the side effects of adrenalectomy. Glucocorticoids (prednisolone sodium succinate 1-2 mg/kg IV) should be given immediately before and after surgery

Table 58-6. Treatment of Hyperadrenocorticism

1. Mitotane (op'DDD, Lysodren, Bristol Meyers)
   A. Induction: 30-50 mg/kg/d PO divided bid for 7-10 d. (For diabetic dogs, decrease dose to 25-35 mg/kg/d and watch for hypoglycemia.)
      (1) Prednisolone 0.2 mg/kg/d is given concurrently.
      (2) Discontinue treatment if lethargy, anorexia, vomiting, or diarrhea develop.
      (3) Monitor ACTH stimulation test. Ideally baseline cortisol and post ACTH cortisol levels should both be between 1-5 μg/dL or 30-150 nmol/L.
         (a) If cortisol levels are too high, continue daily induction dose and recheck ACTH stimulation test in 5-10 d.
         (b) If levels are too low, mitotane must be discontinued until cortisol levels normalize.
   B. Maintenance: 30-50 mg/kg divided into 2-3 doses per week for life
      (1) If clinical signs return, reinduction for 7-10 d is required and maintenance dose is increased by 25%.
2. Other treatments
   A. Ketoconazole
      (1) Begin at low dose (5 mg/kg q 24 h PO for 7 d). If no adverse effects are seen, increase dose to 10 mg/kg PO q 12 h.
      (2) Check ACTH response after 2 wk. If too high, increase ketoconazole to 15-20 mg/kg q 12 h.
   B. L-Deprenyl (Anipryl, Pfizer Animal Health) 1 mg/kg/d PO. Double dose in 2 mo if no improvement seen.
      (1) May not be effective unless posterior pituitary is involved.
      (2) Safe; side effects rare.

and continued orally until normal adrenal function returns. The schedule for oral administration begins at a dosage of 0.5 mg/kg q 12 h for 3 days and tapered over 10 to 14 days to 0.25 mg/kg q 24 h. This dosage is continued for 1 to 3 months until the ACTH stimulation test is normal. Prednisone should not be administered within 24 hours of ACTH testing.

PROGNOSIS

Hypoadrenocorticism has a good prognosis for long-term survival, providing mineralocorticoid and glucocorticoid replacement therapy is continued. Therapy is required for life, and mineralocorticoid dosage may need to be increased over time if hyperkalemia or hyponatremia reoccur. Supplemental glucocorticoids should be given during times of illness or stress.

Hyperadrenocorticism has a guarded prognosis for long-term survival because of the many complications associated with the disease. The average life span following diagnosis is 2 years. Complications include pulmonary thromboembolism, hypertension, congestive heart failure, infection, progression of tumor growth, and recurrence of clinical signs. Animals frequently require adjustments in the dosage of mitotane over time, and ACTH stimulation tests must be monitored every 3 to 6 months.

Pheochromocytoma has a good prognosis, if no metastasis is present, following complete resection of the tumor. Approximately 50% are malignant and carry a grave prognosis if complete surgical resection is impossible.

Adrenalectomy has a good prognosis if the tumor is benign. Invasive adrenal adenocarcinomas carry a grave prognosis because complete surgical resection is not possible.

SUGGESTED READINGS

Bouriad H, Feeney DA, Caywood DD, Hayden DW: Pheochromocytoma in dogs: 13 cases (1980–1985). *J Am Vet Med Assoc* 191:1610, 1987.

Berry CR, Hawkins EC, Hurley KJ, Monce K: Frequency of pulmonary mineralization and hypoxemia in 21 dogs with pituitary dependent hyperadrenocorticism. *J Vet Intern Med* 14:151, 2000.

Burns MG, Kelly AB, Hornof WJ, Howerth EW: Pulmonary artery thrombosis in three dogs with hyperadrenocorticism. *J Am Vet Med Assoc* 178:388, 1981.

Behrend EN, Kemppainen RJ: Medical therapy of canine Cushing's syndrome. *Compend Contin Educ Small Anim Pract* 20:679, 1998.

Kaplan AJ, Peterson ME, Kemppainen RT: Effects of disease on the results of diagnostic tests for use in detecting hyperadrenocorticism in dogs. *J Am Vet Med Assoc* 207: 445, 1995.

Kintzer PP, Peterson ME: Mitotane (o, p-DDD) treatment of 200 dogs with pituitary-dependent hyperadrenocorticism. *J Vet Intern Med* 5:182, 1994.

Kintzer PP, Peterson ME: Treatment and longterm follow-up in 205 dogs with hypoadrenocorticism. *J Vet Intern Med* 11:43, 1997.

Peterson ME, Greco DS, Orth DN: Primary hypoadrenocorticism in ten cats. *J Vet Intern Med* 3:55, 1989.

Rodriguez-Vega GM, Yodice PC, Kaye W: Adrenal insufficiency may be common in critically ill patients with unexplained hypotension or pressor dependency. *Crit Care Med* 27(suppl):A70, 1999.

Roth L, Tyler RD: Evaluation of low sodium: potassium ratios in dogs. *J Vet Diagn Invest* 11:60, 1999.

Scavelli TD, Peterson ME, Matthiesen DT: Results of adrenalectomy for hyperadrenocorticism caused by adrenocortical neoplasia in 26 dogs. *Vet Surg* 15:133, 1986.

59
Pancreatic Disorders: Diabetic Ketoacidosis and Insulinoma

Deborah S. Greco

DIABETES MELLITUS AND DIABETIC KETOACIDOSIS
Introduction

Diabetes mellitus is characterized by reduced or absent insulin secretion from the pancreatic beta cells. Diabetes mellitus has traditionally been categorized as type 1 (exogenous insulin dependent) or type II (non-insulin dependent). Insulin-dependent diabetes mellitus (IDDM) is a diabetic state in which endogenous insulin secretion is never sufficient to support normal glucose physiology and prevent ketone production. Most dogs suffer from type 1 diabetes or IDDM and are prone to diabetic ketoacidosis (DKA) if deprived of exogenous insulin. Most cats suffer from type 2 diabetes mellitus; however, many cats with type 2 diabetes become insulin dependent. Cats often present with mixed hyperosmolar, ketotic syndrome, which may be an end-stage of type 2 diabetes mellitus.[1]

Pathogenesis

Insulin is an anabolic hormone. Insulin deficiency leads to protein catabolism and contributes to weight loss and muscle atrophy. With insulin deficiency, the hormone-sensitive lipase system, which is normally suppressed by insulin, becomes activated. Lipid metabolism in the liver becomes deranged with insulin deficiency and nonesterified fatty acids converted to acetyl-coenzyme A (acetyl-CoA) rather than being incorporated into triglycerides. Acetyl-CoA accumulates in the liver and is changed into acetoacetyl-CoA and acetoacetic acid. Finally, the liver generates ketones including acetoacetic acid, β-hydroxybutyrate and acetone.[2]

Osmotic diuresis caused by glycosuria and ketonuria increases urinary sodium and potassium loss producing hypovolemia and dehydration. Accumulation of ketones and lactic acid in the blood contributes to loss of electrolytes and water. Nausea, anorexia, and vomiting, caused by stimulation of the chemoreceptor trigger zone via ketonemia and hyperglycemia, contribute to the dehydration caused by osmotic diuresis. Dehydration and shock lead to prerenal azotemia and a decline in glomerular filtration rate (GFR). This process results in profound metabolic acidosis. Declining GFR leads to further accumulation of glucose and ketones in the blood. Stress hormones such as cortisol and epinephrine contribute to the hyperglycemia in a vicious cycle. Eventually severe dehydration may result in hyperviscosity, thromboembolism, severe metabolic acidosis, renal failure, and finally death.

Epidemiology

Dogs suffering from diabetes mellitus range in age from 4 to 14 years with a peak incidence at 7 to 9 years. A genetic basis for diabetes mellitus is suspected in the keeshonden. Other commonly affected breeds include miniature and toy Poodles, Dachshunds, Miniature Schnauzers, Beagles, Puliks, Cairn terriers, and Miniature Pinschers.[2] In dogs, females are twice as likely to develop diabetes than are males. In cats, neutered males are 1.5 times more likely than females to develop diabetes mellitus. Risk factors for the development of diabetes mellitus in cats include increased body weight (>6 kg), older age (>8 years) and neutering.[2]

Clinical Signs

Polydipsia and polyuria are the most common clinical signs of diabetes mellitus in dogs and cats.[2] Weight loss is observed more commonly in dogs compared with cats. In some cases, polyphagia is also observed. In dogs, progressive polyuria, polydipsia, and weight loss develop relatively rapidly usually over a period of several weeks. Another common presenting complaint of diabetes mellitus in dogs is acute onset of blindness caused by bilateral cataract formation. Cats will present with chronic complications of diabetes, such as gait abnormalities resulting from diabetic neuropathy, or with chronic gastrointestinal signs such as vomiting, diarrhea, and anorexia.[2]

Physical examination findings of nonketotic diabetes mellitus in cats and dogs are typically nonspecific. The most common physical examination findings in cats are lethargy and depression, dehydration, unkempt haircoat, and muscle wasting.[2] In dogs, the most common physical examination findings are dehydration and muscle wasting or thin body condition. About 25% to 30% of diabetic animals are obese on initial examination; obese diabetic animals are more likely to suffer from non-insulin–dependent diabetes mellitus. Hepatomegaly is observed in both diabetic cats and dogs. Plantigrade rear limb stance resulting from diabetic neuropathy is observed in approximately 10% of diabetic cats. Cataracts are observed in approximately 40% of diabetic dogs.[2]

The most common historical findings in cats with DKA are anorexia, weakness, depression, and vomiting. In dogs, depression, vomiting, and anorexia are the most common historical findings with DKA. Animals suffering from DKA often present in shock. Physical examination findings may include depression, tachypnea, dehydration, weakness, vomiting, and occasionally, a strong acetone odor on the breath. Cats can present recumbent or comatose; this may be a manifestation of severe DKA or mixed ketotic hyperosmolar syndrome. Approximately one third of diabetic cats with DKA will exhibit icterus at presentation. Icterus may be a result of hemolysis, hepatic lipidosis, or acute pancreatitis rather than diabetes mellitus.[3]

Diagnosis

Diabetes mellitus should be diagnosed based on the presence of clinical signs compatible with diabetes mellitus and evidence of fasting hyperglycemia and glycosuria. Common clinicopathologic features of diabetes mellitus in dogs and cats include fasting hyperglycemia hypercholesterolemia, increased liver enzymes (alkaline phosphatase, alanine aminotransferase), neutrophilic leukocytosis, proteinuria, increased urine specific gravity, and glycosuria.[2]

Many cats are susceptible to "stress-induced" hyperglycemia in which the serum glucose concentrations may approach 300 to 400 mg/dL. Renal glycosuria may be found in animals with renal tubular disease and occasionally with stress-induced hyperglycemia. Glycosylated proteins, such as glycosylated hemoglobin and fructosamine, may aid in the diagnosis of diabetes mellitus in cats. Glycosylated hemoglobin is formed by an irreversible, nonenzymatic binding of glucose to hemoglobin. As plasma glucose concentrations increase, hemoglobin glycosylation proportionately increases.[5,6] Serum fructosamine is formed by glycosylation of serum protein such as albumin. The fructosamine concentration in serum is directly related to blood glucose concentration. Serum fructosamine measurement may be beneficial in differentiating early or subclinical diabetes mellitus in the cat from stress-induced hyperglycemia. Normal fructosamine concentrations in dogs and cats should be less than 360 μmol/L.[6]

Common clinicopathologic findings in DKA include all of the above plus azotemia, hyponatremia, hyperkalemia, hyperlipasemia, hyperamylasemia, ketonemia, regenerative or degenerative left shifts, hyperosmolality, ketonuria, bacteriuria, hematuria, and pyuria.[7] Cats in DKA crisis may develop Heinz body anemia.[4]

Treatment of IDDM

Insulin is the primary therapy in IDDM. Human recombinant insulin is the most available insulin preparation on the market and is perfectly acceptable as insulin therapy for all dogs and most cats.[8] Porcine insulin is identical to canine insulin in its amino acid structure and human insulin is very similar to canine insulin. Beef insulin is most similar to cat insulin, differing by only one amino acid in the A chain. Insulin preparations may be short-acting (regular insulin), intermediate (Lente, NPH), or long-acting (Ultralente, PZI). Regular insulin is the most effective insulin for the suppression of ketosis.

Insulin is commercially available in concentrations of 40, 100, and 500 U/mL, which are designated U-40, U-100, and U-500, respectively. One unit of insulin is approximately equivalent to 36 μg.[8] Regardless of the concentration of insulin used for therapy, it is essential to use the appropriate syringe for the concentration of insulin. U-100 insulin syringes are manufactured as low-dose (0.3-mL, 0.5-mL) and 1-mL capacities; U-40 syringes are only available as 1-mL capacity. All insulin syringes are packaged with a fine 27-, 28-, or 29-gauge injection needle. In cats and small dogs (<10 kg), the use of low-dose (0.3- or

0.5-mL) syringes is recommended. These syringes are designed to accurately draw up a small dosage of U-100 insulin without the need for dilution.

Treatment of DKA

Treatment of DKA is outlined in Table 59-1. Key steps in DKA management include: (1) fluid therapy, (2) insulin therapy, (3) electrolyte supplementation (potassium, phosphorus, magnesium), and (4) treatment of metabolic acidosis.

Fluid therapy should begin with 0.9% NaCl supplemented with potassium as soon as insulin therapy is initiated.[7] A large central venous catheter should be used to administer fluid therapy because animals in DKA are severely dehydrated and require rapid fluid administration. Central venous pressure may also be monitored via a jugular catheter to avoid overhydration. In animals treated for DKA, fluid rates are dependent on the severity of dehydration, maintenance requirements, continuing losses (vomiting and diarrhea), and the presence of concurrent disease (congestive heart failure, etc.). Cats with mixed hyperosmolar ketotic syndrome will benefit from judicious fluid therapy because rapid dilution of plasma protein with crystalloid fluid may precipitate or exacerbate cerebral edema.[1]

In dogs, insulin therapy should be initiated as soon as possible using either intravenous (IV) insulin or low-dose intramuscular (IM) methods.[1,9] Table 59-1 outlines the IV insulin fluid rate. A dosage of 2.2 U/kg in dogs or 1.1 U/kg in cats of regular insulin is diluted in 250 mL saline. IV insulin should preferably be administered via a separate peripheral catheter. Approximately 50 mL fluid and insulin is allowed to run through the IV drip set and is discarded because insulin binds to the plastic tubing. The species of regular insulin (beef, pork, or human) does not affect response; however, the type of insulin is important. Regular insulin must be used; *lente, ultralente and NPH should never be given IV*. Using IV insulin administration, blood glucose decreases to below 250 mg/dL by approximately 10 hours in dogs and after about 16 hours in cats.[1,9] Once euglycemia has been achieved, the animal is maintained on subcutaneous regular insulin (0.1-0.4 U/kg, SQ q 4-6 h) until anorexia and the ketosis has resolved. The transition from hospital to home maintenance insulin therapy can be made by using a low dose (1-2 U) of regular insulin combined with the intermediate- or long-acting maintenance insulin (NPH, lente, PZI) at the recommended dosages.[8]

Potassium should be supplemented as soon as insulin therapy is initiated. Although serum potassium may be normal or elevated in animals presenting with DKA, there is actually a total body depletion of potassium. Correction of the metabolic acidosis drives potassium into the intracellular space in exchange for hydrogen ions. Insulin facilitates this exchange; the net effect is a dramatic decrease in serum potassium. The rapid potassium flux must be attenuated with appropriate potassium supplementation in fluids. Refractory hypokalemia may be complicated by hypomagnesemia.[10] Supplementation of magnesium along with

Table 59-1. Stepwise Treatment of Diabetic Ketoacidosis

***STEP ONE:* FLUIDS**

a. Place IV catheter, preferably central venous

b. Fluid rate: Estimate dehydration deficit (%) × BW (kg) × 1000 mL = no. of mls to rehydrate

Estimate maintenance needs: 1 ml/lb/h × no. of hours required to rehydrate (24 h)

Estimate losses (vomiting, diarrhea)

Dehydration deficit + maintenance + losses = no. mL fluid/24 h = hourly fluid rate

c. Fluid composition

Blood Glucose	*Fluids*	*Rate*	*Route*	*Monitor*	*Frequency*
>250 mg/dL	0.9% NaCl	Up to 90 mL/kg/h to rehydrate	IV	Packed cell volume, total solids, Na, K, osmolality	q 4 h
200–250	0.45% NaCl plus 2.5% dextrose		IV		q 2 h
150–200		See above			
100–150	Same	See above		Central venous pressure, urine output	
<100	0.45% NaCl plus 5% dextrose	See above			

***STEP TWO:* INSULIN**

Blood Glucose	*Route*	*Dose*	*Frequency*
>250 mg/dL	IV	1.1 U/kg (C) or hyperosmolar	q 1–2 h
200–250	IV	2.2 U/kg (D)	q 4 h
150–200	IV	0.1–0.4 U/kg	q 2 h
100–150	IV		
<100 IV	SQ		
>250 mg/dL	IM	0.2 U/kg	Hourly
	IM	0.1 U/kg	Hourly
<250 mg/dL	IM	0.1 U/kg	q 4-6 h
	SQ	0.1–0.4 U/kg	q 6-8 h

***STEP THREE:* ELECTROLYTES**

Electrolyte Concentration	*Amount (mEq/L) Added to 1 L Fluids*	*Maximum Rate (mL/kg/h)*
Potassium		
3.5-5.0 mEq/L	20	26
2.5-3.5 mEq/L	40	12
2.1-2.5 mEq/L	60	9
<2.0 mEq/L	80	7
Phosphorus		
1-2 mg/dL	0.01 mmol phosphate/kg/h	Monitor serum phosphorus q 6
<1.0 mg/dL	0.03 mmol phosphate/kg/h	
Magnesium		
<1.2 mg/dL	0.75-1 mEq/kg/d CRI	Use 5% dextrose
	MgCl, $MgSO_4$	Ca and sodium bicarbonate solution

***STEP FOUR:* ACID-BASE BALANCE**

pH	*Bicarbonate Concentration*	*Dose of Bicarbonate*	*Rate*
<7.1	<12 mEq/L	mL IV = 0.1 × BW (kg) × (24 − HCO_3)	over 2 h

potassium as outlined in Table 59-1 may be indicated in cats or small dogs suffering from hypokalemia unresponsive to potassium chloride or potassium phosphate supplementation in fluids.[11]

Serum and tissue phosphorus may also be depleted during ketoacidosis. A fraction of the potassium supplementation should consist of potassium phosphate (one third of the potassium dose as potassium phosphate), particularly in small dogs and cats, which are most susceptible to hemolysis caused by hypophosphatemia.[1,11] Caution should be used because excess supplementation of phosphorus can result in metastatic calcification and hypocalcemia. In cats suffering from DKA, hemolysis may be caused by either hypophosphatemia or Heinz body anemia.

Bicarbonate therapy may be necessary in some patients with blood pH less than 7.1 or if serum HCO_3 is less than 12 mEq/L.[7] Caution is recommended when supplementing with bicarbonate because metabolic alkalosis may be difficult to reverse.

Hyperosmolar Coma

In humans, nonketotic hyperosmolar diabetes is defined by extreme hyperglycemia (serum glucose > 600 mg/dL), hyperosmolality (>350 mOSm/L), severe dehydration, central nervous system depression, and an absence of ketones or metabolic acidosis. Hyperosmolar nonketotic syndrome in dogs and cats is an unusual syndrome characterized by neurologic and gastrointestinal abnormalities such as progressive weakness, anorexia, vomiting, and lethargy.[1] These signs are preceded by the classic signs of polydipsia, polyuria, weight loss, and polyphagia that accompany uncomplicated diabetes mellitus. Physical examination reveals severe dehydration, hypothermia, extreme depression, lethargy, and coma.

In treating hyperosmolar coma, fluid therapy should be administered cautiously by estimating the fluid needs (dehydration deficit) and replacing 80% of the deficit over a 12- to 24-hour period. A lower dosage of insulin (1.1 U/kg/24 h) is recommended and insulin therapy should be delayed until 2 to 4 hours after initiation of fluid therapy.[1]

Iatrogenic Hypoglycemia

Clinical signs of hypoglycemia may be noted with initial insulin therapy due to epinephrine release to counter the hypoglycemia. Nervousness, anxiety, vocalization, muscle tremors, ataxia, and pupillary dilation should alert the owner to the possibility of hypoglycemia. The animal should be offered food and the owner should seek veterinary advice. Late in the course of hypoglycemic shock the animal may become recumbent or comatose, or have seizures. If access to a vein is not readily available, or if the owner is administering therapy, 50% dextrose (Karo syrup, pancake syrup) may be applied to oral mucous membranes using a large syringe. One should caution the owner to pour the syrup on the gums from a reasonable distance to prevent accidental injury from biting. The owner should transport the animal to a veterinarian as soon as possible.

On admission, treatment should consist of administration of a slow IV bolus of 50% dextrose (0.5 g/kg diluted 1:4). Thereafter, a continuous infusion of 5% dextrose should be administered until the animal can be fed. Many animals that experience insulin overdose will suffer cerebral edema and temporary blindness or behavior changes; often these signs are temporary and resolve after several weeks or months. Endogenous glucose stores may have been depleted by the insulin overdose and it may take several days for hyperglycemia to recur. In these cases, insulin therapy should be discontinued until hyperglycemia recurs.

Prognosis

Uncomplicated diabetes mellitus is generally reported to have a good prognosis if reasonable response to management occurs. Cats may be more difficult to maintain disease control; those cats that cannot be regulated have a guarded prognosis. DKA and nonketotic hyperosmolar syndrome carry a guarded to poor prognosis.

INSULINOMA

Pathogenesis and Epidemiology

Insulinomas are tumors that arise from cells referred to as amine precursor uptake and decarboxylation cells (APUD). Other APUDomas include glucagonomas, somatostatinomas, pheochromocytomas, and gastrinomas. Insulinoma is the most commonly recognized APUDoma in the dog; however, there are only three reported cases of beta-cell neoplasia in the cat.[12] Insulinoma occurs most frequently as a single entity but may be part of multiple endocrine neoplasia syndrome (MEN type I), which consists of a pituitary tumor, pheochromocytoma, and APUDoma of the pancreas. Middle-aged to older dogs and cats have been reported to have insulinomas. Dog breeds predisposed to insulinoma include large breed dogs such as standard Poodles, Irish setters, German shepherds, collies, Labrador retrievers, Golden retrievers, and boxers. Two Siamese and one Persian cat have been diagnosed with insulinoma.[12-14]

Clinical Presentation

Clinical signs are caused by excessive insulin secretion for neoplastic beta cells resulting in decreased serum glucose concentrations. Clinical signs include seizures, weakness, ataxia, collapse, exercise intolerance, muscle fasciculations, shaking, abnormal behavior, attitude changes, polyphagia, and trembling. Polyneuropathy has been described in dogs.[15]

The severity and duration of clinical signs are related to the rate of decline in serum glucose concentration, the duration of hypoglycemia, and the absolute serum glucose concentration. Cortisol, glucagon, epinephrine, and growth hormone are released in response to hypoglycemia.

Diagnostic Evaluation

Hypoglycemia is the primary abnormality observed on the serum chemistry profile. Care should be taken to rule out iatrogenic or spurious causes of hypoglycemia including use of a portable glucose monitoring device (results can be 25% below the actual value), old test strips, and delayed separation of serum from red blood cells.[16] Whipple's triad may be used to support a diagnosis of insulinoma. Whipple's triad is composed of (1) symptoms that occur after feeding or exercise, (2) serum glucose less than 50 mg/dL at time of symptoms, and (3) symptoms relieved by administration of glucose.[17]

The best screening test is serum insulin concentration. To document hyperinsulinemia, an animal should be fed a normal meal early in the day then fasted. Glucose should be monitored at hourly intervals until the glucose less is less than 60 mg/dL; a blood sample should then be obtained for insulin and glucose measurement. The animal is then fed small, high-protein meals (1/4 can) hourly over the next several hours. Insulin concentration of greater than 20 µU/mL when serum glucose is less than 60 mg/dL is diagnostic for insulinoma. An insulinoma is probable if serum insulin is in the normal range (5-20 µU/mL) when serum glucose is less than 60 mg/dL. In cases where the insulin concentration is suspect but not diagnostic for insulinoma, an amended insulin/glucose ratio (AIGR) may be used.[12,17]

$$\text{AIGR} = \frac{\text{Serum insulin } (\mu\text{U/mL}) \times 100}{\text{Serum glucose (mg/dL)} - 30}$$

An AIGR above 30 is diagnostic for an insulinoma. Only insulin assays that have been validated for use in the dog and cat should be used for the diagnosis of insulinoma.[18]

Imaging modalities may be supportive in diagnosis. Radiographs are usually not helpful in the diagnosis of insulinoma, but ultrasound of the pancreas may document a large pancreatic beta-cell mass or metastasis to regional lymph nodes or liver. Scintigraphic imaging of the pancreas has also been described for the diagnosis of insulinoma in animals.[19]

Treatment

Hypoglycemia should be treated with 50% dextrose administration. Dextrose may be applied to oral mucous membranes using a large syringe when the animal is stuporous but not having a seizure or if venous access is not readily available. IV treatment should consists of slow IV bolus administration of 50% dextrose (0.5 g/kg) diluted 1:4 with normal saline. This step prevents thrombophlebitis caused by hypertonic dextrose administration. Following bolus loading, a continuous infusion of 2.5% to 5% dextrose should be administered until the animal can be fed. The goal of IV glucose therapy is to stop seizure activity. Administration of higher 50% dextrose doses in an attempt to restore euglycemia may result in rebound hypoglycemia due to provocation of insulin secretion.[12] Refractory seizures should be treated with corticosteroids, such as dexamethasone, and anticonvulsants.

Glucocorticoids may be administered to animals with insulinoma to antagonize the peripheral effects of insulin.[22] Prednisolone (0.5 mg/lb divided bid) may be effective in controlling signs of hypoglycemia by inducing insulin resistance.

An increased prednisolone dosage of 2 to 3 mg/lb/d may be required to control symptoms in advanced cases. Diazoxide, a benzothiadiazide diuretic that inhibits insulin secretion and stimulates gluconeogenesis, has been used to treat canine insulinoma.[12] However, this drug is currently not available.

Recent protocols for treatment of insulinoma include the use of streptozotocin. This agent works by selectively destroying pancreatic beta cells. Because this is a highly nephrotoxic agent, the drug should be administered using saline diuresis protocols similar to those used for other chemotherapeutic agents. Somatostatin analogues, such as octreotide, have been used to inhibit the synthesis and secretion of insulin by beta cells; however, the suppressive effects are variable and the tumors may become refractory.

Exploratory surgery is often indicated to determine the tumor location and distribution.[20] Debulking of the tumors is palliative; many animals can be medically managed for several months to a year even with metastasis. If no tumor is found, a hemipancreatectomy is performed. Dextrose (5%) should be administered IV at a rate of at least twice maintenance before and during surgery to ensure good postoperative pancreatic microvasculature circulation.[12] Postoperative complications include pancreatitis, hypoglycemia (if metastasis is present), and transient diabetes mellitus.[21] One should manage the patient for the first 48 to 72 hours postoperatively as if pancreatitis were present. Water and bland food may be offered on the third day after surgery provided that vomiting is not present.

Prognosis

Prognosis in dogs is guarded to poor; only a few cases of insulinoma have been reported in cats. Of the three cats with beta-cell carcinomas, survival was highly variable, ranging from 5 weeks to 2 years.

REFERENCES

1. Macintire DK: Emergency therapy of diabetic crises: insulin overdose, diabetic ketoacidosis, and hyperosmolar coma. *Vet Clin North Am Small Anim Pract* 25:639, 1995.
2. Plotnick AN, Greco DS: Diagnosis of diabetes mellitus in dogs and cats. Contrasts and comparisons. *Vet Clin North Am Small Anim Pract* 25:563, 1995.
3. Nichols R, Crenshaw K: Complications and concurrent disease associated with diabetic ketoacidosis and other severe forms of diabetes mellitus. *Vet Clin North Am Small Anim Pract* 25:617, 1995.
4. Christopher MM, Broussard JD, Peterson ME: Heinz body formation associated with ketoacidosis in diabetic cats. *J Vet Intern Med* 9:24, 1995.
5. Elliott DA, Nelson RW, Reusch CE, *et al.*: Comparison of serum fructosamine and blood glycosylated hemoglobin concentrations for assessment of glycemic control in cats with diabetes mellitus. *J Am Vet Med Assoc* 214:1794, 1999.
6. Reusch CE, Liehs MR, Hoyer M, Vochezer R: Fructosamine: a new parameter for diagnosis and metabolic control in diabetic dogs and cats. *J Vet Intern Med* 7:177, 1993.
7. Feldman EC, Nelson RW: Diabetic ketoacidosis. *In* Feldman EC, Nelson RW, eds.:

Canine and Feline Endocrinology and Reproduction. Philadelphia: WB Saunders, 1996, p 392.

8. Greco D, Broussard J, Peterson M: Insulin therapy. *Vet Clin North Am Small Anim Pract* 25:677, 1995.
9. MacIntire DK: Treatment of diabetic ketoacidosis in dogs by continuous low-dose intravenous infusion of insulin. *J Am Vet Med Assoc* 202:1266, 1993.
10. Norris CR, Nelson RW, Christopher MM: Serum total and ionized magnesium concentrations and urinary fractional excretion of magnesium in cats with diabetes mellitus and diabetic ketoacidosis. *J Am Vet Med Assoc* 215:1455, 1999.
11. Greco DS: Endocrine pancreatic emergencies. *Compend Contin Educ Pract* 19:23, 1997.
12. Feldman EC, Nelson RW: Beta-cell neoplasia: insulinoma. *In* Feldman EC, Nelson RW, eds.: Canine and Feline Endocrinology and Reproduction. Philadelphia: WB Saunders, 1996, p 422.
13. McMillan FD, Feldman EC: Functional pancreatic islet cell tumor in a cat. *J Am Anim Hosp Asso*, 21:741, 1985.
14. Elie MS, Zerbe CA: Insulinoma in dogs, cats, and ferrets. *Compend Contin Educ Pract Vet* 17:51, 1995.
15. Schrauwen, E, Van Ham L, Desmidt M, *et al.*: Peripheral polyneuropathy associated with insulinoma in the dog: clinical, pathological, and electrodiagnostic features. *Prog Vet Neurol* 7:16, 1996.
16. Simpson KW, Cook A: Hypoglycaemia. *In* Torrance AG, Mooney CT, eds.: BSAVA Manual of Small Animal Endocrinology. Shurdington: Cheltenham British Small Animal Veterinary Association, 1998, p 141.
17. Thompson JC, Jones BR, Hickson PC: The amended insulin-to-glucose ratio and diagnosis of insulinoma in dogs. *N Zeal Vet J* 43:240, 1995.
18. Reimers TJ, Cowan RG, McCann JP, *et al.*: Validation of a rapid solid-phase radioimmunoassay for canine, bovine, and equine insulin. *Am J Vet Res* 43:1274, 1982.
19. Lester NV, Newell SM, Hill RC, *et al.*: Scintigraphic diagnosis of insulinoma in a dog. *Vet Radiol Ultrasound* 40:174, 1999.
20. Matthiesen DT, Mullen HS: Problems and complications associated with endocrine surgery in the dog and cat. *Probl Vet Med* 2:627, 1990.
21. Mehlhaff CJ, Peterson ME, Patnaik AK, *et al.*: Insulin producing islet cell neoplasms: surgical considerations and general management in 35 dogs. *J Am Anim Hosp Assoc* 21:607, 1985.
22. Nelson RW, Foodman MS: Medical management of canine hyperinsulinism. *J Am Vet Med Assoc* 187:78, 1985.

60
Thyroid Disorders

Julia K. Veir and Deborah S. Greco

MYXEDEMA COMA

Myxedema coma is a rare but life-threatening end result of chronic, severe hypothyroidism in dogs. Affected dogs most commonly described in the veterinary literature are middle-aged Doberman pinschers,[2,8,10] but other breeds have been reported as well.[7] Multiple organ systems are involved, including the cardiovascular, respiratory, thermoregulatory, dermatologic, and neurologic systems. Early recognition of the syndrome with appropriate, controlled treatment improves survival in dogs with myxedema coma, although the mortality rate may reach 50%.

Clinical Signs

On physical examination, dogs with classic myxedematous coma have severe hypothermia, bradycardia, decreased amplitude of QRS complexes, thickened, scaling skin, nonpitting edema, hypoventilation, and impaired mentation.[8] The hypothermia may or may not be appropriate for the degree of challenge presented to the dog. It results from a decrease in metabolic rate and dysfunction of the thermoregulatory center of the hypothalamus, resulting in decreased endogenous heat production by the patient.[4] Cardiac signs are manifested by low amplitude complexes on electrocardiographic examination, bradycardia and, sometimes, dilated cardiomyopathy. These can be secondary to lack of stimulation of the sinoatrial cells by thyroid hormone[7] and decreased contractility due to reduced numbers of B receptors on the myocardium. Hyponatremia, a common clinical finding, results from an increase in total body water with a total plasma volume decrease. This is due to decreased delivery of water to the distal tubule of the kidney and a decreased glomerular filtration rate.[4] The increase in total body water, with subsequent decrease in total plasma volume, leads to the classic nonpitting edema found in dogs.[5]

Hypoventilation occurs secondary to reduced response of the respiratory centers to both hypoxia and hypercapnia. The hypercapnia can also contribute to a stuporous or comatose state.[4] Some humans with myxedema coma have pleural effusion secondary to congestive heart failure as well, although this has yet to be reported in the veterinary literature. Since dilated cardiomyopathy has been associated with hypothyroidism in the breeds reported with myxedematous coma, careful evaluation of cardiac function should be performed before aggressive fluid therapy is instituted.[3]

In addition, dogs with myxedema coma usually have a history of muscular weakness secondary to the peripheral myopathy. Dermatologic signs include thickened, scaling skin, diffuse alopecia and, sometimes, nonhealing wounds. Additional clinical findings in dogs include hypercholesterolemia, anemia, hypotension, and hypoglycemia.[12]

Diagnostic Evaluation

Dogs should be evaluated using signalment, history, clinical signs, and supporting clues from initial biochemical profiles and by ruling out other metabolic causes of weakness and bradycardia. However, blood should be drawn in the acute stages for confirmation of hypothyroidism by high endogenous thyroid stimulating hormone (TSH) and low serum total thyroxine (T_4) or low serum free T_4. Endogenous TSH is high in a small number of dogs with nonthyroidal illness; however, combined with clinical signs, response to treatment, and rule out of other differentials for the clinical signs described, a definitive diagnosis can usually be made.

Treatment and Prognosis

Slow, *controlled* rewarming is the mainstay of treatment for hypothermic myxedematous patients. External heat sources such as warm water blankets should be used judiciously because rapid rewarming before adequate thyroid replacement therapy may increase peripheral tissue metabolism without a corresponding response in cardiac output. Slow rehydration with 0.9% NaCl is used to restore plasma volume. It is important to remember that many dogs with myxedema coma have some form of cardiac dysfunction and, therefore, continued monitoring of central venous pressures should be considered to avoid overloading cardiovascular reserve. Respiratory support via mechanical ventilation may be required in the acute phases to compensate for hypoventilation.[4]

Thyroid supplementation must be begun via parenteral routes because oral bioavailability of thyroxine is low and can be slow in onset. Supplementation with intravenously administered levothyroxine should be begun as soon as a clinical diagnosis is made but done judiciously because too rapid restoration of the thyroid concentration can result in increased metabolic demand before hypoxia is resolved, leading to cardiac dysfunction and arrhythmias.[7] After parenteral administration of levothyroxine, oral administration is begun as maintenance therapy as soon as the dog is able to take in solid foods.

Prognosis

Prognosis in humans varies with severity of clinical signs, organ systems involved, and early detection of the myxedematous state. However, mortality rates reach 20% to 30%.[4] In the veterinary literature, few cases have been reported but the success rate seems to be similar.[2,7,8,10]

THYROID STORM

Thyroid storm is a rare but life-threatening complication of hyperthyroidism in humans. The most common cause has been Graves' disease, but other causes of hyperthyroidism (*i.e.*, multinodular goiter, thyroiditis, and overdose of thyroid hormone) have been associated as well.[11] Because most cases of feline hyperthyroidism in veterinary medicine are analogous to toxic multinodular goiter, thyroid storm has not been reported as clinical cases in the veterinary literature. However, it has been associated with radioiodine therapy (I_{131}), an increasingly popular therapeutic choice for hyperthyroidism in cats.

Pathophysiology

The pathophysiology behind thyroid storm is poorly understood. Studies in humans in the late 1980s and early 1990s indicate a rapid rise in free triiodothyronine (T_3) and T_4 concentrations may be the underlying cause. A precipitating cause is usually the reason for decompensation as opposed to severe thyrotoxicosis, in which the primary disease in the only contributing factor. In the normal state of health, the thyroid gland synthesizes and secretes both. The thyroid gland is the only source of T_4 in the body, whereas T_3 comes primarily from peripheral conversion of T_4 to T_3 in the liver and kidneys. Both are usually highly protein bound in the circulation. Only free, nonprotein bound hormone is metabolically active (less than 1%) total hormone.[6] T_3 is the metabolically active form of thyroid hormone. Many human patients with thyroid storm have the same concentration of total circulating hormone as that found in patients with uncomplicated thyrotoxicosis. However, their clinical signs are much more severe. Both T_3 and T_4 concentrations are usually high but not necessarily higher than those found in routine hyperthyroid patients. This has led to speculation that it is actually the rate of rise of free T_3 that is the contributing factor as opposed to absolute values.[1]

Several theories have been proposed to explain the rapid rise in free T_3. A rapid release of all thyroid hormones secondary to massive disruption of thyroid cells, as seen in patients undergoing I_{131} therapy, could overwhelm available protein binding capacity, leading to a rapid rise in free T_3.[11] A second mechanism proposed as a cause for a rapid rise in free T_3 is an acute decrease in total binding capacity as caused by displacement of thyroid hormone by another drug or extrathyroidal illness.[1] A final proposed mechanism is increased sensitivity of tissues to circulating hormone; however, no human or veterinary studies to date have supported this hypothesis.[1]

Clinical Signs

Precipitating events in humans fall into two broad categories: those that cause a rapid rise in thyroid concentration and those that are associated with an acute, extrathyroidal illness. Conditions causing a rapid rise in thyroid hormone concentrations that are commonly seen in veterinary medicine include thyroid surgery, withdrawal of antithyroid drug therapy, and radioiodine therapy. Those conditions that precipitate thyroid storm without causing a rapid rise in thyroid concentrations and are commonly seen in veterinary medicine include diabetic ketoacidosis, infection, and trauma.[4]

Clinical signs can be grouped in two major categories: the classic cluster of signs composing the severe hypermetabolic state and the apathetic state. As stated before, clinical signs are merely exaggerations of the usual clinical signs found in patients with thyrotoxicosis, but evidence of multisystem decompensation and failure separates the two disease states. New onset arrhythmias, severe fever (>41°C [106°F]), and markedly impaired mental status (extreme agitation) are cardinal features of classic thyroid storm in humans. Other features of thyroid storm in humans not usually found in patients with normal thyrotoxicosis include jaundice and hyperkinesis.[4] This state has not been reported in the veterinary literature to date.

The second, more rare condition in humans is the apathetic state. Many features of this syndrome can be found in cats with apathetic hyperthyroidism, including anorexia, stupor, congestive heart failure, and vomiting. In humans, this syndrome is more commonly seen in patients with toxic multinodular goiter, similar to that in cats. Cats with severe pyrexia, inappropriate mentation, and tachyarrhythmias or congestive heart failure should be considered suspect thyroid storm patients if they have a history of untreated hyperthyroidism, recent treatment with I_{131} for hyperthyroidism, or a palpable thyroid slip.

Diagnostic Evaluation

As stated before, laboratory values generally do not differentiate between thyroid storm and severe thyrotoxicosis. Free T_3 and T_4 values in humans overlap between patients with thyrotoxicosis and thyroid storm. Multisystemic decompensation, history of a precipitating event, and supporting laboratory values lead to a clinical diagnosis.

Treatment

The goals of treatment in patients with thyroid storm are 1) to identify and remove the precipitating event, if possible, 2) symptomatically treat the effects of thyroid hormone on tissues and provide supportive therapy, and 3) reduce the activity of thyroid hormone in the patient. Some precipitating events cannot be removed (*i.e.*, I_{131} therapy and thyroid surgery), and a precipitating event often cannot be found. In these cases, symptomatic treatment is begun. Cardiac manifestations should be treated with a β-blocker such as propranolol (Inderal, Ayerst) or calcium channel blocker such as diltiazem (Dilacor XR, Rhone-Poulenc). It should be noted that β-blockers should be used judiciously in patients with evidence of congestive heart failure, because of their negative inotropic effect. Supportive therapy for pyrexia includes appropriate but judicious intravenous administration of fluids and evaporative cooling.

Reduction of thyroid hormone activity can be achieved via several pathways: inhibition of hormone synthesis, blockage of previously synthesized hormone release, prevention of conversion of T_4 to T_3 in the periphery and, if available, direct removal of thyroid hormone from the circulation.[4,11] Inhibition of thyroid hormone synthesis at the level of the thyroid gland is achieved with oral administration of antithyroid drugs (commonly, methimazole or propylthiouracil). In human medicine, propylthiouracil (PTU) is the drug of choice because of its rapid onset of action and prevention of peripheral conversion of T_4 to T_3.[11] However, because of serious side effects of PTU in cats, methimazole would seem to be the preferred drug in veterinary medicine.[9]

Although methimazole (Tapazole, Lilly) blocks production of new thyroid hormone, there can be enough stored thyroid hormone to maintain the concentration for weeks in humans. Prevention stored horomone release of this via administration of a saturated solution of potassium iodide can be used in the acute phases of disease. Prevention of conversion of circulating T_4 to T_3 via high doses of corticosteroids, β-blockers with known membrane stabilizing properties (again with careful consideration of cardiac function), or sodium ipodate is commonly attempted in human patients with thyroid storm. Finally, if available and the above strategies are not successful, direct removal of thyroid hormone from the circulation via plasmapheresis is used in human medicine.[11] However, this technique is not widely available in veterinary medicine, and specific use for this condition has not been reported.

Prognosis

Mortality rates in humans approach 20% to 30% in humans, although this number is lower with early and aggressive recognition and treatment of the state.[11] Since this condition is not commonly recognized in veterinary medicine, no mortality rates have been reported. However, owners of a cat with suspected thyroid storm should be given a guarded prognosis.

REFERENCES

1. Burch HB, Wartofsky L: Life-threatening thyrotoxicosis. *End Metab Clin N Amer* 22:263, 1993.
2. Chastain CB, Graham CL, Riley MG: Myxedema coma in 2 dogs. *Canine Pract* 9: 20, 1982.
3. Fox PR, Sisson DD, Moise NS: Textbook of Canine and Feline Cardiology: Principles and Clinical Practice. Philadelphia: WB Saunders, 1999, 762.
4. Gavin LA: Thyroid crises. *Med Clin North Am* 75:179, 1991.
5. Greco DS: Endocrine emergencies. Part II. Adrenal, thyroid, and parathyroid disorders. *Compend Contin Educ Pract Vet* 19:27, 1997.
6. Guyton AJ, Hall JE: Textbook of Medical Physiology. Philadelphia: WB Saunders, 1991, 873.
7. Henik RA, Dixon RM: Intravenous administration of levothyroxine for treatment of suspected myxedematous coma complicated by severe hypothermia in a dog. *J Am Vet Med Assoc* 16:713, 2000.
8. Kelly MJ, Hill JR: Canine myxedema coma and stupor. *Compend Contin Educ Pract Vet* 6:1049, 1984.
9. Meric SM: Diagnosis and management of feline hyperthyroidism. *Compend Contin Educ Prac Vet* 11:1053, 1989.

10. Noxon JO: Accidental hypothermia associated with hypothyroidism. *Canine Pract* 10:17, 1983.
11. Roth RN, McAuliffe MJ: Hyperthyroidism and thyroid storm. *Emerg Med Clin North Am* 7:873, 1989.
12. Scott DW, Miller WH, Griffin CE: Muller & Kirk's Small Animal Dermatology. Philadelphia: WB Saunders, 1995, 697.

61
Parathyroid Disorders

Kevin A. Hahn

INTRODUCTION

Calcium is involved in many biologic processes, including neuromuscular excitability, membrane permeability, muscle contraction, enzyme activity, hormone release, and blood coagulation. Parathyroid glands maintain serum calcium and phosphorus homeostasis. There are usually four parathyroid glands (one anterior and one posterior to each thyroid gland) that are oblong in shape, caramel colored, and 4 to 6 mm in greatest dimension. The position of the cranial glands is more consistent and usually at the junction of the upper and middle one third of the thyroid gland at the posterolateral aspect at the cricothyroid junction. Parathyroid glands are nourished by the anterior and posterior parathyroid arteries, both of which are branches of the posterior thyroid artery. Parathyroid glands do not receive nourishment from the adjacent thyroid gland.

Parathyroid glands are composed of three histologically distinct cell types. Chief cells are small cells with eosinophilic cytoplasm, clear cells have clear cytoplasm and basal nucleus, and oxyphil cells have brightly eosinophilic cytoplasm with numerous mitochondria. Fat cells make up about 20% to 30% of the adult gland. It is believed that the chief cells are responsible for parathyroid hormone (PTH) production. PTH is an 84-amino acid chain that is cleaved in the liver to its active form, producing a biologically active N-terminal segment and an inactive C-terminal fragment.

Primary control of blood calcium is dependent on (1) PTH secretion, (2) calcitonin secretion, and (3) the presence of cholecalciferol (vitamin D). Secretion of PTH from chief cells is stimulated by low levels of ionized calcium and suppressed by high levels of ionized calcium. PTH protects the body against hypocalcemia through a combination of direct and indirect effects. These are mediated through an intracellular cyclic adenosine monophosphate mechanism at three sites: kidney, bone, and gut. All three sites of calcium homeostasis are believed to be dependent on magnesium. PTH, in concert with calcitriol and magnesium, stimulates osteolysis and release of calcium and phosphorus from bone into extracellular fluid. PTH increases calcium and magnesium reabsorption and increases phosphorus and bicarbonate excretion in the kidney. Phosphorus excretion is increased so that it does not bind to ionized calcium and decrease its concentration. Bicarbonate excretion causes a relative acidosis that results in less protein binding of calcium. PTH indirectly enhances intestinal absorption of calcium by increasing the synthesis of the active form of vitamin D from its inactive form, 25-hydroxyvitamin D in the kidney.

Calcium levels are also controlled by the hormone calcitonin. The primary source of calcitonin is the parafollicular cell population in the mammalian thyroid gland. Calcitonin produces a hypocalcemic effect by decreasing the calcium entry into plasma from the skeleton via temporary inhibition of PTH-stimulated bone resorption. In addition, calcitonin increases the rate of phosphate movement out of plasma into soft tissue and bone. PTH and calcitonin are synergistic in decreasing the renal tubular reabsorption of phosphorus. The level of ionized calcium governs regulation of calcitonin secretion.

The third major hormone involved in the regulation of calcium metabolism is 1,25-dihydroxyvitamin D_3. Ultraviolet irradiation of ergosterol produces vitamin D_2. Vitamin D_2 or D_3 is transformed by the liver to 25-hydroxy-vitamin D and then is actively metabolized in the kidney to 1,25-hydroxyvitamine D. In the skin, ultraviolet light converts 7-dehydrocholesterol to vitamin D_3 (cholecalciferol). The target tissue for this metabolite is the small intestine, where it stimulates calcium and phosphate absorption and increases calcium and phosphate utilization from bone.

Normal serum calcium level in adult companion animals ranges from 8.8 to 10.8 mg/dL. Serum calcium level in immature dogs is approximately 10 to 12 mg/dL. Calcium is present in the serum in two forms. The nondiffusible form is bound to protein (mainly to albumin), constitutes about 45% of the measurable calcium, and is biologically inactive. The ionized form of calcium is biologically active.

PATHOGENESIS

Hypocalcemia

Primary hypoparathyroidism signifies either subnormal amounts of PTH or PTH that cannot react normally with the target cells. Decreased PTH secretion results in hyperphosphatemia, hypocalcemia, and impaired 1,25-dihydroxyvitamin D production. The two most common etiologies of primary hypoparathyroidism are idiopathic atrophy or destruction of parathyroid tissue and iatrogenic secondary to surgical removal of parathyroid tissue (Table 61-1). Idiopathic hypoparathyroidism has been found in mature, small breed female dogs. The clinical manifestations of hypoparathyroidism develop because of reduced bone resorption and reduced calcium levels (4-6 mg/dL). In cats, the most common cause of hypocalcemia is iatrogenic following thyroidectomy with damage to the parathyroid glands.

Secondary hyperparathyroidism may be nutritional or renal in origin. Both conditions result in altered calcium/phosphorus ratios. Nutritional secondary hyperparathyroidism has been reported in a wide variety of species, including the dog, cat, and primate. In nutritional secondary hyperparathyroidism, secretion of PTH increases to compensate for altered mineral levels. Dietary abnormalities

Table 61-1. Causes of Hypocalcemia in Dogs and Cats

Primary hypoparathyroidism
Idiopathic
Post-thyroidectomy
Puerperal tetany
Renal failure
Acute
Chronic
Ethylene glycol toxicity
Acute pancreatitis
Intestinal malabsorption syndromes
Hypoproteinemia or hypoalbuminemia
Laboratory error
Miscellaneous causes
Phosphate-containing enemas
Anticonvulsant medications
Hypomagnesemia

that lead to nutritional secondary hyperparathyroidism are a low dietary calcium level, excessive phosphorus with a normal or low calcium level, and inadequate amounts of vitamin D_3.

Hypercalcemia

Consistent elevation of blood calcium levels (11.5-12.0 mg/dL) indicates potential hypercalcemia. Hypercalcemia can be associated with primary hyperparathyroidism, vitamin D intoxication, malignant neoplasms with osseous metastases, and other malignant neoplasms (pseudohyperparathyroidism) (Table 61-2).

Primary hyperparathyroidism is usually associated with increased PTH hormone secretion from parathyroid tumors. Hormone secretion is autonomous and is usually associated with an adenoma composed of active chief cells.

Pseudohyperparathyroidism is a metabolic abnormality in which parathyroid-like hormone is produced by malignant tumors of nonparathyroid origin. Pseudohyperparathyroidism has been reported in dogs and cats with malignant lymphoma, mammary adenocarcinoma, and apocrine gland adenocarcinoma of the anal sac. Lymphadenopathy or abdominal organomegaly may be present in lymphoma patients.

Table 61-2. Causes of Hypercalcemia in Dogs and Cats

Primary hyperparathyroidism
Hypercalcemia of malignancy
Humorally mediated (lymphoma, apocrine gland adenocarcinoma)
Locally osteolytic (multiple myeloma)
Hypervitaminosis D
Cholecalciferol rodenticides
Excessive supplementation
Hypoadrenocorticism
Renal failure
Granulomatous disease (rare)
Blastomycosis
Nonmalignant skeletal disorder (rare)
Osteomyelitis
Hypertrophic osteodystrophy
Iatrogenic disorder (rare)
Excessive calcium supplementation
Excessive oral phosphate binders
Dehydration (mild hypercalcemia)
Factitious disorder
Lipemia
Postprandial measurement
Young animal (<6 mo)
Laboratory error

Prior to confirming a hypercalcemia diagnosis, total calcium level should be corrected using the following formula in dogs:

$$\text{Corrected calcium (mg/dL)} = \text{measured serum total calcium} - \text{serum albumin (g/dL)} + 3.5$$

EPIDEMIOLOGY

Hyperparathyroidism

Primary hyperparathyroidism is uncommon in dogs and rare in cats. Primary hyperparathyroidism can be caused by a single adenoma, diffuse parathyroid hyperplasia, or parathyroid carcinoma.

Primary hyperplasia is less common than adenomas. Hyperplasia can be due to proliferation of the chief cell or the clear cell. Chief cell hyperplasia is more common than the clear cell form. Chief cell hyperplasia appears microscopically and grossly similar to adenoma because both are composed of the chief cell proliferation. The differentiating factor is that there is more than one diseased gland in cases of hyperplasia. Size cannot be used to determine if a gland is normal or abnormal. In about half the cases, one or two glands are enlarged, and the rest are just slightly enlarged or even normal in size.

Only 3% of hyperparathyroidism cases are caused by parathyroid carcinoma.

The clinical manifestations of parathyroid carcinoma are similar to those caused by adenomas and hyperplasia. PTH is elevated three to four times that of normal. Serum calcium can be greater than 14 mg/dL. Regional and distant metastasis to the lung, liver, and bone may occur.

Secondary hyperparathyroidism is caused by an increased PTH production as a result of decreased levels of calcium associated with end-organ resistance to PTH. Nutritional secondary hyperparathyroidism is caused by a nutritional deficiency of calcium and vitamin D. In most cases, the underlying cause is chronic renal failure, but intestinal malabsorption and lack of vitamin D can also be underlying etiologies.

Hypoparathyroidism

Primary hypoparathyroidism results from an absolute or relative deficiency in PTH secretion. Most cases are classified as idiopathic (*i.e.*, no evidence for trauma, malignant or surgical destruction, or other obvious damage to the neck or parathyroid glands). There may be an immune-mediated component to this disorder.

Iatrogenic hypoparathyroidism following bilateral thyroidectomy is common in cats. This form of hypoparathyroidism may be transient or permanent, depending on the viability of the parathyroid gland(s) saved.

CLINICAL PRESENTATION

Hyperparathyroidism

Clinical presentation varies from asymptomatic to severe systemic illness. Signs in dogs are associated with renal, gastrointestinal, and neuromuscular systems. Renal signs may include polyuria polydypsia, incontinence, dysuria, pollakiuria, and hematuria. Gastrointestinal signs range from inappetence to vomiting and constipation. Neuromuscular signs typically include muscle wasting, weakness, shivering, a stiff gait, and exercise intolerance.

In cats, clinical signs may be anorexia, lethargy, polyuria, polydypsia, hypercalcemia, increased alanine aminotransferase, increased alkaline phosphatase, elevated blood urea nitrogen (BUN), and azotemia. In its mildest form, animals may be asymptomatic; hypercalcemia is discovered only after a serum biochemistry profile is obtained. When signs do develop, they tend to be nonspecific and have an insidious onset. Owners often become aware of specific signs only after hypercalcemia-induced organ system dysfunction occurs.

Hypoparathyroidism

The major clinical signs are directly attributable to hypocalcemia. Neuromuscular signs include nervousness, generalized seizures, focal muscle twitching, rear limb cramping or tetany, ataxia, and weakness. Additional signs may include lethargy, inappetence, intense facial rubbing, and panting. Aggressive behavior and biting or licking at the paws may also be noted. Onset of signs tends to be abrupt and severe, and occurs more frequently during exercise, excitement, and stress. Signs also tend to be episodic; episodes of clinical hypocalcemia are interspersed with relatively normal periods, lasting minutes to days, even though hypocalcemia persists during these "normal" periods.

The most common findings on physical examination are related to muscular tetany. Fever, panting, and nervousness, often to the point of interfering with the examination, are common. Potential cardiac abnormalities include paroxysmal tachyarrhythmias, muffled heart sounds, and weak femoral pulses. Clinical signs in cats include seizures, nervousness, muscle twitching, tetany, ataxia, and weakness. Cataracts have been reported in a few dogs and in one cat.

DIAGNOSTIC EVALUATION

Hyperparathyroidism

Primary hyperparathyroidism is considered when persistent hypercalcemia and normophosphatemia or hypophosphatemia are identified with appropriate clinical signs (Table 61-3). Serum calcium concentration is typically 13 to 16 mg/dL, but can range from 12 to 23 mg/dL. Serum phosphorus concentration is typically less than 4 mg/dL, but can be high in dogs with concurrent renal insufficiency. The common diagnostic approach is to rule out other causes of hypercalcemia, including secondary to hypercalcemia of malignancy, before attempting to document primary hyperparathyroidism.

In dogs with uncomplicated primary hyperparathyroidism, urine specific gravity of less than 1.015 is common. Hematuria, pyuria, bacteriuria, and crystalluria may be found if secondary bacterial cystitis or cystic calculi develop. Uroliths are typically composed of calcium phosphate, calcium oxalate, or mixtures of the two salts. Prolonged (severe) hypercalcemia may cause progressive nephrocalcinosis, renal damage, and azotemia reflected as increased BUN, serum creatinine, and serum phosphorus concentrations. Serum ionized calcium measurement may help differentiate primary hyperparathyroidism-induced from primary renal failure-induced hypercalcemia.

Measurement of serum PTH level helps confirm primary hyperparathyroidism. Radioimmunoassay is the standard methodology used to measure PTH levels. Normal range for PTH is 2 to 13 pmol/L in the dog and cat. PTH is 5 to 100 pmol/L in hyperparathyroidism. A mid-normal to increased serum PTH concentration in a hypercalcemic dog with normal renal function strongly suggests primary hyperparathyroidism. Increased serum PTH concentrations can be found in dogs with renal failure secondary to renal hyperparathyroidism. It is essential that renal function be normal in a hypercalcemic animal if serum PTH concentration is to be considered diagnostic. Alternatively, serum PTH can be evaluated in conjunction with serum ionized calcium concentration, which is typically increased in primary hyperparathyroidism.

Ultrasonography can be used to evaluate parathyroid glands greater than 5 mm diameter. Adenomas appear homogeneous, solid, and hypoechoic. The thyroid appears hyperechoic. Surgical exploration of the neck is ultimately required to establish a diagnosis of primary hyperparathyroidism. Parathyroid hy-

Table 61-3. Differentiating Common Causes of Hypercalcemia

Diagnostic Parameters	Primary Hyperparathyroidism	Renal Secondary Hyperparathyroidism	Pseudohyper-parathyroidism	Neoplastic Osteolysis
Serum calcium	Elevated	Normal to decreased	Elevated	Elevated
Serum phosphorus	Decreased unless uremic; then normal to increased	Increased	Decreased unless uremic; then normal to increased	Frequently increased
Serum alkaline phospha-tase	Normal to increased	Normal to increased	Normal to increased	Normal to increased
Blood urea nitrogen; crea-tinine	Normal unless uremic; then increased	Increased	Normal unless uremic; then increased	Normal unless uremic; then increased
Bone radiographs	Varying degrees of demin-eralization	Varying degrees of demin-eralization	Varying degrees of demin-eralization	Disseminated osteolytic le-sions

perplasia is tentatively diagnosed when more than one parathyroid gland is grossly and microscopically abnormal. Affected glands contain multiple nodules less than 5 mm in diameter, as opposed to adenomas, which consist of a single nodule greater than 5 mm in diameter. The differentiation between hyperplasia and adenoma has important prognostic implications.

Hypoparathyroidism

The relevant biochemical abnormalities are severe hypocalcemia (<6.5 mg/dL) and, in most dogs and cats, hyperphosphatemia (>6 mg/dL). Total protein, albumin, BUN, creatinine, and magnesium concentrations are normal. Diagnosis is made by documenting persistent hypocalcemia and undetectable serum PTH when other causes of hypocalcemia have been ruled out.

Electrocardiographic changes may be observed in patients with hypocalcemia and include prolongation of the ST and QT segments. Sinus bradycardia and wide T waves or T-wave alternans occasionally are seen. Cervical exploration reveals absence or atrophy of the parathyroid glands.

Blood sampling for PTH determination should be performed before initiating therapy. Therapy for hypocalcemia should not be withheld pending the results of this assay. Low or undetectable serum PTH in a hypocalcemic dog or cat strongly suggests primary hypoparathyroidism. Patients with nonparathyroid-induced hypocalcemia have normal or high serum PTH concentrations.

TREATMENT

Hyperparathyroidism

Surgical removal of abnormal parathyroid tissue is the treatment of choice. It is important to evaluate all four parathyroid glands before deciding on which gland(s) to remove. Almost all dogs and cats with primary hyperparathyroidism have a solitary, easily identified parathyroid adenoma. Enlargement of more than one parathyroid gland suggests either multiple adenomas or parathyroid hyperplasia. A thorough presurgical evaluation should rule out secondary causes. A decision to remove three versus four glands should be based on the clinical status and renal function, and on the ability of the owner to treat permanent hypoparathyroidism. If none of the glands appears enlarged or if all appear small, the diagnosis of primary hyperparathyroidism must be questioned; occult neoplasia, ectopic parathyroid tumor, or nonparathyroid PTH-producing tumor should be considered.

Surgical removal of the parathyroid tumor results in a rapid decline in circulating PTH and development of hypocalcemia 1 to 7 days after surgery. The higher the presurgical serum calcium concentration or the more chronic the condition, the more likely clinical hypocalcemia will develop. As a guide, if the serum calcium concentration before surgery is less than 14 mg/dL, the dog or cat should be kept in the hospital for 5 to 7 days and serum calcium monitored twice daily. Treatment for hypocalcemia is not initiated unless serum calcium drops below 8 mg/dL, serum ionized calcium falls below 0.8 mmol/L (3.2 mg/dL), or clinical signs of hypocalcemia develop.

In dogs and cats with serum calcium concentrations greater than 14 mg/dL, vitamin D and calcium therapy should be started immediately after recovery from anesthesia (Table 61-4). In cases with severe hypercalcemia (>18 mg/dL), vitamin D therapy can be initiated 24 to 36 hours before surgery.

The initial management in patients with serum calcium levels greater than 14 mg/dL and increased BUN and creatinine levels is saline-furosemide diuresis. Diuresis expands extracellular fluid volume, increases glomerular filtration rate, decreases calcium reabsorption, and dilutes serum calcium level. Magnesium and potassium levels must be monitored and adjusted if necessary. Other considerations may include mithramycin, which decreases bone resorption by inhibiting osteoclastic activity, or the use of calcitonin, which decreases bone resorption and increases urinary excretion of calcium.

Hypoparathyroidism

Acute therapy to control hypocalcemic tetany includes slow IV administration of calcium (0.25 mmol/kg/h) to effect. Once signs of hypocalcemia are controlled, calcium gluconate should be administered subcutaneous (SQ) every 6 to 8 hours (at the intravenous (IV) dose), and oral calcium and vitamin D therapy initiated. Therapy for postsurgical hypocalcemia includes IV and SQ calcium administration. Some dogs, but more often cats, seem resistant to vita-

Table 61-4. Vitamin D and Calcium Preparations

Preparation	Dose	Maximal Effect	Size
1,25-dihydroxycholecalciferol (active vitamin D_3, calcitriol)	0.03-0.06 mg/kg/d	1-4 d	0.25- and 0.5-mg capsules
Dihydrotachysterol	Initial: 0.02-0.03 mg/kg/d Maint: 0.01-0.02 mg/kg/24-48 h	1-7 d	0.125-, 0.2-, 0.4-, and 0.125-mg capsules, 0.25-mg/mL syrup
Ergocalciferol (vitamin D_2)	Initial: 4000-6000 U/kg/d Maint: 1000-2000 U/kg/d-wk	5-21 d	25,000- and 50,000-U capsules and 8000-U/mL syrup
Calcium carbonate	Dogs: 1-4 g/d Cats: 0.5-1 g/d	40%	350-1500-mg tablets
Calcium gluconate	Dogs: 1-4 g/d Cats: 0.5-1 g/d	10%	325-, 500-, 650-, and 1000-mg tablets
Calcium lactate	Dogs: 1-4 g/d Cats: 0.5-1 g/d	13%	325- and 650-mg tablets

min D in tablet form but respond to the liquid form. The goal of therapy is to maintain the serum calcium concentration within the low-normal range (8-10 mg/dL) until the remaining parathyroid glands regain control of calcium homeostasis. Serum calcium should be measured twice daily and the dose or frequency of SQ calcium administration adjusted to maintain the serum calcium at 8 to 9 mg/dL. SQ calcium should be discontinued by gradually increasing the dosing interval once serum calcium remains greater than 8 mg/dL for 48 hours.

Maintenance therapy should target blood calcium levels in the low-normal range (8-9.5 mg/dL) through daily administration of calcium and vitamin D supplements (see Table 61-4). Ideally, dogs and cats should remain hospitalized until their serum calcium concentration remains between 8 and 10 mg/dL without parenteral support. Thereafter, serum calcium concentrations should be monitored weekly, and the vitamin D dosage adjusted to maintain a serum calcium of 8 to 9.5 mg/dL. Serum calcium concentrations greater than 10 mg/dL are unnecessary to avoid tetany and increase the likelihood of hypercalcemia.

Once serum calcium concentration is stabilized in the low-normal range, attempts can be made to slowly taper the oral calcium and the vitamin D to the lowest effect dose. Most dogs and cats with primary hypoparathyroidism require permanent vitamin D therapy, but the calcium supplement can often be gradually tapered over 2 to 4 months and then stopped. Supplementing the diet with calcium-rich foods (*e.g.*, dairy products) helps ensure adequate calcium intake. Once the dog or cat is stable and maintenance therapy is established, periodic re-evaluation of the serum calcium concentration (*e.g.*, every 3–4 months) is advisable.

PROGNOSIS

Hyperparathyroidism

Removal of a parathyroid adenoma results in a cure, if one normal parathyroid gland remains. The likelihood of persistent or recurrent hyperparathyroidism is high with parathyroid hyperplasia, unless all abnormal parathyroid tissue is removed. Unfortunately, preventing recurrence of hyperparathyroidism often requires removal of all four parathyroid glands, which produces permanent hypoparathyroidism.

Prognosis depends on the severity of renal changes induced by hypercalcemia and on the ability to prevent severe postoperative hypocalcemia. If serious renal damage has not occurred and severe postoperative hypocalcemia is avoided, the prognosis is excellent. Hypercalcemia may recur weeks to months after surgery in dogs and cats with primary hyperparathyroidism if one or more parathyroid glands are left in situ.

Hypoparathyroidism

With owner compliance, proper therapy, and timely re-evaluations, prognosis is excellent.

SUGGESTED READINGS

Bruyette DS, Feldman EC: Primary hypoparathyroidism in the dog. Report of 15 cases and review of 13 previously reported cases. *J Vet Intern Med* 2:7, 1988.

Chew DJ, Nagode LA, Carothers M: Disorders of calcium: hypercalcemia and hypocalcemia. *In* DiBartola SP, ed.: Fluid Therapy in Small Animal Practice. Philadelphia: WB Saunders, 1992, p 116.

Feldman EC: Disorders of the parathyroid glands. *In* Ettinger SJ, Feldman EC, eds.: Textbook of Veterinary Internal Medicine. Philadelphia: WB Saunders, 1994, p 1437.

Feldman EC, Nelson RW: Hypocalcemia and primary hypoparathyroidism. *In* Feldman EC, Nelson RW, eds.: Canine and Feline Endocrinology and Reproduction. Philadelphia: WB Saunders, 1996, p 497.

Peterson ME, James KM, Wallace M, *et al.*: Idiopathic hypoparathyroidism in five cats. *J Vet Intern Med* 5:47, 1991.

Waters CB, Scott-Moncrieff JCR: Hypocalcemia in cats. *Compend Contin Educ Pract Vet* 14:497, 1992.

SECTION IX
Neurologic Disorders

62
Single Seizure, Cluster Seizures, and *Status Epilepticus*

Joane Parent and Roberto Poma

INTRODUCTION

The veterinary literature is scant on the investigation of therapeutic modalities for *status epilepticus* (SE) in dogs or in cats.[1–3] The existing literature is primarily based on human data and/or clinical experience of an author or group of authors. This chapter makes no exception. The management and therapeutic approach to seizure activity in the emergency setting offered herein are based on the literature and our clinical experience.

PATHOGENESIS

Convulsive SE is a life-threatening emergency requiring immediate and vigorous treatment. The operational definition of convulsive SE is the recurrence of convulsive seizures without full recovery of neurological function (including mental status) between seizures, or a single prolonged convulsion.[4] Cluster seizures (CS) are defined as two or more seizures occurring over a 24 hour period between which the patient regains consciousness. Cluster seizures are treated aggressively because they often evolve into SE. A distinction is made between the early stage of SE (<30 minutes) and the later stage (>30 minutes). Within 10 minutes following a single seizure, there is a massive release of epinephrine and norepinephrine into the circulation.[5] This results in an increase in systemic blood pressure, heart rate, and cerebral blood flow. The system responds effectively to the first seizures. In a study of dogs with experimentally induced seizures, it was found that in the early stage of convulsive seizures, cerebral oxygen supply exceeded oxidative demands, and cerebral blood flow kept pace with CO_2 production.[6] In the early or compensated stage of SE, metabolic (hyperglycemia, lactic acidosis), autonomous (salivation, hyperthermia), cardiovascular (increased cardiac output, central venous pressure and heart rate), and cerebral effects (increased blood flow, metabolism, glucose and oxygen utilization) occur but without yet permanent damage.[7] But if the seizures continue, profound deleterious systemic and cerebral changes ensue because increased cerebral demands for oxygen and energy substrate cannot be met. In this late or decompensated stage of SE, the metabolic (electrolytic imbalance, hypoglycemia, metabolic and respiratory acidosis, hepatic and renal dysfunction, coagulopathy, muscular necrosis), autonomous (hyperthermia), cardiovascular (systemic hypoxia, respiratory collapse, cardiac failure, pulmonary edema), and cerebral effects (failure of cerebral autoregulation where cerebral blood flow becomes dependent on systemic blood pressure, hypoxia, increased intracranial pressure, cerebral edema) lead to extreme systemic complications, permanent cerebral damage, and frequently death.[7] Although it was believed that the secondary systemic effects were as detrimental to the brain as the seizures themselves, there is now abundant evidence indicating that the permanent cerebral neuropathologic damage is primarily the result of the sustained seizure activity and not from the systemic abnormalities.[4]

EPIDEMIOLOGY

Little data exists in the veterinary literature on the epidemiology of SE. In one study, a prevalence of 0.44 percent of the total hospital admission was estimated for dogs with either SE or CS.[3] In this study, one-third of the dogs had primary or idiopathic epilepsy, one-third secondary epilepsy, and in the rest of the dogs the cause was undetermined.[3] Generalized convulsive SE is the most common type of SE.

CLINICAL PRESENTATION

The spectrum of clinical symptoms at presentation is wide and the etiology highly variable.[3] The animal may be normal, as in dogs experiencing a first convulsion and having fully recovered at the time of presentation. Other patients are in a post-ictal phase, panting, pacing compulsively, and disoriented, while others are convulsing while being examined. Finally, some patients in the decompensated stage of SE are presented in a coma, with only subtle motor manifestations, such as twitching of the eyelids and face or nystagmoid jerks of the eyes to indicate that seizure activity is still ongoing. If the animal is not actively seizing, it is important to substantiate that a seizure did in fact take place. The clinician should not readily accept from the owner that a seizure has occurred without a detailed description of what was observed. Neck spasms secondary to cervical intervertebral disc extrusion and obsessive/compulsive behaviors are examples of disorders that may occasionally be mistaken for seizure activity. Although most owners recognize a convulsion, veterinarians and owners frequently fail to recognize complex partial seizures as being seizure activity. Following partial seizure activity, the pet is disoriented and uncoordinated sometimes for up to 20 minutes at a time. The owner often reports to the veterinarian only the difficulty in walking. Without questioning the condition of the animal's mental status during the episode, it is not possible for the veterinarian to recognize that a seizure has occurred.

Due to the controversy in veterinary medicine on the classification of seizures,[8] it is necessary to define the seizure type because seizure classification has an impact on the differential diagnosis. The seizure is classified as **generalized** if there is loss of consciousness. Although generalized seizures are most commonly convulsive, non-convulsive generalized seizures do occur but are rare. The seizure is classified as **partial** (with or without secondary generalization) if the patient remains conscious (simple partial seizure) although the mental status may be altered (complex partial seizure). The presence of an aura indicates partial seizure.[8] We distinguish four categories of patients presented for seizure activity:

1. **The patient experiencing a single convulsion, CS, or SE for the first time** with no history of systemic illness. Regardless of the animal's breed, age, and seizure type (partial or generalized), if a detailed history fails to indicate any abnormalities prior to the development of the seizures, if the physical and neurologic examinations are unremarkable and the data base (CBC, chemistry, urinalysis) is within reference range, the animal likely has an idiopathic (unknown) form of epilepsy. Only if the animal develops acute convulsive SE can a toxin be incriminated.
2. **The patient experiencing partial or generalized seizures with a history indicative of a neurologic disorder** days to weeks preceding the onset of seizures. The epilepsy is secondary to an active brain disease, ie, a space-occupying lesion (brain neoplasia, granuloma), an encephalitis, etc.
3. **The patient presented in complex partial status** (eg, continuous twitching of the facial muscles) with no history of previous illness, or neurologic deficits preceding SE. The animal may exhibit facial twitching, head bobbing, or head jerks that may last minutes, days, or months. Pending the severity of the clinical signs and frequency of the episodes, this type of seizure may or may not be treated since they often do not progress into generalized seizures.
4. **The known epileptic patient experiencing CS or SE.** The animal is already on maintenance antiepileptic drugs (AEDs) such as potassium bromide (KBr) and/or phenobarbital (PB). The owner may have administered diazepam in the rectum as an in-home emergency measure.

DIAGNOSTIC EVALUATION

The diagnostic evaluation consists of rapid assessment of the overall condition of the patient, the need for emergency treatment, and integrating this information with the history, seizure pattern, and physical and neurologic examinations to determine a probable cause of the seizures.

One cannot emphasize enough the need for a thorough history of the home behavior to evaluate the animal's mental status prior to seizures or between seizures. Even subtle behavioral abnormalities are important in the diagnosis of active brain diseases. The animal may be more withdrawn, quiet, or disoriented. Observation of the animal's behavior in the hospital environment is insufficient to carry a judgment on the animal's mental status in the few days or weeks preceding the seizures, and even less if the animal is in post-ictal phase, or seizing at the time of presentation. Contrary to secondary epilepsy (neoplasia, encephalitis, etc.), in idiopathic causes of seizures, there are no mental changes.

Upon presentation of the seizing patient, the physical examination is rapidly performed to evaluate the need for emergency treatment. The animal's mental status, capillary refill, respiratory and heart rates, and body temperature are parameters useful to stage the animal's condition. The abnormalities found must be taken in light of the CS or SE. The evaluation of the mental status (by history and examination), the responses to menace gesture and nasal septum stimulation, and the proprioceptive positioning are four tests of the neurological examination that target specifically the cerebral cortex. Bilateral and symmetric neurologic deficits are expected in the animal in the post-ictal phase (e.g., absent menace and nasal septum response bilaterally). Presence of asymmetry in the neurological examination is a strong indicator of focal cerebral disease justifying further diagnostic work up (cerebrospinal fluid and/or magnetic resonance imaging). The neurologic examination should be done with attention to detail especially when performing these tests because the abnormalities may be subtle.

A blood sample should be collected as soon as possible to assess the systemic status of the animal and to rule out life-threatening conditions such as hypoglycemia or hypocalcemia. CBC, serum biochemistry profile, electrolytes, and blood gas analysis determine if concurrent metabolic disorders (ie, insulinoma, hepatic encephalopathy, ethylene glycol toxicity) and acid-base imbalance need to be addressed. If the animal is being treated with AED(s), obtain blood for AED level measurements.

The seizure pattern (age at onset of seizures, seizure type, and seizure frequency) is a crucial element in establishing a differential diagnosis. The recognition that a seizure is partial (eg, aura) at onset implies the presence of a focal cerebral disease even if the seizure generalizes later on. Generalized seizures occur with toxicity, genetic epilepsy, and in reactive (secondary to metabolic diseases) seizures. Toxin-induced seizures rapidly evolve into convulsive SE once the seizures appear. It is the toxin present within the central nervous system (CNS) that leads to seizures. The animal seizes to death or until treatment is applied. There is no recovery time between the seizures. Seizures of metabolic origin, such as hypoglycemia or portosystemic shunt, should be generalized from onset. However, if the metabolic disease has been present for a long duration, brain damage may ensue and the seizures may then be partial with/without secondary generalization. Arrhythmia is a rare, if ever, cause of seizures in the dog but central nervous system diseases may cause cardiac dysfunction.

The combination of history, seizure pattern, and animal's signalment is of extreme diagnostic value. In idiopathic epilepsy, the dog is usually less than three years of age at the first seizure and is otherwise healthy. The seizures are generalized or partial with rapid secondary generalization, and the seizures frequently occur when the animal is asleep or resting. In large breeds of dogs with idiopathic epilepsy, CS becomes increasingly more frequent with occasional subsequent SE. In Pugs, a diagnosis of Pug encephalitis is likely if the animal is young and has a history of abnormal behavior accompanying or preceding the seizures.

TREATMENT

The goal in the treatment of CS and SE is to end all clinical and electrical seizure activity as rapidly and effectively as possible. The treatment becomes a balance between ending seizure activity rapidly while avoiding respiratory and cardiac depression secondary to the anti-epileptic treatment. The therapeutic principle in CS or SE is that the more frequently the animal has seized in a given time, the more drugs, time, and money will be necessary to control the seizures.

General Treatment

Emergency measures include immediate evaluation and correction of the physiologic abnormalities that may be present as a consequence of the CS or SE. These principles include the following:

1. The ABCs of all emergencies (i.e., stabilization of Airway, Breathing, and Circulation).
2. Obtain blood sample for hematology and chemistry profile, and AED serum levels if the animal is treated with PB phenobarbital and/or KBr. Consider sampling for toxicologic analysis and infectious disease titers.
3. Place an intravenous catheter in a large vein and keep it open with saline-based fluids. Avoid dextrose-containing solutions because of the potential precipitation of AEDs. An in-line burette is added to the fluid line and the use of an infusion pump is strongly recommended to control fluid administration rate.
4. A dextrose intravenous (IV) bolus is administered (1 to 5 ml 50% dextrose over 10 minutes) only in documented hypoglycemia. There is evidence that hyperglycemia may exacerbate SE neuronal damage.[9]
5. Hyperthermia (T > 39.5°C) exacerbates neuronal damage and should be rapidly corrected with fans and cold water.
6. Acidosis does not usually necessitate treatment because the pH normalizes quickly once SE is stopped.

Specific Treatment Selected

Status epilepticus treatment is applied to convulsive SE, severe partial SE, and dogs that have had more than one seizure in the last 24 hours. Specific treatment consists of drug administration to stop the seizures. Ideally, the drug selected should be available for parenteral administration, have a high lipid solubility so it penetrates and distributes to the brain rapidly, be stable in solution, not react with plastic sets, not precipitate with other medication, have low toxicity at therapeutic doses, and a rapid and sustained duration of action.[7] No single drug has all features but the combination of diazepam (DZ) and PB has many of the requirements. The following protocol is used in SE management:

1. Initiate AED to stop all gross motor seizure activity or to rapidly reach therapeutic serum levels in the non-seizing dog

   Diazepam IV bolus 0.5–1.0 mg/kg is administered. Rectal DZ is reserved for patients where an IV access cannot be successfully obtained. Wait 5 minutes, and if SE persists, repeat DZ bolus.
2. To prevent recurrence of seizures, a constant rate infusion (CRI) of DZ at

0.5–1 mg/kg/hr is added to the hourly maintenance fluid therapy in the in-line burette. Only 1 to 2 hours of solution is prepared at a time to minimize DZ adsorption to the plastic tubing and its deactivation by light. The CRI with DZ can be continued for a few hours. Once seizure activity has subsided for 4 to 6 hrs, the DZ is gradually withdrawn over as many hours.

3. In most cases, PB is added to the CRI. (Dogs may develop acute refractoriness to DZ.) Most known epileptic dogs are on PB for maintenance therapy and their levels may need adjustments.

   Phenobarbital IV bolus 2 mg/Kg. The bolus can be repeated every 30 minutes to effect for a maximum of 24 mg/kg over a 24-hour period (Table 62-1). The patient should be carefully monitored for cardiorespiratory depression. The PB serum concentration rises approximately 20 umol/L (5 ug/ml) for each 3 mg/kg administered IV.[14]

   Phenobarbital is added to the CRI at a rate of 2 to 10 mg/hr.

4. SE refractive to diazepam and PB.

   a) **Propofol** is the next preferred route. The drug has barbiturate and benzodiazepine-like effects on GABA receptors and can suppress central nervous system metabolic activity. An anticonvulsant effect has been documented in experimentally induced seizures.[10] Its fast clearance and shorter terminal half-life offer advantages over pentobarbital.[1] Although EEG activation after low-dose propofol anesthesia is described in dogs, research suggests that the EEG findings are dose-related.[11]

   Propofol is administered at a dose of 2–8 mg/kg as a slow IV bolus to avoid respiratory depression and cyanosis. A 25% of the recommended dose is administered every 30 seconds until the desired effect is achieved. In cases refractory to repetitive IV boluses, a constant rate infusion may be considered superior. The recommended dose for CRI is 0.1–0.6 mg/kg/minute (see Table 62-1). Use caution with this drug since hypoxemia secondary to apnea and myocardial depression are the primary side effects.

   b) **Isoflurane** anesthesia and **phenytoin** CRI are secondary options for refractive SE management. Isoflurane is reported to suppress drug-induced convulsions in animals.[12] Phenytoin, a potent AED in humans for maintenance and SE treatment, has not been used historically in dogs due to its failure to generate and maintain therapeutic concentrations. It may have its place in SE refractory to other means. Significant brain concentrations have been measured in dogs and cats within 6 minutes of IV administration.[13] The recommended dose is 2–5 mg/kg IV slowly or a CRI of 1–3 mg/kg/hour (see Table 62-1). Phenytoin IV injection must be given slowly (>30 minutes) as it may cause severe hypotension in dogs.[14]

   c) **Pentobarbital** is an anesthetic agent not an AED. Pentobarbital anesthesia may protect the brain during periods of hypoxia induced by the seizures but it has weak antiepileptic effects compared to PB. In humans, simultaneous EEG monitoring is essential to ensure suppression of all

Table 62-1. The Most Common Antiepileptic Drugs Used in the Treatment of *Status Epilepticus* in the Dog with Dosages and Routes of Administration, Half-lives, Onset of Action, and Limitations

	IV Bolus	CRI	Per Rectum	Halflife	Onset of Action	Limitations
Diazepam	0.5–1mg/kg	0.5–1mg/kg/hr	0.5–1 mg/kg	2–4 hours	4 min	Short duration
Phenobarbital	2mg/kg	2–6 mg/kg/hr	N/A	53 hours	15 min	Cardiopulmonary depression
Pentobarbital	3–15mg/kg	5 mg/kg/hr	N/A	8 hours	30 sec	Cardiopulmonary depression
Propofol	2–8 mg/kg	0.1–0.6 mg/kg/min	N/A	1.4 hour	30 sec	Hypoxemia, myocardial depression
Phenytoin	2–5mg/kg	1–3 mg/kg/hr	N/A	Variable	20 min	Hypotension

epileptiform activity. The recommended dose in dogs is 2 mg/kg IV slowly to effect, followed by 5 mg/kg/hr infusion to effect. This dosage results in general anesthesia commonly referred to as barbiturate coma. Pentobarbital may be used to treat on-going SE when all else has failed.

5. In severe CS or SE, dexamethasone 0.25 mg/kg IV is administered once daily for 2–3 days unless an infectious process is suspected.
6. Maintenance oral AED therapy is initiated or resumed as soon as the animal can swallow. Antiepileptic treatment is recommended at the second generalized seizure (regardless of the length of time between seizures) in the young animal (<3 years old).

   Potassium bromide is used as a first line maintenance AED in patients with primary or idiopathic epilepsy. The half-life is long, necessitating a loading dose. Although loading a dose of 600 mg/kg is advocated, 60 mg/kg/day over a 10-day period is preferable to avoid excessive sedation and polydipsia/polyuria. The dose is thereafter reduced to 30 mg/kg q24hrs.

   Phenobarbital can be used as a first line AED when it is crucial to obtain therapeutic serum levels as rapidly as possible. A loading dose of 5 mg/kg q12hrs for 2 days is given to reach therapeutic range followed with a dose of 5–8 mg/kg divided q12hrs.

   If the animal is already treated with PB and/or KBr and has subtherapeutic drug levels, the dose(s) is (are) adjusted. The optimal therapeutic range for PB is 100-130 umol/L (23–28 μg/mL) and for KBr > 20 mmol/L. If used as single therapy, the optimal therapeutic serum level for KBr is 22–30 mmol/L.

   In complex partial SE, oral **clonazepam,** 1–2 mg tablets q8hrs, is recommended if treatment is deemed necessary. In humans, clonazepam has a beneficial effect on partial complex seizures and anxiety or panic disorders. Our personal experience suggests a beneficial effect in some dogs as maintenance therapy. There are no therapeutic reference ranges for the dog. The maximum recommended daily dose is 2 mg q8hrs. Like most AEDs, the drug must be discontinued gradually to avoid withdrawal seizures.
7. The patient is discharged from the hospital after a 24-hour period without seizure.

PROGNOSIS

It is our experience that treatment failure in CS and SE is often related to delayed treatment. It is crucial that AED treatment be early and as aggressive as the patient can tolerate. In a study of dogs with CS or SE, a poor outcome was significantly associated with granulomatous meningoencephalitis, recurrence of seizures after 6 hours of hospitalization, and the development of partial SE.[3] In many large-breed dogs, epilepsy progresses to refractoriness and is more likely to be presented with severe CS or SE.

REFERENCES

1. Steffen F, Grasmueck S: Propofol for treatment of refractory seizures in dogs and a cat with intracranial disorders. *J Small Anim Pract* 41: 496, 2000.
2. Heldmann E, Holt DE, Brockman DJ, *et al:* Use of propofol to manage seizure activity after surgical treatment of portosystemic shunts. *J Small Anim Pract* 40:590, 1999.
3. Bateman SW, Parent JM: Clinical findings, treatment, and outcome of dogs with status epilepticus or cluster seizures: 156 cases (1990-1995). *J Am Vet Med Assoc* 215:1463, 1999.
4. Treiman DM: Generalized convulsive status epilepticus. *In* Engel JR and Pedley TA, eds.: Epilepsy, a comprehensive textbook. Philadelphia: Lippincott-Raven, 1998, p 669, 1317.
5. Simon RP: Physiologic consequences of status epilepticus. *Epilepsia*, 26 (suppl. 1), S58, 1985.
6. Plum F, Posner JB, Troy B: Cerebral metabolic and circulatory responses to induced convulsions in animals. *Arch Neurol* 18:1, 1968.
7. Shorvon SD: Status epilepticus: its clinical features and treatment in children and adults. Cambridge, England: Cambridge University Press, 1994, p. 139.
8. Berendt M, Gram L: Epilepsy and seizure classification in 63 dogs: a reappraisal of veterinary epilepsy terminology. *J Vet Intern Med* 13:14, 1999.
9. Blennow G, Brierley JB, Meldrum BS, Siesjö BK: Epileptic brain damage: the role of systemic factors that modify cerebral energy metabolism. *Brain* 101:687, 1978.
10. Heavner JE, Arthur J, Zou J: Comparison of propofol with thiopentone for treatment of bupivacaine induced seizures in rats. *Br J Anaesthesiology* 71:715, 1993.
11. Kusters AH, Vijn PC, Van den Brom WE *et al:* EEG-burst-suppression-controlled propofol anesthesia in the dog. *Vet Quarterly* 20:105, 1998.
12. KofkeWA, Snider MT, O'Connell BK *et al:* Isoflurane stops refractory seizures. *Anesthesiol Rev* 15:58, 1987.
13. Ramsay RE, Hammond EJ, Perchalski RJ, Wilder BJ: Brain uptake of phenytoin, phenobarbital and diazepam. *Arch Neurol* 36:535, 1979.
14. Boothe DM: Anticonvulsant therapy in small animals. *Vet Clin North Am* 28(2): 411, 1998.

63
Ocular Manifestations of Systemic Disease

Juliet R. Gionfriddo and Cynthia C. Powell

INTRODUCTION

A complete ocular examination should be done in all critically ill patients. A thorough ocular examination of the critically ill patient should include evaluation of both anterior and posterior segments. Magnification (a head loupe or biomicroscope) should be used to evaluate corneal, conjunctival, and scleral integrity and to look for aqueous flare or anterior chamber hemorrhage. Pupillary size and symmetry and pupillary light reflexes (both direct and indirect) must be evaluated in both bright and dim ambient light. Fluorescein dye and Schirmer tear testing should be done in all cases of suspected corneal pathology, and tonometry should be performed on all animals. A Tonopen applanation tonometer works well to measure intraocular pressures (IOPs). Indirect ophthalmoscopy is an efficient way to evaluate the fundus in these patients because it allows for a wider field of view and more rapid scanning of the fundus than direct ophthalmoscopy.

Fundic examination is particularly important in animals suspected of having neuropathies, vasculopathies, immune-mediated diseases, or infectious diseases, because these frequently have ocular manifestations.[1] In viewing the retinal blood vessels, the examiner directly visualizes the systemic vasculature and often can detect vascular problems before they appear systemically. The optic nerve head also should be evaluated carefully because it is a direct extension of the central nervous system and can be an early indicator of intracranial problems.

ASSESSMENT OF VISION

Vision loss may be due to ocular disease and brainstem or cerebral cortical disease. In some critically ill patients such as victims of head trauma, assessment of vision may be challenging. Depressed mentation may interfere with normal responses to visual stimuli. In other animals, positive responses to menacing gestures, the ability to track dropped cotton balls, and the ability to navigate a maze (in both bright and dim light) may help the clinician assess the visual status of the patient. It is important to realize that neither a positive pupillary light reflex (PLR) nor dazzle reflex indicates that the animal is visual. The absence of PLRs can be diagnostic for visual deficits when the loss results from lesions of the afferent arm (retina and optic nerve) of the visual pathway.[2] Testing of the dazzle reflex is accomplished by quickly shining a very bright light in one eye at a time. A normal response is a quick blink. Dazzle is a subcortical reflex; the method tests the integrity of the retina and optic nerve pathways but it does not assess the ability of the brain to "see" the light.[2]

Pupillary Abnormalities

Pupillary abnormalities are common after head trauma and acute brain injury.[2] Bilateral miosis indicates a severe cerebral, subcortical, or midbrain problem.[2,3] Progression from miosis to mydriasis in pupils that are unresponsive to light is indicative of advancing brain disturbance (usually a rising intracranial pressure) and accompanies severe contusion of the midbrain; return of pupils to normal size and responsiveness to light is a favorable prognostic sign.[2,3] Bilaterally dilated and unresponsive pupils or midrange-fixed pupils may indicate bilateral oculomotor nerve dysfunction and may be associated with hemorrhage due to basilar skull fractures.[3] These symptoms may indicate severe, irreversible nerve damage.[3]

Anisocoria in dogs and cats with pigmented irides is pathologic[4] and pupillary asymmetry may be seen in many conditions. Unilateral retinal, optic nerve, and optic tract lesions nearly always lead to mild anisocoria with the more dilated pupil in the affected eye.[4] In Horner's syndrome, the pupil in the affected eye is miotic and the difference between the size of the two pupils is more pronounced in dim light.[4] The presence of Horner's syndrome may indicate head, neck or chest trauma, or neoplasia or middle ear inflammation. Unilateral miosis also may be seen as a consequence of unilateral anterior uveitis.

Abnormalities of Ocular Position

Nystagmus is involuntary, rhythmic, ocular movement in response to head movement.[2] Physiologic nystagmus is induced by slowly moving the head from side to side or up and down. In cases of head trauma, the absence of physiologic nystagmus carries a grave prognosis for the animal, because it indicates severe brainstem injury.[4] Abnormal nystagmus (rhythmic ocular movement that does not correspond to head movement) in patients that are arousable indicates vestibular dysfunction and carries a more favorable prognosis.[4]

Strabismus (deviation of one or both eyes from center) in critically ill patients may be a sign of a brainstem injury or a space-occupying mass, particularly at the level of the medial longitudinal fasciculus (MLF).[2] The MLF interconnects the motor efferents of the nerves innervating the extraocular muscles and thereby it coordinates eye movements.[2]

Lesions of the oculomotor nerve(s) (cranial nerve III) alone may present as a lateral strabismus, whereas lesions of the abducens nerve(s) (cranial nerve VI) lead to medial strabismus. Involvement of all the nerves to the extraocular muscles may cause both external and internal ophthalmoplegia (immobile globe with a midrange, immobile pupil).

OCULAR TRAUMA

The symptoms for which animals with ocular trauma are presented depend on whether the trauma was blunt or sharp and on the severity of the trauma. Blunt trauma may lead to episcleral hemorrhage, hyphema, vitreal hemorrhage, retinal detachment, or proptosis. Emergency therapy for intraocular hemorrhage consists of frequent applications of topical atropine ophthalmic medications (unless IOPs are elevated), topical and systemic antibiotics, and topical or systemic anti-inflammatories. Steroids are the anti-inflammatories of choice unless they are contraindicated either topically (by a corneal ulcer) or systemically (by systemic infection or diabetes mellitus). In such cases, topical and oral nonsteroidal anti-inflammatories may be used.

Retinal detachments may be primary due to blunt trauma or secondary to retinal tears following penetrating trauma. An anti-inflammatory dose of systemic steroids is important therapy in the early stages of exudative retinal detachment.[5] Rapid referral to a veterinary vitreoretinal surgeon may be required to save vision in many cases.[6]

Proptosed globes should be replaced as soon as the patient is stable enough to undergo general anesthesia. The globe should be well lubricated until surgery can be performed. An excellent method of replacement of the globe is shown in Figure 63-1. Systemic anti-inflammatory therapy should be given after globe replacement to decrease swelling and possibly reduce optic nerve inflammation.

INFECTIOUS SYSTEMIC DISEASE

Uveitis is an important component of many infectious systemic diseases in domestic animals (Tables 63-1 and 63-2)[7] and anterior uveitis (iridocyclitis), posterior uveitis (chorioretinitis), or both may be the presenting complaints of these diseases.[1] Clinical signs of anterior uveitis include episcleral and conjunctival hyperemia, blepharospasm, epiphora, cloudy cornea, aqueous flare, and miosis. Animals with chorioretinitis may present with visual disturbances due to fundic abnormalities such as retinal detachments and subretinal debris.

Animals with ocular inflammation should receive aggressive ocular anti-inflammatory therapy. This therapy should include both topical and systemic anti-inflammatory drugs and mydriatics. Steroids should be administered topically unless contraindicated. Systemic, nonsteroidal anti-inflammatory drugs may be given, because in most infectious diseases systemic steroids are contraindicated. In addition, the pupils should be kept dilated with topical atropine ophthalmic medications to alleviate pain and prevent posterior synechiae. The prognosis is usually guarded in these cases but depends on the nature of the infection.

METABOLIC DISEASE

Diabetes Mellitus

In dogs presented for acute vision loss, diabetes mellitus should be considered among the differential diagnoses.[8,9] Vision loss in diabetes mellitus is due

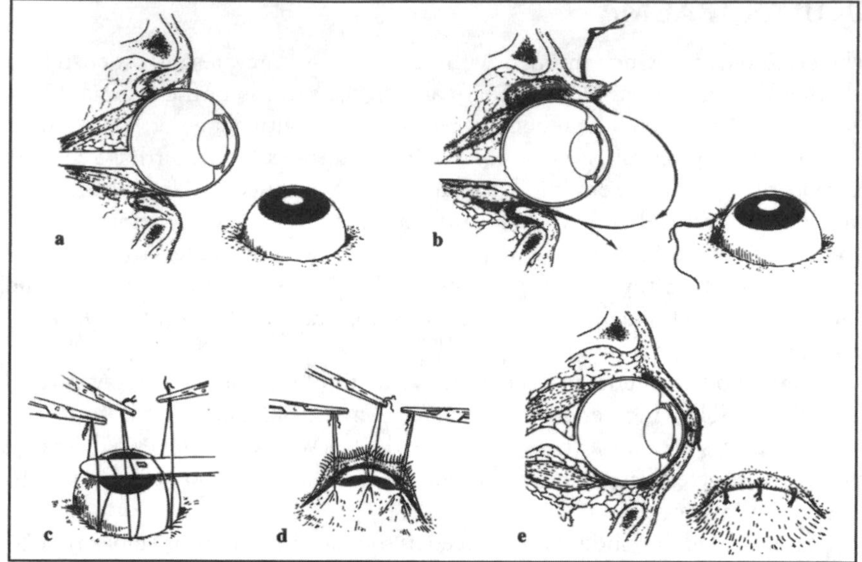

Figure 63-1
Replacement of prolapsed globe. (Reprinted with permission from Severin GA: Veterinary Ophthalmology, 3rd ed. Fort Collins, CO: GA Severin, 1995, p 492). A. Cross-sectional and lateral view of the prolapsed eye. B. Placing the first suture in the eyelid. The eyelid can be pulled away from the globe enough to place the suture. After the suture has been placed the eyelid returns to the edge of the globe. C. Three sutures have been placed. The globe is lubricated with ophthalmic ointment. A Bard-Parker handle is placed between the globe and the sutures. Tension on the sutures will simultaneously apply pressure to the globe and pull the eyelids around the eye. D. The eye is replaced and the sutures are ready for tying. E. The sutures are tied. Additional split-thickness tarsorrhaphy sutures may be placed if needed.

to the rapidly developing, bilaterally symmetrical cataracts that frequently are associated with this disease.[8,9] Cataract development in dogs with diabetes mellitus is attributed to the accumulation of sorbitol within the lens. This leads to increased lenticular osmolarity and consequent inflow of aqueous humor, which disrupts the lens fibers. In addition, biochemical changes occur that lead to altered electrolyte activity and to lens opacification.[9,10]

No available medical treatment reverses diabetic cataracts. In most cases, however, topical anti-inflammatory therapy (either steroidal or nonsteroidal) should be started immediately because, lenticular protein leak leads to lens-induced uveitis. Once uveitis is controlled and the patient's blood glucose is stabilized, the animal may be referred for cataract surgery.

Hypocalcemia

Low serum calcium levels may be due to puerperal tetany, ethylene glycol toxicity, dietary imbalances of calcium and phosphous, or hypoparathyroidism.[1,11,12] Characteristic focal to punctate linear cataracts in the anterior and

Table 63-1. Infectious Diseases Causing or Associated with Uveitis in the Dog

Algae
Prototheca spp.
Bacterial
Brucella canis
Borrelia burgdorferi
Leptospira spp.
Septicemia of any cause
Fungus
Blastomyces dermatitidis
Coccidiodes immits
Cryptococcus neoformans
Histoplasma *capsulatum*
Other mycoses
Parasites
Ophthalmomyiasis interna posterior
Ocular filariasis (*Dirofilaria immitis*)
Ocular larval migrans (*Toxocara* and *Balisascaris* spp.)
Protozoa
Leishmania donovani
Toxoplasma gondii
Rickettsial
Ehrlichia canis or *platys*
Rickettsia rickettsii
Virus
Adenovirus infection
Distemper virus
Herpesvirus
Rabies

Reprinted with permission from: Collins BK, Moore CP: Canine anterior uvea. *In* Gelatt KN, ed.: Veterinary Ophthalmology, 2nd ed. Philadelphia: Lea & Febiger, 1991, p 357.

posterior lens cortex are common ocular manifestations of hypocalcemia in the dog[1,11,12] (Fig. 63-2). The degree and duration of hypocalcemia required to produce these cataracts is unknown, but treatment of the underlying disorder and calcium supplementation will gradually stop the formation of new focal opacities.[1] The existing opacities will not disappear.[1]

Hyperadrenocorticism

Hyperadrenocorticism has been associated with ocular lesions consisting of progressive and nonhealing corneal ulcers that may be presented as emergencies.[1] In one study, 10 of 57 dogs affected with hyperadrenocorticism had unilateral corneal ulcers that were refractory to routine medical or surgical therapy.[13] The etiology of the ulcers was not determined, but the condition may have been due to a combination of retarded healing ability of the corneal epithelium and the presence of keratoconjunctivitis sicca (KCS) in many of the dogs.[13] In such cases, the corneal ulcer also should be treated aggressively with antibacterials, anticol-

Table 63-2. Infectious Diseases Causing or Associated with Uveitis in the Cat

Bacteria
Mycobacterium spp.
Septicemia
Fungus
Blastomyces dermatitidis
Candida albicans
Coccidiodes immits
Cryptococcus neoformans
Histoplasma capsulatum
Other mycoses
Parasite
Ophthalmomyiasis interna posterior
Ocular filariasis (*Dirofilaria immitis*)
Ocular larval migrans (*Toxocara* and *Balisascaris* spp.)
Protozoa
Leishmania donovani
Toxoplasma gondii
Virus
Feline immunodeficiency virus
Feline infectious peritonitis
Feline leukemia (due to its role in producing lymphosarcoma)
Rabies

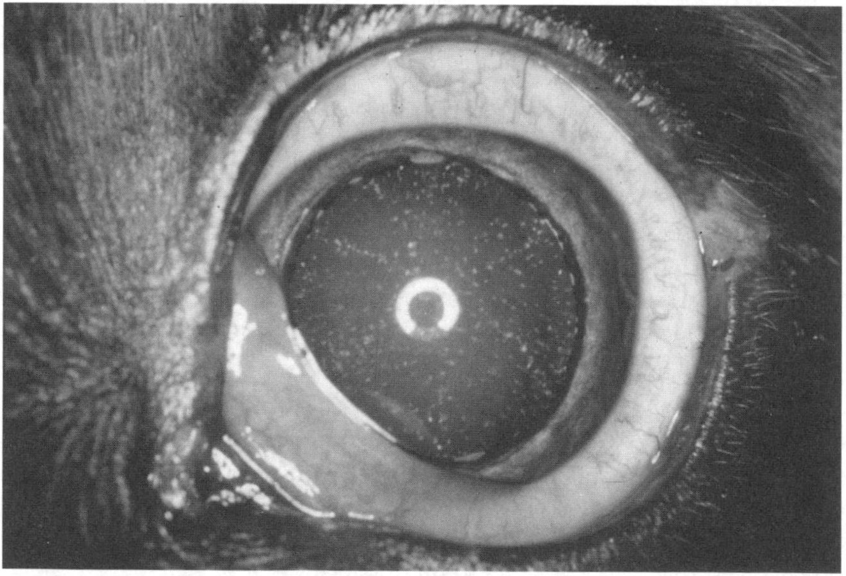

Figure 63-2
Characteristic cataract in a hypocalcemic puppy. The circular, bright area on the central cornea is flash artifact. (Courtesy of Dr. Charlie Martin, University of Georgia.)

lagenase drugs, artificial tears, and cyclosporine ophthalmic ointment (Optimmune). If the cornea is in imminent danger of rupturing, referral for surgical repair is indicated. In the KCS-affected dogs, tear production returned to normal after treatment of the systemic disease.[13]

BLOOD/VASCULAR DISORDERS

Hypertension

Hypertension is associated with renal disease, hyperadrenocorticism, pheochromocytoma, primary aldosteronism, hypothyroidism, and hyperthyroidism in dogs and cats.[15,16] Hypertensive dogs and cats often are brought to clinics as emergencies because these animals may have acute blindness secondary to retinal detachments or posterior segment hemorrhages.[14,15] Sustained elevations of blood pressure cause occlusion and ischemic necrosis of blood vessel walls, leading to serous exudation, hemorrhages, and edema.[15] Treatment of the cause of the hypertension, if known, is important to maintain the blood pressure within normal limits. Often, once the blood pressure is lowered, the retinas reattach and some vision is regained.[14-16] Specific ocular therapy is required if there is concurrent ocular inflammation or glaucoma.[14-16] Topical steroidal or nonsteroidal anti-inflammatory drugs are indicated in the presence of anterior uveitis. Systemic nonsteroidal or steroidal anti-inflammatory drugs may be used in cases of anterior and posterior uveitis. If the animal has refractory, secondary glaucoma and vision loss, enucleation, evisceration, or ciliary body ablation may be indicated to control pain.

Hyperviscosity Syndrome

Hyperviscosity syndrome is caused by elevated levels of immunoglobulins (usually IgM associated with polymerized IgA) in the bloodstream.[1] This syndrome usually is associated with neoplasia (most commonly multiple myeloma), but infectious disorders such as ehrlichiosis may also cause hyperviscosity.[17-19] Ocular pathology in hyperviscosity syndrome may include secondary glaucoma, retinal detachment, anterior uveitis, or retinal hemorrhage.[17] In some cases, however, the presenting complaint may be decreased vision or an abnormal-appearing eye.[17]

The prognosis for return of vision in dogs with retinal detachments due to blood hyperviscosity depends on the chronicity and severity of the underlying disease and the presence of anterior uveitis.[17] In one retrospective study, dogs without anterior uveitis or with medically controlled anterior uveitis regained vision even if their retinas had been detached for months.[17] Therefore, in addition to being treated for the primary disease, dogs presenting with anterior uveitis should be treated aggressively for the uveitis using topical steroids and atropine. For dogs that develop glaucoma secondary to anterior uveitis, the prognosis for return of vision is very poor.[17]

Thrombocytopenia

Animals with platelet counts below 50,000 cells/μL usually have ocular petechiae.[1] Hemorrhages often occur earlier in retinal blood vessels than in mucous membranes; thus the presence of retinal hemorrhages may be an early indicator of thrombocytopenia.[20] An acute loss of platelets is more likely to lead to ocular hemorrhages than a more chronic loss.[20] Therapy is directed at treating the underlying disease and includes transfusions of whole blood or platelet-rich plasma.[1]

Anemia

Severe anemia may lead to fundic changes including retinal hemorrhage, pale retinal vessels, and changes in tapetal reflectivity.[1] Hemorrhage is often seen when the hematocrit drops to 5% to 7% and may be secondary to hypoxia of the vessel walls.[1] Treatment for the anemia will lead to resolution of the hemorrhages, but pigmentation of the fundus may remain in the areas of previous hemorrhage.[1]

Polycythemia

Ophthalmic signs of polycythemia in dogs and cats include engorged and tortuous retinal blood vessels, retinal hemorrhages, and diffuse retinal detachment.[1,21-23] Therapy involves treating the primary cause, and if provided early, may prevent retinal detachments.[1]

Intravenous Fluid Overload

A syndrome of retinal detachment has been identified in animals that have compromised renal function and are being given intravenous fluids.[1] The syndrome begins with multiple, subretinal bullae of clear fluid that coalesce and enlarge to the point that they detach the retina.[1] There are no retinal hemorrhages and the animals are not hypertensive.[1] Decreasing the amount of fluid given or correcting the renal disease will allow the subretinal fluid to be reabsorbed and the retinas to reattach.[1]

Neoplasia

Both primary and metastatic neoplasia may involve the eye. Animals with primary ocular neoplasms may present to emergency clinics as cases of uveitis, intraocular hemorrhages, ocular masses, or vision loss. Primary ocular tumors reported in dogs include limbal (epibulbar) melanomas, anterior uveal melanomas, choroidal melanomas, ciliary body adenomas, carcinomas, medulloepitheliomas, and astrocytomas.[24] The most common secondary ocular neoplasm in dogs and cats is lymphoma, and ocular disease may be the presenting complaint in these cases.[24,25] Secondary glaucoma and keratitis have also been reported in dogs with lymphoma.[24] Numerous other types of malignant tumors (especially adenocarcinomas) are known to metastasize to the eye, and their clinical presentation is similar to those of lymphoma.[24]

SYSTEMIC TOXICITIES

In dogs, administration of **trimethoprim-sulfadiazine (TMS)** and other sulfa drugs (even given at therapeutic levels) may lead to decreased tear production and even to overt KCS.[26,27] Affected dogs may present to emergency clinics with an acute onset of ocular pain, squinting, and mucoid or purulent ocular discharge. Corneal ulcers, which could become infected and deepen, may also be present. Decreased tear production can occur as early as 2 to 3 days after the initiation of sulfonamide treatment, but the average duration of treatment before the onset of KCS usually is much longer (41–91 days).[26,27] Immediate discontinuation of TMS therapy is essential for the return of tear production. In many cases, topical treatment with cyclosporine ophthalmic ointment (a lacrimogenic drug) and a topical triple-antibiotic ophthalmic preparation is indicated. The prognosis is guarded because in some cases TMS may entirely destroy the lacrimal glands and thus there is no response to cyclosporine therapy.[26]

Overdoses of **ivermectin** can lead to blindness in the dog. Blindness usually occurs only in cases of gross overdosing (such as a dog being given oral preparations designed for large animals), but some breeds such as collies are very sensitive to the drug and may develop signs when given a canine therapeutic dose.[28] Other presenting clinical signs of ivermectin toxicity include ataxia, depression, mydriatic pupils, and muscle tremors; blindness may occur, without other neurologic signs.[1] Ophthalmoscopic signs include retinal edema with folds and papilledema.[1] Dogs with ivermectin-induced blindness generally recover vision within 2 to 10 days if given supportive therapy.[1,28,29]

Coumarin toxicity due to consumption of rodenticides may lead to ocular or orbital hemorrhages in many species.[1] Affected animals may present with exophthalmos (due to retrobulbar hemorrhage) and the diagnosis may be confused with that of a retrobulbar abscess or tumor.[1] Treatment of these cases should be directed at protecting the eye from exposure keratitis as well as treating the platelet abnormalities caused by the toxin.

Ethylene glycol toxicity has been reported to cause retinal detachment and blindness in a cat.[30] Toxicity was thought to have been due to crystalization of oxalates within the retina, but it may have been secondary to renal failure associated hypertension.[31]

REFERENCES

1. Martin CL: Ocular manifestations of systemic disease, the dog. *In* Gelatt KN, ed.: Veterinary Ophthalmology, 3rd ed. Philadelphia: Lippincott, Williams & Wilkins, 1999, p 1401.
2. Slatter D: Neuro-ophthalmology. *In* Fundamentals of Veterinary Ophthalmology. Philadelphia: WB Saunders, 1st Ed. 1990, p 437.
3. Mathews KA, Parent J: Head trauma. *In* Mathews KA, ed.: Veterinary Emergency and Critical Care Manual. Guelph, Ontario, Canada: Lifelearn, 1996, p 32.

4. Scagliotti RH: Comparative neuro-ophthalmology. *In* Gelatt KN, ed.: Veterinary Ophthalmology, 3rd ed. Philadelphia: Lippincott, Williams & Wilkins, 1999, p 1307.
5. Severin GA: Veterinary Ophthalmology, 3rd ed. Fort Collins, CO: GA Severin, 1995, p 492.
6. Smith PJ: Surgery of the canine posterior segment. *In* Gelatt KN, ed.: Veterinary Ophthalmology, 3rd ed. Philadelphia: Lippincott, Williams & Wilkins, 1999, p 935.
7. Collins BK, Moore CP: Canine anterior uvea. *In* Gelatt KN, ed.: Veterinary Ophthalmology, 2nd ed. Philadelphia: Lea & Febiger, 1991, p 357.
8. Wyman M, Sato S, Akagi Y, *et al.*: The dog as a model for ocular manifestations of high concentrations of blood sugars. *J Am Vet Med Assoc* 108:1153, 1988.
9. Davidson MG, Nelms SR: Diseases of the lens and cataract formation. *In* Gelatt KN, ed.: Veterinary Ophthalmology, 3rd ed. Philadelphia: Lippincott, Williams & Wilkins, 1999, p 797.
10. Sato S, Takahashi Y, Wyman M, *et al.*: Progression of sugar cataract in the dog. *Invest Ophthalmol Vis Sci* 32:1925, 1991.
11. Bruyette DS, Feldman EC: Primary hypoparathyroidism in the dog. *J Vet Intern Med* 2:7, 1988.
12. Kornegay JN, Greene CE, Martin C, *et al.*: Idiopathic hypocalcemia in four dogs. *J Am Anim Hosp Assoc* 16:723, 1980.
13. Lorenz MD: Diagnosis and medical management to canine Cushing's syndrome: a study of 57 consecutive cases. *J Am Anim Hosp Assoc* 18:707, 1982.
14. Bovee KC, Littman MP, Crabtree BJ: Essential hypertension in a dog. *J Am Vet Med Assoc* 195:81, 1989.
15. Paulsen ME, Allen TA, Jaenke RS, *et al.*: Arterial hypertension in two canine siblings: ocular and systemic manifestations. *J Am Anim Hosp Assoc* 25:287, 1989.
16. Ortega TM, Feldman ED, Nelson RW, *et al.*: Systemic arterial blood pressure and urine protein/creatinine ratio in dogs with hyperadrenocorticism. *J Am Vet Med* Assoc 209:1724, 1996.
17. Hendrix DV, Gelatt KN, Smith PJ, *et al.*: Ophthalmic disease as the presenting complaint in five dogs with multiple myeloma. *J Am Anim Hosp Assoc* 34:121, 1998.
18. Hoskins JD, Barta O, Rothschmitt J: Serum hyperviscosity syndrome associated with *Ehrlichia canis* infection in a dog. *J Am Vet Med Assoc* 183:1011, 1983.
19. Sansom J, Dunn JK: Ocular manifestations of a plasma cell myeloma. *J Small Anim Pract* 34:283, 1993.
20. Breitschwerdt EB: Infectious thrombocytopenia in dogs. *Compend Cont Ed Pract Vet* 10:1177, 1988.
21. Lombard CW, Twitchell M: Tetrology of Fallot, persistent left cranial vena cava, and retinal detachment in a cat. *J Am Anim Hosp Assoc* 14:624, 1978.
22. Crow SE, Allen DP, Murphy CJ *et al.*: Concurrent renal adenocarcinoma and polycythemia in a dog. *J Am Anim Hosp Assoc* 31:29, 1995.
23. Waters DJ, Prueter JC: Secondary polycythemia associated with renal disease in the dog: two case reports and review of the literature. *J Am Anim Hosp Assoc* 24:109, 1988.
24. Miller PE, Dubilzig RR: Ocular tumors. *In* Withrow S, MacEwen EG, eds.: Small Animal Clinical Oncology, 3rd ed. In press.
25. Krohne SG, Henderson NM, Richardson RC, *et al.*: Prevalence of ocular involvement in dogs with multicentric lymphoma: prospective evaluation of 94 cases. *Vet Comp Ophthalmol* 4:127, 1994.

26. Diehl KJ, Roberst SM: Keratoconjunctivitis sicca in dogs associated with sulfonamine therapy: 16 cases (1980–1990). *Prog Vet Comp Ophthalmol* 1:276, 1991.
27. Morgan RV, Bachrach A: Keratoconjunctivitis sicca associated with sulphonamide therapy in dogs. *J Am Vet Med Assoc* 180:432, 1982.
28. Hopkins KD, Marcella KL, Strecker AE: Ivermectin toxicosis in a dog. *J Am Vet Med Assoc* 197:93, 1990.
29. Houston DM, Parent J, Matushek KJ: Ivermectin toxicosis in a dog. *J Am Vet Med Assoc* 191:78, 1987.
30. Barclay SM, Riis RC: Retinal detachment and reattachment associated with ethylene glycol intoxication in a cat. *J Am Anim Hosp Assoc* 15: 719, 1979.
31. Stiles J: Ocular manifestations of systemic disease. The cat. *In* Gelatt KN, ed.: Veterinary Ophthalmology, 3rd ed. Philadelphia: Lippincott, Williams & Wilkins, 1999, p 1448.

64
Myasthenia Gravis

Curtis W. Dewey

INTRODUCTION

Myasthenia gravis (MG) is an autoimmune neuromuscular junction disorder in which antibodies are produced against nicotinic acetylcholine (ACh) receptors of skeletal muscle. The resulting impairment of neuromuscular transmission is clinically manifested as muscle weakness.[1,2] MG is a relatively common immune-mediated disease in dogs, but is infrequently diagnosed in cats. In both species, the variety of clinical forms in which the disease presents can pose a diagnostic challenge to the clinician. In addition to a high index of suspicion, knowledge of the clinical aspects of acquired MG is beneficial to timely diagnosis and therapy.

Abundant information exists concerning the pathophysiology, epidemiology, and diagnosis of MG. However, few clinical data address therapeutic efficacy and overall disease prognosis in dogs. Clinical information regarding acquired MG in cats is even less complete; the incidence of MG appears to be lower and typically less severe, compared with dogs.[1,3-8] Accordingly, most of the information in this chapter focuses on canine MG, with occasional references made to the feline disorder. This chapter reviews the salient clinical features of acquired MG and focuses on aspects of treatment and prognosis.

PATHOGENESIS

The underlying abnormality in MG is a lack of functional ACh receptors at the end-plate regions of skeletal muscle. A heterogeneous group of autoantibodies, primarily of the IgG class, are produced by B lymphocytes, following antigen processing and presentation by macrophages to helper T lymphocytes. The autoantibodies primarily target an extracellular region of the ACh receptor, referred to as the main immunogenic region. Proposed mechanisms for autoantibody impairment of neuromuscular transmission include accelerated endocytosis of antibody cross-linked ACh receptors, complement-mediated destruction of postsynaptic muscle cell membrane adjacent to ACh receptors, decreased synthesis and incorporation of new ACh receptors, and direct interference with ACh receptor function by bound antibody. The decreased number of functional ACh receptors increases the chance of failed neuromuscular junction impulse transmission. Although the thymus is believed to play an integral role in the initiation of the autoimmune response to ACh receptors, the factors responsible for triggering the autoimmune process remain a mystery.[1,2]

EPIDEMIOLOGY

Dog breeds commonly associated with MG include golden retrievers, Labrador retrievers, and German shepherds.[1] Although these breeds may appear overrepresented in disease incidence, their popularity accounts for much of the apparent association with MG. Akitas and terriers appear to have a high breed predilection for developing MG.[5] There have been several reports suggesting a predilection for Abyssinian and Somali cat breeds.[6-8] The existence of breed predilections for canine and feline MG supports the contention that genetic factors play a role in the disease pathogenesis. There is a bimodal age distribution in dogs and cats, with peaks at approximately 3 and 10 years of age. Both males and females are equally likely to develop acquired MG.[1,6] Sexually intact dogs may be slightly less likely to develop MG than spayed and neutered dogs.[5]

CLINICAL PRESENTATION

Common historical complaints offered by owners of myasthenic dogs and cats include swallowing difficulty, vomiting/regurgitation, hypersalivation, coughing, labored breathing, and limb muscle weakness. Owners often report that their dog is vomiting; eliciting a detailed description of the "vomiting" events usually reveals them to be episodes of regurgitation. A history of a "voice change," or change in the quality of the bark or meow, is occasionally elicited from the owner. Some unique features of myasthenic cats that occasionally occur include a dropped jaw and ventroflexion of the neck.[1,6,7]

The concept of a "classic" clinical presentation of the myasthenic patient should be abandoned in light of the recent description of multiple clinical forms of the disease (Table 64-1). The clinical forms of MG have been divided into focal, generalized, and acute fulminating categories.[1,6,9,11] Patients with focal MG exhibit no clinical evidence of appendicular muscle weakness, and typically exhibit clinical signs associated with dysfunction of "bulbar" musculature (*i.e.*, pharyngeal, esophageal, facial, laryngeal muscles). Generalized myasthenics display appendicular muscle weakness, usually in combination with weakness of "bulbar" muscles. Dogs and

Table 64-1. Clinical Forms of Acquired Myasthenia Gravis (MG) in Dogs and Cats

Focal MG—no clinical signs of appendicular weakness
- ➢ Megaesophagus alone
- ➢ Pharyngeal weakness, laryngeal weakness, facial muscle (*e.g.,* blink reflex) weakness, with or without megaesophagus

Generalized MG—clinical signs of appendicular weakness
- ➢ With (usually) or without focal ("bulbar") signs
- ➢ Predominantly/exclusively pelvic limb weakness
- ➢ Approximately equal weakness in thoracic versus pelvic limbs

Acute Fulminating MG—rapid onset and progression of severe weakness
- ➢ Profound "bulbar" and appendicular weakness
- ➢ Acute onset, rapid progression to nonambulatory tetraparesis and respiratory distress
- ➢ Usually fatal

cats that exhibit acute onset and rapid development of severe weakness (typically recumbent with respiratory embarrassment within 72 hours of onset) are designated as having acute fulminating MG. In one study, 36% of the dogs had focal MG, 48% had generalized MG, and 16% had acute fulminating MG.[9] Clinical forms of MG appear to be distributed differently in cats. Focal MG appears to account for only 15% of cases, with the remainder exhibiting appendicular muscle weakness.[6-8] Dogs with generalized MG tend to display predominantly pelvic limb weakness; this peculiarity has not been reported in cats.[1,6-8,9] Acute fulminating MG appears to comprise approximately 15% of feline MG cases.[6,7]

DIAGNOSIS

Essential to a prompt MG diagnosis are a knowledge of the different clinical disease forms and a high index of suspicion. In addition to historical and clinical evidence suggestive of MG, the clinician has available an array of tests that may help confirm the diagnosis. All patients suspected of having MG should have basic blood studies (complete blood count, chemistry profile) and a urinalysis performed. Because of the association between canine MG and hypothyroidism, a resting serum thyroxine (T_4) level should also be obtained in suspect dogs.[1,12] Hypothyroidism in cats is extremely rare. However, evidence suggests that methimazole treatment for hyperthyroid cats is related to the development of MG.[8,13]

Thoracic radiographs are recommended to document megaesophagus, aspiration pneumonia, and mediastinal masses (*i.e.*, thymoma). Megaesophagus is present in over 80% of canine cases (Fig. 64-1).[9] Myasthenic cats are less likely

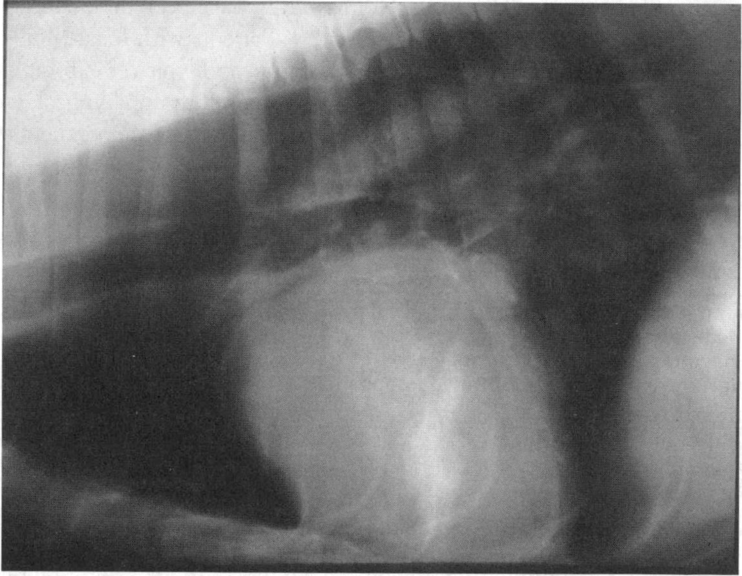

Figure 64-1
Lateral thoracic radiograph of a myasthenic dog with megaesophagus.

to exhibit megaesophagus (about 40%), presumably due to the small proportion of skeletal muscle in the feline esophagus.[6-8] Myasthenic dogs administered barium frequently develop severe aspiration pneumonia shortly following the procedure. In patients with historical/clinical evidence of pharyngeal/esophageal dysfunction, especially with radiographically evident megaesophagus, the author considers barium esophagrams to be contraindicated. Recently, scintigraphy has been used to evaluate esophageal function in myasthenic dogs (Bahr and coworkers, unpublished data). This procedure is safe, easily performed, and provides objective information regarding esophageal function (Fig. 64-2).[1,14]

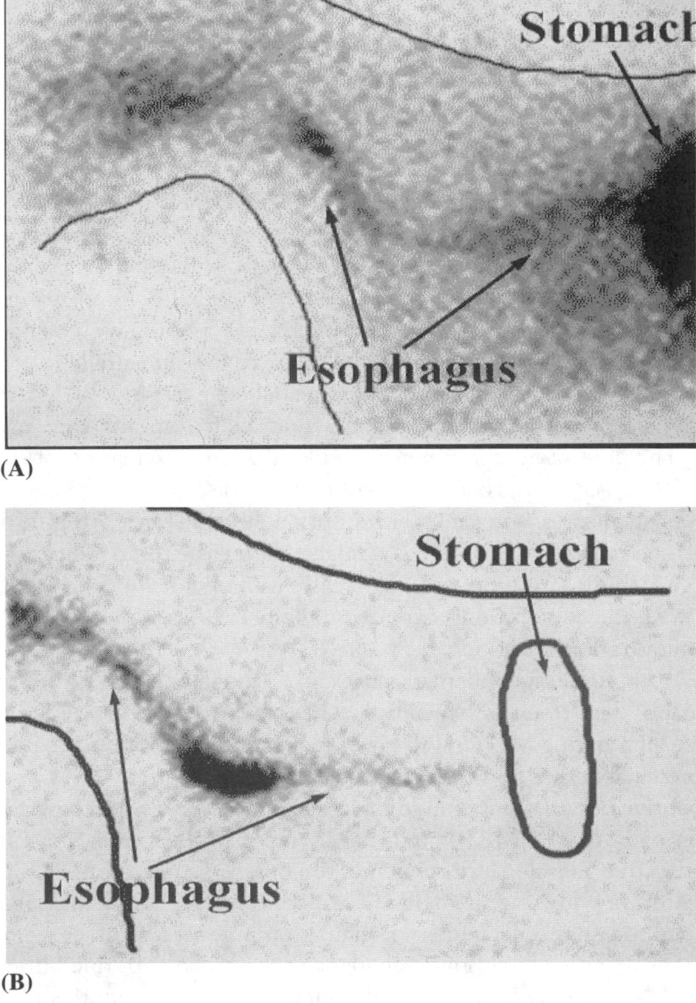

Figure 64-2
Esophageal scintigraphy in a normal (**A**) and myasthenic (**B**) dog. (Courtesy of Dr. Anne Bahr.)

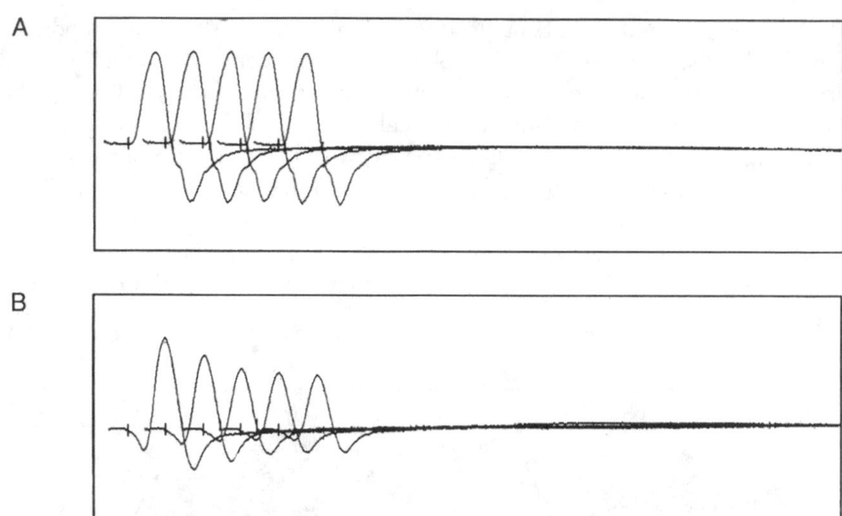

Figure 64-3
Repetitive nerve stimulation. The decremental response shown in (B) supports an MG diagnosis. (Reprinted with permission.[1])

Tests that support the MG diagnosis include edrophonium challenge (tensilon response) test, repetitive nerve stimulation (RNS), and single-fiber electromyography (SF-EMG).[1,2,7] The edrophonium challenge test involves intravenous administration of edrophonium, and observation for an increase in muscle strength. The dose of edrophonium chloride is 0.1 to 0.2 mg/kg for dogs, and 0.25 to 0.50 mg *per cat*.[1,7] To avoid a cholinergic crisis from this drug, the author routinely premedicates with a muscarinic anticholinergic (*e.g.*, atropine or glycopyrrolate) and has one of these drugs available during the test. Due to the subjective nature of this test, it is most useful in cases with obvious appendicular muscle weakness. An unequivocal improvement in ambulatory function after edrophonium administration constitutes a "positive" test result. Although an obviously "positive" edrophonium challenge test result is clinically useful, a "negative" or "questionable" test result is typically not helpful in ruling out MG.[1,7] Patients with acute fulminating MG tend to have "negative" edrophonium challenge test results, presumably due to a lack of available ACh receptors.

Repetitive nerve stimulation involves measuring successive compound muscle action potentials (CMAPs) induced by repetitively stimulating the nerve that supplies that muscle. A decremental response (>10%) is highly supportive of a diagnosis of MG (Fig. 64-3).[1,6,7,9] On occasion, the author has observed a decremental response to facial nerve stimulation in focal MG cases when a limb RNS is normal. The edrophonium challenge test can be performed in conjunction with RNS; normalization of a decremental response after edrophonium chloride administration is interpreted as a "positive" result.[9] SF-EMG is thought

Table 64-2. Treatment Options for Canine and Feline MG

Anticholinesterase Drugs
- Pyridostigmine
- Neostigmine

Immunosuppressive Drugs
- Prednisone
- Azathioprine (dogs)
- Cyclosporine
- Mycophenolate mofetil (dogs)

Thymectomy
- Thymic hyperplasia (not evaluated in dogs and cats)
- Thymoma (not until MG signs controlled)

Nutritional Support
- Elevated feedings
- Gastrostomy tube feedings

Other Therapies
- Plasmapheresis
- Intravenous immunoglobulin
- Immunoadsorption therapy

to be a very specific electrodiagnostic test for human MG. Although successful modification of this test for veterinary use has been demonstrated in normal dogs, no clinical information is yet available for its use in canine or feline MG patients.[1,2,15]

The most specific test for canine and feline MG is an immunoprecipitation radioimmunoassay (RIA), which quantitates serum antibodies directed against the ACh receptor. ACh receptor antibody concentration exceeding 0.6 nM/L for dogs and 0.3 nM/L for cats (the upper limit for "background" or nonspecific binding) is considered diagnostic for MG; false-positive results are rare.[1,4,7,8] Although serum ACh receptor antibody concentrations tend to be lower in focal MG compared to other forms, there is not a consistent relationship between antibody concentration and disease severity among patients. Sequential ACh receptor antibody concentrations measured in an *individual* patient, however, appear to correlate with disease progression/regression.[1,6,7] If a dog or cat is highly suspected to be myasthenic, but has a negative RIA result, one or more of the supplemental diagnostic tests (*e.g.*, edrophonium response test, RNS) should be considered.

TREATMENT

Considering the array of clinical manifestations of acquired MG in dogs and cats, multiple treatment options are available for these patients (Table 64-2). In general, treatment needs to be individualized for the specific myasthenic patient.[3] It is the author's opinion that the majority of myasthenic patients will require immunosuppressive therapy at some point during their treatment regimen, to obtain and maintain adequate control of the disease.

Anticholinesterase Drugs

Anticholinesterase therapy comprises the cornerstone of MG treatment in dogs and cats.[2,3,6,7] Anticholinesterase therapy is most effective in improving ambulatory function in generalized myasthenics. Anticholinesterase drugs have less efficacy in improving esophageal function compared to limb function.[3] It is important to know that cats are more sensitive to anticholinesterase drugs compared to dogs.[7] Anticholinesterase agents prolong the action of ACh at the neuromuscular junction by reversibly inhibiting acetylcholinesterase. Pyridostigmine is the most commonly used anticholinesterase drug. It is administered by mouth or stomach tube at a dosage of 0.5 to 3.0 mg/kg, q 8 to 12 h in dogs and 0.25 mg/kg, q 8 to 12 h in cats. The clinician should start at the low end of the dose and increase as needed (to avoid a cholinergic crisis).[3,7] The response to pyridostigmine is variable and may reflect the availability of ACh receptors in a given patient.[3]

In dogs that are unable to take oral medications (*i.e.*, frequent regurgitation) and do not have a gastrostomy tube in place, injectable neostigmine may be intramuscularly administered (0.04 mg/kg q 6 h).[3] There is no pharmacokinetic information available for the use of neostigmine in cats.

It must be kept in mind that anticholinesterase drugs have no effect on the immune response against the ACh receptors.[3,10]

Immunosuppressive Drugs

Immunosuppressive therapy remains controversial in canine MG due to the susceptibility of myasthenic dogs to develop aspiration pneumonia, which is the main reason for death or euthanasia.[3,9] Immunosuppressive doses of prednisone (2-4 mg/kg/d) may have an adverse effect on neuromuscular transmission in dogs. This effect increases in clinical importance with increasing MG severity.[3,9,16] Adverse effect of glucocorticoids on neuromuscular transmission does not appear to be a major clinical problem in cats.[6,7] In general, immunosuppressive therapy should not be instituted until aspiration pneumonia has been ruled out or resolved. A commitment to close patient follow-up must always accompany the decision to immunosuppress a myasthenic patient.[3]

Prednisone is administered at anti-inflammatory doses (*e.g.*, 0.5 mg/kg, q 12-24 h), gradually building to immunosuppressive levels over 10 to 14 days.[3,16] Persistence of esophageal, pharyngeal, or laryngeal dysfunction because of an unattenuated autoimmune response may also place a patient with MG at constant risk of developing life-threatening aspiration pneumonia. Aspiration pneumonia appears to be a relatively infrequent complication of MG in cats; it has been documented in only 20% of feline MG cases.[6]

Azathioprine (AZA) has demonstrated efficacy in the treatment of human MG, either as an adjunct to prednisone or as a sole immunosuppressive agent.[2,17] AZA use was associated with a positive clinical response and a decrease in ACh receptor antibody concentration (81% reduction) in 4 of 5 dogs in a recent report. Subsequent experience with AZA as a sole immunosuppressive therapy for canine acquired MG has been encouraging. Although AZA appears to be an effective immunosuppressive drug for canine MG, there is a lag time of several weeks from onset of therapy to appreciable clinical effect.[10] Therefore, AZA may not be an optimal drug choice in the severely affected or rapidly worsening dog with MG. AZA is well tolerated in dogs, but patients must be monitored for potential side effect. Side effects of AZA therapy typically resolve with dose reduction or temporary discontinuation of the drug. Cats are more susceptible to severe and potentially irreversible bone marrow suppression from AZA; this drug should be avoided in feline patients.[7,18]

Cyclosporine (Neoral, Novartis Pharmaceuticals) is a lymphocyte-specific immunosuppressive drug that interferes with T-cell activation and proliferation via inhibition of interleukin-2 (IL-2) activity. Cyclosporine appears to be an effective immunosuppressive agent in the treatment of human MG.[2,19] No clinical information is available concerning the use of this drug for canine and feline acquired MG, other than a brief mention of one myasthenic cat that was successfully treated with cyclosporine.[6] Cyclosporine is well tolerated by both cats and dogs and has been used successfully as an immunosuppressive drug for other autoimmune conditions as well as an antirejection agent following renal transplantation.[20] The recommended immunosuppressive dose of cyclosporine (Neoral) in dogs and cats is 2.5 to 5.0 mg/kg, q 12 h, and 0.5 to 2.5 mg/kg, q 12 h, respectively.[20] Cyclosporine may become an attractive immunosuppressive drug choice for canine and feline acquired MG, due to its rapid onset of immunosuppressive activity, lymphocyte specificity, and low incidence of side effects. Unlike humans, dogs and cats do not develop nephrotoxicity or hepatotoxicity from cyclosporine administration.[20]

Mycophenolate mofetil, [(MMF) CellCept, Roche Pharmaceuticals], is currently under investigation as a potential treatment for canine MG.[21] The active compound, mycophenolate (MPA), inhibits the action of inosine monophosphate dehydrogenase (IMPDH), an enzyme necessary for the de novo pathway of guanosine triphosphate (GTP) synthesis. Lack of GTP availability impairs the ability of lymphocytes to synthesize DNA, RNA, proteins, and glycoproteins.[21,22] A dose (oral or through a gastrostomy tube) of 20 mg/kg, q 12 h is currently recommended, based on the available literature and limited case experience. The onset of action of the drug is rapid and appears to exert a clinical benefit within the first week of therapy.

Gastrointestinal side effects (anorexia, vomiting, diarrhea) represent a potential drawback to MMF use, but these side effects tend to resolve with dose reduction or temporary discontinuation of the drug.[21,22] There is considerable variability in the pharmacokinetics of this drug among dogs, when administered orally, and there may also be some level of enterohepatic recirculation of drug.[21,23] Because this drug is eliminated via hepatic glucuronidation and subsequent renal excretion, its use in cats should be avoided until information regarding safety in this species becomes available.

Thymectomy

Thymectomy is an important therapeutic option in human MG. Beneficial effects of thymectomy are most apparent in cases of thymic hyperplasia. Thymoma removal does not consistently improve the myasthenic condition in human beings; in fact, clinical signs of MG occasionally worsen following thymoma removal in people. The main goal of thymoma removal, or thymomectomy, is to remove a neoplastic mass from the thoracic cavity, and not primarily to improve control of MG.[2,3,24,25]

The importance of thymic hyperplasia in canine and feline acquired MG remains to be investigated. Radiographic evidence of thymoma is occasionally found in middle-aged to older myasthenic dogs and cats.[16] In a recent study, radiographic evidence of a mediastinal mass was apparent in only 3.4% of dogs with MG.[5] In contrast, two recent studies of feline MG reported incidences of mediastinal masses of 15% and approximately 26%, respectively.[6,8] In the majority of reported cases concerning thymoma removal in myasthenic dogs, the patients died from aspiration pneumonia in the immediate postoperative period.[3,26] Unless a suspected thymoma is posing an imminent threat to a patient's health, thymoma removal should be avoided in myasthenic dogs until the clinical signs of acquired MG are adequately controlled.

Nutritional Support

Nutritional support (*e.g.*, elevated feeding, stomach tube) should be tailored to the needs of the individual myasthenic patient. Some dogs will do well with elevated feedings. In many cases, however, myasthenic dogs will continue to regurgitate frequently, despite properly performed elevated feedings. Some owners may also have difficulty in consistently feeding their dog in an elevated position. The author frequently advocates placing gastrostomy tubes in myasthenic dogs. The advantages of a gastrostomy tube are numerous, and include ease of administering both caloric and water requirements, improved drug delivery (less likely for drugs to linger in the dilated esophagus or be regurgitated), and decreased risk of aspiration pneumonia. The short anesthetic period required to place a gastrostomy tube appears to be generally well tolerated by most myasthenic patients.[3,16]

Other Therapies

Acute fulminating MG is usually rapidly fatal, despite therapy.[3,6,7,9,11] Plasmapheresis and intravenous immunoglobulin (IVIG) administration are effective short-term treatments in people with acute fulminating MG. Temporary improvement afforded by these modes of therapy provides time for maintenance immunosuppressive therapy (*e.g.*, prednisone, AZA) to take effect. Plasmapheresis and IVIG have been suggested as potential therapies for canine acute fulminating MG. Unfortunately, the expense and equipment requirements associated with these therapies will likely limit their use in canine MG.[3,27,28] Immunoadsorption therapy is a form of plasmapheresis in which the patient's plasma is returned after being passed through a filter that adsorbs IgG. This therapy has recently exhibited efficacy in human acquired MG.[29]

Prognosis

The prognosis is guarded for dogs with acquired MG. In one report, the 1-year mortality rate for canine MG was approximately 60%. Aspiration pneumonia with or without respiratory failure (acute fulminating myasthenics) was the cause of death or euthanasia in all cases.[9] In another study, 10 of the 25 dogs for which follow-up information was available had died or had been euthanized due to pneumonia.[30] The key to successful treatment of the canine myasthenic appears to be prevention or prompt resolution of aspiration pneumonia. Intimately linked to controlling pneumonia in myasthenic dogs is resolution of esophageal, pharyngeal, and laryngeal weakness.[3,16] Although spontaneous clinical remission does occasionally occur in myasthenic dogs with no therapy or with "symptomatic" therapy (pyridostigmine) alone, it does not appear to be a common occurrence. Spontaneous clinical remission of MG is most likely to occur in young dogs without severe pharyngeal/esophageal dysfunction. Waiting for spontaneous clinical remission to occur for extended periods of time may place the patient at continued risk for development of aspiration pneumonia. The clinician should not be lulled into a false sense of security if a generalized canine myasthenic responds favorably in terms of ambulatory function shortly after institution of anticholinesterase therapy. Although some dogs will remain well controlled on pyridostigmine alone, many others will demonstrate a transient improvement in limb muscle function, and subsequently succumb to pneumonia.

Although the use of immunosuppressive therapy in canine acquired MG poses inherent risks, cautious use of such therapy is likely to improve survival in many cases. Since the original report of five MG dogs treated with AZA, data from a number of additional cases have been accumulated. Although the information is preliminary at present, the 1-year mortality rate for canine MG patients treated with AZA appears to be in the vicinity of 20%. The efficacy/inefficacy of other immunosuppressive agents, such as cyclosporine and MMF, remain to be investigated as treatment options for canine MG.

Information concerning long-term prognosis for feline MG is lacking; however, the information available suggests a favorable prognosis in cats treated with a combination of pyridostigmine and glucocorticoids. The favorable prognosis in cats with acquired MG is thought to be due, in large part, to the low incidence of megaesophagus and aspiration pneumonia in feline MG, as compared with the canine condition.[6,7]

With improved early recognition and increased availability of effective treatment options, it is likely that the prognosis of MG in dogs will improve in the future.

REFERENCES

1. Dewey CW: Acquired myasthenia gravis in dogs—part I. *Compend Contin Educ Pract Vet* 19:1340, 1997.
2. Massey JM: Acquired myasthenia gravis. *Neurol Clin* 15:577, 1997.
3. Dewey CW: Acquired myasthenia gravis in dogs—part II. *Compend Contin Educ Pract Vet* 20:47, 1998.
4. Shelton GD, Cardinet GH, Lindstrom JM: Canine and human myasthenia gravis autoantibodies recognize similar regions on the acetylcholine receptor. *Neurology* 38:1417, 1988.
5. Shelton GD, Schule A, Kass PH: Risk factors for acquired myasthenia gravis in dogs: 1,154 cases (1991–1995) *J Am Vet Med Assoc* 211:1428, 1997.
6. Ducotè JM, Dewey CW, Coates JR: Clinical forms of acquired myasthenia gravis in cats. *Compend Contin Educ Pract Vet* 21:440, 1999.
7. Ducotè JM, Dewey CW: Clinical forms of acquired myasthenia gravis and other disorders of the neuromuscular junction. *In* August JR, ed.: Consultations in Feline Internal Medicine, 4th ed. Philadelphia: WB Saunders, 374–380 2001.
8. Shelton GD, Ho M, Kass PH: Risk factors for acquired myasthenia gravis in cats: 105 cases (1986–1998) *J Am Vet Med Assoc* 216:55, 2000
9. Dewey CW, Bailey CS, Shelton GD, *et al.*: Clinical forms of acquired myasthenia gravis in dogs: 25 cases (1988–1995) *J Vet Intern Med* 11:50, 1997.
10. Dewey CW, Coates JR, Ducoté JM, *et al.*: Azathioprine therapy for acquired myasthenia gravis in five dogs. *J Am Anim Hosp Assoc* 35:396, 1999.
11. King LG, Vite CH: Acute fulminating myasthenia gravis in five dogs. *J Am Vet Med Assoc* 212: 830, 1998.
12. Dewey CW, Shelton GD, Bailey CS, *et al.*: Neuromuscular dysfunction in five dogs with acquired myasthenia gravis and presumptive hypothyroidism. *Prog Vet Neurol* 6:117, 1995.
13. Shelton GD, Joseph R, Richter K, *et al.*: Acquired myasthenia gravis in hyperthyroid cats on tapazole therapy [abstract]. *J Vet Intern Med* 11:120, 1997.
14. Mears EA, Jenkins CC: Canine and feline megaesophagus. *Compend Contin Educ Pract Vet* 19:313, 1997.
15. Hopkins AL, Howard JF, Wheeler SJ, *et al.*: Stimulated single-fibre electromyography in normal dogs. *J Small Anim Pract* 34:271, 1993.
16. Dewey CW: Acquired myasthenia gravis in dogs: a clinical perspective. Proceedings of the 17th ACVIM Forum, 1999, 272.
17. Cosi V, Lombardi M, Erbetta A, *et al.*: Azathioprine as a single immunosuppressive drug in the treatment of myasthenia gravis. *Acta Neurol* 15:123, 1993.
18. Rhodes KH: Feline immunomodulators. *In* Bonagura, ed: Kirk's Current Veterinary Therapy XII: Small Animal Practice. Philadelphia, WB Saunders, 1995, p 58.
19. Bonifati DM, Angelini C: Long-term cyclosporine treatment in a group of severe myasthenia gravis patients. *J Neurol* 244:542, 1997.
20. Gregory CR: Immunosuppressive agents. *In* Bonagura JD, ed: Kirk's Current Veterinary Therapy XIII: Small Animal Practice. Philadelphia, WB Saunders, 2000, p 509.
21. Dewey CW, Boothe DM, Rinn KL, *et al.*: Treatment of a myasthenic dog with mycophenolate mofetil. *J Vet Emerg Crit Care* 10:19, 2000.
22. Hood KA, Zarembski DG: Mycophenolate mofetil: a unique immunosuppressive agent. *Am J Health Syst Pharm* 54:285, 1997.

23. Langman LJ, Shapiro AMJ, Lakey JRT, *et al.*: Pharmacodynamic assessment of mycophenolic acid-induced immunosuppression by measurement of inosine monophosphate dehydrogenase activity in a canine model. *Transplantation* 61:87, 1996.
24. Nieto IP, Robledo JPP, Pajuelo MC, *et al.*: Prognostic factors for myasthenia gravis treated by thymectomy: review of 61 cases. *Ann Thorac Surg* 67:1568, 1999.
25. Onoda K, Namikawa S. Takao M, *et al.*: Fulminant myasthenia gravis manifested after removal of an anterior mediastinal tumor. *Ann Thorac Surg* 62:1534, 1996.
26. Atwater SW, Powers BE, Park RD: Thymoma in dogs: 23 cases (1980–1991). *J Am Vet Med* Assoc 205:1007, 1994.
27. Keesey J, Buffkin D, Keba D, *et al.*: Plasma exchange alone as therapy for myasthenia gravis. *Am N Y Acad Sci* 377:729, 1981.
28. Arsura E: Experience with intravenous immunogloblin in myasthenia gravis. *Clin Immunol Immunopathol* 53:5170, 1989.
29. Benny WB, Sutton DMC, Oger J, *et al.*: Clinical evaluation of a staphylococcal protein A immunoadsorption system in the treatment of myasthenia gravis patients. *Transfusion* 39:682, 1999.
30. Bartges JW. Hansen D, Hardy RM: Outcome of 30 cases of acquired myasthenia gravis in dogs (1982–1992) [abstract]. *J Vet Intern Med* 11:144, 1997.

SECTION X
Trauma

65
Abdominal Trauma

Joseph Harari

INTRODUCTION

Abdominal trauma is classified as a blunt or penetrating injury. Common causes include vehicular accidents, firearm injuries, falls, and fights“[1,2] (Table 65-1). Less frequently reported are lesions from inhumane acts or assaults by people. All abdominal structures, as well as supportive musculoskeletal elements, are prone to injury[3] (Table 65-2). Signalment and clinical signs of affected patients are variable, and treatments and prognosis are case dependent. Most, if not all, surgical candidates require thorough preoperative examination, diagnostic evaluations, and medical treatments. Conversely, not all medically managed patients undergo surgery. Sequelae to abdominal trauma involve multiple organ systems (Table 65-3).

Table 65-1. Cause of Abdominal Trauma in Urban Dogs and Cats

Injury	Dog	Cat
Vehicular	13	5
Weapons	33	B
Fights	10	22
Falls	2	19
Burns	36	B
Abuse	10	B

Adapted from Kolata RJ, Kraut NH: Patterns of trauma in urban dogs and cats: a study of 1,000 cases. *J Am Vet Med Assoc* 164:499, 1974.

Table 65-2. Abdominal Injuries of 600 Dogs Injured in Motor Vehicle Accidents

Injured Organ	Number of Dogs
Liver	13
Urinary bladder	9
Diaphragm	9
Kidney	5
Spleen	2
Gastrointestinal	2
Prostate-urethra	1

Adapted ftom Kolata RJ, Johnston DE: Motor vehicle accidents in urban dogs: a study of 600 cases. *J Am Vet Med Assoc* 167:938, 1975.

Table 65-3. Sequelae to Abdominal Trauma

Hernia (abdominal wall, diaphragm)
Visceral contusion, laceration, penetration, rupture, avulsion
Muscular wall contusion, laceration, necrosis, defects
Abdominal effusion(s), pneumoperitoneum
Peritonitis

PATHOGENESIS

Blunt trauma produces crushing, stretching, and shearing forces secondary to changes in speed and deformation of tissue.[4,5] Abdominal injuries result as a consequence of viscera accelerating at a disproportionate rate compared to attachment. Kidneys, intestines, and spleen are vulnerable to shear force injuries. With deceleration, the liver may continue to travel relative to its ligamentous attachments and generates a shear strain that causes transection or laceration of the hepatic parenchyma. Additionally, tearing of mesenteric attachments and vascular elements results in traumatic intra-abdominal hemorrhage. Direct deformation of viscera such as pancreas, liver, spleen, and kidneys can also occur as organs are compressed between the point of impact and vertebrae. Direct compression of the abdomen increases intra-abdominal pressure producing rupture of the diaphragm or hollow organs. Direct high-impact (blunt or penetrating) blows will also destroy the integrity of the supporting abdominal wall musculature (Fig. 65-1).

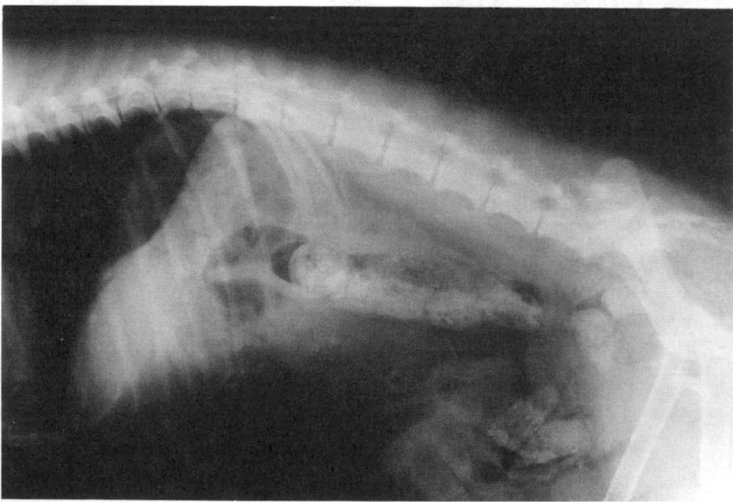

Figure 65-1
Ventral abdominal wall herniation of intestines secondary to vehicular trauma in a dog.

Penetrating injuries involve the transfer of energy to a small tissue area. The velocity of the wound is higher than blunt trauma and varies from low-energy stab wounds to medium/high-velocity gunshot injuries.[5] The energy of the causative agent disrupts and fragments cells and tissues, moving them away from the point of impact. The size of the wound depends on the profile and tumble of the pointed missile and tissue fragmentation. Low-velocity projectiles crush and lacerate tissues. High-velocity missiles also create shock waves that damage tissues away from the missile path and create subatmospheric cavities that suck in external contaminants at exit and entry wounds.[6]

EPIDEMIOLOGY

Age, gender, and breed distribution of animals suffering from abdominal trauma generally reflect regional hospital admission statistics.[4,5] High-rise falls of dogs and cats in New York City have produced surprisingly low rates (15%) of abdominal injury compared to extremity, head, and thoracic lesions.[7,8] Abdominal injuries associated with pelvic trauma (vehicular accidents) have been described, although exact frequencies of injuries are difficult to ascertain.[9]

CLINICAL PRESENTATION

Abnormal clinical findings are variable and may not be evident during the initial presentation. External wounds, bruising, subcutaneous swellings, caudal musculoskeletal, and neurologic injuries are suggestive of abdominal trauma. Umbilical discoloration and detection of a fluid wave (succussion) during abdominal ballottement are characteristics of hemoperitoneum. Clipping of the hair and abdominal palpation confirm abnormal findings not apparent on initial cursory examination. Signs of internal derangement are based on involved organ systems: respiratory distress (diaphragmatic hernia), distended/painful abdomen (hemoabdomen, uroabdomen, bile peritonitis, ruptured bowel), hematuria/anuria (bladder rupture), fever/depression/lethargy (ruptured viscus), and vomiting/hematochezia (gastroenteropathy). Some lesions such as chronic diaphragmatic hernias, autotransplantations of splenic tissue, and periabdominal pellets can be incidental findings long after initial internal injury.

DIAGNOSTIC EVALUATIONS

Four-quadrant abdominocentesis or diagnostic peritoneal lavage are preferred procedures for rapid diagnostic evaluation. Examination of samples for cytology, packed cell volume (PCV), bilirubin, and blood urea nitrogen (BUN) or creatinine are useful diagnostic tests to evaluate intra-abdominal lesions of the liver, biliary tract, spleen, intestines, kidneys, ureter, urinary bladders, and urethra.[9] Paracentesis with catheters and lavage doubles the accuracy (>90%) of simple needle paracentesis, although concern for dilution of postlavage samples has been described.[9,10] With elevations of PCV, amylase, bilirubin, BUN, or creatinine higher than a peripheral blood sample, internal injury should be suspected.

Enteric contents or toxic neutrophils should not be present in evaluation of normal abdominal fluid.

Most imaging studies are based on survey (including serial) or contrast (air, dye) studies; computed tomography and magnetic resonance imaging may prove useful in large clinical centers. Abnormal imaging findings include loss of detail (retroperitoneal space), effusions, unexplained mass effects, abdominal air, loss of body wall integrity, grossly displaced viscera, identification of foreign objects, fractures, and luxations.

TREATMENT

Indications for a surgical celiotomy (diagnostic and therapeutic) or laparoscopy include: (1) progressive abdominal distention or discomfort; (2) progressive hemoabdomen; (3) peritonitis associated with urine, bile and feces; (4) abdominal origin sepsis; (5) progressive patient deterioration with undetermined cause(s); (6) delayed abnormal signs (icterus, respiratory distress, dysuria, vomiting) in a previously injured patient; (7) life-threatening organ dysfunction and (8) body wall defects.

Perioperative medical management of fluid, acid–base, and electrolyte abnormalities is critical. Prophylactic (or therapeutic for known wounds) antibiotic medications should include broad-spectrum antimicrobials such as cephalosporins (cefoxitin), fluoroquinolones (enrofloxacin), potentiated sulfanamides (trimethoprim-sulfadiazine), lincosamides (clindamycin), or nitro-imidazoles (metronidazole).[11] Useful anesthetic regimens include induction or premedications with ketamine/diazepam, oxymorphone/diazepam, low (titrating) doses of propofol, thiopental, and maintenance with isoflurane. Intraoperative epidural lidocaine infusion or preoperative narcotic epidural is recommended to reduce anesthetic and postoperative analgesic requirements.[12] Positive inotropic agents such as dopamine or dobutamine can be used intraoperatively in hypotensive, anuric patients. Postoperative nutritional requirements should be maintained with parenteral or enterostomy (distal to the lesion) support to enhance patient recovery.

Principles for traumatic abdominal surgery include generous exposure and thorough examination of all visceral structures, isolation of affected tissues, lavage with warm isotonic fluids, closure with noncontaminated instruments, and use of synthetic, absorbable monofilament or nonabsorbable sutures (polydioxanone, polypropylene). Surgical treatments are based on the location and severity of the abdominal injuries. Options include hemiorrhaphy, intestinal resection and anastomosis, partial hepatectomy, splenectomy, cholecystectomy or biliary diversion, nephrectomy, ureter/urethral anastomosis, urinary bladder repairs, and open or closed peritoneal drainage. Abdominal wall defects are reconstructed with synthetic meshes, omentum, or muscular flaps.[13]

Circumferential abdominal wrapping has been used in animals with an experimentally created hemoabdomen to limit blood loss and support arterial pressure, and is recommended for patients without diaphragmatic injuries.[4,14] Intra-abdominal hemorrhage may not be controlled by bandage counterpressure and visceral organ blood flow may be deleteriously affected by longterm wrapping.[15]

PROGNOSIS

Recovery is based on the nature of the lesion(s) and the timing and types of medical/surgical interventions. In studies of feline and canine high-rise syndromes, surprisingly, only 10% of cats and 1 of 81 dogs died from their injuries.[7,8] A survival rate of 57% has been documented for patients with hemoperitoneum (severe) requiring blood transfusion and treated medically or surgically.[16] A survival rate of nearly to 80% was reported for open peritoneal drainage for peritonitis associated with naturally traumatic and surgically related abdominal injuries.[17]

REFERENCES

1. Archibald J, Holt JC, Sokolovsky V: Management of Trauma in Dogs and Cats. Santa Barbara, CA: American Veterinary Publications, 1981, 229.
2. Kolata RJ, Kraut NH: Patterns of trauma in urban dogs and cats: a study of 1,000 cases. *J Am Vet Med Assoc* 164:499, 1974.
3. Kolata RJ, Johnston DE: Motor vehicle accidents in urban dogs: a study of 600 cases. *J Am Vet Med Assoc* 167:938, 1975.
4. Wingfield WE: Veterinary Emergency Medicine Secrets. Philadelphia: Hanley & Belfus, 1997, 81.
5. Hoyt DB: Trauma. *In* Greenfield LJ, ed.: Surgery-Scientific Principles and Practice. Philadelphia: JB Lippincott, 1993, p 245.
6. Bebchuk TN, Harari J: Gunshot injuries: pathophysiology and treatments. *Vet Clin North Am Small Anim Pract* 25:1111, 1995.
7. Gordon LE, Thacher C: High-rise syndrome in dogs: 81 cases (1985–1991). *J Am Vet Med Assoc* 202:118, 1993.
8. Whitney WO, Mehlhaff CJ: High-rise syndrome in cats. *J Am Vet Med Assoc* 1987: 191, 1403.
9. Verstraete FJM, Lambrecht NE: Diagnosis of soft tissue injuries associated with pelvic fractures. *Compend Contin Educ Pract Vet* 14:921, 1992.
10. Crowe DT: Diagnostic abdominal paracentesis techniques: clinical evaluation in 129 dogs and cats. *J Am Anim Hosp Assoc* 20:223, 1984.
11. Fossurn TW: Small Animal Surgery. St. Louis: Mosby, 1997, 195.
12. Tranquilli WJ, Benson GJ: Essentials of Small Animal Anesthesia and Analgesia. Philadelphia: Lippincott Williams & Wilkins, 1999, 52.
13. Smeak DD: Abdominal hernias. *In* Slatter D, ed.: Textbook of Small Animal Surgery, 2nd ed. Philadelphia: WB Saunders, 1993, p 433.
14. McAnulty JF, Smith GK: Circumferential external counterpressure by abdominal wrapping and its effect on simulated intra-abdominal hemorrhage. *Vet Surg* 15:270, 1986.
15. Brockman DJ, Mongil CM: Practical approach to hemoperitoneum in the dog and cat. *Vet Clin North Am Small Anim Pract* 30:657, 2000.
16. Mongil CM, Drobatz KJ: Traumatic hemoperitoneum in 28 cases. *J Am Anim Hosp Assoc* 31:217,1995.
17. Greenfield CL, Walshaw R: Open peritoneal drainage for treatment of contaminated peritoneal cavity in dogs and cats. *J Am Vet Med Assoc* 191:100, 1987.

66
Brain Trauma

Curtis W. Dewey

INTRODUCTION

Severe brain injury is associated with a high mortality rate in humans and animals. Death typically results from progressive increases in intracranial pressure (ICP). Brain injury in dogs and cats is most often due to automobile trauma; other causes include missile injuries (*e.g.*, gunshot wounds), animal bites, and falls.[1-3] There is considerable controversy concerning therapy and this field is one of intense research in human neurology/neurosurgery. Little retrospective or prospective clinical data pertain to the treatment of canine and feline brain injury; most of the clinical recommendations in this chapter are based on information from human studies and investigations of experimental brain injury. What constitutes appropriate therapy for the severely brain-injured pet is debatable, but few would argue that treatment needs to be expedient and aggressive if the animal is to survive. The first veterinarian the brain-injured pet encounters after the traumatic incident will likely dictate the eventual outcome for that patient. It is of utmost importance to alleviate brain swelling and prevent damage to vital brainstem structures. Dogs and cats can function well with considerable loss of cerebral tissue, if given time to recover from a severe brain insult.[4] The ultimate goal in brain injury management is to return the patient to the role in society occupied before the injury.

PATHOPHYSIOLOGY OF BRAIN INJURY

Brain injury can be conceptually divided into primary and secondary injury (Table 66-1). Primary brain injury occurs immediately following impact and initiates multiple inflammatory cascades that result in secondary brain injury. Both primary and secondary brain injury contribute to increased ICP.[1-3,5] A basic understanding of the mechanisms of brain tissue damage following injury and ICP dynamics is essential to logical therapy of the severely brain-injured patient.

Primary Brain Injury

This category of injury refers to the physical disruption of intracranial structures that occurs immediately at the time of the traumatic event. Such injury includes direct damage to brain parenchyma, such as contusions, lacerations, and diffuse axonal injury. Damage to blood vessels may result in intracranial

Table 66-1. Primary and Secondary Processes Associated with Brain Injury in Dogs and Cats

Primary Brain Injury
- Direct damage to brain parenchyma
- Direct damage to blood vessels

Secondary Brain Injury
- ATP depletion
- Intracellular accumulation of Na^+ and Ca^{++}
- Increased cytokine production
- Elevated extracellular glutamate
- Oxygen free radical production
- Lactic acidosis
- Nitric oxide accumulation
- Arachidonic acid, kinin, complement, coagulation/fibrinolytic pathway activation

hemorrhage and vasogenic edema. The extent of primary brain injury is a function of the force of impact. Acceleratory and deceleratory forces of both the impacting object(s) and the intracranial contents will affect overall tissue damage. Direct parenchymal damage associated with primary brain injury is beyond the control of the clinician.[1-3,5]

Secondary Brain Injury

Damage caused by the primary brain injury activates a number of interrelated biochemical pathways that act to perpetuate further brain tissue damage and ICP elevation. Adenosine triphosphate (ATP) depletion disrupts cellular ionic homeostasis. Sudden, uncontrolled intracellular influx of sodium (Na^+) and calcium (Ca^{++}) occurs. Cellular swelling (cytotoxic edema) and depolarization result. Uncontrolled depolarization leads to large amounts of glutamate, an excitatory neurotransmitter, to be released into the extracellular environment.[1-3,6,7] Glutamate causes further increase in intracellular Ca^{++} levels. Elevated intracellular Ca^{++} levels activate a number of tissue-damaging pathways, including the arachidonic acid cascade (phospholipase A_2 activation) and the xanthine oxidase (free-radical producing) pathway. Free radical species (*e.g.*, hydroxyl and superoxide radicals) preferentially damage cell membranes containing high levels of polyunsaturated fatty acids (PUFAs) and cholesterol. Iron (Fe^{++}) is a vital cofactor in the xanthine oxidase pathway. Brain tissue is rich in both Fe^{++} and membranes with high levels of PUFAs and cholesterol. Free-radical species are thus particularly damaging to neuronal membranes and probably play a major role in secondary brain injury. Their production is also induced by ischemia, arachidonic acid metabolites, catecholamine oxidation, and activated neutrophils.[1-3,6,7] Other secondary autolytic processes include complement, kinin, and coagulation/fibrinolytic cascades. Tissue damage mediators produced by these various reactions perpetuate their continued production as well as the production of other mediators. Maintenance of an ischemic environment perpetuates tissue-damaging processes and leads to the accumulation of lactic acid (via anaerobic glycolysis). Accumulation of lactic acid leads to further brain tissue damage. Hypotension and hypoxemia can worsen brain ischemia and thereby enhance the biochemical processes responsible for secondary brain injury. The end result of these secondary processes is increased ICP. Unlike primary brain injury, the clinician has some control over secondary brain injury.[1-3,6,7]

ICP DYNAMICS

Intracranial pressure is the pressure exerted by tissues and fluids within the cranial vault. Normal ICP values for dogs and cats range between 5 and 12 mm Hg.[8,9] Cerebral perfusion pressure (CPP) is the principal determinant of cerebral blood flow and hence brain oxygenation and nutritional support. CPP is defined by the following equation:

$$\text{CPP} = \text{MABP} - \text{ICP}$$

where MABP is mean arterial blood pressure.

The normal contents of the cranial cavity include brain parenchyma, blood, and cerebrospinal fluid (CSF). In the normal animal, these components exist in equilibrium with each other and ICP remains within normal limits. Between the MABP extremes of 50 and 150 mm Hg, ICP remains constant. This phenomenon is called *pressure autoregulation*. Pressure autoregulation serves to link systemic blood pressure changes to brain vasculature tone. If MABP rises, vasoconstriction occurs; if MABP falls, vasodilation occurs. In the normal animal, vasoconstriction prevents ICP from rising, and vasodilation prevents ICP from falling. *Chemical autoregulation* refers to the direct responsiveness of cerebral vasculature to $PaCO_2$; elevated $PaCO_2$ levels cause vasodilation, and decreased $PaCO_2$ levels cause vasoconstriction. Both pressure and chemical autoregulation often remain intact in people with severe brain injury; pressure autoregulation may be lost in approximately 30% of patients.[1,3,9-11]

Intracranial hemorrhage and edema can add to intracranial volume. Due to the nonexpansile nature of the skull, one or more cranial cavity components must accommodate the increased volume, or increased ICP will result. This accommodation or volume buffering is accomplished by fluid shifts in the brain vasculature and CSF pathways and is referred to as *intracranial compliance*. Compliance is expressed as the change in volume per unit change in pressure. Intracranial compliance has limitations and decreases as ICP increases. If intracranial volume increases beyond the abilities of compensatory mechanisms, progressively larger increases in ICP result per unit of volume increase, CPP is compromised, and ischemic death of brain tissue occurs. In cases of severe brain injury, intracranial compliance often is quickly exhausted. If MABP decreases (hypotension), the brain vasculature will vasodilate in an effort to preserve blood flow. The increase in blood volume increases ICP, but CPP remains inadequate. In addition, the secondary autolytic processes occurring in the injured brain are enhanced by hypotension and hypoxemia, and further brain injury and edema occur with a resultant rise in ICP.[1,9,10,12-14]

INITIAL ASSESSMENT AND EMERGENCY TREATMENT

Initial evaluation and management of the severely brain-injured patient focuses on correcting life-threatening abnormalities. The clinician must first focus on the ABCs of trauma management (airway, breathing, cardiovascular status). In doing so, the brain will benefit as well as the rest of the patient. Quick assessment tests, including packed cell volume, total solids, blood urea nitrogen, and blood glucose are an important part of the initial patient assessment. Many patients suffering severe brain injury present to the clinician in a state of hypovolemic shock. The clinician should not be in a rush to focus initially on the patient's neurologic status; it may well improve once the shock state is corrected. Remember that traumatized, hypovolemic patients with no appreciable brain injury often exhibit depressed mentation, due primarily to the hypotensive state. Because hypovolemia and hypoxemia are strongly correlated with elevated ICP and increased mortality in human brain injury victims, these two conditions need to be addressed immediately.[1,10,11,15,16]

Fluid Therapy

There is often concern that aggressive intravenous (IV) fluid therapy in the brain-injured patient may increase cerebral edema. Because of this concern, there have been recommendations to volume limit victims of severe brain injury. Such recommendations are not only unfounded, but *strictly contraindicated*. There is no debate over the disastrous consequences to the injured brain if hypotension is allowed to persist. Hypotension has been repeatedly shown to be a reliable predictor of sustained elevations of ICP and increased mortality in brain-injured humans. Blood pressure must be restored to normal levels as soon as possible. A brain-injured person with a systolic blood pressure less than 90 mm Hg is considered hypotensive.[1,10,11,15,16]

Certain volume replacement fluids (hetastarch, hypertonic saline) afford some protection to the edematous brain, even when used in combination with large volumes of crystalloids (lactated Ringer's solution [LRS], 0.9% NaCl). Hetastarch and hypertonic saline can improve MABP and thus CPP without exacerbating brain edema. If the patient is anemic, whole blood or packed red blood cell transfusion may assist in maintaining normovolemia as well as adequate tissue oxygenation. Fluid support may include one or more of the following choices:

- Hetastarch: 10 to 20 mL/kg to effect (up to 30 mL/kg/day) for shock. This can be given as a rapid bolus in dogs; give it in 5-mL/kg increments over 5 to 10 minutes in cats. Hetastarch is the author's fluid of choice in restoring normal blood pressure in the brain-injured victim.[1,15,16-18]
- Hypertonic saline (7%): 4 to 5 mL/kg over 3 to 5 minutes for shock. Although hypertonic saline has been shown to improve MABP and CPP and protect against increased ICP, sodium has recently been implicated as the major osmotic agent contributing to brain edema. Hypertonic saline may have a global protective effect on the brain, but theoretically may lead to increased compromise to focal areas of damaged parenchyma.[1,2,10,15,16,19]

- Dextran 70: 10 to 20 mL/kg (up to 30 mL/kg/day) for shock in dogs. Cats should be administered dextran 70 as 5-mL/kg boluses, given over 5 to 10 minutes, with a maximum of 20 mL/kg. Dextran 70, given as a sole fluid support, has not exhibited beneficial effects demonstrated with hetastarch and hypertonic saline. Therefore, dextran 70 should be considered as an adjunctive fluid therapy choice.[1,15,17,18,20]
- Crystalloids (LRS, 0.9% saline): 90 mL/kg/h (dogs), 60 mL/kg/h (cats) for shock. The "shock dose" of crystalloids should be given to effect, because overhydration producing cerebral edema and increased ICP is a concern during crystalloid administration, If the entire volume is not necessary to restore euvolemia and normal MABP, the fluid administration rate should be tapered when core physiologic goals are met.[1,16]
- Blood products: 4 to 10 mL/kg/h (typically over 4-6 hours) in the stable patient, faster (to effect) if the patient is unstable. Goals of therapy with blood products are a PCV between 25% and 30%, and a plasma albumin level over 2.0 g/dL.[1,17,18]

Oxygenation and Hyperventilation

Hyperoxygenation is recommended for the majority of acutely brain-injured animals. Oxygen status of a severely brain-injured patient can be initially assessed based on breathing rate and pattern, mucous membrane and tongue color, and thoracic auscultation. Pneumothorax and pulmonary contusions are common sequelae of trauma, and need to be addressed, if present. If arterial blood gas analysis is available, the PaO_2 should be maintained at or above 85 mm Hg. Pulse oximeters are extremely useful and relatively accurate estimators of oxygenation status. However, the reliability of pulse oximeters varies with model used and with the PaO_2 level (pulse oximeters may overestimate oxygenation status at lower PaO_2 levels). In general, oxyhemoglobin saturation values (SaO_2) from pulse oximeters should be interpreted as shown in Table 66-2.[1,15,16,21-24]

Patients who are conscious and not obviously deteriorating neurologically should be administered supplemental oxygen (O_2) via face mask, nasal O_2 catheter, or transtracheal O_2 catheter. An O_2 cage is generally ineffective in administering supplemental O_2 to the severely brain-injured patient because such cages do not allow for close patient observation (requires opening the cage door) and maintenance of a high O_2 environment. An inspired O_2 concentration of 40% is provided with flow rates of 100 mL/kg/min and 50 mL/kg/min, respectively, with nasal and transtracheal O_2 catheters. Concentrations of O_2 up to 95% can be delivered with

Table 66-2. Interpretation of Pulse Oximeter Values

SaO_2	PaO_2	Interpretations
>95%	>80%	Normal
<89%	<60%	Serious hypoxemia
<75%	<40%	Lethal hypoxemia

higher flow rates. Nasal O_2 catheters must not be placed farther than the level of the medial canthus (to avoid entering the cranial vault through a fracture site). Inadvertent jugular vein compression should be avoided while during placement of a transtracheal O_2 catheter. Patients who are losing or have lost consciousness should be intubated and ventilated. In the patient with oscillating levels of consciousness, a tracheostomy tube may be indicated for assisted ventilation.[1,15]

Arterial blood gas measurement is the best way to monitor $PaCO_2$ levels. End-tidal CO_2 measurement is a useful monitoring tool, but tends to underestimate the true $PaCO_2$ levels. Ventilatory rates of 10 to 20 breaths per minute should keep $PaCO_2$ levels between 25 and 35 mm Hg. Although this has been the recommended range of $PaCO_2$ levels to prevent excessive brain vasodilation, recent evidence suggests the $PaCO_2$ less than 30 mm Hg may lead to excessive vasoconstriction, with impairment of CPP.[1-3,10,11]

Hyperventilation may be deleterious to patients whose ICP elevation is not due to hypercarbia-induced dilation of brain vasculature. Indiscriminate use of hyperventilation to decrease ICP should be avoided, because excessive vasoconstriction of brain vasculature can decrease CPP.[10,16,25]

SECONDARY ASSESSMENT AND DIAGNOSTIC PROCEDURES

Once normovolemia is restored and oxygenation/ventilation are stabilized, the patient should be carefully assessed for other nervous system injuries (*e.g.*, vertebral fractures/luxations), as well as to other body systems (lungs, abdominal organs, musculoskeletal system). A complete neurologic examination should be performed at this time. Specific medical therapy for brain injury should concomitantly begin with the secondary assessment. Additional blood studies as well as radiographs may be warranted.[10,15]

Imaging of the patient's head is often indicated, especially in animals that fail to respond to aggressive medical therapy or deteriorate after responding to such therapy. Skull radiographs are unlikely to reveal clinically useful information in cases of severe brain injury, but on occasion may reveal evidence of depressed fractures of the calvaria. Computed tomography (CT) is the preferred modality for imaging the head in cases of severe brain injury. CT is preferred over magnetic resonance imaging (MRI) in brain injury cases. CT scans are obtained much more quickly than MRI results (an important advantage in the critical patient scenario), CT is considerably less expensive than MRI, and acute hemorrhage and bone are better visualized with CT than with MRI.[3,10,15]

SPECIFIC MEDICAL THERAPY FOR THE BRAIN-INJURED PATIENT

In addition to fluid and O_2 therapy, a number of medical therapies are recommended for the brain-injured victim. Most of these are controversial and not definitively proven to affect outcome. In addition to these treatments, proper physical therapy and nutritional support are vital to a positive outcome. In the recumbent patient, the head should be kept slightly elevated (15°–30°) to assist in lowering ICP.[8,13,15]

Mannitol (20%–25%)

Once the brain injury victim is hemodynamically stable, mannitol should be considered first-line therapy for decreasing ICP and improving CPP.[1,3,10,15,16,26-29] Mannitol is administered IV over 10–20 minutes at a dosage of 0.5 to 1.0 g/kg. Mannitol is an osmotic diuretic that has demonstrated efficacy in reducing brain edema and ICP in cases of severe brain injury. There are several proposed mechanisms of action by which mannitol decreases ICP, including reflex vasoconstriction of brain vasculature secondary to decreased blood viscosity, reduction of CSF production, scavenging free-radical species, and osmotic transfer of extravascular edema fluid into the intravascular space. The mechanism thought to be primarily responsible for mannitol's most immediate effects on ICP is reflex vasoconstriction. This response is linked to the brain's pressure autoregulation mechanism; it allows for improved CPP at a lower brain blood volume (decreased ICP). The effect of reflex vasoconstriction on ICP occurs within a few minutes, whereas the osmotic action requires 15 to 30 minutes to occur. The effect of mannitol on decreasing brain edema lasts between 2 and 5 hours.

Serum osmolality and electrolytes should be monitored with repeated mannitol use; osmolality should be maintained at or below 320 mOsm/L (to prevent renal failure) and electrolytes should be kept within normal limits. A useful guideline to prevent unwanted side effects after mannitol use is to limit mannitol administration to 3 boluses in a 24-hour period. Because mannitol tends to crystallize at room temperature, it should be warmed to approximately 37°C (99°F) and administered through an in-line filter. Administration of furosemide (2–5 mg/kg) a few minutes before mannitol administration may be synergistic in reducing ICP.[1,3,9,10,15,16,26,27]

A frequently raised concern of mannitol administration is exacerbating hemorrhage due to the osmotic action of mannitol. This concern is unfounded clinically and should be ignored. Another concern of mannitol use in the head trauma victim involves the concept of "reverse osmotic shift." The result of this phenomenon is increased brain edema. With appropriate mannitol use, "reverse osmotic shift" is extremely unlikely to occur.

Glucocorticoids

Despite their traditional role in the treatment of central nervous system trauma, little evidence supports the use of glucocorticoids in victims of severe brain injury.[1,9,1015,16,30] "Standard" dosing protocols of prednisone and dexamethasone are unlikely to benefit brain-injured patients. "High-dose" methylprednisolone therapy should be considered as adjunctive treatment in those patients not responding adequately to appropriate resuscitative (fluid and O_2 therapy) measures and mannitol administration for those who are not hyperglycemic.[1] This protocol involves the IV administration of a 30 mg/kg bolus of methylprednisolone sodium succinate (Solu-Medrol) at time 0, and 15-mg/kg boluses at 2 and

6 hours. These boluses should be given over several minutes. A continuous IV infusion of 2.5 mg/kg/h may then be instituted, depending on the patient's response. Limited evidence of efficacy exists for the "high-dose methylprednisolone" protocol in severe brain injury. The "high-dose" protocol is thought to provide therapeutic benefit via free-radical scavenging action, rather than by activation of steroid receptors.[1,3,9,15,16,30,31]

Because large doses of glucocorticoids can exacerbate hyperglycemia, a blood glucose level should be checked before administering the "high-dose" protocol. Hyperglycemia (>200 mg/dL) has been associated with increased mortality in severely brain-injured people. It is postulated that the provision of extra glucose to the ischemic brain helps to fuel anaerobic glycolysis, which increases brain lactic acid. The increased lactic acid levels cause further brain damage.[11,16,20]

Miscellaneous Therapies

Induction of a barbiturate coma with pentobarbital has been suggested as a "last ditch" effort to decrease metabolic demands of the injured brain, thereby mitigating effects of ischemia and decreasing ICP. In addition to limited evidence of clinical efficacy, induction of a barbiturate coma in a brain-injured patient may be detrimental to survival. Barbiturates may lead to hypotension and/or hypoventilation, both of which will cause increased ICP.[9,10,15,16]

Recent experimental and clinical evidence in human brain-injured patients supports the induction of moderate hypothermia (32°–34°C [89.6°–93.2°F]) as a means to decrease ICP and improve outcome. Although traditionally thought to decrease ICP via decreasing brain metabolic demands, induced hypothermia is now thought to provide beneficial results mainly by inhibiting release of inflammatory cytokines and glutamate.[9,32-34]

Lazaroids, or 21-aminosteroids, are analogs of methylprednisolone that do not activate glucocorticoid receptors. These agents theoretically provide therapeutic free-radical scavenging activity without producing undesirable steroid receptor-mediated side effects. In addition to lazaroids, a number of free-radical scavenging agents have been investigated for potential use in severe brain injury. Examples include dimethylsulfoxide, allopurinol, deferoxamine mesylate, and liposome-encapsulated forms of superoxide dismutase and catalase. Despite experimental evidence of efficacy for these drugs, clinical evidence to support the use of these agents in the brain-injured victim is currently lacking. Similarly, there exists some experimental, yet not clinical, evidence of efficacy for antagonists of opiate and glutamate receptors, as well as several calcium channel blockers.[1,15]

INDICATIONS FOR SURGERY

Surgical intervention should be strongly considered in brain-injured dogs and cats that are deteriorating neurologically despite aggressive medical therapy. Indications for surgical intervention are well defined in the management of human patients with brain injury. The guidelines for when to pursue surgery in brain-injured people center on the presence and extent of intracranial hemorrhage. Measurements of focal hemorrhage and accompanying midline shifts of the falx cerebri from CT images are combined with ICP measurements in making surgical decisions in people with severe brain injury.[35,36]

Historically, surgical intervention has played a relatively minor role in managing brain-injured dogs and cats, due to the belief that clinically significant intracranial hemorrhage is rare in these species. Some evidence suggests that brain-injured dogs and cats may experience surgically manageable intracranial hemorrhage.[37,38] With the increased availability of CT facilities for dogs and cats, surgery may begin to play a larger role in canine and feline brain injury management. Other potential indications for surgery in the brain-injured dog or cat include open skull fractures, depressed skull fractures (with associated neurologic impairment), and retrieval of potentially contaminated bone fragments or foreign material lodged in brain parenchyma.[3,15]

Although surgical removal of focal intracranial hemorrhage is an accepted and proven aspect of management in human brain injury, there is division in the literature concerning the value of craniectomy solely as a decompressive maneuver in the patient demonstrating neurological deterioration despite aggressive medical therapy (*i.e.*, with no evidence of focal intracranial hemorrhage). It has been recently demonstrated in normal dogs and cats, combined craniectomy/durotomy results in dramatic decreases in ICP.[8,9,41] The value of craniectomy/durotomy is unknown in canine and feline brain injury.

PROGNOSIS AND COMPLICATIONS

The prognosis for victims of severe brain injury is considered guarded to poor. However, the recuperative ability of brain-injured dogs and cats is tremendous, and aggressive therapy may be successful in apparently hopeless cases. Predicting the outcome of an individual patient is difficult, but several factors may assist the clinician in estimating prognosis. These factors include level of consciousness, presence or absence of brainstem reflexes, age and general physical status, and presence and extent of other concurrent injuries. A dog or cat that is comatose with absent brainstem reflexes from the time of impact is generally less likely to recover than a patient who is obtunded with intact brainstem function.[1,15,42]

Potential complications associated with brain-injured patients include coagulopathies (*e.g.*, disseminated intravascular coagulation), pneumonia, fluid and electrolyte abnormalities (*e.g.*, central diabetes insipidus), and sepsis. Seizure activity may develop around the time of trauma (suggesting intraparenchymal hemorrhage) or months to years after trauma (development of a glial "scar"-seizure focus). Most of these complications are treatable or preventable.[1,11,15]

REFERENCES

1. Dewey CW: Emergency management of the head trauma patient: principles and practice. *Vet Clin North Am* 30:207, 2000.
2. Proulx J, Dhupa N: Severe brain injury. Part I. Pathophysiology. *Compend Contin Educ Pract Vet* 20:897, 1998.

3. Hopkins AL: Head trauma. *Vet Clin North Am* 26:875, 1996.
4. Sorjonen DC, Thomas WB, Myers LV *et al.*: Radical cerebral cortical resection in dogs. *Prog Vet Neurol* 2:225, 1991.
5. Graham DI, Adams JH, Gennarelli TA: Pathology of brain damage in head injury. *In* Cooper PR, ed.: Head Injury, 3rd ed. Baltimore: Williams & Wilkins, 1993, p 91.
6. Siesjo BK: Basic mechanisms of traumatic brain damage. *Ann Emerg Med* 22:959, 1993.
7. Katagama Y, Maeda T, Koshinaga M, *et al.*: Role of excitatory amino acid-mediated ionic fluxes in traumatic brain injury. *Brain Pathol* 5:427, 1995.
8. Bagley RS: Intracranial pressure in dogs and cats. *Compend Contin Educ Pract Vet* 18:605, 1996.
9. Bagley RS, Harrington ML, Pluhar GE, *et al.*: Effect of craniectomy/durotomy alone and in combination with hyperventilation, diuretics, and corticosteroids on intracranial pressure in clinically normal dogs. *Am J Vet Res* 57:116, 1996.
10. Chestnut RM: The management of severe traumatic brain injury. *Emerg Med Clin North Am* 15:581, 1997.
11. Gruen P, Liu C: Current trends in the management of head injury. *Emerg Med Clin North Am* 16:63, 1998.
12. Bouma GJ, Muizelaar JP, Bandoh K, *et al.*: Blood pressure and intracranial pressure-volume dynamics in severe head injury: Relationship with cerebral blood flow. *J Neurosurg* 77:15, 1992.
13. Fessler RD, Diaz FG: The management of cerebral perfusion pressure after severe head injury. *Ann Emerg Med* 22:998, 1993.
14. Marmarou A, Tabaddor K: Intracranial pressure: physiology and pathophysiology. *In* Cooper PR, ed.: Head Injury, 3rd ed. Baltimore: Williams & Wilkins, 1993, p 203.
15. Dewey CW, Budsberg SC, Oliver JE: Principles of head trauma management in dogs and cats. Part II. *Compend Contin Educ Pract Vet* 15:177, 1993.
16. Proulx J, Dhupa N: Severe brain injury. Part II. Therapy. *Compend Contin Educ Pract Vet* 20:993, 1998.
17. Rudloff E, Kirby R: The critical need for colloids: selecting the right colloid. *Compend Contin Educ Pract Vet* 19:811, 1997.
18. Rudloff E, Kirby R: The critical need for colloids: administering colloids effectively. *Compend Contin Educ Pract Vet* 20:27, 1998.
19. Menzies SA, Betz AL, Hoff JT: Contributions of ions and albumin to the formation and resolution of ischemic brain edema. *J Neurosurg* 78:257, 1993.
20. Young B, Ott L, Dempsey R, *et al.*: Relationship between admission hyperglycemia and neurologic outcome of severely brain-injured patients. *Ann Surg* 210:466, 1989.
21. Aldrich J, Haskins SC: Monitoring the critically ill patient. *In* Bonagura JD, ed.: Kirk's Current Veterinary Therapy XII. Philadelphia: WB Saunders, 1995, p 98.
22. Fairman NB: Evaluation of pulse oximetry as a continuous monitoring technique in critically ill dogs in the small animal intensive care unit. *J Vet Emerg Crit Care* 2:50, 1992.
23. Hendricks JC, King LG: Practicality, usefulness, and limits of pulse oximetry in critical small animal patients. *J Vet Emerg Crit Care* 3:5, 1993.
24. Matthews NS, Sanders EA, Hartsfield SM, *et al.*: A comparison of 2 pulse oximeters in dogs. *J Vet Emerg Crit Care* 5:115, 1995.

25. Yundt KD, Diringer MN: The use of hyperventilation and its impact on cerebral ischemia in the treatment of traumatic brain injury. *Crit Care Clin* 13:163, 1997.
26. Anonymous: The use of mannitol in severe head injury. *J Neurotrauma* 13:705, 1996.
27. Muizelaar JP, Lutz HA, Becker DP: Effect of mannitol on ICP and CBF and correlation with pressure autoregulation in severely head-injured patients. *J Neurosurg* 61: 700, 1984.
28. Allen CH, Ward JD: An evidence-based approach to management of increased intracranial pressure. *Crit Care Clin* 14:485, 1998.
29. Kaufman AM, Cardoso ER: Aggravation of vasogenic cerebral edema by multiple-dose mannitol. *J Neurosurg* 77:584, 1992.
30. Nguyen T, Frank E, Trunkey D: Steroids in central nervous system injury. *Adv Surg* 30:53, 1997.
31. Hall ED: High dose glucocorticoid treatment improves neurological recovery in head-injured mice. *J Neurosurg* 62:882, 1985.
32. Bernard S: Induced hypothermia in intensive care medicine. *Anaesth Intensive Care* 24:382, 1996.
33. Clifton GL: Systemic hypothermia in treatment of severe brain injury: a review and update. *J Neurotrauma* 12:923, 1995.
34. Zornow MH: Inhibition of glutamute release: a possible mechanism of hypothermic neuroprotection. *J Neurosurg Anesthesiol* 7:148, 1995.
35. Bullock R, Teasdale G: Surgical management of traumatic intracranial hematomas. *In* Vinken PJ, Bruyn GW, Klawans HL, eds: Handbook of Clinical Neurology: Head Injury. New York: Elsevier, 1990, p 249.
36. Cooper PR: Post-traumatic intracranial mass lesions. *In* Cooper PR, ed.: Head Injury, 3rd ed. Baltimore: Williams & Wilkins, 1993, p 275.
37. Dewey CW, Downs MO, Crowe DT: Management of a dog with an acute traumatic subdural hematoma. *J Am Anim Hosp Vet Assoc* 29:551, 1993.
38. Dewey CW, Downs MO, Aron DN, *et al.*: Acute traumatic intracranial hemorrhage in dogs and cats: a retrospective evaluation of 23 cases. *Vet Comp Orthop Traumatol* 6:153, 1993.
39. Fisher CM, Ojemann RG: Bilateral decompressive craniectomy for worsening coma in acute subarachnoid hemorrhage: observations in support of the procedure. *Surg Neurol* 41:65, 1994.
40. Gaab MR, Rittieroddt M, Lorenz M, *et al.*: Traumatic brain swelling and operative decompression: a prospective investigation. *Acta Neurochir Suppl (Wien)* 51:326, 1990.
41. Harrington ML, Bagley RS, Moore MP, *et al.*: Effect of craniectomy, durotomy, and wound closure on intracranial pressure in healthy cats. *Am J Vet Res* 57:1659, 1996.
42. Vollmer DG: Prognosis and outcome of severe head injury. *In* Cooper PR, ed.: Head Injury, 3rd ed. Baltimore: Williams & Wilkins, 1993, p 553.

67
Spinal Injury

Curtis W. Dewey

INTRODUCTION

Injury to the spine is common in canine and feline medicine. The most common cause of spinal injury is disk extrusion. This chapter deals with traumatic spinal injury, which is often due to automobile-induced trauma. Other causes of spinal injury include falls, missile injuries (*e.g.*, gunshot wounds), fights with other animals, and blunt trauma from other animals (*e.g.*, kicks). There are many similarities between the pathophysiology and management of the spinal injury patient and the brain injury patient. The uncertain clinical value of the available medical therapies for spinal injury is another theme shared with this aspect of critical care medicine and brain injury. The most important clinical consideration in spinal injury cases, following stabilization of life-threatening associated injuries, is identifying and addressing continued spinal cord compression. The most crucial clinical decision to be made in cases of canine and feline spinal injury is whether to pursue surgical decompression/stabilization or to treat the patient with medical therapy alone. There are no statistically proven "rules" to guide this decision-making process. The mode of therapy for a given patient with a spinal injury should be individualized for that specific patient, and based primarily on logic, with guidance derived from the literature and clinical experience.[1-5]

PATHOPHYSIOLOGY OF SPINAL INJURY

As with brain injury, it is conceptually useful to divide spinal injury into primary and secondary insults. Primary injury is that which is associated with the traumatic incident. However, vertebral instability secondary to vertebral fracture or luxation may produce repeated primary injury. Unlike brain injury, the clinician may be able to prevent repeated primary spinal cord damage. Secondary injury refers to events set in motion by the primary traumatic event. Similar to brain injury, secondary phenomena include continued hemorrhage, edema, tissue damage mediated by free radicals, and excitatory neurotransmitter-mediated damage.[1-4,6,7]

CLINICAL PRESENTATION AND INITIAL MANAGEMENT

Two important management principles should be exercised before transport of the traumatized dog or cat. The first is to avoid injury to transporting personnel.

Because of pain associated with spinal fracture/luxation, even the most docile of pets may attempt to bite anyone who attempts to move the pet. If there is any indication that the animal may bite, that patient should be muzzled. The second important principle is to minimize excessive motion during transport to a veterinary facility. Ideally, the patient should be taped to a flat, firm surface, like a board, to inhibit motion of a potentially unstable vertebral column while moving the patient. An acceptable alternative is to fashion a sling using a towel or blanket. In either case, the author recommends a minimum of three people to effectively and safely transport the patient with spinal injury. One person should focus on keeping the spine immobile, and the other two (or more) work on securing and moving the pet.[1,2,6]

On arrival at the hospital, the ABCs of trauma management (airway, breathing, cardiovascular status) take precedence over neurologic injury. Once life-threatening injuries are either ruled out or effectively treated, the clinician should next focus on the spinal injury. The initial neurologic examination should be brief and should not involve moving the patient until spinal radiographs have been procured. Mental status, cranial nerves, spinal reflexes, and nociception (pain perception) to the limbs can all be assessed in the recumbent, immobilized patient. Assessing voluntary motor function to the limbs may be difficult or impossible with the patient immobilized, but it is not essential at this point of patient assessment. Observing the patient's posture and responses to environmental stimuli will often provide some information regarding both lesion localization and preservation or loss of voluntary motor function. A recumbent pet may demonstrate purposeful limb or tail movement in response to calling his or her name. If apparent voluntary movement of the thoracic limbs, but not the pelvic limbs is noted, a thoracolumbar lesion should be suspected. If the pelvic limb reflexes are intact, the localization can be further refined to the T3-L3 spinal cord segments. Loss of pelvic limb reflexes indicates that the lesion is somewhere from L4 caudally. If the thoracic limbs are held in rigid extension, this may reflect the Schiff-Sherrington syndrome. The clinician must understand that the Schiff-Sherrington syndrome may be helpful in lesion localization, but that it is *not a prognostic indicator*. If no purposeful movement of any of the limbs is noted, a cervical lesion should be suspected. In severe cases, respiratory embarrassment may also be evident with cervical spinal cord injury.[1,2,4-6]

The assessment of pain perception (nociception) is vital in establishing prognosis. Testing for superficial pain perception (response to skin pinching) to the limbs should always be performed first, initially with fingers, then with a hemostat, if there is no conscious response. If the patient indicates a behavioral response to superficial pain testing (*e.g.* cries, bites at the examiner, tries to get away), testing for deep pain perception is superfluous. If superficial pain is absent, the clinician then must check for deep pain perception. The presence or absence of deep pain perception is often the pivotal factor in owner's decisions to pursue costly therapeutic options. The clinician must be able to both properly perform and interpret the test for deep pain perception. Using either the blunt handles of bandage scissors (less likely to damage the skin) or a hemostat, a crushing-type stimulus is applied across the bone of the distal digit. The author will test each digit until a behavioral response is elicited or all digits have been tested. Deep pain perception to the tail is evaluated if there is no response to digital testing. *Deep pain perception and withdrawal reflex are often assessed simultaneously, but they are not the same thing.* If the spinal cord lesion is above the lower motor neuron (LMN) pool necessary for the withdrawal reflex, an intact withdrawal reflex is expected. When testing for pain perception, the clinician is interested in the ascending spinal cord tracts that travel past that LMN pool and past the lesion site to arrive at the brain for interpretation. The most common error made by veterinarians when assessing for deep pain perception is interpreting an intact withdrawal reflex as pain perception. The term "perception" necessitates cerebral recognition, and therefore a behavioral response from the patient. If the patient withdraws the limb being tested, but does not appear to recognize (*e.g.*, no crying, biting at the examiner, trying to get away) that a noxious stimulus is being applied, deep pain perception is assessed as being absent.

A potential pitfall when assessing deep pain perception in a spinal-injured dog or cat is inadvertent movement of the spine while the patient withdraws the leg. If even slight movement of a spinal luxation/fracture occurs coincident with limb withdrawal, the resultant pain that this unintended motion produces may be falsely interpreted as intact deep pain perception to the digits. Having an assistant ensure spinal immobility during assessment of deep pain perception should prevent this misinterpretation.[1,2,6]

DIAGNOSTIC EVALUATION OF THE PATIENT WITH SPINAL INJURY

Basic emergency blood studies should be performed for all spinal injury victims. Thoracic radiographs are often advisable to evaluate for pulmonary contusions and pneumothorax. Spinal radiographs may be obtained with the patient awake, sedated, or anesthetized, depending primarily on the animal's demeanor. The clinician should bear in mind that the awake patient with vertebral instability will contract the paraspinal musculature surrounding the unstable area to minimize movement. Sedation and anesthesia may lessen or eliminate this protective mechanism. Lateral radiographs of the spine should be obtained before ventrodorsal views. Localization of potentially unstable areas of the vertebral column on lateral radiographs will help guide the clinician in preventing movement of those areas while positioning for the ventrodorsal views. As with emergency transport of the spinal injury patient, a minimum of three people should be involved in moving a dog or cat with a potentially unstable spine. The author recommends radiography of the entire vertebral column in spinal injury cases. There may be multiple sites of vertebral fracture or luxation, and this information is best obtained before considering therapeutic options.[1,2,4,6,8]

When considering therapeutic options (discussed below), it is helpful to conceptualize vertebral fracture/luxations using a three-compartment model.

The dorsal compartment includes the spinous processes, dorsal lamina, articular facets and associated pedicles, and soft tissues associated with these structures (*e.g.*, facet joint capsules, interarcuate ligament). The middle compartment includes the dorsal part of the vertebral body, the dorsal annulus fibrosus of the disk, and the dorsal longitudinal ligament. The ventral compartment includes the bulk of the vertebral body (middle and ventral portions), the remainder of the annulus fibrosus, and the ventral longitudinal ligament. If spinal radiographs suggest that only one of the three compartments appears to be damaged, the fracture/luxation is probably stable. If two or all of the compartments are compromised, the fracture/luxation should be considered unstable.[1,2,4,6,8,9]

The degree of vertebral displacement evident on plain radiographs is important clinical information, but does not absolutely correlate with the severity of the spinal insult. Radiographic findings should always be interpreted in the context of the patient's neurologic status. Considerable vertebral displacement can occur in the cervical area with minimal neurologic deficit due to the relatively large vertebral canal/spinal cord ratio in this region. Preservation of neurologic function may occur with complete overriding fracture/luxations of the lumbosacral region due largely to the resistance to compression and stretch of the nerve roots comprising the cauda equina. A complete luxation of vertebral segments can occur at the moment of impact, transecting the spinal cord, and the vertebral segments can "snap back" into near apposition.

In spinal injury cases for which surgery is indicated, the question of whether to perform myelography in addition to survey radiography is often raised. There is always the potential that there may be compressive soft tissue in the vertebral canal (*e.g.*, hematoma, traumatically extruded disk material) that requires myelography or other imaging procedures (*e.g.*, computed tomography [CT], magnetic resonance imaging [MRI]) to be identified. Advanced imaging, such as CT or MRI, are superior imaging choices to plain radiographs and myelography (Fig. 67-1).[1,2,4,5,8-10] If the surgeon is planning a laminectomy in addition to stabilization, the need for myelography is obviated. If only stabilization is planned, there is a risk of missing a compressive lesion (*i.e.*, other than that caused directly by vertebral luxation) if only plain radiographs are obtained before surgery. Until more information is available, the author recommends either performing myelography before surgery or creating a small exploratory laminectomy window at the time of stabilization surgery if myelography has not been performed.

In cases of gunshot injuries to the spine, there is often minimal evidence of vertebral instability on plain radiography. If no bullets or bullet fragments are noted within the vertebral canal, further imaging of the spine is probably unnecessary. The reason for additional imaging (*e.g.*, myelography) is to search for a compressive lesion that may require surgical intervention. Gunshot injuries to the spine in people are usually not managed surgically because surgical intervention does not appear to improve overall outcome.[5] However, the author has operated on several gunshot injuries to the spinal cord in dogs and cats in which a myelogram revealed evidence of active cord compression and swelling (Fig. 67-2). The patients neurologically improved after decompressive surgery.

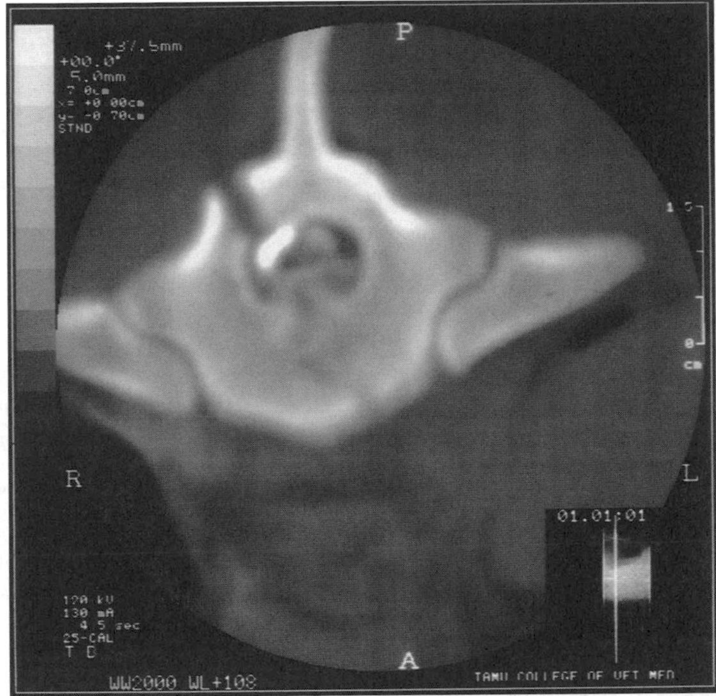

Figure 67-1
Transaxial CT/myelogram image of a T13 vertebral fracture.

Although anecdotal, this experience emphasizes the need to individualize diagnostic and therapeutic decisions for specific case situations.

THERAPY

Medical Therapy

Proper medical therapy of the spinal-injured pet includes preventing motion of the fracture/luxation segments. Minimizing movement of the injured vertebral area is paramount to a successful outcome. If surgical stabilization is not performed, application of an immobilization brace is recommended in cases with suspected vertebral instability. A soft wrap (*e.g.*, cast padding, roll cotton) is applied initially, and a rigid support (*e.g.*, fiberglass, metal bars) is added over that wrap (Fig. 67-3). Even with an immobilization brace, the patient should be confined to a crate for a minimum of 6 weeks. Immobilization braces should be considered adjuncts to confinement therapy, not a method of circumventing confinement therapy. If ambulatory, the animal may be allowed to walk to urinate and defecate, but otherwise should be confined to the crate. Although most dogs and cats with vertebral injuries adapt well to crate confinement, some may require sedation during the confinement period (*e.g.*, oral acepromazine).[1,2,4,21]

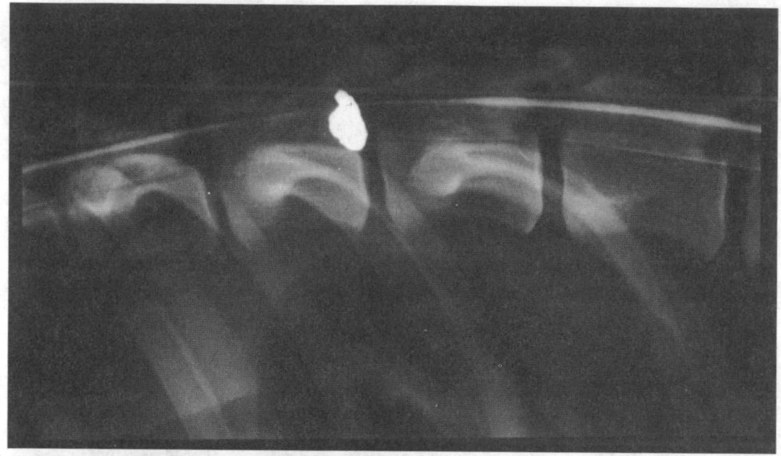

(A)

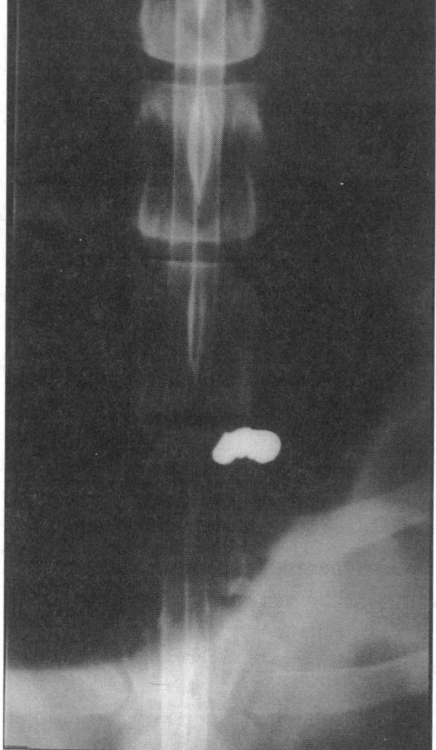

(B)

Figure 67-2
Lateral (**A**) and ventrodorsal (**B**) myelographic views of a spinal gunshot injury in a dog, demonstrating spinal cord swelling.

The high dose methylprednisolone protocol has demonstrated a statistically significant beneficial effect when administered to people with severe traumatic spinal injury. This protocol has also shown promise in experimental animal studies.[1-7,11-17] However, recent evidence challenges the validity of the benefits reported in humans treated with this protocol.[18] All of the "high-dose" protocols

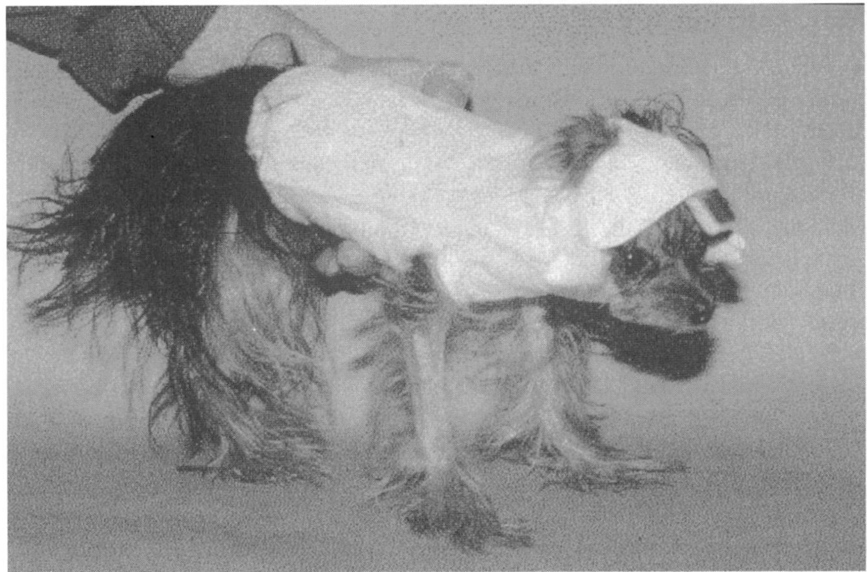

Figure 67-3
Typical immobilization brace for patients with vertebral instability. (Courtesy of Dr. Joan Coates.)

begin with an initial intravenous dose of 30 mg/kg methylprednisolone. The author prefers to administer a 15 mg/kg dose at 2 and 6 hours after the initial dose.[1-7,11-17] The injection should be given over 5 to 10 minutes because rapid injection may occasionally lead to nausea and/or hypotension. This therapy appears to be beneficial only when administered within 8 hours after spinal injury in people. It is suspected that the "window of opportunity" may be shorter in dogs and cats. Because there is some evidence of efficacy, the author promotes the use of "high-dose" methylprednisolone as soon as possible following spinal injury. Treating the spinal injury patient with "standard" doses of prednisone or dexamethasone is ineffective and may harm the patient. Administering superfluous glucocorticoid treatments may increase the likelihood of serious glucocorticoid-mediated side effects, especially if the patient is subsequently treated with the "high-dose" protocol.[1,2,11,16-17,19]

Although mannitol is an effective agent in reducing intracranial pressure in severe brain injury, it does not appear to have any beneficial effect for dogs and cats with spinal injury. Some evidence indicates that administration of mannitol to the patient with spinal injury may be harmful.[6,11,20]

Appropriate bladder management and recumbent patient care (if nonambulatory) are pivotal aspects of treating the spinal-injured dog or cat. The specifics of this maintenance care are beyond the scope of this chapter, but are covered in detail in several excellent review articles.[22-25]

Surgical Therapy

The indications for surgical therapy in the spinal-injured dog or cat are based mainly on clinical judgment rather than statistics. In general, the author recommends surgical intervention if there is moderate to severe displacement of vertebral segments, if the patient is neurologically deteriorating in the face of vertebral instability, or if there is myelographic evidence of spinal cord compression. This clinical decision-making is often tempered by other factors, such as demeanor of the patient and financial abilities of the pet owner.[1,2,4,26-29] Abundant clinical evidence indicates that nonsurgical treatment of dogs and cats with vertebral fracture/luxations is often successful.[26-28] In one retrospective study concerning dogs and cats with vertebral fracture/luxations, no significant difference in outcome was found between those patients treated surgically versus those treated nonsurgically. Patients treated nonsurgically were likely to have a longer recuperative period than the surgically treated animals, but were equally likely to recover function.[26]

Multiple methods are available to stabilize vertebral fracture/luxations. Although some are biomechanically more rigid than others, all are acceptable stabilization methods. The exact mode of stabilization is often determined more by clinician preference and anatomic location of the fracture/luxation than by results of in vitro biomechanical studies. Methods of vertebral fracture/luxation stabilization include modified segmental stabilization ("spinal stapling"), dorsal spinous vertebral body plating, screw or pin vertebral body placement with polymethylmethacrylate (PMMA) bridging, and vertebral body plating.[1,4,6,26,29-35] For cervical fracture/luxations, pin or screw placement with PMMA bridging is often performed (Fig. 67-4). From the T1-12 vertebral segment, the author prefers either using a spinal stapling technique or dorsal spinous process plating (Fig. 67-5). Pins or screws with PMMA bridging is a technique that is readily applied to the remainder of the vertebral column, including fracture/luxations of the lumbosacral junction area (Fig. 67-6). Although technically more demanding than pins/screws and PMMA techniques, vertebral body plating is a very effective and very rigid stabilization method that may be readily applied from the T12 through the L4 (Fig. 67-7). This method is often not used caudal to L4, for fear of damaging the nerve roots contributing to the femoral nerve (L4, L5, L6) during plate application.

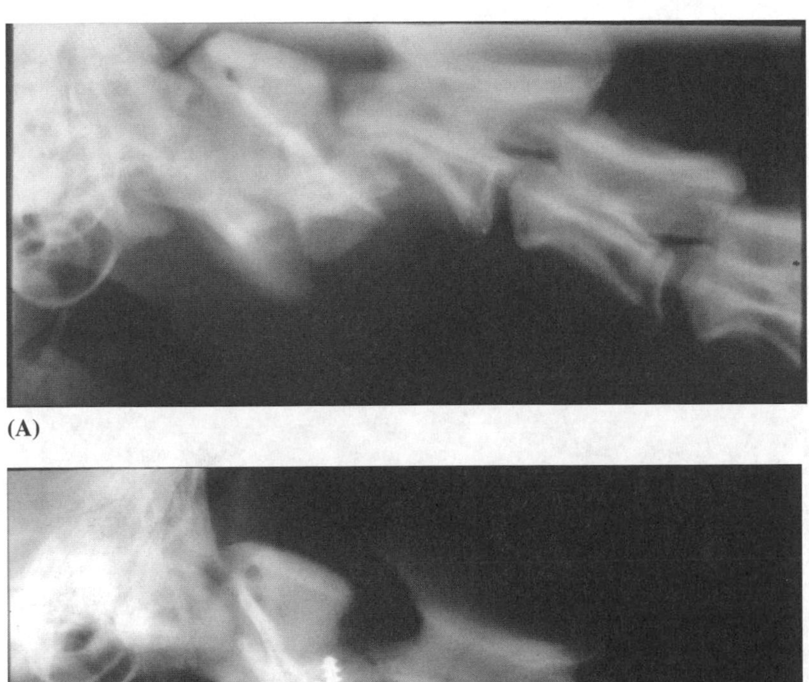

(A)

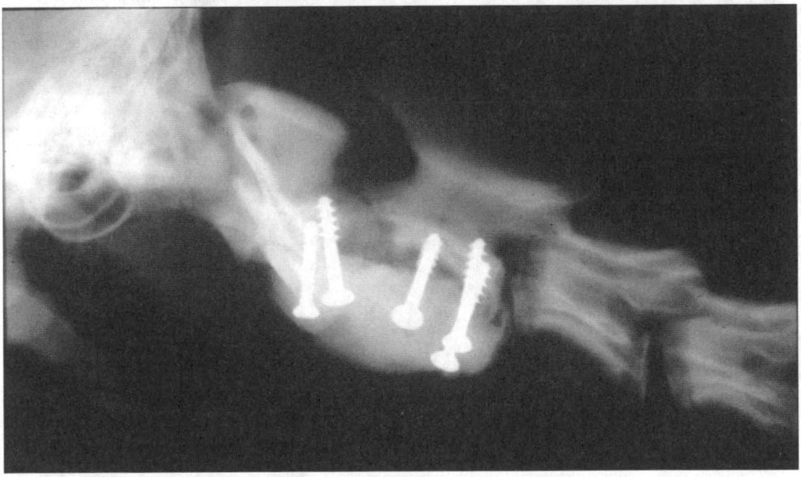

(B)

Figure 67-4
Presurgical (**A**) and postsurgical (**B**) lateral radiographs of a dog with a displaced C2 fracture, stabilized with screws and PMMA.

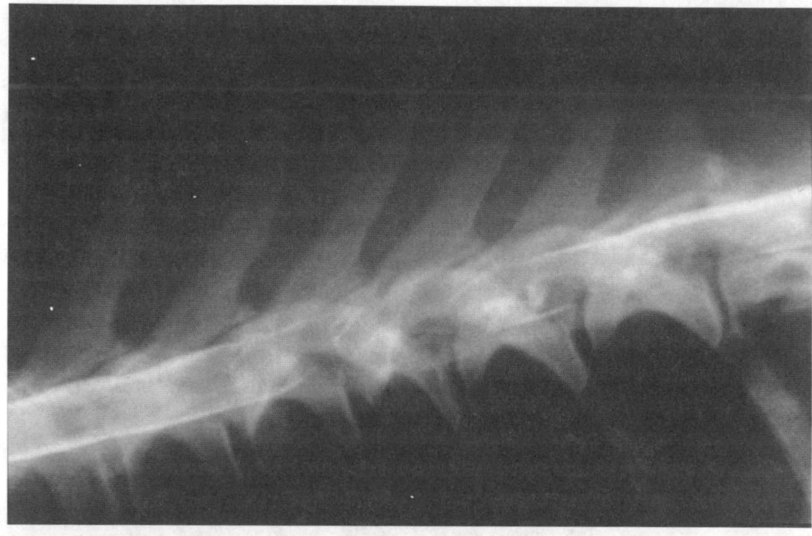

(A)

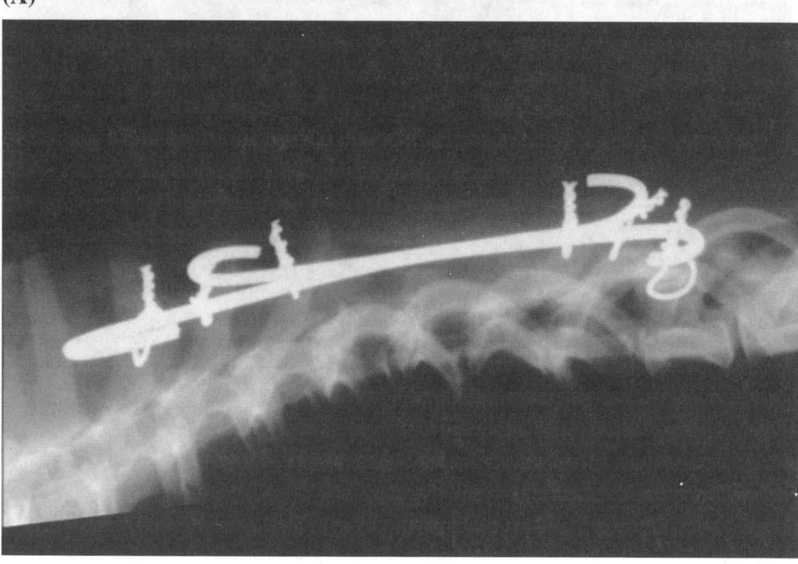

(B)

Figure 67-5
Presurgical (**A**) and postsurgical (**B**) lateral radiographic views of a pathologic compression fracture of T8 in a dog, stabilized with modified segmental stabilization ("spinal stapling").

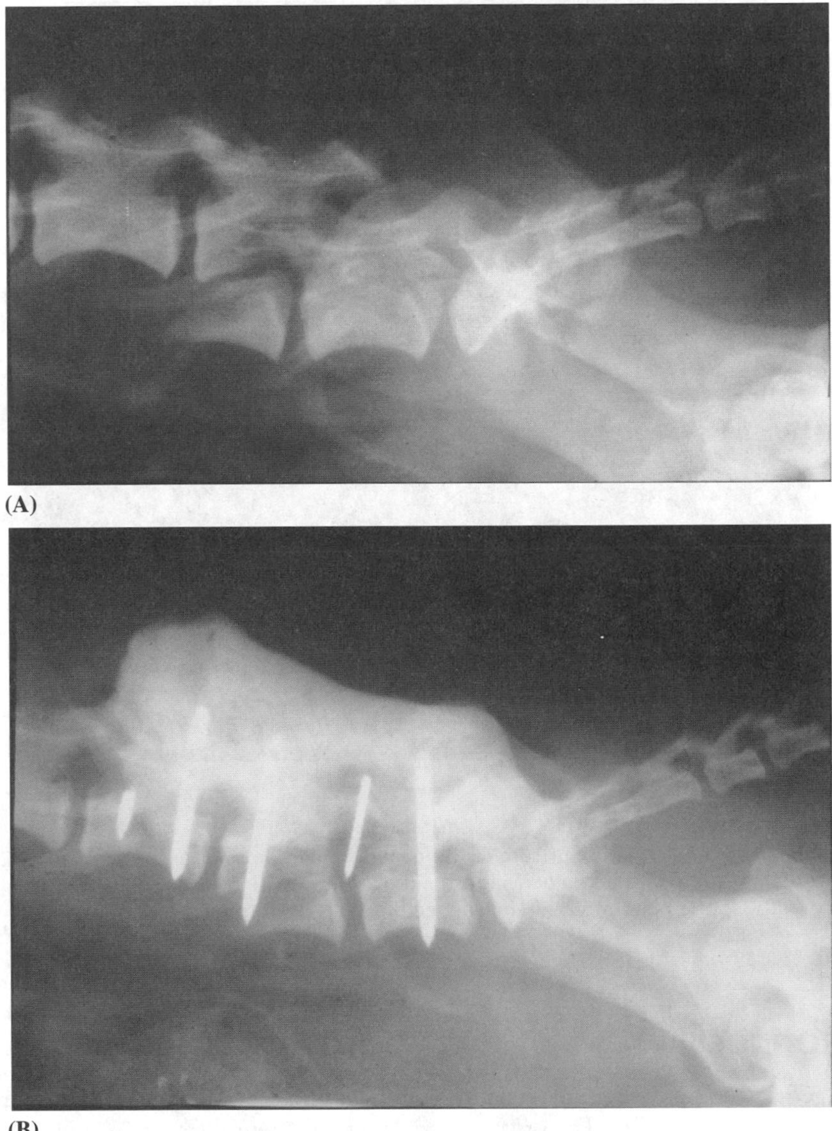

Figure 67-6
Presurgical (**A**) and postsurgical (**B**) lateral radiographic views of a displaced fracture of L6 in a dog, stabilized with pins and PMMA.

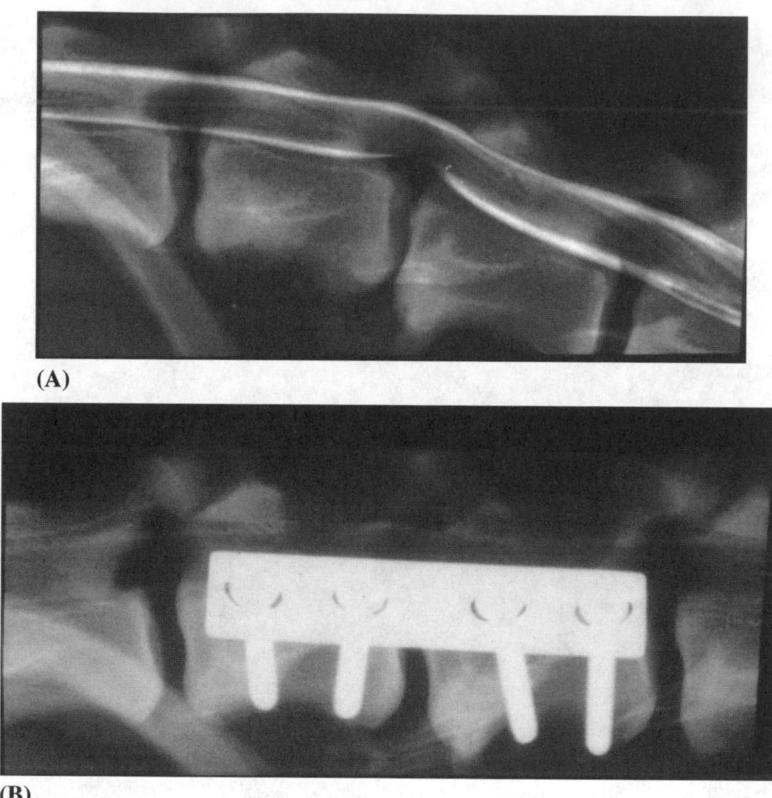

Figure 67-7
Lateral presurgical (**A**) and postsurgical (**B**) myelographic views of a dog with an L1-2 vertebral luxation with accompanying traumatic disk extrusion. The area was stabilized with a bone plate after a hemilaminectomy was performed.

PROGNOSIS

In general, the prognosis for spinal-injured dogs and cats with intact deep pain perception is favorable. The prognosis for functional neurologic recovery in spinal-injured dogs and cats that have lost deep pain perception is unknown. There is extensive data concerning the prognosis for patients with "no deep pain" disk extrusion (approximately 50%).[1,2,29,36] The author's impression is that the prognosis for "no deep pain" victims of exogenous spinal trauma is considerably less than this. If there is complete overlapping (complete luxation) of the vertebral canal evident on radiographs and no deep pain perception is elicited, the prognosis for recovery should be considered extremely poor. In rare instances, the dorsal lamina in the area of luxation fractures off during the traumatic event, effecting a decompression of the spinal cord. In these cases, there may be more hope of recovery.

REFERENCES

1. Bagley RS: Spinal fracture or luxation. *Vet Clin North Am* 30:133, 2000.
2. Bagley RS, Cambridge AJ, Harrington ML, *et al.*: Exogenous spinal trauma: clinical assessment and initial management. *Compend Contin Educ Pract Vet* 21:1138, 1999.
3. Kraus KH: The pathophysiology of spinal cord injury and its clinical implications. *Semin Vet Med Surg Small Anim* 11:201, 1996.
4. Shores A: Spinal trauma: pathophysiology and management of traumatic spinal injuries. *Vet Clin North Am Small Anim Pract* 22:859, 1992.
5. Chiles BW, Cooper PR: Acute spinal injury. *N Engl J Med* 334:514, 1996.
6. Rucker NC: Management of spinal cord trauma. *Prog Vet Neurol* 1:397, 1990.
7. Olby N: Current concepts in management of acute spinal cord injury. *J Vet Intern Med* 13:399, 1999.
8. Brawner WR, Braund KG, Shores A: Radiographic evaluation of dogs and cats with acute spinal cord trauma. *Vet Med* July:703, 1990.
9. Shires PK, Waldron DR, Hedlund CS, *et al.*: A biomechanical study of rotational instability in unaltered and surgically altered canine thoracolumbar vertebral motion units. *Prog Vet Neurol* 2:6, 1991.
10. Fagerlund MKJ: Acute neuroradiology: methods, indications and timing. *Ann Med* 27:657, 1995.
11. Meintjes E, Hosgood G, Daniloff J: Pharmaceutic treatment of acute spinal cord trauma. *Compend Contin Educ Pract Vet* 18:625, 1996.
12. Hall ED: The neuroprotective pharmacology of methylprednisolone. *J Neurosurg* 76:13, 1992.
13. Bracken MB, Shepard MJ, Collins WF, *et al.*: A randomized, controlled trial of methylprednisolone or naloxone in the treatment of acute spinal-cord injury. *N Engl J Med* 322:1405, 1990.
14. Bracken MB, Shepard MJ, Collins WF, *et al.*: Methylprednisolone or naloxone treatment after acute spinal cord injury: 1-year follow-up data. *J Neurosurg* 76:23, 1992.
15. Braughler JM, Hall ED: Effects of multi-dose methylprednisolone sodium succinate administration on injured cat spinal cord neurofilament degradation and energy metabolism. *J Neurosurg* 61:290, 1984.
16. Braughler JM, Hall ED, Means ED, *et al.*: Evaluation of an intensive methylprednisolone sodium succinate dosing regimen in experimental spinal cord injury. *J Neurosurg* 67:102, 1987.
17. Hoerlein BF, Redding RW, Hoff EJ, *et al.*: Evaluation of naloxone, crocetin, thyrotropin releasing hormone, methylprednisolone, partial myelotomy, and hemilaminectomy in the treatment of acute spinal cord trauma. *J Am Anim Hosp Assoc* 21:67, 1985.
18. Hurlbert RJ: Methylprednisolone for acute spinal cord injury: an inappropriate standard of care. *J Neurosurg* 93(suppl 1):1, 2000.
19. Culbert LA, Marino DJ, Baule RM, *et al.*: Complications associated with high-dose prednisolone sodium succinate therapy in dogs with neurological injury. *J Am Anim Hosp Assoc* 34:129, 1998.
20. Hoerlein BF, Redding RW, Hoff EJ, *et al.*: Evaluation of dexamethasone, DMSO, mannitol, and solcoseryl in acute spinal cord trauma. *J Am Anim Hosp Assoc* 19:216, 1983.
21. Patterson RH, Smith GK: Backsplinting for treatment of thoracic and lumbar fracture/luxation in the dog: principles of application and case series *Vet Comp Orthop Traumatol* 5:179, 1992.

22. Jerram RM, Hart RC, Schulz KS: Postoperative management of the canine spinal surgery patient—part I. *Compend Contin Educ Pract Vet* 19:147, 1997.
23. Hart RC, Jerram RM, Schulz KS: Postoperative management of the canine spinal surgery patient—part II. *Compend Contin Educ Pract Vet* 19:1133, 1997.
24. Nicoll SA, Remedios AM: Recumbency in small animals: pathophysiology and management. *Compend Contin Educ Pract Vet* 17:1367, 1995.
25. Taylor RA: Postsurgical physical therapy: the missing link. *Compend Contin Educ Pract Vet* 14:1583, 1992.
26. Selcer RR, Bubb WJ, Walker TL: Management of vertebral column fractures in dogs and cats: 211 cases (1977–1985). *J Am Vet Med Assoc* 198:1965, 1991.
27. Carberry CA, Flanders JA, Dietze AE, *et al.*: Nonsurgical management of thoracic and lumbar spinal fractures and fracture/luxations in the dog and cat: a review of 17 cases. *J Am Anim Hosp Assoc* 25: 43, 1989.
28. Hawthorne JC, Blevins WE, Wallace LJ, *et al.*: Cervical vertebral fractures in 56 dogs: a retrospective study. *J Am Anim Hosp Assoc* 35:135, 1999.
29. Bagley RS, Harrington ML, Silver GM, *et al.*: Exogenous spinal trauma: surgical therapy and aftercare. *Compend Contin Educ Pract Vet* 22:218, 2000.
30. McAnulty JF, Lenehan TM, Maletz LM: Modified segmental spinal instrumentation in repair of spinal fractures and luxations in dogs. *Vet Surg* 15:143, 1986.
31. Blass CE, Seim HB: Spinal fixation using steinmann pins and methylmethacrylate. *Vet Surg* 13:203, 1984.
32. Shores A: Fractures and luxations of the vertebral column. *Vet Clin North Am Small Anim Pract* 22:171, 1992.
33. Blass CE, Waldron DR, Van Ee RT: Cervical stabilization in three dogs using Steinmann pins and methylmethacrylate. *J Am Anim Hosp Assoc* 24:61, 1988.
34. Stone EA, Betts CW, Chambers JN: Cervical fractures in the dog: a literature and case review. *J Am Anim Hosp Assoc* 15:463, 1979.
35. Matthiesen DT: Thoracolumbar spinal fractures/luxations: surgical management. *Compend Contin Educ Pract Vet* 5:867, 1983.
36. Duval J, Dewey C, Roberts R, *et al.*: Spinal cord swelling as a myelographic indicator of prognosis: a retrospective study in dogs with intervertebral disc disease and loss of deep pain perception. *Vet Surg* 25:6, 1996.

68
Respiratory Injury

Elisa M. Mazzaferro

INTRODUCTION

Injury to the respiratory system is often life-threatening and requires immediate veterinary care. Injury can result from penetrating wounds, such as bite wounds, or from malicious projectiles, such as bullets and arrows. Blunt trauma most commonly is associated with motor vehicle accidents, but can also result from a malicious attack or fall from heights.

Injuries to the thorax secondary to trauma can be classified into the following categories: (1) closed versus open, (2) pleural cavity pathology, (3) involvement of the lung parenchyma, (4) involvement of the thoracic wall, and (5) tracheobronchial tree abnormalities (Table 68-1).[1] Cardiovascular abnormalities also are often associated with injury to the thorax, but will be listed as a separate entity for purposes of discussion.

EPIDEMIOLOGY OF RESPIRATORY TRAUMA

Approximately 10% of all dogs and cats presented on an emergency basis have thoracic trauma resulting in respiratory compromise.[2] In several studies evaluating injuries from motor vehicle accidents, thoracic injury is reported to range from 38.9% to 59.5% of presented cases.[3-6] The four most common injuries associated with thoracic trauma include pneumothorax, pulmonary contusions, rib fractures or flail chest, and diaphragmatic hernia. Pulmonary contusions occur in approximately 50% of cases, often in combination with other injuries including rib fractures, flail chest, pneumothorax, hemothorax, diaphragmatic hernia, and myocardial injury.[3] Although it may be simple to discuss injuries as separate entities, they often occur in combination, with multiple injuries contributing to compromised respiratory function.

GENERAL APPROACH TO PATIENTS WITH RESPIRATORY TRAUMA

Trauma to the respiratory system manifests itself as respiratory difficulty. Clinical signs are associated with the location and extent of injury. Injury to the head can result in obstruction of the upper airway secondary to severe epistaxis and pharyngeal collapse. Damage to the lower airways, lung parenchyma, or pleural space often cause restriction to respiration. Space occupying mass within the pleural space that stops complete expansion of the lungs during inspiration

Table 68-1. Common Injuries Associated with Neck and Thoracic Trauma

Subcutaneous emphysema
Tracheal damage/rupture
Rib fractures
Flail chest
Pulmonary contusions
Pneumothorax
Open
Tension
Diaphragmatic hernia
Myocardial injury
Pericardial hemorrhage
Hemothorax
Infection secondary to bite wounds or foreign body

(pneumothorax, pulmonary contusion, hemothorax, diaphragmatic hernia) will result in a rapid shallow restrictive respiratory pattern, open-mouthed breathing, orthopnea (extension of the head and neck and abduction of the elbows away from the thorax), and cyanosis. Open pneumothoraces may have a sucking chest wound that is both visible and audible during inspiration. Patients with flail segments have a paradoxical motion of the chest wall during all phases of respiration.

Diagnostic Evaluation

Physical Examination

Evaluation of the trauma patient begins at presentation. The most important diagnostic tools are the clinician's eyes and ears. Careful observation of the patient's respiratory rate and pattern before handling can aid in the diagnosis of pulmonary injury and assist in localizing the injury to upper versus lower respiratory system. The clinician should observe the patient for evidence of severe inspiratory stridor or epistaxis, which signals damage to the upper airways. Evidence of a sucking chest wound or paradoxical chest wall motion signifies open pneumothorax or flail chest. Sudden changes in the patient's respiratory pattern characterized by more rapid and shallow breathing indicates rapid deterioration. Careful auscultation of both sides of the thorax is necessary to determine if intrapleural problems exist. Muffled heart and lung sounds are apparent in pneumothorax, hemothorax, and diaphragmatic hernia. Increased adventitial sounds or harsh crackles may occur with pulmonary contusions. Percussion with simultaneous auscultation may reveal hyperresonant sounds indicating areas of free air within the pleural space.[46] Primary therapy of respiratory trauma involves rapid patient stabilization followed by continuous monitoring. Patient stabilization must occur before further diagnostics are performed.

Radiography

Thoracic radiographs are an important diagnostic tool in evaluating pulmonary system injury. One of the most important rules in trauma patients is to *delay* radiography until the patient is stable. Many patients with underlying respiratory injury cannot handle the stress of restraint necessary for proper radiography to be performed. Dorsoventral and standing lateral projections may be required to minimize stress and respiratory compromise. DO NOT place the patient in a position that they are not comfortable in maintaining.

PENETRATING INJURIES TO THE NECK AND THORAX

Bite Wounds

Epidemiology

Bite wounds comprise approximately 10% to 15% of veterinary emergencies.[7,8] Approximately one third of bite wounds are associated with head, neck, and thoracic trauma, with half of these directly associated with thoracic injury.[9,10]

Pathophysiology

Bite wounds from animal interactions can cause tremendous damage to skin and underlying structures. Frequently superficial injuries appear relatively innocuous, yet damage to the underlying tissues is severe and can be life-threatening. This is known as the "iceberg effect."[11] Combinations of crush, tear, avulsion, punctures, and lacerations often result from dog bites.[7] In animals, the skin overlying the neck and thorax is freely movable and pliable. This characteristic, combined with shear forces exerted by shaking action during animal attacks, can cause ripping of the underlying muscles, avulsion of the laryngeal or cervical trachea, recurrent laryngeal nerve damage, bony fractures (rib fractures and flail chest), and contusions to the lung parenchyma and myocardium. Damage to the intercostal and internal thoracic arteries and great vessels can also occur, but is uncommon except in projectile injury.

Clinical Presentation

Bite wounds to the head and neck should be carefully evaluated for tracheal disruption or avulsion. The patient presents with severe inspiratory stridor and bruising over the affected areas.[10] Epistaxis and facial swelling can cause occlusion of the upper airways in patients with severe head injuries. Tracheal injury results in air leakage from the injury site. Free air can dissect through tissue planes causing subcutaneous emphysema, pneumomediastinum, and respiratory distress. In some cases, pneumomediastinum may progress to a life-threatening tension pneumothorax. If recurrent larygneal nerve damage is present, a stridorous respiration occurs secondary to laryngeal paralysis.[10]

Diagnostics

Thoracic radiographs are important in documenting pneumothorax, pulmonary contusions, and diaphragmatic hernia. In one study, the most common radiographic findings included subcutaneous emphysema, pneumothorax, pulmonary contusions, and rib separation.[12]

Treatment

The first priority in treatment of bite wounds to the head and neck involves establishing a patent airway and administration of supplemental oxygen (O_2). The mode of supplemental O_2 therapy often depends on the extent of injury and whether concurrent injuries to the thorax and lung parenchyma are present. Supplemental O_2 therapy can be conservative in the form of flow-by, hood, or nasal O_2,[13] or placing the animal in an O_2 cage (delivering 40% O_2). Severe injury with pharyngeal collapse or cervical tracheal disruption may require intubation, tracheostomy, or mechanical ventilation. Rapid induction with a short-acting anesthetic, such as propofol (4-7 mg/kg IV), may be administered to allow endotracheal intubation. Therapeutic thoracocentesis (Fig. 68-1) or placement of a thoracic drain may be required if concurrent pneumothorax is present. Once a patient's condition is stabilized, each wound should be surgically explored, debrided, and copiously flushed to remove residual debris.

All bite wounds should be considered contaminated until proven otherwise. Bacteria commonly identified in animal bite wounds include *Pasteurella multocida*, *Staphylococcus aureus*, *Staphylococcus intermedius*, and *Streptococcus* spp.[7] Coverage with broad-spectrum antibiotics (first- or second-generation cephalosporins such as cefazolin [22 mg/kg IV or IM tid] or cefoxitin [22 mg/kg IV or IM tid]) should begin immediately after initial triage.

Prognosis

The prognosis of patients with bite wounds to the head, neck, and thorax largely depends on the extent of the injury and tissue damage. Between 6% and 25% of animals with thoracic bite wounds die or are euthanized as a result of their injuries.[12,14] Animals that survive to veterinary hospital admission may have survived the critical time period after injury.[1] Potential sequelae of bite wounds include chronic infection, delayed wound healing, systemic inflammatory response syndrome, disseminated intravascular coagulation, and multiple organ dysfunction. Tracheal stenosis may occur long-term after trauma.[7]

Projectile Injury to the Thorax

Epidemiology

The incidence of projectile injuries to the thorax has increased in recent years.[8,15] In one retrospective study, 26% of the projectile injuries involved the thorax.[15]

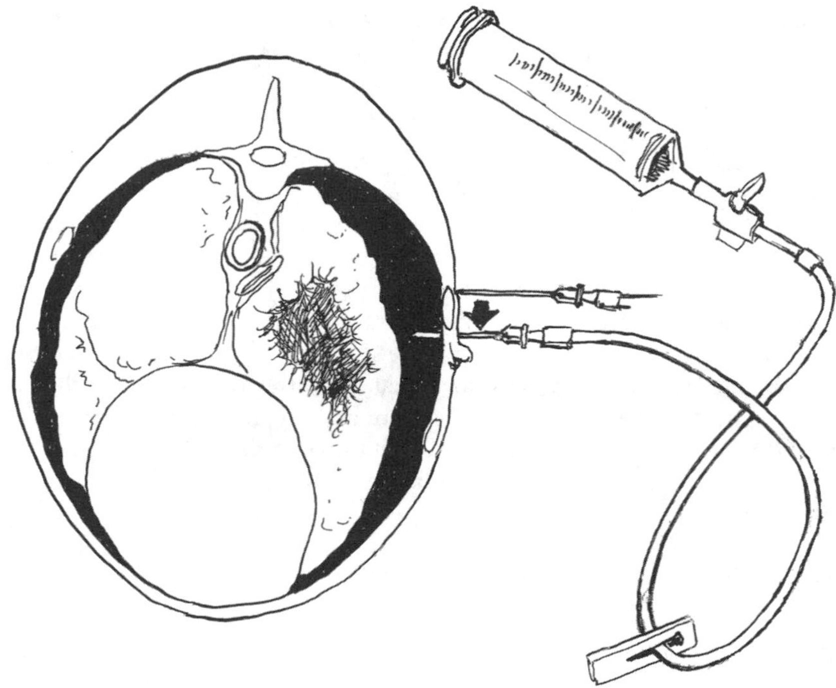

Figure 68-1
Diagnostic and therapeutic thoracocentesis. Following routine aseptic preparation of the skin, a needle is inserted between the seventh and ninth intercostal spaces. The bevel of the needle is positioned toward the thoracic cavity. The needle is then placed parallel with the body wall to avoid lacerating a lung. Always tap both sides of the thorax when treating for pneumothorax or pleural effusion.

Pathophysiology

Projectile penetration of the thorax can cause severe damage to the body wall, lung parenchyma, great vessels, and heart. Acutely, severe hemorrhage from lacerated venae cavae, heart, or aorta can result in severe hypovolemia and hemothorax. Hypovolemia, in turn, decreases cardiac output, further reducing systemic perfusion. Hemothorax also results in inadequate expansion of the lung parenchyma and leads to atelectasis and ventilation-perfusion (V/Q) mismatch. Penetration of the thorax can result in an open sucking chest wound and pneumothorax, further contributing to atelectasis and hypoxemia.

Clinical Presentation

Clinical presentation depends on the location and extent of injury. A patient with pneumothorax or hemothorax will present with a rapid, shallow restrictive respiratory pattern, pale mucous membranes, and tachycardia or bradycardia. Auscultation of the thorax may reveal muffled heart and lung sounds if pneumothorax or hemothorax is present. External bleeding will be apparent at the site of projectile entry. In many cases, hair enters the wound at the site of injury. In some cases a larger exit wound is also apparent.

Treatment

Emergency management of penetrating thoracic injury includes cardiovascular resuscitation using IV fluids, supplemental O_2, and evacuation of free air and blood from the pleural space. In the past, immediate surgical intervention has been advocated to aggressively debride the wound, remove foreign objects (bullet or pellet), and to irrigate the wound to prevent infection.[15] More recently, conservative management of projectile wounds to the thorax has indicated that infection rate is low. One theory is that the speed of the missile, combined with rotation, helps to prevent the dragging of hair and other debris into the thoracic wound. In humans, conservative management and simple reinflation of the lungs using thoracic drainage often results in direct counterpressure and cessation of intrathoracic bleeding.[16,17] Only in rare instances is exploratory thoracotomy required (Table 68-2).

Prognosis

In most cases, projectile injuries to the thorax have a good prognosis provided that adequate care is instituted on presentation.[15] Morbidity and mortality are associated with the extent of injury, involvement of great vessels and heart, and presence of concurrent injuries.[15] When death occurs, it is often associated with laceration of the heart and great vessels. In one study only 1 of 32 dogs with gunshot wounds to the thorax required exploratory thoracotomy. Two deaths occurred in this case series, both due to laceration of great vessels.[15]

Table 68-2. Indications for Thoracotomy Following Thoracic Trauma

Persistent hemorrhage
Pneumothorax that persists after continuous suction from bilateral thoracic drains
Damage to lung parenchyma
Lung torsion
Lung bullae
Lung laceration
Lung abscess
Tension pneumothorax
Severe flail chest with continuous injury to the lung parenchyma
Tracheal avulsion

DAMAGE TO THE LOWER AIRWAY AND LUNG PARENCHYMA

Intrathoracic Tracheal Rupture

Epidemiology

Intrathoracic tracheal rupture is an uncommon sequela to blunt thoracic trauma. It has also been reported to occur secondary to endotracheal intubation. Although rare, several reports in the literature discuss this syndrome.[18-22]

Pathophysiology

Mechanical forces play a role in intrathoracic tracheal rupture. In cats, the distal trachea is fixed in position at the level of the carina; the cranial portion of the trachea is more freely mobile within the thorax. The force of trauma causes hyperextension of the head and neck, which produces instantaneous traction on the trachea producing mechanical rupture at the carina. The surrounding mediastinal tissue and peritracheal tissue allows for continuity of the trachea to be maintained immediately after the injury. Overinflation of high-volume, low-pressure cuffed endotracheal tubes during general anesthesia also can cause tracheal rupture in cats.[22,23]

Clinical Presentation

Most cats with tracheal rupture show mild respiratory distress on initial presentation that resolves without treatment. Within 7 to 14 days the cat represents with severe respiratory distress and coughing. Clinical signs are associated with restrictive respiratory pattern (rapid shallow respirations) and open-mouthed breathing is noted on physical examination. Cyanosis may be present. Thoracic auscultation reveals muffled heart and lung sounds characteristic of pneumothorax.

Diagnostics

Thoracic radiographs reveal loss of tracheal continuity, often at the level of the carina, and an air-filled diverticulum between tracheal rings. Presence of air-filled diverticulum is called "pseudoairway" and suggests chronicity.[21]

Treatment

Therapy involves surgical correction as soon as possible. Techniques for surgical stabilization of the ruptured trachea are discussed elsewhere.[18]

Prognosis

Following surgical stabilization and anastomosis, long-term prognosis for these cats is extremely good.[24] Sequelae following surgical repair includes radiographic narrowing of the thoracic trachea and laryngeal paralysis (likely secondary to recurrent laryngeal nerve dysfunction).

Pulmonary Contusions

Epidemiology

Pulmonary contusion occurs in approximately 50% of thoracic trauma cases and is the most common injury to the respiratory system.[3] Pulmonary contusions often occur in combination with other thoracic injuries including rib fractures, flail chest, pneumothorax, and diaphragmatic hernia.

Pathophysiology

The pathophysiology of pulmonary contusions is well understood.[25] The rib cage can be viewed as a compressible box. Trauma to the thoracic wall produces a compression-decompression class injury.[3] When an animal is struck by an object or motor vehicle, initially the body remains stationary and absorbs the force of impact due to inertial forces. The rib cage on the affected side is compressed towards midline, resulting in severe compression of the underlying lung parenchyma. Elastic recoil of the compressed rib cage occurs just before the animal is thrown away from the site of impact. Recoil of the thoracic cage results in decompression of the affected areas of lung (Fig. 68-2). Rupture of alveoli and adjacent blood vessels occurs, resulting in atelectasis and intra-alveolar and interstitial hemorrhage.[3,26-28] Disruption of blood vessels causes hemorrhage at the affected area followed by leakage of plasma into the surrounding tissues. As the

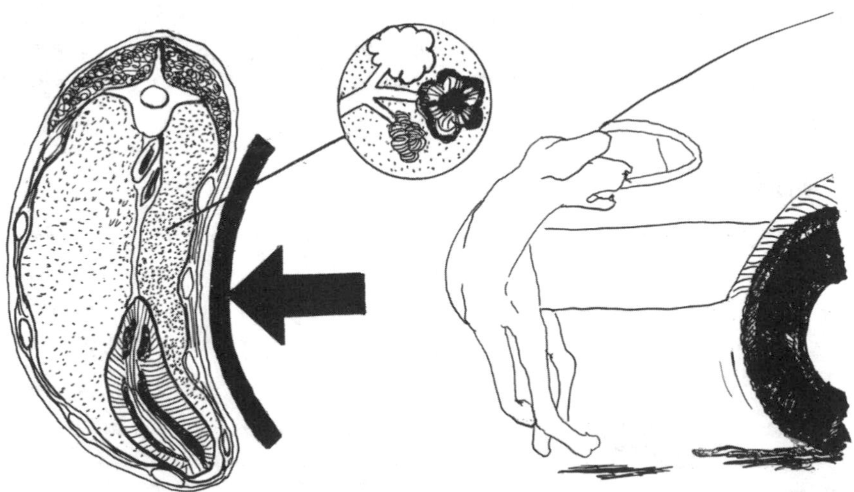

Figure 68-2
Effect of blunt trauma on pulmonary parenchyma. After blunt trauma, elastic recoil of the thoracic cage results in compression of the lung parenchyma, causing three types of injury: atelectasis, hemorrhage, and edema.

affected area becomes filled with fluid, interstitial lymphatic drainage is obstructed. Additionally, damage to lung tissue causes the release of arachidonic acid and lipoxygenase into the affected area. Arachidonic acid serves as a precursor for prostaglandin release leading to inflammation. Lipoxygenase serves as a chemotactic agent for neutrophils and macrophages. Once present, activated neutrophils and macrophages produce lysosomal enzymes and O_2 free radicals, further contributing to tissue injury.

The local tissue response to pulmonary contusion produces impaired O_2 and carbon dioxide (CO_2) diffusion due to an increased diffusion distance across the capillary alveolar membrane. In the early stage of injury, the body response to local vascular injury in the lungs is vasoconstriction. Vasoconstriction is mediated by local pulmonary hypoxia and the presence of vasoactive prostaglandins and leukotrienes.[29] The early effect of pulmonary vascular changes is decreased pulmonary alveolar perfusion, increasing V/Q mismatch. Later in injury, the influx of edema and inflammatory cells into lung interstitium causes a decrease in mechanical compliance of the injured area. Ventilation decreases, resulting in low V/Q mismatch and venous admixture of blood, producing hypoxemia. Progression of the injury can cause severe intrapulmonary shunting and is refractory to supplemental O_2 therapy. In severe cases, hypoxemia (PaO_2 <60 mm Hg), CO_2 retention ($PaCO_2$ >60 mm Hg), intrapulmonary shunting, and pulmonary hypertension with right-sided heart failure occurs.[3,30,31] Hypoxemia may be exacerbated by pain and hypoventilation.

Clinical Presentation

Clinical signs, including hemoptysis, respiratory distress, orthopnea, open-mouthed breathing, and cyanosis may be apparent on presentation, but become progressively worse over time. Physical examination findings include a rapid respiratory rate and moist rales plus increased adventitial sounds on thoracic auscultation.

Diagnostics

Radiography. Radiographic signs are often not apparent hours after injury. Radiographic signs usually develop over 4 to 6 hours after initial presentation.[32] Radiographic features include patchy interstitial and alveolar areas of lung. Depending on the degree of lung injury, the densities may be focal or diffuse in nature. Pulmonary contusion is often observed in combination with other injuries.

Arterial Blood Gas Analysis. The gold standard for determining the degree of respiratory damage is an arterial blood gas. Data obtained from an arterial blood gas can provide useful information regarding the patient's oxygenation (PaO_2) and ventilation ($PaCO_2$) status. Diffusion impairments, often associated with pulmonary contusions, can be evaluated using an alveolar-arterial oxygen gradient (A-a gradient) (Fig. 68-3).[33] Alveolar-arterial O_2 tension gradients can also be used to monitor progression of disease and response to therapy. If an

$A = [(\text{Barometric pressure} - \text{water vapor pressure})FiO_2 - PaCO_2/0.8] - a$

Where: water vapor pressure = 47
$FiO_2 = 0.21$ on room air
$PaCO_2$ = arterial CO_2 tension in mm Hg
0.8 = respiratory quotient
a = PaO_2 = arterial O_2 tension in mm Hg
A = alveolar oxygen tension

Criteria for acute respiratory distress syndrome (ARDS)[33]:
A-a = 0-10: normal
A-a = 10-20: mild impairment of O_2 exchange
A-a = 20-30: moderate impairment of O_2 exchange
A-a > 30: ARDS (severe impairment of O_2 exchange)

Figure 68-3
Calculation of alveolar-arterial O_2 tension gradient (A-a gradient).

arterial blood gas sample cannot be obtained or analyzed, pulse oximetry is a useful tool in determining oxygen status.

Treatment

O_2 Therapy. Animals with pulmonary contusion can rapidly decompensate and become hypoxemic. Hypoxemia is associated with V/Q mismatch, atelectasis, and intrapulmonary shunts. Mild cases of pulmonary contusion can benefit from supplemental O_2 administration via nasal insufflation, hood, or O_2 cage. More severe cases may require mechanical ventilation until the lung parenchyma has had time to heal (Table 68-3).

Fluid Therapy. Fluid therapy in pulmonary injury patients remains a controversial topic. Damage to lung parenchyma and associated capillary beds can allow leakage of crystalloid fluids into the pulmonary interstitial space. Impaired lymphatic drainage associated with tissue swelling and edema decreases removal of crystalloid fluid, thus worsening local edema and tissue function. The judicious use of colloids (*i.e.*, hetastarch) in combination with crystalloids may be used

Table 68-3. Indications for Mechanical Ventilation of the Trauma Patient

Altered level of mentation or unconsciousness
Occlusion of airway due to hemorrhage
Hypoventilation, with $PaCO_2$ >60 mm Hg
Minute volume <150 mL/kg/min
PaO_2 <60 mm Hg on supplemental O_2
Respiratory fatigue
Increased intracranial pressure
Change in mental status
Bradycardia with systemic hypertension following head trauma (Cushing reflex)

to improve tissue perfusion and help retain crystalloids within the vascular space. Ongoing monitoring of patient's respiratory rate and pattern, arterial blood gas analysis, pulse oximetry, arterial blood pressure, and electrocardiograph is essential for monitoring patient response.[3]

Controversial Therapies. A number of controversial therapies have been suggested in patients with pulmonary injury secondary to trauma.[1] The use of steroids has demonstrated equivocal results in numerous studies in both human and veterinary trauma patients.[37-39] Although some studies reported improved survival, others described reduced lung bacterial clearance. The use of steroids in pulmonary injury is not advocated at this time.

Bronchodilators have been recommended for pulmonary injury secondary to trauma. Aminophylline has pharmacologic action characterized by direct relaxation of pulmonary bronchial and vasculature smooth muscle.[26,40] Aminophylline may aid in decreasing the work of respiration by increasing force of diaphragmatic contraction, and has central actions characterized by stimulation of central respiratory centers.[41] However, because bronchoconstriction is not a major factor in the development of pulmonary contusion, the use of bronchodilator therapy probably is unwarranted and has not been proven to be beneficial.[3]

Antibiotics should be used only if bronchopneumonia develops secondary to pulmonary injury. Bronchopneumonia has been observed as a common sequela to pulmonary trauma in humans, but is not appreciated in veterinary medicine.[42] One retrospective study observed a 1% pneumonia rate in canine patients with pulmonary contusion.[28] Frequent turning and patient mobilization aids in preventing atelectasis and the development of pneumonia.

Prognosis

The prognosis for patients with pulmonary injury secondary to trauma largely depends on the degree of initial injury, presence of other injuries, and the hemodynamic status of the patient at the time of presentation.[3] In one retrospective study, the mortality of canine patients with pulmonary contusion was 7%.[3]

DAMAGE TO THE PLEURAL SPACE

Pneumothorax

Epidemiology

Pneumothorax is reported in 13% to 47% of patients with traumatic fractures.[43] Pneumothorax is defined as accumulation of free air within the pleural space. It is classified as open versus closed, depending if the body wall is disrupted from penetrating trauma. Open pneumothorax may be self-limiting if the rent in the thoracic wall is small relative to the size of the glottis, or can become life-threatening if the defect is large relative to the size of the glottis.[44] Closed pneumothorax can be simple and self-limiting or can become rapidly life-threatening in the form of a tension pneumothorax.

Pathophysiology

There are two theories regarding forces involved in creating pneumothorax secondary to trauma. The first theory is that the energy absorbed by the thoracic cage at the time of impact is transmitted to the lungs and causes a rapid compression of air. This results in a rapid, transient increase in airway pressure and shear force damage to the lung parenchyma, which causes air to leak and local tissue failure to occur. The rapid increase in air also causes implosion or rupture of alveoli, allowing air to escape from the lung parenchyma into the pleural space.[1] The second theory is that air and fluid have different densities. Tissues containing air and fluid at the level of the carina differ in their rates of acceleration and deceleration at the time of impact, creating shear forces that mechanically stretch and tear airways, allowing air to escape.[44] This is known as the spalling effect.[1]

The mildest form of pneumothorax is simple closed pneumothorax, in which a small amount of air escapes from the lungs at the time of injury separating the visceral and parietal pleura.[44] Closed pneumothorax typically results from blunt trauma causing mechanical disruption of the trachea, bronchi, pulmonary parenchyma, or esophagus.[24] Collapse of lung parenchyma results in a decrease in tidal volume proportional to the amount of free air within the thorax. Minute ventilation is maintained by a compensatory increase in respiratory rate. Dogs tolerate surprisingly large amounts of free air within their thorax; up to 150% of their calculated tidal volume, before demonstrating signs of respiratory distress.[45] Cardiac output remains unchanged in the face of small volumes of intrapleural air.[45]

In more severe cases of pneumothorax, progressive alveolar collapse produces regions of low V/Q balance and intrapulmonary shunting.[45] Pulmonary vasoconstriction occurs secondary to hypoxemia, which then leads to an increase in pulmonary vascular resistance. Severe, right-sided heart failure can develop, thus reducing cardiac output. Increased intrapleural pressure causes a collapsed venae cavae and impedes venous return to the heart, further decreasing cardiac output.

The most severe form of pneumothorax is a tension pneumothorax. Air escapes from the lungs into the pleural space during inspiration. During exhalation, the area of pulmonary leak collapses, producing a one-way flap, and air is prevented from escaping. The net result is severe trapping of free air within the pleural space. Rapid decline in respiratory function occurs, and the lungs become atelectatic. Increased intrapleural pressure eventually exceeds atmospheric pressure, causing collapse of the venae cavae, and decreased venous return to the right side of the heart.[44] This intensifies a decrease in cardiac output and hypoxemia.

Clinical Presentation

In most cases, the animal presents with few signs of respiratory distress. In more severe cases, the patient presents with a rapid shallow restrictive respiratory pattern. Patients with penetrating thoracic injuries have a sucking sound on

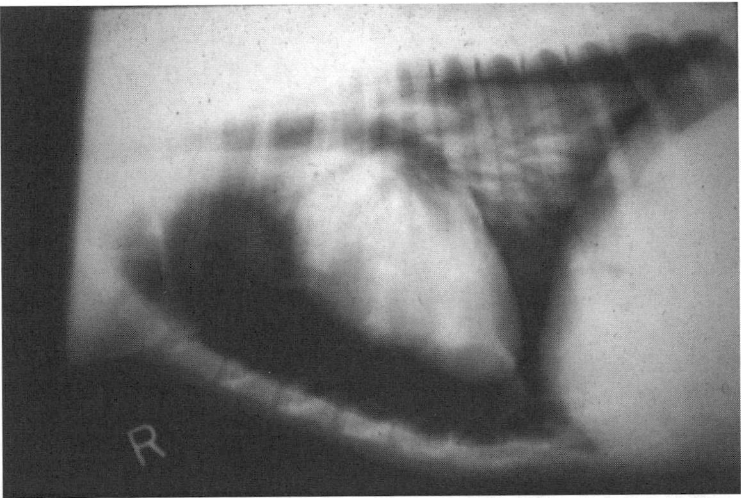

Figure 68-4
Radiograph of pneumothorax presents an example of severe pneumothorax in a dog. The heart is elevated away from the sternum. Lung lobes are atelectic and retracted away from the thoracic wall. Severe subcutaneous emphysema can also be observed.

inspiration as air moves into the thorax. Thoracic auscultation reveals muffled heart and lung sounds, particularly in the dorsocaudal lung fields. Percussion of the thorax will reveal a hyperresonant sound over areas of air accumulation.

Diagnostics

Diagnostic radiographs should only be performed once all systems have been addressed and the patient's condition is determined stabilized. Radiographic features include retraction of the lungs away from the thoracic wall, elevation of the heart away from the sternum on lateral views, and consolidation of the lung parenchyma (Fig. 68-4).

Treatment

Treatment of an open pneumothorax involves placement of a water and airtight seal over the defect, and placing a thoracic drain to keep the pleural space evacuated.[44] The thoracic wound is temporarily closed using a gloved finger or sterile glove. Sterile water-based lubricating gel (K-Y) should be placed over the wound and the overlying fur quickly clipped from the area. Next, the area should receive a quick aseptic scrub. Sterile water-resistant gel is placed *around* the wound and a piece of sterile glove placed over the wound, creating a water and air-tight seal. For a more permanent seal of the thoracic wound, petroleum jelly-impregnated gauze squares are placed over the thoracic wound. A thoracic drain should then be placed to keep the thorax evacuated. Following patient

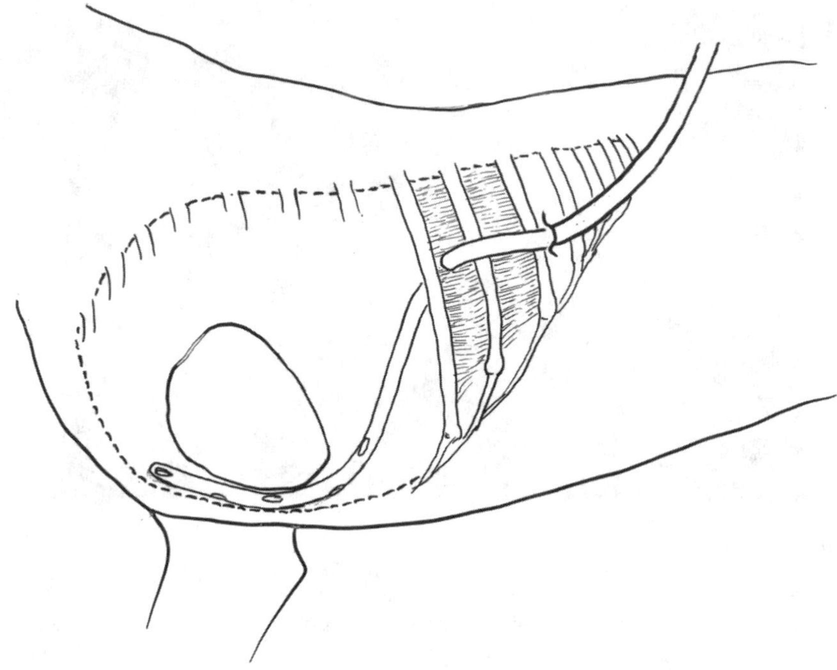

Figure 68-5
Correct placement of a thoracic drain. Following routine aseptic preparation of the skin and injection of local anesthetic, a stab incision is made in the skin at the level of the 10th to12th intercostal space. A trochar is directed cranially, creating a subcutaneous tunnel to the level of the 5th to 7th intercostal space. The trochar then penetrates the intercostal muscles into the pleural space. The thoracic drain is then directed cranioventrally off of the trochar to the 3rd intercostal space. The drain is connected to a closed connection system and secured to the body wall with horizontal mattress and purse-string sutures.

stabilization, the open wound should be surgically explored and debrided of devitalized tissue and debris.

Immediate thoracic drainage via thoracocentesis is necessary with life-threatening pneumothorax. Treatment for simple pneumothorax requires bilateral thoracic drainage (see Fig. 68-1). It was previously thought that the mediastinum in small animals had small fenestrations and freely communicated from side to side. However, the mediastinal tissues may not communicate; therefore, bilateral thoracocentesis after blunt trauma is necessary. In some cases, very little air will be trapped on one side of the thorax, and extremely large amount of air will be found on the other. Therefore, always tap both sides of the thorax in patients with suspected pneumothorax. Placement of a thoracic drain may be necessary if negative pressure cannot be obtained, or if the patient requires frequent thoracocentesis (Fig. 68-5). Immediate thoracic drainage is necessary with life-threatening tension pneumothorax.

Prognosis

The prognosis for pneumothorax is good if diagnosed and managed early in the disease course. Repeated thoracocentesis or continuous air leak following chest drain placement suggests a less favorable resolution. The presence of respiratory difficulty and the need for thoracocentesis are negative prognostic indicators in one retrospective study of veterinary patients with pneumothorax.[43]

Hemothorax

Pathophysiology

Massive hemothorax is uncommon in dogs and cats.[46] In most cases, rupture of the great vessels is a diagnosis made at necropsy because many patients do not survive this type of injury. However, bleeding from smaller arteries such as the intercostal or internal thoracic arteries can be self-limiting.

Clinical Presentation

Clinical signs of hemothorax are identical to those of pneumothorax. Patients will present with a rapid shallow respiratory pattern consistent with a restrictive breathing pattern. Mucous membranes may be pale with a prolonged capillary refill time. Auscultation of the thorax will reveal muffled heart and lung sounds.

Diagnostics

Thoracocentesis reveals the presence of bloody fluid that does not clot within the pleural space. Very large volumes of blood within the pleural space (typically 50–60 mL/kg) are required before respiratory difficulty becomes apparent.[24] Removal of the blood is *unnecessary* in the treatment of hemothorax secondary to trauma unless severe respiratory compromise is noted.

Treatment

Treatment of hemothorax involves rapid infusion of crystalloid fluids or blood products. Hypotensive small-volume resuscitation is advocated for some patients with hemothorax, pulmonary contusions, and head trauma.[31] If more than 10 mL/kg of blood is present within the pleural space secondary to trauma, autotransfusion may be required.[47] If the patient remains unresponsive to medical management, exploratory thoracotomy may be required.[7,48]

Prognosis

Many animals with hemothorax secondary to laceration of the heart, venae cavae, or aorta do not survive transport to the hospital and have a grave prognosis. Stabilized hemothorax has a guarded to good prognosis.

Diaphragmatic Hernia

Epidemiology

About 80% to 85% of diaphragmatic hernias are trauma associated.[49,50] Approximately half of diaphragmatic tears are found on the right side of the diaphragm; 37% are on the left side of the diaphragm. In 4% of cases, multiple tears are present. 38% of cases have concurrent thoracic trauma.[50] However, almost 50% of patients with diaphragmatic hernia have no other apparent injuries.[50]

Pathophysiology

During normal respiration, the glottis remains closed and the lungs remain inflated, both of which counteract changes in intrapleural and intra-abominal pressure gradients. When blunt force, such as during trauma, is applied to the abdomen, the glottis no longer remains closed. This, combined with tense abdominal musculature, results in a large peritoneal-pleural pressure gradient.[49] The majority of the applied force is directed cranially toward the diaphragm, resulting in diaphragmatic rupture at the weakest point.[50] Sliding of peritoneal contents into the thorax depends on the location and size of the rent in the diaphragm. Organs that commonly traverse diaphragmatic hernias include the liver, spleen, small intestine, stomach, and greater omentum.[50]

The presence of abdominal viscera in the thorax decreases both functional lung capacity and cardiac output. Pulmonary compression reduces the number of alveoli available for gas exchange, resulting in areas of low ventilation and hypoxia. Further, other alveoli may become overventilated, resulting in areas of low perfusion.[49] Both result in a decrease in PaO_2. The hypoxemia often worsens due to concurrent pulmonary parenchymal damage, thoracic wall trauma, and pneumothorax.[50] Abdominal viscera within the thorax compress the great vessels such as the venae cavae, resulting in impeded venous return to the right heart, leading to a decrease in cardiac output.[49] This is further complicated in many cases by hemorrhage or hypovolemia.

Clinical Presentation

Clinical signs of diaphragmatic hernia are not pathognomonic. The most common presenting sign is respiratory difficulty, which may resolve with thoracic elevation. The animal may be uncomfortable and develop increased respiratory distress when forced to lie down. Thoracic auscultation reveals muffled lung sounds. Intestinal borborygmi are heard if air-filled intestinal loops are present. Percussion reveals tympanic sounds if gastric entrapment is present. In some cases, cardiac auscultation will reveal increased heart sounds if the heart is displaced laterally within the thorax. The patient's abdomen may appear tucked up and have few structures palpable. Some animals present with gastrointestinal signs such as vomiting undigested food.

Diagnostics

Radiography is the most informative tool to diagnose diaphragmatic hernia. Plain radiographs may reveal the presence of air-filled or soft-tissue densities within the thorax. The heart, lungs, or trachea may be compressed and displaced. The normal contour of the diaphragmatic crura may be absent or not easily visualized. If the rent in the diaphragm is small, or if abdominal viscera freely slide through the diaphragmatic rent, plain radiography may not reveal any abnormalities. The presence of abdominal or thoracic effusion may make visualization of normal structures difficult. In such instances, contrast studies are warranted. A positive contrast gastrogram with barium sulfate can reveal gastrointestinal structures within the thorax. A negative result does not necessarily rule out the presence of a sliding hernia. Contrast gastrography will not reveal if the liver, spleen, or greater omentum are present within the thorax. Positive contrast celiography or double-contrast celiography can also be used to diagnose diaphragmatic hernia.[51]

Treatment

Initial treatment involves stabilization of the patient with fluid support to correct hypovolemia, thoracocentesis to improve ventilation if pneumothorax is present, O_2 to improve oxygenation, and analgesic agents to treat discomfort and pain. Definitive treatment of diaphragmatic hernia is surgical intervention.[50,53,54] If the patient's condition cannot be stabilized, immediate surgical intervention is necessary, particularly if the stomach is entrapped within the thorax or if necrotic viscera are present. General anesthesia in patients with diaphragmatic hernia is often challenging due to hypoxemia, severe V/Q mismatching, hypovolemia, poor cardiac output and hypotension, and the presence of concurrent complicating injuries. Drugs that suppress ventilation or increase heart rate should be avoided.[52,53]

Prognosis

Prognosis for any patient with a diaphragmatic hernia is guarded. The majority of deaths occur within a 24-hour period after surgery.[50,54] The presence of diaphragmatic hernia with concurrent thoracic trauma dramatically increases the incidence of mortality.[55] Usually, death occurs secondary to multiorgan dysfunction.

DAMAGE TO THE THORACIC WALL

Rib Fractures

Pathophysiology

Rib fractures may be noted following any traumatic event. The biomechanics of rib fracture are similar to other diaphysial bones. In general, the structure and support of ribs permit a greater force application prior to fracture injury. It is important to remember that the lung underlying a fractured rib absorbs a significant portion of concussive force generated during the trauma event. Any force severe enough to fracture ribs will cause damage to the underlying lung parenchyma. Whenever a diagnosis of rib fracture is made, the clinician should anticipate the development of pulmonary contusions.

Hypoxemia associated with rib fractures is associated with both damage to the lung parenchyma and pulmonary contusion, with the pain of the fracture causing hypoventilation. Pain associated with rib fractures causes restriction of respiration by reluctance to fully expand the thorax during inspiration.[56] This results in hypoventilation, which can exacerbate hypoxemia secondary to other concurrent thoracic injuries such as pneumothorax or pulmonary contusion.[56,57]

Diagnostics

Open rib fractures may readily be apparent on initial physical examination. In the cases of isolated rib fractures, most are initially overlooked on presentation and are discovered as "incidental" findings on thoracic radiographs once the patient is stabilized.[4]

Treatment

In most cases, rib fractures can be conservatively managed, unless the fractured segment causes continuous trauma to the lung parenchyma.[24] Conservative management of simple rib fractures typically involves supplying supplemental O_2 and to improve ventilation with careful administration of analgesics. Both systemic and local analgesics should be considered. Low-dose morphine (0.25 mg/kg SQ qid) or constant rate infusions of fentanyl (1–5 μg/kg/h) have dramatic analgesic properties without impairing ventilation. Local infusion of lidocaine (total dose 1–2 mg/kg, diluted to a sufficient volume to deliver 0.5 mL at each injection site) and bupivacaine (total dose 1–2 mg/kg, diluted to a volume sufficient to deliver 0.5 mL at each injection site) at the caudal portion of the rib, both dorsal and ventral to the fracture, will provide analgesia and cause marked improvement of ventilation by alleviating patient discomfort.[59]

Flail Chest

Pathophysiology

Flail chest is a severe form of rib fracture in which two or more contiguous ribs are fractured in both a dorsal and ventral location on the same rib thereby causing a freely moving segment of body wall.[60] Previously it was thought that the paradoxical motion of the chest wall resulted in a "to and fro" movement of air within bronchi increasing dead space ventilation, reducing the vital capacity and compliance, and increasing resistance to airflow thus increasing the work of breathing.[56,58,60] The paradoxical motion is now thought to decrease tidal volume. Hypoxemia is more often caused by the underlying pulmonary contusion rather than by the paradoxical motion of the flail segment itself.[1,39]

Treatment

Decreasing pain associated with the flail segment dramatically reduces the work of breathing in patients without the need for surgical intervention.[57,61,62] Local infusion of lidocaine (1–2 mg/kg diluted to a volume sufficient to deliver 0.5 mL at each injection site) or 0.5% bupivacaine (0.5 mL at each injection site) at the caudal border of each fractured rib, above and below each fracture site, and at the caudal borders of the rib cranial to and caudal to the flail segment, will decrease the patient's pain. In many cases, patients with flail chest can be managed conservatively. However, more severe cases have severe underlying pathology and require aggressive treatment, including mechanical ventilation or exploratory thoracotomy. Mechanical stabilization of the flail segment with both internal and external fixation devices has been recommended.[57,60,61] Surgical intervention is warranted only in the most severe cases of flail chest. Criteria for surgical intervention include fractures involving more than five contiguous ribs, flail chest in combination with open pneumothorax, or fracture segments creating continued damage to the underlying tissues.

Prognosis

The prognosis for patients with simple rib fractures and flail chest is good, provided that other severe injuries are not present. Because cost of care is a frequent consideration in veterinary medicine, mortality may be increased in such cases when treatment cost is prohibitive.[56]

REFERENCES

1. Berkwitt L, Berzon JL: Thoracic trauma—newer concepts. *Vet Clin North Am Small Anim Pract* 15:1031, 1985.
2. Kolata RJ, Kraut NH, Johnston DE: Patterns of trauma in urban dogs and cats: a study of 1000 cases. *J Am Vet Med Assoc* 164:499, 1974.
3. Hackner SG: Emergency management of traumatic pulmonary contusions. *Compend Contin Educ Pract Vet* 17:677, 1995.
4. Selcer BA, Buttrick M, Barstad R: The incidence of thoracic trauma in dogs with skeletal injury. *J Small Anim Pract* 28:21, 1987.
5. Tamas PM, Paddleford RR, Krahwinkel DJ: Thoracic trauma in dogs and cats presented for limb fractures. *J Am Anim Hosp Assoc* 21:161, 1985.
6. Spackman CJ, Caywood DD, Feeney DA, *et al.*: Thoracic wall and pulmonary trauma in dogs sustaining fractures as a result of motor vehicle accidents. *J Am Vet Med Assoc* 185:975, 1984.
7. Davidson EB: Managing bite wounds in dogs and cats: part I. *Compend Contin Educ Pract Vet* 20:811, 1998.
8. Kolata, RJ: Management of thoracic trauma. *Vet Clin North Am Small Anim Pract* 11:103, 1981.
9. Kolata RJ: Trauma in dogs and cats: an overview. *Vet Clin North Am Small Anim Pract* 10:515, 1980.
10. Holt DE, Griffin G: Bite wounds in dogs and cats. *Vet Clin North Am Small Anim Pract* 30:669, 2000.

11. Waldron DR, Trevor P: Management of superficial skin wounds. *In* D. Slatter, ed.: Textbook of Small Animal Surgery. Philadelphia, WB Saunders, 1993, p 269.
12. McKiernan BC, Adama WM, Huse DC: Thoracic bite wounds and associated internal injury in 11 dogs and 1 cat. *J Am Vet Med Assoc* 184:959, 1984.
13. Marks SL: Nasal oxygen insufflation. *J Am Anim Hosp Assoc* 35:366, 1999.
14. Cowell AK, Penwick RC: Dog bite wounds: a study of 93 cases. *J Compen Contin Educ Pract Vet* 11:313, 1989.
15. Fullington RJ, Otto CM: Characteristics and management of gunshot wounds in dogs and cats: 84 cases (1986–1995). *J Am Vet Med Assoc* 210:658, 1997.
16. Adkins RB, Whiteneck JM, Woltering EA: Penetrating chest wall and thoracic injuries. *Am Surg* 51:140, 1985.
17. Grimes WR, Deitch EA, McDonald JC: A clinical review of shotgun wounds to the chest and abdomen. *Surg Gynecol Obstet* 160:148, 1985.
18. Lawrence DT, Lang J, Culvenor J, *et al.*: Intrathoracic tracheal rupture. *J Feline Med Surg* 1:43, 1999.
19. Brouwer GJ, Burbidge HM, Jones DE: Tracheal rupture in a cat. *J Small Anim Pract* 25:71, 1984.
20. Feeney DA: What is your diagnosis? *J Am Vet Med Assoc* 175:303, 1979.
21. White RN, Milner HR: Intrathoracic tracheal avulsion in three cats. *J Small Anim Pract* 36:343, 1995.
22. Hardie EM, Spodnick GJ, Gilson SD, *et al.*: Tracheal rupture in cats: 16 cases (1983–1998). *J Am Vet Med Assoc* 214:508, 1999.
23. Manning MM, Brunson DB: Barotrauma in a cat. *J Am Vet Med Assoc* 205:62, 1994.
24. Ludwig, LL: Surgical emergencies of the respiratory system. *Vet Clin North Am Small Anim Pract* 30:531, 2000.
25. Oppenheimer L, Craven KD, Forkert L, *et al.*: Pathophysiology of pulmonary contusion in dogs. *J Appl Physiol* 47:718, 1979.
26. Jones KW: Thoracic trauma. *Surg Clin North Am* 60:957, 1980.
27. Cohn SM: Pulmonary contusion: review of the clinical entity. *J Trauma* 42:973, 1977.
28. Powell LL, Rozanski EA, Tidwell AD, *et al.*: A retrospective analysis of pulmonary contusion secondary to motor vehicle accidents in 143 dogs: 1994–1997. *J Vet Emerg Crit Care* 9:127, 1999.
29. Wagner RB, Slivko B, Jamieson PM, *et al.*: Effect of lung contusion o pulmonary hemodynamics. *Ann Thorac Surg* 52:51, 1991.
30. Fulton RL, Peter ET: The progressive nature of pulmonary contusion. *Surgery* 67: 499, 1970.
31. Zapol WM, Snider MT: Pulmonary hypertension in severe acute respiratory failure. *N Engl J Med* 296:476, 1977.
32. Erickson DR, Shinozaki T, Beekman E, *et al.*: Relationship of arterial blood gases and pulmonary radiographs to the degree of pulmonary damage in experimental pulmonary contusion. *J Trauma* 11:689, 1971.
33. VanPelt DR, Wingfield WE, Wheeler SL, *et al.*: Oxygen-tension based indices as predictors of survival in critically ill dogs: clinical observations and review. *J Vet Emerg Crit Care* 1:19, 1991.
34. Kirby R, Rudloff E: Fluid therapy for the trauma patient. *In* Emergency Care of Trauma Patients, 22nd Annual Waltham Symposium for the Treatment of Small Animal Diseases, 1998, p 44.
35. Thijs LG: Fluid therapy in septic shock. *In* Sibbald WJ, Vincent JL, eds.: Clinical Trials for the Treatment of Sepsis. Berlin: Springer Verlag, 1995, p 167.

36. Bickell WH, Wall MJ, Pepe PE, *et al.*: Immediate versus delayed fluid resuscitation for hypotensive patients with penetrating torso injuries. *N Engl J Med* 331:1105, 1994.
37. Franz JL, Richardson JD, Grover FL, *et al.*: Effect of methylprednisolone sodium succinate on experimental pulmonary contusion. *J Thorac Cardiovasc Surg* 68:842, 1974.
38. Svennevig LG, Bugge-Asperheim B, Bjorgo S, *et al.*: Methylprednisone in the treatment of lung contusion following blunt chest trauma. *Scand J Thorac Cardiovasc Surg* 14:301, 1980.
39. Trinkle JK, Furman RW, Hinshaw MA, *et al.*: Pulmonary contusions—pathogenesis and effect of various resuscitation measures. *Ann Thorac Surg* 16:568, 1973.
40. Crowe DT: Traumatic pulmonary contusions, hematomas, pseudocysts, and acute respiratory distress syndrome. Part I. *Compend Contin Educ Pract Vet* 5:396, 1983.
41. Plumb DC: Aminophylline/theophylline. *In* Veterinary Drug Handbook, 3rd ed. Ames, IA: Iowa State University Press,1999, p 23.
42. Antonelli M, Moro ML, Capelli O: Risk factors for early onset of pneumonia in trauma patients. *Chest* 105:224, 1994.
43. Krahwinkel DJ, Rohrbach BW, Hollis BA: Factors associated with survival in dogs and cats with pneumothorax. *J Vet Emerg Crit Care* 9:7, 1999.
44. Kagan KG: Thoracic trauma. *Vet Clin North Am Small Anim Pract* 10:641, 1980.
45. Bennett RA, Orton EC, Tucker A, *et al.*: Cardiopulmonary changes in conscious dogs with induced progressive pneumothorax. *Am J Vet Res* 50:280, 1989.
46. Brasmer TH: A is for Airway. *In* Piermatti D, ed.: Major Problems in Veterinary Medicine. Vol 2. The Acutely Traumatized Patient. Philadelphia, WB Saunders, 1984, p 85.
47. Crowe DT: Surgical management of thoracic trauma. *I:* Proceedings of the 7th Annual American College of Veterinary Surgeons Symposium, Lake Buena Vista, FL, 1997, p 321.
48. August JR: Dog and cat bites. *J Am Vet Med Assoc* 193:1394, 1988.
49. Levine SH: Diaphragmatic hernia. *Vet Clin North Am Small Anim Pract* 17:411, 1987.
50. Wilson GP III, Hayes HM Jr: Diaphragmatic hernia in the dog and cat: a 25 year overview. *Semin Vet Med Surg Small Anim* 1:318, 1986.
51. Stickle RL: Positive-contrast celiography (peritoneography) for the diagnosis of diaphragmatic hernia in dogs and cats. *J Am Vet Med Assoc* 185:295, 1984.
52. Bednarski RM: Diaphragmatic hernia: anesthetic considerations. *Semin Vet Med Surg Small Anim* 1:256, 1986.
53. Wilson DV: Anesthesia for patients with diaphragmatic hernia and severe dyspnea. *Vet Clin North Am Small Anim Pract* 22:456, 1992.
54. Wilson GP III, Newton CD, Burt JK: A review of 116 diaphragmatic hernias in dogs and cats. *J Am Vet Med Assoc* 159:1142, 1971.
54. DeHoff WD, Greene RW, Greiner TP: Surgical management of abdominal emergencies. *Vet Clin North Am Small Anim Pract* 2:301, 1972.
55. Kraje BJ, Kraje AC, Rohrbach BW, *et al.*: Intrathoracic and concurrent orthopedic injury associated with traumatic rib fracture in cats: 75 cases (1980–1998). *J Am Vet Med Assoc* 216:51, 2000.
56. Anderson M, Payne JT, Mann FA, *et al.*: Flail chest: pathophysiology, treatment and prognosis. *Compend Contin Educ Pract Vet* 15:65, 1993.
57. Hunt CA: Chest trauma?p007,179?the approach to the patient with chest injuries. *Compend Contin Educ Pract Vet* 1:537, 1979.

58. Maloney JV, Schmutzer KJ, Raschke E: paradoxical respiration and pendelluft. *J Thorac Cardiovasc Surg* 41:291, 1961.
59. Mazzaferro EM: Respiratory emergencies. *In* Wingfield WE, ed.: Veterinary Emergency Medicine Secrets, 2nd ed. Philadelphia: Hanley & Belfus, 2000, p 60.
60. McAnulty JF: A simplified method for stabilization of flail chest injuries in small animals. *J Am Anim Hosp Assoc* 31:137, 1995.
61. Bjorling DE, Kolata RJ, DeNovo RC: Flail chest: review, clinical experience, and new method of stabilization. *J Am Anim Hosp Assoc* 18:269, 1982.
62. Thompson SE, Johnson JM: Analgesia in dogs after intercostal thoracotomy: a comparison of morphine, selective intercostal nerve block, and intrapleural regional analgesia with bupivacaine. *Vet Surg* 20:73, 1991.

69
Penetrating Wounds

Michael M. Pavletic

INTRODUCTION

By definition, a *penetrating wound* is one that enters the interior of an organ or cavity. A *perforating wound* is one that enters and exits a given organ or cavity. For the purposes of this chapter, both types of wounds are discussed, because each can occur with the various forms of trauma noted in the veterinary small animal patient.

COMMON TYPES OF PENETRATING WOUNDS

Bite wounds are the most common penetrating wounds noted in veterinary small animal practice. Other penetrating/perforating wounds include projectile wounds (bullets, pellets, arrows), stab wounds (knives, pointed weapons), impalement wounds (sticks, fencing, metallic objects), and migrating objects (plant awns, wood fragments, grass fragments, porcupine quills).

GENERAL FACTORS INFLUENCING THE SEVERITY OF PENETRATING WOUNDS

Energy is imparted to tissues during penetration by a foreign object. In the case of projectile injuries, the velocity and mass of the propelled object, and the tissues affected, will heavily influence the severity of trauma to the patient. This is especially evident when bone is hit by a powerful projectile. The bone absorbs a large portion of the kinetic energy of the bullet. Bone is shattered and fragments of bone are driven into the adjacent tissues. Additional energy is released to the tissues adjacent to the projectile's pathway (cavitation). Frangible projectiles also enhance soft-tissue injury by scattering fragments into the regional tissues.[1]

Bite wounds also can result in massive tissue destruction. Depending on the size of the animals involved, and the body regions attacked, the canine teeth can penetrate deep into the body. Tissues can be torn from the struggle that ensues. Energy also is absorbed as tissues are crushed by the compressive force of the jaws. Circulatory compromise to the tissues, tissue trauma, and contamination from virulent bacteria residing in the oral cavity can result in life-threatening infection.[1,2]

Penetrating objects contaminate tissues not only from topical bacteria and debris on their surface, but also by "dragging" skin surface contaminants into the wound tract. Higher velocity projectiles also create a transient negative pressure during passage, which is capable of sucking contaminants from the entry and exit wounds.[1,2]

Retention of plant material is particularly problematic. For example, penetrating sticks may fragment in the tissues planes. Unless this debris is removed by the surgical exploration of the penetrating wound, the retained plant material commonly will result in recurrent abscess formation, migrating foreign bodies, and draining tracts associated with their retention.[1]

PENETRATING WOUNDS: PERTINENT CLINICAL QUESTIONS

Answers to specific questions pertaining to penetrating wounds will assist the clinician in determining the nature of the injury and what steps are required to care for the patient. These questions include:

1. What was the cause of the penetrating wound?
2. What tissues and body regions are (or possibly are) involved?
3. Is there any portion of the penetrating object retained?
4. When did the injury occur?

The exact characteristics and composition of the penetrating object, the area of impact, and the time between injury and presentation to the hospital are factors that will help determine the appropriate methods of wound management. A detailed history and complete physical examination serve as the "clinical baseline" for the patient. Additional diagnostic tests are often indicated to better assess the (1) nature of the injury, (2) location of a retained object, (3) status of the patient, and (4) selection of the appropriate treatment for the injuries incurred.

Diagnostic Tests

Plain radiographs, contrast studies, ultrasonography, computed tomography (CT), and magnetic resonance imaging (MRI) can be used for noninvasive evaluation of the patient sustaining a penetrating wound. In general, plain radiographs are used to screen a body area to locate retained (radiopaque) penetrating objects. They also are used to assess the condition of regional skeletal tissues, joints, and the thoracic and abdominal cavities for the presence of air/fluid. Contrast fistulograms can be used to assess the course of a draining tract associated with a retained (chronic) foreign body. Occasionally, the injected contrast material will outline the silhouette of a radiolucent object, such as a retained wood fragment. Ultrasound, CT, and MRI can be used to better locate problematic retained foreign bodies and any associated abscess cavity.[1,2] Suspected injuries to the urinary tract can be assessed by lower urinary contrast studies or intravenous pyelography to assess the integrity of the kidneys and ureters.

MANAGEMENT OF SPECIFIC PENETRATING WOUNDS

Urgent/emergent patients will necessarily require immediate medical/surgical attention. In the case of simple penetrating wounds confined to the skin, hypodermis, and underlying soft tissues, surgical cleansing and surgical exploration may be used as a diagnostic and therapeutic approach to the wound. In many acute injuries, radiographs may be followed by exploratory surgery to directly examine injured tissues, remove accessible foreign debris and necrotic tissue, and repair damaged structures.

Bite Wounds

The severity of bite wounds depends on several factors including the size of the attacking animal, the shape and length of the contacting teeth, the size of the injured patient, the area bitten (presence of vital structures, profile of the area bitten), and the amount of energy absorbed. Large predators are capable of grasping large areas of the body. Their mouth may completely envelop large portions of the victimized animal, resulting in massive internal injuries that may not be recognizable on the initial patient examination[1,2] (Fig. 69-1).

In most carnivores, the canine teeth are primarily designed for deep tissue penetration. Larger dogs are capable of generating 450 psi, a crushing force capable of inflicting massive tissue trauma. Circulatory compromise to crushed tissues can result in large areas of tissue necrosis; the severity of tissue injury may not be apparent for up to a week after injury.[1,2]

In smaller predators (the domestic cat), the straight, needle-like teeth can readily penetrate regional tissues. Although the crushing forces generated by a pet cat are not particularly imposing to other cats and dogs, the stiletto-like penetration and local laceration of tissues commonly predisposes the site to infection.[1,2]

Not all bite wounds necessarily result in a penetrating wound. Firm structures located beneath the skin can be punctured, lacerated, and crushed without the presence of an overlying cutaneous puncture wound. Careful palpation of the bite area may alert the clinician to tears and holes to these underlying tissues.[1,2]

Aerobic and anaerobic bacteria that commonly reside in the mouth gain direct access to the body through the penetrating wounds. Tissue trauma punctuated by circulatory compromise form a perfect medium for infection, unless prompt medical/surgical management is instituted.[1,2]

Management Considerations

A complete physical examination is indicated. If a small patient has been lifted and shaken violently, serious internal injuries may be present that are not directly associated with the bite wounds (indirect trauma). A small dog or cat grasped over the lumbar area by a larger animal may have spinal trauma, renal trauma, or traumatic hernias that may be overlooked without close assessment.

Many of the bite wounds seen in a general veterinary practice are comparatively minor wounds with penetration limited to the skin and underlying hypodermal tissues. (This may be a more typical presentation for domestic cat bite

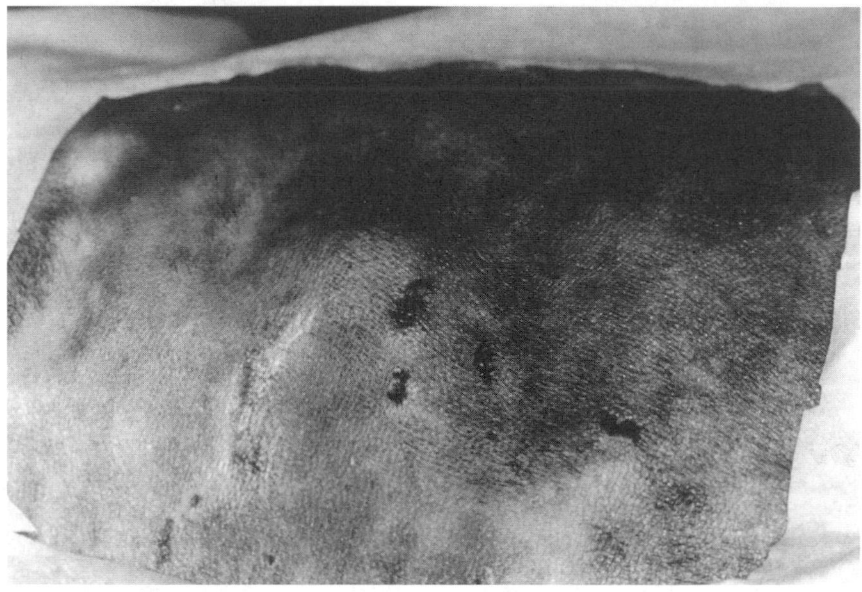

(A)

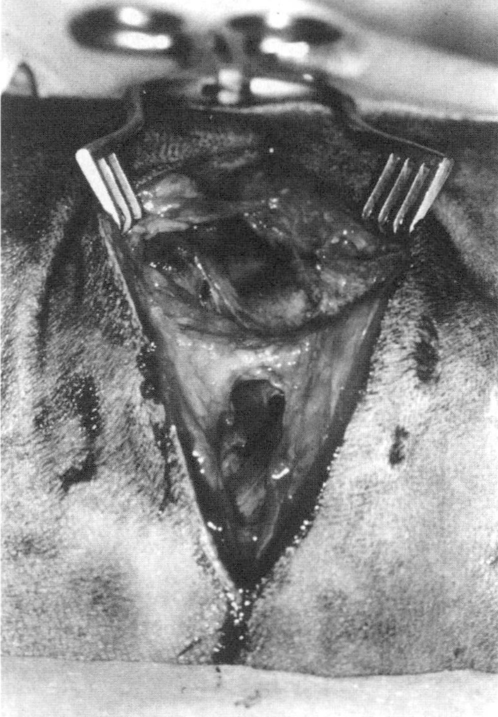

(B)

Figure 69-1
(**A**) Thoracic bite wound. (**B**) The skin was incised, revealing massive soft tissue trauma and a flail chest.

wounds inflicted on another cat or dog.) Many of these wounds may be managed with basic wound care and the prompt administration of a broad-spectrum antibiotic. However, the severity of the underlying tissue trauma can be masked by the comparatively minor appearance of the overlying skin. Practitioners who overlook the more severe nature of these bite wounds can place the patient at serious risk of infection. Clearly, the early institution of the appropriate surgical and medical care can preclude many of the serious complications associated with traumatic bite wounds. To prevent this mistake, a "conservative exploratory" should be considered for most penetrating bite wounds.[1,2]

Temporary Care and the Management of Minor Bite Wounds

Temporary wound care is directed at gently cleaning and protecting the open wound until more definitive wound care can be initiated. Minor bite wounds can be managed in a similar fashion.[1,2]

1. The appropriate use of analgesics will reduce the patient's pain and anxiety before the wounds are cleaned. Lidocaine can be injected around the wound margins to further reduce discomfort during manipulation of the injured area.
2. Puncture and laceration wounds can be temporarily covered with sterile surgical gauze before clipping hair liberally around the traumatized area.
3. Warm sterile saline with the addition of an antimicrobial agent (0.05% chlohexidene solution in 1:40 dilution; 1% povidone iodine solution in 1:9 dilution) may be used both to clean the skin around the immediate area and lavage the wound.
4. Small puncture wounds can be slightly enlarged by trimming the cutaneous margins with a scalpel blade. Slight enlargement of the constricted site will allow the surgeon to better inspect the wound with sterile forceps while facilitating wound lavage. Enlargement of the skin wound also will help to ensure egress of the above solution. Use of an 18-gauge needle and 35-mL syringe is a simple method of pressure lavaging the immediate area. Copious lavage is preferable.
5. A topical antimicrobial ointment can be applied to the wounds, followed by a dressing and outer protective bandage.
6. Broad-spectrum antibiotics should be administered intravenously at presentation in patients with serious bite wound trauma.

Definitive Wound Management

When warranted, definitive wound exploration and repair almost invariably require general anesthesia. Fur should be liberally clipped from the areas to be explored. Bite wounds involving the abdominal/thoracic cavities will require exploration. It must be remembered that the soft, pliable abdominal wall can collapse under the compressive forces of a large, attacking dog. As a result, seemingly short canine teeth can penetrate to the deeper organs from the compressive forces generated by the jaws of a large predator. Penetrating abdominal wounds require a mandatory exploratory laparotomy.[1,2]

Definitive bite wound care would include:

1. Sterile technique is used in all aspects of wound care.
2. Puncture wounds can be uncapped using a scalpel blade to create a 1.0-cm or larger circular opening. Mosquito hemostats can be inserted and opened, serving as a speculum to assess the underlying tissues. If warranted, an incision can be made over the wound for better examination, debridement, and repair. The incision can be extended to an adjacent puncture wound to facilitate the simultaneous management of both wounds. Understanding the general location of major direct cutaneous arteries can help preclude accidental division of these vessels that may be essential to survival of compromised skin.
3. Debridement of hair, tissue debris, and necrotic tissue from the wound site. Expendable muscle tissues, in which viability is questionable, may also be resected. Thoracic wall injuries must be prepared for the possibility that a thoracotomy may be required. Tears to the intercostal musculature may not be readily apparent; during the management of thoracic wall injuries, any "sucking sound" should alert the clinician to air entering the thoracic cavity, necessitating prompt ventilation, pleural space evacuation by thoracocentesis, or the temporary insertion of a thoracostomy tube.
4. Skin viability occasionally is difficult to determine after bite wound trauma. Necrosis may not be evident for 5 to 7 days after injury. If loose skin is present at the site of injury, aggressive debridement may be performed to help prevent the need for additional surgical debridement at a later date. However, a more conservative "wait and reassess" approach is advisable for extremity wounds when skin viability is questionable. The limited skin available on the lower extremities would preclude aggressive debridement unless skin clearly is identified as dead.
5. Wound drainage is essential in bite wound management. The presence of contamination, dead space, and compromised tissues increases the risk of infection unless drainage is established. Vacuum drains, Penrose drains, and, in some situations, open wound management (delayed primary closure, secondary closure, second intention healing) are options for establishing appropriate drainage. Vacuum drains are particularly useful in managing wounds where the use of Penrose drains would be ineffective or contraindicated.

Other Considerations in Bite Wound Management

The head and neck are commonly attacked by predators. The neck is particularly susceptible to serious trauma based on its comparatively narrow silhouette and concentration of vital structures. Of immediate concern are those patients with upper respiratory trauma. Bite wounds to the pharyngeal area may result in laryngeal obstruction as a result of the accumulation of blood, saliva, edema, and crushing of tissues. An emergency tracheotomy may be advisable. It must be kept in mind that tears to the trachea can provide an easy access for temporary tube insertion.[1,2]

The prompt administration of antibiotic therapy (within 1-3 hours of injury) will help reduce the likelihood of infection, when combined with appropriate surgical/medical management of the bite wound patient sustaining significant trauma. Cephalosporins, ampicillin, and penicillin enter the wound within 1 hour. If infection is already present at the time the patient is presented, aerobic and anaerobic cultures are advisable. Representative samples can be obtained from deep within the infected wound by aspiration or at the time of surgical management.[1,2]

Stab Wounds

Although stab wounds from knives or pointed objects (ice picks, sharpened screw drivers, etc.) are uncommon in animals, the author has seen several cases over an extended period of clinical practice. Single- or double-edged cutting blades cut tissues, whereas "picklike" weapons primarily traumatize tissues by piercing through body structures. Unlike bite wounds, there is no crushing component associated with the use of these weapons.

Management

Wounds confined to the soft tissues are managed in a fashion similar to bite wounds. Trauma to tissues generally is modest unless vital structures were targeted. There is no significant crushing effect to the tissues: trauma primarily is confined to the course of the weapon. Penetrating wounds to the abdominal cavity must be explored; penetrating wounds to the thorax may require an exploratory thoracotomy, particularly when faced with massive hemorrhage or pneumothorax, unresponsive to thoracostomy tube placement and emergency medical care.

Impalement Injuries

Common examples of impalement injuries noted by veterinarians have included: (1) animals falling from a height onto a fence or other pointed object; (2) animals pushed, thrown, or propelled into a pointed object; (3) animals that run into an object; and (4) oral impalement secondary to driving a pointed object (usually a stick), carried in the patient's mouth, through the oral/pharyngeal mucosa[1,3] (Figs. 69-2 and 69-3).

Management

Like stab wounds, tissue trauma often is confined to the general path of the object. In those cases of stick (wood) impalement injuries, exploration of the tract is advisable to minimize the likelihood that fragments of organic material are not retained.

Manual debris removal, debridement of traumatized tissues, copious lavage, and appropriate wound closure are performed. Vacuum drain systems are particularly useful to maintain appropriate drainage to the contaminated wound postop-

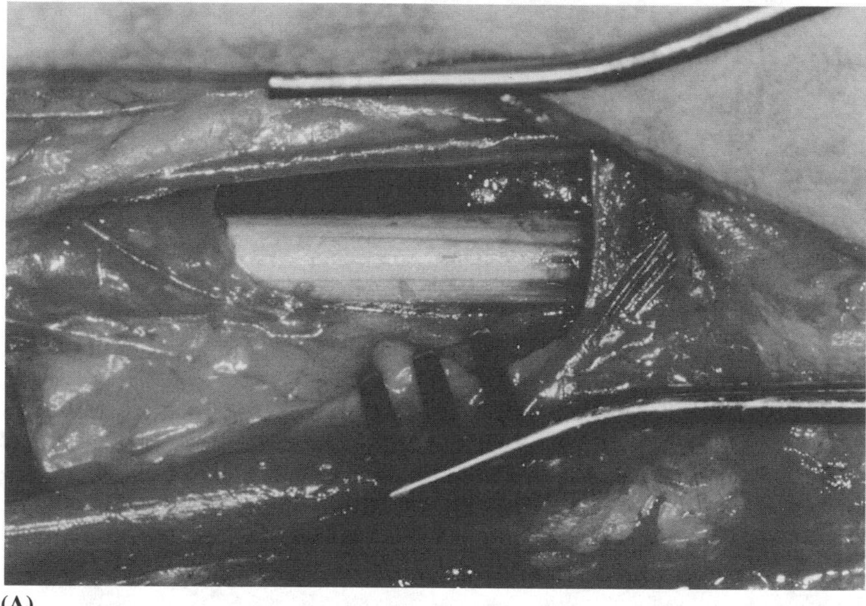

(A)

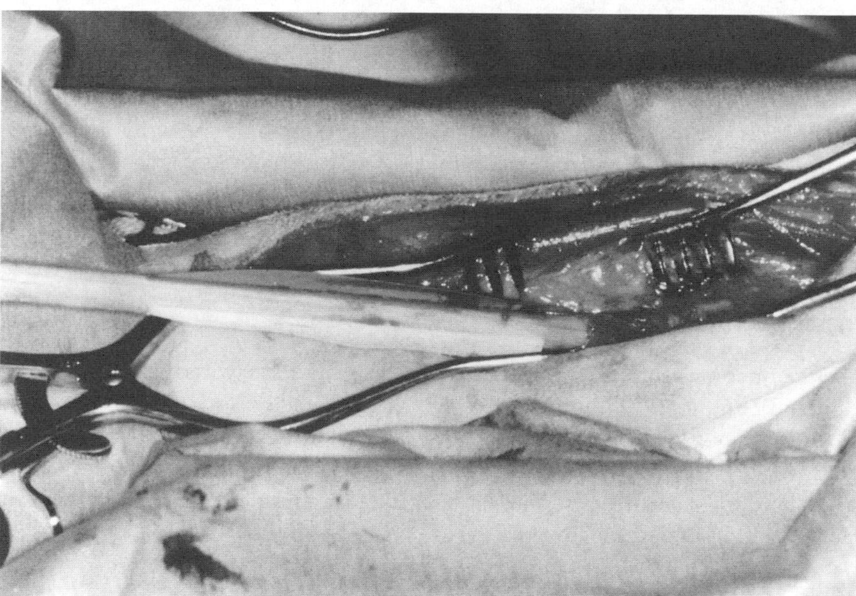

(B)

Figure 69-2
(A) Unusual impalement wound of the pharynx and cervical area. The dog impaled itself on the "nock end" of an arrow as it ran at the projectile embedded in the ground. View of the arrow through a cervical incision. **(B)** The arrow was extracted from the neck. The pharyngeal tear was repaired. The cervical incision was closed after insertion of a vacuum drain.

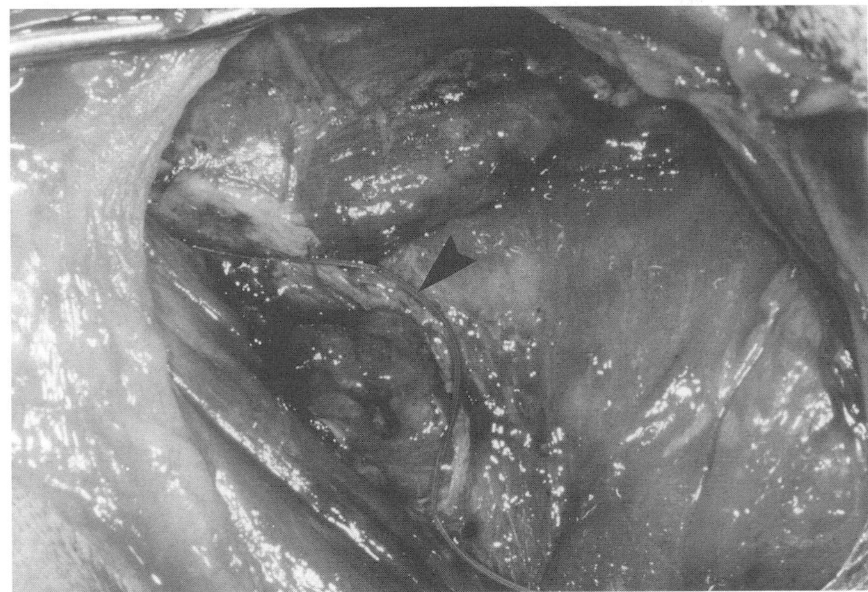

(A)

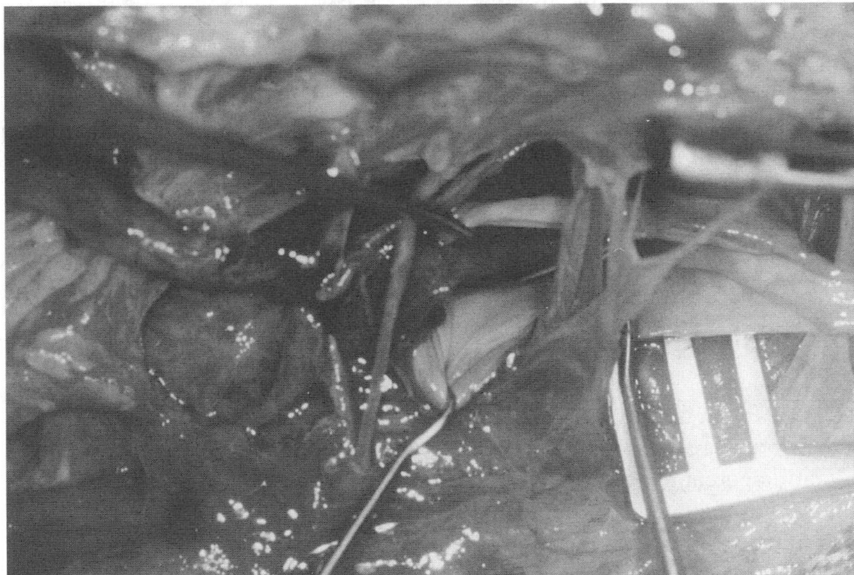

(B)

Figure 69-3
(A) Cervical exploration of an impalement wound, secondary to the dog running with a pine branch in its mouth. The stick was removed by the owner. Note the pine needle in the exploratory area (arrow). **(B)** Skin hooks were used to elevate the pharyngeal mucosa associated with the laceration, prior to debridement and closure.

eratively. Penetrating/perforating wounds to the oral cavity can be particularly problematic. Large tears commonly occur in the pharyngeal mucosa, and the penetrating object can be driven deeply into the cervical tissues. In some cases, a long object can extend into the thoracic inlet or axillary area. Saliva and oral contaminants can drain into cervical tissues, along the course of the foreign object. Care must be taken to identify the oral laceration, and close the defect to limit further contamination at the time of surgery.[1,3]

Miscellaneous Penetrating Wounds

Porcupine Quills

Penetrating wounds secondary to porcupine quills are noted in some areas of North America.[4] Dogs are the primary recipient of quill injuries. Although some owners will attempt to withdraw one or two quills with a pair of pliers, many owners will seek out veterinary assistance, especially when multiple quills are discovered embedded in their pet.

Management. With problematic cases, light anesthesia is advisable because removal of the barbed quill can be difficult and painful. The patient should be closely inspected to locate all quills. The oral cavity also should be closely inspected. Quills vary in length, generally from 2 to 10 cm. Parting the fur for visual inspection, and slowly running your fingers through the fur to identify the exposed point, are useful in detecting the smaller quills. When located, the shaft is grasped at skin level with a hemostat or needle holder. The more superficially embedded quills can be extracted with a firm, quick tug. More deeply embedded quills may require a small skin incision with a # 11 scalpel blade, parallel to the quill shaft, to facilitate their complete removal. Great care is taken to ensure the entire quill shaft is removed. Contrary to popular folklore, cutting a quill does not cause the quill to "deflate," thereby facilitating their removal. Although topical application of an antiseptic to the skin can be justified, few quill sites get infected when the quills are promptly removed.

Retained quills are capable of migrating deep into the body. Although infection can occur in association with retained quills, their migration into deeper body structures can result in more serious complications. The author has removed migrating porcupine quills from the lungs of dogs presenting to the emergency service with "spontaneous" pneumothorax and lung abscess (Fig. 69-4). In one case, postmortem examination of a canine brain abscess revealed a porcupine quill that migrated through one of the foramina of the skull.

Migrating Plant Fragments

Penetrating plant awns, dry grass fragments, and wood fragments occasionally perforate the skin and migrate into the soft tissues. Local abscess formation may herald the presence of the foreign material. In more chronic cases, a tract forms and drains through one or more skin sites. Actinomycosis and other bacterial infections may be associated with the presence of plant material.[1]

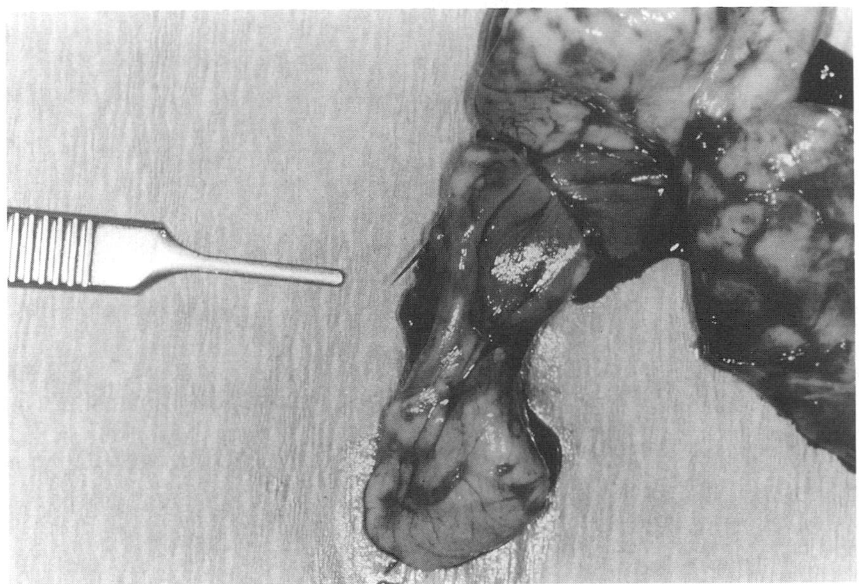

Figure 69-4
Spontaneous pneumothorax associated with a lung abscess. Note the small porcupine quill (pointer) that was recovered from the adjacent lung lobe resected with a surgical stapling device.

Management. Additional diagnostic tests (discussed above) may be performed to locate problematic foreign bodies. Draining tracts can be meticulously dissected out to locate a migrating foreign body. A fistulogram can be useful in highlighting the course of the tract and ensure the patient is appropriately prepared for surgery.[1]

Abscesses can be simple or complex. Whereas a simple abscess is a unilocular swelling, complex abscesses may have multiple abscess pockets, occasionally with interconnecting tracts that drain through one or more skin sites. A granulomatous reaction resulting from these tracts may be noted. Complex abscesses should be cultured for aerobic and anaerobic bacteria, as well as fungal organisms. Biopsies of the tissue also are indicated to rule out other conditions, including neoplasia. When feasible, *en bloc* excision of a complex abscess is a preferred method of managing these problematic wounds.[1]

PROJECTILE WOUNDS

Gunshot Wounds

Gunshot wounds are most commonly associated with rural or inner city areas. Weapons include handguns, rifles, shotguns, and air-powered weapons. Tissue damage depends on several factors, including the kinetic energy (velocity and mass) of the projectile, the amount of kinetic energy absorbed by the body, and the tissues affected. The design of the projectile also influences the severity of trauma.[1,5]

Higher velocity projectiles generate greater kinetic energy; the mass of the projectile also is a factor in determining the severity of trauma and depth of penetration. Most handguns are considered "low- to medium-velocity" weapons (<1000–2000 ft/sec), whereas the higher velocity projectiles are fired from rifles. High-velocity projectiles (>2000–2500 ft/sec) generate considerable kinetic energy, which is capable of damaging tissues a few to several centimeters from the permanent bullet tract, as a result of "cavitation."[1]

Not all the kinetic energy of a high velocity projectile is absorbed. For example, a high-velocity projectile may pass through the relatively elastic skin and muscle of the cranial thigh region, missing major nerves and vessels, before exiting on the opposite side of the limb. Elastic tissues (skin, lung, muscle) can absorb a portion of the kinetic energy released. The intact projectile, losing little velocity, exits the thigh with little loss of its kinetic energy. With limited tissue trauma, this wound can be managed in a more conservative fashion, despite the fact that it would be considered a high-velocity gunshot wound. This is in contrast to a high-velocity round that directly hits the femur (high specific gravity tissue). In this case, the bone absorbs a large portion of the projectile's kinetic energy. The bone shatters, releasing secondary projectiles into the adjacent soft tissues. Similarly, a frangible bullet may collapse and break apart, also creating regional tissue trauma. To salvage the limb, exploratory surgery is required to resect and repair seriously compromised tissues, remove contamination, stabilize the fracture, and establish wound drainage. Intensive postoperative medical/surgical care will be required in most cases. Because of the severity of tissue compromise and contamination, there is an increased likelihood of infection.[1,5]

Lower velocity projectiles, including many handguns and air-powered weapons, generate less kinetic energy and inflict relatively little trauma to soft tissues traversed. Although many low-velocity projectiles are capable of fracturing bone, the severity of trauma is modest compared to the high-velocity injuries. Despite the low velocity and comparatively low mass of air-powered pellets and BBs, these comparatively modest weapons are fully capable of inflicting a serious injury by direct impact with a vital structure. Human and animal fatalities have been reported with injuries sustained from pellet and BB guns.[1,5]

Shotguns are capable of firing a variety of projectiles, including single "deer slugs," darts or flechettes, or variable-sized round pellets. Pellet size depends on the intended game of the "hunter." At close range shotguns are capable of causing massive tissue destruction. Multiple pellets, dispersed in a dense profile, cause a central area of tissue destruction with a smaller halo of pellets at the perimeter. However, at greater distances, the shot pattern widens and the pellet velocity dramatically decreases, with a proportional reduction in destructive capacity. This is best exemplified in dogs where scattered pellets are noted in the dermal, hypodermal, and underlying musculofascial tissue, as an incidental finding on routine radiographs. In most of these cases, the owner was unaware of any injury or disturbance to the pet.[1,5]

Management

Radiographs of the involved areas are indicated to help determine the extent of trauma and path of the projectile. Radiographs of body regions above and below the area affected are indicated when the course of the projectile has not been determined. It must be kept in mind that retained projectiles can migrate. Bullets can shift their in position in soft tissues or body cavities. In humans, bullets have been reported to enter vessels and embolize. Similarly, bullets also have been reported to enter the tracheobronchial tree, only to be coughed up or swallowed by the patient.[1,5]

Projectiles that pass through soft tissues (skin, muscle, and fascia) and are retained in the patient usually are low-velocity projectiles. High-velocity rounds, which maintain much of their velocity on impact, exit canine or feline soft tissues. As a result, it may not be possible to determine the velocity or caliber of any projectile that exits the patient, unless there is historical information pertaining to the weapon.[1,5]

Extensive trauma associated with high-velocity projectiles is most apparent when dense cortical bone is affected. In some cases, high-velocity rounds will shatter dense bone, and still maintain significant mass and velocity to exit the body. The unsuspecting clinician may recognize the injury as a gunshot wound by the presence of fine or coarse metallic fragments (lead core or metallic jacket) on the initial radiographs taken. Both entry and exit wounds can vary in size, depending on ballistics, composition and design of the projectile, and the tissues hit.[1,5]

Low-velocity projectile wounds often require little more than local entry/exit wound care and application of a topical dressing/bandage, when the injury is confined to soft tissues (skin, muscle, fascia). Fractures will require appropriate surgical stabilization. High-velocity wounds, involving skin, muscle, fascia and bone, generally require exploration of the wound for debridement, wound lavage, and fracture management. In some cases, extensively damaged extremities may require amputation. "Through-and-through" high-velocity wounds, confined to skin and muscle, without major structural trauma, may be managed conservatively, unless significant tissue destruction is suspected.[1,5] Systemic antibiotics may be advisable in the face of infection or the likelihood of infection. All penetrating or perforating gunshot wounds to the abdomen must be explored, on presentation. Delays in exploring the abdomen can result in catastrophic peritonitis (Fig. 69-5).

Thoracic wounds usually do not routinely require exploration unless massive hemorrhage or tension pneumothorax persists despite emergency medical care and thoracostomy tube placement. Cervical and cranial gunshot wounds can be problematic due to the concentration of vital structures in these two body regions. Careful examination of the patient and the areas affected is necessary to determine whether exploratory surgery is advisable.[1,5]

Lead poisoning is rarely associated with retention of a projectile in the soft tissues. However, it is advisable to remove lead projectiles from joints, not only because of the risk of degenerative arthritis and infection, but also because of

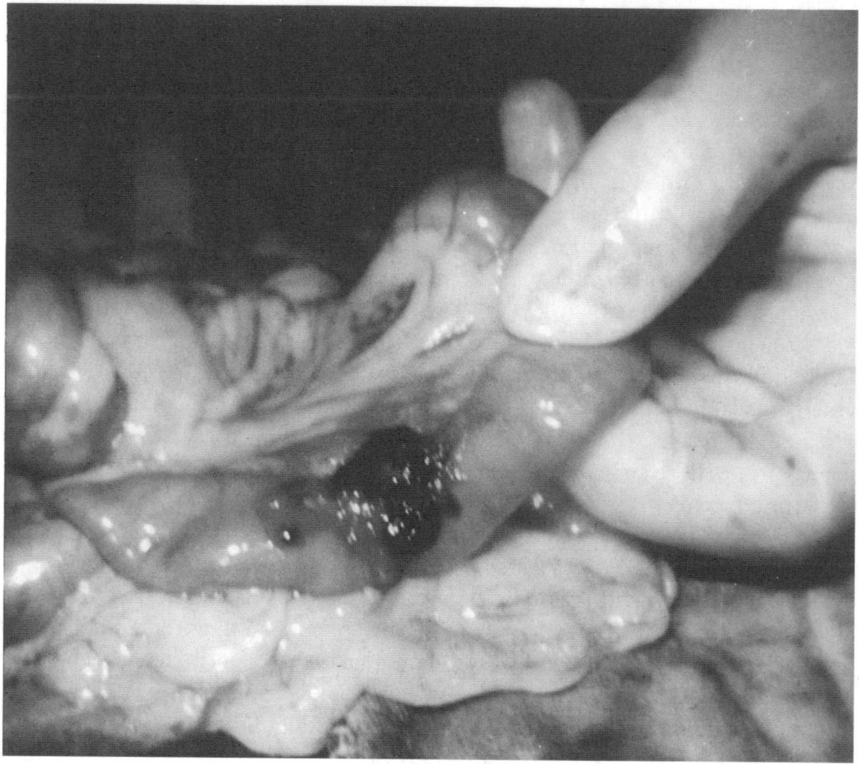

Figure 69-5
Bowel perforation in a cat, associated with a BB fired from an air rifle. Exploratory laparotomy should be performed on all penetrating/perforating abdominal wounds.

the tendency for lead to slowly dissolve in joint fluid. However, not all projectiles are composed of lead: today, steel shot is more commonly used in bird hunting. Air-propelled BBs also are composed of steel. Many jacketed bullets have a lead core encased in brass, cupronickel, or steel.[1,5]

Removal of nonproblematic projectiles, which are not easily accessible, is usually unnecessary. However, there may be occasions in which removal of a projectile is important for legal purposes. Veterinarians must be familiar with the legal ramifications associated with gunshot wounds and the transfer of evidence to legal authorities.[1,5]

Arrow Wounds

Athough far less common that gunshot wounds, arrow wounds are occasionally seen in small animal practice. Arrows are divided into two general categories, based on the type of "point" or "head": field points and hunting points (broad heads). Field points have a pointed, noncutting tip with a diameter comparable to the shaft. Broad heads are hunting arrows with blades designed to cut tissues on impact. Hunting arrows are primarily designed to kill by striking vital organs

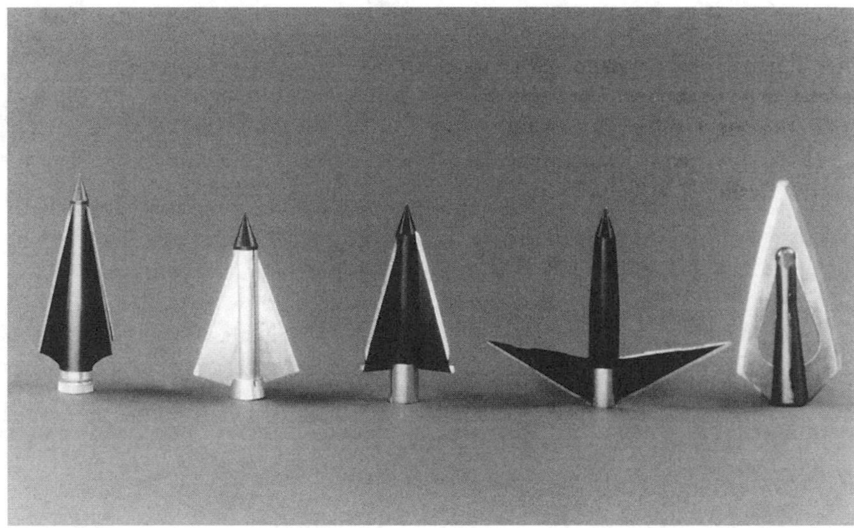

Figure 69-6
Broad heads vary in shape, design, weight, and number of blades (usually two, three, or four). Broad heads are frequently threaded and screwed onto the arrow shaft. The third broad head (from left) has three blades that open in a tripod fashion (fourth from left) on penetration, to enhance its cutting surface area. (From Pavletic MM: Atlas of Small Animal Reconstructive Surgery. Philadelphia, WB Saunders, 1999.)

and cutting major vascular tissues, causing massive hemorrhage (Fig. 69-6). Compared to bullets, arrows are low-velocity weapons that generally cause little peripheral trauma other than the tissues in the path of the arrow head.[1]

The shaft of basic target arrows is composed of cedar, whereas the more expensive arrows are composed of aluminum, carbon fiber, or composites of aluminum, fiberglass, and carbon fiber. The shaft length, weight, and width can vary. Short "bolts" or "quarrels" refer to the shorter arrows fired by cross-bows. Expensive arrows commonly have a threaded tip, thus enabling the hunter to change the broad head when necessary.[1] The surgeon may find it an advantage to unscrew the broad head by holding the head with forceps while untwisting the attached shaft.

Management

Based on the physical examination and radiographic assessment of the patient, the appropriate surgical approach can be determined. In some cases, the concerned owner may have extracted the arrow, making accurate determination of the projectile's pathway more difficult. This is of particular concern for the management of arrow wounds embedded in the thoracic and or abdominal cavities. Arrow retention facilitates surgical exploration of the wound tract, to ensure that no tissue injuries are overlooked. Moreover, there have been reported incidents in humans, in which the presence of the penetrating object has sealed an organ (*e.g.*, heart), thereby limiting leakage of its contents. The animals should be gently restrained to avoid additional tissue trauma associated with jostling of a retained arrow. Long portions of an exposed shaft can be cut with bolt cutters above the entry level of the arrow to facilitate positioning of the patient and minimize movement of the retained projectile. Exposed broad-head arrows oftentimes can be unscrewed from the shaft, as noted above.[1]

Radiographs are useful to determine the nature of a retained arrow head and to determine if fragments of the broad-head blade were broken off in the body. As with other major penetrating/perforating wounds, mandatory exploratory is indicated. Wide, aggressive debridement of arrow wounds generally is not indicated. Although field point arrows lack cutting blades, broad-head arrows can cut or lacerate tissues. After wound lavage and inspection, damaged tissues can be repaired. Drainage can be established with the use of Penrose drains and vacuum drainage systems.[1] In some cases, systemic antibiotics may be indicated, especially in the presence or likelihood of infection.

REFERENCES

1. Pavletic MM: Management of specific skin wounds. *In* Pavletic MM, ed.: Atlas of Small Animal Reconstructive Surgery, 2nd ed. Philadelphia: WB Saunders, 1989, pp 50, 66, 85.
2. Pavletic MM: Bite Wound Management in Small Animals. Lakewood, CO: AAHA Professional Library Series, 1995.
3. Griffiths LG, Tiruneh, R, Sullivan, M, Reid SWJ: Oropharyngeal penetrating injuries in 50 dogs: a retrospective study. *Vet Surg* 29:383, 2000.
4. Grahn BH, Szentimrey D, Pharr JW, *et al.*: Ocular and orbital porcupine quills in the dog: a review and case series. *Can Vet J* 36:488, 1995.
5. Pavletic MM: Gunshot wound management. *Compend Contin Ed Pract Vet* 18:1285, 1996.

70
Burn Injury

Nishi Dhupa

INTRODUCTION

Burn injury in small animals may be seen as a consequence of exposure to sources of heat, caustic household and industrial chemicals, or electric current. Burn trauma may be accidental in nature, or it may be malicious. Direct thermal trauma such as seen in household fires, following contact with scalding liquid such as water or tar, or heated surfaces such as radiators, stoves, or automobile exhaust pipes will result in immediate thermal wounds. Chemical burn injuries will also be immediately apparent. Inappropriate contact with electric heating pads and overexposure to hot air dryers or heat lamps will cause thermal burn injuries with lesions developing over several days.[1] Electrical injuries related to high-voltage current such as seen in lightning strikes will result in immediate burn injury; those associated with low-voltage current such as with young animals chewing electric cords will result in tissue damage that may be immediately visible or may not be apparent for several days.

Iatrogenic causes of thermal injuries are more common. Caution must be exercised when warming anesthetized, debilitated, or pediatric patients with potent external heat sources such as heating pads, hot water bottles, or heating lamps. Considerable heat can be generated by these sources; prolonged contact in combination with local heat retention can produce sizeable full-thickness burns.[1]

Although the skin is most affected, burns affecting greater than 20% of total body surface area (TBSA) will have systemic effects including impaired cardiac, respiratory, and immune function. Management of burn injuries includes both local wound management, as well as the support of vital organ systems. Adjunctive therapies include nutritional support, the provision of analgesia, and, where necessary, of systemic antibiotic therapy.

CLASSIFICATION OF BURNS

The severity of the burn injury is determined by the evaluating the degree or depth of injury as well as the percentage of TBSA involved. In animals, burns are classified as superficial (first degree), partial-thickness (second degree), or full-thickness (third degree), depending on the depth of tissue damage. Superficial burns affect only the epidermal layer of the skin. Partial-thickness burns may be either superficial (involving the epidermis and the superficial dermis) or deep (involving the whole epidermis and mid to deep dermis). Full-thickness burns include the entire epidermis and dermis and may involve underlying structures.[2] Deep burns may result in excessive scar formation and impaired mobility, as well as hair loss.

The percentage of TBSA involved can be estimated by allotment of specific percentages to various body regions (Rule of 9): the head and neck account for 9%, each forelimb for 9%, each rear limb for 18%, and the thorax and abdomen each for 18%.[2]

PATHOPHYSIOLOGY

Thermal injury

Local Burn Injury

Burns occur when thermal energy is applied to tissue. The temperature of the heat source, the duration of contact, and the ability of the tissue to dissipate heat all influence the severity of the burn. The tissue closest to the heat source undergoes complete necrosis. Injured tissue adjacent to the necrotic region has reduced blood flow and intravascular sludging, due to vascular damage as well as release of vasoactive substances. Progressive dermal ischemia in the 24 to 48 hours following initial injury, with convert partial-thickness burns into full-thickness injuries. The tissue furthest from the heat source is characterized by minimal damage and inflammation. Capillaries and venules in this area become highly permeable, leading to marked interstitial edema formation. Where the burn surface area is large, significant fluid and protein shifts may occur, resulting in hypovolemia. Burn tissue also sequesters sodium, which pulls additional water from the circulation.[3]

Systemic Effects

Burns affecting greater than 20% of TBSA will impair cardiac, respiratory, and immune function. Massive fluid shifts and vascular changes result in hypovolemia and circulatory shock. Capillary damage and the release of inflammatory mediators and oxygen free radicals produce leakage of plasma proteins into the burn site. Once hypoalbuminemia develops, generalized soft-tissue edema occurs. Cardiac output falls as a consequence of hypovolemia and shock. Profound hypovolemia will lead to tissue hypoperfusion and impaired delivery of oxygen and nutrients to vital organs. Myocardial depressant factors released from burned tissues, together with the effects of carbon monoxide, may also impair myocardial contractility. This results in multiorgan system dysfunction.[3]

Pulmonary function may be markedly impaired in the burned patient. Truncal burns may result in restriction of ventilation. Respiratory failure results from severe bronchopulmonary injury related to carbon monoxide, cyanide and smoke toxicities. Carbon monoxide combines with hemoglobin causing displacement of oxygen and consequent hypoxemia.[4] Smoke toxicity may cause direct heat-related airway injury, laryngeal edema, and bronchoconstriction. Damage to protective cilia and compromise of surfactant activity leads to atelectasis. Long-term sequelae may include bronchopneumonia and pulmonary fibrosis.[4]

Chemical Injury

The extent of injury caused by a caustic chemical agent depends on the chemical concentration and duration of contact. When strong acids or alkalis contact skin, injury results from thermal energy, coagulation necrosis, vascular thrombosis, and collagen denaturation. Paint solvents, furniture strippers, and concentrated flea dip solutions are also capable of causing superficial and partial-thickness skin injuries.

Electrical Injury

Electric current damages tissue by the conversion of electric energy into heat producing protein coagulation. The severity of electrical injury is related to the type of circuit, voltage, amperage, duration of contact, pathway of current, and tissue resistance. Tissue injury is most severe at the point of contact, where the current density is greatest. This type of injury is responsible for the oral burns seen in most animals treated for electric cord injuries, which are caused by low-voltage (<1000 V) household alternating current (60 Hz). Low-voltage oral burns commonly involve the commissures of the lips, gums, tongue, and palate in small animals.[5] Electrical injury may be associated with the development of pulmonary edema, which may be mediated through a centroneurogenic reflex causing an increased pulmonary capillary hydrostatic pressure. This form of edema has a typical caudodorsal distribution in the lungs of the victim and may have an immediate (within 1 hour) or delayed (24-36 hours) onset. This "neurogenic" pulmonary edema is usually seen with oral electrical burns in young dogs and cats that bite live electric cords.[5] High-voltage (>2000 V) electric current, such as seen with lightning strike or high-tension power transmission lines, may also cause burns. These injuries are uncommon in pets and are usually fatal. The contact or entry point is usually charred and leathery, and the exit wound at the ground point may be "exploded."

DIAGNOSTIC EVALUATION

Thermal Injury

Clinical Presentation

The depth and extent of injury must be assessed to determine prognosis and implement a treatment plan. The full extent of injury may not be apparent for 5 to 7 days until necrotic tissue separates from bordering and underlying viable tissue.[3] Patients with superficial burns have skin that is erythematous, dry to the touch, hyperesthetic, and without blister formation.

Desquamation of the epidermis occurs, followed by development of a thick scab or crust. Healing will occur within 3 to 5 days, with hair regrowth likely.[3] Superficial partial-thickness burns will appear denuded, with exudation, blister formation and pain, and normal resistance to hair pulling. Healing will occur in 10 to 21 days with minimal scarring.[3] Deep dermal partial-thickness burns appear dark or yellow-white, contain ruptured bullae, and have decreased sensation to a pinprick but intact sensation for deep pressure. Healing is prolonged and often results in extensive scar formation and marked contracture of tissues, unless surgical intervention occurs. Significant systemic effects, such as cardiovascular shock, are present.[3] Full-thickness burns appear as charred, leathery, bloodless, hairless lesions (or easily epilated hair) with little or no pain or sensitivity.[3] These wounds heal slowly, by second intention. Surgical intervention, in the form of skin grafting, is often necessary.

It is essential to recognize the signs of "burn shock," which include pale mucous membranes, prolonged capillary refill time, tachycardia, and hypotension. If the hair on the face and mouth are singed or evidence of corneal damage is noted, then smoke inhalation injury should also be suspected.

Laboratory and Radiographic Findings

The hematocrit will be elevated and serum albumin levels will be decreased in a patient with significant plasma loss into burned tissue. Concomitant red cell hemolysis may result in a normal or decreased hematocrit. Loss of fluid from the burn surface may result in hypernatremia ($>$145 mEq/L) and hyperchloremia ($>$110 mEq/L), unless replacement fluids are provided. Tissue necrosis may cause mild hyperkalemia. Poor tissue perfusion and shock in the early postburn period may result in metabolic acidosis.[3] In smoke inhalation injury, thoracic radiographs may reveal interstitial and alveolar patterns consistent with pulmonary edema.[4]

Chemical Injury

The medical history may reveal the nature of the chemical and duration of contact. Burn injury may be mild, appearing as intercellular edema of the skin or separation of the dermis from the epidermis, with pruritis or pain. Deeper tissue destruction resulting in full-thickness burns may be seen with acids and, particularly, strong alkalis. If the agent is unknown, a sample may be submitted for analysis. Where vapor inhalation or consumption of the material is suspected, close attention should be paid to the eyes, and the oral/laryngeal/pharyngeal area.

Electrical Injury

Electrical injury is most commonly seen in young animals. The history may be definitive if the episode is witnessed. More commonly the animal is found collapsed with characteristic oral and cutaneous burns involving commissures of the lips, the dorsum of the tongue, and the hard palate. These tend to be well circumscribed, cold, bloodless, and pale yellow in color. The lesions are also painless. Arcing of the current may result in copper deposits within the burn lesion. The presence of respiratory compromise, characterized by labored breathing, coughing, and fine pulmonary crackles on auscultation, indicates the development of neurogenic pulmonary edema. Thoracic radiographs will reveal a generalized alveolar-bronchial pattern with air bronchograms in the caudal lobes of the lung. This pattern is usually bilateral and symmetrical. Electrocardiography may reveal ventricular arrhythmias. Other clinical signs include grand mal seizures, respiratory and cardiac arrest (particularly with high-voltage injuries), weakness, unconsciousness, transient muscle stiffness, vomiting, or diarrhea.[5]

TREATMENT

General Principles

Wound management involves protection of burned tissue. Debridement of devitalized tissue helps to control infection and provides and environment conducive to healing and surgical closure. Extensive burns may require closure with skin grafts.

Initial Wound Management

Damage to skin and underlying tissue may continue after the initial injury due to the low thermal conductance of skin. If the patient is seen within 2 hours of injury, cold water and saline at a temperature of 3° to 17°C (37°–63°F) can be applied to the wound surface, for at least 30 minutes to decrease heat retention and reduce the depth of tissue injury. Extremities may be cooled by immersion in the cold liquid. Burned tissue must not be packed in ice because this will further compromise tissue viability. After burned tissue is cooled, the hair should be carefully clipped from the burn area. The wound is then examined to assess the depth and extent of damage. Small superficial and partial-thickness burns can be topically covered with a broad-spectrum antibiotic ointment. Burn wounds on lower extremities and the ventral trunk can then be covered with sterile occlusive bandages to protect the tissue from contamination and external trauma. In the case of more extensive wounds, topical agents may be applied without a covering bandage. The topical ointment selected for use should be a broad-spectrum antimicrobial with reasonable penetration into the burn eschar; it should be nonirritating and nontoxic, with minimal systemic absorption. Commonly used agents include silver sulfadiazine (Flint SSD, Flint), nitrofurazone (Furacin, Roberts), povidone-iodine (Betadine, Purdue Frederick) and gentamicin (Garamycin, Schering). The antibiotic ointment should be applied two to three times a day after wound cleaning and debris removal. Wound cleaning, debridement, and bandaging will require the use of sedatives or general anesthesia. Analgesics are an integral part of patient care during the hospitalization period (Table 70-1).

Long-Term Wound Management

Debridement

As full-thickness injuries become more apparent as necrotic tissue separates, serial debridement to remove devitalized tissue may become necessary. If left alone, the necrotic tissue and exudates (known as the burn eschar) will undergo

Table 70-1. Analgesia for Burned Patients

Drug	Dosage
Morphine sulfate (Astramorph, Astra)	Dog: 0.2–0.5 mg/kg SQ, IM, IV, q 2–4 h
Oxymorphone hydrochloride (Numorphan, Dupont)	Dog: 0.05–0.20 mg/kg SQ, IM, IV q 2–4 h Cat: 0.05 mg/kg IV, SQ q 4 h
Butorphanol tartrate (Torbutrol, Fort Dodge)	Dog: 0.1–0.4 mg/kg IM, SQ, IV, PO q 2–5 h Cat: 0.1–0.4 mg/kg SQ q 2–5 h
Ketamine hydrochloride (Vetalar, Fort Dodge)	Dog: 1–2 mg/kg IV, IM, SQ q 1 h or 10 mg/kg q 6 h PO[7] Cat: 1–2 mg/kg IV, IM, SQ q 1 h
Fentanyl, Transdermal (Duragesic, Janssen)	Dog: <20 lb 25 μg/h 25-50 lb 50 μg/h >50 lb 75 μg/h Cat: 25 μg/h per cat

bacterial colonization and predispose to the development of sepsis. Additionally, the persistence of the burn eschar results in impaired granulation bed formation and delayed wound healing.[6] Debridement is particularly important in the management of deep partial- and full-thickness burns. Conservative mechanical debridement involves the immersion of the injured area in water or isotonic saline, or the application of wet-wet dressings. This facilitates the softening and separation of necrotic tissue from the underlying viable tissues. Immersion should be carried out for 20- to 30-minute periods, two or three times daily. Following immersion, loose tissue can be removed with thumb forceps and scissors. The wound is then covered with an antimicrobial ointment. Surgical debridement or wound excision is used to remove the entire burn wound before temporary or permanent surgical closure. After surgical excision, a healthy granulation bed forms within 5 to 7 days. Following this, graft or flap closure is possible. This technique facilitates wound healing and often results in a considerable reduction in morbidity and hospital stay.[6]

Wound Closure

Superficial and partial-thickness burns will re-epithelialize within 3 weeks, whereas deep dermal partial-thickness burns take longer. Full-thickness defects heal by contraction and epithelialization from the wound edges. This process takes a long time, and in the case of large skin defects, will not allow successful closure of the wound. In these cases, autogenous free grafts, axial pattern flaps, and skin advancement techniques are used to provide wound surface coverage.[6] Smaller full-thickness wounds may heal by contracture and re-epithelialization alone, but often the end result is severe scarring and contracture, with possible compromise to function, particularly in areas subject to constant motion.

Specific Treatment

Thermal Injury

Thermal wounds should be managed as described above in the section on wound management. Oxygen supplementation may be necessary in patients with shock or those with inhalational injuries. Aggressive fluid therapy is essential for resuscitation of severely burned animals. Large volumes of fluids may be required to correct losses occurring both from the burned surface as well as into the interstitial space. Initial fluid management involves the use of isotonic crystalloid solutions. Fluid requirements range from 2 to 6 mL/kg body weight multiplied by percent TBSA burned, to be administered in the first 24 hours. One half of the calculated dosage is administered within the first 8 hours to combat the loss of fluid into the interstitium during the phase of rapid edema formation.[2] Additionally, larger "shock doses" of fluids may be given, as needed, for resuscitation. Once capillary microvascular leakage slows after the first 6 to 8 hours, colloids such as dextrans (Gentran-70, Baxter), hetastarch (Hespan, Dupont), and plasma will be retained within the vasculature and can be administered to the patient. Both colloids and blood transfusions are avoided in the first 8 hours because of the risk of extravasation into burn tissue, leading to increased edema formation.[2] For long-term support of volume and colloid oncotic pressure, synthetic colloids can be administered as constant rate infusion at a dosage of 20 mL/kg/d. If serum albumin levels fall below 1.5 g/dL, plasma transfusion should be considered, at a dosage of 0.5 mL plasma × body weight (kg) × percent TBSA burned.

During the chronic phase, maintenance of plasma volume, electrolyte balance, and nutritional requirements must be addressed. Nutritional support is essential to prevent excess protein catabolism and to promote wound healing. Oral, parenteral, or enteral routes may be used, and supplementation should begin within 48 hours of a burn injury. Systemic antibiotic therapy may be indicated for life-threatening pneumonia (in patients with inhalation injury) or sepsis. Antibiotics should be selected and administered on the basis of results of culture and sensitivity of transtracheal washings or wound discharges. Analgesic administration is an integral part of patient management. See Table 70-1 for analgesic options and dosages.

Chemical Injury

Chemical burns caused by acids, alkalis, and household solutions should be lavaged with large volumes of water to return skin pH to normal and limit the extent of injury. Solvents and petroleum products may be washed with strong detergents such as Ivory or Dawn dishwashing liquids. Hot tar may be removed with surface-active agents such as polyoxyethylene sorbitan (Tween 80, Sigma), which is present as an emulsifying agent in Neosporin (Neosporin Plus, Glaxo-Wellcome) and other antibiotic ointments. Alkali-related burns require extensive and prolonged lavage to normalize tissue pH. Neutralizing agents may also be helpful in limiting the extent of injury, following copious lavage. These agents may be applied to the wound surface with gauze sponges for 15 to 20 minutes, and the application may be repeated. Acidic compounds such as sulfuric, nitric, and hydrochloric acids may be neutralized by magnesium hydroxide or sodium bicarbonate solutions. Burns caused by lyes such as sodium hydroxide, potassium hydroxide, ammonia, or lime may be neutralized by weak (0.5%-5.0%) acetic acid or lemon juice.[3] If ocular exposure has occurred, copious lavage with sterile saline solution is recommended. Management of superficial and partial-thickness chemical burns is similar to the management of thermal burns. Deeper necrosis of skin and underlying tissues is best managed by excision and closure unless the minor size of the wound supports healing by secondary intention.

Electrical Injury

If the episode is witnessed the animal must immediately be removed from contact with the electrical source, once the power has been turned off. Local treatment of the burn site includes clipping and cleaning the site and the application of a topical antibacterial agent. Animals should be hospitalized for observation as the onset of respiratory symptoms may be delayed. Oral and cutaneous burns are usually slow to heal. Many mild injuries will slough and heal within 3 weeks without the need for surgical debridement. Oronasal fistulae require surgical closure with mucosal flaps, labial advancement flaps, or skin flaps.[6] Large areas of necrosis will require debridement and eventual surgical closure.

PROGNOSIS

Thermal Injury

Prognosis is reasonably good if the patient survives the first 48 hours. Partial-thickness burns covering less than 15% to 20% TBSA carry a good prognosis because wound treatment and supportive therapy are minimal. Patients with deep partial-thickness and full-thickness wounds involving greater than 20% TBSA usually require intensive supportive therapy and wound management involving lengthy hospitalization and reconstructive surgery. Owners must be counseled about the effects of wound contracture on limb function as well as of the potential cosmetic effects of hair loss. Where full-thickness burns cover over 50% of TBSA, large expenses and intensive nursing should be expected, and the chances of recovery are poor.[3] Euthanasia is a reasonable option in these patients.

Chemical Injury

Mild to moderate chemical burn injury is associated with a more favorable prognosis. Severe chemical burns may cause severe systemic effects including shock and sepsis, as well as significant compromise of function, with a poor prognosis.

Electrical Injury

Animals that survive the initial electrical shock and the first 24 hours usually recover. If oral lesions are severe, healing may result in contracture and scarring of the tongue and lip commissures. Pulmonary edema usually resolves within 2 to 4 days.

REFERENCES

1. Swaim SF, Lee AH, Hughes KS: Heating pads and thermal burns in small animals. *J Am Anim Hosp Assoc* 25:156, 1989.
2. Saxon WD, Kirby R: Treatment of acute burn injury and smoke inhalation. *In* Kirk RW, Bonagura eds.: Current Veterinary Therapy XI. Philadelphia: WB Saunders, 1992, p 146.
3. Lee-Parritz DE, Pavletic MM: Burns. *In* Murtaugh RJ, Kaplan PM, eds.:Veterinary Emergency and Critical Care Medicine. St. Louis: CV Mosby, 1992, p 199.
4. Drobatz KJ, Walker CM, Hendricks JC: Smoke exposure in dogs: 27 cases (1988–1997). *J Am Vet Med Assoc* 215:1306, 1999.
5. Hansen BD, Morgan RV: Electric cord and smoke inhalation Injuries. *In* Morgan RV, ed.: Manual of Small Animal Practice, 2nd ed. Philadelphia: WB Saunders, 1995, p 1357.
6. Pavletic MM: Atlas of Small Animal Reconstructive Surgery, 2nd ed. Philadelphia: WB Saunders, 1999, p 70.
7. Joubert K: Ketamine hydrochloride—an adjunct drug for analgesia in dogs with burn wounds. *J S Afr Vet Assoc* 69:95, 1998.

71
Smoke Inhalation

Kenneth J. Drobatz

INTRODUCTION

Smoke inhalation is a relatively rare occurrence in veterinary emergency and critical care. At the University of Pennsylvania only 27 dogs and 22 cats have been admitted to the Emergency Service with a diagnosis of smoke inhalation/exposure during an approximate 10-year period.[1,2] This relatively infrequent presenting complaint is surprising given the frequency of dwelling fires in an urban environment such as Philadelphia where 1550 fires have been reported to occur in 1996 alone. The spectrum of physiologic compromise that can occur to animals that are exposed to smoke can vary widely. Compounding this is the reported delayed effects that can occur and the complications that skin burns contribute to the respiratory and overall physiologic changes. There is a paucity of information regarding animal smoke exposure in the veterinary clinical literature although numerous animal models of smoke inhalation provide insight into this challenging clinical problem. Though rare, it is important that the veterinary emergency and critical care practitioner be familiar with the pathophysiology, clinical manifestations, therapeutic rationale, and prognosis of this medically challenging condition to optimize outcome in these critically ill animals.

PATHOGENESIS

The components of smoke are complex and are determined by the type of material that is burned, the heat that is generated, and the amount of oxygen (O_2) available during combustion. Extensive reviews have been written regarding the variety of chemicals that may be present in smoke.[3-5] Although extensive knowledge regarding the individual chemicals that may be present and the resultant damage they can induce in the pulmonary tissue is interesting, it is nearly impossible for the clinician to know what the animal has inhaled. Nevertheless, there are three major pathophysiologic insults of smoke inhalation: tissue hypoxia, thermal damage, and pulmonary irritation.

Tissue hypoxia occurs due to decreased inspired O_2 concentration, decreased ability of the blood to carry O_2, decreased tissue perfusion, and disruption of the cells' ability to use O_2. The consumption of O_2 and the production of carbon dioxide (CO_2) during combustion in a closed space can lower inspired O_2 concentration to 15%.[6] In addition, tissue asphyxia occurs due to inhalation of carbon monoxide, cyanide, and the production of methemoglobinemia.[7] The acute decrease in inspired O_2 concentration is the reason many animals lose consciousness at the fire scene. Carbon monoxide also contributes to tissue hypoxia through binding to hemoglobin and decreasing O_2-carrying capacity of the blood. Carbon monoxide competitively binds to hemoglobin with 200 to 250 times the affinity compared to O_2. Other proposed mechanisms of carbon monoxide effects on O_2 delivery and metabolism include a leftward shift of the O_2/hemoglobin dissociation curve, preventing the release of O_2 to the tissues, cardiotoxic effects from binding to myoglobin, and poisoning of the mitochondrial cytochromic oxidase.[8]

Cyanide is produced from the combustion of wool, plastics, polyurethane, silk, nylon, rubber, paper products, and other materials. Cyanide can inhibit tissue aerobic metabolism by binding to the ferric ion on cytochrome-A_3 and also arrests the tricarboxylic acid cycle. As a result, cells generate adenosine triphosphate primarily through glycolysis causing increased production of lactate.

Decreased tissue O_2 delivery may occur due to the formation of methemoglobinemia from heat denaturation of hemoglobin, oxidation of nitrogen, and combustion of nitrites.[7]

In people, the first respiratory signs are typically upper airway signs and may occur within minutes to hours after fire exposure. The upper airway signs may be due to particulates, irritants, or thermal injury. The severity of the upper airway signs may progress over the first 1 to 12 hours due to progressive edema and swelling. Particularly with aggressive fluid therapy, upper airway swelling may progress to complete obstruction necessitating tracheostomy.

Upper airway signs are some of the most common signs noted in dogs and are usually evident at presentation to the emergency hospital. Thermal injury of the pulmonary system is primarily limited to the upper airways due to the high heat capacity of the upper respiratory system. Injury is typically limited to the supraglottic area and larynx. Swelling, inflammation, and edema can progress to the point of complete obstruction of the upper airway. These changes generally occur within the first several hours of smoke exposure, although in a clinical study in dogs, tracheostomy for upper airway injury was necessary between 24 and 72 hours after exposure to fire.[1]

Chemical irritants in smoke include sulfur dioxide, chlorine gas, and acroleins. Irritants cause direct injury to the respiratory mucosa through the production of acid and alkali burns as well as formation of free radicals and protein denaturation (acroleins). They also contribute to respiratory dysfunction by inciting a reflex bronchoconstriction and pulmonary inflammation. The irritants may cause pulmonary injury anywhere along the pulmonary tract. High water-soluble irritants tend to cause upper airway lesions and low water-soluble irritants penetrate to the lower airways and alveoli causing damage. The irritants may also inactivate surfactant within seconds of smoke inhalation causing atelectasis and decreased compliance.[9]

Smoke particulates cause mechanical irritation and reflex bronchoconstriction. Superheated particles contribute to mucosal burn; dissolved irritant gases cause chemical irritation and injury to the respiratory mucosa.

The clinical manifestations of tissue hypoxia are primarily manifested by organs that use large amounts of O_2 including the brain and heart. Neurologic signs can range from mild depression or stupor to coma or seizures. Cardiac manifestations typically manifest as arrhythmias. Tissue hypoxia may occur at the onset of combustion when ambient O_2 in consumed and CO_2 and carbon monoxide are produced. Decreased inspired O_2 (FIO_2) is a likely cause of the immediate mentation changes that occur in these patients. In a study evaluating dogs and cats with smoke exposure, several dogs and cats were reported to have severe mentation changes or loss of consciousness at the fire scene.[1,2] Many of these animals had rapid improvement in mentation on removal from the dwelling and exposure to O_2 supplementation or fresh air. Persistent neurologic changes may occur due to decreased inspired O_2 or decreased tissue O_2 delivery from high concentrations of carboxyhemoglobin or methemoglobin. Altered mentation may persist until carboxyhemoglobin concentrations decrease to a safe level or persist beyond normalization of carboxyhemoglobin concentration if brain tissue hypoxia has been prolonged. Persistent neurologic changes attributed to high carboxyhemoglobin changes in people include personality and memory disturbances, a Parkinson-like disorder, mixed motor and sensory neuropathy, and psychiatric disturbances.[7] In cats and dogs, persistent neurologic changes are noted within the first hours after presentation and range from depressed mentation or gait changes to stupor or coma.[1] Some animals are euthanatized within several hours of presentation due to severe neurologic changes. Long-term persistent neurologic changes have been noted in dogs and include pacing, shaking the head, and acting as if hearing things or just "never acting right" since the exposure to fire.

EPIDEMIOLOGY

The majority of smoke inhalation cases tend to occur in the colder months of the year. This likely reflects the greater frequency of dwelling fires due to space heater accidents, heater malfunctions, and the use of Christmas lights.[1,2] Also, animals have less chance to escape due to closed windows and doors although it has been reported that animals do not always look for an avenue of escape but move to areas of familiarity.[10] The majority of animals that present to the veterinary emergency facility tend to be younger animals with a median age of slightly greater 3 years.[1,2] Experimental models have demonstrated that older dogs tend to do worse than younger ones.[9] It could be that the younger animals are more likely to survive and make it to the emergency hospital.

CLINICAL PRESENTATION

The clinical signs vary depending on the ingredients of the smoke that has been inhaled, the heat of the smoke, and the intensity and duration of the exposure. Animals may present with mild or no obvious clinical signs or have life-threatening respiratory and neurologic abnormalities.

The most common clinical signs in dogs noted at the scene of the fire include stupor or coma (47%), coughing/gagging (35%), and respiratory difficulty

(35%). Other less commonly reported signs include weakness/ataxia, foaming from the mouth, and rubbing at the eyes.

In cats, difficulty breathing (44%), open-mouth breathing (44%), vocalizing (44%), coughing (22%), loss of consciousness (22%), and lethargy (22%) are the most common clinical signs noted at the fire scene.

PHYSICAL EXAMINATION

The physical manifestations of smoke exposure in dogs and cats are a manifestation of tissue hypoxia, thermal damage, and irritation of mucous membranes. Of particular concern are the effects of smoke on the pulmonary and central nervous systems.

Temperature, Pulse Rate, and Respiratory Rate

The majority of dogs and cats have normal rectal temperature and pulse rates. Respiratory rate is usually increased as a result of pulmonary irritation, bronchoconstriction, and hypoxia.

Mucous Membrane Color

Mucous membrane color may vary from normal pink to hyperemic or cyanotic. The more severely affected animals tend to have hyperemic mucous membranes. The hyperemia may be a result of mucous membrane irritation by smoke, carbon monoxide intoxication, and, less likely, by increased CO_2 concentration or cyanide toxicity.

Ocular Changes

Corneal and conjunctival irritation occur commonly in dogs and cats exposed to smoke. This is manifested by conjunctivitis, blepharospasm, rubbing at the eyes, corneal ulceration, and edema.

Skin

The majority of dogs and cats that present with smoke exposure do not have skin burns. Many have a smoky smell that confirms relatively close contact with smoke. Skin burns indicate a close exposure to the fire and possibly greater thermal and smoke exposure for the pulmonary system. Pulmonary effects tend to be worse when smoke inhalation and skin burns occur together and a more serious prognosis is warranted.

Nervous System

Loss of consciousness may occur at the fire scene and is most often due to decreased inspired O_2 concentration from the combustion of material during the fire. Many of these animals regain consciousness once removed from the smoke-filled environment and given supplemental O_2. The majority of dogs and cats are relatively alert or are mildly depressed at presentation to the veterinarian.

More serious nervous system abnormalities can occur and include stupor, coma, disorientation, and ataxia.

Respiratory System

The majority of dogs and cats have an increased respiratory rate. Upper airway sounds occur as a result of mucosa swelling from irritation and thermal injury. Lower airway abnormalities are relatively common and are manifested as increased bronchovesicular sounds and crackles. Expiratory wheezes are heard with small airway narrowing from bronchoconstriction and mucosal swelling. Rarely, localized areas of decreased airway sounds may occur due to small airway obstruction from mucosal swelling, mucosal sloughing, and particulate debris.

DIAGNOSTIC EVALUATION

Evaluation of packed cell volume (PCV), total solids, dipstick glucose, and dipstick blood urea nitrogen are warranted in the more severely affected patients. PCV tends to be higher and blood glucose lower in more severely affected dogs.[1]

Arterial blood gas analysis is invaluable for assessment and monitoring of respiratory function. If arterial blood gases are drawn during O_2 supplementation, the evaluation of the ratio of PaO_2/FIO_2 provides an assessment of the lung's ability to oxygenate the blood. The nadir of this ratio in dogs with smoke inhalation tends to occur between 24 to 48 hours after smoke exposure.[1] A persistent severe base deficit (or high lactate concentration) in the absence of the most common causes of metabolic acidosis (renal failure, poor tissue perfusion, ketoacidosis, and toxin ingestion) suggest possible carbon monoxide, methemoglobinemia, or cyanide intoxication. Co-oximetry provides direct measurement of carboxyhemoglobin and methemoglobinemia, this technology is not commonly available in veterinary medicine. Pulse oximetry is a noninvasive method of assessing oxygenation of hemoglobin. In smoke inhalation where carboxyhemoglobin or methemoglobin may form, pulse oximetry is inaccurate and will overestimate the hemoglobin saturation with O_2.

In animals with ocular signs, evaluation for foreign bodies and corneal ulceration should be performed. Topical ocular anesthesia will decrease blepharospasm and allow exploration under the eyelids and a more detailed evaluation of the cornea. Fluorescein stain should be performed to assess for corneal ulceration. Superficial corneal ulceration occurs frequently in animals exposed to smoke and fire.

Thoracic radiographs provide additional assessment and monitoring of the respiratory system. A variety of abnormalities may be noted including alveolar, interstitial, and peribronchial patterns.[1,2] Rarely, a collapsed lung lobe may occur as result of bronchial obstruction from mucosal swelling, sloughing, and debris. As with most dynamic disease processes, thoracic radiographic changes lag behind the clinical appearance of the animal.

Finally, as with any critically ill animal, a complete blood count, chemistry screen, and urinalysis should be performed.

TREATMENT

The treatment of smoke inhalation is primarily supportive. O_2 supplementation should be administered to any patient showing respiratory or neurologic changes. Administration of 100% O_2 will treat hypoxemia and decrease the elimination half-time of carbon monoxide from 4 hours to 80 minutes.[4]

Hydration with intravenous balanced electrolyte solution should be maintained to avoid drying and thickening of airway secretions. Pulmonary vascular permeability may be increased and overhydration should be avoided to minimize accumulation of pulmonary fluid.

Corticosteroids have been used to decrease airway inflammation in animals with smoke inhalation. The use of corticosteroids in experimental animal models of smoke inhalation and one clinical study in people have had mixed results. Dexamethasone and methylprednisolone decreased mortality in a rat model of smoke inhalation, whereas cortisone and hydrocortisone did not.[11] Dexamethasone given to people with smoke inhalation did not make a difference on any parameter assessed compared to the group that did not receive corticosteroids.[12] In a retrospective study on smoke exposure in dogs, dexamethasone was administered more frequently to dogs that had longer hospital stays and more complicated clinical courses.[1] The retrospective design of the study could not illuminate the cause and effect of this association. In summary, there is no strong evidence for corticosteroid administration in animals with smoke inhalation and is not currently recommended.

Antibiotics are often administered to animals with smoke inhalation. Currently, prophylactic antibiotics are not indicated and antibiotic therapy should be guided by culture and sensitivity. Animals with smoke inhalation that are intubated and receiving positive pressure ventilation may be particularly susceptible to pulmonary infection and should be monitored accordingly. If pulmonary infection is diagnosed, then broad-spectrum antibiotic administration is warranted.

Airway irritation due to particulates and irritants can result in bronchoconstriction. Bronchodilators such as β_2-agonists or phosphodiesterase inhibitors may relieve the bronchoconstriction.

Dogs with severe pulmonary congestion and productive coughing may benefit from nebulization and physiotherapy every 4 to 6 hours. This assists in thinning and clearance of airway secretions. Rarely, bronchial obstruction may occur as a result of airway secretions, debris accumulation, and mucosal swelling. Bronchoscopy and lavage to clear the major airways may be necessary to relieve the obstruction.

Animals with corneal ulceration should have topical broad-spectrum antibiotics applied. If miosis secondary to ciliary spasm is present, topical atropine should be administered as well.

PROGNOSIS

The majority of animals that make it to the veterinary hospital alive do well and survive to discharge. Dogs that are not worse by the second day and have mild respiratory signs will likely remain in the hospital about 2 days. Dogs that have severe signs and have become worse by the second day either die by 72 hours or remain hospitalized for 6 to 7 days before being discharged.[1] Similarly, in a study on cats with smoke exposure, the outcome for cats that survived to be admitted to the veterinary hospital was good with none of the cats dying spontaneously and only two requiring euthanasia due to severe neurologic or respiratory compromise.[2] Overall, the survival rate was 91%. This rate is comparable to the 90% survival rate of humans with smoke inhalation only (no skin burns).[13] When euthanasized animals were excluded, 100% of the cats survived. As in dogs, it appears that if a cat can make it to the hospital alive, there is a good chance that it will survive.

REFERENCES

1. Drobatz KJ, Walker LM, Hendricks JC: Smoke exposure in dogs: 27 cases (1988–1997). *J Am Vet Med Assoc* 215:1306, 1999.
2. Drobatz KJ, Walker L, Hendricks JC: Smoke exposure in cats: 22 cases (1986–1997). *J Am Vet Med Assoc* 215:1312, 1999.
3. Shusterman DJ: Clinical smoke inhalation injury: systemic effects. *Occup Med* 8: 469, 1993.
4. Weiss SM, Lakshminarayan S: Acute inhalation injury. *Clin Chest Med* 15:103, 1994.
5. Orzel RA: Toxicological aspects of firesmoke: polymer pyrolysis and combustion. *Occup Med* 8:414, 1993.
6. Dressler DP: Laboratory background on smoke inhalation. *J Trauma* 19:913, 1979.
7. Bizovi KE, Leikin JD: Smoke inhalation among firefighters. *Occup Med* 10:721, 1995.
8. Piantadosi CA: Carbon monoxide, oxygen transport, and oxygen metabolism. *J Hyperbaric Med* 2:27, 1987.
9. Nieman G, Clark W, Wax S, Webb RW: The effect of smoke inhalation on pulmonary surfactant. *Ann Surg* 191:171, 1980.
10. Tams TR, Sherding RG: Smoke inhalation injury. *Compend Contin Educ Pract Vet* 11, 986, 1981.
11. Dressler DP, Skornik WA, Kupersmith S: Corticosteroid treatment of experimental smoke inhalation. *Ann Surg* 183:46, 1976.
12. Robinson NB, Hudson LD, Riem M, *et al.*: Steroid therapy following isolated smoke inhalation injury. *J Trauma* 22:876, 1982.
13. Venus B, Takayoshi M, Copiozo JB, Mathru M: Prophylactic intubation and continuous positive airway pressure in the management of inhalation injury in burn victims. *Crit Care Med* 9:519, 1981.

72
The Transfusion Trigger

Wayne E. Wingfield

INTRODUCTION

Anemia is commonly seen and whole blood transfusions are often necessary. The goals of transfusion are to reduce mortality and morbidity and improve the functional status that results from anemia and inadequate oxygen (O_2) delivery. Challenges in providing adequate availability of blood to meet the needs of the veterinary patient is often encountered. To optimize use of this valuable resource, we can offer guidelines in providing a transfusion but medical judgments cannot, and should not, be determined solely by algorithms, flow charts, and packed cell volumes (PCVs). These represent laboratory values at which a transfusion is usually reasonable and for which no further justification is necessary.

CLINICAL SIGNS OF ANEMIA

The classic clinical signs of severe anemia include exercise intolerance, respiratory distress, lethargy, hypotension, pale mucous membranes, tachycardia, and impaired consciousness. Most commonly these signs appear when the PCV is dangerously low. Few data are available for animals but in humans, exertional dyspnea does not occur until the hemoglobin concentration Hb falls to less than 7 g/dL.[1] In another study, at Hb levels of less than 6 g/dL, only 54% of patients experienced tachycardia, 32% had hypotension, 35% had impaired consciousness, and 27% had dyspnea.[2] Levels of anemia required to produce symptoms in children are even more severe. Therefore, relying on clinical signs of anemia to guide transfusion decisions likely result in significant undertransfusion of patients. Moreover, relying on clinical signs in the anesthetized animal would obviously be fruitless.

When does one transfuse a patient? What is the transfusion trigger? These are questions pondered for many years. Interestingly, there are few objective data or obvious physiologic end points that can serve as a basis for making transfusion decisions. The "transfusion trigger" is the minimum Hb or PCV (Hb equals one-third PCV) value at which a red blood cell (RBC) transfusion is usually administered. One decision-making factor is the "10/30" rule often cited in human medicine. The origin of this value, an Hb of 10 g/dL and PCV level of 30%, for receiving a transfusion has existed for many years.[3]

At the turn of the last century, human surgeons and anesthetists observed those patients with a Hb less than 10 g/dL did not do well. In 1920, Barcroft[4] noted that tissue oxygenation was a function of Hb, oxygenation of blood by the lungs, and cardiac output (CO). In 1942, Adams and Lundy[5] reported that the effects of anemia on the O_2-carrying capacity of blood result in inadequate transport of O_2 to the tissues. They suggested preoperative transfusion of blood "when the concentration of hemoglobin is less than eight to 10 grams per 100 cubic centimeters." This is the origin of the 10/30 rule and is based solely on clinical experience. When they first addressed the problem of tissue oxygenation as a problem and then provided a Hb range, they established the basis for the current practice and debate.[6] Unfortunately, the 10 g/dL became dogma and was passed on as lore for nearly 60 years. Internists, hematologists, and surgeons supported it. The "transfusion trigger" was established as a Hb of less than 10 g/dL.

Between the 1940s and 1980s considerable effort was directed to improving our understanding of O_2 delivery (DO_2) and oxygen consumption (VO_2) physiology, and at unraveling the many mysteries of O_2 use. Many of these studies became the basis for a physiologic rationale for transfusion therapy.[7] In vitro and animal studies lend support to the concept that DO_2 peaks at a PCV of 30%[8] and 40%.[9-11] During the Korean conflict data demonstrated that a patient's vital signs did not deteriorate if the Hb was approximately 7 g/dL and the blood volume maintained.[12]

It was not until 1988 that the "10/30" rule was seriously questioned. The National Institutes of Health Consensus Conference on Perioperative Red Blood Cell Transfusion lowered the trigger to "7/21".[13] This conference noted there was no single measure serving as an indicator for transfusion and that clinical judgment, expressed as risk assessment, plays a role.[14]

RISKS FROM ANEMIA

The level of anemia at which adverse events occur is needed to develop guidelines for transfusion, but data are limited. Healthy animals subjected to acute hemodilution, tolerate Hb levels between 3 and 5 g/dL. When the Hb is less than 3 g/dL, ischemic electrocardiographic signs, increased lactate production, depressed ventricular function, and death occur.[15,16] Chronic anemia, in theory, is better tolerated than acute anemia because of the opportunity for the oxyhemoglobin dissociation curve to shift toward increased O_2 release (Fig. 72-1). Whether this is true or not is unknown.[15]

Determining the need for erythrocyte transfusion includes the etiology and chronicity of the anemia, the patient's ability to compensate for decreasing O_2-carrying capacity, and tissue O_2 requirements. The animal with less than 33% blood loss is able to compensate for acute blood loss, but the patient with dilated cardiomyopathy may not be able to compensate. Loss of a liter of blood in a fracture site of a 50-kg dog is very different from treating an anemic Toy Poodle undergoing adriamycin treatment for lymphosarcoma. Obviously, no RBC transfusion trigger will be appropriate for all patients!

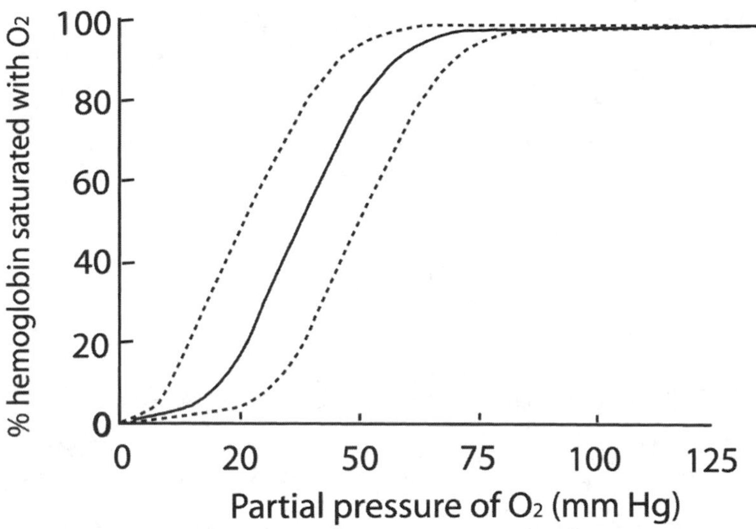

Figure 72-1
The oxyhemoglobin dissociation curve. The solid line represents O_2-binding affinity to the Hb molecule at standard temperature (37°C) and a pH of 7.4. The dashed lines represent hypothetical shifts in the curve; to the right with increased 2,3-diphosphoglycerate (2,3-DPG) levels or decreased temperature or pH; to the left with decreased 2,3-DPG or increased temperature or pH.[17]

PHYSIOLOGY OF ACUTE BLOOD LOSS[17]

The compensatory mechanisms activated by acute blood loss include changes in O_2 transport, CO, VO_2, the kinetics of O_2, and adaptive changes associated with anemia. Early in acute blood loss there is stimulation of the adrenergic nervous system, release of vasoactive hormones, redistribution of fluid from the interstitium to the intravascular space, a shift of fluid from the intracellular to extracellular compartment, renal conservation of water and electrolytes, and hyperventilation. These changes all contribute to an increase in CO, the primary determinant of tissue perfusion.[18]

Hemoglobin is a complex molecule consisting of four globin moieties, each incorporating an iron-containing heme ring where O_2 is bound according to its partial pressure (PO_2). The O_2-binding affinity of Hb is illustrated by the sinusoidal relationship between Hb O_2 saturation and PO_2 (see Fig. 72-1). This relationship, referred to as the oxyhemoglobin dissociation curve, enables both efficient loading in the lungs at high PO_2 and efficient unloading in the tissues at low PO_2 levels. However, the O_2-binding affinity of Hb may be altered by various disease states and may play a significant adaptive role in response to anemia.

The content of oxygen in arterial blood (CaO_2) is described in the following equation:

$$CaO_2 = (1.34 \times [Hg] \times SaO_2) + (0.003 \times PaO_2) \qquad 72\text{-}1$$

The contributions of Hb and the percentage of Hb saturated with O_2 (SaO_2) are described by the first term of the equation and the second term describes the small contribution of O_2 free in the plasma. One gram of Hb can actually bind 1.39 mL O_2 at full saturation.[19] However, a small fraction of the circulating Hb is represented by forms that do not readily bind O_2 (*i.e.*, methemoglobin and carboxyhemoglobin). Thus, 1.34 mL/g more accurately describes the behavior of the pool of circulating Hb.

The amount of O_2 delivered, either to the whole body or to specific organs, is the product of the total blood flow and arterial O_2 content. For the whole body, DO_2 is the product of CO and CaO_2:

$$DO_2 = CO \times CaO_2 \qquad 72\text{-}2$$

When CaO_2 from the first equation is substituted into the second, the resulting equation is:

$$DO_2 = CO \times (SaO_2 \times 13.4^{a} \times [Hgb]) \qquad 72\text{-}3$$

Where, CO is cardiac output in L/min and SaO_2 is the percentage of Hb saturated with O_2. CO, a measure of blood flow to the entire body, is the other major determinant of O_2 delivery. CO may be quantified by multiplying the stroke volume (the difference between end-diastolic volume and end-systolic volume in milliliters) and heart rate (in beats per minute). Stroke volume is influenced by preload (end-diastolic volume affected by filling pressure), afterload (the arterial pressure and resistance encountered during each ventricular ejection), and contractility (the force generated during a contraction).

Oxygen consumption (VO_2) from the microcirculation is a function of CO and the difference in O_2 content between arterial and venous blood:

$$VO_2 = CO \times (CaO_2 - CvO_2) \qquad 72\text{-}4$$

Because CaO_2 and CvO_2 share the same term for Hb binding (Equation 72-1), the equation for VO_2 can be rewritten as:

$$VO_2 = CO \times Hb \times 13.4 \times (SaO_2 - SvO_2) \qquad 72\text{-}5$$

In humans, the normal range for VO_2 is 110 to 160 mL/min/m^2.[b]

The oxygen extraction ration (OER) is the ratio of O_2 to O_2 delivery (VO_2/DO_2). The OER represents the fraction of O_2 delivered to the microcirculation that is taken up into the tissues. Thus only a small fraction of available O_2 is used to support aerobic metabolism. O_2 extraction is adjustable and in conditions where DO_2 is impaired, the OER can increase to 0.5 to 0.6. These adjustments are important in maintaining O_2 uptake when DO_2 is variable. This can be seen by rearranging the equation for OER:

$$VO_2 = DO_2 \times OER \qquad 72\text{-}6$$

---

[a] 10 times 1.34 converts the final result to mL/min.

[b] To be precise, CO is actually cardiac index (CI), which is simply calculated by knowing CO and dividing by the body surface area in meters squared.

In Equation 72-6, when a decrease in DO_2 is accompanied by a proportional increase in OER, the VO_2 remains constant.

In health, the amount of O_2 delivered to the whole body exceeds resting O_2 requirements by a factor of two to four. For example, if we assume a Hb of 15.0 g/dL, 99% saturation of Hb with O_2, and CO of 5 L/min, then DO_2 will be 1032 mL/min. At rest, the amount of O_2 required or consumed by the whole body will range from 200 to 300 mL/min. A decrease in Hb to 10 g/dL results in a DO_2 of 688 mL/min. Despite this 33% decrease in DO_2, there remains a twofold excess of DO_2 compared with consumption. However, a further drop in Hb to 5 g/dL with all other parameters, including CO, remaining constant decreases DO_2 to a critical level of 342 mL/min. Under stable experimental conditions, this dramatic decrease in DO_2 would not affect VO_2; however, below a critical level or threshold of O_2 (DO_2 [critical]), VO_2 decreases with further decreases in Hb (and decreased DO_2). The latter portion of this relationship indicates the presence of tissue hypoxia. Both laboratory and clinical studies have attempted to determine DO_2 [critical]. The most rigorous clinical study found a threshold value of 4 mL/min/kg,[20] whereas other clinical and laboratory studies found values in the range of 6 to 10 mL/min/kg.[20-23]

Oxygen delivery measured for the whole body is a composite for all organs, whose individual anaerobic thresholds may be significantly different from the average DO_2 [critical]. In addition, the anaerobic threshold and associated DO_2 [critical] values will also vary substantially with metabolic rate, some disease states, and perhaps such complex factors as a patient's age or genetic make-up. Once blood is oxygenated, it is distributed to all organs and tissues throughout the arterial tree. Organ blood flow is controlled by arterial tone in medium-sized vessels, which responds primarily to changes in autonomic stimulation and the release of locally generated vasodilating substances. Within organ systems, erythrocytes are carried into a network of capillaries where O_2 is released to the tissues through the thin walls. Once released, O_2 diffuses through the interstitial space, finally finding its way into cells and their mitochondria to be used in cellular respiration. Each of these physiologic mechanisms may be altered in disease states.

A relationship is identified between global DO_2 and VO_2 (Fig. 72-2). VO_2 appears to be both independent of and dependent on blood flow. For example, at a given flow, VO_2 ceases to be flow dependent and achieves a relatively steady state in normal, nonseptic humans. If this critical DO_2 point is assumed to represent tissue perfusion, and can be identified, this information can contribute to the transfusion decision.

Tissue hypoxia (and anoxia) will occur if DO_2 is permitted to decrease to a level at which tissues no longer have enough O_2 to meet metabolic demands. From Equations 72-1 and 72-3, it is apparent that tissue hypoxia may be caused by decreased DO_2 due to decreases in either Hb (anemic hypoxia), CO (stagnant hypoxia), or Hb saturation (hypoxic hypoxia). Each of the determinants of DO_2 has substantial physiologic reserves, thereby enabling the animal body to adapt to significant increases in O_2 requirements or decreases in one of the determinants of DO_2 as a result of various diseases.

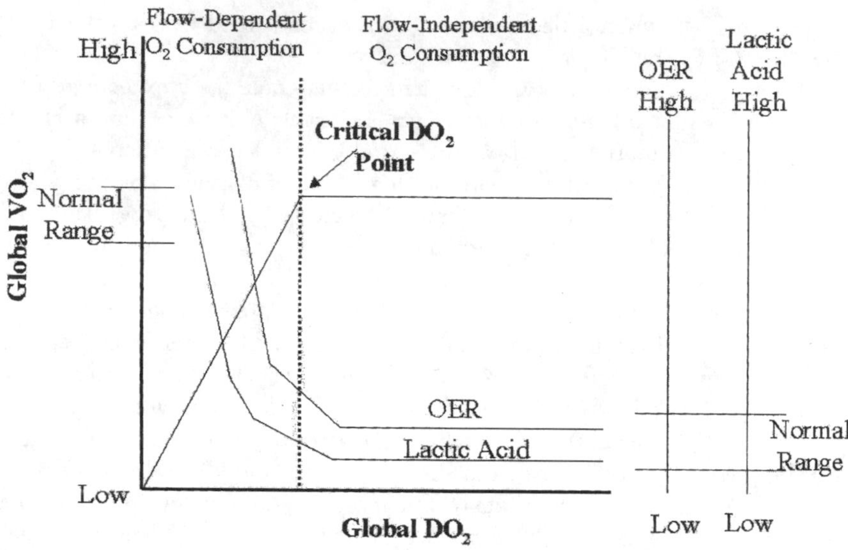

Figure 72-2
Schematic representation of the relationship of oxygen delivery (DO_2), oxygen consumption (VO_2), and tissue perfusion reflected by oxygen extraction ratio (OER) and lactic acid levels. Metabolism appears appropriately aerobic and adequate when VO_2 is independent of DO_2.[6]

Two factors that reflect tissue perfusion begin to change at or near the critical DO_2 point: (1) lactate levels increase and (2) the OER changes its slope. With decreased DO_2, global OER begins to increase. If these parameters and variables are indeed markers of tissue hypoxia, their change from normal implies the presence of inadequate DO_2 to the tissues. In humans it appears that these increases are most useful in trauma and surgery but not sepsis nor acute respiratory distress syndrome. Increases in the OER and lactate values below the critical DO_2 point may be physiologic transfusion triggers.

A physiologically defined end point of poor tissue perfusion appears to be an increase in OER above 0.30, an increased blood lactate level, and a global DO_2 of less than 10 to 12 mL/kg/min in humans. These variables may improve with an increase in inspired O_2, a fluid challenge to increase preload, or other manipulations to increase CO. If OER, DO_2, and lactate levels do not improve with these measures, then the addition of increased O_2-carrying capacity (erythrocytes or erythrocyte substitutes) is indicated.

ADAPTIVE MECHANISMS IN ANEMIA

In anemia, O_2-carrying capacity is decreased but tissue oxygenation is preserved at Hb well below 10g/dL. Adaptive responses include a shift in the oxyhemoglobin dissociation curve, hemodynamic alterations, and microcirculatory alterations. The shift to the right of the oxyhemoglobin dissociation curve in anemia is primarily the result of increased synthesis of 2,3-diphosphoglycerate (2,3-DPG) in erythrocytes.[15] This enables more O_2 to be released to the tissues at a given PO_2, offsetting the effect of the reduced O_2-carrying capacity of the blood. This shift also occurs in vitro with decreases in temperature and pH. Because measurements of Hb O_2 saturation are generally performed on arterial specimens processed at standard temperature and pH, they will not reflect O_2-binding affinity and unloading conditions in the patient's microcirculatory environment, which may be affected by temperature, pH, and a number of disease processes.

The shift in the oxyhemoglobin dissociation curve because of decreased pH is referred to as the Bohr effect. Because changes in pH rapidly affect the ability of the Hb molecule to bind O_2, this mechanism has been postulated to be an important early adaptive response to anemia.[24] However, the equations describing the physical process indicate that a very large change in pH is required to modify the P50 by a clinically important amount (*i.e.*, about 10 mm Hg). As a result, the Bohr effect is unlikely to have important clinical consequences.

Several hemodynamic alterations also occur following the development of anemia. The most important determinant of cardiovascular response is the patient's volume status or more specifically, left ventricular preload. The combined effect of hypovolemia and anemia often occurs as a result of blood loss. Thus, acute anemia may cause tissue hypoxia or anoxia through both diminished CO resulting in stagnant hypoxia and decreased O_2-carrying capacity (anemic hypoxia). The body attempts to preserve DO_2 delivery to vital organs primarily by redistributing the available cardiac output through increased arterial tone. The adrenergic system plays an important role in altering blood flow to and within specific organs.

The renin-angiotensin-aldosterone system is also stimulated to retain both water and sodium. Losses in blood volume of 5% to 15% result in variable increases in resting heart rate and diastolic blood pressure. Larger losses will result in progressive increases in heart rate and decreases in arterial blood pressure accompanied by evidence of organ hypoperfusion. The increased sympathetic tone diverts decreasing CO away from the splanchnic, skeletal, and cutaneous circulation toward the coronary and cerebral circulation. Once vital organ systems such as the kidneys, the central nervous system, and the heart are affected, the patient is considered in hypovolemic shock. The American College of Surgeons Committee on Trauma has categorized the cardiovascular and systemic response to acute blood loss according to degree of blood loss.[25] Many of these responses are modified by the rapidity of blood loss and patient characteristics such as age, concurrent illnesses, pre-existing volume status, and Hb, and the use of medications having cardiac (*i.e.*, β-blockers) or peripheral vascular effects (*i.e.*, antihypertensives).

The compensatory changes in CO have been the most thoroughly studied cardiovascular consequences of normovolemic anemia. When intravascular volume is stable or increases following the development of anemia, increases in CO are consistently reported. Indeed, an inverse relation between Hb and CO has been clearly established in well-controlled laboratory studies (Fig. 72-3).[26]

Researchers have attempted to determine the level of anemia at which CO begins to rise. Reported thresholds for this phenomenon have ranged from 7.0

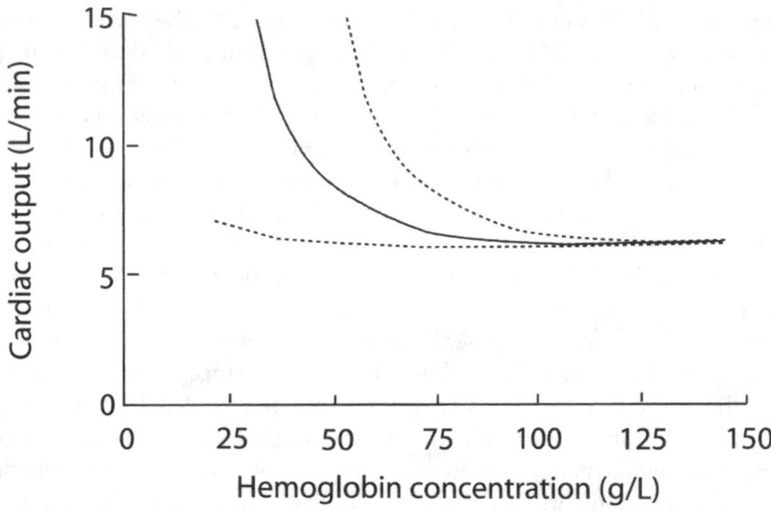

Figure 72-3
The theoretical effect of Hb on CO. The solid curve describes this relation in a healthy adult human. The upper dashed line shows how the cardiac response may be accentuated in a young athlete; the lower dashed line might correspond to poor cardiovascular function.[17]

to 12.0 g/dL.[26,27] Two mechanisms are thought to be principally responsible for the physiologic processes underlying increased CO during normovolemic anemia: reduced blood viscosity and increased sympathetic stimulation of the cardiovascular effectors.[28] Blood viscosity affects both preload and afterload, whereas sympathetic stimulation primarily increases heart rate and contractility. Compared with hypovolemic anemia, in compensation for normovolemic anemia, the effects of blood viscosity appear to predominate.

The interactions between blood flow, blood viscosity, and CO are complex. In blood vessels, blood flow affects whole blood viscosity and, in turn, blood viscosity modulates CO. Under experimental conditions, blood flow in a rigid hollow cylinder is directly related to the fourth power of the diameter and the driving pressure and inversely related to the cylinder length and blood viscosity (Poiseuille-Hagen law).[28] Also, blood viscosity increases as flow decreases because of increasing aggregation of erythrocytes. Thus, viscosity is highest in postcapillary venules where flow is the slowest, and lowest in the aorta where flow is fastest. In postcapillary venules, a disproportionate decrease in blood viscosity occurs as anemia worsens and, as a consequence, venous return is augmented for a given venous pressure. If cardiac function is normal, the increase in venous return or left ventricular preload will be the most important determinant of the increased CO during normovolemic anemia. Decreased left ventricular afterload, another cardiac consequence of decreased blood viscosity, may also be an important mechanism in maintaining CO if ventricular function is impaired.

Anemia causes sympathetic stimulation and increased heart rate.[26,29] This physiologic response is thought to be predominantly mediated by aortic chemoreceptors and release of catecholamines.[10] However, primary laboratory studies and studies of perioperative normovolemic hemodilution and chronic anemia have not consistently demonstrated significant increases in heart rate in response to moderate degrees of anemia. A detailed review indicated significant differences in species response as well as differences between awake and anesthetized patients.[29]

In summary, the anemia-induced increase in CO is more dependent on stroke volume and, to a lesser extent, on heart rate, in most clinical settings. If increased heart rate occurs following normovolemic anemia, one of its major consequences will be to inhibit coronary blood flow by shortening diastole, when the left ventricular myocardium is perfused. The shortening of diastolic filling time alone is usually insufficient to induce myocardial ischemia in normal human subjects. The O_2 supply-demand relationship may also be adversely affected by additional changes to ventricular loading conditions. Sympathetic stimulation may affect CO by enhancing myocardial contractility and increasing venomotor tone. If sympathetic stimulation is significant in the specific clinical setting, then contractility will be increased from stimulation of the β-adrenergic receptors.[29]

Under laboratory conditions there are significant increases in coronary blood flow directly related to the degree of normovolemic anemia. These studies do *not* demonstrate significant shifts in the transmural distribution of coronary flow between endocardium and epicardium in the normal coronary circulation during moderate degrees of anemia. Further, significant alterations in the distribution of flow between major organs following acute hemodilution have also been documented.[10] Disproportionate increases in coronary and cerebral blood flow occur with simultaneous decreases in blood flow to the splanchnic circulation.

The inverse relation between CO and Hb has led investigators to try to find the Hb at which O_2 transport is maximum. In a canine model, Richardson and Guyton[30] established that optimum O_2 transport occurred at a hematocrit of 40% to 60%; others[31-34] have determined that maximum DO_2 occurs at the low end of this range (40%-45%). However, one of the most widely quoted studies[35] reported that peak O_2 transport occurred at a hematocrit of 30% (Hb 10.0 g/dL). Attempting to identify a single Hb that maximizes DO_2 overlooks the large number of factors interfering with adaptive mechanisms in anyone other than healthy young patients with anemia.[17]

INTERACTION BETWEEN PATHOPHYSIOLOGIC PROCESSES AND ANEMIA

A number of diseases that affect either the entire body or specific organs may limit adaptive responses to anemia. Heart, lung, and cerebrovascular diseases have been proposed to increase the risk of adverse consequences from anemia.[13,27,35] Age, severity of illness, and therapeutic interventions may also affect adaptive mechanisms.[17]

The heart, especially the left ventricle, may be particularly prone to adverse consequences of anemia because the myocardium consumes 60% to 75% of all DO_2 delivered to the coronary circulation. Such a high OER is unique to the coronary circulation. As a result, delivery of O_2 to the myocardium primarily increases by increasing blood flow. Moreover, most of left ventricular perfusion is restricted to the diastolic period, and any shortening in its duration (*e.g.*, in tachycardia) constrains blood flow. Moderate anemia is poorly tolerated in perioperative and critically ill human patients with cardiovascular disease.[36] Anemia may also result in significant increases in morbidity and mortality in patients with other cardiac pathologies including heart failure and valvular heart disease, presumably because of the greater burden of the adaptive increase in CO.[37]

During normovolemic anemia, cerebral blood flow increases as Hb decreases. Investigators have observed increases ranging from 50% to 500% of baseline values in laboratory studies.[38-40] Increased cerebral blood flow occurs because of overall increases in CO, which is preferentially diverted to the cerebral circulation. Also, as DO_2 begins to decrease, cerebral tissues extract more O_2 from the blood. A number of factors, including the degree of hemodilution, the type of fluid used for volume expansion, volume status (preload), and the extent of the cerebrovascular disease, can modify global or regional cerebral blood flow during anemia. The laboratory studies suggest that moderate degrees of anemia alone should rarely result in or worsen cerebral ischemia. As a therapy in acute ischemic stroke, hemodilution did not produce a significant overall improvement in clinical outcome.[17] However, because of the large variety of variables that may affect the extent of clinical outcomes, the negative findings may not rule out the possibility of therapeutic benefits.

Changes in O_2 delivery to the brain (as a result of increases or decreases in blood flow) during normovolemic anemia do not uniformly affect various forms of cerebral pathologies. For example, patients with increased intracranial pressure from traumatic brain injury may be adversely affected by increased cerebral blood flow. However, following subarachnoid hemorrhage, mild degrees of normovolemic or hypervolemic anemia may improve overall DO_2, possibly by overcoming the effects of cerebral vasospasm thereby improving cerebral blood flow through decreased viscosity. The effects of moderate to severe anemia in subarachnoid hemorrhage have not been assessed either in laboratory or clinical studies.[17]

Redistribution of CO to the coronary and cerebral circulation during normovolemic anemia results in a shunting of blood away from other organs. In critically ill patients who are affected by a wide variety of pathologic processes this redistribution may result in increased gut ischemia, bacterial translocation, and multisystem organ failure. Critical illness may also tax many of the body's adaptive responses, specifically, cardiac performance that may already be responding to increased metabolic demands.

Currently it is not possible to offer guidelines on how to increase, maintain, or even determine optimum DO_2 in high-risk patients or how transfusion strategies might best be used under these conditions. From the brief review of physiologic principles and the strong consensus in the literature, it is evident that *cardiac function* must be a central consideration in decisions about transfusion in anemia, because of the critical role it plays in ensuring adequate O_2 supply to all vital tissues. Because high-level evidence on the interactions of concurrent diseases and anemia in various patient populations is lacking, an understanding of the physiologic consequences of anemia and of the diseases is useful but not sufficient to guide transfusion practice in specific complex clinical conditions. Clinical and experimental investigation is required to support comprehensive clinical practice guidelines for RBC transfusions.

ERYTHROCYTE ADMINISTRATION

Red blood cells are administered to augment delivery of O_2, not as a therapy for hypovolemia. There is a minimum Hb level for each individual below which organ failure will occur as a result of O_2 deprivation. However, it is impossible to determine this level clinically and establish a specific erythrocyte trigger. The Hb value is not the only factor to consider when deciding whether erythrocyte administration is indicated. Other determinants of tissue DO_2 are the inspired O_2 concentration (FIO_2) and pulmonary gas exchange. Tissue VO_2 must also be considered.

Erythrocytes are not infrequently transfused to promote wound healing and "well-being." However, animal studies, confirmed by observations in postoperative human patients, indicate that normovolemic anemia is not detrimental to wound healing. The critical hematocrit at which anemia may influence tissue repair appears to be approximately 15%.

Hemodilution is used in anesthetized patients continuously monitored to ensure normovolemia and adequate oxygenation. An increased FIO_2 is ordinarily administered. In addition, VO_2 is usually decreased during a properly conducted anesthetic. These conditions do not usually persist beyond the operating room.

In chronic anemia, the patient's symptoms must be considered. When anemia develops slowly, several physiologic adjustments occur. Delivery of O_2 becomes more efficient due to a rightward shift of the oxyhemoglobin dissociation curve. This shift begins at Hb levels of approximately 9 g/dL and is prominent below 6.5 g/dL. It is due primarily to increased synthesis of 2,3-DPG. An increase in 2,3-DPG is unlikely to occur in acute blood loss as this requires 12 to 36 hours. The CO increases as the Hb falls. The increase in CO occurs primarily as a result of decreased viscosity secondary to reduced erythrocyte mass. The exact level where CO increases varies among individuals and in humans is influenced by age. No change is usually seen until the Hb is below 9 g/dL. In some patients, CO does not increase until the Hb falls below 7 to 8 g/dL. In normal adult humans, the increase in CO is due primarily to increased stroke volume. In patients with impaired ventricular function, as well as in children, increased heart rate assumes a more important role.

When all the studies, clinical experience, and individual options are considered, it is difficult to improve on the statement of the National Institutes of Health Consensus Development Conference on perioperative erythrocyte transfusion[13]:

"No single measure can replace good clinical judgement as the basis for decisions regarding perioperative transfusion. However, current experience would suggest that otherwise healthy patients with hemoglobin values of 10 g/dl or greater rarely require perioperative transfusion, whereas those with hemoglobin values less than 7 g/dl will frequently require transfusion of erythrocytes."

WHERE DO THE NEW HEMOGLOBIN SUBSTITUTES COME INTO CLINICAL USAGE?

Beginning in the 1960s, the military and private companies sought to develop a substitute for erythrocytes. The goal was principally to duplicate the O_2-carrying capacity of Hb. Such a substitute promises to improve the shelf-life over erythrocytes, no need for compatibility testing, and therefore immediate availability, and improved safety.

One Hb solution is available for clinical usage in veterinary medicine. Oxyglobin (hemoglobin glutamer-200 [bovine]) is an ultrapurified, polymerized Hb solution of bovine origin (13 g/dL) in modified Ringer's lactate solution. It is stable for at least 2 years when stored under ambient temperatures (2°–30°C). The O_2 saturation pressure (P50) of Oxyglobin is 38 mm Hg (normal dog P50 = 30 mm Hg). This means it has a greater efficiency of releasing O_2 to the tissue relative to Hb in the erythrocyte.[41] The half-life is reported by the manufacturer to be dose dependent and typically 30 to 40 hours at 30 mL/kg in healthy dogs. In a multicenter clinical trial in dogs with moderate to severe anemia (PCV 6%-23%), blood loss, hemolysis, or ineffective erythropoiesis, Oxyglobin showed a positive treatment success.[42] Unfortunately the definition of "success" was defined as not requiring additional O_2-carrying support for 24 hours. Because the half-life exceeds 24 hours, it is no wonder the study showed a treatment success. Very likely these animals required an erythrocyte transfusion as the Hb associated with the RBC has a longer duration of effect.

Oxyglobin in serum may cause artifactual increases or decreases in serum chemistry results. In general, all tests using colorimetric techniques are invalid. Additionally, urine dipstick measurements for pH, glucose, ketones, and proteins are inaccurate due to the gross discoloration of the urine.

When compared to whole blood, Oxyglobin's tissue O_2 tensions in the muscle of dogs is increased compared to stored or fresh erythrocytes.[43] In a study on cats, Oxyglobin solution and autologous blood were equally effective in restoring O_2 transport variables, including heart rate, arterial and venous O_2 content, O_2 extraction, and blood gases.[44]

Currently, there are advantages to use of Oxyglobin in the crisis setting. The substance is readily available, has an excellent shelf-life, provides O_2-carrying capacity in anemia, and improves O_2 transport variables. Drawbacks to its use include the short duration of effect, the interference with biochemical and urologic monitoring parameters, and its expense. Likely this solution will provide a quick fix but will not substitute for transfusion of erythrocytes.[45]

REFERENCES

1. Carmel R, Shulman IA: Blood transfusion in medically treatable chronic anemia: pernicious anemia as a model for transfusion overuse. *Arch Pathol Lab Med* 113:995, 1989.
2. Muller G, N'tial I, Nyst M, *et al.*: Application of blood transfusion guidelines in a major hospital of Kinshasa, Zaire. *AIDS* 6:431, 1992.
3. Zauder HL: Preoperative hemoglobin requirements. *Anesth Clin North Am* 8:471, 1990.
4. Barcroft J: The Respiratory Function of the Blood. Part I: Lessons from High Altitudes. New York: Cambridge University Press, 1925.
5. Adams RC, Lundy JS: Anesthesia in cases of poor surgical risk: some suggestions for decreasing the risk. *Surg Gynecol Obstet* 74:1011, 1942.
6. Greenburg AG: A physiologic basis for red blood cell transfusion decisions. *Am J Surg* 170(6A):44S, 1995.
7. Nunn JF, Freeman J: Problems of oxygenation and oxygen transport during hemorrhage. *Anesthesia* 19:206, 1964.
8. Stehling L, Sauder HL: Acute normovolemic hemodilution. *Transfusion* 31:857, 1991.
9. Robertie PG, Gravlee GP: Safe limits of isovolemic hemodilution and recommendations for erythrocyte transfusion. *Anesth Clin* 28:197, 1990.
10. Chapler CK, Carn SM: The physiologic reserve in oxygen carrying capacity: studies in experimental hemodilution. *Can J Physiol Pharmacol* 64:7, 1986.
11. Winslow RM: A physiological basis for the transfusion trigger. *In* Spiess BD, Counts RB, Gould SA, eds.: Perioperative transfusion medicine. Baltimore: Williams & Wilkins, 1998, p 27.
12. Crosby WH: Misuse of blood transfusion. *Blood* 13:1198, 1958.
13. National Institutes of Health Consensus Conference. Perioperative red blood cell transfusion. *JAMA* 260:2700, 1988.
14. Greenburg AG: Alternatives to conventional uses of blood products. Critical care: state of art. *Soc Crit Care Med* 14:325, 1992.
15. Rodman T, Close HP, Purcell MK: The oxyhemoglobin dissociation curve in anemia. *Ann Intern Med* 52:295, 1960.
16. Wilkerson DK, Rosen AL, Sehgal LR, *et al.*: Limits of cardiac compensation in anemic baboons. *Surgery* 103:665, 1988.
17. Hébert PC, Hu LQ, Biro GP: Review of physiologic mechanisms in response to anemia. *Can Med Assoc J* 156: S27-40, 1997.
18. Stehling L, Simon TL: The red blood cell transfusion trigger: physiology and clinical studies. *Arch Pathol Lab Med* 118, 429, 1994.
19. Zander R: Calculation of oxygen concentration. *In* Zander R, Mertzlufft F, eds.: The Oxygen Status of Arterial Blood. Basel: S. Karger, 1991, p 203.
20. Ronco JJ, Fenwick JC, Tweeddale MG, *et al.*: Identification of the critical oxygen delivery for anaerobic metabolism in critically ill septic and nonseptic humans. *JAMA* 270:1724, 1993.

21. Shibutani K, Komatsu T, Kubal K, *et al.*: Critical level of oxygen delivery in anesthetized man. *Crit Care Med* 11:640, 1983.
22. Nelson DP, Samsel RW, Wood LDH, *et al.*: Pathological supply dependence of systemic and intestinal oxygen uptake during endotoxemia. *J Appl Physiol* 64:2410, 1988.
23. Nelson DP, King CE, Dodd SL, Schumacker PT, *et al.*: Systemic and intestinal limits of oxygen extraction in the dog. *J Appl Physiol* 63:387, 1987.
24. Welch HG, Meehan KR, Goodnough LT: Prudent strategies for elective red blood cell transfusion. *Ann Intern Med* 116:393, 1992.
25. Alexander RH, Ali J, Aprahamian C, *et al.*: Advanced Trauma Life Support: Program for Physicians, 5th ed. Chicago: American College of Surgeons, 1993.
26. Welch HG, Meehan KR, Goodnough LT: Prudent strategies for elective red blood cell transfusion. *Ann Intern Med* 116:393, 1992.
27. Woodson RD, Auerbach S: Effect of increased oxygen affinity and anemia on cardiac output and its distribution. *J Appl Physiol* 53:1299, 1982.
28. Tuman KJ: Tissue oxygen delivery: the physiology of anemia. *Anesth Clin North Am* 9:451, 1990.
29. Spahn DR, Leone BJ, Reves JG, *et al.*: Cardiovascular and coronary physiology of acute isovolemic hemodilution: a review of nonoxygen-carrying and oxygen-carrying solutions. *Anesth Analg* 78:1000, 1994.
30. Richardson TQ, Guyton AC: Effects of polycythemia and anemia on cardiac output and other circulatory factors. *Am J Physiol* 197:1167, 1959.
31. Fan FC, Chen RYZ, Schuessler GB, *et al.*: Effects of hematocrit variations on regional hemodynamics and oxygen transport in the dog. *Am J Physiol* 238:H545, 1980.
32. Jan KM, Heldman J, Chien S: Coronary hemodynamics and oxygen utilization after hematocrit variations in hemorrhage. *Am J Physiol* 239:H326, 1980.
33. Jan KM, Chien S: Effect of hematocrit variations on coronary hemodynamics and oxygen utilization. *Am J Physiol* 233:H106, 1977.
34. Messmer K, Lewis DH, Sunder-Plassmann L, *et al.*: Acute normovolemic hemodilution. *Eur Surg Res* 4:55, 1972.
35. American College of Physicians. Practice strategies for elective red blood cell transfusion. *Ann Intern Med* 116:403, 1992.
36. Carson JL, Duff A, Poses RM, *et al.*: Effect of anaemia and cardiovascular disease on surgical mortality and morbidity. *Lancet* 348:1055, 1996.
37. Kobayashi H, Smith CE, Fouad-Tarazi FM, *et al.*: Circulatory effects of acute normovolemic hemodilution in rats with healed myocardial infarction. *Cardiovasc Res* 23: 842, 1989.
38. Kimura H, Hamaaki N, Yamamoto M, *et al.*: Circulation of red blood cells having high levels of 2,3-bisphosphoglycerate protects rat brain from ischemic metabolic changes during hemodilution. *Stroke* 26:1431, 1995.
39. Reasoner D, Ryu K, Hindman B, *et al.*: Marked hemodilution increases neurologic injury after focal cerebral ischemia in rabbits. *Anesth Analg* 82:61, 1996.
40. Yanaka K, Camarata P, Spellman S, *et al.*: Optimal timing of hemodilution for brain protection in a canine model of focal cerebral ischemia. *Stroke* 27:906, 1996.
41. Rentko V: Practical use of blood substitute. *In* Bonagura JD, ed.: Kirk's Current Veterinary Therapy XIII. Philadelphia: WB Saunders, 2000, p 424.
42. Rentko V, Wohl, J, Murtaugh R, *et al.*: A clinical trial of a hemoglobin-based oxygen carrier (HBOC) fluid in the treatment of anemia in dogs. *J Vet Intern Med* 10: 177, 1976.

43. Standl T, Horn P, Wilhelm S, *et al.*: Bovine hemoglobin is more potent than autologous red blood cells in restoring muscular tissue oxygenation after profound isovolumetric hemodilution in dogs. *Can J Anaesth* 43:714, 1996.
44. Walton RS: Polymerized hemoglobin versus hydroxyethyl starch in an experimental model of feline hemorrhagic shock. Proceedings of the 5th IVECC Symposium, San Antonio, TX, 1996.
45. Muir W (Moderator): Tissue in desperate need of oxygen: roundtable on transfusion triggers. *Vet Forum* April:50, 1999.

73
Myocardial Injury

Adam J. Reiss and Wayne E. Wingfield

INTRODUCTION

Thoracic injury is frequently noted following trauma in small animals. Blunt force injury to the chest can produce cardiovascular lesions including myocardial contusion, pericardial tear, interatrial and interventricular septal perforation, and cardiac rupture. Penetrating injuries to the myocardium of small animals are rare in clinical veterinary medicine. Primary cardiac injury is not a prerequisite for injury-induced myocardial dysfunction. Autonomic imbalance, ischemia, reperfusion injury, electrolyte derangements, and acid-base abnormalities may all account for arrhythmias in traumatized animals.

The first reports in the human literature of myocardial injury secondary to blunt thoracic trauma appeared in the 1920s.[1,2] The next 70 years produced numerous papers and editorials that discuss the classification, incidence, diagnosis, clinical significance, and need for treatment. Cost-cutting efforts in our human health care system have resulted in strong disagreement concerning the diagnosis and treatment of myocardial injury.[3,4] Most clinicians still question whether we know the incidence and clinical significance of myocardial injury caused by blunt thoracic trauma. It is theorized that the true incidence of myocardial injury may be higher than that reported because of lack of recognition and pre-hospital death.

ETIOLOGY AND MECHANISM OF INJURY

Thoracic trauma is common in dogs injured by automobiles.[18-21] Currently, the exact mechanism of cardiac injury following trauma is unknown but most likely remains multifactorial in origin. Research in humans has shown that a direct thoracic blow can result in up to a 50% alteration in thoracic diameter.[1] The elastic nature of the thorax subjects its contents to compressive, concussive, and penetrating injuries.[5,7,11] The severity of injury caused by trauma is affected by the rate and magnitude of the impacting force and the volume of soft tissue absorbing that force.[1,19] Other factors influencing the severity of injury include the position of the animal relative to the direction of the traumatic force and whether or not the animal is aware of the impending event and is able to initiate a protective response.[19]

The most common mechanism of compressive cardiac injury in dogs is secondary to lateral chest compression.[5,11] It has been proposed that distortion of the thoracic cage results in a rise in intrathoracic and intracardiac pressures that causes shearing stresses within the myocardium powerful enough to result in contusions. Pandian et al.[14] measured intracardiac pressures before, during, and after cardiac trauma. They found significant increases in left and right end-diastolic pressures and decreases in left ventricular systolic and aortic pressures following myocardial injury. Although these intracardiac pressure changes were significant, they did not result in significant changes in peripheral pressures.[14]

Rapid elevations in blood pressure during chest and/or abdominal compression have also been suggested to result in shearing injury to the myocardium.[7,22] In addition, the suspended position of the heart within the thoracic cavity subjects it to potential concussive injury from forceful contact with the ribs, sternum, and vertebrae when rapid acceleration or deceleration occurs.[5,7,11,13]

Other conditions associated with trauma and shock (metabolic acidosis, hypoxia, and catecholamine release) can injure the myocardium and predispose the heart to the development of arrhythmias.[6-8,12] Neurogenic injuries have also been implicated as a cause of myocardial injury and arrhythmias.[6,15] Experimentally, myocardial injury may be related to excessive sympathetic stimulation.[6,15] This observation is supported by noting a similar distribution of myocardial injury and the anatomic distribution of the adrenergic nerve supply to the heart.[6,18]

Injury to the right ventricle may indirectly play an important role in the development of functional abnormalities of the left ventricle.[1] Direct injury to the right ventricle results in decreased ejection fraction and increased afterload. This results in a leftward shift of the interventricular septum.[1] The septal shift markedly decreases the preload and compliance of the left ventricle, resulting in depression of left ventricular ejection fraction and impending pump failure.[1]

PATHOPHYSIOLOGY OF ARRHYTHMIC FORMATION

(See Chapter 31.)

Pathology

Pandian et al.[14] correlated histopathology areas with areas of injury found during echocardiographic examination in 25 dogs with induced blunt chest trauma. In this model, the impact was randomly delivered to either the right or left thorax and resulted in different areas of myocardial injury. When the trauma was delivered to the left side of the chest, abnormalities were located primarily in the craniolateral wall of the left ventricle; right-sided chest trauma produced septal and right ventricular wall damage. Pathologic findings were characterized by localized edema, ecchymosis and intramyocardial hematoma formation. No evidence of injury to the valves or coronary arteries was identified on gross pathologic evaluation. The area of myocardial contusion was often transmural, with the epicardial surface being more severely affected.[14]

Multiple clinical reports have described similar gross and microscopic pathologic findings following traumatic injury to the heart.[1,6,15,22-24] Radioactive labeled microsphere perfusion studies have shown that regional myocardial blood flow remains normal in the contused region, and thus hypoperfusion or ischemia does not appear to be responsible for impairment of function in these areas.[14]

EPIDEMIOLOGY

In the veterinary literature, Selcer et al.[18] evaluated 100 automobile injured dogs with radiographic evidence of skeletal trauma for concurrent thoracic trauma. Within 12 hours of admission and before anesthesia, thoracic radiographs, lead-II electrocardiogram (ECG), and an arterial blood gas sample were obtained from each patient. A 17% incidence of cardiac arrhythmias in dogs sustaining skeletal injury was found. The incidence of cardiac arrhythmias increased to 30% in animals with skeletal injury and evidence of any other identifiable thoracic pathology. In this study, 14 of the 17 dogs that developed arrhythmias had orthopedic trauma localized caudal to the 10th thoracic vertebra. Selcer also found that thoracic injury was not recognized on routine physical examination in 45 of 57 (79%) dogs in the study, suggesting a large number of undiagnosed injuries.[18] The reported incidence of human myocardial injury with blunt thoracic trauma ranges from 8 to 95%.[2,3,25,26] The wide range in the incidence of these injuries may be due to the variation in diagnostic modalities and criteria used to identify them.[1,3,9,13,14,21,24,27,30]

DIAGNOSIS

The possibility of myocardial injury should be considered in dogs that are struck by motor vehicles and have the following associated injuries: 1) fractures of extremities, the spine or pelvis; 2) external evidence of thoracic trauma; 3) radiographic evidence of chest trauma such as pulmonary contusions, pneumothorax, hemothorax, diaphragmatic rupture, and rib or scapular fractures; and 4) neurologic injury.[5,6,15-18]

The search for a single, noninvasive, sensitive, and specific modality to identify myocardial injury due to trauma is an active area of scientific investigation. Currently, a combination of tests is used to diagnose traumatic myocardial injury.[2,28] An understanding of the injury mechanism, the awareness of associated injuries, and a high index of suspicion are essential in making a diagnosis.[31] In humans, the most commonly used tests to diagnose myocardial injury include the ECG, thoracic radiographs, echocardiogram, and serum myocardial isoenzyme/protein analysis. A prospective study of 71 human patients in a level-one trauma center evaluated the predictive values of these modalities and found the ECG echocardiogram, creatine phosphokinase-myocardial band CPK-MB, and troponin-T to have poor sensitivity but high specificity (Table 73-1).[30] At present, the diagnostic gold standard in identifying myocardial injury is the gross or histologic examination of the heart.[30]

A lead-II ECG should be performed on examination and repeated at set intervals (every 12 to 24 hours) as a minimum cardiac database in dogs.[5,6,18] Continuous ECG provides valuable information on arrhythmia initiation and temporal changes in arrhythmogenic location. It is important to note that ECG abnormalities may not be apparent for up to 48 hours after trauma in dogs.[5-7,16]

Table 73-1. Sensitivity and Specificity of Selected Diagnostic Tests Used to Identify Myocardial Injuries

Diagnostic Method	Sensitivity	Specificity
Echocardiogram	0.12	0.98
ECG	0.38	0.93
CPK-MB > 4%	0.12	0.96
Troponin T > 0.2ug/L	0.27	0.91

ECG = electrocardiogram; CPK-MB = percent creatine phosphokinase due to myocardial band. Adapted after Fulda et al.[33]

In a prospective study of 92 human patients with evidence of chest trauma, Fabian et al.[10] demonstrated that 91% of their patients developed arrhythmias within 48 hours. Echocardiographic examination should be considered within the first 48 hours of injury in severely traumatized dogs with a poor response to resuscitative efforts or evidence of external thoracic injuries, even if no ECG abnormalities are observed. In dogs, echocardiography can identify and localize the structural and functional abnormalities of myocardial contusion due to blunt chest trauma.[15] The distinctive echocardiographic features of regional myocardial contusion in the dog include 1) increased end-diastolic wall thickness, 2) impaired contraction, indicated by decreased percent systolic wall thickening and decreased percent systolic ventricular dimension change, 3) increased echogenicity, and 4) localized areas of echolucency consistent with intramural hematomas.[14]

Historically, the isoenzyme used to identify myocardial necrosis in humans is creatinine phosphokinase-myocardial band CPK-MB. Several human clinical studies have demonstrated that CPK-MB isoenzyme measurement is not sensitive, specific, nor predictive of functional cardiac abnormalities.[1,10,29,31] A recent meta-analysis found that abnormal CPK-MB in conjunction with abnormal ECG correlated directly with complications that required treatment.[36] This combination of diagnostics has not yet been evaluated in veterinary medicine.

There have been several recent reports concerning cardiac specific proteins in the diagnosis of myocardial injury in humans. These proteins form a complex which is located on the thin filament of the contractile apparatus in both striated and skeletal muscle tissues.[27,37-39] Troponin consists of three proteins, each identified by a single letter, T, I, and C.[37,40] The isoforms of the troponin proteins expressed in cardiac muscle are different from those in skeletal muscle.[27,37-40] In both humans and dogs, troponins can be detected in the circulation within hours of myocardial injury and a high concentration has been shown to be present for up to 7 days.[17,41,42] O'Brien et al. demonstrated high concentrations of cTnT in the canine heart.[42,43] Release of cTnT by injured myocytes resulted in increases of 1000 to 10,000 fold of cTnT in the peripheral blood within 3 hours of injury.[42,43] The elevations in cTnT were highly correlated to infarct size.

Using animal models, O'Brien was also able to determine that cTnT was an effective biomarker in patients with doxorubicin cardiotoxicosis, traumatic injury, and cardiac puncture.[42] Cummings et al. demonstrated a similarly concentration of cTnI in a canine heart model post-infarction but found that this elevation did not correlate well with subsequent infarct size.[41] Recently, normal cTnI values (0.0–0.07 ng/ml; mean, 0.02 ng/ml) for dogs have been reported.[44] In addition to establishing a normal cTnI range for dogs, the authors found a high cTnI concentration of 0.08 to >50 ng/ml in five dogs with known cardiac disease and trauma, suggesting that a cTnI concentration of >0.07 ng/ml can be correlated with myocardial damage.[44] Although these cardiac specific markers are extremely sensitive and specific for myocardial injury as well as appearing to be of greater diagnostic value than CPK-MB, their clinical value has yet to be demonstrated in injured human and veterinary patients.[27,39]

Other modalities used in the diagnosis of myocardial injury in humans include nuclear cardiography. Nuclear cardiography can be used to simultaneously assess ventricular function, the direction and magnitude of cardiac shunts and to map myocardial perfusion.[32,33] The benefits of nuclear cardiography include a short study acquisition time, noninvasiveness, and it can be performed in an awake animal.[34] It appears that nuclear studies are more sensitive than thoracic radiographs in evaluating cardiac injuries since functional changes of the myocardium often precede changes in cardiac size and shape.[35] Measurement of left ventricular ejection fractions by radionuclide ventriculography has been shown to correlate well with cardiac output measured by thermodilution and M-mode two-dimensional echocardiography in healthy anesthetized dogs.[32] Disadvantages include the limited availability of nuclear studies, interference in image acquisition associated with arrhythmias, and performance of first-pass and gated studies must account for the overlap of the right and left sides of the heart.[34]

TREATMENT

Treatment is typically aimed at suppressing life-threatening arrhythmias that occur secondary to myocardial injury. Antiarrhythmic therapy is recommended in patients with arrhythmias such as multiform premature ventricular contractions, ventricular tachycardia and in those in which R-on-T phenomenon is detected.[7,8,12,16] Treatment may also be indicated if the ventricular rate exceeds 130 to 160 bpm in dogs[7,8]; it is certainly required when arrhythmias are accompanied by clinical evidence of low cardiac output.[8] The choice of specific antiarrhythmic agent lies with the clinician, and depends on the type of arrhythmia and the clinician's experience.

Lidocaine is the drug of choice for the urgent treatment of hemodynamically significant ventricular arrhythmias. It is administered as a slow intravenous bolus (2 mg/kg). If the arrhythmia is controlled with lidocaine bolus, a constant rate infusion (50–80 μg/kg/minute) is administered for antiarrythmic effect. The half life of lidocaine in dogs is extremely short (~9 minutes). Occasionally, supplemental small boluses are required to more quickly reach steady state levels.

Procainamide can also be used intravenously to control ventricular arrhythmias at a dose of 6 to 8 mg/kg given over five minutes. This drug can also be administered as a constant rate infusion of 25 to 50 μg/kg/minute.

Some ventricular tachyarrhythmias appear to be adrenergically mediated and thus will respond to intravenous administration of a short-acting β-blocking drug like esmolol (0.1–0.5 mg/kg slowly over 5 minutes). If this controls the arrhythmia, oral administration of propranolol (0.3–1.0 mg/kg PO q8h) may be used.

Magnesium chloride (25–40 mg/kg intravenously) may be used to control refractory ventricular tachyarrhythmias. The drug is diluted in saline and administered over 20 to 60 minutes. Synchronized DC cardioversion (0.5–1 J/kg) after heavy intravenous sedation can be considered in hypotensive patients with rapid ventricular rhythms that do not respond to drug therapy.

Dogs that have been properly volume expanded but remain in a state of low cardiac output without an arrhythmia require inotropic support. While inotropic drugs have been associated with injury extension in under-perfused myocardium, normal blood flow to contused myocardium has been demonstrated and should preclude further injury secondary to use of this class of drugs.[1,14]

Animals with a suspected myocardial injury often require anesthesia for correction of other injuries. If a patient with a myocardial injury must undergo anesthesia, drugs should be selected that are least likely to induce arrhythmias.[3,7,45]

PROGNOSIS

The clinical significance of myocardial injury is controversial. A literature search revealed no prospective studies that investigated the incidence, severity, and need for therapeutic intervention of traumatic myocardial injury in dogs. While the advent of noninvasive technologies may assist in diagnosing these injuries, the search for a single, noninvasive diagnostic modality to detect myocardial injury is not concluded. For now, the diagnosis of myocardial injury will rely on an organized approach that uses multiple diagnostic modalities. In the future, the application of immunodiagnostics such as the troponin assay may assist in early identification of myocardial injury in dogs and provide clinical information regarding expected outcome.

REFERENCES

1. Roxburgh JC: Myocardial contusion. *Injury* 27:603, 1996.
2. Helling TS, Duke P, Beggs CW, *et al.*: A prospective evaluation of 68 patients suffering blunt chest trauma for evidence of cardiac injury. *J Trauma* 29:961, 1989.

3. Paddleford RR: Anesthetic considerations for the high risk patient requiring a short anesthetic procedure. *In* Proceedings, Annu Meet Am Anim Hosp Assoc 1995, 21.
4. Beresky R, Klingler R, Peake J: Myocardial contusion: when does it have clinical significance? *J Trauma* 28:64, 1988.
5. Alexander JW, Bolton GR, Koslow GL: Electrocardiographic changes in nonpenetrating trauma to the chest. *J Am Anim Hosp Assoc* 11: 160, 1975.
6. Macintire DK, Snider TG: Cardiac arrhythmias associated with multiple trauma in dogs. *J Am Vet Med Assoc* 184:541, 1984.
7. Murtaugh RJ, Ross JN: Cardiac arrhythmias: pathogenesis and treatment in the trauma patient. *Comp Cont Educ Pract Vet* 10:332, 1988.
8. Abbott JA: Traumatic myocarditis. *In* Bonagura JD, ed.: Current Veterinary Therapy XII. Philadelphia: WB Saunders, 1995, 846.
9. Shorr RM, Crittenden M, Indeck M, *et al.*: Blunt thoracic trauma. *Ann Surg* 206: 200, 1988.
10. Fabian TC, Cicala RS, Croce MA, *et al.*: A prospective evaluation of myocardial contusion: correlation of significant arrhythmias and cardiac output with cpk-mb measurements. *J Trauma* 31:653, 1991.
11. Hunt C: Chest trauma—specific injuries. *Comp Cont Educ Pract Vet* 624:624, 1979.
12. Wingfield WE, Henik RA: Treatment priorities in cases of multiple trauma. *Sem Vet Med Surg (Small Anim)* 3:193, 1988.
13. Pearce W, Blair E: Significance of the electrocardiogram in heart contusion due to blunt trauma. *J Trauma* 16:136, 1976.
14. Pandian N, Skorton DJ, Doty DB, *et al.*: Immediate diagnosis of acute myocardial contusion by two-dimensional echocardiography: Studies in a canine model of blunt chest trauma. *J Am Coll Cardiol* 2:488, 1983.
15. King JM, Roth L, Haschek, WM: Myocardial necrosis secondary to neural lesions in domestic animals. *J Am Vet Med Assoc* 180:144, 1982.
16. Buffum RK, Dodd RR: Cardiac arrhythmia following chest trauma in the dog. *Canine Pract* 5:30–36, 1978.
17. Madewell BR, Nelson DT, Hill K: Paroxysmal atrial fibrillation associated with trauma in a dog. *J Am Vet Med Assoc* 171:273, 1977.
18. Selcer BA, Buttrick M, *et al.*: The incidence of thoracic trauma in dogs with skeletal injury. *J Small Anim Pract* 28:21, 1987.
19. Kolata RJ: Trauma in dogs and cats: an overview. *Vet Clin North Am Small Anim Pract* 10:515, 1980.
20. Kolata RJ, Johnston DE: Motor vehicle accidents in urban dogs: a study of 600 cases. *J Am Vet Med Assoc* 167:938, 1975.
21. Kolata RJ, Kraut NH, Johnston DE: Patterns of trauma in urban dogs and cats: a study of 1,000 cases. *J Am Vet Med Assoc* 164:499, 1974.
22. Pretre R, Chilcott M: Blunt trauma to the heart and great vessels. *N Engl J Med* 336 9:626, 1997.
23. Olsovsky MR, Wechsler AS, Topaz O: Cardiac trauma: diagnosis management and current therapy. *Angiology* 48:423, 1997.
24. Boba A: Cardiac contusion as a primary clinical entity. *Am J Emerg Med* 13:105, 1995.

25. Feghali N, Prisant M: Blunt myocardial injury. *Chest* 108:1673, 1995.
26. Norton MJ, Stanford GG, Weigelt JA: Early detection of myocardial contusion and its complications in patients with blunt trauma. *Am J Surg* 160:523, 1994.
27. Ferjani M, Droc G, Dreux S, *et al.*: Circulating cardiac troponin T in myocardial contusion. *Chest* 111:427, 1997.
28. Dowd MD, Krug S: Pediatric blunt cardiac injury; epidemiology, clinical features, and diagnosis. *J Trauma* 40:61, 1996.
29. Mucha P: Blunt myocardial injury and myocardial contusion. *In* Cameron JL, ed.: Current Surgical Therapy, 6th ed. St. Louis: Mosby, 1998, 1004.
30. Fulda GJ, Giberson F, Hailstone D, *et al.*: An evaluation of serum troponin T and signal-averaged electrocardiographic abnormalities after blunt chest trauma. *J Trauma* 43:304, 1997.
31. Spackman CJA, Caywood DD, Feeny DA *et al.*: Thoracic wall and pulmonary trauma in dogs sustaining fractures as a result of motor vehicle accidents. *J Am Vet Med Assoc* 185:975, 1984.
32. Sisson DD, Daniel GB, Twardock AR: Comparison of left ventricular ejection fractions determined in healthy anesthetized dog by echocardiography and gated equilibrium radionucleotide ventriculography. *Am J Vet Res* 50:1840, 1989.
33. Cwajg E, Cwajg J, He ZX, *et al.*: Gated myocardial perfusion tomography for the assessment of left ventricular function and volumes: comparison with echocardiography. *J Nuc Med* 40:1857, 1999.
34. Daniel GB, Bright JM: Nuclear Imaging, computed tomography, and magnetic resonance imaging of the heart. *In* Fox PR, Sisson D, Moise NS, eds.: Textbook of Canine and Feline Cardiology, 2nd ed. Philadelphia:WB Saunders, 1999, 193.
35. Daniel GB, Kerstetter KK, Sackman JE, *et al.*: Quantitative assessment of surgically induced mitral regurgitation using radionuclide ventriculography and first pass radionuclide angiography. *Vet Radiol Ultrasound* 39:459, 1997.
36. Maenza RL, Seaberg D, D'Amico F: A meta-analysis of blunt cardiac trauma: ending myocardial confusion. *Am J Emerg Med* 14:237, 1996.
37. Brown CS, Bertolet BD: Cardiac troponin. *Chest* 111:2, 1997.
38. Adams JE, Bodor GS, Davila-Roman VG, *et al.*: Cardiac troponin I; a marker with high specificity for cardiac injury. *Circulation* 88:101, 1993.
39. Mair P, Mair J, Koller J, *et al.*: Cardiac troponin T release in multiply injured patients. *Injury* 26:439, 1995.
40. Adams JE: Utility of cardiac troponins in patients with suspected cardiac trauma or after cardiac surgery. *Clin Lab Med* 17:613, 1997.
41. Cummins B, Cummins P: Cardiac specific troponin-I release in canine experimental myocardial infarction: development of a sensitive enzyme-linked immunoassay. *J Mol Cell Cardiol* 19:999, 1987.
42. O'Brien PJ, Dameron GW, Beck ML, *et al.*: Cardiac troponin T is a sensitive biomarker of cardiac injury in laboratory animals. *Lab Anim Sci* 47:486, 1997.
43. O'Brien PJ: Deficiencies of myocardial troponin-T and creatinine kinase MB isoenzyme in dogs with idiopathic dilated cardiomyopathy. *Am J Vet Res* 58:11, 1997.

44. Sleeper MM, Clifford CA: Cardiac troponin I levels in healthy dogs and dogs with heart disease. *In* Proceedings, Internatl Vet Emerg Crit Care Symp 2000, 803.
45. Harvey RC, Short CE: The use of isoflurane for safe anesthesia in animals with traumatic myocarditis or other myocardial sensitivity. *Canine Pract* 10:18, 1983.

SECTION XI
Toxicology and Environmental

74
Bites and Stings

Terry W. Campbell

INTRODUCTION

Pet dogs and cats that are victims of stings from bees, wasps, hornets, and ants or bites from spiders are rarely presented to veterinarians for medical care. Owners do not typically seek veterinary advice even when they have witnessed the bite or sting because the lesions are usually mild and seldom have a fatal result. Only serious cases are seen, therefore, the incidence of these bites and stings is unknown.

ARTHROPODS

Animals of the class Arachnida include the order Araneae (spiders) and the order Scorpionida (true scorpions). Spiders have two jaws (chelicerae) with fangs that deliver venom produced by glands in the cephalothorax to the bite. Most native species of biting North American spiders cause little harm to dogs and cats. The lesion caused by the bite is mild and little more than a local swelling that resolves in a few days. Spider bites primarily occur on prehensile areas, such as the face and forepaws. A few spiders, the black widow (*Latrodectus* spp.) and the brown recluse (*Loxosceles* spp.) may cause more serious bites that require medical attention.

There are more than 1500 species of scorpions worldwide and most are capable of inflicting painful stings without systemic effects. Scorpions of the family Buthidae are capable of producing fatal neurotoxicosis to humans.[1] Most of the scorpions in North America belong to the family Vejovidae and the only scorpion of medical interest in North America is the bark scorpion, *Centruroides sculpturatus*.[2]

Black Widow Spiders (*Latradectus* spp.)

Black widow spiders occur throughout North America. Five species occur in the United States and they inhabit every state but Alaska. They are found in woodlands and crevices of buildings. Their funnel-shaped webs are located close to the ground and often in areas where outside lighting attract insects. The webs can be found under stones and logs and in rodent burrows, barns, and sheds. Adult females (15-mm body size with a 40-mm leg span) are twice the size of the males.[3-5] Only the females are capable of causing envenomation to animals.[5] The coloration of the black widow spider varies with the species. The most common species, *L. mactans*, has a globose, shiny black abdomen with an hourglass-shaped red to orange marking on the underside of the abdomen. Immature female black widow spiders have equal potential for envenomation as the adult. Immature females have a colorful pattern of red, brown, and beige on the dorsal surface of the abdomen, but they may not have the classic hourglass-shaped markings. Male black widow spiders are smaller than the females and are usually unable to penetrate the skin when they bite.

Normally, bites from black widow spiders are not painful and like those of other biting spiders, the lesions are minimal. However, severe reactions can occur. Humans bitten by black widow spiders often experience an initial painless or pinprick sensation that develops into a local swelling with redness within 20 to 30 minutes.[4,5] Fang marks 1 to 2 mm apart with a central pale region (halo) surrounded by a red border are common in humans suffering from black widow spider bites.[2] These minor cutaneous lesions may also be found on animals bitten by black widow spiders. Other clinical signs in humans include edema, urticaria, and local lymphangititis.[6] Humans suffering from latrodectism may experience a dull, crampy pain around the bite and affected limb and if bitten in the lower extremity, abdominal cramping may occur.[2,6] Clinical signs of generalized involvement may develop within minutes after an animal has been bitten. The severity of the clinical signs in animals varies and includes pain at the site of the bite and rigid abdominal muscles with abdominal pain. Clinical signs of severe systemic involvement include hypersalivation, diarrhea, tonic-colonic convulsions, flaccid paralysis, and death in 1 to 4 days.[7] The local wound may appear as a jelly-like edema around the bite. Extreme pain may associated with the bite wound, especially when the area is manipulated and may spread to regional lymph nodes. Mortality from black widow bites is very low.

The venom contains a combination of enzymes and nonproteinaceous compounds. It contains a peptide that is a neurotoxin (α-latrotoxin) that destabilizes nerve cell membranes and causes release of acetylcholine and norepinephrine from synaptic vesicles at the neuromuscular junction leading to excessive muscle depolarization.[2] The neuronal calcium channel toxin in the black widow spider venom has specific action on ion channels and neurotransmitter receptors and is responsible for the painful cramping spasms of abdominal muscles.[8]

The diagnosis of a black widow spider bite is based on the presence of the spider and appropriate clinical signs. Treatment depends on the severity of the systemic involvement. Routine wound care is given to the bite wound. Systemic effects (*i.e.*, hypertension, tachycardia, and vomiting) of the spider venom indicate the need for intravenous access, oxygen therapy, and cardiac monitoring. Fluid therapy is given to patients in shock or suffering from hypotension. Animal studies indicate that high extracellular calcium antagonizes the ability of the venom to cause the release of neurotransmitters; however, the intravenous use of a 10% calcium gluconate solution to relieve the muscle cramping in humans is relatively ineffective.[6] Use of a specific Latrodectus antivenin is also controversial. In humans, there is a risk of an IgE-mediated hypersensitivity reaction associated with the equine origin antivenin. Therefore, the antivenin is usually reserved for use in severe, life-threatening envenomations and must be given as soon as possible, that is, within 30 to 60 minutes of the bite.[2]

Brown Recluse Spider (*Loxosceles* spp.)

There are 10 species of brown recluse spiders in the United States and most are found in the southern and midwestern states. Six species are known to cause necrotic arachnidism in humans.[2] *Loxosceles reclusa* has the widest distribution.[2] These spiders are nocturnal. Brown recluse spiders are small spiders (10-mm body with thin 25-mm legs).[9] These spiders vary in body color, but most are brown with a violin-shaped marking on the dorsal surface of the cephalothorax. Brown recluse spiders can be found outdoors under stationary objects, such as woodpiles and rocks. They can also be found indoors and often inhabit basements and dark undisturbed areas of buildings.

Bites from brown recluse spiders are noted for their dermonecrotic effects that result in a slow-healing ulcerative lesion. Most bites from brown recluse spiders that affect humans are often unnoticed, are painless, or are associated with a mild localized stinging sensation.[3,10] The venom involved is a complex blend of protein toxins that include sphingomyelinase D, an enzyme responsible for dermonecrosis and hemolysis.[3,9,10] The site of the bite may become red with a blanched center and the lesion may be pruritic. Within a few hours, a blister (hemorrhagic vesicle) may form. In humans, a cyanotic bulla or ecchymosis surrounded by blanching and edema ("halo" lesion) often develops and spreads peripherally. After 7 to 14 days, pain at the site of the bite may be present and the bulla may rupture, creating a central eschar that develops into a necrotic ulcer.[2] Similar lesions may occur in animals and complete healing may require 8 or more weeks.[7,11] Systemic effects to bites from these spiders are rare. Systemic involvement includes fever, vomiting, diarrhea, hematuria, hemoglobinuria, icterus, convulsions, coma, and death.[12]

The diagnosis of a brown recluse spider bite is based on the presence of the spider and appropriate clinical signs and lesions. Most diagnoses are presumed.

Routine wound management for the bite and prophylactic antibiotics are usually indicated. If the bite is recognized early, the area can be infiltrated with 2% lidocaine solution. Fluid therapy for shock and hypotension should be provided to those animals with systemic manifestation of bites. Surgical excision of necrotic tissue can be performed with chronic lesions. Dapsone is frequently recommended in the treatment of these bites in humans because it inhibits neutrophil activity.[2] Studies with guinea pigs and rabbits using dapsone in the treatment of brown recluse spider bites are inconclusive.[9,12,13] In human medicine, serious complications, such as hemolysis, aplastic anemia, agranulocytosis, hypersensitivity, and toxic epidermal necrolysis can occur with dapsone treatment.[2]

Scorpions

Scorpions are typically brown in color and have a flat body with eight legs. They have two lobster-like pincers and a segmented tail. The tail is usually held upward and forward over the body and terminates in a venomous stinger. A pair of poison glands at the base of the stinger produces the venom. There are approximately 40 types of scorpions in North America; however, the sting of most is painful, but not fatal to humans and their pet dogs and cats. Scorpions that live in the arid southwestern United States, especially *Centruroides sculpturatus*, tend to be the most dangerous. *C. sculpturatus*, called the bark scorpion, is approximately 1.5 inches long and has a yellow cephalothorax, a tubercle at the base of its stinger, and slender pincers.[11] The end of the tail contains a curved, hollow stinging apparatus for injecting the venom. This scorpion is nocturnal and hides in moist, cool areas, such as under rocks, bricks, and wood, during the day.

The incidence of scorpion stings involving domestic animals is unknown because the lesions rarely require medical care and are difficult to differentiate from wasp and bee stings. The stings by most North American scorpions do not produce a major medical concern. Localized erythema, edema, and pain that subside in a few hours characterize most scorpion stings. Scorpion venom is a complex, water-soluble, antigenic poison made of mucopolysaccharides, hyaluronidase, phospholipase, serotonin, histamine, protease inhibitors, histamine-releasing factors, and neurotoxins.[14,15] The neurotoxin is the more medically significant component of scorpion venom. More severe envenomation, such as those from *C. sculpturatus*, may cause an excitatory neurotoxicity. The neurotoxins in the venom of *C. sculpturatus* activate the sodium channels causing prolonged action potentials, depolarization of the presynaptic terminal, and spontaneous overstimulation of the sympathetic and parasympathetic nervous system.[2,15]

The clinical signs of parasympathetic involvement of envenomation by *C. sculpturatus* include constricted pupils, hypotension, bronchial constriction, bradycardia, atrioventricular block, and cardiac arrest.[2,11] Parasympathetic stimulation also leads to excessive lacrimation, bronchial secretions, urination, defecation, and salivation.[11] Hypertension, bradycardia, vasoconstriction, pulmonary edema, and hyperglycemia (inhibition of insulin) are indicative of overstimulation of α-receptors of the sympathetic nervous system.[2,11,16] Overstimulation of β-receptors is indicated by hypertension, tachycardia, arrhythmia (cardiac excitability), vasodilation, and bronchial relaxation.[2,16] Mydriasis and piloerection also indicate sympathetic involvement.[11,16] Death can result from respiratory failure, cardiac conduction disturbances, and severe hypertension. Severe reactions to scorpion stings may resemble organophosphate toxicity or respiratory distress.[11]

The hemodynamic effects of scorpion envenomation occur in two phases, the inotropic phase and the hypokinetic phase.[18,19] The first phase is indicated by increased systemic vascular resistance, blood pressure, and left ventricular contractility. Therefore, vasodilators (*i.e.*, prazosin and captoprol) are indicated for the treatment of the first phase of the hemodynamic effects of scorpion envenomation. The second hemodynamic phase of scorpion envenomation is indicated by hypotension, shock, and impaired ventricular contractility. This phase requires fluid replacement therapy and the use of inotropic agents, such as dobutamine.

Diagnosis of scorpion stings is based on the identification of the scorpion and appropriate clinical signs.

Most scorpion stings do not require treatment. Any treatment provided is directed by the clinical signs or by providing general supportive care. Treatment can be difficult owing to the ability of the scorpion venom to stimulate both sympathetic and parasympathetic branches of the autonomic nervous system. Veterinarians in emergency situations commonly use corticosteroids, but their use with scorpion stings appears to be of little benefit.[17]

A species-specific antivenin for *Centruroides* scorpions derived from goat serum is available.[2] The use of antivenins in human medicine is controversial because of the inherent risk of an acute life-threatening or delayed serum sickness reaction.[2] There has been little use of scorpion antivenin in veterinary medicine.

INSECTS

Hymenoptera (Bees, Wasps, Hornets, Ants)

Bees (family Apidae) have barbed stingers that are actually modified ovipositors. The barbed stinger sticks in the skin and the attached venom sac is pulled out of the bee's abdomen when the bee is either pulled off or attempts to fly away. Muscles attached to the venom sac constrict to pump venom into animal for 2 to 3 minutes after it has detached from the bee. Honeybees (*i.e.*, Italian bee, *Apis mellifera ligustica*, and German bee, *Apis mellifera mellifera*) in the United States tend not to sting unless disturbed. However, the Africanized bees in the southwestern United States are more aggressive and more of a threat to humans and animals. The African honeybee, *Apis mellifera scutellata*, was introduced into Brazil in the 1950s and has gradually moved north, eventually inbreeding with the honeybees in the United States.[20] These Africanized honeybees are found in Texas, California, Arizona, and other isolated areas of the southern United States.[21] They are more aggressive, attack in swarms, and deliver more stings per victim than the native or domestic honeybees. Caged or chained animals are susceptible to severe attacks by Africanized bees.

Yellow jackets, wasps, and hornets (family Vespidae) tend to be more aggressive than bees. These insects have barbless stingers and each individual is able to inflict many stings. Yellow jackets tend to be commonly involved with the stinging of dogs and cats because they nest in the ground. Wasps and hornets tend to nest in higher structures, such as trees and shrubs. The rates of yellow jacket stings increase during late summer and early fall.[21] This phenomenon is referred to as "yellow jacket delirium" and suggests that these insects are more aggressive during this time of year perhaps as they prepare for winter.

Five species of fire ants (*Solenopsis invicta* is the most prevalent) have been introduced in the southeastern part of the United States. Fire ants tend to swarm quickly onto their victim and each ant is capable of delivering many stings. Fire ant mounds are domed patches of earth that can be up to 1 foot tall. Because fire ants do not denude the vegetation associated with their mounds, victims of fire ant stings often do not realize that they are standing in the middle of a fire ant mound.[21]

The venom in stings from Hymenoptera insects contains a mixture of enzymes, peptides, and biologically active amines. Each type of insect venom is a unique mixture of these chemicals. The venom from bees and wasps is primarily made of proteins (*i.e.*, phospholipase A_2, hyaluronidase, mast cell degranulation peptide, acid phosphatase, histamine, meltin, and apamin).[22-24] The hyaluronidase, histamines, and hemolysins in bee venom cause toxic and hemolytic effects in dogs.[23,25] Venom from fire ants is 95% peperdine alkaloids and 5% protein (with bactericidal and fungicidal properties).[21,22]

The clinical signs associated with stings from insects can range from mild to severe depending on the type of venom, location of the sting, number of stings, and sensitivity of the animal receiving the sting. Most lesions caused by insect stings are located on exposed areas of the head and feet because dense fur protects animals from insect stings. Stings on the mouth and tongue are common. Small, localized areas of erythema associated with pain are the most common lesions presented to veterinarians. Larger local reactions are associated with immunologic responses. Examples of such reactions would be facial or limb swelling associated with an insect sting. These lesions can persist for days. In dogs, fire ant stings often produce local reactions with swelling and erythema developing at the site of each sting within 15 minutes.[26] The lesions develop into bright erythematous pruritic papules within 6 hours. The site of the stings appears normal after 24 hours in most cases. These lesions differ from those in humans where pustules at the site of the fire ant sting may persist for several days. The formation of urticaria indicates a superficial systemic allergic reaction to the insect sting.

Anaphylaxis is a severe systemic allergic (antigen-induced IgE-mediated) reaction to insect stings where release of chemical mediators damage blood vessels and smooth muscles. Symptoms of anaphylaxis will occur within 15 minutes of the stinging incident. Anaphylaxis in dogs is indicated by swelling at the site of the sting, vomiting, defecation, urination, muscular weakness, respiratory depression, and convulsions.[22] Death in dogs may occur within an hour of the onset of clinical signs. Anaphylaxis in cats is indicated by pruritis, dyspnea, salivation, incoordination, and collapse. The lung is the shock organ of the cat, so anaphylaxis produces pulmonary hemorrhage and edema.[22] Massive envenomation from insect stings may cause the animal to become depressed and febrile. This systemic toxic reaction to the stings may result in clinical signs of neurologic involvement (*i.e.*, ataxia, facial paralysis, and seizures) or hemorrhagic disorder (*i.e.*, dark brown vomitus, hematuria, and bloody feces).

The diagnosis of insect stings is usually made following a witnessed insect attack. Most dogs or cats stung by insects are not presented for veterinary care. Insect stings must be differentiated from punctures, snakebites, abscesses, and other lesions that may resemble a sting.

The majority of insect stings that result in small local reactions will resolve without treatment. The stinger of bees should be removed quickly and application of a cold compress may provide local comfort. Topical and oral analgesics, such as nonsteroidal drugs, may help to relieve the discomfort associated with a sting. Antihistamines and corticosteroids may be used in stings causing pruritis or urticaria. The pustules caused by fire ant stings usually resolve without treatment.

Insect stings associated with severe local or systemic immunologic reactions should be treated with aggressive fluid therapy, antihistamines (*e.g.*, diphenhydramine at 2-4 mg/kg, IM, bid), epinephrine (IM or SQ), and possibly corticosteroids (*e.g.*, prednisolone at 1 mg/kg, bid tapered over a 5-day period). Anaphylaxis should be treated quickly. Epinephrine (0.5-1.0 mL of a 1:1000 solution) should be given subcutaneously and repeated at 10- to 20-minute intervals.[22] If it is necessary to give epinephrine intravenously, it should be diluted to a 1:10,000 solution. Shock volumes of intravenous crystalloid fluids are needed to combat the vascular collapse.

Biting Flies

Biting flies rarely cause reactions in dogs and cats that require veterinary medical attention. Flies that are capable of inflicting serious bites include black flies (family Simuliidae), horseflies (*Tabanus*), and deer flies (*Chrysops*).

Lesions associated with fly bites vary from the more common mild local wheal or papule to rare systemic reactions.[27] Bites from black flies tend to concentrate on the hairless skin of the head, abdomen, ears, and legs. The resulting papules, crusts, and ulcers are often intensely pruritic. Bites from horseflies and deer flies are less severe.

Most reactions to fly bites will resolve without treatment in a few hours. Local analgesia can be use to relieve some of the discomfort. Large local lesions are likely associated with an immune reaction and may be treated with antihistamines and corticosteroids.

POISONOUS LIZARDS AND TOADS

Gila Monster (*Heloderma suspectum*) and Mexican Beaded Lizard (*H. horridum*)

Gila monsters are large (18-24 inches or 46-61 cm), heavy-bodied lizards. They have short stout legs and a thick tail. They have small beadlike scales on the back with spots of black and yellow, orange, or pink. The face is black. The related Mexican beaded lizard is similar in appearance to the Gila monster. These lizards live in arid and semiarid regions in the southwestern United States and Mexico. They are primarily nocturnal and nonaggressive.

Envenomations from these lizards are rare. They have modified salivary glands lying along the underside of the lower jaw that produce the venom. The venom is not injected like that of a snake, but flows into the open wound via grooved teeth as the lizard chews. The *Heloderma* venom contains a neurotoxin, hyaluronidase, vasoactive peptides, and arginine esterases.[11] The venom also contains a heat-stable, noncholinergic, nonhistaminic smooth muscle-stimulating factor.

Pain usually occurs within minutes of a bite from one of these lizards. Other clinical signs may include increased salivation, lacrimation, urination, and defecation. Severe reactions include a rapid fall in blood pressure, congestion of blood in the lungs, retrobulbar hemorrhage, and a life-threatening hypotensive crisis.[11]

Because the pain associated with a bite from a Gila monster or Mexican beaded lizard may be intense, pain management is often indicated. However, the primary danger is hypotension and intravenous fluid therapy should be initiated whenever envenomation from one of these lizards has occurred. Electrocardiographic monitoring of the heart is also indicated. Routine wound management should be applied to the bite. Because anaphylactic reactions to *Heloderma* venom are rare, use of antihistamines or corticosteroids is of little value.[11]

Toad (*Bufo marinus* and *B. alvarius*) Poisoning

The two species of toads that commonly cause toxicoses in dogs and cats in the United States are the marine giant or cane toad (*Bufo marinus*) and the Colorado River toad (*B. alvarius*). The marine toad is a large (4-9 inches or 10-24 cm), brown to yellow-brown, round bodied toad with enormous paratoids (glands located on the dorsum of the head and neck of toads) extending down the sides of the body. The marine toad is found in south Texas, Florida, and Hawaii. It was introduced in Florida and Hawaii in an attempt to control beetles that damage sugarcane. The Colorado River toad is a large (3-7 inches or 7-18 cm) olive to dark brown toad with relatively smooth and shiny skin. The belly is cream-colored. The elongate parotoid glands touch the prominent cranial crests. These toads have one or two white warts at the corners of the mouth. The Colorado River toad ranges from extreme southeast California to extreme southwest New Mexico and into Mexico. Both toads are primarily nocturnal.

The milky secretions from the parotoid glands of these toads, especially that of the marine toad, is highly toxic. The toxic components of this secretion include catecholamines, epinephrine, norepinephrine, dopamine, and serotonin.[28] It also includes bufagenins and bufotoxins, which are steroids with digitalis-like effects, and bufotenine, which is a pressor substance.[28-32]

The milky secretions from the parotoid glands will burn the eyes and inflame the skin; however, serious intoxication occurs when the toxin enters the mouth. Dogs are more commonly affected than cats, most likely because they tend to lick or pick the toad up in their mouths. The most common clinical signs of toad poisoning in dogs include neurologic disorders, hyperemia of the oral mucous membranes, ptyalism, recumbency, tachypnea, and vomiting.[28] Seizure activity is the most common neurologic disorder observed with toad poisoning, but dogs and cats may also be presented with ataxia, nystagmus, extensor rigidity, opisthotonos, or in a stupor or coma.[28-30,33] The oral mucous membranes of affected dogs are often brick red. Cardiac arrhythmias are relatively uncommon despite the cardioactive bufagenins and bufotoxins.[28] Because *Bufo* toads hibernate during cold weather, most cases of toad intoxication occur during the spring and summer.

The mortality rate for dogs suffering from toad intoxication from *B. marinus* has been previously reported to be 100% in Florida and 5% in Hawaii for untreated cases.[29,33] However, a recent study has shown that the mortality rate for Florida dogs suffering from intoxication from *B. marinus* is low (*i.e.*, 4%) with proper treatment.[28] Most dogs suffering from toad poisoning do not exhibit cardiac abnormalities; however, cardiac monitoring using an electrocardiogram is indicated in dogs with severe neurologic disorders, such as stupor and coma, or tachycardia or dysrhythmias.[28] Rinsing of the oral cavity with water for at least 5 minutes should be performed as soon as possible. For dogs with known cases of toad poisoning, their owners should be instructed to flush out the mouth of their conscious dog with running tap water before transporting the animal to the veterinary hospital. Dogs with severe intoxication and neurologic disorders should be transported immediately for veterinary care. Dogs exhibiting status epilepticus or unconsciousness should be treated with a diuretic, such as furosemide (1-2 mg/kg or 0.45-0.9 mg/lb, IV) and a hyperosmolar agent, such as mannitol (250-1000 mg/kg or 114-455 mg/lb, IV). Diazepam (0.5 mg/kg or 0.23 mg/lb, IV) can be given to dogs with minor seizure disorders and muscle rigidity.[28] Severely affected dogs should be maintained with a balanced crystalloid electrolye solution. Most dogs with toad intoxication do not require hospitalization and are often released after rinsing the oral cavity and identification of a stable patient with a physical examination.

REFERENCES

1. Sofer S: Scorpion envenomation. *Intensive Care Med* 21:626, 1995.
2. Farhat BW: Arachnidism. *Top Emerg Med* 22:1, 2000.
3. Allen C: Arachnid envenomations. *Emerg Med Clin North Am* 10:269, 1992.
4. Johnson L: Toxic bites and stings. *In* Schwartz GR, Cayten CG, Mangelsen MA, Mayer TA, Hanke BK, eds.: Principles and Practice of Emergency Medicine, vol. II. 3rd ed. Philadelphia: Lea & Febiger, 1992.
5. Stack LB: Images in clinical medicine. *Latrodectus mactans*. *N Engl J Med* 336:1649, 1997.
6. Maretic Z: Latrodectism: variations in clinical manifestations provoked by *Latrodectus* species of spiders. *Toxicon* 21: 457, 1983.
7. Murphy MJ: A Field Guide to Common Animal Poisoning. Ames, IA: Iowa State University Press, 1996, 130.
8. Uchitel OD: Toxins affecting calcium channels in neurons. *Toxicon* 35:1161, 1997.
9. Hobbs GD, Anderson AR, Greene TJ, Yearly DM: Comparison of hyperbaric oxygen and dapsone therapy for *Loxosceles* envenomation. *Acad Emerg Med* 3:758, 1996.
10. Otten EJ. Venomous animal injuries. *In* Rosen P, Barkin RM, eds.: Emergency Medicine: Concepts and Clinical Practice, 3rd ed. St. Louis, MO: Mosby-Year Book, 1992, p 1.
11. Peterson ME, Meerdink GL: Bites and stings of venomous animals. *In* Kirk RW, ed.: Current Veterinary Therapy X. Philadelphia: WB Saunders, 1985, p 177.
12. Barrett SM, Romine-Jenkins M, Fisher DE: Dapsone or electric shock therapy of brown recluse spider envenomation. *Ann Emerg Med* 24:21, 1994.
13. King LE, Rees RS: Dapsone treatment of a brown recluse bite. *JAMA* 250:648, 1983.

14. Bawaskar HD, Bawaskar PA. Scorpion envenoming and the cardiovascular system. *Trop Doct* 27:6, 1997.
15. Sofer S: Scorpion envenomation. *Intensive Care Med* 21:626, 1995.
16. Tarasiuk A, Sofer S: Effects of adrenergic-receptor blockade and ligation of spleen vessels on the hemodynamics of dogs injected with scorpion venom. *Crit Care Med* 27: 265, 1999.
17. Abroug F, Novira S, Haguiga H, *et al.*: High-dose hydrocortisone hemisuccinate in scorpion envenomation. *Ann Emerg Med* 30:23, 1997.
18. Tarasiuk A, Sofer S, Huberfelo S, Scharf M: Hemodynamic effects following injection of venom from the scorpion *Leirus quinquestriatus*. *J Crit Care* 9:134, 1994.
19. Gueron M, Adolph RJ, Grupp IL, *et al.*: Hemodynamic and myocardial consequences of scorpion venom. *Am J Cardiol* 45:979, 1980.
20. Shumacher MJ, Egen NB: Significance of Africanized bees for public health. *Arch Intern Med* 155:2038, 1995.
21. Greco LK: Hymenoptera stings. *Top Emerg Med* 22:37, 2000.
22. Cowell AK, Cowell RL: Management of bee and other Hymenoptera stings. *In* Kirk RW, ed.: Current Veterinary Therapy XII. Philadelphia: WB Saunders, 1995, p 226.
23. Wysoke JM, Bland van-den Berg P, Marshall C: Bee sting haemolysis, spherocytosis, and neural dysfunction in three dogs. *Afr Vet Assoc* 61:29, 1990.
24. Salluzzo RF: Insect and Spider Bites. Emergency Medicine. A Comprehensive Guide. 4th ed. New York: McGraw-Hill, 1996.
25. Noble SJ, Armstrong PJ: Bee sting envenomation resulting in secondary immune-mediated hemolytic anemia in two dogs. *J Am Vet Med Assoc* 214:1026, 1999.
26. Rakich PM, Latimer KS, Mispagel ME, Steffens WL: Clinical and histologic characterization of cutaneous reactions to stings of the imported fire ant (*Solenopsis invicta*) in dogs. *Vet Pathol.* 30:555, 1993.
27. Scott DW, Miller WH, Griffin CE: Muller & Kirk's Small Animal Dermatology, 5th ed. Philadelphia: WB Saunders, 1995, p 457.
28. Roberts BK, Aronsohn MG, Moses BL, *et al.*: *Bufo marinus* intoxication in dogs: 94 cases (1997–1998). *J Am Vet Med Assoc* 216:1941, 2000.
29. Palumbo NE, Perri SE: Toad poisoning. *In* Kirk RW, ed.: Current Veterinary Therapy VII. Philadelphia: WB Saunders, 1983, p 160..
30. Peterson ME: Toad venom toxicity. *In* Tilley LP, Smith FWK, eds.: The 5 Minute Veterinary Consult. Baltimore: Williams & Wilkins, 1997, p 1108.
31. Kwan T, Pauisco AD, Kohl L: Digitalis toxicity caused by toad venom. *Chest* 102: 949, 1992.
32. Butler VP, Morris JF, Akizawa T, *et al.*: Heterogenicity and lability of endogenous digitalis-like substances in the plasma of the toad, *Bufo marinus*. *Am Phys Soc* 271: 325, 1996.
33. Knowles RP. The poison toad and the canine. *Vet Med Small Anim Clin* 59:38, 1964.

75
Reptile Envenomations

Wayne E. Wingfield

Young primates appear to be born with only three inborn fears—
of falling, snakes, and the dark.
Carl Sagan[1]

Snakes first appeared in the late Cretaceous period; venomous snakes evolved about 50 million years later in the Miocene epoch. Nearly 3000 species of snake exist and about 10% to 15% of these are venomous. They inhabit all types of terrain, including fresh and salt water, and are active during both day and night. Their inability to raise their body temperature above ambient levels, however, restricts their activity to a fairly narrow range, about 25° to 35°C (77°–95°F). All snakes are carnivorous, and the venom apparatus evolved for the purpose of obtaining food. The toxin and toxic apparatus are quite varied from class to class. For example, the rattlesnake has modified salivary glands and maxillary teeth and uses this system primarily to obtain food.

Most venomous reptile injuries are considered emergencies and require immediate attention. The purpose for this chapter is to acquaint the veterinarian with reptile envenomations from reptiles found in the United States.

IDENTIFICATION OF VENOMOUS SNAKES

Two principles should be kept in mind in the identification of venomous snakes: (1) only experts should handle live snakes, and (2) even dead snakes can envenomate careless handlers. It is not difficult to differentiate between pit vipers and harmless snakes (Fig. 75-1). Pit vipers, as their name implies, have a characteristic pit found midway between the eye and the nostril on both sides of the head. This pit is a heat-sensitive organ that enables the snake to locate warm-blooded prey. Other identifying characteristics of the pit viper include a triangular-shaped head, the presence of an elliptical pupil, the arrangement of subcaudal plates, the tail structure, and the presence of fangs (Fig. 75-2). Although characteristic, they may be inconsistent. An individual's characteristic will vary with the age of the snake, time of the year, and the condition of the tail and mouth parts. One should never attempt to identify pit vipers by color or skin patterns.

Coral snakes can be readily identified by their color and pattern (Fig. 75-3). At first glance they resemble one of several varieties of kingsnake found in the

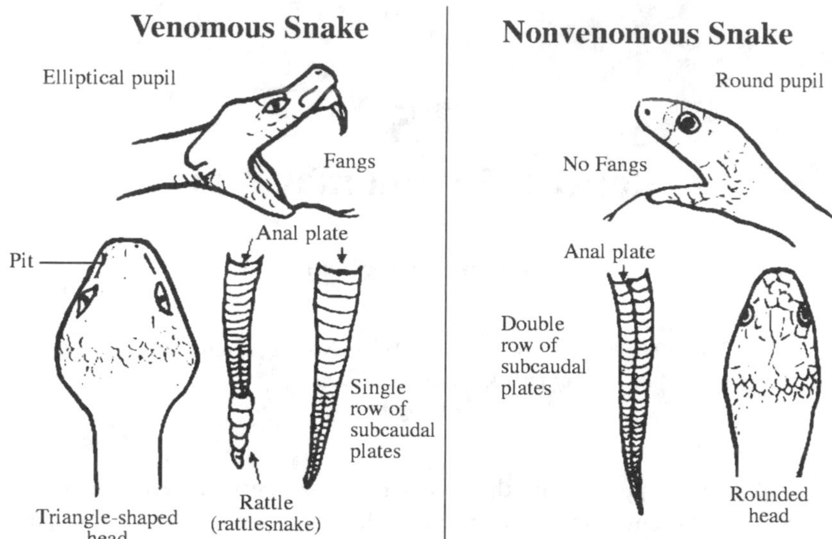

Figure 75-1
Identification of venomous snakes.

southern United States. The coral snake can be differentiated from the kingsnake by two characteristics: (1) the nose of the coral snake is black, and (2) the red and yellow bands are adjacent on the coral snake but separated by a black band on the kingsnake. The popular rhyme in the identification of the coral snake goes as follows:

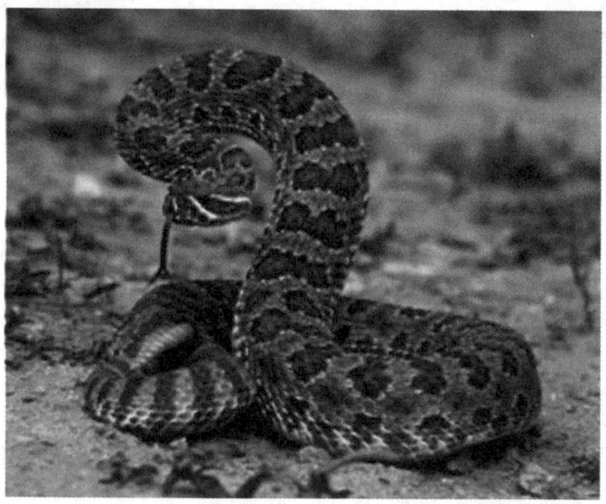

Figure 75-2
Prairie rattlesnake in a strike posture.

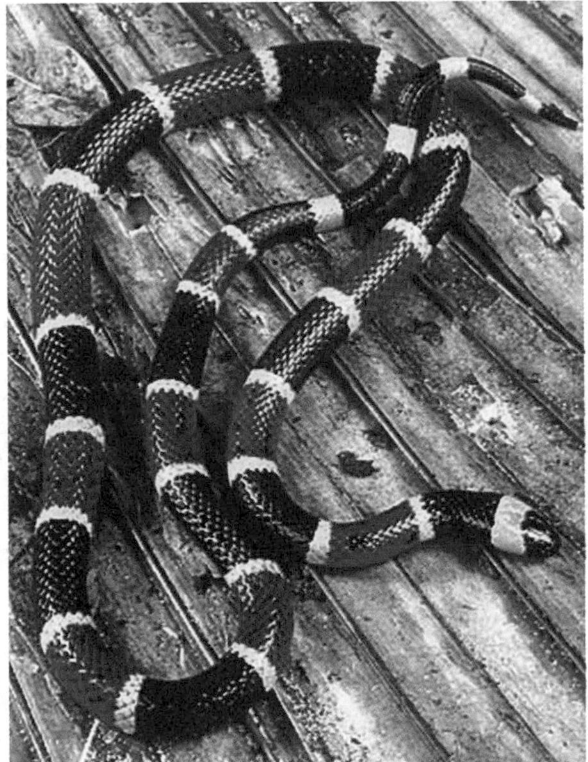

Figure 75-3
The eastern coral snake. Notice the black nose and the red band next to the yellow band.

Red next to yellow, kill a fellow
Red next to black, venom lack (or friend of Jack)

The eastern coral snake is found in North Carolina, South Carolina, Florida, Louisiana, Mississippi, Georgia, and Texas. The western coral snake is native to Arizona and New Mexico. Both species are quite shy unless handled. The eastern coral snake has proven deadly in humans, whereas there is no record of human fatalities from the western species.

EPIDEMIOLOGY

Fourteen families of snakes are known worldwide; five of these contain venomous species. The five venomous families include Colubridae, Hydrophidae, Elapidae, Viperidae, and Crotalidae. The Colubridae, although comprising 70% of all species of snakes, have few venomous members, such as the boomslang and bird snake. The Hydrophidae include sea snakes. The Elapidae are more common and include the cobras, kraits, mambas, and coral snakes. The Viperidae, or true vipers, are represented by Russell's viper, the puff adder, the Gabboon viper, the saw-scaled viper, and the European viper. The Crotalidae or pit vipers are sometimes considered a separate family or a subfamily of the Viperidae. The Elapidae and Crotalidae contain the venomous snakes seen in the United States. Among the pit vipers are found the most common American venomous snakes, such as rattlesnakes, water moccasins, copperheads, bushmasters, and the fer-de-lance.[2,3]

Venom Characteristics

Snake venoms are highly complex mixtures of at least 8 to 30 identified active components consisting of neurotoxins, hemotoxins, cardiotoxins, cryotoxins, and others; the exact composite is species specific.[4] The primary function of reptile venom is directed toward the rapid and effective procurement of food. A significant number of individual peptides and proteins in the venom of pit vipers act as predigestants and thereby initiate the chemical breakdown of prey prior to actual ingestion.[5] Pit viper envenomations are classically associated with hematologic sequelae but also contain variably active neurotoxic components. Similarly, coral snakes (and elapid venoms in general) are predominantly neurotoxic, but also possess cardiotoxicity.[5]

The toxic components of snake venom can be classified into four broad categories: enzymes, polypeptides, glycoproteins, and compounds of low molecular weight. These components can also be classified as protein and nonprotein compounds (Table 75-1). Proteins, which account for most of the toxic manifestations, make up 90% to 95% of venom. These manifestations or symptoms can generally be classified as local or systemic.[4]

Toxic effects of various venoms result from combined effects of enzymes,

Table 75-1. Examples of Compounds Identified in Snake Venoms[3]

Component	Examples
Nonprotein components	**5%-10%**
Metals	Copper, zinc, sodium, magnesium
Free amino acids	Glycine, valine, isoleucine
Peptides	Pyroglutamylpeptide
Nucleosides	Adenosine, guanosine, inosine
Carbohydrates	Neutral sugars, sialic acid
Lipids	Phospholipids, cholesterol
Biogenic amines	Spermine, histamine, serotonin
Protein components	**90%-95%**
Enzymes	Proteolytic enzymes, collagenase, phospholipase-A, nucleotidase, hyaluronidase, acetylcholinesterase, amino acid oxidase
Polypeptides	Crotoxin, cardiotoxin, crotamine

polypeptides, and probably to a lesser degree, nonprotein components. The local effects are generally caused by enzymatic action on the various cellular and noncellular structures in the victim's tissues. These enzymes cause coagulation, anticoagulation, cell lysis, hemorrhage, hemolysis, and the destruction of nucleic acid, mitochondria, and other organelles.

It is known that several animal venoms, such as those from snakes, are potent neurotoxic compounds and that their main component is a specific phospholipase A_2 (PLA_2). Snake venom PLA_2 stimulates the hypothalamic-pituitary-adrenal (HPA) axis.[6] There are PLA_2-dependent mechanisms responsible for several symptoms of inflammatory stress induced neurotoxemia.[6] PLA_2 can inhibit the electron transfer at the level of cytochrome C and render mitochondrial-bound enzymes soluble. It can hydrolyze the phospholipids in the nerve axons, break down acetylcholine vesicles at the myoneural junction, cause myonecrosis, and cause lysis of erythrocyte membranes.[7,8] The polypeptides are structurally smaller, but are more rapidly absorbed and account for the venom's systemic effects on the heart, lungs, kidneys, and presynaptic and postsynaptic membranes.

The components of venom include more than 30 enzymes that act singly or in combination to break down connective tissue, perforate capillary walls, destroy erythrocytes, degrade fibrinogen, inhibit coagulatory function, disrupt neuromuscular transmission, and initiate proteolysis. At least four types of coagulant activity, two subsets of anticoagulant mechanisms, and fibrinogenolytic effects have been identified in Crotalidae venom.[5] The efficacy with which these enzymes act in immobilizing and incapacitating the normal prey species is a testimonial to the destructive effects they can exert on animal recipients.[4]

There is tremendous interspecific and intraspecific snake venom variability.[9] Several rattlesnake envenomations appear to exhibit species-specific clinical syndromes. Timber rattlesnake (*Crotalus horridus*) envenomations typically present with severe thrombocytopenia and prolonged prothrombin times attributed to the presence of crotalacytin (a venom unique to this species) and thrombin-like serine proteinase in humans.[10] The Timber rattlesnake in humans often results in myokymia, an unusual form of muscle fasciculation.

Bites from the canebrake rattlesnake (C. *horridus atricaudatus*) often result in significant elevation of serum creatinine kinase consistent with rhabdomyolysis in humans; the neurotoxin, dubbed "canebrake toxin" is antigenically identical to neurotoxins of the South American rattlesnake (C. *durissus terrificus*) and the Mohave rattlesnake (C. *scutulatus*), both of which have rhabdomyolysis associated with their envenomations.[11] The principle neurologically active component of the Mohave rattlesnake venom is Mohave toxin, with two venom subtypes identified as types A and B. Type A has a presynaptic nerve action that is responsible for the significant neurologic effects typically associated with bites from this reptile. Type A is the largest component of Mohave toxin. Type B has primarily hemotoxic effects due to the small amount of Mohave toxin present.[12]

In general, pit viper venoms act directly and immediately on blood vessel endothelium, and they are primarily dispersed through slow-moving lymphatic fluid channels. Coral snake venom tends to quickly disperse through the bloodstream. It is associated with predominantly neurotoxic effects such as muscular transmission anomalies, bulbar paralysis, and respiratory depression in humans.[4] The biochemical profile of an individual snake's stored venom may be influenced by the season of the year, age, size, and general condition. Physical factors determining the amount of venom injected include motivation (fear, anger), recent feeding, fang-tissue contact time, injection site, number of bites, and snake size.

The mechanism for delivering the venom is fairly standard for snakes. It consists of two venom glands, hollow to grooved fangs, and ducts connecting the glands to the fangs. The glands, which evolved from salivary glands, are located on each side of the head above the maxillae and behind the eyes. Each gland has an individual muscle and nerve supply that allows the snake to vary the amount of venom injected into the victim. The venom duct leads from the rostral portion of the gland along the maxilla to the fang. Pit vipers have fangs that are large rostral maxillary teeth. These teeth are hollow and rotate outward from a resting position to a striking position. The coral snake has fixed, hollow, maxillary teeth that are much smaller than those of pit vipers. The fangs of most snakes are shed and replaced regularly, and it is not unusual to see snakes with double fangs on one side of the mouth.[2,3]

Depending on the species of snake involved, the toxic effects may be local, systemic, or both. Local envenomation can cause serious systemic problems (*i.e.*, intravascular coagulopathies, pulmonary edema, and shock). The animal victim's autopharmacologic response to envenomation may also add to the problems. The enzymes in the venom may trigger release of bradykinin, histamine, and serotonin, which may cause an anaphylactoid reaction. These effects may occur over several days and range from minimal pain to multisystem failure and death.

Occurrence

There is a paucity of information regarding the number of domestic animals bitten by reptiles in the United States. In humans, approximately 7000 to 8000 (roughly 4/100,000 population) cases of venomous snakebite are reported annually and these result in 12 to 20 mortalities (0.002%) and about 200 morbidities.[9,13] These demographics are more meaningful when compared with statistics from abroad. Australia records 1000 to 3000 envenomations per year with an accompanying 21% mortality rate.[14] The African continent claims one million envenomations, with a 20% mortality annually.[15] The prevalence of venomous snakebite in Thailand is 12/100,000 and in Papua New Guinea about 250/100,000.[16] Thus, the United States has a much less urgent snakebite problem in humans than many other global regions.

At least one species of venomous snake occurs in the 48 contiguous United States, with the exceptions of Maine and Delaware.[17] Venomous snakes are not native to Alaska nor Hawaii. Over 70% of snakebites in humans occur in the southeast, with North Carolina leading the nation. Other states with high incidence include Texas, Florida, Arizona, South Carolina, and Georgia. The data reflect a greater number of snake species and population sizes.[18,19] Of the nearly 300 species of serpent native to North America, only 20 are considered sufficiently venomous to be a hazard to humans (and animals) and they are divided into two major taxonomic groups. The first is the Crotalidae, or pit vipers, which accounts for nearly 99% of all envenomations. This group contains the rattlesnakes (genera *Crotalus* and *Sistrurus*) and moccasins (genus *Agkistrodon*), the latter including the copperhead and the cottonmouth. Nearly all fatalities in humans are associated with rattlesnakes; the majority are associated with the eastern diamondback (*Crotalus adamanteus*), the largest North American pit viper and a species capable of delivering up to 700 mg venom with a single bite.[9] The copperhead (*Agkistrodon contortix*) by contrast, is regarded as possessing the least virulent venom of native pit vipers; yet it is a species most often implicated in human envenomations over its broad range.[18,20] Clinical reviews in human medicine support a general "dry bite" rate (no evidence of clinical envenomation) in North American pit vipers of about 20% to 25%, ascribed in part to the snake's control over venom injection.[21,22]

The second major group of venomous North American snakes are representatives of the family Elapidae, the eastern (*Micrurus fulvius*) and western (*Micruroides euryxanthus*) coral snakes, with such notorious Old World members as cobras, kraits, and all of Australia's land-based venomous fauna. The eastern coral snake is responsible for many serious envenomations, whereas the western species has not been linked with medically significant sequelae. Historically, these snakes have been credited with a more crude, "less efficient" envenomation apparatus than their pit viper counterparts, with a corresponding dry bite rate of 25% to 40%.[23] This should not belie the fact that these reptiles will aggressively and energetically defend themselves when threatened.[22]

The Gila monster (*Heloderma suspectum*) (Fig. 75-4) is native to portions of the American Southwest; it and the closely related beaded lizard (*Heloderma horridum*) are the only two species of venomous lizard in the world. Unlike pit vipers and coral snakes, these animals have a constant flow of venom from lower jaw glands into their saliva; any tissue contact may result in an envenomation. The reported rate in humans is 70%.[24]

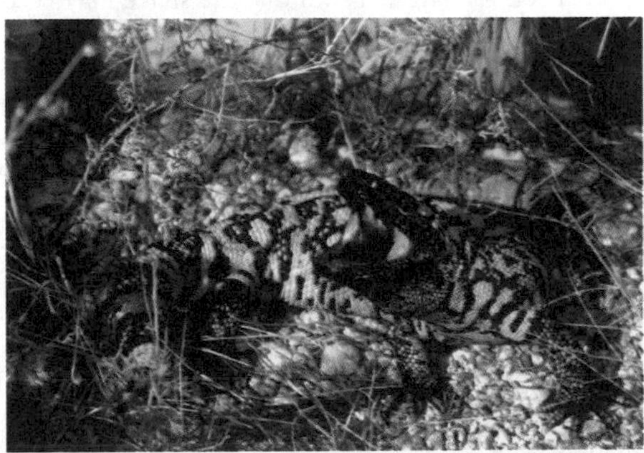

Figure 75-4
The reticulated Gila monster, *Heloderma suspectum.*

A major problem has recently arisen in the United States. In the past, zoos, research centers, and herpetologists have kept exotic venomous snakes and have thus put themselves at risk of envenomation. Today, however, hundreds of people are raising deadly venomous snakes that are not native to the United States. They place themselves, their family (including pets), and the general public at risk.

CLINICAL PRESENTATION

History

Information about the snakebite should include the time elapsed since the bite, the circumstances surrounding the bite, the number of bites, whether first aid was administered, the location of the bite, and any clinical signs noted. If possible, information regarding the medical history of the animal should be obtained to be aware of pre-existing cardiovascular, hematologic, renal, or respiratory problems.

If at all possible, the snake should be identified, but this is not easy to accomplish. The presence of pits is the most consistent feature of the pit viper and the color pattern will help identify the coral snake. In cases of exotic or unknown snakes when the identity of the snake is unknown, most large cities have either zoos or herpetologic societies whose members can be called on to positively identify the specimen. When doubt exists, clinical signs should be observed and supportive therapy given until an identification is made.

Physical Examination

The clinical signs associated with venomous snakebite vary considerably and depend on several factors. In humans, it is reported that 30% to 50% of venomous snakebites result in little to no envenomation. Some reports suggest the snake can control the amount of venom injected and in biting a human (and animal), prey much too large to swallow, the snake may become confused or frightened. However, the snake may inject up to 90% of the contents of the gland for the same reasons. Whether or not it can control the amount of venom injected is a topic of discussion amongst handlers, herpetologists, and scientists.

Other factors that may influence the effects of snakebite are the age, health, and size of the snake; the relative toxicity of the venom; the condition of the fangs; whether the snake has recently fed; whether the snake is injured; the size and age of the victim; the anatomic location of the bite; and the previous health problems of the victim.[25]

Local signs associated with envenomation include fang marks resembling puncture wounds (as opposed to superficial scratches and tears from nonvenomous species), the number of which may be variable. Pain and swelling are the most consistent signs associated with pit viper envenomation (Fig. 75-5). In coral snake envenomation, close examination of the upper and lower lip may identify subtle bite wounds.[26] The amount of pain and swelling are likely related to the amount of venom injected or the amount of swelling present. Subcutane-

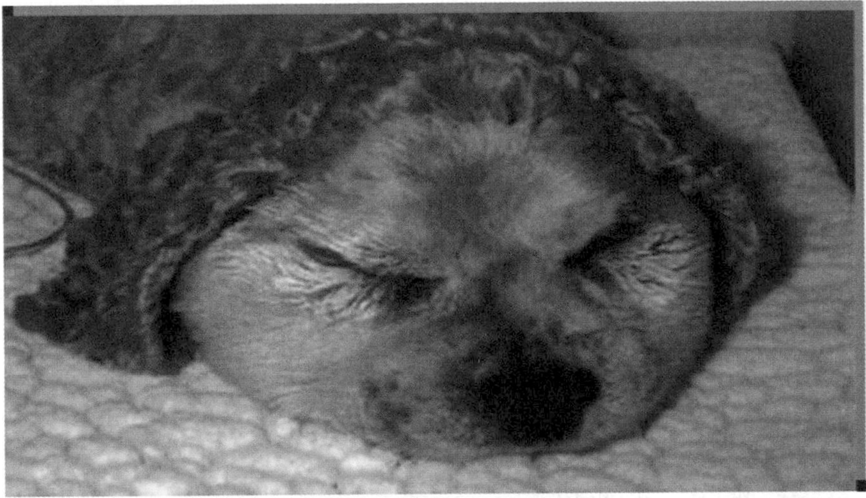

Figure 75-5
Severe facial swelling following rattlesnake envenomation in a dog.

ous edema surrounds the bite, begins early (10-20 minutes), and becomes quite diffuse. Most authorities agree that if specific signs are absent 30 minutes after the bite, envenomation is absent or minor.[9,13] Interestingly, compartment syndromes have not been described even with severe edema in humans. With bite wounds to the extremity, the circumference at the site of the bite and adjacent area should be measured and recorded. These data aid in objectively estimating both the spread of the venom and effect of the antivenin. Petechia, ecchymosis, and serous or hemorrhagic bullae are other local signs (Fig. 75-6).

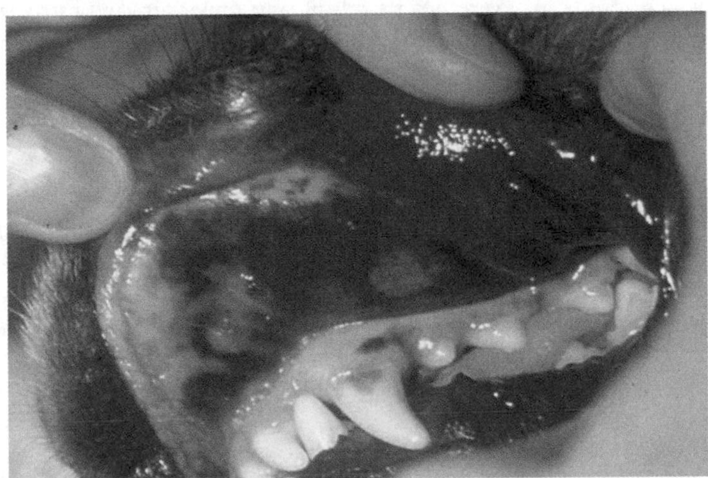

Figure 75-6
Edema and ecchymoses in the buccal mucosa of the dog seen in Figure 75-5.

Systemic signs include nausea and vomiting, bradycardia or tachycardia, hypotension, oliguria or anuria, paresthesias, seizures, fasciculations, and coma. Severe envenomations in humans present with multisystem complications of third-spacing, lactic acidosis, hemoconcentration, hemorrhage, hypovolemic shock, pulmonary edema, and cardiovascular collapse.[27-29] In dogs with coral snake envenomation, lethargy, lower motor neuron weakness (8 of 9 dogs) and cardiac arrhythmias (2 of 9) dogs are reported.[26]

Coral snake bites present in a clinical fashion that is markedly different from those of pit vipers. Delayed presentation symptoms, in some cases up to 12 hours, is the rule in humans. Once present, however, they often herald a precipitous clinical decline. Local signs are frequently sparse with minimal swelling and erythema found in only 50% of cases in one large (human) series.[30] Local signs may also include blood oozing and paresthesias at the bite site. There is usually some sign of broken skin because the snake typically hangs on and envenomates with a chewing motion.[22,30] Systemic signs include nausea and vomiting, hypersalivation, ptosis, generalized weakness, depressed reflexes, respiratory distress, and respiratory depression.

Controversy exists regarding the species resistance or susceptibility to snakebite. Rumor states that the cat is more resistant than the dog. Perhaps this refers to the agile, quick nature of the cat. The Arizona Poison Control reported that cats receive 50% of their bites to the head and 40% to the forelimbs, and that body bites were the most lethal.[31] Similarly, 70% of the snakebite wounds in the dog were to the head, yet less than 1% were lethal.[31] Swine are rumored to be resistant to snakebite likely because of the slow absorption of venom from fat. Contrary to popular belief, the horse is very susceptible to the effects of pit viper venom. Considerable morbidity is associated with envenomation in the horse. A retrospective study of horses poisoned by prairie rattlesnakes showed a death rate of 18% among acutely affected horses.[32] Horses are typically bitten on the muzzle, which results in severe head swelling and upper airway obstruction. In the horse there is an additional debilitating and fatal complication observed following snakebite from the prairie rattlesnake. This complication is acute or chronic myocardial failure due to necrosis of the cardiac muscle.[32]

DIAGNOSTIC EVALUATION

Clinical signs of pit viper envenomation usually develop within 10 to 15 minutes. Using a combination of clinical signs, time of the year, geographic locality, reptile identification, and witnesses to the bite, the diagnosis is usually straightforward. Initial laboratory studies from 100 dogs bitten by the prairie rattlesnake (*C. viridis viridis*) included thrombocytopenia (44 of 50), leukocytosis (37 of 70), and prolonged activated clotting time (8 of 86).[33] Hypokalemia is also reported to occur with rattlesnake envenomation.[34]

A retrospective study of 28 cases of rattlesnake bites in dogs indicated an association of envenomation with echinocytosis; 25 of 28 (89%) had echinocytosis within 24 hours of being bitten. These abnormal cells were described as type III echinocytes and interestingly these resolved within 48 hours of the bite

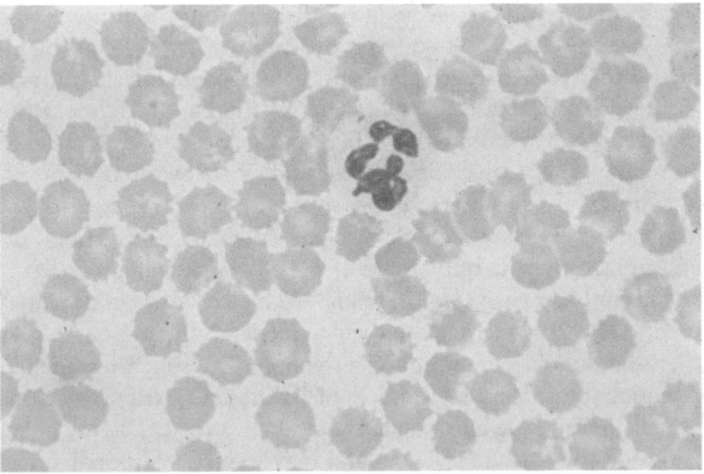

Figure 75-7
Type III echinocytosis seen with rattlesnake envenomation in the dog.

(Fig. 75-7).[34] Erythrocyte morphologic changes were produced in vitro after addition of western diamondback rattlesnake (C. *atrox*) venom to canine, feline, equine, and human blood. These changes were characterized by a dose-dependent echinocytosis. The dose was comparable to *in vivo* envenomation. In an effort to define the mechanisms of echinocytes formation, it was noted that addition of ethylenediaminetetraacetic acid prevented formation of echinocytes *in vitro*. This suggested a change in calcium or a metalloprotein participated in the formation of echinocytes. PLA_2, a calcium-dependent enzyme in snake venom, may be responsible for echinocytic transformation via the production of lysolecithin, a known echinocytic agent.[35] Other potential mechanisms of echinocytic change included erythrocyte cation loss and erythrocyte adenosine triphosphate (ATP) depletion. In canine blood mixed with venom, erythrocyte sodium and potassium concentrations were consistently less than those of controls.[35] This was likely a result of membrane alteration produced by the actions of PLA_2.[35] Careful examination of a blood smear soon after admission will confirm envenomation if type III echinocytes are represented by nearly every red blood cell.

TREATMENT

First Aid

Most authorities agree that too much time is spent administering first aid in the field. Reported field maneuvers encompass such varied forms as tourniquet application, suction devices, high voltage, electrotherapy, and even gasoline ingestion.[4] Other different therapies for snake envenomation have been described in the ancient and modern literature. The fact that many snakes do not envenomate their victims when they bite has helped support the use of whiskey, clam juice, or split chickens.[25]

The best intervention is safe and rapid transport to a definitive care center. Following snakebite, four basic concepts are kept in mind. First, the estimated time of arrival to a veterinary hospital must be considered in instituting first aid measures. If a dog is bitten a few blocks away, the care is different than for a victim on the side of a mountain that is hours away. Second, the spread of venom should be retarded if possible. Several methods for slowing the spread can be instituted. The animal's excitement, physical activity, movement of the bitten area, and depth of the bite all influence the spread of the venom. Calm the animal and immobilize the bitten area. If signs of envenomation occur, a constricting band applied tightly enough to impede lymph flow, but not arterial flow, can be used.[36] The constricting band will impede lymphatic outflow, which is the main dissemination route for pit viper venom; it is much less useful in coral snake envenomations, because the venom has rapid distribution through the bloodstream.[22] Incising the bite wound should be avoided. The use of an ice bag does not impede the spread of venom and may induce additional vasoconstriction leading to necrosis at the wound and further tissue destruction. Initial reports of favorable response to electrotherapy in pit viper envenomations have not been replicated.[37,38]

Third, when feasible, the snake should be identified or brought to the veterinary hospital with the victim. This is risky because there are reports of humans being envenomated from apparently dead snakes. It is noteworthy that many snakebite victims sustained envenomation when attempting to kill the reptile and that reflexive jaw musculature action can result from "dead," even decapitated, specimens. Snakes can and do bite through cloth sacks, so choice of a transport container should take this fact into account.[4] Fourth, the animal victim should be carefully observed on the way to the veterinary hospital. Shock and tissue swelling are common. Additionally, the potential for airway obstruction is very real when the animal has sustained a bite wound on the head or neck (Table 75-2).

Emergency Care of Snakebite

By the time the snakebitten animal arrives at the veterinary hospital, the venom may have already caused much damage both locally and systemically. On arrival, the veterinarian must be prepared to support the respiratory and cardiovascular systems. A team approach in managing the victim is strongly encouraged. While one team member is obtaining a history, another is inserting an intravenous (IV) catheter and collecting blood samples, another is taking vital signs, and another is preparing IV fluids and possibly obtaining antivenin.

Laboratory analysis consists of a complete blood count, examination of a blood smear for type III echinocytosis, a blood urea nitrogen (BUN) and creatinine, electrolytes, activated clotting time and total platelet count, and urinalysis for protein, blood, and glucose. Ideally, collecting samples for prothrombin time (PT), partial thromboplastin time (APTT), and fibrin degradation products (FDP) will better define the presence or absence of disseminated intravascular

Table 75-2. First Aid for Snakebite[24]

1. Move the victim from the vicinity of the snake. Injured or cornered snakes will inflict multiple bites.
2. Calm the animal. If the bite is on the head or neck, remove the animal's collar.
3. Identify or secure the snake if this can be done safely. Do not handle the snake.
4. Immobilize the involved extremity.
5. If no signs of envenomation are present, transport the animal to a veterinary hospital.
6. If signs of envenomation are present, apply a constricting band in cases of extremity bites. This band should be approximately 1 inch wide and should be applied 2 to 4 inches above the bite. It should be loose enough to admit a finger between the skin and band. Do not apply a constricting band if more than 30 minutes have elapsed since the bite occurred. Do not remove the constricting band until examined by a veterinarian. Frequently check distal pulses and loosen the band as necessary to maintain circulation.
7. If more than 1 hour from a veterinary facility, and within 15 minutes of the bite, suction should be performed using a commercial extractor (available at most sporting goods stores). Avoid surgical incision of the bite wound.
8. An ice bag wrapped in a towel can be applied to the swollen area to help alleviate pain. Under no circumstances should the area be packed in ice or immersed in ice water.
9. Wash the bite area with soap and water.
10. The airway, breathing, and circulation should be continuously monitored.
11. Transport the victim to the nearest veterinary hospital as soon as possible.

coagulopathy (DIC). In snakebite, DIC can be initiated through direct enzymatic activation of factor X.[39]

Ideally, two large-bore peripheral IV lines should be established—one for the administration of crystalloid or colloid solutions and the other for antivenin and adjunctive treatments. Oxygen is administered via a facemask or nasal oxygen catheter.

Snakes do not harbor *Clostridium tetani* as part of their normal oral flora. Traditional envenomation treatment protocols have advocated broad-based antibiotics for coverage of gram-negative bacteria, but this may not bear up under investigational scrutiny. Clark and coworkers[40] showed a very low incidence of infection in a prospective study evaluating rattlesnake envenomations that were otherwise treated with standard antivenin and surgical interventions in people. A review of a large series of (presumed) exclusively pit viper envenomations in Ecuador revealed abscess formation to be almost completely confined to those humans receiving broad-based antibiotics as part of their treatment regimen when compared to their variable matched controls who did not receive antibiotics.[41] A study focusing on incidence of wound infection from nonvenomous snake species similarly concluded that use of prophylactic antibiotics was not warranted.[42] The decision to include antibiotics remains a clinical judgment.

A fair amount of controversy surrounds the general medical management of envenomation. The use of commercial antivenin is the center of the controversy for dogs and cats. Fort Dodge Laboratories produces a polyvalent antivenin from equine serum that is used by many veterinarians. Wyeth-Ayerst Laboratories (Philadelphia) produces the commercial antivenin for the North American rattlesnake and eastern coral snake. The Crotalidae is a composite of antibodies to four species of New World pit vipers: (1) *Crotalus adamanteus* (eastern diamondback rattlesnake), (2) C. *atrox* (western diamondback rattlesnake), (3) C. *durissus terrificus* (tropical rattlesnake), and (4) *Bothrops atrox* (fer-de-lance). The coral snake antivenin is specific for bites from the eastern coral snake (*Micrurus fulvius*) and its Texas subspecies (M. *f. tenere*); it is ineffective for bites from the western coral snake (*Micruroides euryxanthus*), for which no specific antivenin has been developed, and for which no case fatalities in humans have been reported.[23] One report on use of antivenin in coral snake bites of dogs reported a single case of anaphylaxis.[24] Bites by copperheads in humans usually cause a moderate amount of edema but do not usually require antivenin.[25,43]

The Wyeth-Ayerst antivenins are produced from equine serum using batch techniques and consistently contain only 10% IgG that is specific for venom antibodies; the remainder is essentially nonimmunoglobulin proteins and nonspecific IgG.[44] The high allergenicity of these preparations is probably caused by glycosolated IgG as well as the horse serum components in the product. Equine immunoglobulin fixes human (animal) complement, triggering inflammatory pathways of the complement cascade, which may result in circulatory collapse.

There are two pertinent categories of hypersensitivity reactions to equine antivenin preparations. The first is an immediate reaction (type I) that manifests with urticaria, angioedema, laryngeal and bronchial spasm, respiratory distress, tachycardia, hypotension, shock, and cardiac dysrhythmias. The second is a delayed reaction (type III), termed serum sickness, that is characterized by the formation of antigen-antibody complexes and a state of antigen excess. It presents with malaise, arthralgias, urticaria, fever, and pruritis.

The decision to use antivenin in the dog and cat certainly has no objectivity at present. Once again, the veterinarian is faced with having to resort to human medicine for guidelines. Inclusion criteria in humans for antivenin vary regionally, but some national trends have emerged. Moderate to severe envenomations marked by hypotension, shock, progressive clinical status deterioration, increased swelling and ecchymoses, severe coagulopathies, hemorrhage states, respiratory distress, and tissue necrosis are all candidates for antivenin treatment.[4,13] The absence of pain, swelling, ecchymoses, systemic symptoms, fasciculations, and abnormal laboratory values within 30 to 60 minutes of a pit viper bite would preclude the use of antivenin.[4] A bite from the copperhead (A. *contortix*) usually does not require antivenin.[9,23] Water moccasin (A. piscivorous) bites are considered intermediate in severity between rattlesnake and copperhead bites, and they are variably treated with antivenin (in humans) based on initial and serial evaluations. All eastern coral snake bites (humans) should be treated with specific antivenin.[23]

Each vial of Wyeth-Ayerst antivenin is reconstituted from its lyophilized form with 10 mL normal saline, sterile water, or 5% dextrose-water (D5W). The shelf-life of the dry product is less than 5 years; reconstituted solutions should be used within 12 hours.[9] Antivenin is always administered *intravenously*, never intramuscularly or subcutaneously; it is never injected into a digit. Animal studies indicate that up to 85% of IV antivenin may accrue at the bite site.[9,23] There is no proven benefit to subcutaneous administration of antivenin at the bite site itself.[25]

Antivenin is most beneficial when given within 4 hours of the snakebite, although clinical efficacy has been demonstrated to extend past 24 hours.[9] High serum levels of antivenin in humans have been demonstrated up to 5 days after treatment. These levels gradually declined over the next 25 days, but were still detectable at low levels even 4 months after administration.[a] Hackett and colleagues[33] provide the only objective data regarding effectiveness of rattlesnake antivenin in veterinary species (dog) bitten by the prairie rattlesnake (*C. viridis viridis*). In this report there where two statistically significant differences between dogs treated with antivenin versus those not treated with antivenin: (1) on day 2 following antivenin administration, the platelet count was higher and (2) the number of days hospitalized was no different yet the client's bill was statistically higher! All other available references in veterinary medicine were simply anecdotal and contained no data for recommending antivenin for the rattlesnake. Interestingly, most animals only receive one vial of antivenin, no matter the size of the dog or cat. One must wonder whether a single vial is an adequate dosage.

Experimental antivenin has been produced for Gila monster envenomation but is not commercially available.[25] Fortunately, envenomation in humans, and likely in animals, responds well to supportive treatment. The reptile often leaves teeth in the bite wound due to their apparently rather loose attachment. These are often so small they are not readily visualized on radiography. Gila monsters are renowned for their bulldog-like grip and are often difficult to remove once firmly attached. Because venom is effectively introduced through pumping action of the jaw musculature, rapid removal of the reptile is greatly desired. Various methods are described, including submersion in cold water, application of heat to the jaws, mechanical prying with pliers or similar instruments, and even decapitation.[44,45]

Advances in Antivenin Research

Russell and coworkers[46] purified the Wyeth-Ayerst Crotalidae antivenin by isolating the Fab fragment via affinity chromatography. With this substance they showed a significant improvement over the parent form in a mouse model. This essentially pure IgG antibody specifically directed against snake venom proteins removed the large burden of foreign material key to the emergence of type III

[a] It is important to realize that most humans receive approximately 10 vials of antivenin as compared to most domestic animals receiving only one vial.

reactions; however, a purified form has not been introduced for clinical use.[25] Ovine and avian Fab products have recently been investigated and these essentially remove the danger of allergic response to equine products.[47,48] An ovine-based antivenom for *Micrurus* (coral snake) species is under development in the United Kingdom. This substance will neutralize both neurotoxic and cardiotoxic components of the venom.[25] The potential for effectively treating envenomation without repercussion of allergic reaction could dramatically change current therapeutic methodology. Unfortunately, the expense involved with the newer Fab antivenoms will preclude use in domestic animals for the foreseeable future.

Adjunctive Therapy for Snakebite

Considerable debate among veterinarians still rages regarding appropriate adjunctive treatment in snakebite. Unquestionably, IV crystalloid administration is indicated to avert onset of shock. The controversies develop when one discusses use of antihistamines, corticosteroids, and dimethyl sulfoxide (DMSO).

The concern in the use of antihistamines is their potential for inducing hypotension. Because hypotension is a hallmark sign of envenomation, one should follow the principle that IV fluid therapy is begun and then antihistamines can be administered. The tissue injury associated with envenomation surely induces release of histamine and thus the rationale for their use. Interestingly, use of antihistamines in human medicine seems more for prophylaxis before administration of antivenin. In the study by Hackett and colleagues,[33] 55% of the dogs bitten by a rattlesnake received antihistamines as part of their therapy. No adverse responses were noted. An interesting secondary effect of the antihistamine is that it will make the animal drowsy and this may allow the animal to rest more comfortably.

Corticosteroids were administered to 83% of dogs bitten by a rattlesnake.[33] Again, no adverse responses were reported. As mentioned above, PLA_2 is a key enzyme in inflammation and is present in snake venom. Interestingly, PLA_2 can be inhibited by corticosteroids (dexamethasone).[49]

There is little available literature to refute use of corticosteroids. In rodents, corticosteroids are of no help and may even be harmful.[50] Although it is tempting to hypothesize that rodents, being natural prey of pit vipers, may have a naturally selected immunologic defense mechanism that is impaired by corticosteroids, no such situation likely exists for the dog, cat, or human. The only two studies examining the use of corticosteroids in dogs provide equivocal results but there is no evidence of a detrimental effect.[51,52] Currently there seems to be little evidence to support the use of corticosteroids in snakebite. Unfortunately, the use of corticosteroids is so ingrained in some treatment regimes that they are likely given only under the old guise that "no dog should die without the benefit of the administration of a corticosteroid"!

Dimethyl sulfoxide is often used in veterinary medicine under the pretense of reducing tissue edema. Little objective data are available to substantiate this fact. Of greater concern is that DMSO can increase absorption of venom and may potentiate the ongoing hemolytic process.[53] Thus, there seems to be no reason to use DMSO in the acute phase of envenomation.

PROGNOSIS

Little information is available to provide objective data on the prognosis following snakebite. In the report of Hackett and coworkers,[33] small dogs stayed longer in the hospital yet the average stay of all dogs was only 24 hours. In this study of 100 dogs, only one death occurred and this animal did receive antivenin as part of its treatment. Emphasizing the species differences to envenomation, Dickinson and colleagues[53] report a mortality rate of 18.5% in 32 horses poisoned by the prairie rattlesnake. Kremer and coworkers[26] reported one death in 9 cases (11%) of coral snake envenomation in the dog. This one death was attributed to anaphylaxis from the antivenin.

If type III echinocytes are present, the animal should be admitted to the hospital for fluid therapy, close observation, and possible antivenin administration. The swelling is painful and these animals will benefit from analgesic administration. Nonsteroidal drugs should be used cautiously because of potential exacerbation of gastrointestinal bleeding in a clinical setting highlighted by coagulopathies. For similar reasons, aspirin and antiplatelet drugs should be avoided. Diazepam to calm the animal may be useful but is relatively contraindicated in envenomations involving the coral snake (and possibly the Mohave rattlesnake) because of the primarily neurotoxic venom effects and potentiation of respiratory depression.[4] Opiates titrated to effect seem reasonably safe and successful in pain attenuation.

Any patient bitten by the eastern coral snake or a Mojave rattlesnake is at risk for developing severe neurologic sequelae that may not become manifest for many hours. As a result, they should be admitted to the hospital where laboratory tests and monitoring can be performed. Antivenin treatment should be initiated at the earliest onset of symptoms. These animals may require use of a ventilator, invasive cardiovascular monitoring, and even dialysis.

REFERENCES

1. Sagan C: The Dragons of Eden. New York: Random House, 1977.
2. Minton SA, Minton R: Venomous Reptiles. New York: The Scribner Printing Office, 1980.
3. US Department of the Navy, Bureau of Medicine and Surgery: Poisonous Snakes of the World. Washington, DC: US Government Printing Office, 1968.
4. Radidis PM: Medical treatment of reptile envenomation: a review of the current literature. *Top Emerg Med* 22:16, 2000.
5. Chippaux JP, Williams V, White J: Snake venom variability: methods of study, results and interpretation. *Toxicon* 29:1279, 1991.
6. Chisari A, Spinedi E, Voirol MJ, *et al.*: A phospholipase A2-related snake venom (from *Crotalus durissus terrificus*) stimulates neuroendocrine and immune functions: determination of different sites of action. *Endocrinology* 139:617, 1998.

7. Tu A. Venoms: Chemistry and Molecular Biology. John Wiley & Sons: New York. 1977.
8. Tu AT. Reptile venoms and toxins. The Handbook of Natural Toxins, vol 5. New York: Marcel Dekker, 1991.
9. Russell FE: Snake venom poisoning in the United States. *Am Rev Med* 31:247, 1980.
10. Bond GR, Burkhart KK: Thrombocytopenia following Timber rattlesnake envenomation. *Ann Emerg Med* 30:40, 1997.
11. Carroll RR, Hall EC, Kitchens CS: Canebrake rattlesnake envenomation. *Ann Emerg Med* 30:45, 1997.
12. Clark RF, Williams SR, Nordt S, *et al.*: Successful treatment of crotalid induced neurotoxicity with a new polyspecific crotalid FAB antivenom. *Ann Emerg Med* 30: 54, 1997.
13. Johnson CA: Management of snakebite. *Am Fam Physician* 44:174, 1991.
14. White J: Envenoming and antivenom use in Australia. *Toxicon* 36:1483, 1998.
15. Chippaux JP: The development and use of immunotherapy in Africa. *Toxicon* 36: 1503, 1998.
16. Chanhome L, Cox WJ, Wilde H, *et al.*: Venomous snakebite in Thailand: medically important snakes. *Mil Med* 163:310, 1998.
17. Conant R, Collins JT: Reptiles and Amphibians of Eastern/Central North America, 3rd ed. Boston: Houghton-Mifflin, 1998.
18. Moorman CT, Moorman LS, Goldner BD: Snakebite in the tarheel state. *N C Med J* 53:141, 1992.
19. Pernell TC, Baba SS, Merideth JW:. The management of snake and spider bites in the southeastern United States. *Am Surg* 53:198, 1987.
20. Burch J, Agarwal R, Mattox KL, *et al.*: The treatment of Crotalid envenomations without antivenom. *J Trauma* 28:35, 1988.
21. Smith AS, Figge HL: Treatment of snakebite poisoning. *Am J Hosp Pharm* 48:2190, 1991.
22. Tennant A: A Field Guide to Snakes of Florida. Houston: Gulf Publishing Company, 1997.
23. Kitchens CS, Van Mierop LHS: Envenomations by the eastern coral snake. *JAMA* 258:165, 1987.
24. Hooker KR, Caravati ED: Gila monster envenomation. *Ann Emerg Med* 24:731, 1994.
25. Otten EJ: Venomous animal injuries. *In* Rosen P, Barkin R, eds.: Emergency Medicine: Concepts and Clinical Practice, 4th ed. Philadelphia: Mosby, 1998, p 924.
26. Kremer KA, Schaer M: Coral snake (*Micrurus fulvus fulvus*) envenomation in five dogs: present and earlier findings. *J Vet Emerg Crit Care* 5:9, 1995.
27. Pernell TC, Baba SS, Merideth JW: The management of snake and spider bites in the southeastern United States. *Am Surg* 53:198, 1987.
28. White RR, Weber RA: Poisonous snakebite in central Texas: possible indications for antivenin treatment. *Am Surg* 5:466, 1991.
29. Wingert WA, Chan C: Rattlesnake bites in southern California and rationale for recommended treatment. *West J Med* 148:37, 1988.
30. Kitchens CS, Van Mierop LHS: Envenomations by the eastern coral snake. *JAMA* 258:165, 1987.
31. Garland T: Recognition and treatment for snake bites. Proceedings 18th ACVIM, Seattle, WA, 2000, p 48.
32. Dickinson C: Envenomations. Proceedings 18th ACVIM, Seattle, WA, 2000, p 158.

33. Hackett TB, Wingfield WE, Mazzaferro E, *et al.*: Clinical experience with prairie rattlesnake (*Crotalus viridis viridis*) envenomation: 100 dogs 1989–1998. Proceedings 17th ACVIM, Chicago, IL, 1999, p 720 (abstract).
34. Brown DE, Meyer DJ, Wingfield WE, *et al.*: Echinocytosis associated with rattlesnake envenomation in dogs. *Vet Pathol* 31:654, 1994.
35. Walton RM, Brown DE, Hamar DW, *et al.*: Mechanisms of echinocytosis induced by *Crotalus atrox* venom. *Vet Pathol* 34:442, 1997.
36. Burgess JL, Dart RC, Egen NB: Effects of constriction bands on rattlesnake venom absorption: a pharmokinetic study. *Ann Emerg Med* 21:1086, 1992.
37. Dart RC, Gustafson RA: Failure of electrical shock treatment for rattlesnake envenomation. *Ann Emerg Med* 20:659, 1991.
38. Howe NR, Meisenheimer TL: Electric shock does not save snake bitten rats. *Ann Emerg Med* 17:254, 1988.
39. Bateman SW, Mathews KA, Abrams-Ogg ACG: Disseminated intravascular coagulation in dogs: review of literature. *J Vet Emerg Crit Care* 8:29, 1998.
40. Clark RF, Selden BS, Farbee B: The incidence of wound infection following crotalid envenomation. *J Emerg Med* 11:583, 1993.
41. Jorge MT, Ribiero LA, da Silva ML, *et al.*: Microbiological studies of abscesses complicating *Buthrops* snakebite in humans: a prospective study. *Toxicon* 32:743, 1994.
42. Weed HG: Nonvenomous snakebite in Massachusetts: prophylactic antibiotics are unnecessary. *Ann Emerg Med* 22:220, 1993.
43. Whitley RE: Conservative treatment of copperhead snakebites without antivenin. *J Trauma* 41:219, 1996.
44. Hooker KR, Caravati ED: Gila monster envenomation. *Ann Emerg Med* 24:731, 1994.
45. Hertschel S: Near death from a Gila monster bite. *Emerg Nurse* 12:259, 1986.
46. Russell FE, Sullivan JB, Egen NB, *et al.*: Preparation of a new antivenin by affinity chromatography. *Am Soc Trop Med Hyg* 34:141:1985.
47. Dart RC, Sefert SA, Carroll L, *et al.*: Affinity purified mixed monospecific crotalid antivenom ovine Fab for the treatment of crotalid venom poisoning. *Ann Emerg Med* 30:33, 1997.
48. Carroll SB, Thalley BS, Theakston RD, *et al.*: Comparison of the purity and efficacy of affinity purified avian antivenom with commercial equine Crotalid antivenom. *Toxicon* 30:1017, 1992.
49. Lilja I, Dimberg J, Sjodahl R, *et al.*: Effects of endotoxin and dexamethasone on group I and II phospholipase A2 in rat ileum and stomach. *Gut* 35:40, 1994.
50. Russell FE, Emery JA: Effects of corticosteroids on lethality of *Ancistrodon contortrix* venom. *Am J Med Sci* 241:507, 1961.
51. Allam MW, Weimer D, Lukens FDW: Comparison of cortisone and antivenin in the treatment of Crotaline envenomation. Publication 44, AAAS, *Science* 393-397, 1956.
52. Deichmann WB, Radomski JL, Farrell JJ: Acute toxicity and treatment of intoxications due to *Crotalus adamanteus*. *Am J Med Sci* 236:204, 1958.
53. Dickinson CE, Traub-Dargatz JL, Dargatz DA, *et al.*: Rattlesnake venom poisoning in horses: 32 cases (1973–1993). *J Am Vet Med Assoc* 208:1866, 1996.

76
Ethylene Glycol Toxicity

Craig B. Webb

INTRODUCTION

Ethylene glycol is one of the most common, and frequently fatal toxicants encountered in veterinary medicine. Several studies indicate that mortality estimates as high as 70%.[1] Ethylene glycol constitutes the main ingredient (95%) of most brands of antifreeze, as well as being a component of many paints, windshield wiper fluids, and polishes. The low minimum lethal dose (1.4 mL/kg in the cat, and 4.4-6.6 mL/kg in the dog), easy accessibility (*i.e.*, garage floor, spills), palatability, and lack of owner awareness all help contribute to the prevalence of this intoxication.[1]

PATHOGENESIS

Ethylene glycol is rapidly absorbed from the stomach with peak plasma levels occurring 2-3 hours after ingestion. Approximately 50% of the ingested compound is excreted unchanged in the urine. Ethylene glycol causes symptoms of gastrointestinal and central nervous system (CNS) toxicity (depression, ataxia, and vomiting). But it is the hepatic metabolism of ethylene glycol to toxic by-products that accounts for the severity of patient presentation and the rapid progression to death. Ethylene glycol is first converted to glycoaldehyde by the enzyme alcohol dehydrogenase (ADH) (Fig. 76-1). This is the rate-limiting enzymatic step and serves as the target for specific antidote administration. ADH requires nicotinamide adenine dinucleotide (NAD) as a cofactor. Aldehyde dehydrogenase, another NAD-requiring enzyme, converts glycoaldehyde to glycolic acid. Glycolic acid is then converted into glyoxalic acid by the enzyme lactate dehydrogenase, and further metabolism of glyoxalic acid produces oxalic acid, glycine, and formic acid.[2] Oxalic acid combines with calcium in the blood to form a soluble calcium oxalate complex. This complex is filtered by renal glomeruli, and subsequently forms predominantly monohydrate calcium oxalate crystals in the urine.[3]

Ethylene glycol and glycoaldehyde are direct CNS depressants; the accumulation of toxic metabolites disrupts glucose, serotonin, and amine metabolism to the brain.[2] Elevated plasma concentrations of glycolic acid results in severe metabolic acidosis (the pH of a 2% aqueous solution of glycolic acid is 2.16). The accumulation of glycolic acid and oxalic acid leads to a significantly elevated anion gap.

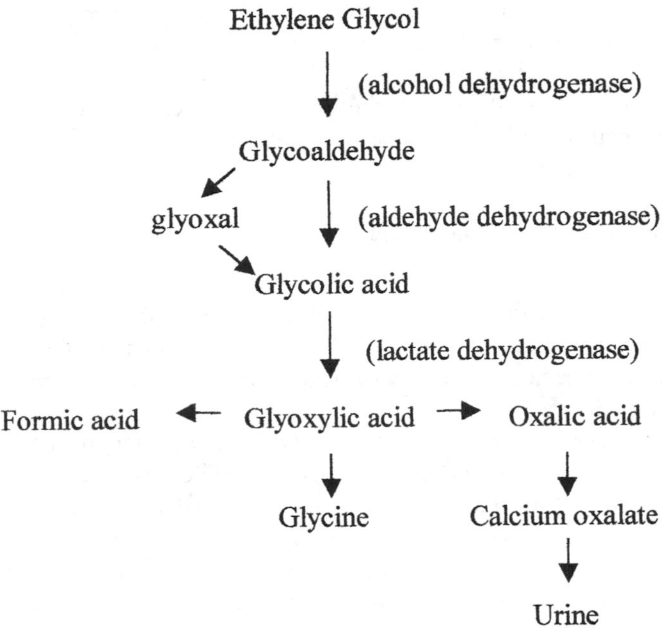

Figure 76-1
Metabolic pathway of ethylene glycol.

CLINICAL PRESENTATION

The emergent presentation of a dog or cat suffering from ethylene glycol intoxication varies with the amount ingested and time elapsed since ingestion. The severity and progression of symptoms mirror the metabolism of the parent compound.

Three phases are used to describe the progression of symptoms. During the first phase (30 minutes to 12 hours after ingestion) animals appear obtunded and are often ataxic with muscle fasciculations, and decreased withdrawal and righting reflexes. Hyperosmolar serum results in an osmotic diuresis and stimulates thirst such that animals are dehydrated, polyuric, and polydypsic. These symptoms correspond to the presence of the parent compound and glycoaldehyde, whose plasma concentration peaks approximately 6 to 12 hours after exposure. CNS signs usually abate toward the end of phase one as the ethylene glycol and glycoaldehyde are further metabolized or excreted.

Animals entering the second phase (8–24 hours after ingestion) demonstrate mental dullness, anorexia, and pulmonary congestion. Often the only clinical signs of phase two intoxication are tachypnea and tachycardia.

Phase three symptoms (24–72 hours after ingestion) are indicative of acute oliguric renal failure; animals exhibit signs of uremic gastritis (anorexia, vomiting, ptyalism, oral ulceration), severe acidosis with an elevated anion gap, azotemia, uremia, polydipsia, and isosthenuria. Ethylene glycol metabolites are directly toxic to renal epithelial cells, resulting in tubular necrosis. Patients may be seizuring, obtunded, or in a coma.[4]

Cats seem to move through the different phases of intoxication over a briefer time course, with phase three and fatalities occurring as soon as 12 to 15 hours after ingestion.[5]

DIAGNOSTIC EVALUATION

A history of possible exposure often accompanies the patient to the emergency room. A relatively acute onset of severe illness and characteristic symptoms in a previously healthy animal, should alert the clinician to the possibility of toxicant ingestion. The time of year (late fall through spring) may also raise the clinician's index of suspicion.

The changes seen on a complete blood count, chemistry panel, and urinalysis are not specific for ethylene glycol ingestion. There is a commercial colorimetric spot test kit available for the detection of ethylene glycol[a] in blood or urine within 12 to 24 hours of ingestion. Propylene glycol can result in a false-positive test result. This is important if drugs using propylene glycol as a vehicle (*i.e.*, diazepam) or an ingredient (*i.e.*, activated charcoal) are used prior to testing.

The ethylene glycol molecule is slightly smaller than albumin (MW 62,000 daltons) and osmotically active. Serum osmolality (normally 280–310 mOsm/kg) can increase significantly just 1 hour following ingestion, along with an abnormally elevated osmolar gap.[b] Metabolism of ethylene glycol to the organic acids, glycolic acid and oxalic acid, results in severe metabolic acidosis (consumption of plasma bicarbonate) and an elevated anion gap (unmeasured anion accumulation) within 1 to 3 hours after ingestion.[c] By 36 to 48 hours following ethylene glycol ingestion (12 hours in the cat) the glomerular filtration rate is decreasing and azotemia occurs. Phosphorus, potassium, and glucose are usually elevated. Calcium levels are usually decreased as this molecule combines with oxalate to form monohydrate calcium oxalate crystals. Phosphorus is initially elevated because it is often added to many antifreeze solutions as a rust retardant. Later this elevation in phosphorus is secondary to renal failure.[6]

The elevated serum osmolality and concurrent osmotic diuresis frequently lead to isosthenuric urine (1.008–1.012). Precipitation of monohydrate calcium oxalate crystals can be observed in urine within 3 to 6 hours after ingestion (Fig. 76-2). Both monohydrate and dihydrate birefringent forms of calcium oxalate may eventually be present. Monohydrate crystals often appear as dumbbells or "coffin" shaped; dihydrate crystals may have the classic "Maltese cross" shape.

[a] EGT Test Kit, PRN Pharmacal, Inc., Allelic Biosystems Ethylene Glycol Test Kit, 5830 McAllister Ave., Pensacola, FL 32524

[b] Osmolar gap = measured osmolarity - calculated osmolarity (normally <10 mOsm/kg)
Calculated osmolality = 1.86 (Na+K) + glucose/18 + BUN/2.8 + 9

[c] Anion gap = (Na+K) − (HCO_3+Cl) (normally 10–15 mEq/L)

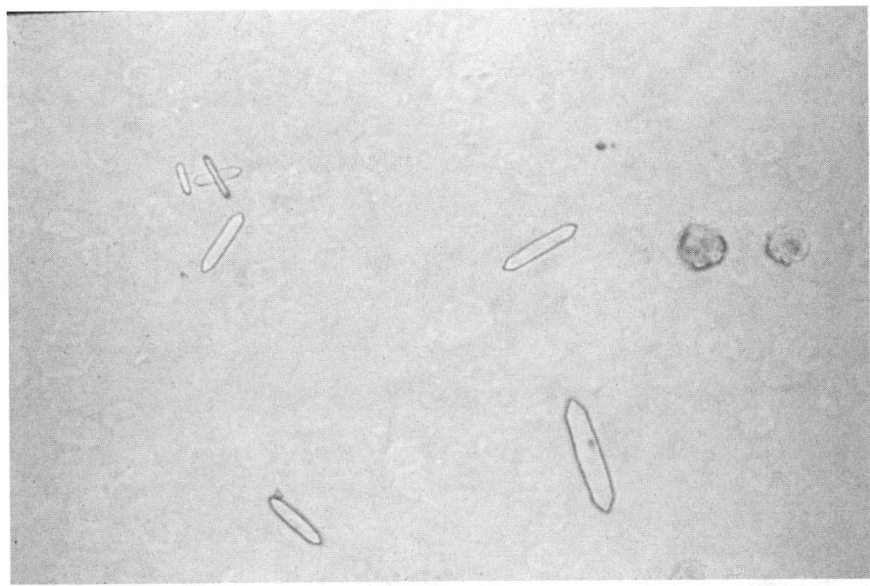

Figure 76-2
The "coffin"-shaped crystal of monohydrate calcium oxalate associated with ethylene glycol toxicity.

An active sediment (granular casts and renal epithelial cells) may be seen depending on the amount of tubular damage present. Some antifreeze manufacturers are adding fluorescent compounds to their formulations, so that illuminating a patient's urine with a Wood's lamp may yield positive results in cases of questionable intoxication.

Ultrasound examination may provide support for the diagnosis of ethylene glycol toxicity and prognostic information. The usual observation is that of increased renal cortical echogenicity. Within 4 to 8 hours after ingestion, the echogenicity of the renal cortices is greater than that of the liver and may be equal to the spleen. With progression of the disease, the renal medullae increase in echogenicity, and eventually the echogenicity of the cortices surpasses that of the spleen. Finally, areas of relative lucency appear at the corticomedullary junction and within the central medullary region (Fig. 76-3). This creates a "halo" sign, which corresponds to clinical anuria and a grave prognosis.[7]

Histolopathology reveals acute tubular necrosis and intratubular calcium oxalate crystal deposition. The ultrasonographic changes correspond to calcium oxalate crystal deposition, but changes in kidney echogenicity to not correlate to chemistry abnormalities such as elevated blood urea nitrogen (BUN) and creatinine.[7] A polarized light source may be used to better visualize the crystal deposition. A postmortem renal calcium tissue concentration of greater than 2000 ppm (normal is 50–200 ppm) is highly suggestive of ethylene glycol nephrotoxicity.[8]

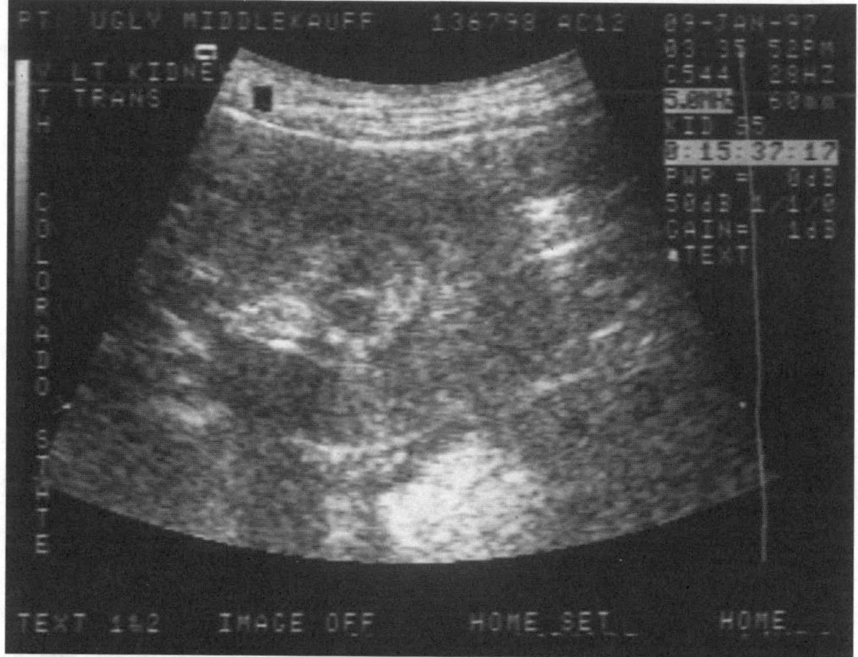

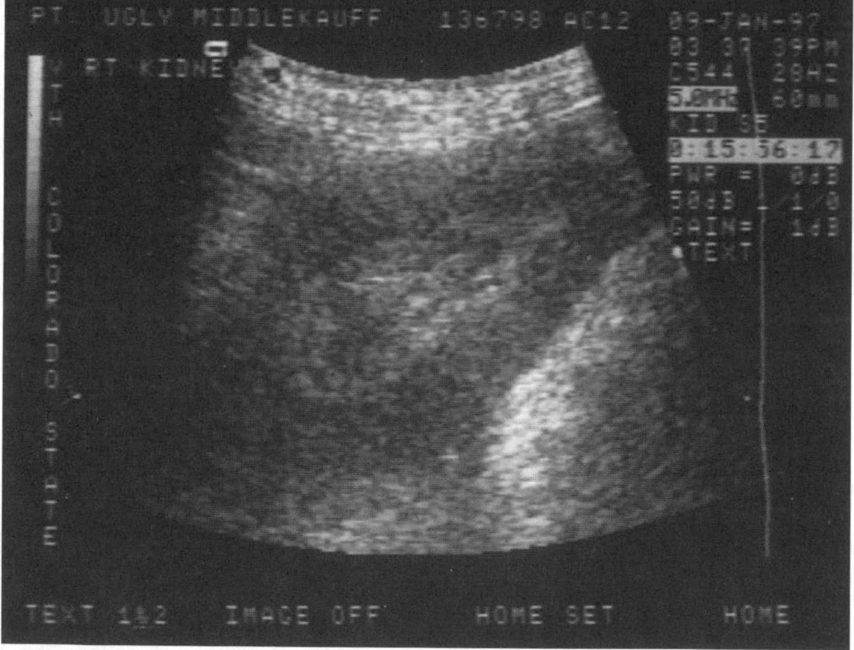

Figure 76-3
Ultrasonographic images of the left kidney from a dog with ethylene glycol intoxication. Sagittal and transverse images show a decrease in corticomedullary differentiation and a hyperechoic "rim" or "halo" sign within the kidney parenchyma.

TREATMENT

If the patient presents within 4 to 6 hours of ingestion and is alert with an intact gag reflex, emesis should be induced (apomorphine hydrochloride 0.02-0.04 mg/kg deposited in the conjunctival sac). Activated charcoal[d] can then be administered (via stomach tube) in an attempt to absorb additional toxicant.

The specific antidotes used for ethylene glycol ingestion are aimed at inhibiting the enzyme ADH, and blocking the conversion of ethylene glycol to its more toxic metabolites. Ethanol is a competitive inhibitor of ADH, and various protocols use ethanol administration for dogs presenting within 12 hours of ethylene glycol ingestion.[e] The time it takes for hepatic metabolism of ethylene glycol, and the toxicity of its metabolites, dictates that blood levels of ethanol remain elevated for at least 48 hours (detectable levels of ethylene glycol can persist in the serum and urine this long). Common side effects of ethanol ingestion include CNS depression, an increase in serum osmolality, hypothermia, and osmotic diuresis. These effects are particularly severe in cats.[9]

4-Methylpyrazole[f] (4-MP) is also used to inhibit ethylene glycol metabolism by forming a noncovalent complex with ADH and its coenzyme NAD. In dogs, 4-MP (as a 5% solution) is given initially as a 20 mg/kg IV dose, followed 12 and 24 hours later with a dose of 15 mg/kg, and a final dose of 5 mg/kg 36 hours after initiation of treatment.[10] The distinct advantage of 4-MP as an antidote is avoidance of the ethanol side effects. Studies comparing the response to treatment suggest 4-MP is a more effective antidote than ethanol.[11] The response to treatment is best if 4-MP is initiated within 5 hours following ethylene glycol ingestion. Mortality increases significantly with any longer delay between exposure and treatment.[12] 4-MP is currently not recommended in cats; cats do not respond to dosages of 4-MP that are used for dogs. As described earlier, cats exposed to ethylene glycol deteriorate more rapidly than dogs, and the minimal lethal dose of ethylene glycol is lower in felines. Cats metabolize ethylene glycol less efficiently than dogs (the V_{max} for ADH is lower in cats than in dogs), and a variety of other metabolic differences may help to explain the disparity between the two species. Higher doses of 4-MP may be required in cats and studies are currently underway investigating this possibility.[12]

Hemodialysis or peritoneal dialysis are potentially beneficial in decreasing toxicant concentrations for up to 24 hours after ingestion. If successful, these techniques give the patient's kidneys additional time for repair and compensation, but often the renal damage is irreversible, and the outcome unavoidable.

[d] Acta-Char 1-4 g/kg, Charcodote 6–12 mL/kg

[e] 5% alcohol in 5% dextrose at 22 mL/kg IV q 4 h for 24 hours, then q 6 h for 24 hours
5.5 mL/kg of 20% ethanol IV q 4 h for 5 treatments, then q 6 h for 4 treatments
20% ethanol as a continuous rate infusion (CRI) at 1.4 mL/kg/h (dogs), 1.25 mL/kg/h (cats)
5% ethanol as a CRI at 5.5 mL/kg/h

[f] 4-MP or fomepizol, Antizol-Vet, Orphan Medical Inc., 13911 Ridgedale Dr., Suite 250, Minnetonka, MN 55305

PROGNOSIS

Prognosis depends, in part, on the amount of ethylene glycol ingested, the prompt presentation of the pet by the owner, and the timely recognition and treatment of the problem by the veterinarian. If therapy is initiated within 8 hours and the dog is not yet azotemic, the prognosis is considered fair to good. In one survey of 37 dogs treated with 4-MP, only 1 of 21 azotemic dogs survived. By comparison, 16 of 16 nonazotemic dogs survived.[1] For cats, the prognosis must always be considered grave because studies have documented a fatality rate of 97% or above. Although rarely measured, concentration of glycolic acid in the urine seems to correlate with mortality.

REFERENCES

1. Connally HE, Thrall MA, Forney SD *et al.*: Safety and efficacy of 4-methylpyrazole for treatment of suspected or confirmed ethylene glycol intoxication in dogs: 107 cases (1983–1995). *J Am Vet Med Assoc* 209:1880, 1996.
2. Bahri LE: 4-Methylpyrazole: an antidote for ethylene glycol intoxication in dogs. *Compend Contin Educ* 13:1123, 1991.
3. Hewlett TP, Jacobsen D, Collins TD, *et al.*: Ethylene glycol and glycolate kinetics in rats and dogs. *Vet Hum Toxicol* 31:116, 1989.
4. Grauer GF, Thrall MA, Henre BA, *et al.*: Early clinicopathologic findings in dogs ingesting ethylene glycol. *Am J Vet Res* 45:2299, 1984.
5. Thrall MA, Grauer GF, Mero KN: Clinicopathologic findings in dogs and cats with ethylene glycol intoxication. *J Am Vet Med Assoc* 184:37, 1984.
6. Thrall MA, Grauer GF, Dial SM: Antifreeze poisoning. *In* Bonagura JD, ed.: Current Veterinary Therapy XII. Philadelphia: WB Saunders, 1995, p 232.
7. Adams WH, Toal RL, Breider MA: Ultrasonographic findings in dogs and cats with oxalate nephrosis attributed to ethylene glycol intoxication: 15 cases (1984–1988). *J Am Vet Med Assoc* 199:492, 1991.
8. Braselton WE, Slanker MR: The use of kidney calcium concentrations for the postmortem diagnosis of ethylene glycol toxicosis. ACVIM Abstract. *J Vet Intern Med* 4:132, 1990.
9. Dial SM, Thrall MA, Hamar DW: Comparison of ethanol and 4-methylpyrazole as treatments for ethylene glycol intoxication in cats. *Am J Vet Res* 55:1771, 1994.
10. Dial SM, Thrall MA, Hamar DW: 4-Methylpyrazole as treatment for naturally acquired ethylene glycol intoxication in dogs. *J AmVet Med Assoc* 195:73, 1989.
11. Grauer GF, Thrall MA, Henre BA, *et al.*: Comparison of the effects of ethanol and 4-methylpyrazole on the pharmacokinetics and toxicity of ethylene glycol in the dog. *Toxicol Lett* 35:307, 1987.
12. Connally HE, Hamar DW, Thrall MA: Inhibition of canine and feline alcohol dehydrogenase activity by fomepizole. *Am J Vet Res* 61:450, 2000.
13. Dial SM, Thrall MA, Hamar DW: Efficacy of 4-methylpyrazole for treatment of ethylene glycol intoxication in dogs. *Am J Vet Res* 55:1762, 1994.

77
Adverse Reactions to Therapeutic Drugs in the CCU Patient

Dawn Merton Boothe

INTRODUCTION
Adverse Drug Events

An adverse drug event (ADE) is any undesirable reaction to therapy with a drug. ADEs can be classified as type A or type B.[1,2] Type A ("augmented") ADEs generally result from plasma drug concentrations that exceed the maximum therapeutic range or, less commonly but equally undesirable, decrease below the therapeutic range. If the clinician is familiar with the drug and the patient, type A events are largely predictable and, with proper precautions, often avoidable. The type A ADE generally is manifested as an exaggerated, but "normal" or expected pharmacologic response. The response might be the primary or targeted response (*e.g.*, bradycardia in a patient receiving propranolol to slow sinus tachycardia) or secondary but untargeted response (*e.g.*, bronchospasms due to nonselective β-blockade effects of propranolol). Type A ADEs include therapeutic failures resulting from subtherapeutic drug concentrations (*i.e.*, underdosing of an antimicrobial). Some drugs also cause ADEs unrelated to their pharmacologic response. These events usually reflect damage to target cells and will be referred to as cytotoxic ADEs. Cytotoxic ADEs are perhaps best exemplified by hepatic necrosis induced by acetaminophen. Often it is the metabolite of the drug rather than the drug itself that causes cytotoxicity. In such cases, drugs that induce metabolism, particularly in the liver (*e.g.*, phenobarbital) may increase the risk of toxicity, whereas drugs that decrease metabolism (*e.g.*, cimetidine) or scavenge oxygen radicals (*e.g.*, *N*-acetylcysteine or *S*-adenosylmethionine) may reduce the risk of toxicity.[3,4]

Type A ADEs are less likely or more avoidable for drugs characterized by a wide safety margin (*e.g.*, most antibiotics), drugs for which the clinical response is easily detected (*e.g.*, gas anesthetics), or drugs that are monitored to ensure that concentrations are within the therapeutic range (*e.g.*, selected antibiotics, cyclosporine, cardiac drugs, and anticonvulsant drugs). Many type A ADEs can be avoided by choosing alternative (safer or more effective drugs), by minimizing the risk of drug interactions, or by modifying the dosing regimen of a drug to accommodate disease or drug-induced changes in drug disposition that might lead to ADE.

The organs most susceptible to type A ADEs are those subjected to the greatest exposure or concentration of the drug. Thus, the organs with the greatest blood flow (*e.g.*, the heart and central nervous system [CNS] during physiologic responses to hypovolemia) and those organs capable of drug concentration (*e.g.*, organs of elimination [liver and kidney]) are most vulnerable to ADEs caused by systemic drugs. Highly metabolic organs are vitally dependent on energy (oxygen) delivery and thus are also at greater risk. Adverse reactions to any drug should be anticipated following absolute (miscalcuation) or relative (due to changes in drug disposition) overdosing (see final section of this chapter and Table 77-1).

Type B ("bizarre") ADEs are neither dose nor concentration dependent. As a result, these events are not predictable and are largely unavoidable. They occur in a small percentage of the population receiving the drug. Generally, their incidence, indeed their existence, often is not documented until well after the drug has been approved. In addition, because their cause is not well understood, treatment of type B ADEs is generally limited to symptomatic therapy. Examples of type B ADEs include drug allergies or idiosyncrasies. Many of these ADEs ultimately may be genetically based, but the cause has yet to be identified and thus the reaction cannot be predicted. As with type A events, type B ADEs may reflect a reaction to the parent drug or its metabolite. The organs most susceptible to damage by type B ADEs tend to be the organs that contain tissues that act as haptens for drug-induced allergy (*e.g.*, skin, blood-forming units), tissues that filter and trap immune complexes (*e.g.*, glomerulus and joints), or tissues that contain large numbers of mast cells (gastrointestinal [GI] and liver in the dog, lung in the cat).

The clinical manifestations of allergic drug reactions vary with the type of reaction and the body system targeted. Previous exposure to the drug must occur or therapy must have been sufficiently long (*i.e.*, 10–14 days) for an allergic response to develop. Drugs generally are too small to be sufficiently antigenic. Rather, drugs generally act as haptens, covalently combining with a body tissue that then becomes antigenic. As a result, the allergic response may be directed toward the drug or tissue. Type I reactions (immediate or anaphylaxis) are IgE-mediated and result from the release of chemical mediators (*e.g.*, histamine, serotonin, eicosanoids) released from tissue mast cells or basophils. The reaction occurs within minutes after administration of the drug and will occur regardless of the dose given. Clinical manifestations generally include nausea, vomiting, circulatory collapse, tachycardia, pulmonary edema, and neurologic signs. Urticaria and angioedema may also be evident. Clinical signs may be species dependent, depending on the "shock" organ of the species. The shock organ generally is the organ in which mast cells occur in greatest numbers. In the dog, the shock organ tends to be the liver and GI tract; in the cat, the shock organ generally is the lung. Sometimes the exact antigen that causes anaphylaxis is not known. Treatment of drug-induced anaphylaxis is directed toward preventing the physiologic response to mediator release (*i.e.*, epinephrine and antihistamines) and preventing further histamine release (*e.g.*, epinephrine and glucocorticoids,

Table 77-1. Treatment of Adverse Reactions Caused by Therapeutic Agents

Drug	Antidote	Treatment
Acetaminophen and phenacetin	β-Acetylcysteine	150 mg/kg loading dose, orally or IV, then 50 mg/kg q 4 h for 17–20 additional doses
Amitraz	Atipamezole	50 µg/kg IM. Signs should reverse in 10 min. Repeat q 3–4 h as needed. Can follow with 0.1 mg/kg yohimbine IM q 6 h.
	Yohimbine	Dogs 0.11 mg/kg IV slowly. Cats 0.5 mg/kg IV slowly
Amphetamines	Chlorpromazine	1 mg/kg IM, IP, IV; administer only half dose if barbiturates have been given; blocks excitation. Higher doses (10–18 mg/kg IV) may be beneficial if large volumes are consumed. Treatment of increased intracranial pressure may be indicated (mannitol, furosemide).
	Urinary alkalinization: Ammonium chloride	100–200 mg/kg/d divided q 8–12 h (contraindicated with myoglobinuria, renal failure, or acidosis).
Antitussives	Naloxone	If narcotic (*e.g.*, hydrocodone, codeine)
Aspirin	No specific antidote (see NSAIDs)	Acute toxicosis: Urinary alkalinization, other supportive therapy. Doses of 50 mg/kg/d (dog) and 25 mg/kg/d (cat); 7 mL/kg/d bismuth subsalicylate (dogs and cats) may be toxic.
Atropine, Belladonna alkaloids	Physostigmine	0.1–0.6 mg/kg (do not use neostigmine).
Barbiturates	Doxapram	2% solution. Give small animals 3–5 mg/kg IV only (0.14–0.25 mL/kg) repeated as necessary. Consider yohimbine, tolazoline. Urinary alkalinization.
Barium, bismuth salts	Sodium sulfate/magnesium sulfate	20% solution given orally. Dosage: 2–25 g.
Bromides	Chlorides (sodium or ammonium salts)	0.5–1.0 g daily for several days; hasten excretion.
Cholinergic agents	Atropine sulfate	0.02–0.04 mg/kg, as needed.

Table 77-1. (continued)

Drug	Antidote	Treatment
Cholinesterase inhibitors	Atropine sulfate	Dosage is 0.02–0.04 mg/kg, repeated as needed for atropinization. Repeat in decreasing doses (cut by half). Treat cyanosis or dyspnea (oxygen) if present first. Atropine blocks only muscarinic effects. Atropine in oil may be injected for prolonged effect during the night. *Avoid atropine intoxication!* Organophosphate inhibition tends to be irreversible; organocarbamate tends to be reversible.
	Pralidoxime chloride (2-PAM)	5% solution; 20–50 mg/kg IM or by slow IV (0.2–1.0 mg/kg) injection (maximum dose is 500 mg/min), repeat as needed 2–3 times. Do not treat again if no effect. 2-PAM alleviates nicotinic effect and regenerates cholinesterase. Morphine, succinylcholine, and phenothiazine tranquilizers are contraindicated.
	Diphenhydramine	1–4 mg/kg IM, PO q 8 h. To block nicotinic effects.
Cocaine	No specific antidote	Chlorpromazine (up to 15 mg/kg; may lower seizure threshold, use cautiously); fluids; metoprolol or propanolol to treat cardiac arrhythmias (see chocolate poisoning); phentolamine or sodium nitroprusside if β-blockers cause hypertension; lidocaine (in lieu of β-blockers to control cardiac arrhythmias; see chocolate poisoning).
Coumarin-derivative anticoagulants	Vitamin K_1	Give 3–5 mg/kg/d with canned food. Treat 7 days for warfarin-type, treat 21–30 d for second-generation anticoagulant rodenticides. Oral therapy is more efficacious than IV.
	Whole blood or plasma	Blood transfusion, 25 mL/kg.
Curare	Neostigmine methylsulfate	Solution: 1:5000 or 1:2000 (1 mL = 0.2 or 0.5 mg/mL). Dose is 0.005 mg/5 kg, SQ. Follow with IV injection of atropine (0.04 mg/kg).
	Edrophonium chloride Artificial respiration	1% solution; give 0.05–1.0 mg/kg IV.

Digitalis glycosides, oleander	Potassium chloride	Dog: 0.5–2.0 g, orally in divided doses. In serious cases, administer as diluted solution given IV by slow drip (ECG control is essential).
	Diphenylhydantoin	25 mg/min IV control is established.
	Propranolol (β-blocker)	0.5–1.0 mg/kg IV or IM as needed to control cardiac arrhythmias (ECG control is essential).
	Atropine sulfate	0.02–0.04 mg/kg as needed for cholinergic control.
Heparin	Protamine sulfate	1% solution; give 1.0–1.5 mg to antagonize each 1 mg of heparin; slow IV injection. Reduce dose as time increases between heparin injection and start of treatment (after 30 min give only 0.5 mg). Note that overdose of protamine may contribute to anticoagulant effects.
Iron		Sodium bicarbonate: 1% for lavage.
	Sodium thiosulfate (arsenic)	10% solution given orally (0.5–3.0 g for small animals. Followed by lavage or emesis. Protein (*e.g.,* evaporated milk, egg whites). Tannic acid or strong tea.
	Dimercaprol	10% solution in oil; give small animals 2.5–5.0 mg/kg IM (0.025–0.05 mg/kg) q 4 h for 2 d, then bid for the next 10 days or until recovery. *Note:* In severe acute poisoning 5 mg/kg dosage should be given only for the first day.
	D-Penicillamine (Cuprimine7, Merck & Co.)	Developed for chronic mercury poisoning, now seems most promising drug; no reports on dosage in animals. Dosage for humans is 250 mg PO, q 6 h for 10 d (3–4 mg/kg).
	Succimer	10 mg/kg PO q 8 h for 10 d.
	N-acetylcysteine	140–280 mg/kg PO then 70 mg/kg PO q 6 h for 3 days (IV administration okay in vomiting dogs).
Iron salts	Deferoxamine	Dose in dogs is 25–50 µg/kg/M

Table 77-1. (continued)

Drug	Antidote	Treatment
Ivermectin	Physostigmine	0.06 mg/kg IV very slowly; actions should last 30–90 min.
	Picrotoxin (GABA antagonist)	Use is controversial. May cause severe seizures. Other treatment may include epinephrine, and, if the product causing toxicosis is Eqvalen, an antihistamine to counteract polysorbate 80 (releases histamine in dogs), and atropine.
Local anesthetics	Methylene blue	1% solution (maximum concentration), give by *slow* IV injection, 8.8 mg/kg; (0.9 mL/kg) repeat if necessary. To prevent fall in blood pressure in case of nitrite poisoning, use a sympathomimetic drug (ephedrine or epinephrine). (Not recommended for cats). Methylene blue can cause methemoglobinemia in the absence of Heinz body formation.
Morphine and related drugs	Naloxone chloride (Narcan7, Endo)	0.02–0.04 mg/kg IV. Repeat as needed. Do not repeat if respiration is not satisfactory.
	Levallorphan tartrate (Lorfan7, Roche)	Give IV, 0.1–0.5 mL of solution containing 1 mg/mL. *Note:* Use either of the above antidotes only in acute poisoning. Artificial respiration may be indicated. Activated charcoal is also indicated.
	Diphenhydramine HCl	For CNS depression, 2–5 mg/kg IV for extrapyramidal signs.
Narcotics	Naloxone	Vomiting indicated only if patient sufficiently alert. Dogs: 0.02–0.04 mg/kg IV; repeat as needed. Cats: 0.05–0.1 mg/kg IV; repeat as needed. Other supportive therapy may include anticonvulsants (especially for meperidine), fluid therapy.
NSAIDs	Sucralfate	500–1000 mg PO q 8 h.
	Misoprostol	3–5 µg/kg q 8–12 h.
	Omeprazole	0.7 mg/kg q 24 h (dog); alternative: ranitidine or famotidine (dog and cat).

Phenothiazine	Methylamphetamine	0.1–0.2 mg/kg IV; also transfusion. Available only in tablet form.
Pyrethrins, pyrethroids	No specific antidotes	Supportive therapy may include treatment of anaphylaxis, atropine (not a specific antidote; indicated only to control parasympathetic signs), fluids and muscle relaxants such as methocarbamol.
Tricyclic Antidepressants	No specific antidote	Supportive therapy should target 1) seizures (diazepam, phenobarbital, or general anesthesia with pentobarbital or short-acting thiobarbiturates; or, if unsuccessful, 2) neuromuscular blockade with pancuronium [0.03–0.06 mg/kg IV] or vecuronium [10–20 µg/kg IV in dogs or 20–40 µg/kg in cats]); 3) cardiotoxicity (see toad poisoning): propanolol, lidocaine (quinidine, procainamide, and disopyramide are contraindicated); 4) sodium bicarbonate (1–3 mEq/kg).
Vitamin K antagonist	Fresh whole blood	To replace deficient coagulation factors. Additional therapy should support hypovolemic shock (care with colloids such as Hetastarch, which may act as anticoagulants).
	Vitamin K_1	Oral preferred to injectable unless contraindicated: 1–5 mg/kg q 24 h for 1–3 wk, depending on rodenticide, based on one-stage prothrombin time. Testing should occur 48–72 hours after vitamin K therapy is completed and retested, if normal, 2–3 d later. If OSPT is prolonged, therapy should continue for another 1–3 wk.
Zinc	Chelation therapy (see lead poisoning)	Calcium EDTA, succimer. Other supportive therapy includes fluid therapy, and antisecretory drugs such as ranitidine, famotidine, or omeprazole to decrease oral absorption of zinc.

ECG indicates electrocardiographic; NSAID, nonsteroidal anti-inflammatory drug; OSPT, TCA, tricyclic antidepressant.

possibly antihistamines). Supportive therapy is also indicated. Treatment on a preventive basis will help decrease the manifestations of anaphylaxis by decreased mast cell response.

Drugs associated with type I allergic reaction in people include penicillins, angiotensin-converting enzyme (ACE) inhibitors (particularly in the first 3 weeks of therapy), nonsteroidal anti-inflammatories (NSAIDs), and opioids. Some drugs can cause an anaphylactic-like reaction (anaphylactoid) that is similar to anaphylaxis but is not mediated by IgE (*i.e.*, is not allergic or immune-mediated). Selected drugs can cause direct mast cell degranulation. Generally these drugs are cationic (basic) and include opioids (morphine), polymixin, radiographic contrast materials, thiacetarsamide, amphotericin B, and others. Hyperosmolar solutions such as mannitol can also cause direct mast cell degranulation. Anaphylactoid reactions tend to be somewhat related to dose; administration of a small test dose may help detect the likelihood of occurrence. Decreasing the rate of drug administration, as well as previously described prophylactic measures are indicated.

Type II reactions (cytotoxic) occur as blood cells become lysed and removed from circulation. Lysis occurs due to binding either directly by IgG or IgM. Complement may or may not be activated. Either stem cells in the bone marrow or mature circulating cells may be targeted. Red blood cells, leukocytes, and platelets may be targeted resulting in hemolytic anemia, agranulocytosis and leukopenia, thrombocytopenia, or any combination thereof.

Type III drug reactions (immune complex disease or serum sickness) is induced by antigen—antibody complexes involving either IgG or IgM and compliment activation. Circulating antigen—antibody complexes may be filtered by and lodged in the vasculature of a number of organs including the kidney, CNS, or the peripheral vasculature. Clinical signs generally refer to the predominant organ affected but also include fever and lymphadenopathy. The Arthus reaction is a variation of the type III reaction and is manifested as swelling and pain at the site of drug administration. Among drug reactions in veterinary medicine, the potentiated sulfonamides are probably the most well-recognized cause of type III immune-mediated drug reaction.[5]

Type IV drug reactions (delayed hypersensitivity, cell-mediated) reflect cellular response at the site of the antigen. Lymphocytes and macrophages infiltrate the site and cause mediator release, which perpetuates the inflammatory response.

The critical care patient is predisposed to ADEs, particularly type A, for a variety of reasons (see Chapter 78). Using a systems-based approach, this chapter will address the role of therapeutic agents in causing ADEs.[6] Those ADEs that are most likely to lead to intensive care or to occur in patients medicated in intensive care will be emphasized. Treatment of drug-induced adverse reactions often is symptomatic. For some drugs, however, specific antidotes may be useful for decreasing the severity of side effects (see Table 77-1).

KIDNEY

Predisposing Factors

The kidney is vulnerable to drug-induced toxicity (Table 77-2)[9] because it receives a large proportion (25%) of the cardiac output, progressively concentrates drugs in the glomerular filtrate, and passively resorbs drugs (further increasing tubular exposure). Additional predisposing factors include the presence of drug-metabolizing enzymes that can generate potentially toxic metabolite, and the high metabolic state of the kidney, which renders it susceptible to the effect of the role that extrarenal factors.[7,8]

Specific cellular or subcellar sites of nephrotoxins injury is frequently not known. Usually a toxin affects more than one type of renal tissue because of the high drug concentrations to which the kidney is exposed. The glomerulus is susceptible to direct nephrotoxicity as well as indirect toxicity such as that caused by immunologic injury.[7] Many nephrotoxins cause predominantly proximal tubular damage. This is expected because blood flow is greatest in the renal cortex where the proximal tubules are located. Variations in proximal tubular susceptibility to toxins may reflect different tubular functions.[7,9]

Nephrotoxic Drugs

Aminoglycosides

Aminoglycosides remain an important part of antimicrobial therapy, and this is particularly true for CCU patients. The mechanism of nephrotoxicity is not completely understood.[10–14] The aminoglycosides induce a glomerular and (principally) tubular nephrotoxicity that is largely reversible unless allowed to progress to an irreversible state. Toxicity results from active uptake into the renal tubular cell and disruption of cellular lysosomes. As with uptake into the bacterial cell, nephrotoxicity may be related to the number of positively charged amino groups on the drugs.[15] Uptake of aminoglycosides may be related to the amount of phosphatidylinositol in the cell membrane, which is disproportion-

Table 77-2. Selected Drugs Associated with Nephrotoxicity

Aminoglycosides
ACE inhibitors
Amphotericin B
Cephaloridine
Cisplatin (metabolites?)
Cyclosporin A (humans)
Methoxyflurane
NSAIDs
Radiocontrast agents (high osmolality)
Sulfonamides
Thiacetarsamide
Tetracyclines

ately higher in renal cortex and cochlear tissues.[16] Impaired synthesis of protective vasodilatory renal prostaglandins by the aminoglycoside may be important to nephrotoxicity development. The initial decrease in glomerular filtration that accompanies aminoglycoside therapy may be associated with the inability of the kidney to vasodilate in response to vasoconstrictor actions such as that signaled by angiotensin II.

Avoidance of aminoglycoside nephrotoxicity is handicapped by the lack of a sensitive, specific indicator of renal damage. Renal damage is first indicated by increased excretion of brush-border enzymes such as alanine aminopeptidase and alkaline phosphatase, but their release is not specific for renal toxicity. Decreased renal concentrating ability, proteinuria, and cast formation are followed by a reduction in glomerular filtration rate and azotemia. These indices are insensitive indicators because major damage has and will continue to occur by the time these abnormalities are evident. Changes in aminoglycoside clearance may be the earliest indicator of nephrotoxicity.[16,17] More recently, spot checks of urine creatinine to γ-glutamyl transferase activity has been suggested as a method to detect or monitor aminoglycoside nephrotoxicity.[18]

Studies that have focused on aminoglycoside toxicity in dogs and cats have used dosing intervals that range from 12 hours to constant intravenous (IV) infusion. Recent studies have supported a 24-hour dosing interval (administering the total daily dose once a day) for aminoglycoside therapy to enhance safety with no loss of efficacy.[19] Some patients (*e.g.*, dogs <14 days of age, patients with diabetes mellitus or hypothyroidism) are protected against aminoglycoside (gentamicin)-induced nephrotoxicity because renal accumulation in the cortical tissues is limited.[20,21] The risk of toxicity with aminoglycoside therapy is likely to be greater if any condition inhibits renal prostaglandin formation.[15,22] Metabolic acidosis (or an acidic urine pH) will also predispose the patient to aminoglycoside nephrotoxicity because drugs are ionized and attracted to the anionic changes of cell membranes.[23] Renal damage may continue after the drug has been discontinued (or reduced) as the tubules eliminate accumulated drug.

Heparin is a predictable and potent inhibitor of aldosterone secretion in human patients, causing natriuresis and the potential for hyperkalemia, particularly in predisposed patient.[34,35] The effects of heparin on the RAA system may be responsible for the antihypertensive effects of heparin.[36] Gentamicin has caused symptomatic hypomagnesemia, hypocalcemia, and hypokalemia; the magnitude appears to be related to the total cumulative dose and is more likely in geriatric patients.[37] The mechanism may involve, in part, inhibition of hormone-mediated (*e.g.*, arginine vasopressin, calcitonin, parathyroid hormone) magnesium uptake in the distal convoluted tubules.[38] Immediate and transient renal calcium and magnesium wasting are evident in normal humans within 5 hours after gentamicin administration.[39] It is not clear if other aminoglycosides cause the same effect.

Aminoglycoside-induced nephrotoxicity is best avoided and can be minimized by using the least nephrotoxic yet most effective aminoglycoside (*e.g.*, amikacin rather than gentamicin); maintaining patient hydration; modifying dosing regimens based on minimal inhibitory concentration (MIC) data, therapeutic drug monitoring (TDM), or serum creatinine concentrations; maximizing peak plasma disappearance curve (PDC) while ensuring that trough PDC drops below 2 μg/mL by using once-daily therapy when appropriate; using combination antimicrobial therapy, particularly with synergistic antibiotics; and avoiding use of other nephrotoxic or nephroactive drugs, including antiprostaglandins and furosemide. Ticarcillin can be used to bind aminoglycosides in patients accidentally overdosed (protection may reflect chemical binding or sodium loading associated with the administration of ticarcillin[24]), although overdosing may not a problem as long as the drug is not dosed again. If the source of infection is in the urinary tract, aminoglycosides are likely to be safer (and more effective) in an alkaline PH that decreases renal tubular cell uptake of aminoglycosides. Interestingly, morning as opposed to evening administration may be safer.[25] The role of prostaglandin analogues supplementation (*i.e.*, misoprostol) in the prevention or treatment of aminoglycoside toxicity has not yet been established. A study of gentomicin nephrotoxicity in dogs found no renoprotective effects of misoprostol.[26]

NSAIDs

NSAIDs inhibit synthesis of renal prostaglandins and may lead to deterioration of renal function in patients whose kidneys are physiologically stressed.[27,28] Analgesic nephropathy is associated with long-term use (or abuse) of high NSAIDs doses. The syndrome is more common in human patients, probably because therapy with NSAIDs is prolonged, often occurs without physician supervision, and is more common in geriatric patients, who are afflicted with reduced renal function. Animals predisposed to developing analgesic nephropathy include geriatric animals, animals afflicted with conditions that impair renal blood flow (*e.g.*, cardiac, renal, or cirrhotic liver disease), animals subjected to a hypotensive state (*e.g.*, prolonged anesthesia without fluid support), and animals receiving nephroactive or nephrotoxic drugs in addition to the NSAID.[29] Interstitial nephritis is a less common syndrome associated with NSAID use in human patients that may occur in animals. The cause of this syndrome appears to be a cell-mediated allergic response. Loss of renal prostaglandins may potentiate the disease as inflammation progresses unchecked.

Drugs that are protective of cyclooxygenase I (COX-1) (see discussion of GI drugs) are not necessarily renoprotective; species differences also are likely to result in different risks of NSAID-induced neprhotoxicity.[30] Most species appear to express COX-1 constitutively in the renal vasculature and collecting ducts, species differences are exhibited particularly for cyclooxygenase II (COX-2) expression in the kidney. COX-2 expression occurs in the renal vasculature of the glomeruli and in the smooth muscle and endothelium of the interlobular vessels. In dogs, COX-2 is consitutively expressed in the thick ascending loop of Henle and in the macula densa.[30] COX-2 expression is markedly increased by hypovolemia and by ACE inhibitors in the presence of factors that predispose the patient to renal dysfunction. Thus, the use of COX-1 selective drugs may not prevent the risk of NSAID-induced nephrotoxicity. Maintenance of hydration, fluid therapy, and avoidance of nephroactive drugs are prudent actions in the CCU patient receiving any NSAID therapy.

Recent studies focusing on the nephrotoxic effects of NSAIDs indicate that the deleterious effects of NSAIDs on renal function may be counteracted with the prostaglandin-E_1 (PGE_1) analog, misoprostol.[31] Misoprostol has been cited for its immunomodulatory, cytoprotective, and vasodilatory effects in many tissues and is being studied for its efficacy in a variety of renal conditions. It has been used clinically in patients suffering from clinical conditions associated with peripheral or renal vasoconstriction. It may prove beneficial for preventing or reducing cyclosporine-induced nephrotoxocity,[32] a syndrome that is unusual in dogs, perhaps because of a difference in pattern of COX isoform activity. However, controversy exits regarding the effects of misoprostol on renal function. These effects may be dose related, with natriuresis, diuresis, and vasodilation occurring at low doses, and vasoconstriction and impaired salt and water excretion occurring at high doses. Misprostol may become a drug important to the management of a variety of acute and chronic renal disorders, and in particular, drug-induced nephropathies.

Other Drugs

Cisplatin is a recognized nephrotoxic antineoplastic drug. Nephrotoxicity in humans has been largely reduced by the use of diuretics coupled with fluid therapy. However, electrolyte disturbances characterized by hypomagnesemia, hypocalcemia, hypokalemia, and hypophosphatemia remain common in human patients. Nephrotoxicity induced by cisplatin appears to be diurnally influenced, with the risk of toxicity reduced with morning administration.[33]

Iodinated radiocontrast agents that are diatrizoate derivatives are almost entirely eliminated by the kidney by glomerular filtration. Characterized by a high osmolality (>1200 mOSm/L), they are potentially nephrotoxic due to changes in renal hemodynamics as well as direct tubular injury. Nephrotoxicity is more likely to occur in patients predisposed due to altered renal function (*i.e.*, heart failure, diabetes mellitus [humans] or receiving other nephroactive or toxic drugs).[40] Radiocontrast media is associated with a 50% incidence of acute renal failure in human patients with pre-existing renal insufficiency. Risk may be minimized with preinfusion and postinfusion of a cocktail comprised of saline, mannitol, bicarbonate, and furosemide.[41]

LIVER

Predisposition to Drug-Induced ADEs

The liver is vulnerable to ADEs (Table 77-3) because it receives a large portion of the cardiac output, is a "portal of entry" for orally administered drugs, is the major site of (potentially toxic) metabolite formation and drug excretion, and, as a highly metabolic organ, is susceptible to toxicities that induce hypoxia,

Table 77-3. Selected Drugs Associated with Liver Toxicity*

Acetaminophen
Anabolic steroids†
Aspirin
Carprofen
Deoxycholic acid
Diazepam (cats)
Etodolac (author's experience)
Glucocorticoids
Griseofulvin (cats)
Halothane (?)
Ketoconazole
Mebendazole
Meclarsamide
Megestrol acetate (cats)
Methoxyflurane
Methotrexate
Mibderone
Oxibendazole
Phenobarbital
Phenytoin
Primidone
Sulfonamides
Thiacetarsamide

* Many other drugs that are metabolized by the liver are potentially hepatotoxic because of the production of phase I reactive metabolites.
† Particularly methylated steroids, *e.g.*, stanazolol.

interactions with enzymes, or loss of energy substrates.[42–45] The risk of drug-induced hepatotoxicity is increased by dietary imbalance (high fat, low protein), concurrent administration of drugs (see Chapter 78), or presence of disease- or age-induced alteration in drug metabolizing enzymes or blood flow.[45,46] Histologic lesions caused by drug toxicity are rarely specific for that drug, but can be caused by a variety of drugs or disorders.[42,43]

Any drug metabolized by the liver can cause hepatic injury if sufficient reactive metabolites are produced. The larger the dose and the longer the exposure, the greater the risk. A drug that is renally excreted might be preferred in patients at risk for developing hepatotoxicity. Treatment of drug-induced liver disease is generally primarily supportive. Because reactive metabolites are often the cause of disease, or exacerbate disease, use of compounds that help prevent metabolite damage to the liver should be considered. Specific examples include *N*-acetylcysteine, an intracellular form of glutathione; ascorbic acid, an antioxidant drug; and *S*-adenolslymethionine, a compound that contributes to a number of methylation reactions in the body as well serves as an oxygen radical scavenger.[47]

Hepatotoxic Drugs

Anticonvulsant Drugs

Dogs receiving chronic therapy with liver metabolized anticonvulsant agents are at risk for drug-induced hepatotoxicity. The causes of hepatotoxicity include both direct effects as well as (for selected drugs such as phenobarbital) the sequelae of drug interactions. Although most dogs receiving chronic anticonvulsant therapy can be expected to develop abnormalities in serum biochemistries and hepatic function tests,[48,49] only about 15% of dogs on long-term anticonvulsant therapy are at risk for developing serious hepatotoxicity. This risk is greatly increased if drug concentrations approach the maximum therapeutic range. For example, phenobarbital concentration greater than 35 μg/mL for long time periods places the patient at risk for drug-induced hepatotoxicity.[50] Clinical laboratory tests associated with toxicity include changes in serum alkaline phosphatase, alanine transaminase, and aspartate transferase values; and changes in tests indicative of hepatic function, such as increased serum bile acid concentrations, decreased serum albumin, blood urea nitrogen, and cholesterol concentrations. Serum bilirubin is not a sufficiently sensitive indicator of phenobarbital-induced drug toxicity. Phenobarbital-induced hepatotoxicity appears reversible if therapy is discontinued prior to development of hepatic fibrosis.[45] Potent enzyme inducing drugs that undergo phase I metabolism by the liver (*e.g.*, carprofen, acetaminophen) should be avoided in a critical care patient that is receiving phenobarbital therapy.

Diazepam has been associated with hepatotoxicity in cats.[51,52] Manifestations include vomiting, depression, jaundice, lethargy, and acute death. Clinical laboratory tests associated with diazepam toxicity include increased serum alanine transaminase, aspartate transferase, and alkaline phosphatase activities and increased bilirubin. Toxicity does not appear to be associated with the dose nor duration of therapy. Toxicity has not been experimentally induced, suggesting that the reaction is idiosyncratic (*i.e.*, unpredictable).

Analgesic Drugs

Acute hepatic necrosis has been reported as an adverse effect to carprofen in dogs. Approximately 2 years after its approval, reports of GI toxicity led Pfizer to address concerns regarding side effects in a technical report.[53] Of the 4 million dogs receiving carprofen, an incidence of 0.18% suspected side effects was reported, with 0.052% involving the liver. Side effects associated with the liver were responsible for 29% of carprofen ADEs reported to Pfizer. Although 33% of animals affected in initial reports were Labrador retrievers, this number was not corrected for the prevalence of this breed. Hepatopathy has been diagnosed in all breeds of dogs receiving carprofen and at least 70% of afflicted animals were considered geriatric, suggesting that geriatric animals are predisposed. Because lesions appear to occur within the first several weeks of therapy, evaluation (clinical laboratory tests indicative of hepatic damage and hepatic function) prior to and sequentially within the first several months of therapy is prudent, particularly in geriatric animals. Use of other highly protein-bound drugs, including other NSAIDs, should be avoided. Although liver disease induced by carprofen can be lethal, discontinuation of the drug can lead to complete resolution of biochemical abnormalities. Use of hepatoprotective agents such as *N*-acetylcysteine or *S*-adenosylmethionine should prove beneficial during initial hepatic damage. Etodolac probably does not offer a reduced risk of hepatotoxicity.

Acetaminophen is a predictable hepatotoxin in the cat.[54] Methemoglobinemia is the predominant manifestation of acetominophen toxicity. The majority of acetaminophen is normally conjugated to glucuronide, with a smaller portion undergoing drug metabolism to both nontoxic and toxic metabolites. Generally, the toxic metabolites are removed by glutathione conjugation. Because the cat is deficient in glucuronyl transferase, a larger proportion of acetaminophen is shunted to formation of toxic metabolites that rapidly deplete glutathione.[55,56] Toxic metabolites accumulate and cause acute hepatic necrosis and systemic methemoglobinemia. Treatment is oriented toward supplementing glutathione by the administration of *N*-acetylcysteine, a glutathione precursor that can penetrate cell membranes. The use of cimetidine, a potent drug-metabolizing enzyme inhibitor, in the treatment of acetaminophen toxicity is controversial but warrants consideration.[57]

Miscellaneous Drugs

Sulfonamides can cause toxicity of multiple organs including the liver,[5,56] probably due to an allergic reaction. In one report, the duration of therapy before hepatotoxicity developed ranged from 4 to 30 days and the dose ranged from 18 to 53 mg/kg every 12 hours.[56] Because the reaction is largely unpredictable, the prudent clinician will anticipate ADEs in patients receiving sulfonamides. Their use in CCU patients is not contraindicated, but use in immune-mediated disorders should be reconsidered.

Heparin (both low-molecular-weight and fractionated products) causes increased serum alanine transaminase and aspartate transaminase in up to 93% of human patients receiving heparin therapy. Increases peak approximately 7 days into therapy and then return to normal, with no obvious detrimental clinical sequelae. Heparin will also interfere with and falsely increase bile acids.

GASTROINTESTINAL

Orally administered drugs are capable of causing nausea or vomiting simply due to irritation of the GI mucosa. Many IV drugs will also cause nausea or vomiting, particularly if given rapidly, because of stimulation of the chemoreceptor triggering zone (CRTZ). A number of drugs are recognized for their tendency to stimulate the CRTZ regardless of the route of administration. Examples include digoxin, anticancer drugs, and most opioids.[59]

NSAIDs

Among the drugs most commonly causing GI disease are the NSAIDs. GI ulceration is the most common NSAID-induced toxicity in humans and animals, in part due to inhibition of cyclooxygenase. This enzyme occurs in at least two forms: an inducible form (COX-2), produced by stimulation of mononuclear phagocytic cells with bacterial lipopolysaccharides,[60,61] and a constitutive form (COX-1).[62,63] Virtually all tissues express COX-1 under basal conditions.[62] Studies indicate that constitutive prostaglandins mediated by COX 1 are largely responsible for basal homeostatic mechanisms. PGE_2 mediated by COX-1 is present in all areas of the GI tract and is expressed over 2-fold compared to COX-2 in selected areas.[64,65] NSAIDs inhibit epithelialization and angiogenesis, actions mediated by COX-2-generated PGE_2 in the GI tract.[66] NSAIDs that nonselectively inhibit COX appear to be associated with a greater risk of GI ulceration. Because COX-2 expression occurs in selected areas of the spinal cord, where it may be a key mediator of transmission of pain, the use of COX-2 selective (or COX-1 sparing) drugs for control of pain in the critically ill patient is reasonable. However, their use is not without risk; in the gastroinestinal tract, COX-2—mediated prostaglandins mediate healing. Human CCU patients are predisposed to GI ulceration; by 72 hours after admission, 90% have developed gastric erosions.[67] Thus, care must also be taken with NSAIDs, even those that are COX-1 protective. The role of COX-2 in renal homeostasis has been previously discussed.

Carprofen (United States), etodolac (United States), and meloxicam (Canada) are NSAIDs with relative selectivity for COX-2 (*i.e.*, COX-1 protective) that are approved for use in animals in North America. Although data clearly suggest that carprofen and etodolac are less likely than aspirin to cause GI ulceration.[68] discriminating which among these drugs is safer can be difficult. In a canine-derived in vitro platelet and macrophage systems, the COX-1/COX-2 ratio (the concentration of drug necessary to inhibit 50% or 80% of COX-1 compared to the concentration necessary to inhibit COX-2) was markedly high for carprofen[69] suggesting that it might be the safest at maintaining platelet function. Although in vitro data regarding COX selectivity should be interpreted cautiously, the safety of carprofen compared to etodolac and meloxicam is also supported by toxicity data accompanying package inserts.

In human patients, NSAID-induced GI ulceration is often managed empirically with either an H_2-receptor antagonist or proton pump inhibitor. Prevention includes combination therapy with a proton pump inhibitor and misoprostol, or the use of an NSAID that is selective for COX-2.[70] Prophylactic therapy is recommended in patients predisposed to develop complications. A clinical trail in human patients with GI ulceration receiving either H_2-receptor antagonists, proton pump inhibitors, or misoprostol, revealed that each was effective in preventing ulceration, although misoprostol was the only prophylactic agent that reduced ulcer complications.[71] Double doses of H_2-receptor antagonists were necessary for gastric but not duodenal ulcers. Although misoprostol was effective at any dose studied, it was more effective for gastric ulcers when given three times rather than twice a day. Misoprostol has also proven useful for prevention of NSAID-induced ulceration in dogs and cats.[72]

CNS AND SPECIAL SENSES

Because of its role in integrating body systems, toxic injury to the brain often causes pansystemic consequences. The high metabolic rate and marked dependency on nutritional support renders neurons highly susceptible to damage by drugs that affect CNS metabolism (*e.g.*, drugs that cause hypoglycemia, hypoxia).[73] Some CNS toxicities may not be apparent until age-related attrition of neurons leads to decompensation. Delayed manifestations occur when neuronal reserves no longer compensate for the abnormalities. The longer time between cause and effect decreases the likelihood of recognizing the relationship between exposure and neurotoxicity.[73] The blood—brain barrier limits the incidence of adverse reactions in the CNS. However, increased barrier permeability, such as might occur in pediatric patients, or with trauma or disease, predisposes animals to CNS reactions.

All CNS-active drugs are likely to cause CNS signs if overdosed. Drugs that can induce seizures in epileptic patients, and that should therefore be avoided, include phenothiazines,[74] butyrophenones, and tricyclic antidepressants (TCAs).[75] Metaclopramide potentially may lower seizure threshold.[76,77] Dexamethasone and other glucocorticoids appear to have an antiepileptic effect on experimentally (picrotoxin)-induced seizures (in the hippocampus[78]); other steroids (adrenal or sex) appear to potentiate seizure activity (e.g., limbal),[84] particularly with chronic use.[80] Glucocorticoids may contribute to CNS damage due to accumulation of glutamate.[81] Because of their effects on cellular homeostasis and free-radical oxygen formation, glucocorticoids potentiate neurodegeneration and neurodegradative events such as seizures and hypoglycemia.[82]

The CNS toxicity of ivermectin, and to a lesser degree, milbemycin occurs due to blockade of γ-aminobutyric acid-receptor interactions.[83–85] The toxicity has been well documented in sensitive breeds such as collies and Australian shepherds, perhaps because of greater permeability in the blood–brain barrier. Doses as little as 100 μg/kg can cause toxicity in these breeds. However, toxicity will occur in any animal that is sufficiently overdosed. Clinical signs include emesis, diarrhea, salivation, fever, disorientation, ataxia, trembling, seizures, depression, coma, and blindness. Clinical signs may not occur for 2 to 3 days. Picrotoxin (1 mg/min for 8 minutes) and physostigmine (1 mg IV) have been recommended as antidotes; however, picrotoxin is also associated with toxicities (seizures) and its effective use is not recommended unless the patient is comatose. Supportive therapy is also indicated.

Other non CNS active drugs may produce CNS effects when toxic systemic doses are reached. Among its many toxicities, digoxin also causes neurologic effects, including malaise and drowsiness.[59] Benzyl alcohol, a common preservative found in drugs, can cause CNS toxicity, particularly in cats. Glucuronide deficiency in cats results in accumulation of benzoic acid (a phase I metabolite of benzyl alcohol). Although generally present in safe concentrations, toxicity can occur following a single dose of 0.3 to 0.45 g/kg/d or administration of 50 to 100 mL/kg lactated Ringer's solution containing 1.5% benzyl alcohol (1.5 g/dL). Benzoic acid is a preservative used in pet foods and toxicity may occur with consumption of diets containing 0.2% or more of benzoic acid. Clinical signs include hyperesthesia, ataxia, muscle fasciculations of the head and neck, aggression, salivation, depression, respiratory failure, coma, and death. Toxicity results from the accumulation of a phase I metabolite, benzoic acid.[86]

The relatively standard use of enrofloxacin IV in dogs and cats may increase the incidence fluorinated quinolone-induced CNS side effects including potentiation of seizures. The mechanism of action appears to be inhibition of GABA-receptor interactions and may (jury is still out regarding this fact) be facilitated by the presence of NSAIDs.[87] High doses are therefore to be avoided particularly in predisposed patients. Enrofloxacin has recently been associated with acute retinal blindness in cats. Ocular safety of ciprofloxacin, which varies from enrofloxacin only by the lack of an ethyl group, has been documented in a number of laboratory animals. However, the association with blindness at doses of 20 to 50 mg/kg has led manufacturers of the drug to warn against using the drug at doses higher than 5 mg/kg twice daily in cats. Although a higher dose is likely to be safe in many cats, acquisition of informed consent by the owner may be wise.

Several other antibiotics are associated with CNS toxicity in people.[88] These include the β-lactams with imipenem and cefazolin being the most epileptogenic (Table 77-4). The aminoglycosides cause peripheral neuromuscular blockade by interfering with calcium-mediated acetylcholine release. This effect is potentiated in the presence of other neuromuscular blockaders and anesthetics.

The TCAs and other antidepressants can cause a variety of CNS disorders by virtue of their inhibitory effect on CNS neurotransmitters. Because these transmitters often modulate the normal physiology of multiple body systems, the clinical manifestations of reactions to these drugs can be diverse and subtle. Manifestations related to the CNS include seizures, change in behavior, and depression. Acute poisoning with TCAs is common in human patients (accidental or intentional) and appears to be a significant problem in animals.[89] Symptoms in humans vary and are complex. Excitement and restlessness may be accompanied by myoclonus or tonic-clonic seizures. Coma may rapidly develop, associated with depressed expiration, hypoxia, hypothermia, and hypotension.[90,91] Anticholinergic effects include mydriasis, dry mucosa, absent bowel sounds, urinary retention, and cardiac arrhythmias, including tachycardia. Clinical signs reported after accidental ingestion in animals[89] include hyperexcitement and vomiting as early manifestations, followed by ataxia, lethargy, and muscular tremors. Bradycardia and other cardiac arrhythmias occur later. These later signs occurred shortly before death in experimental animal models of TCA toxicosis.[89]

Treatment for TCA toxicosis is supportive, including respiratory (intubation) and cardiovascular support. Gastric lavage with activated charcoal can be used early. Emetics probably should be avoided because of the risk of aspiration pneumonia in seizing animals (some antiemetics may further predispose the ani-

Table 77-4. Selected Drugs Associated with Adverse Reactions of the CNS

Drug	Manifestation
Amitraz	Sedation, ataxia, muscle weakness
Aminoglycosides	Neuromuscular blockade
Antidepressants	Hyperexcitability, depression, aggression, seizures, ataxia
Antihistamines	Sedation; excitement
Benzyl alcohol	Hypersynthesis, ataxia, aggression, depression, coma (cat)
β-Lactams	Lowered seizure threshold, ataxia (cefazolin and imipenem)
Bismuth	Lethargy, somnolence
Butyrophenones	Lowered seizure threshold
Enrofloxacin	Seizures, exacerbated by coadministration of NSAIDs; dizziness
Erythromycin	Seizures, others
Glucocorticoids	Lowered seizure threshold with long-term therapy (?)
Griseofulvin	Ataxia, seizures
Hexachlorophene	Neuropathy
Ivermectin	Depression, lethargy, seizures, etc
Lidocaine	Seizures
Metoclopramide	Hyperexcitability, may lower seizure threshold (controversial)
Metronidazole	Ataxia, nystagmus, seizures
Milbemycin	Depression, lethargy, seizures, etc
NSAIDs	Nonseptic meningitis (naproxen); exacerbates seizures caused by fluorinated quinolones
Opioids	General CNS depression
Phenobarbital	Hyperexcitability; depression
Phenothiazines	Lowered seizure threshold
Quinolones	Seizures, etc
Sulfonamides	Aseptic meningitis
Vincristine	Neuropathy

mal to seizures). Short-acting barbiturates (or similar drugs) without pre-atropinization are preferred for anesthetic control during gastric lavage. Cathartics (sorbitol or sodium sulfate [Glauber's salt]) can be beneficial. Pharmacologic interventions for cardiac arrhythmias have not been well established. Alkalinization (sodium bicarbonate sufficient to maintain blood pH above 7.5; 2–3 mEq/kg over 15–30 minutes IV) may prevent death by increasing protein binding and increasing cardiac automaticity (due to potassium shifts).[89] Cardiac drugs, including antiarrhythmics and digoxin, are contraindicated in human patients. Phenytoin may provide antiarrhythmic effects and, in human patients, is useful for treatment of seizures.[90,91] This latter effect is not likely to occur safely in animals. Diazepam is indicated for acute management of seizures. The β-adrenergic receptor antagonists and lidocaine may be useful.[90,91] The risk of tonic-clonic seizures is increased in human patients, particularly at high doses.

INTEGUMENT

The skin is the organ most commonly manifesting drug reactions in people.[92] Both type A and type B reactions occur in the skin (Table 77-5). Although the reactions are generally mild, they can become life-threatening. Equally important, these manifestations may also be a prelude to a severe manifestation and thus should be followed closely. Drug-induced skin reactions may be a manifestation of an allergic response or an autoimmune disease that targets the skin. Of the type B reactions, all subtypes of allergic reactions (*i.e.*, types I-IV) can involve the skin. Dermatologic manifestations of type I hypersensitivity occur at mucocutaneous junctions (including mucous membranes of the eyes, moth, nose, lips or tongue), or may present as pruritus, flushing, erythema, urticaria. Angioedema is the most life-threatening because of the risk of upper airway obstruction. Treatment includes epinephrine (for acute respiratory distress), antihistamines, and glucocorticoids. Skin lesions reflecting ADEs include wheal and flare reactions, erythema, blisters, lichenoid lesions, purpura, changes in pigmentation, necrosis, pustular lesions, and changes in hair growth. The most common reactions are erythematous macular or papular rashes that resolve even if untreated in several days.

Life-threatening drug-induced reactions that occur in the skin of people include the Stevens-Johnson syndrome (SJS), toxic epidermal necrolysis (TEN), hypersensitivity syndrome, serum sickness, vasculitis, and angioedema. Lesions of SJS and TEN may be hard to differentiate; SJS may be a milder form of TEN. Both appear as "scalded-skin" and reflect a cell-mediated cytotoxic reaction. The diseases are characterized by irregularly shaped blistering with poorly defined borders and extensive detachment of the epidermis. Both TEN and SJS tend to affect the trunk. Mucous membranes are frequently involved and patients are generally febrile, particularly with TEN. The presence of neutropenia is interpreted as having a poor prognosis in human patients suffering from TEN. Treatment of TEN includes management protocols similar to that for extensive burns; infection with *Staphylococcus aureus* (which by itself can cause a "skin-scalding" lesion) is likely to complicate therapy. Drugs associated with TEN and SJS in humans include sulfonamides, anticonvulsants, allopurinol, oxicams, and (less frequently) other NSAIDs. A small number of human patients have developed skin necrosis with both unfractionated and low-molecular-weight heparins. Lesions are similar to toxic epidermal necrolysis and can be lethal. The cause is unknown.[93]

HEMATOLOGIC DYSCRASIAS

The absence of universally standardized definitions of an ADE complicates recognition of hematologic disorders induced by drugs. The criteria for drug-induced

Table 77-5. Examples of Drugs Associated with Adverse Dermatologic Reactions

Drug	Lesion
Ampicillin	Fixed drug eruption
Anticancer drugs	Alopecia
Bromide	Pruritus
Coal-tar shampoos	Generalized eczema
Chloramphenicol	Purpura, TEN
Diethylcarbamazine	Eczematous dermatitis, pruritus
Erythropoietin, human recombinant	Skin or mucocutaneous lesions
Flea collars	Generalized exfoliation
5-Flurocytosine	Eczematous dermatitis
Glucocorticoids	Alopecia, hyperpigmentation
Gold-containing drugs	Alopecia (dog), pruritus, pemphigus vulgaris-like reaction
Griseofulvin	Eczematous dermatitis
Hetacillin	Alopecia (cat)
Levamisole	Drug eruptions
Lime sulfur dips	Generalized exfoliation
Neomycin (topical)	Generalized eczema
Phenothiazine derivatives	Erythematous dermatitis
Phenytoin	Alopecia
Prednisone	Alopecia (dog)
Quinidine	Generalized exfoliation
Sulfonamides	Eczematous dermatitis
Tetracyclines (oral)	Urticaria, angioedema
Thiabendazole	Pemphigus vulgaris-like reaction
Thiacetarsamide	Fixed drug eruption
Vitamin K (IV)	Urticaria, angioedema

hematologic disorders have been described for human medicine and are based on cell count, assessment of time to onset after drug exposure, and time to resolution of signs after the drug has been discontinued, and the course of the reaction.[94] Both immunologic and nonimmunologic (toxic) damage can occur to the bone marrow or mature circulating cells. The reaction may be either to the parent drug or its metabolites. Toxic responses of the blood can reflect impaired bone marrow production (erythropoiesis) or damage to the circulating cells (hemoglobin, *e.g.*, methemoglobinemia or Heinz body formation; Table 77-6).

Bone marrow suppression can result in pancytopenia or may target only a single cell line (*i.e.*, anemia, leukopenia, or thrombocytopenia).[95] Discerning an

Table 77-6. Examples of Drugs Associated with Hematologic Disturbances

Drug	Manifestation
Acetaminophen	Methemoglobinemia (especially cats)
Anticancer drugs	Bone marrow suppression*
Azo dye (urinary antiseptics)	Methemoglobinemia (cats)
Benzocaine (and related drugs)	Methemoglobinemia (cats)
Chloramphenicol	Bone marrow suppression
Cimetidine	Thrombocytopenia
Coumarin derivatives	Coagulation dysfunction
Erythropoietin (human recombinant)	Anemia
Estrogens	Bone marrow suppression
Griseofulvin	Bone marrow suppression
Heparin	Thrombocytopenia, platelet dysfunction, coagulation dysfunction
Methimazole	Methemoglobinemia
Methylene blue	Methemoglobinemia (cats)
NSAIDs	Platelet dysfunction
Phenobarbital	Neutropenia
Phenylbutazone	Bone marrow suppression
Propylthiouracil	Methemoglobinemia
Ranitidine	Anemia

* Bone marrow suppression might be manifested as anemia, leukopenia or thrombocytopenia, or any combination thereof.

immunologic basis can be difficult particularly if the antibodies involved have not been identified. Drugs most commonly associated with nonimmune-mediated bone marrow suppression include most cancer chemotherapeutic agents because of their predictable effects on DNA and cell division (see Chapter 82). Other drugs associated with nonimmune-mediated bone marrow dyscrasias include phenylbutazone, estrogen derivatives, and chloramphenicol.[96] Phenobarbital has caused leukopenia and other hematologic disorders when used to treat epilepsy; white cell counts normalize once the drug is discontinued. Captopril also has been reported to cause pancytopenia in the dog.[97]

Malfunction of the red blood cells may occur as a result of methemoglobinemia in cats. Methemoglobinemia occurs following chemical oxidation of the heme irons of hemoglobin (valance change from 2+ to 3+). Both oxygen content of the blood decreases and the oxygen dissociation curve shifts to the left. Heinz bodies represent a continuum of oxidative stress to red cells. The Heinz body may be preceded by methemoglobinemia but this is controversial. Heinz bodies appear to be covalently bound to the inner surface of red blood cells and may lead to premature splenic phagocytosis, impaired passive ion transport, changes in osmotic pressure, hyperpermeability, and intravascular hemolysis.[98] Drugs reported to cause methemoglobinemia in the cat include urinary antiseptics containing methylene blue or azo dyes, acetaminophen and related compounds, benzocaine, DL-methionine, and propylthiouracil.[99–101]

Human recombinant erythropoietin and granulopoietin have been used to treat anemias associated with chronic renal disease and leukopenia induced by disease (*i.e.*, parvovirus) or drugs (*i.e.*, anticancer drugs) in dogs and cats. Unfortunately, these proteins are foreign and antibodies may develop after 10 to 14 days, destroying not only the exogenous drug but also endogenous factors.[102–103]

Drugs that affect hemostatic components include all NSAIDs, anticoagulants such as warfarin derivatives, and heparin (these generally reflect a relative overdose). The impact of COX-2 selective NSAIDs on hemostatic function has yet to be well described, but the risk of thrombosis may be increased. Use of COX-1 selective products may predispose the coagulation cascade towards thrombogenesis.[62] This may be the reason that glucocorticoids, which are COX-1 protective, predispose some patients to thrombogenesis. In contrast, aspirin, which is characterized by a high selectivity (in humans) for COX-1 compared to COX-2, will predispose the patient to bleeding disorders and are recognized for their ability to impair thromboxane synthesis, the prostaglandin responsible for platelet aggregation. The use of COX-1 protective drugs may reduce the risk of impaired platelet function because platelet aggregation is mediated by COX-1 prostaglandins. The use of drugs that primarily target COX-2 selective drugs may predispose the CCU patient to thrombosis.

At high doses, heparin is antithrombotic. Thrombocytopenia has been reported in 5% to 30% of human patients receiving heparin and is more likely to occur with bovine as opposed to porcine preparations.[93,104,105] Both type I (A) and type II (B) ADEs causing thrombocytopenia have been described. Several days of therapy are necessary for type I to occur; it resolves once therapy is discontinued. Type I may occur less frequently with low-molecular-weight heparins. Type II occurs in fewer people, is more severe, and is characterized by a longer time to onset (6–10 days). Type II may be an allergic response to the secondary and tertiary structures of heparin.[103] As with type I thrombocytopenia, the incidence of type II is likely to be less with low-molecular-weight heparins.

Hemorrhage is the major complication of heparin therapy, occurring in 18% to 22% of human patients receiving heparin.[98] Hemorrhage is less likely to occur with low dosages and constant IV infusion (as opposed to intermittent IV administration).[106] The incidence of hemorrhage can be reduced by (1) confirming the need for therapy, (2) using the appropriate dose and frequency, (3) avoiding combination therapy with other antihemostatic drugs, including aspirin and other salicylates, and (4) monitoring the effects of therapy with clotting or coagulation tests. At higher doses, activated partial thromboplastin time (APTT) can be useful for assessing the likelihood of hemorrhage. Monitoring APTT is less useful when low doses of heparin are given. Heparin is contraindicated in the bleeding patient and in those with disseminated intravascular coagulopathy (DIC) unless replacement blood or plasma therapy is given. Excessive therapy (theoretically) might be treated with protamine sulfate, a compound that complexes with heparin. It is dosed according to the amount of heparin to be neutralized, but it also can contribute to hemorrhage and thus seldom is used to treat heparin overdose.

CARDIOTOXICITIES

A number of drugs cause direct or indirect ADEs involving the heart (Table 77-7).[107] Doxorubicin is an anthracycline antibiotic used as an antineoplastic agent. It is capable of causing acute and chronic cardiomyopathy. The acute form is manifested as electrocardiographic changes that are not life-threatening and a potentially life-threatening reduction in ejection fraction that can lead to congestive heart failure within 24 hours after a single dose.[108] The chronic form is manifested as congestive heart failure and the risk increases as the total dose accumulates. In humans, the mortality can reach up to 50% following administration of doses as low as 250 mg/m^2. Cardiotoxicity may not occur until several years after therapy has been completed. Cardiotoxicity in humans might be reduced by coadministration of an iron chelator (dexrozoxane) and carvedilolol, an α- and β-adrenergic drug also characterized by oxygen radical scavenging ability.[109]

Digitalis intoxication most commonly reflects improper use, including errors in dosing. Signs of toxicity are more easily recognized than are signs of efficacy, contributing to the perceived narrow therapeutic margin that likely would be

Table 77-7. Drugs Associated with Cardiotoxicity

Antibacterial antibiotics
Aminoglycosides (calcium related, selected species)
Erythromycin (torsades de pointes)
Chloramphenicol, tetracycline (direct negative inotrope, selected species)
Neoplastic agents
5-fluouracil (myocardial ischemia)
Cyclophosphamide (hemorrhagic necrosis at high doses)
Doxorubicin, daunorubicin (acute and chronic congestive heart failure)
Centrally acting drugs
TCAs
General anesthetics
Opioids
Phenothiazines
Local anesthetics (conduction in excitable tissues)
Catecholamines and related drugs
Miscellaneous
Digoxin
Antiarrhythmics
Antihistamines (selected H_1-antagonists: terfenadine, astemizole)
Cisapride (torsades de pointes)

larger with proper use. Serious toxic effects of digitalis are due to altered electrical activity: changes in intracellular calcium, sodium, and potassium and, thus, the electric potential formed across the cell membrane.[59,110] Digitalis causes an increase in automaticity and ectopic beats. Direct toxicities occur when cellular calcium markedly increases. Dysrhythmias tend to worsen as calcium increases. Increased calcium results in afterdepolarization-mediated automaticity.[111] In the atrium, digoxin shortens the action potential, predisposing it to atrial fibrillation.[111] Because the mechanism of toxicity (automaticity) is the same as the mechanism of positive inotropic effects, which occurs at higher digoxin concentrations, the safety margin of the glycosides becomes more when it is used as a positive inotrope. The negative chronotropic effects of digoxin also can directly slow sinus nodal activity leading to heart blockade.

Toxic effects with digitalis are frequent and can be lethal if allowed to persist. Dogs with severe cardiomegaly and congestive heart failure are probably at greater risk of developing ectopic ventricular arrhythmias. Other factors predisposing to digoxin toxicity include but are not limited to hypokalemia, hypercalcemia, hypomagnesemia, hypothyroidism, acid-base imbalances, and abnormal renal function.[59] Combination therapy with other drugs also predisposes the patient. Selected digoxin preparations also are more likely to cause toxicity because of differences in absorption.

The cat is more sensitive to digoxin than the dog. The most frequent cause of digoxin toxicity is probably overdosing. The potential for toxicity is increased with hypokalemia. This may occur, for example, if the patient is also receiving diuretic therapy that causes potassium loss (furosemide, thiazides, and other "nonsparing" diuretics).

The treatment of cardiac glycoside intoxication includes (1) discontinuation of digitalis therapy for at least one drug elimination half-life; (2) discontinuation of potassium-depleting diuretics; (3) administration of phenytoin, which blocks atrioventricular nodal effects of digitalis (bradyarrhythmias), lidocaine (for ventricular arrhythmias), and oral potassium supplementation (*e.g.*, potassium chloride), if hypokalemia exists.[110] Atropine may be useful to treat sinus bradycardia, and second- or third-degree heart block induced by cholinergic augmentation. Procainamide also has been shown experimentally to be useful for treatment of digoxin-induced ventricular arrhythmias in the canine heart when plasma drug concentrations approximate 8 to 12 μg/mL.[112,113]

Fatal toxicities to theophylline can occur usually during chronic oral or rapid IV administration. Tachycardia and CNS signs (restlessness, hyperexcitability, sensory disturbances) can be correlated to increased plasma concentrations. Local GI irritation and nausea, vomiting, and diarrhea may occur with oral administration. These can be avoided by administering the drugs with food.

PULMONARY TOXICITY

Pulmonary toxicities are of greater concern in human medicine. Although compounds toxic to the lungs can arrive by hematogenous route, most pulmonary toxicities result from direct exposure of the respiratory tract through the naso-

Table 77-8. Resource Sites

ASPCA/National Animal Poison Control Center	800-548-2423/900-680-0000 www.napcc.aspca.org/prevent.htm
$30.00 per case unless supported by sponsor $20.00 for first 5 min; $2.95 for each additional minute	
Adverse Reaction Reporting	
Food and Drug Administration	888-FDA-Vets www.cvm.fda.gove/fda/ade96/adeindex.html
US Pharmacopeia	800-487-7776 www.usp.org/ptractrep/vprp.thm
National Pesticide Telecommunications Network	800-858-7378 www.ace/orst.edu/info/nptn (topically applied external parasiticides)
USDA Veterinary Biologics Hotline	800-752-6255 www.aphis.usda.gov/vs/cvb/ic/docs/aivform.pdf

pharyngeal or oropharyngeal airways and subsequently the tracheobronchial tract and alveoli.[78] Gaseous and particulate toxicants are most common. Acute pulmonary toxicity generally is not caused by therapeutic agents in humans. Macrophage clearance of drugs in the lungs may be accompanied by macrophage death and may be accompanied by the release of inflammatory mediators, which can damage surrounding cells and contribute to toxic effects of a drug. Compounds that cause pulmonary injury in humans due to the inflammatory response tend to be toxins rather than drugs.[78] However, selected drugs are noted for their potential to cause or exacerbate pulmonary disease. Examples include bronchoconstriction induced by nonselective β-adrenergic drugs or NSAIDs. Anecdotal reports suggest that bromide used as an anticonvulsant in cats may cause bronchial asthma associated with eosinophilic infiltrates.

REFERENCES

1. Lawson DH, Richared RME: Clinical Pharmacy and Hospital Drug Management. London: Chapman and Hall, 1982, 211.
2. Griffin JP, Darcy PF: A Manual of Adverse Drug Interactions, 2nd ed. Chicago: Billing and Sons, 1979, 4.
3. Ariens EJ, Simonis AM, Offermeier J: Introduction to General Toxicology. New York: Academic Press, 1976, 79.
4. Mitchell JR, Smith CV, Lauferburg BH, *et al.*: Reactive metabolites and the pathophysiology of acute lethal cell injury. *In:* Mitchell JR, Homing MG, eds. Drug Metabolism and Drug Toxicity. New York: Raven Press, 1984, p 301.
5. Cribb A: Adverse reactions to sulphonamide and sulphonamide-trimethoprim antimicrobials: clinial syndromes and pathogenesis. *Adverse Drug React Toxicol Rev* 15:9, 1996.
6. Boothe DM: Drug-induced diseases. *In:* Boothe DM, ed.: Small Animal Clinical Pharmacology and Theraputics. Philadelphia: WB Saunders, 2001.
7. Hook JB, Hewitt WR: Toxic responses of the kidney. *In:* Klassen CD, Amour

MO, Doull J, eds.: Toxicology: The Basic Science of Poisons, 3rd ed. New York: Macmillan, 1985, p 310.

8. Bennett WM: Drug interactions and consequences of sodium restriction. *Am J Clin Nutr* 65(2 suppl):678S, 1997.
9. Engelhardt JA, Brown SA: Drug-related nephropathies. Part II: Commonly used drugs. *Comp Cont Educ* 9:281, 1987.
10. Brown SA, Bansanti JA, Crowell WA: Gentamicin-associated acute renal failure in the dog. *J Am Vet Med Assoc* 186:686, 1985.
11. John JF: What price success? The continuing saga of the toxic:therapeutic ratio in the use of aminoglycoside antibiotics. *J Infect Dis* 158:1, 1988.
12. Moore RD, Lietman PS, Smith CR: Clinical response to aminoglycoside therapy: importance of the ratio of peak concentration to minimal inhibitory concentration. *J Infect Dis* 155:93, 1987.
13. Powell SH, Thompson WL, Luthe MA, *et al.*: Once-daily vs continuous aminoglycoside dosing: efficacy and toxicity in animal and clinical studies of gentamicin, netilmicin and tobramycin. *J Infect Dis* 147:918, 1993.
14. Maller R, Ahrne H, Lausen I, *et al.*: Once- versus twice-daily amikacin regimen: efficacy and safety in systemic Gram-negative infections. *J Antimicrob Chem* 31:939, 1993.
15. Neu HC: Principles of antimicrobial use. *In:* Brody TM, Larner J, Minneman KP, Neu HC, eds.: Human Pharmacology: Molecular to Clinical. St. Louis, Mosby, 1994, p 616.
16. Riviere J, Spoo W: Aminoglycosides. *In:* Adams R, ed.: Veterinary Pharmacology and Therapeutics. Ames, IA: Iowa State University Press, 1995.
17. Frazier DL, Aucoin DP, Riviere JE: Gentamicin pharmacokinetics and nephrotoxicity in naturally acquired and experimentally induced disease in dogs. *J Am Vet Med Assoc* 192:57, 1988.
18. Grauer GF, Greco DS, Behrend EN, *et al.*: Estimation of quantitative enzymuria in dogs with gentamicin induced nephrotoxicosis using urine enzyme/creatinine ratios from spot urine samples. *J Vet Intern Med* 9:324, 1995.
19. Gilbert DN, Lee BL, Dworkin RJ, *et al.*: A randomized comparison of the safety and efficacy of once-daily gentamicin or thrice-daily gentamicin in combination with ticarcillin-clavulanate. *Am J Med* 105:182, 1998.
20. Cowan RH, Jukkola AF, Arant BS: Pathophysiologic evidence of gentamicin nephrotoxicity in neonatal puppies. *Pediatr Res* 14:1204, 1980.
21. Brown SA, Nelson RW, Moncrieff CS: Gentamicin pharmacokinetics in diabetic dogs. *J Vet Pharmacol Ther* 14:90, 1991.
22. Boothe DM: Effects of drugs on endocrine testing. *In:* Current Veterinary Therapy (XII), Small Animal Practice. Philadelphia: WB Saunders, 1995, p 339.
23. Hsu CH, Kurtz TW, Easterling RE, *et al.*: Potentiation of gentamicin nephrotoxicity by metabolic acidosis. *Proc Soc Exp Biol Med* 146:894, 1974.
24. Ohnishi A, Bryant TD, Branch KR, *et al.*: Role of sodium in the protective effect of ticarcillin on gentamicin nephrotoxicity in rats. *Antimicrob Agents Chemother* 33:928, 1989.
25. Bleyzac N, Allard-Latour B, Laffont A, *et al.*: Diurnal changes in the pharmacokinetic behavior of amikacin. *Ther Drug Monit* 22:307, 2000.
26. Davies C, Forrester SD, Troy GC, Saunders GK, Shell LG, Johnston SA. Effects of a prostaglandin E1 analogue, misoprostol, on renal function in dogs receiving nephrotoxic doses of gentamicin. *Am J Vet Res* 1998 Aug;59(8):1048–54.
27. Angio RG: Nonsteroidal antiinflammatory drug-induced renal dysfunction related to inhibition of renal prostaglandins. *Drug Intell Clin Phar* 21:954, 1987.

28. Dunn JM, Simonson J, Davidson EW, *et al.*: Nonsteroidal anti-inflammatory drugs and renal function. *J Clin Pharmacol* 28:524, 1988.
29. Selig CB, Maloley PA, Campbell JR: Nephrotoxicity associated with concomitant ACE inhibitor and NSAID therapy. *South Med J* 83:1144, 1990.
30. Khan KN, Venturini CM, Bunch RT, *et al.*: Interspecies differences in renal localization of cyclooxygenase isoforms: implications in nonsteroidal antiinflammatory drug-related nephrotoxicity. *Toxicol Pathol* 26:612, 1998.
31. Fullerton T, Sica DA, Blum RA: Evaluation of the renal protective effect of misoprostol in elderly, osteoarthritic patients at risk for nonsteroidal anti-inflammatory drug-induced renal dysfunction. *J Clin Pharmacol* 33:1225, 1993.
32. John EG, Fornell LC, Radhakrishnan J, *et al.*: The effect of prostaglandin E1 analog misoprostol on chronic cyclosporin nephrotoxicity. *J Pediatr Surg* 28:1429, 1993.
33. To H, Kikuchi A, Tsuruoka S, *et al.*: Time-dependent nephrotoxicity associated with daily administration of cisplatin in mice. *J Pharm Pharmacol* 52:1499, 2000.
34. Oster JR, Singer I, Fishman LM: Heparin-induced aldosterone suppression and hyperkalemia. *Am J Med* 98:575, 1995.
35. Aull L, Chao H, Coy K: Heparin-induced hyperkalemia. *DICP: Ann Pharmacother* 24:244, 1990.
36. Susic D, Mandal AK, Jovovic D, *et al.*: Antihypertensive action of heparin: role of the renin-angiotensin aldosterone system and prostaglandins. *J Clin Pharmacol* 33:342, 1993.
37. Kes P, Reiner Z: Symptomatic hypomagnesemia associated with gentamicin therapy. *Magnes Trace Elem* 9:54, 1990.
38. Kang HS, Kerstan D, Dai L, Ritchie G, Quamme GA. Aminoglycosides inhibit hormone-stimulated Mg2+ uptake in mouse distal convoluted tubule cells. *Can J Physiol Pharmacol* 2000 Aug;78(8):595–602.
39. Elliott C, Newman N, Madan A. Gentamicin effects on urinary electrolyte excretion in healthy subjects. *Clin Pharmacol Ther* 2000 Jan;67(1):16–21.
40. Goldstein RS, Schnellmann RG: Toxic responses of the kidney. 417–442.
41. Louis BM, Hoch BS, Hernandez C, Namboodiri N, *et al.*: Protection from the nephrotoxicity of contrast dye. *Ren Fail* 1996 Jul;18(4):639–46.
42. Ockner RK: Drug-induced liver disease. *In:* Zakim D, Boyer TD, eds.: Hepatology: A Textbook of Liver Disease. Philadelphia: WB Saunders, 1982, p 691.
43. Plaa GL: Toxic responses of the liver. *In:* Klassen CD, Amour MO, Doull J, eds.: Toxicology: The Basic Science of Poisons, 3rd ed. New York: Macmillan, 1985, p 286.
44. Lee WM: Review article: drug-induced hepatotoxicity. *Aliment Pharmacol Ther 7*: 4775, 1993.
45. Bunch SE: Hepatotoxicity associated with pharmacologic agents in dogs and cats. *Vet Clin North Am Small Anim Pract* 23:659, 1993.
46. Schenkers B: Drug disposition and hepatotoxicity in the elderly. *J Clin Gastroenterol* 18:232, 1994.
47. Lopez PM, Finana IT, De Agueda MC, Sanchez EC: Protective effect of melatonin against oxidative stress induced by ligature of extra-biliary duct in rats: comparison with the effect of S-adenosyl-L-methionine. *J Pineal Res.* 28:143, 2000.
48. Bunch SE, Conway MB, Center SA, Castleman WL, *et al.*: Toxic hepatopathy and intrahepatic cholestasis associated with phenytoin administration in combination with other anticonvulsant drugs in three dogs. *J Am Vet Med Assoc* 1987 Jan 15;190(2):194–8. No abstract available.
49. Bunch SE, Castleman WL, Baldwin BH, Hornbuckle WE, Tennant BC. Effects

of long-term primidone and phenytoin administration on canine hepatic function and morphology. *Am J Vet Res* 1985 Jan;46(1):105–15.
50. Dayrell-Hart B, Steinbarg SA, Van Winkle TJ, *et al.*: Hepatotoxicity of phenobarbital in dogs: 18 cases. *J Am Vet Med Assoc* 199:1060–1066, 1991.
51. Elston TH, Rosen D, Rodan I, *et al.*: Seven cases of acute diazepam toxicity. *Proc Am Anim Hosp Assoc* October:343, 1993.
52. Center SA, Elston TH, Rowland PH, *et al.*: Fulminant hepatic failure associated with oral administration of diazepam in 11 cats. *J Am Vet Med Assoc* 209:618, 1996.
53. Update: Three years (1997–1999) of U.S. Clinical Experience with Rimadyl (carprofen). Pfizer Animal Health. Technical Bulletin December 2000.
54. Oehme FW: Aspirin and acetaminophen. *In:* Kirk R, ed.: Current Veterinary Therapy Small Animal Practice X. Philadelphia: WB Saunders, 1986, p 188.
55. Welch RM, Conney AH, Burns JJ: The metabolism of acetophenetidin and N-acetyl-p-aminophenol in the cat. *Biochem Pharmacol* 15:521, 1966.
56. Court MH, Greenblatt DJ: Molecular basis for deficient acetaminophen glucuronidation in cats. An interspecies comparison of enzyme kinetics in liver microsomes. *Biochem Pharmacol* 53:1041, 1997.
57. Savides MC, Oehme FW, Leipold HW: Effect of various antidotal treatments on acetaminophen toxicosis and biotransformation in cats. *Am J Vet Res* 46:1485, 1985.
58. Twedt DC, Diehl KJ, Lappin MR, *et al.*: Association of hepatic necrosis with trimethoprim sulfonamide administration in 4 dogs. *J Vet Intern Med* 11:20, 1997.
59. Kelly RA, Smith TW: Pharmacologic treatment of heart failure. *In:* Hardman JG, Limbird LE, eds.: Goodman and Gilman's The Pharmacological Basis of Therapeutics, 9th ed. New York: McGraw Hill, 1995, p 809.
60. Masferrer JL, Zweifel BS, Seibert K, Needleman P. Selective regulation of cellular cyclooxygenase by dexamethasone and endotoxin in mice. *J Clin Invest* 1990 Oct; 86(4):1375–9.
61. Fu JY, Masferrer JL, Seibert K, Raz A, Needleman P. The induction and suppression of prostaglandin H2 synthase (cyclooxygenase) in human monocytes. *J Biol Chem* 1990 Oct 5;265(28):16737–40.
62. Crofford LJ, Oates JC, McCune WJ, *et al.*: Thrombosis in patients with connective tissue diseases treated with specific cyclooxygenase 2 inhibitors. A report of four cases. *Arthritis Rheum* 43:1891, 2000.
63. Cryer B, Dubois A. The advent of highly selective inhibitors of cyclooxygenase—a review. *Prostaglandins Other Lipid Mediat* 1998 Aug;56(5–6):341–61.
64. Kargman S, Charleson S, Cartwright M, Frank J, *et al.*: Characterization of Prostaglandin G/H Synthase 1 and 2 in rat, dog, monkey, and human gastrointestinal tracts. *Gastroenterology* 1996.
65. Mizuno H, Sakamoto C, Matsuda K, Wada K, Uchida T, *et al.*: Induction of cyclooxygenase 2 in gastric nucosal lesions and its inhibition by the specific antagonist delays healing in mice. *Gastroenterology* 1997 Feb;112(2):387–97.
66. Hudson N, Balsitis M, Everitt S, Hawkey CJ. Angiogenesis in gastric ulcers: impaired in patients taking non steroidal anti-inflammatory drugs. *Gut* 1995 Aug; 37(2):191–4.
67. Marino PL: The ICU Book. Philadelphia: Lippincott Williams & Wilkins, 1997, 95.
68. Reimer ME, *et al.*: The gastroduodenal effects of buffered aspirin, carprofen and etodolac in health dogs. *J Vet Intern Med* 13:472, 1999.

69. Ricketts AP. Lundy KM. Seibel SB: Evaluation of selective inhibition of canine cyclooxygenase 1 and 2 by carprofen and other nonsteroidal anti-inflammatory drugs. *Am J Vet Res* 59:1441, 1998.
70. Tseng CC, Wolfe MM: Nonsteroidal anti-inflammatory drugs. *Med Clin North Am* 84:1329, 2000.
71. Rostom A, Wells G, Tugwell P: The prevention of chronic NSAID induced upper gastrointestinal toxicity: a Cochrane collaboration metaanalysis of randomized controlled trials. *J Rheumatol* 27:2203, 2000.
72. Villar D, Buck WB, Gonzalez JM: Ibuprofen, aspirin and acetaminophen toxicosis and treatment in dogs and cats. *Vet Hum Toxicol* 40:156, 1998.
73. Sipes IG, Dart RC: Toxicology. *In:* Brody TM, Larner JL, Minneman KP, eds.: Human Pharmacology: Molecular to Clinical. St. Louis: Mosby, 1998, p 861.
74. Logothetis J: Spontaneous epileptic seizures and electroencephalographic changes in the course of phenothiazine therapy. *Neurology* 17:869, 1967.
75. Spigset O, Hedenmalm K, Dahl ML, *et al.*: Seizures and myoclonus associated with antidepressant treatment: assessment of potential risk factors, including CYP2D6 and CYP2C19 polymorphisms, and treatment with CYP2D6 inhibitors. *Acta Psychiatr Scand* 96:379, 1997.
76. al-Tajir G, Chandler CJ, Starr BS, *et al.*: Opposite effects of stimulation of D1 and D2 dopamine receptors on the expression of motor seizures in mouse and rat. *Neuropharmacology* 29:657, 1990.
77. Hyser CL, Drake ME Jr: Myoclonus induced by metoclopramide therapy. *Arch Intern Med* 143:2201, 1983.
78. Duport S, Stoppini L, Correges P: Electrophysiological approach of the antiepileptic effect of dexamethasone on hippocampal slice culture using a multirecording system: the Physiocard. *Life Sci* 60:PL251, 1997.
79. Roberts AJ, Keith LD: Corticosteroids enhance convulsion susceptibility via central mineralocorticoid receptors. *Psychoneuroendocrinology* 20:891, 1995.
80. Rosen JB, Pishevar SK, Weiss SR, *et al.*: Glucocorticoid treatment increases the ability of CRH to induce seizures. *Neurosci Lett* 174:113, 1994.
81. Stein-Behrens BA, Lin WJ, Sapolsky RMJ: Physiological elevations of glucocorticoids potentiate glutamate accumulation in the hippocampus. *Neurochemistry* 63: 596, 1994.
82. McIntosh LJ, Sapolsky RM: Glucocorticoids may enhance oxygen radical-mediated neurotoxicity. *Neurotoxicology* 17(3-4):873, 1996.
83. Neer TM: Drug-induced neurologic disorders. *Proc Amer Coll Vet Intern Med* 9: 261, 1991.
84. Pullium JR, Seward RL, Henry RT, *et al.*: Investigating ivermectin toxicity in collie dogs. *Vet Med* 80;3340, 1985.
85. Tranquili WJ, Paul AJ, Todd KS: Assessment of toxicosis induced by high dose administration of milbemycin in collies. *Am J Vet Res* 52:1170, 1991.
86. Cullison RF: Toxicosis in cats from use of benzyl alcohol in lactated Ringer's solution. *J Am Vet Med Assoc* 182:61, 1983.
87. Halliwell RF, Davey PG, Labert JJ: The effects of quinolones and NSAIDS upon GABA-evoked currents recorded from rat dorsal root ganglion neurones. *J Antimicrob Chemother* 27:209, 1991.
88. Thomas RJ: Neurotoxicity of antibacterial therapy. *South Med J* 87:869, 1994.
89. Johnson LR: Tricyclic antidepressant toxicosis. *Vet Clin North Am Small Anim Pract* 20:393, 1990.
90. Baldessarini RJ: Drugs and the treatment of psychiatric disorders: psychosis and

anxiety. *In:* Hardman JG, Limbird LE, eds.: Goodman and Gilman's The Pharmacological Basis of Therapeutics, 9th ed. New York: McGraw-Hill, 1995, p 402.

91. Baldessarini RJ: Drugs and the treatment of psychiatric disorders: depression and mania. *In:* Hardman JG, Limbird LE, eds.: Goodman and Gilman's The Pharmacological Basis of Therapeutics, 9th ed. New York: McGraw-Hill, 1995, p 431.
92. Wokenstein P, Revus J: Drug-induced severe skin reactions. Incidence, management and prevention. *Drug Saf* 13:56, 1995.
93. Freedman MD: Pharmacodynamics, clinical indications, and adverse effects of heparin. *J Clin Pharmacol* 32:584, 1992
94. Benichou C, Celigny PS: Standardization of definitions and criteria for causality assessment of adverse drug reactions. Drug-induced blood cytopenias: report of an International Consensus Meeting. *Nouv Rev Fr Hematol* 33:257, 1991.
95. Stroncek DF: Drug induced immune neutropenia. *Transfus Med Rev* VII:268, 1993.
96. Watson ADJ: Chloramphenicol toxicosis in cats. *Am J Vet Res* 89:1199, 1978.
97. Holland M, Stobie D, Shapiro W: Pancytopenia associated with administration of captopril to a dog. *J Am Vet Med Assoc* 1996.
98. Bloom JC, Brandt JT. Toxic Responses of the Blood. In: Klaasen CD (ed): Casarett and Doull's Toxicology. The Basic Science of Poisons. 6th ed. McGraw Hill, NY, 2001, pp 389–418.
99. Boothe DM: Drug therapy in cats. Mechanisms and avoidance of adverse drug reactions. *J Am Vet Med Assoc* 196:1297, 1990.
100. Wilkie DA, Kirby R: Methemoglobinemia associated with dermal application of benzocaine cream in a cat. *J Am Vet Med Assoc* 192:85, 1988.
101. Peterson ME, Horvitz AI, Leib MS: Propylthiouracil-associated hemolytic anemia, thrombocytopenia and antinuclear antibodies in cats with hyperthyroidism. *J Am Vet Med Assoc* 184:806, 1984.
102. Cowgill LD, Polzin DJ, Osborne CA, *et al.*: Results of recombinant human erythropoietin clinical trial. Proceedings of the 12th American College of Veterinary Internal Medicine Forum. 12:490, 1994.
103. Cowgill L: CVT update: use of recombinant human erythropoietin. *In:* Bonagura J, ed.: Current Veterinary Therapy XII. Philadelphia: WB Saunders, 1995, p 961.
104. Shumate MJ: Heparin-induced thrombocytopenia. N Engl J Med 333:1006, 1995.
105. Greinacher A, Michels I, Schäfer M, *et al.*: Heparin-associated thrombocytopenia in a patient treated with polysulphated chondroitin sulphate: evidence for immunological crossreactivity between heparin and polysulphated glycosaminoglycan. *Br J Haematol* 81:252, 1992.
106. Grodman-Gross CA, Sastri SV: Heparin-associated hematomas: possible allergic reaction. *DICP: Ann Pharmacother* 21:180, 1987.
107. Ramos KS, Chacon E, Acosta D: Toxic responses of the heart and vascular systems. *In:* Klaassen CD, ed.: Casarett and Doull's Toxicology. The Basic Science of Poisons, 5th ed. New York: McGraw Hill, 1996, p 487.
108. Chabner BA, Allegra CJ, Curt GA, *et al.*: Antineoplastic agents. *In* Hardman JG, Limbird LE, eds.: Goodman and Gilman's The Pharmacological Basis of Therapeutics, 9th ed. New York: McGraw Hill, 1995, p 1233.
109. Matsui H, Morishima I, Numaguchi Y: Protective effects of carvedilol against doxorubicin-induced cardiomyopathy in rats. *Life Sci* 65:1265, 1999.
110. Adams RH. Digitalis and vasodilator drugs. *In:* Adams R, ed.: Veterinary Pharmacology and Therapeutics. Ames, IA: Iowa State University Press, 1995, p 451.
111. Roden DM. Antiarrhythmic drugs. *In:* Hardman JG, Limbird LE, eds.: Goodman

and Gilman's The Pharmacological Basis of Therapeutics, 9th ed. New York: McGraw Hill, 1996, p 839.

112. DeRick A, Belpaire FM, Bogaert MG, *et al.*: Pharmacokinetics of digoxin. *Am J Vet Res* 39:811–818, 1978.
113. Endou K, Yamamoto H, Sata T: Comparison of the effects of calcium channel blockers and antiarrhythmic drugs on digitalis-induced oscillatory afterpotentials on canine Purkinje fiber. *Jap Heart J* 28:719, 1987.
114. Hashitmoto : Comparative study using other canine arrhythmia models and the new antiarrhythmic drugs propafenone, tocainide and SUN 1165. Heart Vessels 1:29, 1985.

SUGGESTED READINGS

Bryant DH: Drug-induced pulmonary disease. *Med J Aust* 156:802, 1992.

Bushby SRM: Sulfonamide and trimethoprim combination. *J Am Vet Med Assoc* 176: 1049, 1980.

Campbell K, Chambers MD, Davis CA, *et al.*: Effects of trimethoprim/sulfamethoxazole on thyroid physiology in dogs. *Proc Am Coll Vet Dermatol* 11:15, 1995.

Hawkins C, Hanks GW: The gastroduodenal toxicity of nonsteroidal anti-inflammatory drugs: a review of the literature. *J Pain Symptom Manage* 20:140, 2000.

Hornych A: Role of prostaglandins in drug nephrotoxicity. *Contrib Nephrol* 42:220, 1984.

Jones RD, Baynes RE, Nimitz CT: Nonsteroidal anti-inflammatory drug toxicosis in dogs and cats: 240 cases (1989–1990). *J Am Vet Med Assoc* 201:475, 1992.

Kourounakis PN, Tsiakitzis K, Kourounakis AP, *et al.*: Reduction of GI toxicity of NSAIDs via molecular modifications leading to antioxidant drugs. *Toxicology* 144: 205, 2000.

Miller LJ: Adverse effects of angiotensin converting enzyme inhibitors. *Drug Saf* 7:14, 1992.

Munger MA: Renal functional alterations induced by angiotensin-converting enzyme inhibitors in heart failure. *Ann Pharmacol* 27:205, 1993.

Pedersoli WM: Serum fluoride concentration, renal and hepatic function test results in dogs with methoxyflurane anesthesia. *Am J Vet Res* 38:949, 1977.

Raynaud JP: Thiacetarsamide (adulticide) versus melarsomine (RM 340) developed as macrofilaricide (adulticide and larvicide) to cure canine heartworm infection in dogs. *Ann Rech Vet* 23:1, 1992.

Roberts SM, Lavach JD, Macy DW, *et al.*: Effect of ophthalmic prednisolone acetate on the canine adrenal gland and hepatic function. *Am J Vet Res* 45:1711, 1984.

Wallace JL: Distribution and Expression of COX isoenzymes, their physiological roles, and the categorization of nonsteroidal anti-inflammatory drugs. *Am J Med* 107:11s, 1999.

Young DS: Effects of Drugs on Clinical Laboratory Tests, 3rd ed. Washington DC, American Association for Clinical Chemistry, 1990.

78

Changes in Drug Disposition and Drug Interaction

Dawn Merton Boothe

THE CRITICAL CARE PATIENT AT RISK

A variety of factors that may produce adverse drug events (ADEs)[1-4] are present in the CCU patient. Physiologic and pathologic responses to illness or injury may profoundly affect drug disposition and response to the drug. Drugs active in the cardiovascular and central nervous systems (CNS) may present the greatest risk because these vascular responses prioritize blood (and drug) delivery to these organs; additionally, derangements of these systems are often rapidly fatal. The critical patient also is likely to be simultaneously receiving two or more drugs that might negatively interact. Anticipating and thus preventing ADEs is facilitated by an understanding of drug disposition and its changes in the critical patient. This chapter will focus on some of these changes, the role of drug interactions as the cause of an ADE, and methods by which clinicians might accommodate for these changes through modification of the dosing regimen.

Drug Movement and Disposition

The pharmacologic response to a drug reflects drug concentration at the tissue site, which in turn tends to be linearly related to plasma drug concentrations (PDCs). A dosing regimen generally is designed to achieve, but not exceed, a targeted therapeutic range during a specific time interval. The range is characterized by a peak (maximum effective) and trough (minimum effective) PDC. Peak and trough PDCs achieved following administration of a drug reflect the cumulative effect of several drug movements that determine drug disposition.[5] These movements include absorption from the site of administration (most commonly the gastrointestinal [GI] tract) into systemic circulation, distribution from circulation into and back from body tissues, and removal of the drug from the body by either metabolism or excretion. Each movement is affected by a number of host and drug factors. Drug factors include drug chemistry (*e.g.*, lipid solubility, molecular size, and pKa), whereas host factors include local (*e.g.*, environmental pH, surface area) as well as systemic (*e.g.*, motility, blood flow) effects.

Gastrointestinal absorption is determined principally by GI pH, motility, epithelial permeability, surface area, and blood flow. Rate and extent of intramuscular (IM) or subcutaneous (SQ) absorption reflects drug molecular weight, lipid solubility, and regional blood flow to the site of administration. Drugs must be distributed from the central "compartment" to extracellular or intracellular tissues and then back. Both rate and extent of drug distribution are affected by the size of the compartment to which the drug will be distributed (the volume of distribution, Vd), the extent to which the drug is bound to plasma proteins (principally albumin, generally lipid-soluble drugs), regional blood flow to organs (tissues), and binding of drug to tissues. Water-soluble drugs generally are distributed only to extracellular fluid (ECF; Vd generally ≤0.3 L/kg), whereas lipid-soluble drugs tend to be distributed to total body water (Vd generally ≥0.6 L/kg).

Drugs must be eliminated from the body to avoid accumulation. Drug elimination occurs through drug metabolism or excretion. The major site of drug metabolism is the liver. Hepatic blood flow, intrinsic (cytochrome P-450) metabolism, and binding to plasma proteins variably affect drugs metabolized by the liver. Most drug metabolism occurs in two phases, each catalyzed by specific enzymes. Phase I enzymes chemically change and often inactivate the drug. However, the drug often remains or becomes more active following phase I metabolism. Of greater concern is the formation of reactive metabolites that may be more toxic than the parent drug. Accumulation of toxic phase I metabolites by the liver predisposes the liver to drug-induced toxicity. Phase II drug-metabolizing enzymes (glucuronidases, glutathione transferases) generally inactivate the drug or its metabolites and often are important to removal of toxic drug metabolites. Although most metabolism occurs in the liver, a number of tissues (*e.g.*, skin, lung, intestinal tract, kidney) are capable of drug metabolism, which may predispose each organ to drug toxicity. Renal excretion represents the most important mechanism by which drugs or metabolites are irreversibly cleared from the body. Renal excretion is determined by renal blood flow, glomerular filtration (a passive, inefficient process), protein binding (protein-bound drugs will not be filtered), active tubular secretion (a very rapid, efficient process that is not affected by protein binding), and passive tubular resorption of the drug back into circulation. Passive resorption prolongs drug half-life; its rate and extent is determined by lipid solubility, molecular size, and drug ionization, which in turn is dependent on urinary pH and drug pKa. A drug that is unionized (*e.g.*, a weakly acidic drug in an acidic environment) is more diffusible and more likely to be reabsorbed, whereas an ionized drug (a weakly acidic drug in a basic environment) is more likely to be excreted. Biliary drug excretion is an inefficient route of drug excretion but is clinically relevant in part because of the potential of the drug to undergo enterohepatic circulation. In such situations, the GI tract is re-exposed to the drug multiple times and the elimination of the drug is slowed.

Drug Disposition and the Dosing Regimen

A dosing regimen (comprised of a route, dose and interval) is designed to achieve and maintain targeted PDC throughout the dosing interval.[5] The dose of the drug necessary to achieve a given target is determined by the volume of tissue that will dilute the drug (Vd), and, for nonintravenous drugs, the bioavailability of the drug (how much of the drug reaches systemic circulation). For intravenous (IV) drugs, compared to the normal patient, dose modification generally can be in proportion to changes (from normal) in Vd (*e.g.*, increased with edema or decreased with dehydration). The interval of a dosing regimen is based on the acceptable change in PDC (*i.e.*, the difference between peak and trough PDC) and the rate of drug elimination from the body, commonly assessed as drug elimination half-life. For drugs whose pharmacologic effects require the continued presence of the drug (*e.g.*, anticonvulsants, opioid analgesics, time-dependent antibiotics), the dosing interval is largely based on the drug elimination half-life. For drugs characterized by "residual" pharmacologic effects (*e.g.*, anti-inflammatories, hormonal agents, concentration-dependent drugs), the interval is frequently longer than the elimination half-life and often is based on convenience.

Drug elimination half-life is the time necessary for 50% of a drug to be eliminated from the blood. Most commonly, it is determined by the rate of removal of active drug or metabolites by the liver or kidney. Elimination half-life is indirectly proportional to the clearance capacity of organs of elimination. However, clearance is not the sole parameter that affects elimination half-life. To be eliminated, a drug must be in circulation. Thus, the Vd of a drug will directly affect elimination half-life. A drug whose Vd has increased is distributed to more tissues and becomes less accessible to the organs of elimination. Its elimination half-life subsequently is prolonged. The traditional response to prolonged elimination half-life as a result of decreased clearance of a drug (*e.g.*, hepatic or renal disease) is to decrease the dose of a drug. Although this response might be correct for drugs that accumulate (see below), for many drugs, decreasing the dose will increase the risk of therapeutic failure because the PDC never achieves therapeutic concentrations. For drugs that do not accumulate, rather than reducing the dose, the interval of a dosing regimen should be prolonged to accommodate for an increase in elimination half-life. Examples include opioids, antibiotics, and many cardiac drugs.

Accumulation occurs when a drug is given at a dosing interval that is shorter than its elimination half-life. In such cases, at least half—and often much more—of the previous dose remains in the body by the time the next dose is given. Drugs given in such a fashion will accumulate until ultimately, at steady-state, PDC will be some magnitude greater than that following the first dose. The magnitude in accumulation increases with the difference between the interval and the elimination half-life. Bromide (with a 24-day half-life) given every 12 hours is an extreme example of a drug that markedly accumulates (see below). For drugs that accumulate, a decrease (or increase) in PDC requires a proportional change in either dose or interval.

Full response to a drug will not occur until steady-state, the point at which accumulation is complete because drug elimination from the body (drug output) and drug dosing (drug input) are equal. At that point, maximum accumulation of the drug will have occurred. For all drugs, steady-state is reached at three to five drug half-lives. For drugs with a long half-life, therapeutic response or risk of toxicity cannot be fully evaluated until steady-state has been reached. Many drugs with a very short half-life are given as a constant IV infusion (*e.g.*, dopamine, anesthetic agents, and diazepam); steady-state is usually rapidly reached and a loading dose may not be necessary. For bromide, steady-state is not reached for 2 to 3 months and a loading dose is often given. Note that for drugs given at a dosing interval that precludes elimination (*e.g.*, an antibiotic with an elimination half-life of 4 hours, given at 12-hour dosing intervals), "steady-state" never actually occurs. Such drugs are characterized by an increased risk of reaching both toxic (shortly after dosing) and subtherapeutic (just before the next dose) levels during a dosing interval. For such drugs, shortening the dosing interval such that fluctuations are minimized rather than increasing (risking toxic concentrations) or decreasing (thus risking subtherapeutic concentrations) the dose may be more appropriate.

Maintenance doses of drugs that accumulate are designed to target therapeutic PDC at steady-state. Because the time to steady-state may be unacceptably long (*i.e.*, anticonvulsants), both a loading dose and a maintenance dose might be given. A loading dose is associated with a greater risk of adverse reactions because it is designed to rapidly achieve targeted PDC. Simplistically, the loading dose equals the sum of all doses given as steady-state is reached, less the amount eliminated. Realistically, it is calculated from the targeted drug concentrations, the Vd of the drug, and for non-IV drugs, the bioavailability (F) of the drug. The difference between the loading and maintenance dose reflects the difference between the dosing interval and time to steady-state. Thus, for bromide (elimination half-life of about 3 weeks), a single dose of 450 mg/kg should target the minimum end of the therapeutic range (1 mg/mL), which is then maintained by a twice daily maintenance dose of 15 mg/kg. For phenobarbital (half-life of approximately 54-72 hours), the loading dose is 12 to 18 mg/kg compared to a maintenance dose of 2 to 3.5 mg/kg twice daily. The maintenance dose of the drug is intended to maintain what the loading dose achieved (*i.e.*, PDC). If it fails to do so, PDC will continue to increase or decrease until steady-state is achieved at 3 to 5 drug half-lives after the new maintenance dose was begun.

Elimination half-life also is an important consideration to resolution of ADEs resulting from drug overdosing. Supportive therapy in overdose cases must be continued until drug concentration has decreased below the toxic range and the organ has had an opportunity to be repaired. Following one, two, three, and five elimination half-lives, 50%, 75%, 87.5%, and 99% of the drug will be eliminated, respectively, from the body. However, elimination of 99% of the drug may not be enough if the overdose was great. Additionally, if the mechanisms of excretion (especially hepatic metabolism) have been saturated such that elimination is no longer first order (*i.e.*, constant percent eliminated per unit time) but becomes zero order (*i.e.*, constant amount eliminated per unit time), elimination half-life can no longer predict PDC. Finally, changes in the organ of elimination induced by disease may further prolong the elimination half-life.

Changes in Drug Disposition in the Critical Care Patient

Changes in drug disposition in the critical care patient that may result in ADEs must also consider species differences. Differences in physiology renders the cat more susceptible than the dog to a number of drug adversities and the critical care clinician should be aware of these differences as drugs and dosing regimens are selected for feline critical patients.[6–12] Differences in age also must be considered. Both the pediatric[13–22] and geriatric[23–28] patients are characterized by changes in disposition that complicate design of dosing regimens compared to young adult animals. Pregnancy complicates drug therapy due to unique changes in drug disposition of the mother[29–31] and the fetus[32] or neonate.[33,34] The impact of disease adds an additional level of complication. Cardiac,[35] liver,[36–41] and renal[42,43] diseases are of greatest concern because of their potential impact on many drug movements. However, other diseases can cause changes in selected drug movements (*e.g.*, GI disease and drug absorption;[44] thyroid disease and drug metabolism;[45] multiple diseases that alter serum proteins[46]). The role of drug interactions in complicating the proper design of dosing regimens for the critical care patient is discussed later in this chapter.

Changes in Drug Absorption

Decreased longitudinal smooth muscle motility (peristalsis) induced by disease or drugs will decrease movement of drug into the intestine and thus prolong time to peak absorption. However, extent of drug absorption is not likely to be affected. Likewise, because the surface area of the small intestine is so large, increased peristalsis will minimally affect rate or extent of drug absorption. Drugs that slow peristalsis or enhance segmentation (*e.g.*, opioid analgesics) may enhance absorption of luminal contents. Undesirable toxins or degradative products (*e.g.*, parvovirus, bacterial diarrheas) may subsequently be absorbed and such drugs should be avoided. Changes in permeability (as might occur with any inflammatory disease of the GI tract) may increase drug absorption resulting in higher peak and greater extent of absorption. Drugs that normally are not absorbed (*e.g.*, aminoglycosides) may reach systemic circulation in such cases and caution is recommended with oral administration of potentially toxic drugs. On the other hand, permeability changes may be sufficient to present a barrier to drug diffusion (*e.g.*, edema, inflammatory debris). Both rate and extent of drug absorption can be decreased in such a situation.

Parenteral administration often is the preferred route of drug administration in the critical patient in part to avoid factors that might impair the rate and extent of drug delivery to plasma. Absorption from SQ sites is generally slower than that from IM sites; peak PDCs are likely to be lower. Drug absorption from IM and SQ routes can be profoundly affected by decreased regional blood flow associated with hypotension (*e.g.*, dehydration or other causes of hypovolemic shock, cardiogenic shock) or hypothermia (*e.g.*, puppies). Volume replacement and return to normothermia should occur before drug absorption from peripheral sites is reliable. Rectal administration can be a viable route of administration for many drugs.[47] Advantages include easy access and bypassing (to a large degree) first-pass metabolism associated with oral drugs. However, the drug must be dissolved and thus administered as a solution or rectal suppository. Intraosseous administration may be a viable alternative to rapid drug delivery in pediatric patients.[48,49] Intrathecal administration is a rarely used method of direct drug delivery to cerebrospinal fluid. Note that drug does not necessarily gain access to brain tissue with this route. Bypassing the blood–cerebrospinal fluid barrier renders the patient at greater risk to drug-induced neurologic toxicities. Aerosolization can be a powerful tool for facilitating drug distribution to the upper airways or lungs. Attention must be given to the proper selection of an aerosolizer that will generate particles of the proper size necessary for deposition in the targeted airways. Rapid and shallow breathing decreases the proportion of drug that reaches the lower airways. Aerosolization generally should be accompanied by systemic therapy. Transdermal drug delivery may be an effective alternative route of drug delivery to critical care patients. Administration of fentanyl safely and effectively via a transdermal delivery system has been documented in both dogs and cats.[50] In human medicine, formulation of drugs in a phosphatidyllethicin-organic matrix gel and subsequent topical administration has proven to be an important alternative method of delivery for drugs that cannot be given by other routes. The use of such agents is becoming increasingly popular in veterinary medicine.

Drug Distribution

Drug distribution in the critical patient can be affected due to changes in Vd or protein binding. Changes in protein binding are relevant only for drugs highly (>80%) protein bound. Changes in PDC can be expected to change proportionately but indirectly with Vd. Accumulation of fluid (edema, ascites) or loss of fluid (due to dehydration, hyponatremia, etc.) and subsequent resolution (treatment of accumulated fluids with diuretic therapy, or rehydration) can cause Vd to fluctuate by more than 30%. However, the impact of changes in Vd on PDC varies with the lipid solubility of drugs. Lipid-soluble drugs distribute to total body water, and dosing on a milligram per kilogram basis will minimize the impact of fluid shifts on PDC. Dose modification for water-soluble drugs is more complicated. Fluid shifts can be profound in states of hypovolemia, causing a reduction in total body water with marked contraction of the ECF compartment. If ECF is contracted more than total body water, PDC of water-soluble drugs (distributed only to ECF) will be higher unless the milligram per kilogram dose is appropriately decreased. Physiologic responses during hypotension cause more blood (and thus drug) to be delivered to the brain and heart, increasing the risk of cardiac or neurologic ADEs, again requiring a decrease in dose. Fluid accumulation (edema, pediatric patients, fluid therapy) will require the opposite response. The milligram per kilogram dose may need to be increased for water-soluble drugs to compensate for increased fluid volumes. One notable exception exists: accumulation of fluids in discreet compartments such as ascites. Water-soluble drugs may not be distributed to the ascitic compartment. Increasing the dose of drug to accommodate this compartment or failure to dose on a lean body weight (excluding the compartment) may result in drug overdose. Because Vd directly (and proportionately) affects elimination half-life, dosing intervals also may need to be decreased or prolonged by 25%, depending on the fluid shifts. However, changes in half-life due to changes in Vd may be offset by changes in half-life due to changes in clearance.

Changes in protein binding can impact drug distribution in the critical patient. Highly protein-bound drugs (>80% bound) often do not distribute as rapidly as unbound drugs and response to therapy may be prolonged (*e.g.*, anticonvulsants). A disease-induced decrease in serum albumin or the presence of endogenous compounds (*e.g.*, bilirubin, uremic toxins) or exogenous compounds (*i.e.*, other highly protein-bound drugs) can cause displacement of a drug from its binding sites. The greater the normal percent protein binding of the drug, the greater the risk of toxicity if the percent bound changes. For example, displacement of only 1% of a drug 99% protein bound doubles the pharmacologically active concentration of the drug. For some drugs, clearance (*e.g.*, hepatic or glomerular filtration) of the displaced drug may increase, ultimately "normalizing" PDC. However, even for these drugs, an initial period of increased risk of toxicity may occur. Doses of highly protein-bound drugs may need to be decreased.

Cranial trauma causes unique changes in drug distribution. Following cranial trauma, the blood–brain barrier becomes permeable to small molecules normally excluded by the brain. Maximal permeability occurs several days after the injury. Increased drug distribution into the brain increases the risk of neurologic ADEs. Drugs might exacerbate the pathophysiologic sequelae of cranial trauma by contributing to hemorrhage (*e.g.*, mannitol), hypoxia (*e.g.*, sedatives), or hyperglycemia.

Drug Metabolism

The liver is the predominant site of drug metabolism. As with other hepatic functions, drug metabolism appears to be preserved until moderate to severe liver disease has developed. Unlike the kidney, no single diagnostic test can provide a reasonable estimate of changes in the drug metabolic capacity of the liver.[51] Generally, if liver dysfunction is sufficient that serum albumin and urea nitrogen concentrations are decreased and serum bile acids are increased, a proportional decrease in drug metabolism should also be anticipated.[39–41] Prolongation of the dosing interval is the most appropriate modification in the dosing regimen when elimination half-life is prolonged by decreased hepatic clearance, although a decrease in dose might also be indicated for drugs that accumulate (see previous discussion). The patient with portosystemic shunting presents unique considerations regarding drug administration. Hepatic drug metabolism is likely to be decreased in such patients and longer dosing intervals are indicated. Drugs characterized by a high hepatic extraction will largely bypass the liver, depending on the fraction of blood bypassing the liver. Intervals of such drugs should be prolonged, but because the drugs normally are very rapidly eliminated, doses might also be decreased. Certainly oral doses of such drugs must be decreased to account for decreased first-pass metabolism. The proportional decrease might be estimated by the fraction of blood shunted around the liver.

Drug Excretion

Conditions that are accompanied by decreased renal blood flow (dehydration, hypovolemia, cardiac dysfunction) will result in decreased glomerular filtration and active tubular secretion. Dosing intervals of renally excreted drugs that are potentially toxic should be prolonged. Only the percent of clearance of the parent drug (or active metabolites) by the kidney should be modified. Serum creatinine or creatinine clearance can be used to estimate the degree of renal dysfunction and decreased drug clearance. For drugs that do not accumulate, the interval should be proportionately prolonged; for drugs that do accumulate, either the interval or the dose can be modified. As renal function improves, doses may need to be readjusted to compensate for improved renal clearance. Therapeutic drug monitoring should be used whenever possible to guide changes in dosing regimens in critical care patients.

DRUG INTERACTIONS

Drug interactions occur whenever the action of one drug is modified by the presence of another, concurrently administered drug. Their incidence increases with the number of drugs included in the preparation and with the duration of treatment.[52] Drug interactions may occur before or after the drug is absorbed. Factors at the site of drug administration might also interact with a drug, altering its disposition.[11]

Pharmaceutical Drug Interactions

Pharmaceutical drug interactions[11] occur prior to the administration or absorption of a drug. Interactions can occur between two drugs, or a drug and a carrier (solvent or vehicle), receptacle (including IV tubing), or the environment in which it is administered (*i.e.*, gastric environment).[54–57] In human medicine, pharmaceutical interactions most frequently result from the addition of drugs to IV fluid preparations. In veterinary medicine, this is most likely to occur in the critical care environment where IV administration and multiple drug administration are common. Drug incompatibilities can change the chemical or physical nature of a drug. Incompatible reactions can reflect degradation due to changes in pH, binding by drugs with different charges or other molecular interactions, changes in temperature, or exposure to ultraviolet radiation.[58]

Intravenous Preparations

Table 78-1 lists examples of drug interactions in solution.[53] Drugs that are unstable generally have a short shelf-life when in solution. Reconstituted parenteral solutions should always be labeled with the new expiration date and used with strict adherence to the product label instructions after reconstitution. If directed by the label, refrigeration or freezing can prolong the shelf life. However, it is risky to assume that cold storage will prolong the shelf-life of the drug unless efficacy has been documented. Freezing can increase the degradation

Table 78-1. Examples of Drug Interactions in Solution

Drug or Drug Class	Incompatible Drugs	Other Risks
Amino acid solutions	Many drugs	
Aminoglycosides	Semisynthetic β-lactams, heparin Many others; check manufacturer's label	Adsorbs to glass; use plastic for monitoring
Aminophylline	Do not mix with other drugs	
Amphotericin B	Use only 5% dextrose (even for diluent although manufacturer suggests sterile water) Do not mix with other drugs	Light exposure
Ampicillin sodium	Selected diluents and drugs Check manufacturer's label	
Atropine sulfate	Bicarbonate, methicillin, promazine, warfarin, others	
β-Lactams		
Cephalosporins	Many drugs, depending on specific antimicrobial. Check manufacturer's label	Check manufacturer's recommendations regarding stability on reconstitution
Penicillins	As above; aminoglycosides	
Bicarbonate	Many drugs	
Buprenorphine	Do not mix with dimenhydrinate, pentobarbital	
Butorphanol	Do not mix with diazepam	
Blood, red blood cells	Any IV solution except 0.9% saline	
Calcium-containing solutions	Many drugs	
Calcium disodium EDTA	Do not mix with many drugs including dextrose, metal salts	
Chloramphenicol	Many drugs	See also Table 78-3
Carbenicillin disodium	Do not mix with many drugs	
Cefazolin	Do not mix with any other drug	
Cephalothin	Do not mix with any other drug	

Table 78-1. (continued)

Drug or Drug Class	Incompatible Drugs	Other Risks
Diazepam	Cloudiness when mixed with many other drugs indicates precipitation that will include drug. Potency may be reduced.	Adsorbs to IV tubing and plastic containers Protect from light
Digitoxin (not digoxin)	Calcium, epinephrine, vitamin B complex	
Diphenhydramine	Furosemide, methylprednisolone, pentobarbital	
Dobutamine	Alkaline solutions Bicarbonate, heparin, insulin, others	Check manufacturer's label re: discoloration
Doxycycline	Selected drugs including lidocaine, heparin, isoproterenol, vitamin B complex	
Doxyrubicin		Avoid prolonged contact with aluminum
Epinephrine	Calcium-containing solutions; ampicillin; other penicillins, pentobarbital, prochlorperazine Others	
Erythromycin	Several drugs including selected cephalosporins, chloramphenicol, heparin, tetracyclines, and vitamin B complex	
Flunixin meglumine	Most solutions	
Furosemide	Acidic solutions will cause hydrolysis. Precipitates when combined with many drugs	Yellow discoloration. Protect from light.
Gentamicin	Many drugs including dopamine, furosemide, heparin (see also β-lactams, amphotericin B	
Glycopyrrolate	Alkaline solutions. Avoid diluting with saline or bicarbonate for IV infusion. Other drugs	Is a strongly acidic solution
Heparin	Many drugs	Strongly acidic solution Slight yellow discoloration is okay

Table 78-1. (continued)

Drug or Drug Class	Incompatible Drugs	Other Risks
Hydrocortisone	Acid pH will cause hydrolysis	Use proper dilution volume to avoid precipitation
sodium esters	Incompatible with many selected drugs	
Imipenem		Do not freeze
Insulin	Check package label regarding diluents and refrigeration needs. Mixing lente insulins is okay, but mixing regular with lente will alter kinetics. Incompatible with many drugs.	Binds to IV tubing, selected types of glass and plastics.
Iron dextran		Oxytetracycline, sulfonamides
Kanamycin		See gentamicin, aminoglycosides
Ketamine		Barbiturates, diazepam
Lidocaine		Alkaline solutions Loss of drug when stored in PVC bags (absorption to PVC)
Magnesium sulfate		Many drugs including calcium containing drugs, sodium bicarbonate, tetracyclines, others
Mannitol		Blood, strongly acidic or alkaline solutions Crystallization of high (25%) concentrations in glass containers generally can be redistributed by warming. Crystallization in plastic solutions difficult to resolve.
Methylprednisolone	Normosol-R, Normosol-M	Avoid diluting with a volume that is too small; precipitation may occur otherwise.
Metronidazole		Reconstituted lyophilized product very acidic and must be buffered with bicarbonate. Ready-to-use product requires no additional handling. Light sensitive; however, discoloration induced by light not accompanied by loss of potency. Do not freeze

Table 78-1. (continued)

Drug or Drug Class	Incompatible Drugs	Other Risks
Metoclopramide	β-Lactams, erythromycin, sodium bicarbonate Protect from light	
Morphine	Many drugs	
Multiple vitamin	Bicarbonate, selected cephalosporins Complexes aminophylline, others	Lack of potency loss has only been documented 8 hours after dilution.
Nitrofurantoin	Many drugs	
Oxytetracycline	See tetracycline	
Oxytocin	Do not mix with any other drug	Refrigerate at <25°C. Do not freeze
Penicillin-G	See also β-lactams Polyethylene glycol Prochlorperazine, pentobarbital, sulfadiazine Others	Rapidly inactivate in pH <6–7 or >8
Pentobarbital	Acid pH Many drugs	Prepared as extremely alkaline solution.
Phenobarbital	Many drugs, especially acidic solutions	
Phenylephrine	Penicillin, pentobarbital, phenobarbital, phenytoin, Sodium bicarbonate	
Phenytoin	Do not mix with any other drug or IV solution	
Phytonadione	Do not mix with ascorbic acid, barbiturates, phenytoin	
Potassium chloride	Do not mix with amphotericin B	
Pralidoxime chloride (2-PAM)	Reconstitute with sterile water only. Do not mix with any other drug	
Procaine	Many solutions, especially alkaline	
Procainamide	Dextrose	Light yellow but not amber discoloration okay.
Prochlorperazine	Many drugs; do not mix in same syringe	
Promazine	Many drugs	
Promethazine	Selected drugs	

Table 78-1. (continued)

Drug or Drug Class	Incompatible Drugs	Other Risks
Protein hydrolysate	Many drugs	
Propofol	Do not mix with other drugs	
Propranolol	Rapidly decomposes in alkaline solution	
Ringer's lactate	Alcohol in 5% dextrose, epinephrine, oxytetracycline, sodium bicarbonate, sulfadiazine	
Sodium bicarbonate	Many drugs: check package insert	
Sodium iodide	Several drugs	
Sodium succinate	Selected drugs	
Sulfonamides, sodium salts	Many drugs	
Tetracycline	Highly acidic solution may render incompatible with many drugs. Discoloration in multiple electrolyte solution does not indicate potency loss	Dark solution indicates decomposition.
Thiopental	Many drugs	
Vancomycin	Selected drugs	
Vitamin B complex	Magnesium sulfate, erythromycin, selected others	
Warfarin	Many drugs	

From Boothe DM: Factors affecting drug disposition. *In:* Boothe DM: Small Animal Clinical Pharmacology and Therapeutics. Philadelphia: WB Saunders, 2001. King JC: Guide to Parenteral Admixtures. St. Louis, MO: Pacemarq; and Papich MG: Incompatible critical care drug combinations. *In:* Bonagura JD, ed.: Current Veterinary Therapy XII, Small Animal Practice. Philadelphia: WB Saunders, 1995, p 194.

(*e.g.*, ampicillin), crystallization (*e.g.*, heparin, dobutamine, furosemide) or precipitation (*e.g.*, insulin) of drugs. Refreezing of a previously frozen and defrosted solution increases the risk of efficacy loss. The proper reconstituting fluid should be used to avoid inactivation of drugs. For example, amphotericin B should be diluted only with 5% dextrose because precipitates will otherwise form; whole blood or packed red blood cells should be diluted only with 0.9% saline to avoid damage to infused cells. Changing the pH of a solution by improperly diluting it or mixing it with another drug can be risky. The release of some types of insulin is pH dependent; diluting insulin with a solution other than that provided by the manufacturer may change the pH and thus rate of insulin release.

The pH of a solution may be needed to keep the active drug dissolved or stable; changing the pH may result in precipitation or loss of stability. For example, acid-labile drugs (*e.g.*, penicillins) can be destroyed in low pH solution. Drugs prepared as an acid salt (*e.g.*, lidocaine hydrogen chloride) or in acidic solutions (*i.e.*, sodium heparin) should not be combined with alkaline solutions (*i.e.*, sodium bicarbonate). Examples of commonly used drugs that can be mixed safely in IV solutions include glucocorticoids, propranolol, fluorinated quinolones, and vitamin B complex.

Drugs can bind to and inactivate one another, often due to ionic attractions. Calcium in solution will precipitate if combined with solutions containing carbonates (*e.g.*, sodium bicarbonate). Heparin is incompatible with many drugs such as aminoglycoside and β-lactam antibiotics. Thus, saline rather than heparin might be used to maintain patency of catheters through which drugs will be administered. If present in sufficiently high concentrations, penicillins (weak acids) will bind to and inactivate aminoglycosides (weak bases) and fluorinated quinolones.[59,60] In fact, ticarcillin can be therapeutically used to bind gentamicin in cases of life-threatening overdose; protection may also reflect sodium loading.[61] Although plasma concentrations following therapeutic dosing of either drug probably do not achieve concentrations necessary to inactivate aminoglycosides as a once daily dosing regimen of aminoglycosides becomes more generally acceptable, the risk of aminoglycoside inactivation by a penicillin may become greater.

Often, a drug interaction involving IV solutions can be detected by a visual change in the appearance of the drugs. Discoloration, cloudiness, and formation of precipitate are indications of an interaction and use of the drug should be reconsidered. If the drug has simply recrystallized, gently warming the solution may result in re-dissolution without loss of efficacy. However, not all interactions will result in a physical change of the appearance. Likewise, the change in physical appearance of a drug combination does not necessarily indicate that the activity of the drug has been changed. For example, diazepam has been mixed with other preanesthetics with no observable (reported) change in drug efficacy, despite a cloudy discoloration. Whereas a pink discoloration of dopamine indicates inactivation, discoloration of dobutamine does not preclude efficacy if the drug is used within 24 hours. Slight yellow discoloration of procainamide is acceptable; dark discoloration indicates a loss of efficacy. Prudence suggests that any physical change in the character of a drug be reason to not use the drug in a critical patient.

Several drugs can bind to receptacles. For example, lipid-soluble drugs (*e.g.*, diazepam) can bind to plastic containers; insulin binds to selected glasses and many plastics including polyethylene and polyvinyl; aminoglycosides bind to glass. Binding to catheters and IV lines can be minimized by flushing each new system with a sufficient volume of solution (50 mL) before administering the drug. Drugs packaged in brown bottles (*e.g.*, diazepam and furosemide) are protected from UV lighting and protection should be continued if transferred to another vial.

Oral Preparations

Drug interactions can change the diffusibility, dissolution rate and particle size of orally administered drugs (Table 78-2). Many drugs bind luminal contents (Table 78-3) and oral absorption is impaired.[62] On the other hand, the oral absorption of selected drugs is enhanced in the presence of food. The effect of food is most important for concentration dependent antimicrobials (*e.g.*, fluorinated quinolones) whose efficacy is enhanced by high PDCs, drugs with a narrow therapeutic window, and for drugs with a steep dose–response curve because a small change in plasma drug concentration can cause profound differences in response to the drug. Food can alter splanchnic blood flow, gastric motility (and thus mixing and drug dissolution as well as gastric emptying), and gastric secretions. Changes in gastric secretions can alter gastric pH, which can change the percent of ionized and thus diffusible drug. The net effect of food on drug absorption depends on the pKa of the drug; whether or not the drug is labile to the effects of pH and enzymes; and the absorption site of the drug (*i.e.*, stomach versus intestine).[62]

Drug–drug interactions in the GI tract can inactivate or prevent absorption of drugs. Sucralfate, cimetidine, aluminum hydroxide, and Kaopectate are examples of drugs that will bind to and prevent the absorption of many drugs. Other

Table 78-2. Examples of Drug–Food Interactions

Decreased absorption
Ampicillin
Erythromycin (film-coated tablets)
Lincomycin
Rifampin
Sulfafurazole
Tetracyclines
Theophylline
Delayed absorption
Cefaclor
Cephalexin
Cimetidine
Digoxin
Fluorinated quinolones
Metronidazole
Enhanced absorption
Diazepam
Erythromycin
Griseofulvin (fats)
Imidazoles (decreased pH)
Metaprolol
Propranolol

From Toothaker RD, Welling PG: The effect of food on drug bioavailability. *Annu Rev Pharmacol Toxicol* 20:173, 1980, and Boothe DM: Factors affecting drug disposition. *In:* Boothe DM: Small Animal Clinical Pharmacology and Therapeutics. Philadelphia: WB Saunders, 2001.

Table 78-3. Highly Protein-Bound Drugs

Weak acids (albumin)
NSAIDs
Coumarin derivatives
Antibiotics
Doxycycline/minocycline
Anticonvulsants
Valproic acid
Phenytoin
Diazepam
Behavior-modifying drugs
Cardiac drugs
Digitoxin
Diuretics
Furosemide
Weak bases (α-glycoproteins)
Cardiac drugs
Propranolol
Lidocaine (some species)
Tricyclic antidepressants

From Boothe DM: Factors affecting drug disposition. *In:* Boothe DM: Small Animal Clinical Pharmacology and Therapeutics. Philadelphia: WB Saunders, 2001.

drugs alter the rate of absorption by altering gastric motility (see pharmacokinetic interactions). To minimize these effects, none of these drugs should be given simultaneously with another orally administered drug.

Pharmacokinetic Drug Interactions

Drug interactions that occur inside the body may be life-threatening. Pharmacokinetic interactions occur when one drug alters the disposition of another drug.[63] Each stage of disposition of a drug—absorption, distribution, metabolism, or elimination—can be altered by another drug.

Absorption

Absorption of one drug may be hindered due to changes in the drug's passage through biologic phases, and by changes in local pH, the integrity of biologic membranes, regional blood flow and, in the case of orally administered drugs, GI motility. All of these changes can be induced by a concurrently administered drug. Antisecretory drugs may decrease the proportion of a weak acid that is orally absorbed as gastric pH is increased, thus decreasing the absorption of weak acids. Similarly, the efficacy of sucralfate, which requires activation by an acidic environment, may be decreased if administered at the peak antacid effect of an antisecretory drug. Sucralfate and cimetidine are examples of drugs that bind to and prevent the absorption of other drugs causing a pharmaceutical interaction (see above). Likewise, tetracycline and enrofloxacin are bound by divalent or trivalent cations that might be found in antacids or foods. Drugs that alter gastric motility might alter the rate of oral drug absorption. Most drugs are absorbed from the small intestine. Administration of anticholinergics will decrease gastric emptying, allowing a longer time to elapse before a drug moves to the small intestine. Although extent of absorption may not be affected, peak PDCs may be lower. Metoclopramide and cisapride (or other prokinetics) should hasten gastric emptying, which may decrease dissolution of some drugs. Increasing motility of the small intestine is less likely to alter the oral absorption of drugs because the surface area is so large it is difficult to manipulate. A few drugs alter drug absorption by causing malabsorption or altering gastric blood flow.

Distribution

Pharmacokinetic drug interactions that alter drug distribution usually result from competition for protein-binding sites between two or more concurrently administered drugs. Because protein binding is reversible, the drug with the highest affinity for protein (usually albumin) will displace a drug with less affinity (see Table 78-3). If a highly (>80%) protein-bound drug is displaced by only a small fraction, the amount of unbound, pharmacologically active drug will markedly increase, and the risk of toxicity is initially increased. However, increased hepatic clearance of the unbound drug may ultimately counter the increased PDCs and the risk of toxicity may decrease as steady-state concentrations are reached. Most drug interactions involving protein binding involve competition for albumin-binding sites because it is the most common binding protein, particularly for weak acids. Lipoproteins, globulins (increased with acute phase protein increase), and to a lesser extent, albumin, bind to weak bases (*e.g.*, bupivacaine, lidocaine; see Table 78-3). Because nonsteroidal anti-inflammatory drugs (NSAIDs) are generally more than 90% protein bound, even slight displacement of the drug from its binding sites can result in toxic concentrations.

Use of drugs that alter drug distribution to peripheral organs can alter drug delivery to the organs. For example, drug therapy in the CCU patient may be ineffective if the patient is hypovolemic. It should be expected that drug distribution to peripheral organs is likely to increase as the management of a critical patient progresses and physiologic responses to shock and the like are medically resolved. Rarely, drug interactions can occur at the tissue site. For example, drugs can compete with one another at tissue-binding sites. Quinidine will increase digoxin toxicity because it displaces digoxin from cardiac tissues; in contrast, hypokalemia facilitates binding of digoxin to cardiac tissue, thus enhancing digoxin cardiotoxicity.

Metabolism

Pharmacokinetic drug interactions (Table 78-4) frequently alter the metabolism of a concurrently administered drug.[64–68] Most of the interactions result from modulation of hepatic (phase 1) drug-metabolizing enzymes. Many drugs cause the induction of microsomal enzyme activity (see Table 78-4). The rate of metabolism and clearance of concurrently administered drugs that are metabolized by the liver may thus be increased. The usual sequelae of enzyme induction is increased clearance and decreased pharmacologic response. Occasionally, tox-

Table 78-4. Examples of Inducers and Inhibitors of Drug Metabolizing Enzymes

Inducers
Chlorinated hydrocarbons
Griseofulvin
Phenobarbital (and other barbiturates)
Phenylbutazone
Phenytoin
Rifampin
Inhibitors
Chloramphenicol
Cimetidine
Fluorinated quinolones
Ketoconazole
Phenylbutazone
Prednisolone
Quinidine
Theophylline

From Boothe DM: Factors affecting drug disposition. *In:* Boothe DM: Small Animal Clinical Pharmacology and Therapeutics. Philadelphia: WB Saunders, 2001.

icity is enhanced because of increased production of a toxic metabolite, or in the case of prodrugs, the concentration of the pharmacologically active drug is increased. Enzyme induction is probably important in the pathogenesis of hepatotoxicity induced by several drugs (*e.g.*, anticonvulsants) and in the therapeutic failure (reflecting subtherapeutic concentrations) that accompanies some drugs (*e.g.*, anticonvulsants). Several days to weeks of drug administration generally are required for induction to occur. Induction is usually accompanied by increased hepatic RNA and protein synthesis and an increase in hepatic weight. Phenobarbital is one of the most potent microsomal enzyme inducers known and can enhance the hepatotoxicity of other hepatotoxic drugs. Likewise, it will increase the formation of and response to prodrugs and decrease the effect of other drugs metabolized by the liver as clearance of these drugs is increased.[52,63,69]

Drug-induced enzyme inhibition (see Table 78-4) may also occur, although it is probably not as clinically significant as induction.[70] Generally, clearance of a concurrently administered liver metabolized drug is prolonged when an enzyme inhibitor is also administered. The potential for toxicity or an exaggerated pharmacologic response is increased. In contrast to induction, inhibition may rapidly occur. Often inhibition reflects competition for the same metabolic enzymes. Chloramphenicol and cimetidine are examples of potent microsomal enzyme inhibitors.[52,63,69] Coadministration with potentially toxic drugs that are also metabolized by the liver should be done cautiously. Prodrugs (*e.g.*, enalapril; primidone in dogs) are less likely to be activated. Fluorinated quinolones such as enrofloxacin can increase theophylline plasma concentrations to toxic levels, presumably due to impaired theophylline clearance.[52,63,69] Ketoconazole impairs the hepatic elimination of several drugs. Drug-induced inhibition of drug metabolism can be used for therapeutic benefit. Enzyme inhibition has been used clinically in cats suffering from acetaminophen toxicity. Because acetaminophen is metabolized by phase I enzymes to a toxic metabolite (which overwhelms glutathione scavenging activity), cimetidine might be used to decrease the production of the potentially fatal toxic metabolite, although the efficacy is controversial.[71–73] The combination of cilastin with imipenem is another example of drug inhibition used therapeutically; cilastin inhibits renal tubular drug metabolism of imipenem, thus reducing its hepatotoxicity while prolonging its drug elimination half-life. Alcohol and 4-methylpyrazole competitively inhibit alcohol dehydrogenase, the drug-metabolizing enzymes that convert ethylene glycol to its lethal metabolites. Nutrition, sex, age, species differences, and other factors can influence how drug-metabolizing enzymes respond to drugs.

Drug clearance may also be affected by drugs that change hepatic blood flow. However, this interaction is significant only for drugs that are characterized by extensive and rapid hepatic clearance (*e.g.*, propranolol, lidocaine) and probably is not clinically relevant at this time.

Excretion

Pharmacokinetic drug interactions may alter urinary excretion due to changes in glomerular filtration or competition between the drug for active tubular secretion. Competition for carrier proteins responsible for active tubular secretion usually involves acidic drugs (Table 78-5). Probenecid is still occasionally used to prolong the elimination of an expensive penicillin because it competes with the penicillin for a carrier protein. Renal excretion may also be affected by drugs that alter urinary pH and tubular resorption. Changes in urinary pH conducive to formation of a greater proportion of unionized drug (*e.g.*, an acidic urinary pH and an acidic drug) will encourage tubular reabsorption of a drug, thus decreasing its clearance and prolonging its elimination half-life (Table

Table 78-5. Drugs That Compete for Tubular Secretion

Anions (acidic drugs)
Penicillins
Cephalosporins
Probenecid
Sulfonamides
Aspirin
Furosemide
NSAIDs
Phase II metabolites (glucuronic acids, glycine and sulfate conjugates)
Cations (basic drugs)
Procainamide
Dopamine
Trimethoprim
Several opioid agents

From Boothe DM: Factors affecting drug disposition. *In:* Boothe DM: Small Animal Clinical Pharmacology and Therapeutics. Philadelphia: WB Saunders, 2001.

Table 78-6. Drugs Capable of Changing Urine pH

Urinary acidifiers
Ascorbic acid
Methionine
Sodium acid phosphate
Ammonium chloride
Urinary alkalinizers
Sodium bicarbonate, citrate, and acetate
Carbonic anhydrase inhibitors

From Boothe DM: Factors affecting drug disposition. *In:* Boothe DM: Small Animal Clinical Pharmacology and Therapeutics. Philadelphia: WB Saunders, 2001.

78-6).[52,63,69] For example, overdosing of some drugs (*e.g.*, strychnine) can be treated by hastening elimination with urinary acidifiers.

Pharmacodynamic Drug Interactions

Pharmacodynamic drug interactions occur when one drug directly alters the chemical or physiologic response to another drug. Pharmacodynamic interactions can enhance the response of a drug due to additive or synergistic effects either at the same receptor (*e.g.*, the permissive effect of glucocorticoids on β-adrenergic receptors); intracellular site (*e.g.*, epinephrine and theophylline in bronchial smooth muscle), or at different sites but with the same physiologic reaction (*e.g.*, hypokalemia induced by cardiac glycosides and diuretics; many interactions of antibiotics). Pharmacodynamic interactions may decrease the response of some drugs due to competitive antagonism at the same receptor site (*e.g.*, anticholinergics such as atropine and anticholinesterases, or atropine and metoclopramide or cisapride) or due to antagonistic responses mediated at distant, but physiologically related, sites. Antagonistic pharmacodynamic interactions have been used therapeutically, for example, oxymorphone reversal with naloxone, and xylazine and other chemical sedative reversals with tolazoline or yohimbine.

The most familiar pharmacodynamic interactions are probably those that act in an additive or synergistic manner to augment response to a drug. Augmentation can occur through different mechanisms of action (*i.e.*, controlling vomiting by combining a drug active at the chemoreceptor triggering zone with a drug that acts peripherally, controlling seizures by combining phenobarbital with bromide, controlling tachycardia by combining diltiazem with digoxin). Less commonly, augmentation may occur through similar actions at a receptor site; more often, drugs will compete with one another at the same receptor, thus resulting in antagonism. Often, these actions are desirable and are frequently the target of combined drug therapy, for example, atropine to treat organophosphate toxicity, or reversal agents for opioids and anesthetic agents. The use of butorphanol, a mixed opioid analgesic that acts as an agonist at kappa receptors, but an antagonist at mu receptors may reduce the efficacy of a simultaneously administered pure opioid such as fentanyl. This effect may be desirable if attempting to reverse the sedative effects of the pure opioid, but may be undesirable if control of pain is reduced. Interestingly, the combination of fentanyl, a pure mu agonist, and buprenorphine, a partial mu agonist/antagonist may have synergistic analgesic effects rather than the antagonistic effects that might be expected. Antagonistic pharmacodynamic responses can also occur though different receptor sites or different mechanisms. The combination of a "bacteriostatic" antibiotic with a "bactericidal" antibiotic might be considered as an example. Other examples include the prokinetic effects of cisapride and metoclopramide being ameliorated by anticholinergics; the effects of sucralfate being reduced in the presence of high gastric pH induced by antisecretory drug; and calcium-containing solutions not being combined with blood or blood components because the loss of anticoagulant effects will increase the risk of microthrombi formation in the transfused blood.

The prudent clinician will remember that if a drug combination may augment a pharmacologic response, it may just as easily augment an ADE. For example, drugs that impair renal prostaglandin synthesis (*e.g.*, NSAIDs, angiotensin-converting enzyme inhibitors, aminoglycosides) should be used in combination cautiously because their combination increases the risk of renal failure. Likewise, ulcerogenic drugs (NSAIDs, glucocorticoids) enhance the risk of GI ulceration when used in combination.

The number of drugs that might interact with one another is large and extensive. Clinicians treating critical care patients should be familiar with the risks associated with those drugs commonly found in their CCU environment and should review the package inserts and accompanying information when using a drug with which he or she is not thoroughly familiar.

REFERENCES

1. Ariens EJ, Simonis AM, Offermeier J: Introduction to General Toxicology. New York: Academic Press, 1976, 79.
2. Lawson DH, Richared RME: Clinical Pharmacy and Hospital Drug Management. London: Chapman and Hall, 1982.
3. Mitchell JR, Smith CV, Lauferburg BH, *et al.*: Reactive metabolites and the pathophysiology of acute lethal cell injury. *In:* Mitchell JR, Homing MG, eds.: Drug Metabolism and Drug Toxicity. New York, Raven Press, 1984, p 301.
4. Klassen DC: Principles of toxicology. *In:* Klassen CD, Amour MO, Doull J, eds.: Toxicology: The Basic Science of Poisons, 3rd ed. New York: Macmillan, 1985, p 11.
5. Boothe DM: Principles of Drug Therapy. *In:* Boothe DM. Small Animal Clinical Pharmacology and Therapeutics. WB Saunders, Philadelphia, 2001, p 3–17.
6. Peters EL, Farber TM, Heider A, *et al.*: The development of drug-metabolizing enzymes in the young dog. *Fed Proc Am Soc Biol* 30:560, 1971.
7. Baggott JD: Principles of drug disposition in domestic animals. The Basis of Veterinary Clinical Pharmacology. Philadelphia: WB Saunders, 1977, p 73.
8. Wilcke JR: Idiosyncrasies of drug metabolism in cats. *Vet Clin North Am Small Anim Pract* 14:1345, 1984.
9. Boothe DM: Drug therapy in cats: mechanisms and avoidance of adverse drug reactions. *J Am Vet Med Assoc* 196:1297, 1990.

10. Boothe DM: Drug therapy in cats: recommended dosing regimens. *J Am Vet Med Assoc* 196:1845, 1990.
11. Boothe DM: Factors affecting drug disposition and extrapolation of dosing regimens. *In:* Boothe DM. Small Animal Clinical Pharmacology and Therapeutics. WB Saunders, Philadelphia, 2001, p 18–40.
12. Court MH, Greenblatt DJ: Molecular genetic basis for deficient acetaminophen glucuronidation by cats: UGT1A6 is a pseudogene, and evidence for reduced diversity of expressed hepatic UGT1A isoforms. *Pharmacogenetics* 10:355, 2000.
13. Stolk JM, Smith RP: Species differences in methemoglobin reductase activity. *Biochem Pharmacol* 15:343, 1966.
14. Sheng H-P, Huggins RA: Growth of the beagle: changes in the body fluid compartments. *Proc Soc Exp Biol Med* 139:330, 1972.
15. Heimann G: Enteral absorption and bioavailability in children in relation to age. *Eur J Clin Pharmacol* 18:43, 1980.
16. Hellmann J, Vannucci RC, Nardis EE: Blood-brain barrier permeability to lactic acid in the newborn dog: lactate as a cerebral metabolic fuel. *Pediatr Res* 16:40, 1982.
17. Reiche R: Drug disposition in the newborn. *In:* Ruckesbusch P, Toutain P, Koritz D, eds.: Veterinary Pharmacology and Toxicology. AVI Publishing, 1983, p 49.
18. Rane A, Wilson JT: Clinical pharmacokinetics in infants and children. *In:* Gibaldi M, Prescott L, eds.: Handbook of Clinical Pharmacokinetics. New York: ADIS Health Science Press, 1983, p. 142.
19. Morselli PL, Morselli RF, Bossi L: Clinical pharmacokinetics in newborns and infants: age-related differences and therapeutic implications. *In:* Gibaldi M, Prescott L, eds.: Handbook of Clinical Pharmacokinetics. New York:, ADIS Health Science Press, 1983, p 99.
20. Green TP, Mirkin BL: Clinical pharmacokinetics: pediatric considerations. *In:* Benet LZ, Massoud N, Gambertoglio JG, eds.: Pharmacokinetic Basis for Drug Treatment. New York: Raven Press, 1984, p 269.
21. Poffenbarger EM, Ralston SL, Chandler ML, *et al.*: Canine neonatology. Part I. Physiological differences between puppies and adults. *Compend Contin Educ* 12: 1601, 1990.
22. Boothe DM, Tannert K: Special considerations for drug and fluid therapy in the pediatric patient. *Compend Contin Educ Pract Vet* 14:313, 1991.
23. Ehrnebo M, Agurell S, Jalling B, *et al.*: Age differences in drug binding by plasma proteins: studies on human fetuses, neonates and adults. *Eur J Clin Pharmacol* 3: 189, 1973.
24. Massoud N: Pharmacokinetic considerations in geriatric patients. *In:* Benet LZ, Massoud N, Gambertoglio JG, eds.: Pharmacokinetic Basis for Drug Treatment. New York: Raven Press, 283–310, 1984.
25. Ritschel WA: Gerontokinetics: The Pharmacokinetics of Drugs in the Elderly. Caldwell, NJ: Telford Press, 1988, 1.
26. Aucoin DP: Drug therapy in the geriatric animal: the effect of aging on drug disposition. *Vet Clin North Am Small Anim Prac* 19:41, 1989.
27. Feely J, Coakley D: Altered pharmacodynamics in the elderly. *Clin Pharm* 6:269, 1990.
28. Sheaker S, Bay M: Drug disposition and hepatotoxicity in the elderly. *J Clin Gastroenterol* 18:232, 1994.
29. Papich MG, Davis LE: Drug therapy during pregnancy and in the neonate. *Vet Clin North Am Small Anim Pract* 16:525, 1986.

30. Nau H: Clinical pharmacokinetics in pregnancy and periatology. II. Penicillins [review]. *Dev Pharmacol Ther* 10:174, 1987.
31. Krauer B, Krauer F: Drug kinetics in pregnancy. *In:* Gibaldi M, Prescott L, eds.: Handbook of Clinical Pharmacokinetics. New York: ADIS Health Science Press, 1991, p 1.
32. Levy G: Pharmacokinetics of fetal and neonatal exposure to drugs. *Obstet Gynecol* 58(suppl):9S, 1981.
33. Welsch F: Placental transfer and fetal uptake of drugs. *J Vet Pharmacol Ther* 5:91, 1982.
34. Rasmussen F: Excretion of drugs by milk. *In:* Brodie BB, Gilette JR, eds.: Handbook of Experimental Pharmacology, vol 28: Concepts in Biochemical Pharmacology, Part I. New York: Springer-Verlag, 1979, p 390.
35. Benowitz NL: Effects of cardiac disease on pharmacokinetics: pathophysiologic considerations. *In:* Benet LZ, Massoud N, Gambertoglio JG, eds.: Pharmacokinetic Basis for Drug Treatment. New York: Raven Press, 1984, p 89.
36. Wilkinson GR, Branch RA: Effects of hepatic disease on clinical pharmacokinetics. *In:* Benet LZ, Massoud N, Gambertoglio JG, eds: Pharmacokinetic Basis for Drug Treatment. New York: Raven Press, 1984, p 49.
37. Kawata S, Imai Y, Inada M, *et al.*: Selective reduction of hepatic cytochrome P450 content in patients with intrahepatic cholestasis. *Gastroenterology* 92:299, 1987.
38. Blaschke TF: Protein binding and kinetics of drugs in liver diseases. *In:* Gibaldi M, Prescott L, eds: Handbook of Clinical Pharmacokinetics. New York: ADIS Health Science Press, 1989, p 126.
39. Boothe DM, Brown SA, Jenkins WL, *et al.*: Disposition of indocyanine green in dogs with experimentally-induced dimethylnitrosamine hepatotoxicity. *Am J Vet Res* 53:382, 1992.
40. Boothe DM, Jenkins WL, Brown SA, *et al.*: Antipyrine and caffeine disposition kinetics in dogs with progressive dimethylnitrosamine-induced hepatotoxicity. *Am J Vet Res* 55:254, 1994.
41. Boothe DM: Effects of hepatic disease on drug disposition. *In:* Current Veterinary Therapy XII, Small Animal Practice. Philadelphia, WB Saunders, 1995, 758.
42. Riviere JE: Calculation of dosage regimens of antimicrobial drugs in animals with renal and hepatic dysfunction. *J Am Vet Med Assoc* 185:1094, 1984.
43. Brater DC, Chennavasin P: Effects of renal disease. Altered pharmacokinetics. *In:* Benetz LZ, Massoud N, Gambertoglio JG, eds.: Pharmacokinetic Basis for Drug Treatment. New York: Raven Press, 1985, p 149.
44. Nimmo WS: Drugs, diseases and altered gastric emptying. *Clin Pharmacokin* 1:189, 1976.
45. Eichelbaum M: Drug metabolism in thyroid disease. *Clin Pharmacokin* 1:339, 1976.
46. Belpaire FM, DeRick A, Dello C, *et al.*: Alpha 1-acid glycoprotein and serum binding of drugs in healthy and diseased dogs. *J Vet Pharmacol Ther* 10:43, 1987.
47. Mealey KL, Boothe DM: Bioavailability of benzodiazepines following rectal administration of diazepam in dogs. *J Vet Pharmacol Ther* 18:72, 1995.
48. Otto CM, Kaufman GM, Crowe DT: Intraosseous infusion of fluids and therapeutics. *Compend Contin Educ* 11:421, 1989.
49. Fiser DH: Intraosseous infusion. *N Engl J Med* 322:1579, 1990.
50. Franks JN, Boothe HW, Taylor L, *et al.*: Evaluation of transdermal fentanyl patches for analgesia in cats undergoing onychectomy. *J Am Vet Med Assoc* 217:1013, 2000.

51. Morgan DJ, Smallwood RA: Hepatic drug clearance in chronic liver disease: can we expect to find a universal, quantitative marker of hepatic function? *Hepatology* 10:893, 1989.
52. Griffin JP, D'Arcy PF: A Manual of Adverse Drug Interactions, 2nd ed. Chicago: Billing and Sons, 1979, 3.
53. Boothe DM: Factors affecting drug disposition. *In:* Boothe DM: Small Animal Clinical Pharmacology and Therapeutics. Philadelphia: WB Saunders, 2001.
54. Ansel HC: Ointment, creams, lotions and other dermatological preparations. *In:* Introduction to Pharmaceutical Dosage Forms, 2nd ed. Philadelphia: Lea & Febiger, 1976, p 301.
55. Idson B: Vehicle effects in percutaneous absorption. *Drug Metab Rev* 14:207, 1983.
56. Boothe DM: Topical drugs: component interactions, vehicles and the consequences of alterations. *Dermatol Rep* 6:1, 1987.
57. King JC: Guide to Parenteral Admixtures. St. Louis, MO: Pacemarq.
58. Papich MG: Incompatible critical care drug combinations. *In:* Bonagura JD, ed.: Current Veterinary Therapy XII, Small Animal Practice. Philadelphia: WB Saunders, 1995, p 194.
59. Wallace SM, Chan LY: In vitro interaction of aminoglycosides with beta-lactam penicillins. *Antimicrob Agents Chemother* 28:274, 1985.
60. Eliopoulos GM, Moellering RC: Antimicrobial combinations. *In:* Lorian V (ed): Antibiotics in Laboratory Medicine (4th ed). Williams and Wilkins, 1996, pp 333–396.
61. Gilbert DN, Lee BL, Dworkin RJ, Leggett JL, Chambers HF, *et al.*: A randomized comparison of the safety and efficacy of once-daily gentamicin or thrice-daily gentamicin in combination with ticardillin-clavulanate. *Am J Med* 1998 Sep;105(3):182–91.
62. Toothaker RD, Welling PG: The effect of food on drug bioavailability. *Annu Rev Pharmacol Toxicol* 20:173, 1980.
63. Pond SM: Pharmacokinetic drug interactions. *In:* Benet LZ, Massoud N, Gambertoglio JG, eds.: Pharmacokinetic Basis for Drug Treatment. New York: Raven Press, 1984, p 49.
64. Hostetler KA, Wrighton SA, Molowa DT, *et al.*: Coinduction of multiple hepatic cytochrome P-450 proteins and their mRNAs in rats treated with imidazole antimycotic agents. *Mol Pharmacol* 35:279, 1988.
65. Ohnhaus EE, Taras G-E, Park BK: Enzyme-inducing drug combinations and their effects on liver microsomal enzyme activity in man. *Eur J Clin Pharmacol* 24:247, 1983.
66. Bresnick E: The molecular biology of the induction of the hepatic mixed function oxidases. *In:* Schenkman JB, Kupfer D, eds.: Hepatic Cytochrome P-450 Monooxygenase System. New York: Pergamon Press, 1982, p 99.
67. Snyder R, Remmer H: Class of hepatic microsomal mixed function oxidase inducers. [Review] *Pharmacol Ther* 7:203, 1979.
68. Schenkman JP, Kupfer D: Hepatic Cytochrome P-450 Monooxygenase System New York: Pergamon Press, 1982, 99.
69. Vessey DA: Hepatic metabolism of drugs and toxins. *In:* Zakim D, Boyer T, eds.: A Textbook of Liver Disease. Philadelphia: WB Saunders, 1982, p 197.
70. Netter KJ: Inhibition of oxidative drug metabolism in microsomes. *In:* Schenkman JB, Kupffer D, eds.: Hepatic Cytochrome P-450 Monooxygenase System. New York: Pergamon Press, 1982, p 99.

71. Zed PJ, Krenzelok EP: Treatment of acetaminophen overdose. *Am J Health Syst Pharm* 1999 56:1081, 1999; quiz 1091.
72. Al-Mustafa ZH, Al-Ali AK, Qaw FS, *et al.*: Cimetidine enhances the hepatoprotective action of N-acetylcysteine in mice treated with toxic doses of paracetamol. *Toxicology* 121:223, 1997.
73. Burkhart KK, Janco N, Kulig KW: Cimetidine as adjunctive treatment for acetaminophen overdose. *Hum Exp Toxicol* 14:299, 1995.

SUGGESTED READINGS

Boothe DM: Effects of drugs on endocrine testing. In Current Veterinary Therapy (XII), Small Animal Practice, pp 339–346. Philadelphia, WB Saunders Co, 1995.

Ohnishi A, Bryant TD, Branch KR, *et al.*: Role of sodium in the protective effect of ticarcillin on gentamicin nephrotoxicity in rats. *Antimicrob Agents Chemother* 33: 928, 1989.

Savides MC, Oehme FW, Leipold HW: Effect of various antidotal treatments on acetaminophen toxicosis and biotransformation in cats. *Am J Vet Res* 46:1485, 1985.

Shecter RD, Schalm CW, Kanek JJ: Heinz-body hemolytic anemia associated with the use of urinary antisepics in the cat. *J Am Vet Med Assoc* 162:37, 1983.

Shifrine M, Munn SL, Rosenblatt LS, *et al.*: Hematologic changes to 60 days of age in clinically normal beagles. *Lab Anim* 23:894, 1973.

Smith HW: The development of the flora of the alimentary tract in young animals. *J Pathol Bacteriol* 90:495, 1965.

Stern A: Drug metabolism in renal failure. *Compend Cont Educ* 5:913, 1983.

Van Thiel DH, Hassanein T: Assessment of liver function: the current situation. *J Okla State Med Assoc* 88:11, 1995.

Uber WE, Brundage RC, White RL, *et al.*: In vivo inactivation of tobramycin by piperacillin. *DICP* 25:357, 1991.

79
Rodenticides

J. Michael Walters

INTRODUCTION

Rodenticide toxicosis commonly occurs in veterinary medicine, accounting for a significant number of the poisonings in companion animals. It is more common in dogs than in cats, likely due to cats' discriminating palate and, in the case of the anticoagulant rodenticides, a decreased sensitivity. The common types of rodenticides include anticoagulant compounds, cholecalciferol, bromethalin, strychnine, and zinc phosphide. The less common types of rodenticides include pyriminil, Red squill, thallium, arsenic, phosphorous, α-naphthyl-thiourea (ANTU), norbromide, barium, and sodium monofluoracetate (compound 1080). Among the anticoagulant rodenticides, further stratification occurs by a division into first-generation (warfarin and dicoumarol) and second-generation ("super-warfarin") anticoagulants (brodifacoum, bromadiolone, chlorophacinone, coumafuryl, difenacoum, difethalone, and diphacinone). Second-generation anticoagulant rodenticides are more effective because they have a longer half-life and are more highly protein bound. Because the majority of intoxications occurring in companion animals involve the common types of rodenticides listed above, this chapter is devoted to their pathophysiology, historical findings, clinical presentation, and treatment protocols.

ANTICOAGULANT RODENTICIDES

Pathophysiology

The anticoagulant rodenticides inhibit vitamin K 2,3-epoxide reductase and vitamin K quinone reductase in the liver, preventing the reduction of inactive vitamin K_1 (vitamin K quinone). The result is the prevention of carboxylation of the calcium binding sites on clotting factors II, VII, IX, and X.[1-5] The interference with vitamin K 2,3-epoxide reductase in the biochemical lesion of importance, hindering the "recycling" of active vitamin K quinone and a depletion of the vitamin K-dependent clotting factors II, VII, IX, and X.[1,2,4,7] This clotting factor depletion slows the extrinsic, intrinsic, and common pathways in the clotting cascade with resultant uncontrolled hemorrhage.[1,2,4] The circulating half-lives of factors II, VII, IX, and X in the dog are 4.1, 6.2, 13.9, and 16.5 hours, respectively.[1,2,4] Factor VII has the shortest half-life and is the first to be depleted, affecting the extrinsic branch of the clotting cascade and causing a prolongation of the prothrombin time (PT).[2] As the other clotting factors become affected, other coagulation tests, such as activated partial thromboplastin time (APTT) and activated clotting time (ACT), are prolonged.[2] This indirect mode of action explains the lag time that is observed between the ingestion of the rodenticide and the onset of clinical signs.[1,2,4] Clinical signs may take days to manifest themselves.[1,2]

History

There is no sex, age, or breed predelection.[2] Owners may observe dyspnea, lethargy, cough and hemopytsis, pale mucous membranes, lameness, epistaxis, hyphema, melena, ecchymotic hemorrages or bruising, collapse, anorexia, and hematuria.[1-5] In many cases anorexia, lethargy, and dyspnea may be the only clinical signs of note.[1] Historical considerations should include the use of anticoagulant rodenticides in the environment, evidence of consumption (*e.g.*, chewed bait containers, blue-green pellet fragments in stool or vomitus, spilled baits), season (a higher incidence in the spring and fall), and a repeated historical ingestion of second-generation anticoagulant rodenticides.[1-4] The relative toxicity varies depending on the type, chemical makeup of the rodenticide and type and mass of animal that ingests the bait.

Physical Examination

Clinical signs may be occult for as long as 1 to 2 days after ingestion.[1-4] The most common physical findings are respiratory distress or tachypnea, cough, upper respiratory stridor, pale mucous membranes, muffled heart or lung sounds, lethargy/weakness, evidence of external or internal hemorrhage (*e.g.*, hemoptysis, melena, epistaxis, subcutaneous hemorrhages, hemorrhage from venopuncture sites, and hematoma).[1-4,9,10] Other, less obvious signs include abdominal distention due to hemorrhage effusion, generalized pain, fever, or lameness.[1] On occasion, onset may be so quick as to find the animal dead.[1] These sudden deaths may be attributable to sudden, catastrophic hemorrhage into the pericardium, lungs, thorax, mediastinum, abdomen, or brain.[1] Close inspection of stool may reveal blue-green bait fragments.[2]

Diagnostic Evaluation

A presumptive diagnosis may be made on a history of exposure, consistent physical findings, and laboratory findings.[1] Supportive laboratory findings include decreased packed cell volume (PCV) and prolonged clotting times (ACT, PT, and APTT).[1-6,8-10] Another test of coagulation is the PIVKA test (proteins induced by vitamin K antagonists or absence) that has been reported to be more sensitive than PT in detecting subclinical clotting abnormalities. However, the window within which PIVKA is prolonged while PT is normal is narrow.[2] Therefore, it seems unlikely that an animal would be presented with a anticoagulant rodenticide toxicity where both tests would not be prolonged.[2] PT is the first coagulation parameter to be prolonged and it is not unusual to have hemorrhaging dogs with PT more than 100 seconds and APTT more than 300 seconds.[2]

Anemia, thrombocytopenia, and hypoproteinemia will vary in severity.[2] Other laboratory abnormalities include positive fibrin degradation products and hyperfibrinogenemia.[2] Abnormal radiographic findings showing pleural effusion, pulmonary infiltrates, widened mediastinum, and extraluminal tracheal compression may be noted.[2] A differential diagnosis at this point should include disseminated intravascular coagulation (DIC), congenital coagulopathy, trauma, hemangiosarcoma, renal failure, hepatic failure, and thrombocytopathy.[2]

Treatment

For the symptomatic animal, treatment goals include providing replacement clotting factors to prevent further blood loss, replenish vitamin K_1 stores, replenish red blood cells in the face of an anemia, and supportive care.[2] Vitamin K_1 is indicated in all cases of intoxication.[1-6,8-10] Vitamin K has no direct effect on coagulation and new clotting factor synthesis takes 6 to 12 hours to occur.[1,4] A loading dose of 2.5 to 5.0 mg/kg PO, followed by 2.5 to 5.0 mg/kg divided q 8 to 12 h for a minimum of 5 days or up to 6 weeks depending on the type of toxin ingested.[1-4,9,10] Whenever possible, the oral administration of vitamin K_1 is recommended owing to its increased bioavailability.[1-4] This bioavailability can be enhanced by a fatty meal.[2] It should be remembered that activated charcoal can interfere with the absorption of vitamin K_1; therefore, an initial dose administered subcutaneously (SQ) may be used.[1] If the case demands, higher loading doses of vitamin K_1 (4-5 mg/kg) can be used with lower subsequent doses.[2] SQ vitamin K_1 can be used if oral preparations cannot be tolerated.[2] Intravenous (IV) administration should be avoided due to the risk of anaphylaxis and intramuscular (IM) administration due to the risk of hematoma formation.[1-4] The second-generation rodenticides may require vitamin K_1 therapy for as long as 6 weeks.[1-4]

Fresh-frozen plasma (FFP) is a ready source of clotting factors and should be used if the animal is not anemic.[1-3] Whole, fresh blood may not have enough plasma to provide adequate clotting factors.[2] If the animal is anemic, then whole blood, perhaps with additional FFP, or packed red blood cells (PRBC) are indicated.[2] Hemoglobin substitutes are a new and novel method in the treatment of anemia. The advantages of using a hemoglobin glutamer include ready accessibility, 3-year shelf-life, no risk of disease transmission, no need to type or crossmatch, and no risk of transfusion reaction such as those to preformed alloantibodies to RBC antigens. Disadvantages to a hemoglobin glutamer include discolored urine, sclera, and mucous membranes; interference with some serum chemistry values; potential for volume overload due to its colloidal effects; and a short half-life (18-42 hours for Oxyglobin versus 21-42 days for whole or PRBC). A dosage range of 5 to 30 mL/kg, not to exceed 10 mL/kg/h as been used in the treatment of anemia in dogs. It is not approved by the Food and Drug Administration for the use in cats.

Treatment response should be monitored by using clotting times with PT being the preferred method; protocols vary as to the frequency of testing.[1,2] The PT should return to normal within 1 hour of administration of FFP or whole

Table 79-1. Drugs That Increase the Sensitivity to Vitamin K Rodenticides[2]

Chloramphenicol
Trimethoprim-sulfa
Neomycin
Tetracycline
Ibuprofen
Ketoprofen
Phenylbutazone
Cimetidine
Quinidine

blood.[2] If vitamin K_1 alone is used, PT should be reassessed at 12 to 24 hours.[2] A PT should be rechecked 2 to 4 days after the cessation of vitamin K_1 treatment.[1,2] Under special circumstances, a lactating bitch may ingest a vitamin K antagonist rodenticide. Although there are no data to prove that these rodenticides pass into the milk in dogs, data in lactating women support the passage of warfarin into the milk.[3] Puppies and kittens are likely more sensitive because of their reduced hepatic metabolism of the drug.[3] If the lactating animal is nursing, the puppies or kittens should be weaned, if possible, and treated with 2.5 to 5 mg/kg, vitamin K_1, PO, divided q 8 to 12 h for 2 to 3 weeks or should be allowed to nurse, treated as above, with the therapy continued for at least 1 week after the mother's treatment is stopped.[3] If the intoxicated animal happens to be pregnant, the pups may not be able to eliminate the toxin *in utero*.[3] Therefore, the bitch should be treated using the above protocol until she whelps and the offspring treated for at least 1 week or until their coagulation profile normalizes.[3] Many drugs increase the sensitivity to anticoagulant rodenticides.[2] A partial list of commonly used drugs of veterinary interest can be found in Table 79-1.

Certain colloid products have been associated with an induced coagulopathy and should be used with caution in intoxicated animals.[2] Heparin, which may be used for the treatment of DIC, may worsen the hemorrhage and, therefore, should be avoided.[2] There are other forms of vitamin K (vitamin K_3) that should *not* be used in treatment of vitamin K antagonist rodenticide, because they require hepatic metabolism to become active.[2]

Prognosis

A favorable prognosis includes an early return to normal clotting times, early detection of intoxication, and a 48-hour survival time.[2] Unfavorable prognostic indicators include hemorrhage into the lungs or brain and delayed presentation.[2]

CHOLECALCIFEROL

Cholecalciferol [CCF 0.075%] rodenticides have been marketed under the brand names Quintox (Bell Laboratories), Rampage (Ceva Laboratories), Ortho Rat-B-Gon, and Ortho Mouse-B-Gon (Chevron Chemicals).[1,6,10] Intoxication in dogs is most commonly reported in adults dogs (>1 year of age) and juvenile cats

(<1 year of age).[1,6] In cats, this increased sensitivity may be due to the indiscriminate feeding habits of young cats and a dose-response effect due to smaller body size or an increased sensitivity to CCF or its metabolites.[1] There is no sex predilection and the overall incidence of toxicity is unknown.[1,5] Animals with preexisting renal disease are at increased risk.[1] The LD_{50} of the 100% technical grade material has been reported as 88 mg/kg; however, a toxicity can occur with dosages as little as 2 to 3 mg CCF/kg body weight.[1]

Pathophysiology

Calcium homeostasis is under strict control of calcitonin, parathyroid hormone (PTH), and vitamin D metabolites.[1] These hormones regulate the ionized calcium concentration through control of intestinal uptake, renal excretion, and skeletal mobilization of calcium.[1] PTH increases serum calcium via activation of osteoclasts and lowering in bone resorption.[1,6,10] Calcitonin acts as an antagonist to PTH by inhibiting osteoclasts and lowering serum calcium levels.[1,6,10] Vitamin D and its metabolites increase intestinal absorption of calcium, stimulate bone resorption, and increase renal tubular resorption of calcium.[1,6,10] As a fat-soluble vitamin, CCF is absorbed into the lymphatics via chylomicrons.[1,6,10] In the liver, CCF is further metabolized to 25-hydroxycholecalciferol (25-OH-D_3), which is the major metabolite during vitamin D_3 excess.[1,6,10] Further metabolism occurs in the kidney, where 25-OH-D_3 is converted to calcitriol (1,25-$(OH)_2$-D_3).[1,6,10] Cholecalciferol and 25-OH-D_3 have limited biologic activity, whereas calcitriol has the most potent biologic activity by enhancing bone resorption and intestinal calcium transport.[1,6,10] The result of excess vitamin D_3 ingestion is hypercalcemia (>12 mg/dL) and dystrophic calcification of tissues.[1,6,10]

Clinical Presentation

Clinical signs can be divided into four main categories: neurologic, cardiovascular, renal, and gastrointestinal.[1,6,10] Clinical signs typically develop within 12 to 36 hours after ingestion of CCF.[1,6,10] Common clinical signs include the vomiting, depression, anorexia, polyuria, polydipsia, and diarrhea with or without hematochezia/melena.[1,6,10] The presence of blood in the stool may mislead the clinician to the diagnosis of anticoagulant rodenticide.[1] Uncommon clinical signs include bradycardia, cardiac arrhythmias, and shock.[1] These cardiac arrhythmias result from changes in membrane stability and excitability, a slowing of conduction, and a decreased automaticity, which is reflected by prolongation of the PR interval and QT shortening.[6] As the hypercalcemic state worsens, ventricular fibrillation may result from the conduction impairment or direct myocardial necrosis secondary to dystrophic mineralization.[6] A persistent hypercalcemia can result in dystrophic calcium deposition occurring in the kidneys resulting in worsening of renal insufficiency.[1] However, acute renal failure can occur without calcium deposition.[1] Biochemical alterations include marked hypercalcemia (>12 mg/dL), hypoproteinemia, hyperphosphatemia, glucosuria, variable urine cytologic changes, possible metabolic acidosis, and azotemia.[1,6] A differential diagnosis list should include juvenile hyercalcemia, paraneoplastic syndrome, primary renal failure, hypoadrenocorticism, hemoconcentration, and primary hyperparathyroidism.[1,6] The associated metabolic acidosis will cause an increase in ionized caclium (physiologically active) via a hydrogen ion-induced displacement of calcium from albumen.[1]

The diagnosis of CCF rodenticide toxicity depends on a history of potential exposure, appropriate clinical signs, and the development of hypercalcemia plus the ancillary indicators of hyperphosphatemia and azotemia.[1,6] Hypercalcemia and hyperphosphatemia typically develop with 12 to 24 hours.[1,6] Azotemia may be either renal or prerenal in origin.[1,6] Urinalysis results may show hyposthenuria, proteinuria, and glucosuria.[1,6] Urine sediment changes are variable. Radiographic and ultrasound studies may show mineralization of the kidneys.[1,6,10]

Treatment

Current treatment recommendations from the ASPCA National Animal Poison Control Center (ASPCA NAPCC) include the following: decontamination via an emetic, if exposure is less than 4 hours—hydrogen peroxide 1 T/15 lb, maximum 3 T; apomorphine 0.04 mg/kg SQ or administered subconjunctively to effect and repeated doses of activated charcoal, 6 to 12 mL/kg as a slurry or 1 to 2 g as a capsule or powder, PO, q 8 to 12 h for 2 to 3 doses. Laboratory monitoring including baseline calcium (Ca), phosphorus (P), blood urea nitrogen (BUN), creatinine (Cr); a complete blood count and serum chemistry is recommended in older animals or those with pre-existing disease. If Ca, P, BUN, and Cr are within normal limits on presentation, monitor Ca, P, BUN, Cr q 12 h for at least 4 days. The P concentration tends to elevate before Ca. Treatment can be discontinued if all monitored parameters remain normal for 96 hours. If Ca, P, BUN, and Cr are abnormal on presentation, hypercalcemic management is required. Monitor the Ca × P product, if greater than 60, then soft-tissue mineralization is likely to occur. (Be sure to convert both Ca and P units to mg/dL before calculating the Ca × P product.)

Two protocols are recommended to treat hypercalcemia. The preferred protocol involves the use of pamidronate disodium. Pamidronate (Aredia) is a bisphosphonate that is used in human medicine for the treatment of hypercalcemia of malignancy. Normal saline (IV) is the fluid of choice. Dehydration should be corrected, then forced diuresis at twice maintenance until Ca levels begin to drop. Furosemide is dosed at 2.5 to 4.5 mg/kg PO, SQ q 6 to 18 h or via continuous IV infusion; avoid thiazide diuretics becuase they inhibit calceuresis. Dexamethasone 1 mg/g IV, SQ q 6 h or prednisone at 2 to 3 mg/kg PO, SQ q 12 are also administered. Pamidronate can be given at 1.3 to 2 mg/kg, diluted in 250 mL normal saline and administered IV over a 2-hour period.[11] The second protocol is essentially the same as above except for the use of calcitonin instead of pamidronate. Salmon calcitonin (Calcimar) is dosed at 4 to 7 IU/kg SQ q 8 h.[11] The hypercalcemia management using the alternative method is considered less desirable because calcitonin is inconsistent in its ability to lower calcium, and some dogs become refractory to its effects.

Once calcium levels have stabilized, the patient can be weaned off IV fluid support. Ca, P, BUN, and Cr are monitored at least every 24 hours. If BUN and Cr remain elevated, continued treatment for acute renal failure is indicated.[11] If Ca levels start to rise, reinstitute fluid therapy and consider repeat pamidronate dosing. This can be expected to occur with 5 to 7 days after the initial dose, if it occurs at all.[11] In most cases, a single dose of pamidronate is all that is required.[11] A change to oral medications can be made as long as the patient remains normal, has a good appetite (poor appetite can be an early indicator of a rise in Ca), and serum Ca, P, BUN, and Cr concentrations remain within normal limits. Aluminum hydroxide (Amphogel) at 60 mg/kg PO q 8 h can be used if P values remain elevated.[11] Monitor Ca and P for 5 to 7 days after values return to normal, then two to three times a week for 2 weeks and then 1 month after exposure.[11]

BROMETHALIN

Bromethalin is a newer, nonanticoagulant rodenticide introduced in 1985.[1,5,10] It was introduced as a 0.01% based, single-feeding rodenticide under the trade names of Vengeance, Trounce, Assault, Hot Shot, and Sudden Death Mouse Killer.[1,5] Bromethalin-based rodenticides are a pelleted, tan or green, grain-based product packaged as 0.75- to 1.5-oz packs. Biterex (denatonium benzoate) has been recently added to bromethalin bait to deter human consumption (Biterex is also found in other rodenticides).[10] This substance does not interfere with its toxicity as a rodenticide but does make the bait bad tasting, making it difficult for humans to consume a toxic dose.[10] The reported LD_{50} for technical grade bromethalin in cats is reported as 1.8 mg/kg, and 4.7 mg/kg in dogs.[1,5] The minimum toxic dose is reported as 16.7 g/kg in dogs and 3.0 g/kg in cats.[1,5,10] The minimum lethal dose bait in cats is 4.5 g/kg and 25.0 g/kg in dogs.[1,5]

Pathophysiology

The mechanism of action is specifically unknown. It is thought to uncouple oxidative phosphorylation in brain and liver and acts as a neurotoxin.[1,5,10] This leads to a decreased production of adenosine triphosphate (ATP), a diminished activity in Na^+/K^+ ATPase and a subsequent fluid accumulation resulting in cerebral edema.[1,5,10] The cerebral edema ultimately causes an increase in cerebrospinal fluid (CSF) pressure, an increased pressure on nerve axons, and a decreased nerve impulse conduction.[1,5,10]

Clinical Signs

Clinical signs are variable and can present as an acute or chronic syndrome.[1,5,10] Higher doses may present as a more acute onset of signs within 24 hours of ingestion.[1,5,10] Signs include muscle tremors, hyperexcitability, paddling, hyperesthesia, hyperthermia secondary to excess muscle activity, and seizures.[1,5,10] Doses less than the LD_{50} of bait produce a toxic syndrome that is characterized by a lower onset, 24 to 96 hours.[1,5,10] Clinical signs include hind limb ataxia or paresis with or without central nervous system depression.[1,5,10] The most common clinical signs reported to the ASPCA NAPCC include vomiting, ataxia, seizures, tremors, depression, coma, and mydriasis.[1] It becomes apparent that bromethalin toxicosis can mimic a wide variety of disease processes.

Diagnosis

The diagnosis of bromethalin toxicity is entirely dependent on the history of exposure and subsequent development of appropriate clinical signs.[1,5,10] Chemical conformation of bromethalin residues is not widely available.[1,5,10] It can be detected in liver, kidney, and brain tissues but has limited clinical utility.[1] It should be considered as differential diagnosis for cases of cerebral edema and posterior paresis.[5,10]

Treatment

Because there are no reliable methods to detect bromethalin residues, prevention of further absorption from the gastrointestinal tract through decontamination via emetics, activated charcoal, and cathartics becomes extremely important.[1,5,10] Bromethalin absorption is rapid; peak levels occur in less than 4 hours in experimental studies in rats, and excretion is very slow with a plasma half-life of 5.6 days.[1] Supportive care methods are equally important. Methods to decrease the CSF pressure such as mannitol and corticosteroids may be needed for many days, although their effectiveness is under question.[1,5,10] The prognosis for their patients is guarded to poor depending on their presence of clinical signs and the time interval since exposure.[1,5,10]

STRYCHNINE

Strychnine has been largely replaced by zinc phosphide since 1990, but is provided as a historical reference and the possibility that it may be encountered on a rare occasion. It was available under numerous brand names for the control of mice, rats, gophers, and moles. Strychnine is a plant alkaloid derivative found in the seeds of the *Strychnos nux vomica*, a tree native to India.[10] It was introduced in Germany in the 16th century for the control of rats and is still reported today with some 186 exposures reported in 1994.[10]

Pathophysiology

Toxic amounts are rapidly absorbed in the gastrointestinal tract.[10] The primary effect is an antagonizing of inhibitory neurotransmitter, glycine, at the postsynaptic spinal cord motor neurons leading to uncontrolled excitation of spinal cord reflexes.[2,10]

Clinical Signs

Generalized seizures may occur within 15 to 30 minutes of exposure.[10] Seizures may be clonic at first, progressing to tonic with time.[10] All voluntary muscles contract and respiration is impaired.[10] Seizure episodes may occur repeatedly, followed by periods of remission and may be precipitated by sensory stimulus.[5,10]

Classically, a sawhorse stance is described.[2] Secondary hyperthermia can occur as affected animals remain conscious throughout the events.[2]

Diagnosis

History of exposure is the chief diagnostic coupled with compatible clinical signs.[2] Detection of strychnine in vomitus, gastric contents, lavage fluid, and urine will help confirm exposure.[2] Laboratory findings include elevated lactic acid concentrations, increased serum creatine phosphokinase values, and myoglobinuria.[2]

Treatment

The primary management is the prevention or control of convulsions.[2,10] Emesis is contraindicated due to rapid onset of clinical signs and sensitivity to external stimulus precipitating seizures with possible aspiration of stomach contents.[2,10] Activated charcoal can be used if clinical signs are minimal or absent, but should be withheld until seizures are controlled.[2,10] Control of seizures is achieved using barbiturates, such as phenobarbital, or benzodiazapines like diazepam. Diazepam is reported to be preferred in humans because it does not potentiate postictal depression.[10]

Once the animal is anesthetized, gastric lavage and administration of activated charcoal can be performed, with or without a cathartic.[2] Muscle relaxants such as glycerol guaiacolate (100 mg/kg as needed) or methocarbamol (55-220 mg/kg IV, as needed, not to exceed 330 mg/kg/d) may be used to reduce the reliance on barbiturates.[2] In some cases, general anesthesia and mechanical ventilation may be needed.[2] Supportive care via IV fluids to maintain urine output and prevent renal damage from myoglobinura is often needed.[2] Acidification to enhance renal excretion of strychnine is *not* recommended.[2] Prognosis is good if clinical signs are caught early and adequate supportive care is provided for 24 to 48 hours.[2]

ZINC PHOSPHIDE

Zinc phosphide has largely replaced strychnine as a rodenticide.[10] Phosphides are used throughout the world in protect grains from rodents and other pests.[10] On contact with moisture or acid, phosphides form phosphine gas, which is thought to be responsible for their toxic effects.[10] Besides zinc compounds, aluminum and magnesium phosphide can also be found.[10]

Pathophysiology

Phosphides are rapidly broken down in the acid environment of the stomach to release phosphine gas.[2,5,10] The exact mechanism is unclear, but phosphine has been shown to block cytochrome c, inhibiting oxidative phosphorylation and therefore energy production within the cell, resulting in cell death.[2,5,10] There is also a direct irritant effect on the gastrointestinal tract and lungs.[2,5,10] In humans, hypotension and shock are common features in serious cases.[10] Additionally, myocardial injury, arrhythmias, tachypnea, cyanosis, and adult respiratory distress syndrome are reported.[10]

Clinical Signs

Acute onset of emesis, depression, tremors, and weakness progress rapidly to recumbency.[2] Pulmonary edema develops over time.[2] Routine laboratory findings are not helpful.[2] Phosphine gas is heavier than air and has an odor described as rotten fish.[10] This can not, unfortunately, be used as a diagnostic aid.[10]

Treatment

If the exposure is caught early, the treatment is decontamination, with or without activated charcoal/cathartics. Oral administration of 5% sodium bicarbonate may limit acid hydrolysis of zinc phosphide in the stomach, but the efficacy is uncertain.[2] Symptomatic and supportive care remains the mainstay of treatment.[2]

REFERENCES

1. Dorman DC: Toxicology of selected pesticides, drugs and chemicals. Anticoagulant, cholecaliferol, and bromethalin-based rodenticides. *Vet Clin North Am Small Anim Pract* 20:339, 1990.
2. Poppenga RH: Rodenticide toxicosis in dogs and cats. *Compend Standards of Care Emerg Crit Care Med* 2:5, 2000.
3. Lawrence JF, Murphy MJ: CVT Update: anticoagulant rodenticides. *In* Bonagura JD, ed.: Kirk's Current Veterinary Therapy XII. Philadelphia: WB Saunders, 1995, p 228.
4. Murphy MJ, Gerken DF: The anticoagulant rodenticides. *In* Kirk RW, ed.: Kirk's Current Veterinary Therapy X. Philadelphia: WB Saunders, 1989, p 143.
5. Carson, TL: Bromethalin poisoning. *In* Kirk RW, ed.: Kirk's Current Veterinary Therapy X. Philadelphia: WB Saunders, 1989, p 147.
6. Dorman DC, Beasley VR: Diagnosis and therapy for cholecalciferol toxicosis. *In* Kirk, RW, ed.: Kirk's Veterinary Therapy X. Philadelphia: WB Saunders, 1989, p 148.
7. Peterson J, Streeter V: Laryngeal obstruction secondary to brodifacoum toxicosis in a dog. *J Am Vet Med Assoc* 208:352, 1996.
8. Petrus DJ, Henik RA: Pericardial effusion and cardiac tamponade secondary to brodifacoum toxicosis in a dog. *J Am Vet Med Assoc* 215:647, 1999.
9. Murphy MJ: CVT Update: Rodenticide toxicosis. *In* Bonagura JD, ed.: Kirk's Current Veterinary Therapy XIII. Philadelphia: WB Saunders, 2000, p 211.
10. Metts BC, Stewart NJ: Rodenticides. *In* Haddad LM, Shannon MW, Winchester JF, eds.: Clinical Management of Poisoning and Drug Overdose. Philadephia: WB Saunders, 1998, p 864.
11. ASPCA National Animal Poison Control Center Recommended Management of Calciptriene (Donovex®) Ingestion in Dogs, Revised September, 1999.

80
Accidental Hypothermia

Wayne E. Wingfield

INTRODUCTION

Accidental hypothermia is defined as a state of body temperature that is below normal in a homeopathic animal.[1] The normal body temperature for a dog is greater than 37.5°C (99.5°F)[a] and for a cat, 37.8°C (100.0°F). When the animal is unable to maintain thermal homeostasis after prolonged exposure to cold, hypothermia results. In more moderate environmental conditions, hypothermia may be a manifestation of disease processes that alter normal thermoregulation[2] or may inadvertently develop with anesthetic[3] or antiphlogistic drugs. Table 80-1 provides guidelines on how the severity of hypothermia can be graded.[4]

Core body temperature is a measure central body temperature away from the vasoconstrictor effect of peripheral vasculature. It can be measured rectally,[b] esophageally, from the tympanic membrane of the external ear, or from a central intravenous (IV) catheter equipped with an electronic thermistor.

PATHOGENESIS

An animal maintains its body temperature by balancing heat loss from the skin and lungs and heat production from the skeletal muscle and liver.[5] Heat production increases with food ingestion, muscular activity, fever, and acute exposure to cold. When preshivering muscle tone increases as a result of hypothermia, heat production can double. With cold exposure and shivering, maximal heat production lasts only a few hours because of fatigue and glycogen depletion.[6]

When an awake animal is exposed to the cold, it will attempt to conserve heat via behavioral changes (seeking shelter or curling up into a ball). Physiologic responses include piloerection and peripheral vasoconstriction. The trapping of air next to the skin as well as shunting blood away from the periphery provides thermal insulation. Heat loss from the body is primarily from four mechanisms: convection, conduction, radiation, and evaporation. In animals, most heat loss is from convection and conduction. In contrast, in humans, radiation heat loss accounts for 55% to 65% and conduction accounts for 2% to 3% (but may increase to 5 times with wet clothing and 25 times in cold water).[7] Conduc-

[a] Formula for converting Celsius to Fahrenheit: F = (C × 1.8) + 32. Formula for converting Fahrenheit to Celcius: C = (F − 32) ÷ 1.8.

[b] Note: Rectal temperature can be falsely low if the thermometer is in cold feces.

Table 80-1. Guidelines for Grading the Severity of Hypothermia in the Dog and Cat

Core Temperature	Severity of Hypothermia
32°–37° (90°–99°F)	Mild
28°–32° (82°–90°F)	Moderate
<28°C (82°F)	Severe

tion and convection normally account for about 15% of heat loss in people, but convective losses increase with shivering. Respiration and evaporation account for the remainder of heat loss in people with 2% and 9% lost in heating inspired air, and 20% to 27% lost to insensible evaporation from the skin and lungs.[8] With increasing subcutaneous fat thickness there is greater insulation and slower loss of heat.

Heat production may involve voluntary muscle activity (*i.e.*, shivering). Shivering thermogenesis increases the basal metabolic rate two to five times. This shivering also increases oxygen (O_2) consumption and is modulated by the hypothalamus and spinal cord. The hypothalamus orchestrates nonshivering heat conservation and dissipation. Serotonergic and dopaminergic neurons appear to be pivotal.[9] They exert immediate control through the autonomic nervous system and delayed control through the endocrine system. Thermal suppression or activation of the sympathetic nervous system with cold-induced norepinephrine release also occurs. Cold stimulates the hypothalamus to release thyrotropin-releasing hormone. This activates the pituitary, which releases thyroid-stimulating hormone, and results in the release of thyroxine from the thyroid.

With mild hypothermia (see Table 80-1), vasoconstriction, shivering, and nonshivering basal and endocrinologic thermogenesis generate heat. As the core temperature drops to moderate levels, a progressive drop in basal metabolic rate occurs without shivering thermogenesis. Finally, in severe hypothermia, autonomic and endocrinologic mechanisms for heat conservation become inactive.[10]

Predictable cardiovascular responses to hypothermia occur. After an initial tachycardia, a progressive bradycardia develops. The pulse usually decreases by 50% at 28°C (82°F). This bradycardia results from decreased spontaneous depolarization of the cardiac pacemaker cells. As a result, the bradycardia is usually refractory to atropine. There will also be a decrease in mean arterial pressure, respiratory rate, and cardiac output.[11] Increased blood viscosity and increased afterload secondary to peripheral vasoconstriction, and capillary sludging of blood further reduce the cardiac output.

Because the conduction system of the heart is more sensitive to cold than the myocardium, cardiac cycle prolongation occurs (lengthening of the PR, QRS, and QT intervals).[12] Atrial irritability is a feature of early hypothermia. As the body temperature drops, ventricular irritability increases and the animal is predisposed to premature ventricular contractions, tachycardia, and fibrillation. Hypothermia causes a decrease in transmembrane resting potential, which decreases the threshold for ventricular dysrhythmias. When core body temperature is below 28°C (82°F), ventricular fibrillation is common and tends to be unresponsive to electrical defibrillation.[13]

In humans, the Osborn (J) waves are potentially diagnostic but not prognostic. This secondary wave is positive and follows the S wave. It is most commonly seen in leads aVL, aVF, and the left precordial leads. They appear at any temperature less than 32°C (90°F). These abnormal waves appear to be a result of hypothermic ion flux alterations, with delayed depolarization or early repolarization of the left ventricular wall.[14] Unfortunately, the Osborn wave is rarely recognized in small animals.[13]

Following removal from the cold, there is often a further decline in an individual's core temperature. This phenomenon is called "afterdrop." Two processes that contribute to afterdrop are simple temperature equilibration across a gradient and circulatory changes.[15] Countercurrent cooling of the blood, which is perfusing cold tissues, results in a decline in temperature until the gradient is eliminated.

Active external rewarming of the extremities will obliterate peripheral vasoconstriction and reverses arteriovenous shunting.[16] Warm bath immersion rewarming causes a 30% fall in mean arterial pressure, coupled with a 50% decline in peripheral vascular resistance.[17]

Core temperature afterdrop is clinically relevant when treating animals with a large temperature gradient between core and the peripheral tissues. Major afterdrops also occur in severely hypothermic animals if frostbitten extremities are thawed before thermal stabilization.

Exposure to cold will induce a diuresis regardless of the animal's state of hydration. In hypothermia, renal blood flow is reduced by 50% at 27° to 30°C (81°–86°F) resulting in part from reduced tubular reabsorption[18] and depressed production of antidiuretic hormone. These events are a direct consequence of the hypervolemia induced by early vasoconstriction. After the initial diuresis, renal blood flow and glomerular filtration rate decrease as the cardiac output decreases.[4]

With hypothermia there is also depressed central nervous system (CNS) function. With severe hypothermia there is disproportionately higher redistribution of blood flow to the brain. Like the heart, the brain has a critical period of tolerance to hypothermia. There are temperature-dependent neural enzyme systems that are unable to function. The most obvious change is a decreased level of consciousness, which culminates in coma. Cerebral metabolism in humans decreases 6% to 7% for each degree Celsius decline in temperature. Significant changes in the brain's electrical activity begins below 33.5°C (92°F) and the electroencephalogram is flat at 19° to 20°C (66°–68°F).[19] In fact, an animal may appear to be dead with severe hypothermia. The decreased cellular metabolism allows the animal to meet metabolic demands for a short period, even in the presence of bradycardia, asystole, and ventricular fibrillation. In dogs, O_2 consumption is decreased to 50% when the temperature is 30°C (86°F) and to 16% of normal at 23°C (73°F).[20] Delivery of O_2 is slowed by a combination of alveolar hypoventilation, decreased oxyhemoglobin dissociation, and sludging of blood.

Respiration is initially stimulated by hypothermia. This is followed by a progressive decrease in respiratory minute volume, which is proportional to the decreasing metabolism. Carbon dioxide production will decrease 50% with an 8°C (10.8°F) fall in body temperature.[21] Other respiratory effects of hypothermia include the development of respiratory acidosis with carbon dioxide retention, viscous bronchorrhea, decreased ciliary motility, and noncardiogenic pulmonary edema.[22]

Electrolyte changes in hypothermia are unpredictable. As hypothermia progresses, the serum concentration of sodium tends to decrease and potassium increases. This is likely due to decreased enzymatic activity of the cell membrane's sodium–potassium pump. Total body sodium and potassium are close to normal.

Decreasing body temperature has complex effects on blood coagulation. In dogs with decreased splenic perfusion induced by hypothermia, there is a reduction in circulating white blood cells and platelets.[23] With hypothermia there is a platelet dysfunction which occurs.[24] Disseminated intravascular coagulopathy may also occur in severe hypothermia. Interestingly, in humans, hypothermia prolongs the coagulation times (activated partial thromboplastin time and prothrombin time) even with normal levels of clotting factors.[25] Standard clotting tests that are run in the laboratory at 37°C (98.6°F) will not reflect the effects of hypothermia on the enzymes of the clotting cascade.

Hypothermia also has exocrine and endocrine effects on the pancreas. Mainly there is a decrease in insulin production. Hyperglycemia may result but this is often short-lived as the shivering animal readily consumes this glucose. The end result is that the animal is often normoglycemic.

EPIDEMIOLOGY

Many variables contribute to the development of hypothermia. Exposure to extreme cold, age, health, nutritional condition, medications, trauma, and mobility (Table 80-2). All these factors result in either an increased heat loss, decreased heat production, or loss of thermostability.

Undoubtedly the occurrence of hypothermia is grossly underestimated. Few days go by that an animal under prolonged anesthesia is not found to be mildly or moderately hypothermic during the postoperative interval. Smaller animals are more susceptible to hypothermia because of their greater body surface/mass ratio. Too, hypothermia is geographically and seasonally pervasive.

CLINICAL PRESENTATION

When exposure is obvious, the diagnosis is simple. Because standard mercury thermometers can only measure temperatures as low as 34°C (93°F), severe hypothermia can easily be overlooked. A history of environmental exposure, trauma, illness, the patient's age, and anesthesia or drug administration is helpful. Early clinical signs are vague and include mental dullness, abnormal and ataxic gait, shivering, and lethargy. With moderate hypothermia, muscle stiffness without shivering is usually seen. In severe hypothermia the animal may be mistaken as

Table 80-2. Factors Predisposing Animals to Hypothermia

Decreased Heat Production	Increased Heat Loss	Impaired Thermoregulation
Trauma	Trauma	Central failure (CNS trauma, toxins, metabolic, hypothalamic disease, cerebellar lesions, neoplasia)
Immobility	Immobility	Peripheral failure (acute spinal cord injuries, neuropathies, diabetes)
Anesthetic agents	Anesthetic agents	Overwhelming sepsis
Malnutrition	Environmental exposure	Cardiopulmonary disease
Cardiopulmonary diseases	Surgery	Uremia
Endocrine disorders	Size of the animal	Hypotension and hypovolemia
CNS lesions that impair thermoregulation	Toxins (ethylene glycol, barbiturates, carbon monoxide, vasodilator drugs)	
Patient's age (neonates and aged)	Iatrogenic (heat stroke treatment, cold infusions	

dead. The heart sounds are often inaudible, respiratory movements are difficult to detect, and the pupils are fixed and dilated. Extraordinary attempts to detect vital signs should include an electrocardiogram (ECG) and measurement of tidal volume and blood pressure. An often-heard comment about hypothermia is "the hypothermic animal is not dead until it is warm and dead!"

Laboratory assessment of the hypothermic animal is often confusing and misleading. The patient's packed cell volume (PCV) may be deceptively high as a result of the decreased plasma volume. As a general rule, the PCV should increase 2% for each 1°C (1.8°F) fall in temperature.[26] A normal PCV in a moderate to severely hypothermic patient should raise suspicion for acute blood loss or suggest a pre-existing anemia. Leukopenia and thrombocytopenia have been observed in hypothermia but generally are reversed with rewarming. A normal white blood cell (WBC) count does not exclude infection, especially if the animal is debilitated or at each age extreme. Splenic, hepatic, and splanchnic sequestration decreases leukocyte and platelet counts in hypothermia.

Frequent assessment of serum electrolytes is essential during rewarming. Unfortunately there appears to be no safe predictor of their values or trends.[27] Changes will occur in both membrane permeability and in the sodium–potassium pump. The animal's pre-existing physiologic status, the severity and chronicity of hypothermia, and the method of rewarming will alter the serum electrolyte values.[28]

Plasma potassium levels are independent of the primary hypothermic process. Hyperkalemia is often a consequence of metabolic acidosis, rhabdomyolyis, and occasionally renal failure. Importantly, hypothermia enhances the cardiac toxicity and obscures the premonitory ECG changes often seen with hyperkalemia.

Hypokalemia is most commonly seen with chronic hypothermia in humans.[27] It appears to result from potassium entering the muscle, not a kaliuresis. The paradoxical decline in serum potassium level despite a decreasing serum pH is caused by intracellular pH fluxes greater than extracellular pH fluxes.[29] If the serum potassium is less than 3 mEq/L, the addition of 20 to 30 mEq/L potassium chloride to the crystalloid fluid may reduce the gastrointestinal ileus or congestive heart failure of rewarming.

Blood urea nitrogen (BUN) and creatinine levels are seen with pre-existing renal disease or decreased renal clearance. Because of hypothermic fluid shifts, the PCV and the BUN levels are poor indicators of the animal's hydration status.

Blood glucose may provide a subtle clue to the type of hypothermia. Acute hypothermia initially elevates the glucose through catecholamine-induced glycogenolysis, diminished insulin release, and inhibition of cellular membrane glucose carrier systems. On the other hand, subacute and chronic hypothermia induce glycogen depletion leading to hypoglycemia. Symptoms of hypoglycemia are often masked by hypothermia. A cold-induced renal glycosuria does not imply hyperglycemia. Should hyperglycemia persist during rewarming, hemorrhagic pancreatitis or diabetic ketoacidosis should be suspected. Animals with diabetes must be actively rewarmed past 30°C (86°F) because insulin is ineffective below that temperature.

Traditionally, arterial blood gas (ABG) values are adjusted for body temperature based on the concept that pH values at normal temperatures are also appropriate for hypothermia. Currently, the correction of ABGs for temperature is unnecessary as a guide to therapy.[30] When blood cools, the arterial pH increases and the PCO_2 falls. This is due to the direct effect of temperature on both the dissolution of hydrogen ions and gas pressures in the watery solution. Because water dissociates less readily at a lower temperature than at a higher one, the pH of neutrality is higher at 30°C (86°F) than at 37°C (98.6°F). Thus, a pH of 7.4 and a PCO_2 of 40 mm Hg at a temperature of 37°C (98.6°F) are physiologically equivalent to a pH of 7.5 and a PCO_2 of 30 mm Hg at a temperature of 30°C (86°F). Correcting the ABG value to normal values by the analyzer induces a relative respiratory acidosis. This acidosis depresses cerebral and coronary blood flow and cardiac output and increases the occurrence of ventricular fibrillation.[30] Because the arterial PCO_2 decreases with the temperature, the animal would be inappropriately hypoventilated to maintain bicarbonate content in the blood at normothermic levels. In fact, there is normal alveolar ventilation and acid–base balance at any temperature when the uncorrected pH and PCO_2 are maintained at 7.4 and 40 mm Hg.[26] To accurately interpret uncorrected ABGs, the values should be compared to normal values.[30]

The use of uncorrected ABG values to guide resuscitation is called the alpha stat or ectothermic strategy.[26] This approach optimizes enzymatic function, preserves the normal distribution of charged metabolic intermediates, and maintains cellular waste disposal.[31] Gradual correction of acid–base abnormalities is prudent, because the respiratory and renal components of the bicarbonate buffering system become progressively more efficient as body temperature returns to normal.

Hypothermia, like hypocapnia and alkalosis, shifts the oxyhemoglobin dissociation curve to the left, resulting in decreased O_2 release from the hemoglobin into the tissues at a lower PO_2. For example, at 27°C (81°F), the saturation of hemoglobin is 100% at a partial pressure of 59 mm Hg. Vasoconstriction, a ventilation-perfusion mismatch, and increased blood viscosity are additional impediments to tissue oxygenation.

Unlike hibernating animals, dogs and cats lack the protective vasomotor ability to alternately vasoconstrict and vasodilate the peripheral tissue to ensure perfusion. A physiologic increase in coagulation occurs with hypothermia, and a disseminated intravascular coagulation-type syndrome is reported in humans.[32] The cause may be catecholamine or steroid release, simple circulatory collapse, or release of tissue thromboplastin from cold, ischemic tissue.[33]

Coagulopathies develop in hypothermic animals because the enzymatic nature of the activated clotting factors are depressed by the cold.[34] Because the kinetic tests of coagulation are performed in the laboratory at normal body temperature, there will be a disparity between the in vivo clinically apparent coagulopathy and the deceptively "normal" prothrombin time (PT) or activated partial thromboplastin time (APTT). The only effective treatment is rewarming, not the administration of clotting factors.[35]

DIAGNOSTIC EVALUATION

An adequate history includes available information regarding pre-existing cardiac, pulmonary, neurologic, or endocrine disease. Information regarding the duration of exposure should also be recorded. The goals to emphasize prior to transporting the animal to the hospital would include rescue, examination, insulation, and rapid transport.

With a history of exposure to environmentally cold temperatures, prolonged anesthesia, trauma, or severe illness, a diagnosis of hypothermia is suspected. Early clinical signs are vague but include lethargy, dullness, shivering, and an impaired gait. With moderate hypothermia the dog or cat may have muscle stiffness without evidence of shivering. In severe hypothermia the animal may appear dead. Respiration and heart sounds are difficult to detect and the pupils are fixed, dilated, and slowly responsive. Before pronouncing the animal dead, serious attempts at detecting vital signs should be undertaken. These attempts would include an ECG, echocardiography, and plethesmography to detect respiratory movements.

Severe hypothermia is easily overlooked. This is because standard rectal thermometers only measure temperatures to about 34°C (93°F). Electronic thermistors are used to measure core temperature in the esophagus or rectum. Infrared tympanic thermometers will also accurately read low core temperatures.[c]

[c] Infrared tympanic thermometers require some practice by the user to ensure at least 25% of the tympanum is scanned at the time the temperature is measured by the device. Falsely low temperatures may result from operator error.

Importantly, rectal temperatures tend to lag behind core (esophageal or tympanic temperatures).

Perform a complete physical examination and record vital signs, time of day (you will need the time to determine how rapidly an animal is being rewarmed), and core body temperature. A continuously reading electronic thermometer is used to trend the body temperature over time. If the animal is unresponsive and not shivering, presume the animal is in severe hypothermia. At core temperatures below 32°C (90°F), one should expect an irritable myocardium, a temperature gradient between core and peripheral tissues, and relative hypovolemia.

Careful assessment to ensure a patent airway and monitoring the respiratory rate are necessary. In severe hypothermia, respiratory rates are significantly depressed and the animal may appear to be apneic. Additionally, peripheral pulses will be difficult to palpate when the animal is vasoconstricted with extreme bradycardia. At least 1 minute should be expended in palpating and auscultating for a pulse and heart sounds. The extreme bradycardia in severe hypothermia should provide adequate cardiac output to meet the animal's depressed metabolic demands. Continuous ECG monitoring is used to monitor for arrhythmias. If no evidence of perfusion exists, cardiopulmonary resuscitation (CPR) should be initiated. The presence of ventricular fibrillation should be followed by electrical defibrillation at 2 joules/kg up to 200 joules.[36] If defibrillation is unsuccessful, active rewarming is begun and CPR is continued. Interestingly, defibrillation attempts are usually unsuccessful until the body temperature is above 28° to 30°C (80°–82°F).[37]

Once hypothermia is confirmed, core temperature and an ECG are continuously monitored. A urinary catheter is placed to monitor fluid shifts. Ideally, a centrally placed arterial catheter is used to monitor blood pressure. It is not unusual to see a continued drop in body temperature (afterdrop) following removal of the animal from the cold environment. This is due to continuing conduction of heat from the warmer core to colder surface layers. With increasing return of cold blood from the peripheral tissues there is also a resultant drop in temperature. Sudden death may result from afterdrop.

Laboratory minimum database parameters include PCV (PCV increases 2% for each 1°C [1.8°F] decline in temperature), total solids, BUN, blood glucose, serum electrolytes, and at least a urine specific gravity. Hypothermia masks the potassium-induced changes in the ECG. Empirical use of potassium in the fluids may produce toxicity in the animal as it is rewarmed. Hyperkalemia is especially dangerous with metabolic acidosis, rhabdomyolysis, or renal failure.[26] Likewise, cold-induced glycosuria does not indicate the presence of normoglycemia.[26] If the patient's condition warrants, a biochemical and clotting profile, complete blood count, and ABG analysis are recommended.

Coagulopathies often develop in hypothermia despite the presence of normal levels of clotting factors.[32] In vivo, cold directly inhibits the enzymatic reactions of the coagulation cascade.[25] This is not detected by a deceptively normal PT or APTT. Both tests are run at normal temperatures. As the body temperature drops, platelet activity declines with a decreased production of thromboxane B_2

by platelets during hypothermia. Cold induces decreased bone marrow activity and sequestration of blood in the liver and spleen thus further reducing the platelet count. Hypercoagulability and thromboembolism is also possible in hypothermia.

Hypothermia, like hypocapnia and alkalosis, shifts the oxyhemoglobin dissociation curve to the left. This results in decreased O_2 release from hemoglobin into tissues at a lower PO_2. For example, at 27°C (80.6°F) the saturation of hemoglobin is 100% at a PO_2 of 59 mm Hg. Vasoconstriction, a ventilation-perfusion mismatch, and increased blood viscosity are additional impediments of tissue oxygenation.[26] Metabolic causes of acidosis include generation of lactate with muscle shivering and decreased tissue perfusion. Additionally, hepatic metabolism is impaired and there is decreased acid excretion. Dehydration and fluid sequestration are common following lengthy exposure to cold.[27] This necessitates the use of bladder catheters for monitoring urine output in the hypothermic patient.

Traditional blood gas analysis adjusts the sample to body temperature. More recently, it is suggested the unadjusted results are more useful in assessing the acid–base status of animals.[31,38] Unfortunately, there are no reference values for blood gas analysis at lower temperatures. Therefore, it is best to correct the sample to body temperature with the goal of maintaining the pH and PCO_2 within normal ranges for your hospital. If there is a severe respiratory or metabolic acidosis, ventilator care or cautious administration of sodium bicarbonate is indicated. The amount of bicarbonate to administer can be determined with the following formula:

$$\text{Bicarbonate to administer (mEq)} = \text{Body weight (kg)} \times 0.4 \times [(12 - \text{Patient bicarbonate})]/3^{d}$$

TREATMENT

Treatment of animals with hypothermia is directed to rewarming, preventing further heat loss, supporting vital organs, and preventing complications.

Volume Resuscitation

Patients with moderate or severe hypothermia are usually dehydrated. Rapid volume expansion is critical. Fluids should be heated to 40° to 42°C (104°-106.8°F) to lessen the worsening of hypothermia during rapid volume infusions. Caution should be exercised in using large fluid volumes through a central venous catheter. This may result in myocardial thermal gradients and cardiac irritability. The quantity of fluids to administer is controversial. In all likelihood, one should reduce recommended shock fluid volumes by half (normal shock volumes: dog = 50–90 mL/kg/h; cat = 44 mL/kg/h).

[d] By correcting the bicarbonate to 12 mEq/L instead of normal values you are less likely to overcorrect and induce an alkalosis. To further prevent the development of this iatrogenic alkalosis, only 1/3 of the calculated mEq is administered.

Hypothermia normally induces increased naturesis. Pre-existing gastrointestinal losses or medical therapies (*e.g.*, furosemide) also contribute to sodium loss. The fluid selected should be a balanced crystalloid solution to which at least 2.5% dextrose is added. Ringer's lactate solution should be avoided because the cold liver inefficiently metabolizes lactate.[4]

Rewarming

The three rewarming methods used in treating hypothermia are passive rewarming, active external rewarming, and core rewarming. In passive rewarming the animal is wrapped in dry blankets and the intrinsic heat production (shivering) corrects the hypothermia. With shivering there is significant oxygen consumption.

In moderate hypothermia (28°–32°C; 82°–90°F) rapid active external rewarming is indicated. Hot water bottles, circulating hot water blankets, radiant heat, and other exogenous heat sources are added to the blankets used with passive rewarming techniques. Ideally, these heat sources should only be applied to the thorax and the extremities are kept cool to allow the heart to warm and better prepare to perfuse the extremities. Under no circumstances are these external heating devices allowed to contact the patient's skin. Because the patient's skin is vasoconstricted, it is unable to conduct heat away and burn injuries are common.

Active rewarming is the direct transfer of exogenous heat to the patient. A number of techniques used in active rewarming. The administration of heated, humidified air or O_2 by mask or endotracheal tube will rewarm the airways. In humans, no induced dysrhythmias are recognized during endotracheal intubation of hypothermic patients.[27] Preoxygenation prior to intubation will help prevent dysrhythmias. Commercially available heating nebulizers and ventilators require modification to allow the inhalant to reach 40° to 45°C (104°–113°F). Airway rewarming raises the body temperature at an average of 1° to 2°C each hour. It eliminates respiratory heat loss and is a useful adjunct to other rewarming techniques.[39]

Cardiovascular instability and decompensation require rapid rewarming of the core temperature. There are reports of active rewarming with sudden vasodilation leading to severe shock. A canine model comparing cardiac bypass, peritoneal lavage, and active external rewarming (AER) shows that more crystalloids and bicarbonate are required for resuscitation for the AER group.[40] In humans, the largest afterdrop occurs when using a heating pad[41] or hot bath immersion[42] for AER. With AER there are increased peripheral metabolic demands and the ventricular dysrhythmia threshold decreases because of the myocardial temperature gradients.[43] If AER is chosen for rewarming a moderate or severe hypothemia patient, it should be combined with active core rewarming (Fig. 80-1).

Peritoneal lavage using heated (40°–45°C; 104°–113°F) crystalloid dialysate at a dose of 10 to 20 mL/kg is an option for treating severe hypothermia and no perfusion.[40] This is facilitated by placing two abdominal catheters with outflow suction. The rewarming rates with this technique range from 2° to 4°C

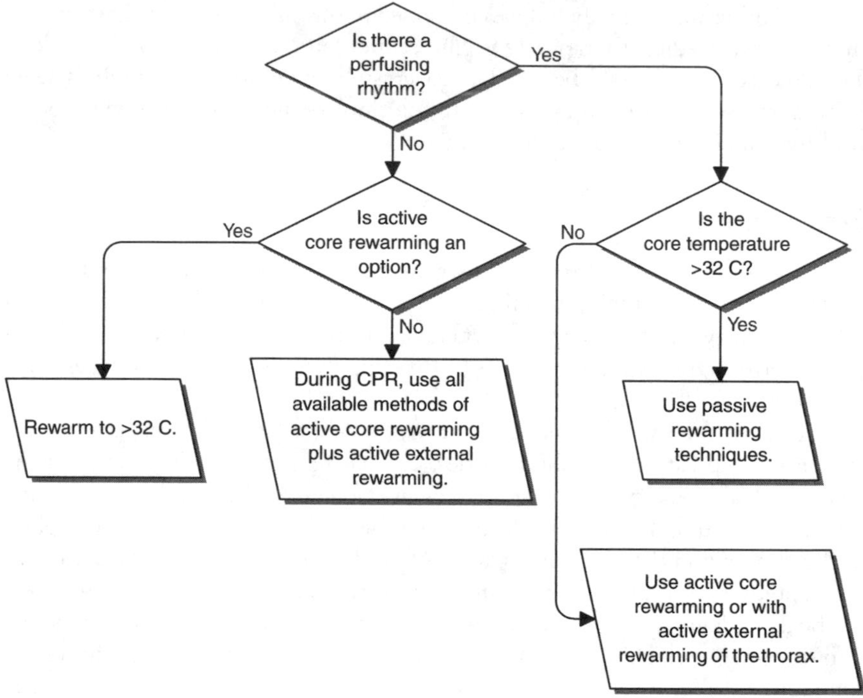

Figure 80-1
Algorithm for selecting a rewarming technique based on the animal's core temperature.

per hour. Ancillary benefits from this technique include direct hepatic rewarming, adjustment of serum potassium concentration, and discovery of occult hemoperitoneum.[26]

Closed pleural irrigation through large-bore thoracostomy tubes may also be considered. Sterile saline is warmed to 40° to 42°C (104°-107.6°F) and infused through one tube while active suction is placed on the second tube. Mediastinal heat transfer is more strategically placed and rewarming approximates that seen with peritoneal lavage.

Gastric, colonic, and urinary bladder irrigation is reported.[4] The amount of surface area in these organs limits their usefulness for heat exchange. These approaches are complicated with electrolyte fluxes, cardiac irritation from orogastric intubation, and the risk of organ perforation.

Pharmacologic Therapy

Target organs and systems become progressively less responsive to medications as the core temperature falls. Liver metabolism is decreased, whereas protein binding increases.[44] As a result, large quantities of insulin or digoxin are ineffective at lower temperatures but can produce a toxic result as rewarming progresses.

During rewarming, excessive pharmacologic manipulation of the vasoconstricted and depressed cardiovascular system should be avoided.[45] Infusions of low doses of catecholamines are indicated in patients who have lower blood pressure than would be expected for the degree of hypothermia and who are not responding to rewarming and crystalloid administration.

The most effective ventricular antiarrhythmic drug in dogs at low temperature is bretylium tosylate (American Regent Laboratories, Inc., Shirley, NY) at an IV dosage of 10 mg/kg. This increases the ventricular arrhythmia threshold despite increasing catecholamine levels. Its protective effect is most likely due to an alteration of the electrophysiologic properties of cardiac tissue and not adrenergic blockade.[13]

With hypothermia the signs and symptoms of infection are often masked. During hypothermia the migration of neutrophils and bacterial phagocytosis are defective. Empirical antimicrobial prophylaxis is frequently warranted.

Animals unresponsive to rewarming may have cerebral edema. The increased intracranial pressure is likely secondary to a combination of edema, osmotic gradients associated with glucose levels, or ischemic injury. Treatment consists of osmotic diuresis using mannitol and use of furosemide. There is no evidence that corticosteroids affect cerebral edema in hypothermia.

PROGNOSIS

Because of the variability in an animal's physiologic responses, outcome is difficult to predict. The type and severity of the underlying or precipitating disease process is the major determinant. Patient age in humans is not a predictor of mortality.[27] In humans, predictors of outcome include prehospital cardiac arrest, a low or absent blood pressure, elevated BUN, and the need for endotracheal or nasogastric intubation. Grave prognostic indicators include evidence of thromboembolism, severe hyperkalemia, and significantly elevated ammonia levels.[46]

Otherwise healthy animals who have mild accidental hypothermia, 32° to 37°C (90°-99°F), usually rewarm easily. With more severe hypothermia the animal must be examined for the presence of underlying medical disorders. Rewarming of all animals below 32°C (90°F) requires continuous temperature and ECG monitoring.

REFERENCES

1. Virtue RW: Hypothermic Anesthesia. Springfield, IL: Charles C. Thomas, 1955, p 3.
2. Ferguson J, Epstein F, Van de Leuv J: Accidental hypothermia. *Emerg Med Clin North Am* 1:619, 1983.
3. Waterman A: Accidental hypothermia during anesthesia in dogs and cats. *Vet Rec* 96:308, 1983.
4. Dhupa N: Hypothermia in dogs and cats. *Compend Contin Educ Vet* 17:61, 1995.
5. Adams T: Carnivores, protection against hypothermia. *In* Whittow GC ed.: Comparative Physiology of Thermoregulation. New York: Academic Press, 1971, p 158.

6. Granberg PO: Human physiology under cold exposure. *Arctic Med Res* 50:23, 1991.
7. Harnett RM, Pruitt JR, Sias FR: A review of the literature concerning resuscitation from hypothermia. Part II. Selected rewarming protocols. *Aviat Space Environ Med* 54:487, 1983.
8. Jolly BT, Ghezzi KT: Accidental hypothermia. *Emerg Med Clin North Am* 10:311, 1992.
9. Myers RD: Serotonin and thermoregulation: old and new views. *J Physiol* 77:505, 1981.
10. Pozos RS, Israel D, McCutcheon R, *et al.*: Human studies concerning thermal-induced shivering, postoperative "shivering," and cold-induced vasodilatation. *Ann Emerg Med* 16:1037, 1987.
11. Harari A, Regnier B, Rapin M, *et al.*: Hemodynamic study of prolonged deep accidental hypothermia. *Eur J Intensive Care Med* 1:65, 1975.
12. Bashour TT, Gualberto A, Ryan C: Atrioventricular block in accidental hypothermia: a case report. *Angiology* 40:63, 1989.
13. Orts A, Alcarez C, Delaney KA, *et al.*: Bretylium tosylate and electrically induced cardiac arrhythmias during hypothermia in dogs. *Am J Emerg Med* 10:311, 1992.
14. Ilia R, Ovsyshcher I, Rudnik L, *et al.*: Atypical ventricular tachycardia and alternating Osborn waves induced by spontaneous mild hypothermia. *Pediatr Cardiol* 9:63, 1988.
15. Webb P: Afterdrop of body temperature during rewarming: an alternative explanation. *J Appl Physiol* 60:385, 1986.
16. Mittleman KD, Mekjavic IB: Effect of occluded venous return on core temperature during cold water immersion. *J Appl Physiol* 63:2375, 1988.
17. Hayward JS, Eckerson JD, Kemna D: Thermal and cardiovascular changes during three methods of resuscitation from mild hypothermia. *Resuscitation* 11:21, 1984.
18. Segar WE, Riley PA, Barlia TG: Urinary composition during hypothermia. *Am J Physiol* 185:528, 1956.
19. Fitzgibbon T, Hayward JS, Walker D: EEG and visual evoked potentials of conscious man during moderate hypothermia. *Electroencephalogr Clin Neurophysiol* 58:48, 1984.
20. Churchill-Davidson HG, McMillan IK, Melrose DG, *et al.*: Hypothermia: experimental study of surface cooling. *Lancet* 2:1011, 1953.
21. Kiley JP, Eldridge FL, Millhorn DE: Respiration during hypothermia: effect of rewarming intermediate areas of ventral medulla. *J Appl Physiol* 59:1423, 1985.
22. O'Keeffe KM: Treatment of accidental hypothermia and rewarming techniques. *In* Roberts JR, Hedges JR, eds.: Clinical Procedures in Emergency Medicine. Philadelphia: WB Saunders, 1985.
23. Villalobos TJ, Adelson E, Riley PA, *et al.*: A cause of the thrombocytopenia and leukopenia that occurs in dogs during deep hypothermia. *J Clin Invest* 37:1, 1958.
24. Valeri CR, Cassidy G, Khuri S, *et al.*: Hypothermic-induced reversible platelet dysfunction. *Ann Surg* 205:175, 1987.
25. Reed RL II, Bracey AW Jr, Hudson JD, *et al.*: Hypothermia and blood coagulation: dissociation between enzyme activity and clotting factor levels. *Circ Shock* 32:141, 1990.
26. Danzl DF, Pozos RS: Accidental hypothermia. *N Engl J Med* 331:1756, 1994.
27. Danzl DF, Pozos RS, Auerbach PS, *et al.*: Multicenter hypothermia study. *Ann Emerg Med* 16:1042, 1987.
28. Koht A, Cane R, Cerullo LJ: Serum potassium levels during prolonged hypothermia. *Intensive Care Med* 9:275, 1983.

29. Boelhouvver RU, Bruining HA, Ong GL: Correlations of serum potassium fluctuations with body temperature after major surgery. *Crit Care Med* 15:310, 1987.
30. Delaney KA, Howland MA, Vassallo S, *et al.*: Assessment of acid-base disturbances in hypothermia and their physiologic consequences. *Ann Emerg Med* 18:72, 1989.
31. White FN: A comparative physiological approach to hypothermia. *J Thorac Cardiovasc Surg* 82:821, 1981.
32. Patt A, McCroskey BL, Moore EE: Hypothermia-induced coagulopathies in trauma. *Surg Clin North Am* 68:775, 1988.
33. Carden DL, Nowak RM: Disseminated intravascular coagulation in hypothermia. *JAMA* 247:2099, 1982.
34. Rohrer MJ, Natale AM: Effect of hypothermia on the coagulation cascade. *Crit Care Med* 20:1402, 1992.
35. Reed RL 2d, Johnson TD, Hudson JD, *et al.*: The disparity between hypothermic coagulopathy and clotting studies. *J Trauma* 33:465, 1992.
36. Tacker WA Jr, Babbs CF, Abendschein DR , *et al.*: Transchest defibrillation under conditions of hypothermia. *Crit Care Med* 9:930, 1981.
37. Lloyd EL: Hypothermia: the cause of death after rescue. *Alaska Med* 26:74, 1984.
38. Swaim, JA: Hypothermia and blood pH: a review. *Arch Intern Med* 148:1643, 1988.
39. Lloyd EL: Equipment for airway warming in the treatment of accidental hypothermia. *J Wilderness Med* 1:330, 1991.
40. Moss JF, Haklin M, Southwick HW, *et al.*: A model for the treatment of accidental severe hypothermia. *J Trauma* 26:68, 1986.
41. Harnett RM, *et al.*: Initial treatment of profound accidental hypothermia. *Aviat Space Environ Med* 51:680, 1980.
42. Hayward JS, Eckerson JD, Kemna D: Thermal and cardiovascular changes during three methods of resuscitation from mild hypothermia. *Resuscitation* 11:21, 1984.
43. Gregory RT, Doolittle WH: Accidental hypothermia. II. Clinical implications of experimental studies. *Alaska Med* 15:48, 1973.
44. Wong KC: Physiology and pharmacology of hypothermia. *West J Med* 138:227, 1983.
45. Chernow B, Lake CR, Zaritsky A, *et al.*: Sympathetic nervous system "switch off" with severe hypothermia. *Crit Care Med* 11:677, 1983.
46. Hauty MG, Esrig BC, Hill JG, *et al.*: Prognostic factors in severe accidental hypothermia: Experience from the Mt. Hood tragedy. *J Trauma* 27:1107, 1987.

81
Hyperthermia

J. Michael Walters

INTRODUCTION

Hyperthermia is defined as an elevation in body temperature. It can be characterized as pyrogenic hyperthermia (fever) and nonpyrogenic hyperthermia.[1] The primary difference between pyrogenic and nonpyrogenic hyperthermia is the presence or absence of a fully functional thermoregulation mechanism.[1] In the case of fever, endogenous or exogenous pyrogens act on the anterior hypothalamus to raise the set point to a higher temperature.[1] Nonpyrogenic hyperthermia occurs when the thermoregulation mechanisms and heat dissipating systems are unable to compensate for the heat-producing mechanisms, leading to an increased body temperature *above the set point*.[1] Common causes of nonpyrogenic hyperthermia include heatstroke, excessive exercise, seizures, hypothalamic lesions, thyrotoxicosis, and malignant hyperthermia.[1] This chapter considers the nonpyrogenic syndrome of heatstroke and briefly discusses malignant hyperthermia.

HEATSTROKE

Heatstroke is a common pathologic state caused by an excessive elevation in body temperature.[1,2] It is a commonly recognized syndrome in dogs, especially those who live in hot, humid environments.[1,2] A brief overview of thermoregulation may help the reader further understand the mechanisms of thermoregulation.

Body heat is produced by three primary processes: basal metabolism, muscular activity, and the assimilation of food (oxidative metabolism).[1] Body heat is dissipated by several methods including radiation of infrared heat, conduction, convection, and evaporation.[1] A very small amount heat is lost through the excretion of stool and urine.[1] The majority of heat loss in dogs and cats is through radiant heat and evaporate cooling via the respiratory tree.[1]

The thermoregulation centers are located in the anterior hypothalamic preoptic region.[1] Thermoregulation can be thought of as simply a balance between heat loss and heat generation mechanisms.[1] The narrow range in which body temperature is maintained is referred to as the *set point*.[1] Depending on the temperature of the body, homeostatic mechanisms will either activate heat-generating (shivering, increased voluntary activity, catecholamine release, peripheral vasoconstriction) mechanisms or heat-dissipating mechanisms (peripheral vasodilation, increased respiratory rates, panting).[1]

Heatstroke is a multifactorial, complex pathophysiologic state that results in a direct thermal injury to body tissues exposed to the excessive temperature.[1] Enzymatic alterations and denaturation of proteins occurs at a critical temperature of 43°C (109°F).[1,2] At or above this temperature, cell membrane integrity, organ deterioration, and dysfunction are consistent occurrences.[1] Predisposing factors to heatstroke include a lack of acclimatization, excessive environmental humidity, water deprivation, drug administration, obesity, concurrent or occult cardiovascular disease, exercise, central nervous system (CNS) disease, and previous heatstroke episodes.[1] Brachycephalic breeds are more susceptible to heatstroke, as are dogs with underlying upper airway disease such as laryngeal pararlysis.[1,2] The most common historical finding in dogs suffering heatstroke are those that are confined in a sealed automobile, even for the shortest of times.[1]

Pathophysiology

The multisystemic effects of heatstroke are primarily due to direct thermal effects on body systems.[1] Common systems effected include the (1) CNS, (2) gastrointestinal (GI), (3) cardiovascular, (4) hepatobiliary, (5) renal/urologic, (6) hematologic, and (7) muscular.[1,2]

The effects of excessive heat on the CNS are primarily neuronal injury and cell death with subsequent cerebral edema.[1] In addition, localized areas of intraparenchymal hemorrhage may occur, which can lead to seizures.[1] Cerebellar dysfunction can occur as a consequence of heatstroke and may effect the animal throughout its life.[1] Another potential consequence of heatstroke is damage to the thermoregulatory centers in the hypothalamus with a predisposition to subsequent hyperthermic episodes.[1]

The GI effects of heatstroke include ulceration secondary to ischemia and profuse, hematochezia/melena.[1] These conditions are often associated with endotoxemia and the development of the systemic inflammatory response syndrome (SIRS).[1,2] Direct thermal injury may also cause severe or fatal hepatic injury.[1]

Hyperthermia leads to increased cardiac output, concurrent hypoxia due to increased metabolic demands, decreased systemic vascular resistance, and hypovolemia, secondary to dehydration.[1,2] Myocardial injury will often lead to tachyarrhythmias and cardiogenic shock.[1]

The most profound, and often most life-threatening, effects of heatstroke and thermal injury are to the renal system.[1] Acute renal failure is common, especially in the dehydrated animal.[1] Rhabdomyolysis, due to muscle necrosis, is common and can exacerbate the acute tubular necrosis via dehydration, hypoperfusion, and pigment despostion.[1]

The hematologic effects of heatstroke include hemoconcentration secondary to dehydration, leukocytosis due to catecholamine release, anemia due to blood loss, and coagulopathies.[1,2] Excessive heat results in direct destruction of clotting factors or in decreased hepatic synthesis of clotting factors.[1] Megakaryocytes appear to be especially sensitive to hyperthermia; therefore, thrombocytopenia is a common finding.[1] Thrombocytopenia associated with thermal injury to megakaryocytes may take several days to become apparent and should not be confused with the thrombocytopenia seen earlier in the disease course.[1] This early thrombocytopenia is likely due to a consumptive process secondary to GI bleeding.[1] Disseminated intravascular coagulation (DIC) may develop at any time during the heatstroke event.[1] The contributing factors include the previously mentioned clotting factor destruction or synthesis failure, disruption of vascular endothelium, vascular sludging secondary to shock, and the consumption of clotting factors with GI hemorrhage.[1]

Hyperthermia also has profound effects of the acid–base status. Most often a mixed derangement with a respiratory alkalosis, because of panting, coupled with metabolic acidosis, due to excess muscular activity and shock, is seen.[1]

Clinical Presentation

A presumptive diagnosis of nonpyrogenic hyperthermia should be made when presented with an animal with a body temperature greater than or equal to 40.7°C (106°F) with no obvious evidence of infection.[1] Pyrogenic hyperthermia is a result of a change in the thermoregulatory set point; therefore, dogs with fever will not necessarily present with panting hypersalivation (heat dissipating).[1] Animals with heatstroke will have excessive panting, dark, often brick red mucous membranes in an attempt to decrease their body temperature.[1]

The most common clinical signs reported by owners include collapse, vomiting, ataxia, hypersalivation, diarrhea, loss of consciousness, seizure, listlessness, and muscle tremors.[2] Less commonly reported signs include hematuria/pigmenturia, cyanosis, altered level of consciousness, epistaxis, swollen tongue, head tremors, dilated pupils, stridorous respirations, and vocalizing.[2]

A thorough history to reveal a predisposing cause in the animal's ability to dissipate heat is helpful.[1] Causes can include being locked in a car on a hot day, forced exercise in high ambient temperatures, underlying diseases such as laryngeal paralysis, upper airway disease, neurologic dysfunction, cardiovascular disease, a previous hyperthermia/heatstroke episode, hyperthyroidism, drug administration that may alter thermoregulation, brachycephalic conformation, water or salt depletion, and having a thick hair coat.[1,2]

Common physical examination findings are elevated rectal temperatures, ranging from 40.5° to 43.0°C (104.9°-109.4°F), altered mental status, hyperemic mucous membranes, increased respiratory effort, weak or irregular femoral pulses, and cutaneous or mucosal petechiae, and cortical blindness.[2]

A complete blood count (CBC), serum biochemistry panel, urinalysis, serial blood gas determinations, and serial coagulation profiles should be performed in all animals presenting with heatstroke.[1,2] Serum biochemistries reflect serious, multiorgan dysfunction. Common findings are elevation in blood urea nitrogen (BUN) and creatinine (Cr) as seen with acute tubular necrosis.[1,2] Hepatic injury is evident with elevations in aspartate transaminase (AST), alanine transaminase (ALT), and bilirubin.[2,5] Rhabdomyolysis may cause marked increases in creatinine phosphokinase and AST. Blood glucose is often extremely low, although this is an inconsistent finding.[2,5]

The CBC often reflects severe dehydration through elevations in packed cell volume (PCV) and total protein.[2,5] Evidence of DIC is often present (thrombocytopenia, increased fibrin degradation products [FDPs], prolonged prothrombin time [PT], and activated partial thromboplastin time [APTT]).[2,5]

Blood gas analysis is often variable. In the early stages of heatstroke, animals may pant without affecting alveolar ventilation.[5] As the heat stress progresses, respiratory effort becomes more pronounced and a respiratory alkalosis develops.[5] As the hyperdynamic phase of heatstroke progresses to vasomotor collapse, metabolic acidosis results from increased lactic acid accumulation.[5]

The presence of renal casts and glucosuria in the face of low or normal blood glucose may indicate significant renal tubular damage.[5] Myoglobinuria is suggestive of rhabdomyolysis and can lead to an exacerbation of acute tubular necrosis.[5]

Treatment

The goal of heatstroke treatment is early recognition and the institution of cooling measures.[1,2,4,5] Actual treatment of the heatstroke victim should be begin with the first telephone call by the owner, the first responder.[1] Owners should be instructed to spray their pet with cool, not cold water, before the animal is transported to the veterinary hospital.[1] Have the owner take advantage of enhanced radiant and convection cooling by keeping the car windows open or the air conditioner on maximum during their trip.[1] On arrival, the most important aspect of treatment is to lower core temperature.[1,2,4,5]

It is equally important not to overcool the pet.[5] The cooling end point is to reduce core temperature to 39°C (103°F) over a period of 30 to 60 minutes.[4] Cooling is stopped at 39°C (103°F) to avoid shivering as the cooling process continues.[5] In addition, cerebral edema is a common complication in heatstroke and can lead to hypothalamic thermoregulation dysfunction, impairing the animal's homeostatic mechanisms.[5] Continued core temperature monitoring is imperative to avoid iatrogenic hypothermia.[2,5] Evaporative cooling is enhanced by using a fan during the cooling process.[5] In one study, iatrogenic hypothermia was associated with a worse outcome in dogs treated for heatstroke.[2] The cause of this poor outcome could not be determined, whether it was a cause or did it effect the outcome by enhancing such things as poor perfusion, hypothalamic dysfunction, and so forth.[2] Cold water and ice water baths should be avoided because they may actually slow the core cooling process. Shivering and peripheral vasoconstriction lessen the heat loss.[4,5] Other methods that lower body temperature without causing peripheral vasoconstriction are massage, cool intravenous (IV) fluids, gastric lavage with cool or cold slurries, and cold water enemas.[5] Several studies have been performed to look at more advanced, central cooling methods: iced gastric lavage, high-frequency jet ventilation, and iced peritoneal lavage.[6-8] In the case of iced gastric lavage and iced peritoneal lavage, no real advantage could be found over a noninvasive, peripheral cooling method.[6,8] In the study of high-frequency jet ventilation, the authors felt that further study is warranted, even though no difference is found in survival rates when compared to peripheral cooling.[7] Clearly, the cornerstone of the treatment remains rapid recognition and peripheral cooling.[1,2,4-8]

Intravenous fluid resuscitation to correct hypovolemia and support cardiac output are instituted during the cooling process.[1,2,4,5] Judicious use of IV fluids is warranted with care given to avoid fluid overload.[5] Early in the heatstroke event, fluid deficits are minimal and there is an increase in cardiac output. Large volumes of IV fluids may actually lead to fluid overload and worsening of pulmonary or cerebral edema. Fluid needs of the patient presented with heatstroke are individual and needs to be balanced with treatment response, central venous pressure (CVP), electrolyte balance, acid–base imbalance, blood pressure monitoring, lung auscultation, and urine output rather than a strict fluid volume end-point goal.[5] Dogs with severe upper airway obstruction either owing to concurrent laryngeal paralysis or subsequent laryngeal edema or comatose animals require supplemental oxygen therapy, possible endotracheal intubation or emergency tracheostomy.[1,4,5]

The use of antipyretic drugs such as dipyrone, aspirin, flunixin meglumine, carprofen, and etodolac is *contraindicated*.[1,2,4,5] Remember, heatstroke is a form of *nonpyrogenic* hyperthermia and has a normal hypothalamic thermoregulation set point.[1,2,4,5] These drugs will alter the hypothalamic temperature set point resulting in iatrogenic hypothermia.[1,2,4,5] The use of corticosteroids in the treatment of heatstroke and concurrent shock remains controversial and may actually exacerbate certain complications such as gastric ulceration and ischemic injury to the kidneys.[2,4,5] The treatment of cerebral edema by using corticosteroids is equally controversial and needs to be balanced with their risk.[5] Dantrolene sodium, a skeletal muscle relaxant known to be effective in the treatment of malignant hyperthermia in humans and swine, also does not appear to enhance passive cooling in experimental heatstroke studies performed in dogs and swine.[9,10]

The complications encountered during the treatment of heatstroke are variable. Temperatures at or above 43°C (109°F) often result in irreparable organ damage, uncoupling of oxidative phosphorylation, cell membrane dysfunction, and enzymatic denaturation.[1,2,4,5] Kidney damage is common due to direct thermal injury, decreased renal blood flow, hypotension, myoglobinuria, and renal vessel thrombosis (due to DIC) resulting in acute renal failure and acute tubular necrosis.[1,2,4,5] Direct thermal injury is also responsible for GI ulceration, disruption to the mucosal barriers, and bacterial translocation, leading to bacteremia, SIRS, and sepsis.[5] Hepatic injury is also common as is evident by increased ALT, AST, and bilirubin levels.[1,2,4,5] By far, the most common complication is DIC. DIC should be assumed in all cases of heatstroke before it is proven. Widespread thermal injury to endothelial cells and cellular necrosis lead to global inactivation and consumption of platelets and clotting factors.[5] The classic signs of DIC, thrombocytopenia, prolonged PT and APTT, and the presence of FDPs, are often seen.[5] A proactive rather than a reactive treatment protocol is essential for successful treatment of DIC in addition to all the common complications.

Patient monitoring should be aggressive and continual and is required for several days.[1,2,4,5] Blood pressure, CVP, urine output via closed collection system, electrocardiogram, as well as monitoring abnormal serum biochemical and CBC findings are essential.[4,5]

Restoration of fluid volume, improved glomerular filtration rate, improved renal blood flow, electrolyte balance, broad-spectrum, nonnephrotoxic antibiotics, fresh-frozen plasma, and seizure control are all considerations in the treatment of heatstroke.

Prognosis

The overall prognosis is guarded to grave depending on the presence or absence of underlying disease entities or complications.[4] Mortality rates seem proportional to duration and intensity of the hyperthermia and the time required to achieve normothermia.[1,2,4] Dogs who survive may have permanent damage to thermoregulatory systems or permanent nephrologic injury, resulting in a predisposition to hyperthermia and diabetes insipidis.[4] Heatstroke holds a guarded to poor prognosis with a high morbidity and mortality rate.[1,2]

MALIGNANT HYPERTHERMIA

First reported in humans in 1960, malignant hyperthermia (MH) was not reported in swine until 1970.[11] MH is a potentially life-threatening pharmacogenic myopathy that is most commonly reported in humans and swine.[11] MH has been reported in other species including dogs, cats, horses, birds, deer, and other wild species.[11] In wild species MH is known as capture myopathy.[11] Volatile inhalant anesthetics can initiate MH, and halothane is the most potent trigger agent relative to the other anesthetic gases.[11]

Pathophysiology

This syndrome is characterized by a rapid rise in body temperature that, if not treated, rapidly leads to death.[11] Animals that are prone to MH can be anesthetized safely by avoiding trigger agents and prophylactic treatment with dantrolene given prior to anesthesia.[11] The occurrence of MH is associated with a sudden increase in oxygen requirement by striated muscle, thus causing an increase in lactate production.[11] Metabolic acidosis is accompanied by muscle contraction, sympathetic activation, and increased muscle cellular permeability.[11] Initially, serum magnesium, calcium, phosphorus, and potassium concentrations are increased.[11] This is followed by a decrease in potassium and calcium concentraton.[11] Myoglobinuria often appears shortly after this finding and many animals die at this point unless intervention occurs.[11] It appears that individuals who develop MH have difficulty in regulating calcium ion concentration in muscle tissue as a result of altered cell membrane permeability.[11] In humans, MH is a genetically linked trait.

Clinical Presentation

Clinically, MH is characterized by a rapid onset of tachycardia, hyperthermia, muscle rigidity (extensor muscles), tachypnea with progression to dyspnea, and finally apnea.[11] Rapidly increasing end-tidal carbon dioxide concentration is the most revealing of impending MH.[11] In later stages, tachycardia is accompanied by dysrrhythmias that lead to bradycardia and finally cardiac arrest.[11]

Prevention and Treatment

The drug most commonly used to prevent and treat MH is dantrolene (Dantrium, 2-5 mg/kg IV).[11] This is a muscle relaxant that also an antipyretic.[11] It suppresses calcium ion release but does not appear to inhibit uptake of calcium by muscle cell tissures.[11] Symptomatic care, as with other forms of hyperthermia, are necessary.[11] Rapid cessation of inhalant anesthesia, changing the anesthetic machine to a "clean" machine, administration of 100% oxygen, and body cooling are all methods used to diminish the effects of MH.[11]

REFERENCES

1. Ruslander D: Heatstroke. *In* Kirk RW, Bonagura JD, eds.: Kirk's Current Veterinary Therapy XI. Philadelphia, WB Saunders, 1992, p 143.
2. Drobatz KJ, Macintire DK: Heat-induced illness in dogs: 42 cases (1976–1993). *J Am Vet Med Assoc.* 209:1894, 1996.
3. Ellis FP: Heat illness. II. Pathogenesis. *Trans R Soc Trop Med Hyg* 70:412, 1977.
4. Bücheler J: Heatstroke and hyperthermia. *In* Tilley LP, Smith FWK Jr, eds.: The 5 Minute Veterinary Consultant. Baltimore: Williams & Wilkins, 1997, p 640.
5. Hackett T: Heatstroke. *In* Wingfield WE, ed.: Veterinary Emergency Medicine Secrets. Philadelphia: Hanely & Belfus, 1997, p 40.
6. White JD, Kamath R, Nucci R, *et al.*: Evaporative versus iced peritoneal lavage treatment of heatstroke: comparative efficacy in a canine model. *Am J Emerg Med* 11:1, 1993.
7. Barker WJ, Amsterdam JT, Syverud SA, *et al.*: High-frequency jet ventilation cooling in a canine hyperthermia model. *Ann Emerg Med* 15:680, 1986.
8. Syverud SA, Barker WJ, Amsterdam JT, *et al*: Iced gastric lavage for the treatment of heatstroke: efficacy in a canine model. *Ann Emerg Med* 14:424, 1985.
9. Amsterdam JT, Syverud SA, Barker WJ, *et al.*: Dantrolene sodium for the treatment of heatstroke: lack of efficacy in a canine model. *Am J Emerg Med* 4:399, 1986.
10. Zuckerman GB, Singer LP, Rubin DH, *et al.*: Effects of dantrolene on cooling times and cardiovascular parameters in an immature porcine model of heatstroke. *Crit Care Med* 25:135, 1997.
11. Riebold TW: Swine Anesthesia. *In* Thurmon JC, Tranquilli WJ, Benson GJ, eds.: Lumb and Jones' Veterinary Anesthesia. Baltimore: Williams & Wilkins, 1996, p 642.

82
Toxicology of Antineoplastic Treatments

Kenneth M. Rassnick

INTRODUCTION

Chemotherapy is associated with a wide range of adverse effects. Although this chapter cannot be completely inclusive of all potential toxicities associated with antineoplastic treatments, it should serve as a basis from which clinicians can develop experience with the various drugs used in veterinary oncology. Whenever unusual symptoms develop subsequent to the administration of chemotherapy, the clinician should be suspicious of a potential chemotherapy-associated toxicity and should consult a veterinary oncologist or human textbook for a more complete description.

GASTROINTESTINAL TOXICITY

Chemotherapy-induced gastrointestinal (GI) toxicity can be debilitating and potentially life-threatening. Symptoms may include nausea, anorexia, vomiting, and diarrhea. Certain chemotherapeutic agents have a higher incidence of adverse GI effects (Table 82-1), but all drugs should be considered to have the potential to cause GI toxicity in an individual patient. Additionally, it is important to recognize that GI symptoms associated with fever are a more serious problem because they can be the first signs of sepsis.

The mechanisms by which antineoplastic agents cause GI toxicity are multifactorial and involve (1) direct damage of GI mucosa, (2) stimulation of the chemoreceptor trigger zone (CRTZ) and medullary emetic center via stimulation of various neurotransmitter receptors, and (3) local GI tract irritation to stimulate gut neurotransmitter receptors and subsequent activation of the vomiting center via vagus and sympathetic nerves. Neurotransmitters include serotonin, dopamine, histamine, and norepinephrine among others. Serotonin released from enterochromaffin cells of the GI tract seems to be important in the pathophysiology of acute vomiting; whereas other neurotransmitters may be more important in the delayed GI adverse effects of chemotherapy.

Vomiting *during* chemotherapy administration is uncommon with the exception of cisplatin, dacarbazine, streptozotocin, and occasionally doxorubicin, actinomcyin, and cyclophosphamide. Most veterinary patients experience *delayed* vomiting, beginning 2 to 5 days after treatment, when desquamation of the intestinal crypt cells begins. Anorexia is a common sequela to chemotherapy in cats, especially after receiving vincristine, and may be related to its peripheral

Table 82-1. Emetic Potential of Chemotherapy Drugs

High	Moderate	Low
Cisplatin	Actinomycin	Bleomycin
Dacarbazine	Carboplatin	Chlorambucil
Streptozotocin	Cytosine arabinoside	CCNU
	Doxorubicin	Cyclophosphamide
	Etoposide	Ifosfamide
	Methotrexate	L-asparaginase
	Mustargen	Melphalan
	Procarbazine	Mitoxantrone
	Vinblastine	5-Fluorouracil
	Vincristine	

neurotoxic effects on the GI tract leading to a paralytic ileus. Diarrhea usually occurs several days after chemotherapy and is related to damage to rapidly dividing mucosal epithelial cells. Most drugs can cause diarrhea; common examples are doxorubicin, vincristine, cisplatin, and methotrexate. Very rarely, pancreatitis subsequent to chemotherapy is the cause of emesis. Doxorubicin, L-asparaginase, azathioprine, methotrexate, and prednisone have all been implicated in causing pancreatitis in veterinary patients.

Management of chemotherapy-induced GI toxicity includes restriction of oral intake, parenteral fluid support, and antiemetics. Prophylactic antibiotics are not routinely instituted but the clinician should always monitor a vomiting chemotherapy patient for fever because the occurrence of GI toxicity and neutrophil nadir are often overlapping. Should imminent sepsis be suspected, systemic antibiotic therapy is indicated. Nutritional support should always be considered in patients experiencing severe or prolonged GI toxicity secondary to chemotherapy because malnutrition may adversely affect survival and quality of life.

Generally, replacement fluids such as lactated Ringer's are administered. For dogs that are hospitalized within 36 hours of receiving cisplatin, 0.9% NaCl is the fluid of choice; if any active drug remains in the body, the high chloride environment is protective against the nephrotoxic effects of the drug.

Metoclopramide (Reglan, Robins) is the author's first choice for vomiting chemotherapy patients. This is a GI promotility drug that also has central antiemetic effects via dopaminergic receptor antagonism. A constant rate infusion of metoclopramide at 2.2 mg/kg IV over 24 hours is preferable; however, injectable doses can be given at 0.05 to 0.1 mg/kg q 6 to 8 h IM or SQ. Prokinetic effects of metoclopramide are particularly effective for GI toxicity secondary to vincristine administration because the drug can cause hypomotility and ileus.

For animals that have persistent vomiting despite therapy with metoclopramide, phenothiazine antiemetics such as chlorpromazine (Thorazine, SmithKline Beecham, 0.5 mg/kg q 6 h SQ) can be used. These antiemetics act centrally to block dopamine in the CRTZ as well as the emetic center and peripheral receptors.

The introduction of serotonin receptor antagonists (odansetron, Zofran, Glaxon Wellcome, 0.5–1.0 mg/kg q 12–24 h PO or IV; dolasetron, Anzemet, Aventis, 0.6–1 mg/kg q 24 h PO or IV) has resulted in a significant improvement in the control of chemotherapy-induced GI toxicity in human and veterinary cancer patients.[1] Although the benefit to patients is substantial, serotonin antagonists are expensive. Improving the control of vomiting with these drugs may reduce hospitalization costs and make these drugs an attractive choice of antiemetic therapy.

Butorphanol (Torbugesic, Fort-Dodge, 0.4 mg/kg IM) has been shown to be effective in controlling vomiting in dogs given cisplatin.[2] Butorphanol is administered once during the cisplatin infusion protocol; an additional treatment with butorphanol may prove beneficial for dogs exhibiting severe nausea or acute vomiting within 6 to 12 hours of receiving the drug.

As with vomiting, any animal with diarrhea following chemotherapy should be monitored for fever and septicemia. Mild diarrhea can be treated symptomatically and most often resolves in a few days. However, if diarrhea is profuse or nonresponsive to conservative management, hospitalization is recommended to provide IV fluid replacement.

Treatment with doxorubicin in dogs is associated with a unique hemorrhagic colitis. Hemorrhagic colitis may respond well to bismuth subsalicylate (Pepto-Bismol, Proctor & Gamble, 1 T/15 lb q 8 h or 1 tablet/15 lb divided q 12 h). Loperamide (Imodium, Janssen, 0.08 mg/kg q 6 h PO) is a potentially effective nonspecific antidiarrheal agent for diarrhea secondary to chemotherapeutic agents.

Finally, opportunistic infections secondary to alteration of GI flora following chemotherapy should be considered in patients with diarrhea nonresponsive to previously mentioned therapy. For patients, with colitis, treatment with metronidazole (Flagyl, Searle, 15 mg/kg q 12 h PO) or sulfasalazine (Azulfidine, Pharmacia Corp, 10–15 mg/kg q 6–8 h PO) is often helpful; but for those with small bowel diarrhea, underlying infections with salmonella or campylobacter should be considered.

HEMATOLOGIC TOXICITY

Adverse effects on the bone marrow are major dose-limiting aspects of anticancer therapy. The most chemosensitive cells in the bone marrow are the proliferating hematopoietic precursors and progenitors that are beginning to commit to a particular lineage, but are still immature. Hematopoietic stem cells are largely nonproliferating and are relatively resistant to chemotherapy toxicity. Similarly, the more differentiated cells are also nonproliferating and are unaffected by anticancer drugs. This pool provides mature cells to the circulation for 5 to 10 days.

The life span of neutrophils in circulation is approximately 6 hours. For this reason, neutrophil nadirs occur most commonly 5 to 10 days after chemotherapy. One notable exception is carboplatin, a commonly used drug that can cause profound neutropenia 7 to 28 days after treatment. The life span of platelets is approximately 5 to 6 days and the nadir occurs 1 to 2 weeks after treatment. Thrombocytopenia is rarely severe enough to cause spontaneous bleeding unless coupled with problems such as gram-negative septicemia, disseminated intravascular coagulation, or vasculitis. Because normal erythrocytes survive much longer (dogs, 110–120 days; cats, 70 days), anemia after chemotherapy is uncommon and rarely a clinical problem. Hydroxyurea, the drug of choice for treatment of polycythemia vera and chronic myelogenous leukemia in dogs and cats, is one drug that can potentially cause severe anemia.

Neutropenia

Anticancer drugs vary in their potential to suppress the bone marrow (Table 82-2). As previously mentioned, the neutrophil nadir generally is 5 to 10 days after chemotherapy. The risk of sepsis is high in patients with absolute neutrophil counts less than 1000 cells/μL. Although possible, it is unusual to see clinical problems in animals with more than 1000 neutrophils/μL.

The primary source of infection is most often the GI tract. Chemotherapy-induced mucosal damage allows invasion by opportunistic gram-negative bacteria such as *Escherichia*, *Klebsiella*, and *Pseudomonas*. Gram-positive cocci and, less commonly, anaerobic organisms may also be involved.

The manifestations of neutropenia can range from nonclinical to life-threatening, so all animals treated with chemotherapy agents should be considered at

Table 82-2. Classification of Antineoplastic Agents by Degree of Myelosuppression When Used as Single Agents

Severe (<1000 neutrophils/μL)	Moderate (1000-2000 neutrophils/μL)	Mild-None (>2000 neutrophils/μL)
Carboplatin	Actinomycin	Bleomycin
CCNU	Cisplatin	Chlorambucil
Cyclophosphamide	Cytosine arabinoside	Corticosteroids
Doxorubicin	Dacarbazine	L-Asparaginase*
Mitoxantrone	Etoposide	Vincristine*
	Hydroxyurea	
	Ifosfamide	
	Melphalan	
	Mustargen	
	Procarbazine	
	Vinblastine	
	5-Fluorouracil	

* When used in combination, moderate-to-severe myelosuppression may occur presumably due to delayed hepatic clearance of vincristine.

risk for developing neutropenia. Clinical signs associated with neutropenia and sepsis may include fever, weakness, shaking, brick-red mucous membranes, tachycardia, tachypnea, coughing, vomiting, and diarrhea. Many of the cardinal signs of inflammation may be absent due to insufficient numbers of neutrophils to participate in the inflammatory process. Even bacterial pneumonia may not be evident on radiographs when a patient is severely neutropenic.

For the purposes of management, neutropenia is classified as afebrile and febrile. Afebrile patients are generally asymptomatic. If the absolute neutrophil count is below 1000 cells/μL, prophylactic antibiotic therapy should be initiated. If a patient is showing vague, nonspecific signs such as diminished appetite or lethargy and the count is 1000 to 2000 neutrophils/μL, prophylactic antibiotics are also advised. However, underlying causes for these symptoms such as GI toxicity (see previous section) or tumor progression should also be investigated. The author generally uses sulfadiazine-trimethoprim (Tribrissen, Schering, 15 mg/kg q 12 h PO) for 5 to 7 days as an empirical broad-spectrum antibiotic. Owners should monitor rectal temperature (q 12 h × 48 h) and if fever develops or patient condition deteriorates, more aggressive diagnostics and therapy are recommended.

As a general rule, pyrexia in a patient after chemotherapy should be attributed to septicemia. Minimum database should include a thorough history and physical examination, complete blood count, platelet count, serum biochemistry profile, and urinalysis. Caution is advised when evaluating potentially neutropenic chemotherapy patients with complete blood counts performed on in-house hematology analyzers. Results from dogs with severe neutropenia may not correlate with those evaluated by reference methods used by clinical pathology laboratories. They may be grossly inaccurate and patient status may be interpreted erroneously.[3] Without supporting history or physical examination findings, thoracic radiographs are generally of low yield but can be considered. Blood cultures may be performed in febrile, neutropenic patients. However, definitive culture results take many days and knowing the colony flora is unlikely to make an impact on initial treatment because broad-spectrum antibiotics should be immediately used. Even with a comprehensive evaluation, an infectious organism may only be demonstrated in 50% of patients.

Fever in a neutropenic patient constitutes a medical emergency. Hospitalization for IV fluid support and antibiotics is recommended. Antibiotics should be administered IV to avoid limitations of poor absorption across the intestinal epithelium. A large number of highly effective antibiotics are currently available for use and it is difficult to recommend specific treatments for initial therapy. Febrile neutropenia is life-threatening: polymicrobial, broad-spectrum antibiotics should be administered. Table 82-3 is provided as a guide for potential drug combinations recommended by the author and other veterinary oncologists.

Granulocyte colony-stimulating factor (G-CSF) is a hematopoietic growth factor that regulates the production, maturation, and function of cells of the neutrophil lineage. The primary use of G-CSF has been to administer it 24 to 48 hours following highly myelosuppressive chemotherapy. When given before the onset of neutropenia, G-CSF may decrease the duration and depth of the

Table 82-3. Guidelines for Managing Patients with Febrile Neutropenia

1. Place aseptic catheter.
2. Begin IV fluids.
3. Discontinue anticancer drugs:
   a. If receiving corticosteroids—gradual taper or consider physiologic doses depending on duration and dosage currently being administered.
4. Start empirical antibiotics:
   a. Aminoglycoside or fluoroquinoline.
      and
   b. Cephalosporin or extended-spectrum penicillin.
5. Treat until neutrophil count returns to normal and patient is clinically normal (usually 72–96 h).
6. Discharge with broad-spectrum oral antibiotics:
   a. Sulfadiazine-trimethorprim.
      or
   b. Fluoroquinolone and penicillin or cephalosporin.

neutropenia period. It has been proposed that the administration of G-CSF to neutropenic patients that are already febrile might speed neutrophil recovery and reduce the overall duration of antibiotic therapy and hospitalization. However, data from human literature do not show a consistent and clinical benefit, so G-CSF is not recommended as an adjunct to empirical antibiotic therapy.[4] Also, currently only recombinant human granulocyte colony-stimulating factor (rhG-CSF) is available for use in veterinary patients. When administered to dogs, rhG-CSF will cause neutralizing antibodies to be produced and ultimately neutrophil counts will decrease. However, this only seems to be a clinical problem if prolonged courses (*i.e.*, >3 weeks) of rhG-CSF are administered.[5] The author does recommend use of rhG-CSF (Neupogen, Amgen, 5 μg/kg q 24 h SQ) for veterinary patients that have been inadvertently overdosed and when the duration of neutropenia is expected to be prolonged.

CARDIAC TOXICITY

Cardiotoxicity is associated with the anthracycline drugs doxorubicin, epirubicin, and daunorubicin. Doxorubicin is one of the most widely used anticancer drugs in veterinary medicine. Although not precisely defined, a safe cumulative dosage range for doxorubicin in dogs is thought to be 180 to 240 mg/m^2 body surface area. However, cardiac abnormalities can occur in dogs that receive much lower doses.[6] Electrocardiographic, echocardiographic, and histologic changes have all been reported in cats receiving doxorubicin. However, clinical cardiac disease does not seem to be a problem.[7]

Doxorubicin-induced cardiotoxicity is classified into acute and chronic toxicity. Acute cardiotoxicity is uncommon but may occur during rapid IV infusion of doxorubicin and is characterized by vasodilation, hypotension, collapse, and arrhythmias. This uncommon toxicity is related to histamine-mediated catecholamine release that can occur during rapid infusion of the drug (see Hypersensitivity Reactions).

Chronic toxicity is the most common and clinically important form of doxorubicin-induced cardiotoxicity. The cause is multifactorial; however, a large body of evidence points toward free radical-mediated myocyte damage. Free radicals such as superoxide anion, hydroxyl radical, and hydrogen peroxide are generated during the reduction of doxorubicin. These highly reactive molecules cause cellular injury through lipid peroxidation of cellular, mitochondrial, and nuclear membranes and subsequent disruption of enzymatic respiration and DNA damage.[8] The myocardium in dogs, and humans, is especially sensitive to myocyte damage by free radicals because the myocardium possesses lower concentrations of catalase, one of the major scavengers of free radicals. Iron needs to be present for free radical generation to occur. Dexrazoxane (Zinecard, Pharmacia & Upjohn) is an iron chealator and has been used to reduce the cardiac toxicity of doxorubicin.[9] Treatment with dexrazoxane does not afford any benefit once cardiac damage has occurred.

Clinical signs of cumulative doxorubicin-induced cardiotoxicity may develop from days to months following the last dose. Electrocardiographic abnormalities may include arrhythmias and conduction disturbances. Cardiotoxicity may culminate in dilated cardiomyopathy with decreased fractional shortening observed on echocardiography. Clinical signs of doxorubicin-induced cardiomyopathy may include tachycardia, tachypnea, weakness, cough, and other signs consistent with heart failure.

Therapy of anthracycline-induced cardiac arrhythmias and cardiomyopathy is limited to conventional therapies for other types of cardiomyopathies and heart failure. Effective long-term treatment of heart disease in dogs resulting from doxorubicin is difficult and the overall prognosis is generally very poor.

HYPERSENSITIVITY REACTIONS

Several chemotherapeutic agents can induce hypersensitivity reactions. These include L-asparaginase, doxorubicin, etoposide, and taxanes (paclitaxel, docetaxel). Idiosyncratic allergic reactions can potentially occur with any of the other available anticancer drugs.

L-Asparaginase is a polypeptide of bacterial origin, displaying multiple antigenic sites that can stimulate production of IgE or other immunoglobulins. These immunoglobulins can mediate an acute type I anaphylactic reaction. Delayed reactions occurring from a few hours to several days can also be seen. IM or SQ administration are associated a decreased incidence of allergic reactions compared to IV or intraperitoneal administration. Patients that experience a hypersensitivity reaction to L-asparaginase should not receive any more drug because subsequent doses will result in more severe allergic reactions.

Doxorubicin induces a hypersensitivity reaction especially if administered too quickly. Also, a higher frequency of acute reactions has been documented when using a generic doxorubicin product.[10] Hypersensitivity reactions related to doxorubicin are not immunologically mediated; instead, the drug induces direct mast cell degranulation and histamine release. This can be minimized if the drug is given as a slow infusion (1 mg/min) or with pretreatment with dexamethasone (Azium, Schering, 0.5–1 mg/kg IV) and diphenhydramine (Benadryl, Parke-Davis, 2.2 mg/kg IV).

Paclitaxel contains Chremophor EL and etoposide contains polysorbate 80 as vehicles to enhance water solubility. These carriers are thought to be the cause of hypersensitivity reactions; however, the drugs themselves may also play a role. The exact mechanism has not been well studied. Clinicians should be aware that reactions are not immunogenic and can occur after the first dose. Premedication with dexamethasone and diphenhydramine is necessary to prevent potentially life-threatening reactions with these drugs.[11,12]

Clinical signs of hypersensitivity include pruritis, urticaria, cutaneous erythema, agitation, head shaking, facial edema, vocalization, injection site discomfort, and occasionally vomiting and diarrhea. This can progress to respiratory distress, hypotension, and collapse if medical intervention is not initiated. If a patient exhibits any signs that can be attributed to a hypersensitivity reaction after returning home, owners are advised to have the animal evaluated and treated immediately. If the reaction develops during the infusion or while the patient is in the hospital, administration of the drug is immediately discontinued and treatment with IV dexamethasone and IM diphenhydramine instituted. If an animal develops a severe anaphylactoid reaction, treatment should also include IV epinephrine (0.1–0.5 mL of a 1:1000 solution) and IV fluids at shock doses to prevent development of hypotension. Patients should be closely monitored for response to therapy. If clinical signs do not completely resolve, repeat injections of diphenhydramine are recommended.

NEUROLOGIC TOXICITY

Toxicity affecting the nervous system in dogs and cats has been primarily associated with 5-fluoruracil (5-FU). Cisplatin can cause acute seizures and vincristine is associated with a peripheral neuropathy, but these are very rare complications in veterinary patients.

Clinical signs of 5-FU toxicity include death, seizures, blindness, hyperexcitability, disorientation, tremors, collapse, ataxia, and vomiting. Signs may develop within 45 minutes to 48 hours after exposure. Because 5-FU is a component of solutions and creams used topically in human patients with cancer, accidental ingestion may occur. Ingestion of more than 20 mg/kg was associated with development of toxicosis in dogs.[13] 5-FU is absolutely contraindicated in cats due to extreme sensitivity that leads to death.

PULMONARY TOXICITY

This complication is extremely rare in veterinary patients. Cisplatin given at standard canine dosages will cause acute pulmonary vasculitis in cats. Cats will develop fulminate, fatal pulmonary edema 48 to 96 hours after receiving cisplatin.[14] Due to this significant toxicity, cisplatin is contraindicated in cats.

Hydroxyurea is the drug of choice for polycythemia vera. A potential, but rare, complication of hydroxyurea in cats is methemoglobinemia and hemolytic anemia with Heinz bodies. Signs of methemoglobinemia include dyspnea and dark mucous membranes, and in the few cats reported, occur within 24 hours of receiving the drug.[15]

Finally, bleomycin can produce interstitial pneumonia and pulmonary fibrosis in dogs receiving large cumulative doses. This adverse effect is rare because bleomycin is not commonly used in veterinary patients.

REFERENCES

1. Ogilvie GK: Dolasetron: a new option for nausea and vomiting. *J Am Anim Hosp Assoc* 36:481, 2000.
2. Moore AS, Rand WM, Berg J, *et al.*: Evaluation of butorphanol and cyproheptadine for prevention of cisplatin-induced vomiting in dogs. *J Am Vet Med Assoc* 205:441, 1994.
3. Bienzle D, Stanton JB, Embry JM, *et al.*: Evaluation of an in-house centrifugal hematology analyzer for use in veterinary practice. *J Am Vet Med Assoc* 217:1195, 2000.
4. Ozer H, Armitage JO, Bennett CL, *et al.*: 2000 update of recommendations for the use of hematopoietic colony-stimulating factors: evidence-based, clinical practice guidelines. *J Clin Oncol* 18:3558, 2000.
5. Henry CJ, Buss MS, Potter KA, *et al.*: Mitoxantrone and cyclophosphamide combination chemotherapy for the treatment of various canine malignancies. *J Am Anim Hosp Assoc* 35:236, 1999.
6. Mauldin GE, Fox PR, Patnaik AK, *et al.*: Doxorubicin-induced cardiotoxicosis. Clinical features in 32 dogs. *J Vet Intern Med* 6:82, 1992.
7. O'Keefe DA, Sisson DD, Gelberg HB, *et al.*: Systemic toxicity associated with doxorubicin administration in cats. *J Vet Intern Med* 7:309, 1993.
8. Shan K, Lincoff AM, Young JB: Anthracycline-induced cardiotoxicity. *Ann Intern Med* 125:47, 1996.
9. Herman EH, Ferrans VJ: Preclinical animal models of cardiac protection from anthracycline-induced cardiotoxicity. *Semin Oncol* 25:15, 1998.
10. Phillips BS, Kraegel SA, Simonson E *et al.*: Acute reactions in dogs treated with doxorubicin: increased frequency with the use of a generic formulation. *J Vet Intern Med* 12:171, 1998.
11. Long HJ: Paclitaxel (Taxol): a novel anticancer chemotherapeutic drug. *Mayo Clin Proc* 69:341, 1994.
12. Hohenhaus AE, Matus RE: Etoposide (VP-16): retrospective analysis of treatment in 13 dogs with lymphoma. *J Vet Intern Med* 4:239, 1990.
13. Dorman DC, Coddington KA, Richardson RC: 5-Fluorouracil toxicosis in the dog. *J Vet Intern Med* 4:254, 1990.

14. Knapp DW, Richardson RC, DeNicola DB, *et al.*: Cisplatin toxicity in cats. *J Vet Intern Med* 1:29, 1987.
15. Watson ADJ, Moore AS, Helfand SC: Primary erythrocytosis in the cat: treatment with hydroxyurea. *J Small Anim Pract* 35:320, 1994.

SECTION XII
The Veterinary Critical Care Unit

83
Equipping an Emergency/Critical Care Veterinary Hospital

Wayne E. Wingfield

INTRODUCTION

The explosion of veterinary emergency clinics and now 24-hour critical care facilities during the past 10 years has led our profession to significant improvement in our ability to help the ill and injured animal. As a result of this improvement, patient survival is increased and client awareness and appreciation acknowledged. Simultaneously, the explosion in monitoring technology provides us with the ability to identify and follow physiologic parameters in emergency patients. Undoubtedly, the veterinarian is challenged to keep pace with the development and application of this technology. This is especially true in the busy emergency/critical care hospital. Cost and even medicolegal implications tend to be competing priorities and further muddy the waters when deciding what equipment is most useful in the emergency setting.

Important parallels can be drawn between development of monitoring technology and microprocessors. As the veterinarian tours down the many aisles of technology displayed at the large meetings, it is important to constantly ask "What technology will be developed next week that will make this week's technology obsolete?" Purchasing and equipping a veterinary emergency/critical care facility is not cheap! When identifying needs and purchasing monitoring equipment, one must be ever mindful of the need to upgrade hardware and software prior to committing to the purchase.

To *monitor* means to measure or observe a physiologic parameter either continuously or intermittently. The device may provide a snapshot in time or may allow trending to detect deterioration, tracking of improvement, or measurements of the effects of interventions.[1] Monitoring parameters such as clinical observation, routine vital sign measurement, and electrocardiographic (ECG) monitoring are basic requirements in the practice of emergency/critical care medicine. Regardless of the sophistication of the equipment, there is no substitute for appropriately trained and experienced emergency/critical care veterinarians and technicians in assessing and monitoring the acutely ill emergency patient.

There are five important questions to ask with respect to monitoring, and thus equipping, a veterinary emergency/critical care facility: (1) Which physiologic parameters are important indicators of a patient's medical status or progression? (2) What technology monitors that parameter? (3) Can the monitoring device be relied on to monitor that parameter with precision and accuracy given the animals of varying size, disposition, and cooperation? In other words, are there limitations to the technology? (4) How far is the animal's owner prepared to go and how skilled is the veterinarian in accepting the responsibility for more sophisticated monitoring? (5) Does the standard of care demand a certain level of monitoring?[2]

Recently, the American Animal Hospital Association (AAHA)[3] and the Veterinary Emergency and Critical Care Society (VECCS)[4] have provided important guidelines for emergency/critical care hospitals in veterinary medicine. The remainder of this chapter will attempt to summarize these guidelines. A complete set of the guidelines can be obtained by contacting AAHA and VECCS (http://www.veccs.org/guidelines.html).

VETERINARY EMERGENCY HOSPITALS

Veterinary emergency hospitals must be full-service hospitals. They must provide professional diagnostic and emergency treatment during hours when local veterinary facilities are normally closed. These hospitals must provide adequate space, staff, equipment, and material for professional diagnosis, emergency treatment, and surgery of critically ill or injured animals.

Personnel

At least two veterinarians with alternating shifts must be available to operate an emergency veterinary hospital. Alternatively, one veterinarian on a permanent basis, relieved by services of part-time veterinarians, will suffice. Each emergency hospital will have well-trained, auxiliary personnel available at all times. The personnel of an emergency hospital must be well-trained in the diagnosis and care of critically ill or injured animals, presurgical preparation, surgical assisting procedures, and actual nursing care.

Observation of critically ill or injured animals, recovery area care, care after the animal is returned to a cage, and proper use of bedding and control of heat loss are extremely important. All personnel must be thoroughly familiar with emergency procedures for the resuscitation of animals in a state of shock or respiratory, or cardiopulmonary arrest. This will include the proper administration and use of oxygen (O_2), anesthetics, endotracheal tubes, and monitoring and resuscitative equipment. All personnel will be familiar with the limitations of certain drugs, proper use of fluid therapy, advantages and limitations of certain crystalloid fluids, and proper use of hematogenous and synthetic colloids.

Personnel in an emergency hospital will be thoroughly familiar with emergency equipment, interpretation of results, troubleshooting, and limitations. Emergency equipment will include imaging devices, especially radiographic equipment. More and more the use of diagnostic ultrasound is encouraged to quickly seek the answer to questions of cardiac structure, function, and disease as well as identifying fluid, air, calculi, thrombosis, mass lesions, intestinal obstruction, pancreatitis, neoplasia, and urologic structure and abnormalities.

Other equipment will include a mobile, accessible, well-stocked crash cart. In this cart will be emergency drugs, resuscitation equipment, thoracocentesis setups, needles, syringes, and catheters. Sterile surgical packs that include needle holders, towel clamps, mosquito hemostats, Metzenbaum scissors, sharp-sharp scissors, Bard-Parker knife blade holder, at least one no. 10 blade, at least one Carmalt and Allis tissue forceps, thumb forceps, 4 × 4 gauze sponges, and towels should be available. Drugs available in the crash cart include epinephrine, atropine, magnesium chloride, sodium bicarbonate, lidocaine, bretylium tosylate, and naloxone. Drugs that must be readily available include 50% dextrose, analgesics (preferably morphine or fentanyl), diazepam, an antihistamine, O_2, and possibly corticosteroids (methylprednisolone and dexamethasone). Crystalloids (Normosol-R, 0.9% sodium chloride, 0.45% sodium chloride with 2.5% dextrose), hematogenous (fresh-frozen plasma and whole blood) and synthetic colloids (hetastarch or dextran-70), and possibly a hemoglobin-based O_2 therapeutic must be readily available.

Transfer of Patients

Most veterinary emergency hospitals are not equipped to provide additional care for animals. Thus, most will be released to the owner or be taken to another veterinary hospital for continuity of care. To maintain professional collegiality the veterinary staff and personnel at the emergency hospital must cooperate to accomplish a successful transfer of the emergency patient to the client's home or to another veterinary hospital. Additionally, the receiving hospital veterinarian and staff must cooperate with the emergency staff to accomplish a successful transfer. The receiving hospital will receive written notice of all procedures, drugs administered, complications, client and patient data, and recommendations provided to the client via a copy of the patient's medical record. If the animal is returned to the owner, written instructions are provided, and the veterinarian will answer all questions before discharging the animal. Additionally, the emergency veterinarian will provide the client with recommended contact information should complications or questions arise.

Examination Facilities

Examination facilities are necessary for the complete physical examination of patients. History taking, physical examination, minor therapy, ophthalmic or otoscopic examination, and client education are all activities that require a designated space. Admission to the hospital, dismissal from the hospital, and outpatient treatment are several intended functions of an examination room.

Equipment

The minimum equipment in each examination room will include an examination table that is easily sanitized and has a fluid-impervious surface. There will also be a stethoscope and a set of scales for recording an accurate weight for each patient. Additionally, there will be a thermometer, preferably infrared, or electronic capable of measuring body temperatures ranging from 21.1° to 44.4°C (70°–112°F). Each examination room should also include an otoscope with a variety of sized cones and a direct ophthalmoscope or indirect ophthalmic lens with a light source. To facilitate handwashing between each patient, a sink must be located in, or convenient to, each examination room. A radiographic view box must be located in, or convenient to, each examination room.

The size of the examination room should be no smaller than 80 square feet. This will allow the veterinarian, patient, client, and assistant to move easily in the room. The room must be kept clean and professional and should be attractive in appearance.

Medical Records

A detailed, legible, individual record must be maintained for every patient. It is recommended that letter-sized records be in place or electronic data storage be used. These records serve as a basis for planning patient care and promote communication among members of the hospital staff and referring or regular veterinarian. The records furnish documentary evidence of the patient's illness, hospital care, and treatment and serve as a basis for review, study, and evaluation of medical care rendered by the veterinarian and the hospital.

Personnel and Procedures

There must be an established system of medical record keeping within the veterinary emergency hospital. Each animal must have a separate medical record. However, the medical record for a litter may be recorded either on the dam's record or on a litter record until the individual animals are permanently placed or reach the age of 3 months.

These records communicate valuable information; they must be legible. The patient identification used will follow through all areas of the hospital on other records (*i.e.*, radiographs, laboratory, ultrasound, and necropsy records). All medical records will be kept long enough to comply with federal, state, provincial, or local regulations (usually 3–10 years). A copy of the medical record must be sent to the primary care veterinarian in a timely manner for inclusion in the patient's medical record. The veterinary staff will record sufficient information in the history and examination portions of the record to justify the tentative diagnosis and to warrant the treatment. No prescribed coding is required, but the hospital director should require meticulous recording of information. Where abbreviations are used, application of AAHA standard abbreviations is encouraged. The author of all medical record entries must be legibly identified (*i.e.*, full name, code number, employee number, or initials).

Each emergency hospital must maintain records in such a fashion that any veterinarian coming into the hospital may, by reading the medical record of a particular patient, be able to proceed with the continuity of care and treatment of this animal. Consent forms will be used when animals are admitted to the facility and will be considered a part of the medical record.

Medical Records Equipment

No particular filing equipment or system is required, but the hospital director will review the medical record filing system for ease of retrieval cross-referenced information. Whichever system is chosen, it must be adequate for the case load and for staff use. Although there are no structural specifications for housing records, there must be adequate space for reception, filing, and clerical operations necessary for both admission and discharge of patients.

Structure of the Medical Record

The structure of the medical record is either problem or source oriented. The problem-oriented veterinary medical record (POVMR) format is strongly recommended. Each medical record must clearly reflect the date, initial problem, pertinent history, examination findings, plan for treatment and care, and should note the veterinarian's impression for a prognosis. The medical record should clearly reflect a tentative diagnoses or rule-outs. Use of a cost-estimate sheet is encouraged. This sheet should break down all costs as close as can possibly be ascertained. The cost estimate should be signed by both the veterinarian and client. One copy will remain with the medical record and the second will be given to the client. The record must reflect written discharge instructions to be given to the client.

Patient Information. Each animal must be properly identified. The following identification will be recorded accurately on each patient's medical record: patient's name (ID number if applicable), species, breed, date of birth, sex, color, and/or markings.

Client Information. Each client must be identified properly. The owner's name, address, home, and alternate telephone numbers will be recorded accurately within each patient's medical record. The name, address, and telephone number of the client's primary care veterinarian should be entered into the medical record. Other useful data may include the name of the person who referred the client or other reason for selecting the facility.

Chief Complaint. The complaint is an important part of the medical history and must be included. Observations made by the client about signs exhibited by the patient, which may be important clues to the identification of the illness and its underlying causes, should compose the balance of the history. A problem is entered on the medical record only if it can be defined by objective data.

Medical History. A thorough medical history will be documented. Several problems may be present, though the owner may have noticed only that one for which the animal was presented to the veterinarian. It is important to both problem definition and treatment to acquire and record as complete a medical history as possible, including all previous illnesses, injuries, surgeries, radiographs, vaccinations, laboratory tests, most recent body weight, anthelmintics administered, and current medical/surgical/cancer regimens.

Physical Examination. A report of physical examinations must be written. All patients must be given an appropriate physical examination before all medical or surgical procedures. A systematic procedure of examination should be followed. Current body weight will be recorded in the medical record. The record must accurately reflect the findings (both normal and abnormal) for each system examined. If a system is not examined, it should be noted on the physical examination report.

Progress Notes. Records of treatment, both medical and surgical, must minimally reflect all procedures performed in chronological order and in the context of the medical or surgical problem to which they pertain. The record of medical treatment will include identification of each medication given in the hospital, together with the date, dosage, route of administration (when more than one route is acceptable), frequency, and duration of treatment. The individual administering the medications should be identified with each treatment. All medications dispensed or prescribed must be recorded on the medical record, including directions for use and quantity. Any changes in medications or doses, including changes made by telephone, also must be recorded on the patient's chart or record. Client waivers or deferrals of recommended care must be noted on the progress notes. Client communication, including recall or recheck recommendations made to the client, also must be noted on the progress notes.

Surgical Record. An accurate summary of all surgical procedures including identity of the surgeon must be kept in the patient's medical record.

Necropsy Reports. If a necropsy is performed, the gross findings will be accurately recorded, tissues to be submitted for histopathology noted, and samples taken for additional diagnostic tests (*i.e.*, cultures, titers, parvovirus, ethylene glycol, and so forth) will be written into the record.

Problem List or Index. A problem is anything that interferes with the patient's well-being and requires management or further evaluation. This may be a clinical sign, physiologic abnormality, physical finding, abnormal laboratory test result, or a diagnosis. A separate listing of the patient's problems must be maintained and can serve as the index or table of contents for the entire record. Each problem or diagnosis will be listed chronologically and will represent the current health status of the animal. In the traditional, source-oriented medical record, this list is called the diagnostic summary index; in the POVMR, it is called the master problem list.

Diagnostic Reports. The patient's permanent record will contain a report of all laboratory tests conducted, significant abnormal conditions detected, and results of all biopsy specimen evaluations. Diagnostic reports, including histopathologic, cytologic, and ECG evaluations, must be written on the patient's record or on a separate form and included in the patient's record. Diagnostic imaging evaluations must be noted in the medical record or on a separate form attached to the patient's record and should include the part imaged, special techniques, and a diagnostic record of findings. The record should contain a cross-reference so that the patient's imaging files may be easily located. The practice of filing radiographic films separate from the patient's medical record should be encouraged.

Consultation. Professional consultation reports must be summarized, included in the patient's record, or written on a separate form attached to the patient's record. Telephone or on-site consultations with other professionals also must be recorded, showing the consultant, date, and recommendations from the consultation.

Prognosis. In complex or serious cases, a prognosis must be made and recorded following a thorough examination and tentative diagnosis. The probable outcome must be described with that term which best explains the case. Usually one of the following applies: good, fair, guarded, or grave.

Pharmacy

Veterinary emergency hospitals will provide for storage, safekeeping, and use of drugs in accordance with federal, state, and provincial regulations. The pharmacy is where drugs are stored, secured, and prepared for internal use or dispensing. Internal controls should be in effect for substances that can be abused as well as those items regulated by federal, state, or provincial regulations. The hospital director is responsible for maintenance of the pharmacy and required records of controlled substances. A separate, accurate, and properly cross-referenced log must be maintained for all controlled drugs used and dispensed. The logs should not be stored in the locked cabinet used to store those drugs to which it applies. Each hospital director must ensure that all records comply with federal, state, or provincial regulations. In the United States, this includes but is not limited to the following: (1) initial inventory, (2) biennial (every 2 years) inventory, and (3) balance on hand. Documentation must be retained for the full statute of limitations as established by federal, state, or provincial regulations.

Adequate quantities of drugs and supplies must be available at all times. The hospital director will ensure that all outdated drugs are returned or disposed of in accordance with federal, state, provincial, and local regulations.

When dispensing medication, each label will include the following formatted information: be typed or printed (clear tape should be placed over the label to preserve it), be permanently affixed to the container, include expiration (if appropriate), include warning labels (if appropriate). Each label must have recorded thereon the following information: client's name, patient's name, date, name of the drug, usage directions including route of administration, quantity dispensed, hospital's name, address, and telephone number including area code, and the name of the veterinarian dispensing the drug. If a child-resistant container is declined by the client, it must be noted on the patient's medical record.

Drugs will only be dispensed or administered on the order of a licensed veterinarian.

Each dose of any medication administered, dispensed, or prescribed will be recorded on the medical record, including usage directions, quantity, and number of refills. Telephone calls changing medications or dosages also must be recorded on the medical record. If clients bring their animal's medications to the hospital, these drugs should not be administered unless they can be identified. Orders to administer these medications should be given by the veterinarian in charge of the animal. Any drugs that are not used should be stored and returned to the client on the discharge of the animal from the hospital. Hazardous medications (*e.g.*, chemotherapeutic medications) will be handled in accordance with federal, state, or provincial regulations. Drugs used in euthanasia procedures must be stored in a locked cabinet. It is recommended that these agents be identified and segregated.

Equipment

Equipment must include cabinets or shelf units for storage of drugs and supplies; shelves for reference materials; clean surfaces for drug preparation; fixed, lockable units for safekeeping of all controlled drugs; and a refrigerator for those products that require refrigeration. Proper storage of drugs must not allow for any cross-contamination, but it should permit all preparations to be readily and easily located. One of several storage systems may be used: alphabetical, by usage, or by type. All dispensed or repackaged medications must be in approved, child-resistant containers unless otherwise requested by the client or if the drug packaging precludes it from being dispensed in such a container. The container must in no way alter the drugs being dispensed and must be moisture resistant.

Each pharmacy must contain at least one reference text, formulary, or compendium of pharmaceuticals that is current (within 3 years) and provides the necessary information on drugs, chemicals, and biologicals in use within the hospital or dispensed for use by the client. Current antidote information should be readily available for emergency reference in addition to the telephone number of a poison control center. The client should be made aware of possible adverse drug reactions and the proper procedure to follow if problems should occur. Staff education about adverse reactions and contraindications for the use of all drugs, chemicals, and biologicals used within the hospital is encouraged.

Laboratory

Clinical pathology services are necessary for the proper diagnosis and treatment of many diseases. Whether the procedures are performed within or outside the hospital will be determined by the services available, economics, proximity of the hospital to outside laboratories, and qualifications of such laboratories to handle animal samples. Ideally, when an outside laboratory is used, an American College of Veterinary Pathology diplomate should be affiliated with the laboratory, especially for histopathologic services. Results of life-dependent procedures should be available within a few hours after sample collection. Blood gas and electrolytes results should be available within 1 hour. The choice of procedures used with any particular patient is a professional decision.

Pathology services available must include the following: hematology and serology, blood chemistry analysis, blood gases, urinalysis, including urine sediment examination, microbiology, culturing, and antibiotic sensitivity, parasitologic examinations (fecal, blood, and skin), exfoliative cytology, histology or histopathology, toxicology, blood medication and hormone levels, and fluid analysis (including composition analysis, cultures, and cytology).

Specimen Data

Each specimen must be identified with the identification of the patient.

Necropsy Data

Each necropsy procedure and record thereof must be thorough and detailed. Tentative diagnosis, where appropriate, will be recorded promptly in the patient's medical record. The final report will be made a part of the patient's medical record.

The hospital director is responsible for the accuracy of tests performed both in and outside the hospital. The director or a practice associate must be fully aware of all techniques used within the hospital to train personnel, monitor the performances of personnel, and perform basic tests in emergency situations. Pathology services are an essential component to the practice of quality veterinary medicine and must be readily available. Reference range values must be available for all laboratory tests performed by both in-house and external laboratories.

Outside laboratory logs must reflect the following data: data from specimen, date of sample collection, identity of outside laboratory, tests required, date results received, and date results are communicated to the emergency veterinarian. Reports of all pathology services and examinations must be made part of the patient's medical record.

Quality Control Program

All in-house laboratory services performed must be carried out by competent personnel using approved standard laboratory procedures. The quality control system within the pathology laboratory will be designed to ensure medical reliability of laboratory data. For in-hospital laboratory procedures, equipment must be operated and evaluated according to the manufacturer's recommendations and have a written protocol of operation. A record of the quality control tests and maintenance procedures performed on all laboratory equipment will be maintained.

For outside laboratory procedures, a current letter from the outside laboratory should be available ensuring that a quality control program is in effect. The outside laboratory should participate at least annually in proficiency surveys or reference sample services covering all types of analyses performed to verify competence.

Equipment

Instrumentation for tests performed on the premises must be adequate. The minimum equipment must include the following: microhematocrit, microscope (binocular preferred), clinical centrifuge, refractometer, refrigerator, glucometer or blood glucose determination strips, cytologic stains, activated clotting time tests, and an ethylene glycol test kit.

If the services of an outside laboratory are not used, the following equipment and necessary supplies must be available: hemocytometer or electronic cell counter, incubator (37°C), blood chemistry analyzer, in-house serology kits, electrolyte and blood gas equipment, lactate analyzer, and coagulation assay equipment.

A continuous record should be maintained on the daily submission of specimens. Each specimen should be numbered or otherwise properly identified. Each specimen should be identified with laboratory number. In each laboratory, a separate laboratory log should be maintained in which all laboratory tests are recorded chronologically as conducted or reported. In-office laboratory logs must reflect the following information: data from specimen, date of sample collection, identification of personnel performing tests, and the tests requested.

Diagnostic Imaging

The emergency veterinary hospital must have the capacity to generate quality radiographic images on the premises. Diagnostic imaging exists to aid in the accurate diagnosis and evaluation of medical and surgical problems and to assist in determining an appropriate course of management.

Personnel and Procedures

Radiographic equipment will be operated only by persons aware of all hazards (actual and potential) to themselves, assisting personnel, patients, and other nearby individuals. Educational information must be available to all staff concerning radiation safety. Documentation of a radiation safety program must be on file. Radiation safety procedures must be in compliance with all federal, state, provincial, or local regulations.

Monitoring of Exposure. Dosimeter monitoring of exposure levels must be provided for all personnel working with or near an x-ray generator. The individual badge will be worn near the collar on the outside of the leaded apron. Records of the exposure results must be maintained indefinitely and be readily available. Exposure results must be communicated to each of the staff.

Inspections. Machines must be inspected in accordance with federal, state, provincial, or local regulations. Results of inspections must be posted. Hospital personnel must be made aware of the medical and legal importance of proper image identification and of organized storage of these imaging records. A special file of images on specific conditions or examples of normal structures can be used for comparative and demonstration purposes. Use of skeletal models is encouraged. If images are retained, they must be in compliance with federal, state, provincial, or local regulations. Images of patients must be identified properly and filed for easy location and retrieval.

Processing. An automatic processor must be well maintained and capable of good-quality film processing. A regular cleaning schedule should be established and documented. A regular maintenance schedule should be established and documented.

Imaging Log. An imaging log must be maintained and must include the following information: date, owner and patient identification, area imaged, views taken, and technician/veterinarian identification. The other factors logged should include the following: species and breed, date of birth or age, time, kVp, mA, thickness of the area radiographed, use of a grid, and level of sedation (awake, sedated, anesthetized). All films taken must show evidence of collimation. Lead gloves, aprons, and thyroid collars (shields) must be tested yearly for effectiveness.

Equipment

Cassettes loaded with film must be stored in a manner to protect them from unintended exposure. Two or more of each size of cassette used should be available. Radiopaque characters will be used to identify right (R) and left (L) sides of the patient. Permanent identification of each image is required and must occur prior to processing. Minimal image identification must include date, patient identification, and hospital identification. Additionally, owner name and patient date of birth or age should be included.

Measuring calipers to determine accurately the thickness of the part being radiographed must be used to reduce nondiagnostic exposures. All personnel must wear protective apparel while in the room during exposure. Protective equipment must include leaded aprons, gloves, and thyroid collars (shields). At least two aprons, two pairs of gloves, and two thyroid shields must be available. They must be in safe condition and properly cared for to ensure a reasonable life. All protective apparel must meet federal, state, provincial, or local regulations. Proper safelights with lamps of correct wattage must be mounted at the recommended distance from work areas. The color of safelight filters depends on the type of films being used.

Radiograph Machine. The hospital must have the capacity to generate quality radiographic images on the premises. All regulatory agencies require a total of 2.5 mm of aluminum equivalent filtration in the x-ray beam. It must be within, above, or part of the collimator. The x-ray machine, generator, tube, and tube stand must have a capacity that is adequate to produce consistent films of diagnostic quality.

The x-ray table must be large enough to accommodate the largest patient seen by the practice positioned for a ventrodorsal view of the pelvis and femurs. Adequate working space around three sides of the table must be provided. A balanced combination of film and imaging screens should be used. A rare-earth high-speed system is recommended to reduce radiation exposure.

A reliable exposure chart (technique chart) must be available near the x-ray controls and should be used by all personnel. The radiographic machine must have an adjustable collimator or a series of attachable cones to restrict the size and shape of the primary x-ray beam to the size of the cassette being used.

Positioning devices and tie-downs must be provided and should be used when radiographing anesthetized patients so that personnel are not needlessly exposed. High-speed film and imaging screen systems must be used unless the x-ray machine has an attainable output of 300 mA at 125 kVp. Grids, either fixed or moving (Bucky), must be available for use. Alignment of a grid with central rays of the x-ray beam is easier to maintain if the grid is mounted under the table top in conjunction with a tray for holding and centering the cassettes. Any new grid purchased for "fixed" operation should have aluminum interspaces, not fiber.

At a minimum, two radiographic view boxes will be present; one of these should be in surgery. Use of surgical suite viewers must be restricted to surgical cases and not as the site for routine study and film interpretation.

Diagnostic Ultrasonography. If ultrasonography services are provided, equipment for this imaging modality must be a type that is appropriate for patients imaged. It is recommended that the machine used be equipped to record the study as it is being performed.

State-of-the-Art Diagnostics. If computed tomography scanning, nuclear magnetic resonance imaging, or other computerized imaging methods are used, all procedures and safety aspects of their operation must be in compliance with current laws and medical practice.

Structure

It is desirable to have a separate room devoted to radiography; however, it may serve other purposes provided it is not the major surgery room. It is recommended that the x-ray controls, at least the exposure control device, be located outside the radiographic room. Whenever possible, x-ray personnel should be behind a lead shield or screen or outside the room during the exposure. The protective barrier effect of the walls and doors should be such that adjacent occupied areas will not receive radiation above recommended levels. Room structure, shielded control booth, or other restrictive barriers must comply with federal, state, provincial, or local radiation safety regulations.

The darkroom must be light tight and sufficient in size. The light-tight darkroom should be painted a light color to enhance safelight effectiveness. The darkroom must be adequately ventilated in compliance with federal, state, provincial, and local regulations.

It is suggested that anesthesia or sedation be used whenever possible for comfort, safety, and minimizing stress for the patient and the safety of the personnel performing the radiographic procedures. Image-amplified fluoroscopy is the only type of fluoroscopy advisable in the practice of veterinary medicine. It is advisable to refer the patient to an institutional facility or to a veterinary radiologist who has access to these special units. It is recommended that lead glasses be used when extensive radiographic procedures are performed (*e.g.*, fluoroscopy).

Anesthesiology

Anesthesia services must include performance of routine preanesthetic examinations and exercise of proper safeguards in selection and use of anesthetics. Although the type of anesthesia for each procedure is left to the discretion of the attending veterinarian, the continued study, evaluation, and use of newer and safer anesthetic agents and equipment are recommended.

Personnel and Procedures

Anesthesia services must be provided. These services will include routine preanesthetic examination and awareness of proper anesthetic safeguards in selection and use. Anesthetic agents should be administered by a veterinarian or by persons trained in their administration and under supervision of an on-premises veterinarian. Administration will be in compliance with federal, state, provincial, or local regulations.

A preanesthetic examination must be performed on the day of the administration of any premedication or the induction of the anesthetic. There must be a notation of the veterinarian's findings (both normal and abnormal) for each system examined. Cardiac, respiratory, arterial blood pressure, or other electronic monitors must be used. A consent form for anesthesia or surgery will be available and used in all cases where a general anesthetic is required.

During anesthesia, some method of respiratory monitoring will be used, such as observing chest movements, watching the rebreathing bag, or using a respiratory monitor. When endotracheal tubes are used, they must remain in place during recovery from anesthesia until appropriate protective reflexes have returned to lessen the occurrence of aspiration pneumonitis.

In the event of cardiopulmonary arrest, standard procedures for cardiac resuscitation will be followed using drugs and equipment to be found in an emergency cabinet, on a crash cart, or on an emergency tray. Doses and dosages must be printed for all emergency drugs or be readily available in chart form.

An anesthesia and surgical log must be maintained but they can be combined. The anesthesia log must contain the following information: date, patient identification, preanesthetic agent, anesthetic agent, the volume drawn and amount used, the surgical procedure, duration of the anesthetic, and duration of the surgery.

Surgery/Anesthesia Mortality Record

A log of hospital mortalities related to surgery or anesthesia must be complete and readily accessible. The record must show the following information: date, patient and client identification, type of anesthesia and equipment used, preoperative condition of patient, cause of death (if known), and all applicable diagnostic laboratory tests.

Equipment

All equipment needed for the administration of local and general anesthesia must be readily available and in good repair. The anesthetic area must have emergency lighting available. The anesthetic area will contain the following: preanesthetic agents, induction anesthetic agents for intravenous (IV) administration, anesthetic and preanesthetic antagonists (as appropriate), appropriately sized endotracheal tubes and tube adapters, antiseptic agent for venipuncture preparation, sterilized needles and syringes, a stethoscope, a blanket to retain an animal's body heat, a machine for the administration of gaseous anesthesia that includes a canister containing a fresh agent to absorb carbon dioxide, gaseous agent for the induction and maintenance of general anesthesia, an O_2 source and a device for administration of the O_2, a gas scavenging system that complies with federal, state, provincial, and local regulations, and a rebreathing bag or similar device for monitoring respiration.

Support Equipment

Emergency medications and equipment required in the event of a cardiopulmonary arrest must be available (may be located in the operating room). IV catheters, administration sets, IV fluids or other cardiovascular support medications (plasma expanders, whole blood) must be readily available. Some means of assisting ventilation, either manual or mechanical, must be readily available during general anesthesia. The anesthetic area must contain the following: an electronic respiratory monitor (it is recommended that monitoring equipment be in proportion with the anesthetic case load and anesthetic equipment available), the ability to monitor end-tidal carbon dioxide is recommended (especially in the case of the 24-hour critical care facility), an ECG or heart monitor, temperature monitor, esophageal stethoscope, pulse oximeter, and blood pressure monitor (direct or indirect).

Structure

The emergency veterinary facility must contain an area for the administration of general anesthesia. A recovery area outside the operating room or a recovery room where the patient can be observed closely until appropriate protective reflexes have returned will be available.

Surgery

A separate room for aseptic surgical procedures must be provided.

Definitions

- *Surgery:* The act of incising living tissue; an operative procedure; and/or a room or facility where an operative procedure is done (*i.e.*, the operating room).
- *Aseptic surgery:* Surgery performed in ways or by means sufficiently free from microorganisms so that significant infection or suppuration does not occur.
- *Minor surgery:* Any surgical intervention that neither penetrates and exposes a body cavity nor produces permanent impairment of physical or physiologic function. Examples are superficial wound suturing and cutaneous biopsy.
- *Major surgery:* Any surgical intervention that penetrates and exposes the body cavity; any procedure that has the potential for producing permanent physical or physiologic impairment; or any procedure associated with extensive transection or dissection of tissue.

Personnel and Procedures

All surgeries must be performed by a licensed veterinarian.

Preparation of Patient. A standard, accepted procedure must be used to prepare the patient for surgery. All personnel assisting in the presurgical preparation of the patient must be aware of the danger and sources of bacterial contamination. They must be adequately trained and under the direct supervision of a veterinarian.

Surgical Attire. Surgical assistants and the surgeon must be properly attired with cap, mask, sterile gown, and sterile gloves when major surgery is performed. Surgeons, surgical assistants, and operating room attendants will wear a surgical cap and mask at all times while in the surgical suite. All scalp and facial hair must be completely covered by the cap and mask. Operating room attendants should remain outside of the sterile field. The sterile field is the area above the sterile drapes on the operating table and adjacent instrument trays. The sterile field extends from the edges of these drapes in a vertical plane to the ceiling.

Sterility. Surgical procedures require the use of sterilized instruments, gowns, towels, drapes, and gloves as well as clean caps and masks. Sterile surgical packs will be used for each patient. Surgical packs must be steam or gas sterilized. A regular maintenance program for autoclaves and other sterilizing equipment must be instituted. Employee training must be adequate for the proper operation of the equipment and awareness of any malfunction that may occur. When gas or steam sterilization procedures are used, sterility indicators will be in evidence on the exterior surface of each unit. When large surgical bundles (gowns, drapes, instrument packs) are sterilized, monitors that verify appropriate steam temperature and time must be used in the center of each pack. A pressure of 15 lb at

106.9°C (250°F) for 15 minutes is sufficient to kill both spore-forming and non-spore-forming bacteria. However, penetration of steam into large surgical bundles will be slower, so at least 30 minutes must be allowed for sterilization. The drapes, laparotomy sheets, towels, gauze sponges, suture materials, and gowns to be sterilized must be properly wrapped. The contents of the bundles must be in good repair, cleaned or laundered, dried, wrapped, and sterilized as outlined. Surgical packs will be dated with the date on which they were sterilized. If not used within 30 days, packs must be resterilized before use. Shelf-life may be extended by using alternative wraps, such as double wrap, steri-peel, and dust covers. Single-use sterile surgical gloves must be used. Cold sterilization solution must be changed in accordance with manufacturer's recommendations. The use of cold sterilization should be limited to those instruments used in minor surgical procedures or those that cannot be steam sterilized.

Surgical Patients

Every patient presented for surgery must have a documented presurgical examination immediately before the procedure. There must be a notation of the findings (both normal and abnormal) for each system examined. The following factors must be addressed: positive patient identification, satisfactory immunization history, history of possible complicating problems, general physical examination or anesthetic risk assessment, laboratory evaluation (as indicated), radiographic evaluation (as indicated), and indication or reason for surgical procedure(s).

Every patient with unexpected reactions associated with surgery should be evaluated by applicable diagnostic procedures—clinical pathology, histopathology, microbiology, necropsy, and toxicology.

When a surgical assistant is working within the sterile field. The individual will wear the same attire as the surgeon. The assistant must have a functional knowledge of aseptic surgery and know the names and application of surgical instruments and suture material.

Equipment

Dry heat and gas sterilizers are useful in the preparation of surgical instruments. Special care must be taken when using gas sterilization to ensure that the procedure does not in any way present a risk to personnel or patients. Gas sterilization procedures must be in compliance with federal, state, provincial, and local regulations. Steam under pressure is best for sterilization of gowns, gloves, towels, laparotomy sheets, and gauze sponges. Any autoclave-type apparatus equipped with a pressure gauge must maintain steam at a pressure high enough and for a period long enough to kill all bacteria and their spores. Brushes used for scrubbing surgeon's hands must be thoroughly washed and sterilized. Reusable caps and masks should be laundered after each day's use. Disposable caps, masks, and scrub brushes are preferred.

Equipment that must be present in the operating room will include the following: surgical light of adequate candle power to illuminate the surgical field (preferably the type of lamp that is completely enclosed to avoid dust accumulation), instrument table(s) constructed of impervious material, surgical table(s) constructed of impervious material, IV fluid hanger(s), a gas anesthetic machine capable of being able to provide respiratory assistance with a vaporizer(s) compatible with the gaseous agent(s) used, a bucket receptacle of impervious material (kick bucket, preferably mobile), supply of O_2, battery-operated or alternate power supply emergency lighting, and adequate drugs for emergency use readily available in an accessible emergency box or designated place (may be located in the anesthetic induction area). Equipment that must be present in the operating room includes the following: thick pads on the surgery tables for comfort and alleviation of possible injury to patients, a temperature control pad must be available and used, radiographic viewer limited to surgical use, a wall clock, electronic respiratory monitor, electrocardiograph or heart monitor, suction apparatus, and an IV pump. The operating room should include an electrosurgical unit.

Proper scavenging of all excess anesthetic waste gases must be provided in accordance with all federal, state, provincial, and local regulations. Equipment that will be present in the surgical preparation area includes the following: surgical instrumentation must be properly cleaned, in good repair, and sufficient in number and variety to match the requirements of the surgical case load, O_2, anesthetic machine, gas scavenger system, emergency drugs, endotracheal tubes, instruments used for intubation, clippers with a surgical blade or other accepted means of hair removal, and a vacuum device to remove loose hair clipped from the patient.

Equipment that must be components of the scrub area will include the following: knee-, elbow-, electric eye-, or foot-operated hot and cold water taps, deep sink made of impervious material, foot- or elbow-operated or automatic soap dispenser.

Structure

Surgical Preparation Room. Preoperative preparation must be performed outside the operating room. The preparation room should be a separate room convenient to the operating room and well lit. Floors, walls, and countertops should be of smooth, impervious material that is easily cleaned. This room may double as a laboratory, scrub room, treatment room, or extra examination room.

Operating Room. The operating room must be a separate, closed, single-purpose room for only aseptic surgical procedures. An aseptic surgical suite can be located anywhere in the hospital, provided it is convenient to the recovery rooms and the prep room. It should be out of traffic areas. The operating room must be so constructed and equipped that cleanliness can be easily maintained. Flooring must be of an impervious material. Walls and ceilings must be of a washable, impervious material. Doors must be well fitted and should be wide enough to permit passage of patients. These doors must be kept closed and traffic into the surgical suite kept to a minimum. A viewing window will reduce the need for support personnel to open the door to see into the room. Telephones in the operating room may promote excessive traffic and, therefore, should not be located in that room. Telephones used as voice-activated intercoms are permitted, provided that they do not result in excessive operating room traffic and a compromised surgical environment. The operating room should have positive pressure airflow to avoid contamination.

Scrub Area. The scrub area must be of adequate size to permit the installation and operation of any standard type knee-, elbow-, electric eye-, or foot-operated, deep scrub sink of impervious material. The surgical scrub sink must be located outside of the surgical suite and in an area immediately adjacent to the surgical suite. It may be part of a preparation room or treatment room. The scrub area should be protected from contamination.

Nursing Care

Personnel and Procedures

Nursing care must be provided and must include the provision of diagnostic, presurgical, surgical, and recovery procedures as well as custodial care. A job description should delineate functions, responsibilities, and desired qualifications for each position of nursing service. All patient care provided by the nursing staff will be under the supervision of a veterinarian.

Each patient will be positively and properly identified (sufficient to differentiate between two like animals) during their hospital stay. Each medication will be entered on the patient's medical record showing date, name of drug, type, dose, route of administration (when more than one route is acceptable), and frequency of administration. All referred patients (ECG, internal medicine, and so forth) must have a summary of results, interpretations, diagnosis, and treatment recommendations returned to the referring facility for inclusion in the patient's file.

The practice staff must demonstrate humane care of animals and provide for the care and prevention of animal abuse or neglect of patients. Nursing personnel will ensure that all animals are individually housed unless otherwise requested by owner and approved by the veterinarian. Nursing personnel will be trained to know the proper maintenance of optimum body temperature of all patients and to ensure patients' comfort and cleanliness, ensure that water and food is withheld or provided when required, be trained in the proper restraint and handling of patients, and therapeutic bathing and dipping. Proper protective apparel must be worn by all personnel performing therapeutic bathing and dipping.

Nursing notes must be recorded in the patient's medical record. All personnel must be trained and routinely monitored to ensure that medications are administered in accordance with the directions of the veterinarian. Accurate and complete records must be kept by personnel administering any kind of medication. Assignments must be made so that one person is responsible for the proper observation of each anesthetized patient. Nursing personnel must be trained in the proper use of O_2 and anesthetics, placement of endotracheal tubes, and use of monitoring, and resuscitative equipment.

Nursing personnel must be capable of performing an ECG for purposes of monitoring or diagnostic testing, be trained to assist in the resuscitation of patients, and the proper method of handling animals found in a state of shock or respiratory or cardiac collapse. Nursing personnel must be trained in the proper establishment, monitoring, and administration of fluid therapy.

Nursing personnel must be trained in the principles of contagious nursing care. Proper handwashing between patients is considered to be the most effective way to prevent cross-contamination. The nursing staff must be familiar with the proper handling and disposal of all waste materials and the cleaning and disinfection of compartments, exercise areas, and runs. If external exercise areas exist, and cannot be easily cleaned, all fecal waste must be removed promptly.

When and if animals with contagious diseases are hospitalized, ideally, they must be housed in a separate, single-purpose isolation room. Proper attire must be used for handling animals with contagious diseases. Proper attire includes disposable or easily disinfected gowns, disposable foot coverings or a means of disinfecting footwear, and disposable gloves. All contaminated materials must be double-bagged or decontaminated before removal from the area where a patient with infectious disease is housed or examined. The biomedical waste must be disposed of in accordance with federal, state, provincial, and local regulations. If a single-purpose isolation room exists, only the equipment and material for the care and treatment of the current patient within the isolation room may be kept therein. Twenty-four-hour nursing care or observation must be available for hospitalized patients.

Equipment

Emergency veterinary hospitals must have on-site access to an ECG or transtelephonic ECG transmitter, a means by which an O_2-enriched environment can be created must be in evidence within the facility, a water blanket or other means of maintaining body temperature must be available, fluid monitors, such as burettes or fluid chambers, or infusion pumps must be available. A method for the indirect monitoring of arterial blood pressure should be available.

Structure

There are no specific ward requirements; however, all animal-holding areas must be secure, escape-proof, and easily cleaned. Runs or exercise areas must be available, maintainable, secure, escape-proof, and adequate in relation to the normal caseload. The facility must provide cages or runs that are large enough to permit the largest patient admitted to the facility to turn about freely and to easily stand, sit, and lie in a comfortable, normal position. All runs should be sloped and individually drained to prevent cross-contamination. If drained by a common trough, the trough *must* be covered. Concrete floors and runs must be well sealed, clean, and in good repair. Cage doors and run gates must be clean and in good repair. All cages and runs must be constructed in such a way that contamination from one animal to the next is controlled at all times. The partitions between the runs should be of solid construction and impervious material to a minimum height of 48 inches above the finished floor. Nose-to-nose contact above the partitions can be prevented by not housing large-breed dogs in adjacent runs.

Continuing Education

A medical library consisting of basic textbooks and current periodicals must be provided. The professional library must include current books, periodicals, and other multimedia materials appropriate to the needs of the staff. It is recommended that the library be conveniently located so that hospital staff can easily enter, quickly refer to relevant medical literature, and return to work. The library should offer seating and writing surfaces for more leisurely research but also should be capable of supporting audiovisual equipment.

REFERENCES

1. Phillips GD, Runciman WB, Isley AH: Monitoring in emergency medicine. *Resuscitation* 18(suppl):S21, 1989.
2. Murphy MF: Monitoring the emergency patient. *In* Rosen P, ed.: Emergency Medicine: Concepts and Clinical Practice. Philadelphia: Mosby, 1998, p 119.
3. American Animal Hospital Association (AAHA) Emergency and Critical Care Standards and Accreditation Manual. Denver, CO: AAHA, 2000, p 1.
4. Recommendations for Veterinary Emergency and Critical Care Facilities. San Antonio, TX: Veterinary Emergency and Critical Care Society (VECCS), 2000, p 1.

SUGGESTED READINGS

Baker SJ, Tremper KK: Pulse oximetry: applications and limitations. *Int Anesthesiol Clin* 25:155, 1987.

Bateman SW, Mathews KA, Abrams-Ogg, AC, *et al.*: Evaluation of point-of-care tests for diagnosis of disseminated intravascular coagulation in dogs admitted to an intensive care unit. *J Am Vet Med Assoc* 215:805, 1999.

Buck WB. A poison control center for animals: liability and standard of care. *J Am Vet Med Assoc* 203:1118, 1993.

De Jong JR, Ros HH, De Lange JJ: Noninvasive continuous blood pressure measurement during anesthesia: a clinical evaluation of a method commonly used in measuring devices. *Int J Clin Monit Comput* 12:1, 1995.

Gattinoni L, Brazzi L, Pelosi P, *et al.*: A trial of goal-oriented hemodynamic therapy in critically ill patients. *N Engl J Med* 333:1025, 1995.

Grosenbaugh DA, Gadawski JE, Muir WW: Evaluation of a portable clinical analyzer in a veterinary hospital setting. *J Am Vet Med Assoc* 213:691, 1998.

Hannah HW: Malpractice—the higher standard of skill and care. *J Am Vet Med Assoc* 165:880, 1974.

Hannah HW: Diagnosis—what is the standard of care? *J Am Vet Med Assoc* 181:664, 1982.

Hannah HW: Practice standards and the standard of skill and care. *J Am Vet Med Assoc* 188:497, 1986.

Hannah HW: The standard of care—some legal considerations. *J Am Vet Med Assoc* 200: 610, 1992.

Hannah HW: Establishing the standard of care. *J Am Vet Med Assoc* 208:1034, 1996.
Hannah HW: Practice standards—by law, by regulation, by code of ethics, by association's guidelines, or not at all? *J Am Vet Med Assoc* 214:638, 1999.
Herrick JB: Food for thought for food animal veterinarians: standard of care. *J Am Vet Med Assoc* 198:1348, 1991.
Sepien RL, Rapoport GS: Clinical comparison of three methods to measure blood pressure in nonsedated dogs. *J Am Vet Med Assoc* 215:1623, 1999.
Severinghaus JW: Oximetry: what does it tell you? ASA *Annual Refresher Course Lectures* 266:1, 1991.
Tremper KK, Barker SJ: Pulse oximetry. *Anaesthesiology* 70:98, 1989.

84
Staffing the Intensive Care Unit

Lesley G. King and Leslie Carter

INTRODUCTION

The subspecialty of intensive care medicine has grown in sophistication in response to demands from the public and from within the profession. With increasing public education about advanced techniques now available for patient care, and with the expanding accessibility of monitoring and therapeutic equipment, it is clear that the CCU is poised to become a fixture in referral veterinary hospitals of the future. Specialists in other fields, particularly surgeons, realize that the availability of a well-staffed, well-equipped, state-of-the-art CCU can enhance their success and can permit them to pursue more challenging cases, while concurrently decreasing the demands on their time for the postoperative care of their sickest patients. It is also becoming evident that the CCU can more than support itself financially and could be a significant income source for the specialty practice.

It is true to say that you can have the best equipment and physical set-up in the world, but if you do not have the right staff, then you do not have a CCU. As CCUs become a desired part of academic veterinary hospitals and specialty practices, the need for a thoughtful staffing plan becomes paramount. Before considering the issues involved in staffing, it is necessary to define what we mean by the term "critical care unit." The small animal CCU and its staff should ideally:

- Focus on the sickest patients, predominantly high-risk medical and surgical patients
- Operate 24 hours a day, 7 days a week
- Be equipped to provide optimal state-of-the-art monitoring and therapy
- Be prepared to accept referrals of critical patients and new patient admissions at any time, and be prepared for all possible immediate crisis needs of patients in the unit
- Prioritize communication within the CCU staff, and between the CCU staff and the admitting doctors, clients, and referring veterinarians

The unit specifically dedicated to critical/intensive care differs from the emergency room in that there are fewer non–life-threatening emergency patients, and therefore less dilution of staff away from critically ill cases. In comparison with the emergency room, there is usually a much smaller caseload. A long-term (days, maybe weeks) focus on individual patients blends the immediate need to stabilize and support body systems with the requirement to establish a concrete diagnosis. During the course of a pet's CCU stay, strong bonds often develop between the clinical staff and the pet owner, bearing in mind that owners of CCU patients tend to be extremely committed, dedicated, intense, and willing to commit tremendous financial and emotional resources to the care of their critically ill dog or cat. The clinical course of the small animal CCU patient is often complex, dynamic, frustrating, and extremely challenging.

The staff of the CCU consists of a team of doctors and nurses working together side by side. It is impossible to overemphasize the importance of a well-trained nursing staff in the smooth running of the unit. The nursing staff must implement most aspects of patient care and should be encouraged to demonstrate initiative and a logical, critical thought process. Effective and timely communication between clinicians and nurses is therefore a vital component of patient care in the CCU. Every effort must be made to include nurses in the decision-making process and to communicate the rationale behind treatment decisions.

When making decisions about staffing the CCU, a number of issues must be considered:

- Is 24-hour staffing necessary?
- What is the ideal staff/patient ratio?
- Should staff be specially certified/trained?
- Should residents/trainees be used for staffing?
- What is the best way to retain qualified staff and prevent burnout?

IS 24-HOUR STAFFING NECESSARY?

Because CCU patients are the sickest, most heavily instrumented, most dynamic, and at the highest risk, it is axiomatic that the CCU must be staffed with nursing 24 hours a day. These are not patients that can be left unattended overnight. The need for veterinarians to be physically present 24 hours a day varies with the type and number of cases. In general, if the veterinarians' shifts do not extend through the full 24-hour period, then a veterinarian must be available at all times to answer questions and respond to changes in clinical status of patients immediately. Although many questions can be answered on the telephone, it is often necessary for the veterinarian to return to the CCU if a change in the patient's condition mandates a doctor's attention immediately.

The ongoing demands of these patients around the clock tend to create a high stress level for the clinician in a CCU that is not staffed with qualified doctors 24 hours a day. By definition the CCU clinician is responsible for critically ill patients whose conditions can change unpredictably within minutes or hours. Frequently, a long workday is followed by a night of interrupted sleep troubleshooting changes in a patient's condition. Although many CCU clinicians are "adrenaline junkies," this lifestyle inevitably takes its toll, often resulting in burnout. In addition, the absence of an overnight doctor can add considerably to the stress of the night shift nurses, who must cope on their own, and may feel guilty if circumstances require frequent calls to the doctor during the night. There can be little doubt that the ideal small animal CCU should aim toward the standards set in human hospitals, with 24-hour coverage by doctors as well as nurses. Staffing at this level allows development of a "shift" system, permitting clinicians to leave the hospital at the end of the day knowing that their patients are taken care of, thereby reducing stress levels, producing career longevity, and ultimately improving patient care.

One potentially useful option if an emergency room exists in the same hospital is to have the emergency clinicians troubleshoot the CCU patients overnight. This solution works only if the emergency clinicians are not overwhelmed with their own emergency patients, if the emergency room and CCU are located close to each other, and if there is exceptionally good communication between the CCU and emergency room clinicians.

When staffing a CCU, it must be remembered that one week represents $7 \times 24 = 168$ hours. To staff a unit round the clock with just one nurse or one doctor at a time, each working 40 hours a week, it is necessary to budget at least 4 individuals (160 hours). Ideally, considering vacations and sick days, 4.5 or 5 nurses, working with 4.5 or 5 doctors are needed to provide "one-deep" round the clock coverage. Recognizing that with current staff availability it is very difficult to fill positions with qualified individuals, most CCUs compromise staffing numbers at the expense of staff stress and a high turnover rate.

WHAT IS THE IDEAL STAFF/PATIENT RATIO?

The ideal ratio of staff to patients largely depends on the intensity of patient management. The sickest animals that are being managed with the most intensive instrumentation and support may require a 1:1 ratio of nurses and clinicians per patient. The best examples of this type of patient include ventilator patients, those on peritoneal dialysis, or animals that are dynamically changing from hour to hour, such as the hypotensive patient in septic shock. Sometimes the most demanding patient can be the not-so-sick animal with severe diarrhea that repeatedly soils its bedding, lines, and catheters, requiring frequent time-consuming cleanups and bandage changes. More routine patients may require less intensive attention.

Currently, a reasonable average ratio of nursing staff to patients in the state-of-the-art small animal CCU is about 1:3, depending on the level of care being provided. It is optimal to ensure that at least two nurses are always on duty, because two pairs of hands are usually necessary for catheter placement, patient restraint, or to run a cardiac arrest. This ratio will certainly continue to decrease as the intensity of monitoring and therapeutic protocols continues to increase.

The number of clinicians required per shift varies depending on the patient load and the experience level of the clinicians. Many of the same considerations apply to the doctors as to the nursing staff: one critical patient can consume one clinician to the exclusion of all else. Therefore an ideal goal is to try to staff the CCU with a minimum of two doctors per shift, at least during the day, to make sure that all of the patients are being adequately cared for even if one patient is demanding all of the attention of one doctor.

IS SPECIALLY CERTIFIED STAFF AN ASSET?

Specialty certification is available for both clinicians and nurses in the field of emergency and critical care. Achieving Board Certification or Veterinary Technician Specialist status requires a great deal of commitment and a lot of work, but it is valuable not only in terms of personal satisfaction, but also for the quality of patient care and for the advancement of the field of emergency and critical care medicine.

ACVECC Board Certification

The American College of Veterinary Emergency and Critical Care is a specialty organization that promotes advancement and high standards of practice for veterinarians involved in veterinary emergency and critical care.[1] The organization also establishes requirements for advanced training in the field, monitors residency training programs, and examines and certifies veterinarians as specialists. In addition, the ACVECC exists to encourage research and to promote communication and dissemination of knowledge relating to emergency and critical care.

Although individuals can, of course, practice intensive care medicine without board certification, and many do it well, in general there is no guarantee of the quality of training that uncertified individuals have received. In contrast, veterinarians who are board certified by ACVECC have passed a rigorous testing process that ensures that their knowledge base and level of practice reach the highest standards. The CCU that is staffed with Diplomates of ACVECC can be expected to function at a state-of-the-art level. It is likely that Diplomates of ACVECC will lead advancements and the generation of new knowledge in intensive care medicine in the future.

AVECCT Certification

The veterinary technician is an integral part of the veterinary health care system. As a response to the rapid growth in knowledge and technology in veterinary medicine and the trend toward specialization in veterinary nursing, the Academy of Veterinary Emergency and Critical Care Technicians (AVECCT) was formed in the mid 1990s with the goals of promoting consumer protection, professionalism, and excellence in veterinary emergency and critical care nursing through the following objectives[2]:

- Promote advancement and high standards of practice for those individuals involved
- Establish education and experience prerequisites leading to certification in the specialty
- Examination and certification of veterinary technicians as specialists
- Encourage research and other contributions to knowledge
- Promote continuing education and dissemination of knowledge

Certification by AVECCT is a mechanism of validating the knowledge and skills required for the competent practice of veterinary emergency and critical care nursing. AVECCT is the first veterinary technician specialty organization to be recognized by the North American Veterinary Technicians Association. The veterinary technician who becomes certified by AVECCT as a Veterinary Technician Specialist (Emergency and Critical Care) demonstrates superior knowledge in the care and management of the critically ill patient. Candidates must meet extensive experience and credential requirements to qualify for AVECCT certifying examination. Further information may be obtained from the AVECCT website at http://veccs.org/technicians/index.cfm.

SHOULD RESIDENTS BE USED AS A MEANS OF STAFFING?

There is a significant temptation to solve staffing problems by using residents or trainee nurses as a means to cover hours. The advantages of this approach are that residents can often be hired relatively inexpensively compared with board-certified specialists, and there is usually a large pool of excellent candidates applying for entry into residency programs. The presence of one or more residents can stimulate discussion, growth, and ongoing learning within a group. Individuals graduating from a residency program can provide a pool from which to hire qualified CCU staff in the future.

Although this solution to the staffing problem seems attractive, it also has some drawbacks. Most importantly, the residency training program is definitively a training position, and during at least the first half of the program residents require significant teaching time from the supervising clinician before becoming a staffing asset. The requirements for a residency in ACVECC are quite rigidly structured, including significant overlap of clinical duty with the supervising clinician, daily rounds, and weekly didactic sessions.[4] These requirements therefore limit the usefulness of residents for covering hours and can add to the workload of the supervising Diplomates.

Thus, residents should only be used as a means of staffing if the supervising clinicians are willing to devote a considerable amount of time to teaching and discussing cases and the literature. This is emphasized in the ACVECC Training and Application Guidelines, which state that: "A Residency Training Program in the American College of Veterinary Emergency and Critical Care is an intensive postgraduate training program, designed to prepare an individual for Examination for Board Certification in this Specialty, and for a career as a specialist in Emergency and Critical Care." The goals of the residency training program include[4]:

- Development of a critical thought process and use of the problem-based approach to patient care
- Development of clinical skills and expertise in emergency and critical care
- Development of a critical understanding of the current veterinary and human literature and proficiency in library research skills

- Demonstration of an ability to teach, communicate, and effectively present information
- Demonstration of exceptional ethical standards and ability to act as a professional role model

HOW TO RETAIN QUALIFIED STAFF AND PREVENT BURNOUT?

The CCU is a place where the staff often work hard, take their work home with them, and experience intense "highs" when they pull off a "save," balanced by "lows" when all of their best efforts are unsuccessful.[5] Clients are also highly stressed, often distressed or aggressive because they are under intense strain, and this further adds to the difficulties of working with critically ill patients. The more stressful the environment, the more likely that burnout will occur, and the higher the staff turnover rate. Recent studies of cortisol levels in human CCU physicians and nurses revealed that cortisol levels were often high even though the staff did not have a conscious perception that they were stressed.[6] Interestingly, the stress response did not abate until individuals had more than 8 years of experience. It is likely that the same findings would be true in the veterinary CCU.

Staff stress can be managed and minimized by attention to the following measures:

- Adequate staffing to ensure that veterinarians and nurses all feel that they can do a good job taking care of every case for which they are responsible. Because the CCU staff is exceptionally devoted to the care of the most needy patients, the staff is likely to experience a considerable amount of stress if they are too busy to do their best for each animal. Clearly, the unit cannot always be staffed to cope with occasional exceptionally busy times, but efforts should be made to ensure that the unit is adequately staffed to cope with a typical number of patients, most of the time. Adequate numbers of nurses should be scheduled to achieve optimal coverage for projected nurse/patient ratios. Ideally, at least one of those nurses per shift should be specialty trained or AVECCT certified, especially during training of new nurses. The addition of minimally qualified personnel or volunteers, who can keep on top of tasks such as cleaning and stocking can help to protect the time of the qualified nursing staff, freeing them to focus on patient care. Using on-call or short-notice staff during exceptionally busy times or unexpected staff absenteeism may also ameliorate stress.
- Adequate time off and reasonable hours are a priority in dealing with staff stress. Clinicians and nurses may have invested many hours in one individual patient, and it is important to ensure that qualified patient care providers are available to take over when they leave. Knowing that the animal is in trusted hands allows clinicians and nurses to leave their patient concerns at work, rather than taking them home. Scheduling presents an opportunity to help manage staff stress. Many people prefer to work longer hours (10–12) per shift to have longer breaks between work "weeks." Others (with child

care issues, for instance) may prefer 8-hour shifts. Although overnight shifts are undesirable to many, some may prefer and thrive in that shift. Individual needs for flexibility may be accommodated so long as the overall needs of the unit are not compromised. No individual should be scheduled to work longer than is reasonable to expect effective productivity. If shift rotation is necessary, it should be done slowly by phase delay (morning to afternoon to night) rather than phase advance (night to afternoon to morning).[3] Maintaining consistency while incorporating 8-, 10-, and 12-hour shifts with or without rotations, presents a creative challenge, but is rewarded by increased productivity of a satisfied staff.

- An open forum must be available for discussion of problem patients or situations, to promote communication and help to resolve misperceptions regarding patient care decisions. Simple misunderstandings can often build into serious problems that could have been easily resolved if they had been addressed right away. Facilitating communication between shifts is imperative to keep the team unified and focused on common goals. Mechanisms for facilitating intrashift communication include e-mail, a communication log or message board, and regularly scheduled meetings.
- Provision of ongoing training and continuing education. This is of particular importance for the nursing staff, to ensure that stress is not resulting from a lack of knowledge of disease processes, protocols, equipment or a lack of understanding of management strategies. For example, management of a ventilated patient can be a stressful prospect for a nurse who is not comfortable making decisions about ventilator settings, but satisfying for a well-trained nurse who is comfortable and challenged by this type of patient. Attendance at high-quality continuing education presentations obviously allows career development, but also promotes networking with colleagues in the same field, facing the same problems.

REFERENCES

1. American College of Veterinary Emergency and Critical Care Constitution. Available on-line at http://veccs.org/acvecc/bylaws.html.
2. Academy of Veterinary Emergency and Critical Care Technicians Constitution and Bylaws. Available through the Veterinary Emergency and Critical Care Society.
3. Battaglia A, ed.: Small Animal Emergency and Critical Care: A Manual for the Veterinary Technician. Philadelphia: WB Saunders, 2001, p 343.
4. American College of Veterinary Emergency and Critical Care Training and Application Guidelines. Available on-line at http://veccs.org/acvecc/guidelines.html.
5. Brackenridge S: Stress: causes and consequences; Stress management and coping techniques; and Alleviation of stress in veterinary critical care. *In* Proceedings of the International Veterinary Emergency and Critical Care Symposium, San Antonio, TX, 1996, p 369.
6. Fischer JE, Calame A, Dettling AC, *et al.*: Experience and endocrine stress responses in neonatal and pediatric critical care nurses and physicians. *Crit Care Med* 28:3281, 2000.

85
Staff Relations and Work/Life Balance

Ashley Harvey, Dana Durrance, Greg Conger, and Sara Sugerman

INTRODUCTION

The demands placed on the veterinary team in veterinary critical care settings can be extraordinary. Survival strategies used in adapting to chronic crisis intervention (*e.g.*, ignoring needs for food, rest) can significantly affect long-term professional and personal life. Just as stress can facilitate a staff to be more efficient during crises and enhance mental alertness, it can also exacerbate a tense situation and lead to sleepless nights, depression, and use or abuse of alcohol and drugs. When stress depletes personal resources and well-being, staff may be prevented from recovering and regaining control.

A comprehensive list of exactly how stress manifests in our lives does not exist. Each person experiences a unique and specific stress response. Effects may be physiologic (*e.g.*, peptic ulcers), psychological (*e.g.*, depression), or cognitive (*e.g.*, memory inhibition), or include inappropriate verbal responses such as exaggerated anger, and behavioral responses such as drug and alcohol use or abuse. Prolonged stress can lead to burnout, a syndrome that includes pervasive emotional exhaustion, decreased productivity, and depersonalization of clients and fellow team members.[1] Any member of the veterinary critical care team is at risk for burnout, which may last from just a few days or weeks to months or even years.[2] One researcher estimates stress-related mental and emotional crises lead to a loss of 73 working days in a year in an average veterinary practice with 10 employees.[3] These figures are startling considering that one or two absent employees on any given day in a 10-person practice can create role overload and leave the staff struggling for balance.

Clearly, stress and burnout are significant dangers to staff relations if not taken seriously. Although no one solution exists to prevent stress and burnout, a cohesive staff working together in a supportive environment is vital. This chapter offers strategies in three broad categories that can be used to create a cohesive and supportive veterinary team: strategic planning, conflict resolution, and stress management.

The authors would like to acknowledge the editorial contributions of Leslie Carter, MS, VTS (Emergency and Critical Care).

STRATEGIC PLANNING

Strategic planning in veterinary medicine is often thought of as a business function related to increased growth and profit. One might wonder how strategic planning relates to the practice of veterinary emergency and critical care medicine. Here it will be considered as a method of improving teamwork. Development and regular discussion of a strategic plan can help a veterinary staff create a healthy atmosphere, where communication, team support, and stress management are priorities.

In an environment where efficiency can mean the difference between life and death, people need to communicate well and work as a team. Retaining good employees in highly stressful work settings requires employers to provide not only adequate compensation, but a work environment where staff members feel engaged, important, appreciated, and personally invested.[4,5] The following strategic planning process has been used successfully in a busy small animal emergency hospital. Although the focus is primarily on improving teamwork, it will likely lead to increased growth and profit.

The strategic planning process serves a variety of functions: building and strengthening the team; identifying strengths and weaknesses of the practice; developing concrete plans to address weaknesses; increasing staff engagement through their participation in future-planning; creating an ideal vision of the practice; establishing short- and long-term goals; and providing an opportunity for the staff to discuss the practice outside the clinic, away from the pressures of a medical environment.

The strategic planning process described here can be accomplished in 2 to 3 hours. Meeting in a "retreat" format at a location away from the hospital not only provides a fresh look at the practice but also makes the planning process more interesting (not "just another staff meeting"). Employees should be paid for their time at the meeting. Providing meals presents additional opportunities for team-building and discussion of ideas presented during the planning process. The following is a brief description of each step of the strategic planning process.

Step One: Icebreaker

Beginning the retreat with a short activity encourages people to talk and think creatively, and helps them feel more comfortable with one another (*e.g.*, group problem-solving activity, puzzle). The reader is referred to a variety of good books describing icebreaker activities.[6–9]

Step Two: Vision

In this portion of the process, participants take 5 minutes to write down their vision of the practice at its very best in the next 3 to 5 years. Then, each person reads his or her vision aloud and a facilitator leads the group in forming a common vision for the practice. Using a chalkboard or a large flipchart allows everyone to see the vision develop. This same process can be used to write a mission statement that clearly states the mission, or purpose, of the practice

Table 85-1. Sample Mission Statement

Animal Emergency Care Center is dedicated to providing comprehensive, compassionate emergency care for dogs, cats, birds, and exotic animals to the Colorado Springs metro area. In addition to offering state of the art emergency and critical care for animals, Animal Emergency Care Center seeks to educate its clients and provide them with complete information and compassionate support during what is often a crisis situation. Animal Emergency Care Center also strives to provide a supportive, friendly, and challenging team-oriented work environment.

(Table 85-1). When employees co-create the practice vision and mission they are more likely to be invested in the practice and to work to see their vision come to fruition. The process of creating a common or shared vision and mission also encourages teamwork and open communication.[5,10]

Step Three: Identifying Strengths and Weaknesses

In this activity, staff members write down three strengths of the practice and how they are accomplished and three weaknesses of the practice and suggestions for improving each weakness. It is important to emphasize that it is not a forum for complaining, rather an opportunity to brainstorm solutions for identified problems. Steps four and five make the solutions concrete.

Step Four: Developing a Plan of Action

When participants have completed brainstorming practice problems and ideas for solving them (using a flipchart or chalkboard), a facilitator helps the group divide problems/solutions into two lists: "little or no cost" and "significant cost" ideas. Then the group looks at each "little or no cost" item and creates concrete goals. For example:

Problem: Critical care treatments are administered late.
Goal: Administer all treatments on time.

The group then uses the suggestions that participants have brainstormed to identify tasks for accomplishing each goal. The facilitator asks for volunteers for each task and has them identify a target date for completion of the task. For example:

Suggestion: Create and use a white board chart on the wall listing all critical care treatments and what time they need to be administered.
Tasks:

Buy whiteboard	Sam	March 1
Create template	Jake	March 3
Write template on board and hang board	Sara & Pat	March 7
Train staff to use board (at staff meeting)	Jan	March 9

The facilitator should take note of who has volunteered for projects, and encourage those who have not volunteered to do so. By the end of the problem-solving session every person should have at least one task to work on. Encouraging people to work in pairs or groups on larger tasks further enhances team-building. As staff members work on their tasks and feel the importance of their involvement in the practice, they become more invested in solving the practice's problems.

After "little or no cost" items have been discussed, the group prioritizes "significant cost" ideas. After the retreat, the practice owner or manager is primarily responsible for budgeting and purchasing "significant cost" items as funds permit. Purchasing prioritized equipment shows employees that their ideas and input have resulted in tangible improvements in the practice.

Step Five: Follow-up

Follow-up is a crucial part of strategic planning. One staff member volunteers to compile all of the information generated from the "significant cost" and "little or no cost" lists, with task, names, dates, and so forth, and presents a copy to each employee at the next staff meeting. At that meeting and every meeting thereafter, someone (usually the practice manager or owner) asks the following questions of each "Little or no cost" goal:

- How is this task coming along? Is it completed? (If completed, put a big check mark by it, and have everyone applaud!)
- What is getting in the way of completing this task? What information or resources do you need to complete it? Is there anything you need from me?
- Who will help (name of person who volunteered to do the task) do this?

The manager/owner then reports on the status of each "significant cost" goal. Providing consistent follow-through on tasks demonstrates to employees that their efforts are valuable and subsequently encourages involvement in future projects. This highlights the importance of regularly scheduled meetings (Table 85-2 lists ideas). A thank-you note sent by the manager/owner for exceptional efforts further reinforces feelings of employee appreciation and engagement.

Thoughtfully implemented strategic planning improves employee engagement in the practice, as well as communication and initiative. Although strategic planning can serve as a profit building activity, it can also significantly enhance teamwork—the cornerstone of effective functioning in emergency and critical care environments.

CONFLICT RESOLUTION

Conflict in the workplace is a fact of life. In critical care settings; staff conflict is not only inevitable, but if is often exacerbated by the stressful nature of the work. No one can prevent conflict from occurring—it is the natural result of different people, personalities, genders, ethnicities, backgrounds, educations, and cultures interacting on a regular basis. What can be controlled is *how* conflict

Table 85-2. Ideas for Monthly Staff Meetings

- Come to the staff meeting prepared with an agenda.
- Serve refreshments.
- Pay employees for their time at the meeting.
- Ask whoever is late to buy refreshments for next meeting.
- Invite a guest speaker to present continuing education (*e.g.,* a radiologist to teach something new about interpreting radiographs; an anesthesiologist to talk about new drugs, etc.).
- Ask a staff member to pick an area of interest, do a little research, and present it to the rest of the staff (*e.g.,* how to place a jugular catheter).
- Have weekly rounds to discuss particularly challenging cases. The discussion can focus on medical aspects or other aspects such as difficult clients or sadness of staff about an animal's death.
- Review task sheets generated by strategic planning to see what has been accomplished. Thank and applaud those who have diligently and consistently worked on tasks.
- Surprise and delight the staff . . . take them to the mall, give each $50 and tell them they have 1 hour to spend it on *themselves.*
- Invite open discussion: "How are things going? Any concerns, ideas, questions?"
- Ask each staff member to "brag" about someone on staff—describing something exceptional someone did.

is dealt with. The strength of most veterinary staffs can be measured by how conflict is handled and resolved.

The Systemic Nature of Conflict

It is important to recognize the systemic nature of conflict in veterinary critical care settings. *Systems theory*[11] is a metaperspective used by mental health professionals in family therapy[12] and organizational settings.[13] Systems theory suggests that problems do not exist in an individual alone, but in the interactions between individuals. In a veterinary practice, team members exhibit mutual influence. Each member's behavior affects every other member. We often see another person's part in the problem yet fail to see how we may play a role. As we come to understand systems theory, we learn that problems occur in complex cycles in which the problem behavior may have been introduced by one individual, but gets reinforced and maintained by everyone.

To more fully understand the systemic nature of conflict, two sample problem cycles are "mapped" below. In the first conflict (Fig. 85-1), a veterinarian attempts to delegate a task to a technician and fails. Bob is a veterinarian of 10 years who has worked in an emergency clinic for 1 month, and Jennifer is a technician who has worked there for 3 years. Bob thinks the conflict is Jennifer's responsibility because she lacks initiative and Jennifer thinks that this is Bob's problem because he is overbearing. Unless they recognize that the problem resides in the interaction between them, they are likely to repeat this problem

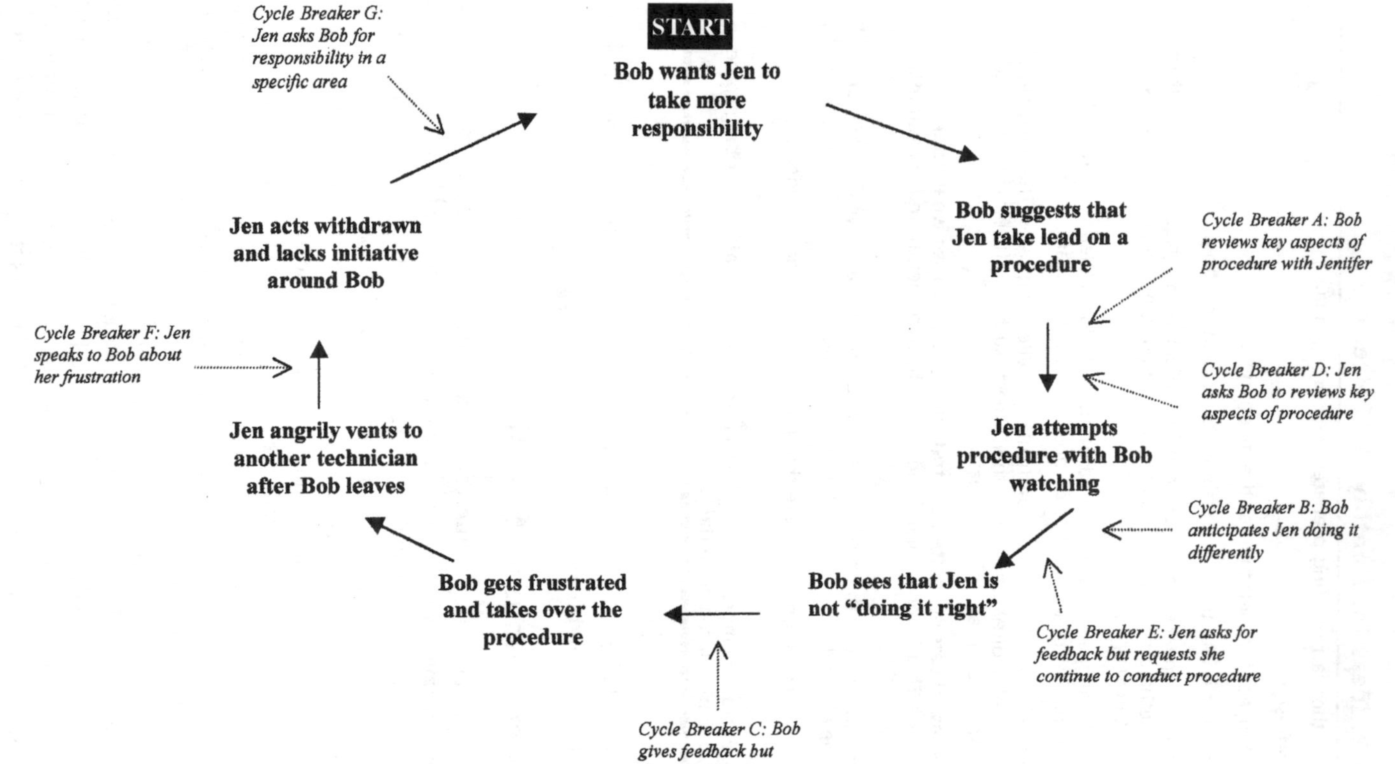

Figure 85-1
Mapping a problem cycle gives insight into the cyclical nature of conflict and the methods both parties can use to "break" the cycle.

cycle and eventually develop negative beliefs about one another. In actuality, both Jennifer and Bob could take actions that would "break" this problem cycle. Cycle breakers for Bob might be asking Jennifer how she usually handles it and sharing what he sees as the key aspects of the procedure (A), recognizing that there may be more than one way to conduct a procedure and anticipating individual differences (B), or giving Jennifer encouragement and constructive feedback instead of taking over (C). Cycle breakers for Jennifer might include asking Bob to review what he thinks are key aspects of the procedure and agreeing on a method (D), soliciting feedback but requesting that Bob allow her to conduct the procedure (E), sharing her frustration with Bob in a constructive manner (F), or asking Bob for responsibility in an area in which she feels more competent (G).

In the second problem cycle (Fig. 85-2), a clinician and technician are in conflict regarding management of a patient's pain. The technician thinks the animal is in pain and that medication should be altered. The clinician disagrees with the technician, and inadvertently minimizes the technician's concern. The technician then avoids interacting with the clinician. Cycle breakers for the clinician include requesting the technician's input as the animal is recovering (A), asking the technician for more detailed information when the technician expresses concerns (B), taking the time to share his rationale with the technician and engaging in discussion (C), and seeking continuing education on pain management for himself and staff (D). Cycle breakers for the technician include gently but directly telling clinician how her concerns feel minimized (E), seeking continuing education on pain management and offering to present material gained to rest of staff (F), and suggesting regular case rounds in which technicians and clinicians can collaboratively engage in treatment planning (G).

Gender Issues and Conflict

Gender is becoming increasingly recognized as contributing to conflict in workplace settings. Whether or not gender roles are innate or learned continues to be debated in the social sciences. Research does suggest that the differences between men and women are less pervasive than the portrayal in the popular media, and that notable within-gender variability exists.[14] However, stereotypical gender traits often exert a subtle influence, especially in relational contexts in the home or workplace. Stereotypical masculine traits include being self-reliant, assertive, a leader, a risk-taker, dominant, individualistic, competitive, ambitious,[15] in control, and unemotional (except displays of anger).[16] Stereotypical feminine traits include being yielding, sensitive to the needs of others, understanding, compassionate, soft-spoken, gentle,[15] relationship focused, covert, passive,[16] caretaking, and nurturing.[17]

In an ideal setting, veterinary professionals would refrain from reinforcing stereotypical gender behaviors, and instead allow each individual a full range of emotions, behaviors, and opportunities. However, veterinary professionals and staff will vary widely in their adherence to or divergence from stereotypical gender behaviors. Traditional beliefs can be surprisingly influential. Take, for exam-

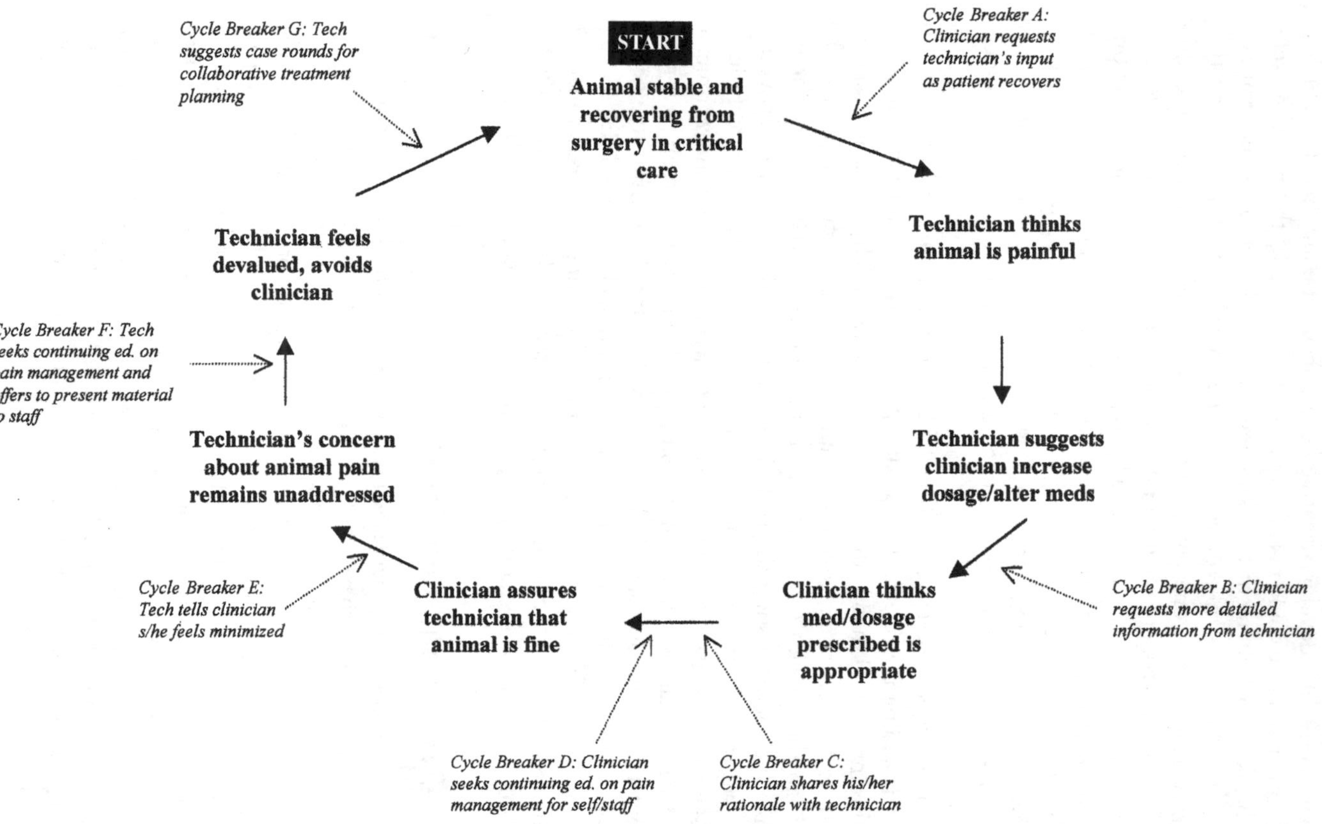

Figure 85-2
Problem cycle in which technician and clinician disagree on management of patient pain. Cycle breakers are indicated.

ple, the stereotypical masculine trait of being unemotional. Both male and female staff members may be more alarmed or unsettled by male tears, and male staff may be less likely to cry in front of coworkers than their female counterparts. With regard to the stereotypical feminine traits of being passive and accommodating, it may be less likely (or less well received) for female staff members to exhibit anger, assert needs and desires, or ask for a raise. At times, it is these underlying gender expectations of others and ourselves that can impede workplace communication and effective teamwork.

Methods to Conflict Resolution

Common staff conflicts in critical care settings are included in Table 85-3. Regardless of the initial cause, behind most conflicts are people who feel hurt or affected in some way. Discerning *why* feelings are hurt facilitates conflict resolution.[18] Most conflicts result from miscommunication. They often begin as minor issues and escalate into full-blown problems. The key is to identify at which point the miscommunication occurred and clear up any and all misunderstandings that followed. The single most important factor in successful conflict resolution is a positive attitude and sincere willingness of all involved parties to work through the problem. No conflict resolution technique in the world will be effective without sincerity and open, honest communication.

Given the stressful environment of a critical care facility, it is essential that staff conflicts be addressed as soon as possible. The verbal skill of immediacy (commenting on the unspoken thoughts or feelings being shared at the moment) is particularly useful. For example:

Table 85-3. Common Staff Conflicts in Critical Care Settings

- Differences in opinion about patient status, patient care, pain control, or timing of euthanasia
- Power differences between and among veterinarians, technicians, and support staff
- Differing levels of experience/tenure between and among veterinarians, technicians, and support staff
- Lack of uniform policies across all shifts (wearing gloves, wrapping catheters, how clinicians/technicians/support staff interact, etc.)
- Scheduling conflicts
- Unclear or unrealistic expectations
- Conflicts between different shifts—people can feel "ownership" over a patient and may blame/judge other shifts if the patient dies or if they perceive inadequate care
- "Us versus Them" philosophy—the perception that one shift or job is the hardest and most stressful (often becomes a destructive cycle of "we work harder than you because . . . "). This can include conflicts about the delegation of assigned duties (support staff wishing they could do more medical/technical procedures, etc.).
- Lack of follow-up or communication between shifts

Pat: "Jan, I get the impression that you are angry with me about something. Can you tell me what it is?"
Jan: "Pat, to be honest, I felt angry and criticized when you snapped at me when we were placing the catheter in that cat."
Pat: "I am sorry about that, I was just stressed because I'm behind with my treatments and was feeling rushed. After we've administered the 3:00 o'clock treatments, could we take a few minutes to talk?"
Jan: "That would be great."

If left unresolved, it is easy to see how this simple miscommunication between Jan and Pat could escalate into a bigger conflict. Jan could assume that Pat is rude, critical, and abrasive. She might also assume that Pat doesn't care about her feelings and that Pat has a low opinion of her technical skills. Without knowing why Jan is angry, Pat could assume that Jan is unfriendly, distant, and uncooperative. Both could continue these negative assumptions and develop new conflicts over time. The end result could be quite damaging. With other misunderstandings driving the conflict, both Jan and Pat could end up quitting their jobs from this one simple miscommunication.

Beyond immediacy, successful conflict resolution requires risk and commitment. It takes courage to share true feelings with others, particularly if those feelings might be judged as negative (*e.g.*, anger, resentment, jealousy, guilt, embarrassment, insecurity). It also takes commitment when the conflict is long-standing or complicated. Owners and managers can help to model this behavior by personally addressing conflicts with commitment and honesty. Setting a standard for others to follow is invaluable (*e.g.*, refusing to participate in gossip, giving other team members the benefit of the doubt, and using immediacy before making harmful assumptions). Other strategies for resolving staff conflicts in critical care include:

1. If in doubt, ask. Never assume anything about what a person is thinking or feeling. Give people a chance to explain or apologize for what they meant or said before escalating the interaction.
2. Clarify expectations of each staff members' duties and roles. Expectations must be made overt and discussed frequently.
3. Use "I" statements to prevent others from getting defensive (*e.g.*, "Pat, I need to feel that my work is respected and I feel criticized when you are abrupt with me during procedures," versus "Pat, you need to stop being so abrupt with me during procedures.").
4. Be flexible in managing patient care. Maintain a certain standard of care, but recognize that individuals may have different approaches and that the same result may be achieved through a different process.
5. Allow time for people to vent frustrations, feelings, and concerns before moving to problem-solving. Ensure that those feelings are acknowledged in some way. Without proper acknowledgement, people are generally not ready to let go of their emotions and move towards problem-solving.
6. Try asking these questions to resolve conflict[19]:

   a. What is the underlying conflict separate from the individuals?
   b. Why is this issue important to the people involved?
   c. Do other people subtly contribute to the conflict?
   d. What does each person want or need? What might they need to give up?
   e. Do my own biases affect how I see this conflict?
   f. What needs to change to resolve the conflict?
   g. How do the employees view the problem?
   h. What should happen if a resolution doesn't occur?
7. Instigate a policy that all employees must treat each other with civility and respect. Inability to meet such requirements should result in:
   a. A prompt managerial response or investigation
   b. Appropriate warnings as needed
   c. Dismissal of employees who cannot act civilly and respectfully
8. Solicit the facilitation skills of an organizational consultant or outside mediator. Conflict resolution is an advanced communication skill that can be developed over time.

In the short term, it is often easier to dismiss conflicts and assume that they will "blow over" especially when time is so limited. However, taking time to effectively address conflict will be well worth the effort expended.

STRESS MANAGEMENT

Personal strategies for managing stress in the workplace are critical. However, changing the person is not a panacea; a flexible and adaptable workplace is also crucial in reducing stress.[4] In current society, one of the primary tasks being demanded of the workplace is to facilitate, rather than hinder, work/life balance. Historically, Americans worked primarily to ensure survival and often worked at the same job their entire lives. Today, many American workers have multiple jobs during their professional lives and people are no longer living for their jobs. Rather than just surviving, people are seeking personal fulfillment from their jobs and from their lives.[20] Additionally, the number of women in the workforce is increasing, particularly in the veterinary profession.[21] Like most traditionally male professions, many veterinary practices have been built on a family structure consisting of a bread-winning father and a stay-at-home mother,[22] with the female managing childcare and household responsibilities, and frequently providing paid or unpaid support in the veterinary practice. Currently, dual-earner and single-parent families far outweigh families in which one person works and the other manages the household[23]; instead, most employees are juggling multiple responsibilities in addition to their paid jobs.

In light of all of this, it is surprising that Americans are working more now than ever. Due to the decrease in paid time off, sick leave, personal days, and holidays, Americans today are working the equivalent of an extra month each year as compared to their counterparts 20 years ago.[24] Even "Generation Xers," (those born between 1965 and 1985)[25] who are sometimes portrayed in the media as "slackers" are not logging any fewer hours than young workers 20 years ago.[26] Thus, employers are shifting their focus from finding ways to encourage employees to work longer hours to finding ways to retain good employees. Nowhere is this more needed than in the veterinary profession, in which burnout and staff turnover have become epidemic for many veterinary practices.[27,28]

Like all employers, veterinary practice owners need to meet the needs of contemporary veterinarians, technicians, and staff. Extrinsic rewards such as a competitive salary and benefits are always important, but veterinary team members are also seeking intrinsic rewards such as feeling valued and essential to the veterinary hospital and the larger community. Employees are more likely to stay in jobs that are supportive and empowering.[26] Veterinary practice owners must work not only to improve staff relations, but also to increase family-friendliness in the workplace. However, changing attitudes toward work have posed enormous dilemmas for practice owners and their staff. Owners and managers are struggling to meet staff needs while at the same time delivering high-quality medicine and building a financially successful practice. While veterinarians and technicians are questioning how much effort to "give" to their jobs, practice owners are wondering how much they should "bend" to meet the needs of their employees.

Critical care work is highly demanding, and if anything, the demands are increasing. Veterinary professionals in critical care are experiencing "intensity inflation"; the number of procedures that can be done for each patient has increased, entailing more equipment, expertise, and time—without a corresponding increase in staff. When jobs are this demanding, it is crucial that they be high quality (offering autonomy, learning and advancement opportunities, and meaning) and supportive (offering flexibility, mentoring, supervisor support, positive coworker relations, respect, and an absence of discrimination and favoritism). In fact, the quality of workers' jobs and the supportiveness of their workplaces are the most powerful predictors of productivity, more so than money or benefits.[26] If jobs are difficult and demanding but of low quality and support, then employees experience higher levels of negative spillover from work into their lives off of the job—affecting their personal and family life. Then, when workers are burned-out and have insufficient time for themselves and their families, and work puts them in a bad mood, this spills back over into job performance, creating a counterproductive cycle. Work and family used to be thought of as separate spheres. However, current research recognizes that family issues will spill over into and affect work performance, and vice versa.[23]

Fostering Family-Friendly Work Environments

In organizations in which family-friendly policies have been enacted, the benefits have proven numerous. "Family-friendly" policies certainly help parents with children, but also benefit employees with varying household units, family forms, and lifestyles. Family-friendly policies help businesses stay competitive with other employers and thus improve both recruitment and retention.[29] Morale and productivity are improved and absenteeism is reduced.[29] Furthermore, organi-

Table 85-4. Examples of Family-Friendly Policies

- ***Time Management***

  Flexible hours

  Compressed weeks (*e.g.,* four 10-h days)

  Job sharing

  Alternative work schedules (required to work core hours only)

  Able to bank leave to take sabbaticals or extended leaves

  Adequate vacation time

  On-Site Support

  Mentoring

  Personal counseling (employee assistance programs)

  Free work and family seminars

  Staff/family social functions

  Access to ongoing staff development funds

  Discounts on services

  Assistance with moving, relocation, including spouse relocation

  Work-site neck and back massages

- ***Family-Related Resources***

  Maternity/paternity leave

  Accommodations for nursing mothers

  Referral service for child and elder care

  Sick days to care for ill family members

- ***Financial***

  Investment plans

  Profit-sharing

  Pretax flexible spending accounts (medical and child care)

  Pet insurance

zations with family-friendly policies have also shown increased profits.[30,31] Examples of family friendly policies are given in Table 85-4. Flexibility in scheduling and time management has some of the most positive effects of all of the family-friendly policies, namely, less distress at work and fewer physical symptoms. In negotiating specific aspects of work/life balance with their employers, veterinary professionals are encouraged to do the following: approach their employers with plenty of lead time, present several detailed options, and look for "win-win" situations. Strategies veterinary practice owners or supervisors can use when negotiating work/life balance include: suggest a brainstorming session with the veterinary team to realize the impact on other team members and to find win-win scenarios, and suggest trying out proposed changes for a period of time and then re-evaluating.

Additional On-the-Job Strategies

Given these extraordinary stressors, there are strategies staff can implement into their work lives to promote a healthy lifestyle (Table 85-5). Chief among them is acknowledging and honoring grief. Veterinarians encounter more death than any other medical professionals, five times the rate of their physician counterparts.[32] This statistic is likely even higher in veterinary critical care settings, which consistently respond to devastating traumas such as brain and spinal cord injuries, as well toxicologic and environmental injuries. Attending to the patient's physical pain and the client's emotional pain can tax the resources of an already stressed staff. Furthermore, the need for debriefing about these experiences is often not acknowledged. Instead, the implicit rule is "I should be able to handle this." This mantra often leads to feelings of being used, overwhelmed, isolated, inadequate, and out of control. Perhaps the greatest gifts staff members can give to one another with regard to grief are opportunities for cathartic sharing of thoughts and feelings and a perception of social support. Although a full discussion of grief is beyond the scope of this chapter, it is critical to give ourselves, our clients, and our coworkers permission to grieve.

Creating a purposeful ending can help to draw closure to a case, day, week, or year. A purposeful ending is a vehicle for honoring efforts, grieving losses, and saying thank you. It can take the form of thoughts, actions, or events, and can be created in many ways using the creativity and ideas of the veterinary staff. Examples include donating to an animal-related organization, saying a prayer, sending a collective thank-you letter to all clients, instigating a "memorial day" to honor special animals who have died, and even actions as simple as completing casenotes and putting away files. Ideally, purposeful endings are implemented regularly and are accomplished through the development of ongoing patterns or rituals that signal work is truly over.

Many who work in critical care tend to be highly driven overachievers with a strong innate desire to help others. As a result, some feel guilty about leaving at the end of a shift or feel responsible for critical patients even when they are

Table 85-5. Stress Management Strategies

- Make sure to have adequate coverage so that all staff have time for meals, personal breaks.
- Create consistent yet flexible scheduling (fewer days with longer hours) and variable schedules for those who prefer it.
- Regularly debrief. Debriefing is a conversation designed to assist the participants of a stressful situation in coping with the emotional responses that sometimes surface after intense cases.[34] Debriefing can also be used in regular staff meetings to promote discussion and provide ongoing support.
- Use humor to restore perspective, achieve balance, and promote self-care.
- Seek support from friends, family, and mental health professionals when appropriate.
- Take a brisk walk around the outside of the hospital. As little as 6 minutes of aerobic exercise can reduce anxiety.[35]

not working. Developing a personal philosophy of detached concern[33] is essential for keeping emotionally draining work from interfering with family/home time. Detached concern entails a commitment to providing the best medical care, yet sufficiently detaching to have sound judgment and awareness of the need for self-preservation. Detached concern is challenging to achieve and is realized by attending to personal grief work as well accepting the normal limitations of any given helping situation.

Another strategy for managing stress in the critical care environment is to redefine the idea of "success." Success does not have to be limited to a healthy, happy animal walking out the front door. Given the prevalence of death in the critical care environment, success can be defined in many ways. It may mean helping to ease the pain of an animal before it dies, or ensuring that the animal does not die alone. A compassionate, loving, client-present euthanasia may be viewed as a success knowing that the animal is no longer suffering and that the owner was able to say good-bye.

The demands placed on the staff in a critical care facility are enormous. It is not surprising that many veterinary teams experience conflict, dissatisfaction, and stress at some time. Clear communication is critical in addressing these challenges. Communication skills are as "learnable" as those required in treating critical patients. Veterinary professionals and staff cannot afford to wait until a "slower time" in the future to address long-standing conflict, instigate strategic planning, or reduce work-related stress. Too frequently, that slower time never comes. When used on an ongoing basis, strategic planning, conflict resolution, and stress management can create and sustain an engaged, energized critical care team.

REFERENCES

1. Maslach C, Jackson SE, Leiter, MP: Maslach burnout inventory. *In* Zalaquett CP, Wood RJ, eds.: Evaluating Stress: A Book of Resources, 3rd ed. Lanham, MD: The Scarecrow Press, 1997, p 191.
2. Pines AM, Aronson E, Kafry D: Burnout: From Tedium to Personal Growth. New York: The Free Press, 1981.
3. Dale C: Helping those you manage to give of their best. *Practice* 19:392, 1997.
4. Maslach C, Leiter MP: The Truth About Burnout: How Organizations Cause Personal Stress and What to Do About It. San Francisco: Jossey-Bass, 1997.
5. Kouzes J, Posner BZ, Peters T: The Leadership Challenge. San Francisco: Jossey-Bass, 1996.
6. Cain JH: Teamwork and Teamplay. Dubuque, IA: Kendall-Hunt, 1998.
7. Nilson C: Team Games for Trainers. New York: McGraw-Hill, 1993.
8. Rohnke K: Silver Bullets. Hamilton, MA: Project Adventure, 1984.
9. Rohnke K: Cowstails and Cobras II: A Guide to Games, Initiatives, Ropes Courses and Adventure Curriculum. Dubuque, IA: Kendell-Hunt, 1989.
10. Kouzes J, Posner BZ: Encouraging the Heart: A Leader's Guide to Rewarding and Recognizing Others. San Francisco: Jossey-Bass, 1999.
11. Von Bertalanffy L: General Systems Theory. New York: Braziller, 1968.
12. Bowen M: Family Therapy in Clinical Practice. New York: Jason Aronson, 1978.
13. Sager RR, Wiseman KK, eds.: Understanding Organizations: Applications of Bowen

Family Systems Theory. Washington DC: The Georgetown University Family Center, 1982.
14. Lott B: Dual natures or learned behavior: the challenge to feminist psychology. *In* Hare-Mustin R, Marecek J, eds.: Making a Difference: Psychology and the Construction of Gender. New Haven: Yale University Press, 1990, p 65.
15. Bem SL: The measurement of psychological androgyny. *J Consult Clin Psychol* 42: 155, 1974.
16. Tannen D: You Just Don't Understand: Women and Men in Conversation. New York: Ballantine Books, 1991.
17. Gilligan C: In a Different Voice: Psychological Theory and Women's Development. Cambridge, MA: Harvard University, 1982.
18. Lagoni L, Durrance D: Connecting With Clients: Practical Communication Techniques in 15 Common Situations. Lakewood, CO: AAHA, 1998.
19. Craig M: Resolve staff conflicts. *Vet Econ* 40:40, 1999.
20. Manning G, Curtis K, McMillen S, eds.: Building Community: The Human Side of Work. Cincinnati: Thomson Executive Press, 1996.
21. Brown JP, Silverman JD: The current and future market for veterinarians and veterinary medical services in the United States. *J Am Vet Med Assoc* 215:161, 1999.
22. Slater MR, Slater M: Women in veterinary medicine. *J Am Vet Med Assoc* 217: 472, 2000.
23. Williams J: Unbending Gender: Why Family and Work Conflict and What to do About It. New York: Oxford University Press, 2000.
24. Bravo E: The Job/Family Challenge: Not for Women Only. New York: John Wiley & Sons, 1995.
25. Blanken RL, Liff A: Facing the future: Major trends and issues affecting associations. *Am Soc Assoc Exec* January 1999:77.
26. Bond JT, Galinsky E, Swanberg JE: The 1997 National Study of the Changing Workforce. New York: Families and Work Institute, 1998.
27. Zuziak P: Stress and burnout in the profession (part 1): veterinary practitioners dragged through traumatic times. *J Am Vet Med Assoc* 198:521, 1991.
28. Myers W: Cultivating technicians. *Vet Econ* 40:30, 1999.
29. Kimball G: Twenty-first Century Families: Blueprints to Create Family-Friendly Workplaces, Schools, and Governments. Chico, CA: Equality Press, 1998.
30. Pfeffer J: The Human-Equation: Building Profits by Putting People First. Boston: Harvard Business School, 1998.
31. Friedman D, ed.: Linking Work-Family Issues to the Bottom Line: The Work-Family Issues and the Work Ethic Institute Conference Proceedings (#962). New York: The Conference Board Publishers, 1991.
32. Hart LA, Hart BL: Grief and Stress from so Many Animal Deaths. *Companion Anim Pract* 1:20, 1987.
33. Lief HO, Fox DC: Training for Detached Concern in Medical Students. *In* Lief HI, Lief VI, Lief NR, eds.: The Psychological Basis of Medical Practice. New York: Harper & Row, 1963, p 12.
34. Zunin LM, Zunin HS: The Art of Condolence. New York: Harper Perennial, 1991.
35. Petruzzello SJ, Landers DM, Hatfield BD, *et al.*: A meta-analysis on the anxiety reducing effects of acute and chronic exercise: outcomes and mechanisms. *Sports Med* 11:143, 1991.

86
The Human-Animal Bond

Dana Durrance, Ashley Harvey, and Greg Conger

INTRODUCTION

You have likely seen it hundreds of times in your professional life. You look into the eyes of a person who loves a companion animal, and you see the essence of the human-animal bond. The veterinarians who share in the power of this bond understand what they are witnessing—friendships that transcend time and a love and loyalty unlike any other. In recent decades, veterinarians have seen the relationships between humans and animals intensify in response to societal changes within family structures and support systems. Divorced, widowed, never-married, and childless people make up larger segments of the population in western society than ever before. For many children and adults, companion animals are a primary source of emotional and social support. Pets are often thought of as children, best friends, partners, confidantes, as well as sources of unconditional love and companionship.[1] At our institution, these highly attached pet owners are called "bond-centered families."[2]

According to marketing studies, veterinarians are most often compared to pediatricians, because they both care for the most helpless members of the family—those who cannot speak or make decisions for themselves.[3] As a result, veterinarians are considered to be part of a family's "health care team" (*e.g.*, pediatrician, family physician, family dentist, family veterinarian), and veterinarians find themselves having to care for the human family members as well as the pets. This is the essence of "bond-centered practice,"[4] that is, comprehensive veterinary care that goes beyond the level of quality medicine. A bond-centered practice is one in which the medical needs of animals and the emotional needs of owners are simultaneously addressed.

Given the deep attachments in these bond-centered families, it is no surprise to find that amidst a pet's critical illness, injury, or death, you see not only an animal in a medical crisis, but a pet owner in an emotional crisis. Because most veterinary schools offer little or no training in human crisis intervention, this chapter discusses the basic ideas and strategies that you can use when helping clients with the crisis-related situations encountered in the emergency setting.

THE CRITICAL CARE ENVIRONMENT

You know the daily challenges of working in critical care settings. Unpredictable work hours, going from calm to crisis in a matter of seconds, and experiencing emotional highs and lows are all part of the territory. Added to that is the stimulus overload (lights, alarms, animals vocalizing) and people experiencing emotions in a heightened state of arousal. All of these factors contribute to a work environment that is primed for stress. Communicating effectively with clients in this type of setting requires skill and commitment. The goal is to intervene quickly, decisively, and calmly. To effectively assist a person in crisis, it is important to understand how crisis affects human behavior.

CHARACTERISTICS OF CRISIS

Although some people function effectively in a crisis, many respond in ways that can be upsetting and frightening to watch. Common characteristics of crisis include feeling panicked, angry, confused, or out of control; having difficulty recalling information; and experiencing distortions in time and having tunnel vision. People in crisis may experience a breakdown in their normal coping mechanisms. It is not unusual for a person in crisis to display symptoms of shock, anger, anxiety, and even hysteria. Some people in the acute stage of a crisis can display intense emotion and erratic behavior, and become demanding, unreasonable, or obnoxious.[5] Clients may even disclose irrelevant personal information to gain leverage, attempting to elicit greater empathy from others so they will work harder to create the desired outcome. These behaviors are often unconscious and are not meant to be manipulative; rather, they are evidence of intense feelings of desperation.

Additionally, many people in crisis experience feelings of grief and loss (or the anticipation of loss). Grief affects people in a variety of ways and can manifest itself on many levels—intellectual, emotional, physical, social, and spiritual (Table 86-1). It is important to note that grieving people, like those in crisis, can appear irrational or difficult. Understanding the ways in which grief affects your clients will go a long way toward helping you to communicate and support them with their emotions. Once you have the sufficient knowledge to understand *why*

Table 86-1. Manifestations of Grief

Although grief responses differ from one person to another, there are many predictable manifestations of grief before, during, and after the loss.
Physical: crying, numbness, a lump in the throat, stomach ache or nausea, overwhelming fatigue, sleeping disturbances
Intellectual: denial, inability to concentrate, confusion, hallucinations, or a need to reminisce
Emotional: sadness, anger, depression, guilt, anxiety, or a desire to blame others
Social: isolation, alienation, greater dependency on others or rejection of others
Spiritual: bargaining with God to prevent loss or renewed or shaken religious beliefs

Adapted from Lagoni L, Butler C, Hetts S: The Human-Animal Bond and Grief. Philadelphia: WB Saunders, 1994.

your clients behave the way they do, you can reframe "difficult" clients into "grieving" clients.[4]

RESPONDING TO CLIENTS IN CRISIS

When assisting clients in crisis, your goal is to sufficiently stabilize the situation so that clients can achieve the following: communicate needs, understand information, and make short-term plans. To effectively stabilize people in crisis, it is essential to communicate that you are on their side. Providing a calm, caring, and confident demeanor is mandatory. Because crisis situations often make people feel helpless, it is important that you create ways to empower clients as soon as possible. Giving clients small choices such as asking them if they would like to sit down, or call a friend are simple, yet important ways to start the de-escalation process. It is also important to provide structure through your use of verbal and nonverbal communication.[4] Effective communication allows you to provide a framework for interacting with clients, enabling you to better support them and facilitate problem resolution.

Nonverbal Skills

One of the quickest and easiest ways to assist a client in crisis is to *structure the environment*. Adapt the physical space in your hospital to allow for comfortable seating, a quiet/private space for clients and families, easy telephone access, and boxes of tissues in the waiting/examination rooms. By creating a calm environment free from noises, distractions, and other intrusions, you will assist a client's physical and psychological needs by making the individual feel safe and grounded. Encouraging clients in crisis to sit down or even take a drink of water can help them remember to breathe—something many people in crisis forget to do. You can also structure the environment in such a way as to minimize any discomfort or anxiety for the animal. Using soft fleeces, thick pads, and comfortable exam rooms will be appreciated by your patients and clients alike.

When supporting a client in crisis, use good *attending behaviors* such as making eye contact, keeping an open posture, and nodding to acknowledge what the client is saying. This can lower the client's anxiety level by conveying trust and caring. If you assume a calm, open, and friendly demeanor, clients will be reassured that you are the person they can count on to help them through their crisis.

Use *touch* appropriately to provide comfort and reassurance. A light touch on the shoulder can take the place of words when no words seem to fit or say enough. Touch can also be used to help physically guide or stabilize someone who may be feeling faint, or needs gentle encouragement to sit down or move from a certain spot. This also works well with clients who, in the midst of crisis, refuse to let go of their animals for treatment. Make sure to use touch respectfully and be aware of gender and cultural differences. "Safe" areas to touch include shoulders, arms, and sometimes hands. If you are uncertain as to a client's response to touch, an alternate choice is to touch the client's animal with great sensitivity and care.

Verbal Skills

When assisting clients in crisis, it is essential that you *acknowledge* the client's emotions ("Mary, I can see how much you love Biscuit and how terrified and shocked you are about this accident. We will do our very best to save his life."). Acknowledging also alleviates client anxiety by letting clients know that you do not judge them. Clients may be struggling with guilt for ending an animal's life or for feeling that they are putting their animal through too much. To acknowledge emotions accurately, it is essential to listen carefully and pay attention to any statements clarifying needs or goals (*e.g.*, "I have to be with Biscuit as soon as possible! He needs to know I haven't abandoned him."). Acknowledging also means using concrete terms to describe an animal's illness, injury, or death (e.g., "Biscuit's injuries are severe and we may need to talk about helping him to die" versus "letting him pass away."). Using concrete terms helps to break through the shock so that clients can accept the reality of the situation and move on to other decisions that need to be made. When using concrete language, make sure to convey compassion and sensitivity through a gentle voice tone and appropriate touch.

A key component in acknowledging is *paraphrasing*. A paraphrase is a restatement of the client's communication to test your understanding and often begins with "It sounds like . . . " "You're feeling . . . " "I can hear that . . . " or "I'm hearing you say. . ."

Asking open-ended questions allows you to gain valuable insight into the circumstances of the client's crisis and helps identify any obstacles to decision-making. Specific questions about what you observe or perceive can greatly reduce confusion and future stress (*e.g.*, "How can I support you best right now?" or "What are your hopes for Biscuit right now?"). Questions can help you obtain important facts concerning the relationship between the client and animal, the client's perception of the animal's medical condition, the client's support system, and specific information about other issues currently facing the client. When asking questions it is important to be selective and precise because people in crisis are not always thinking clearly. Help your clients assess and prioritize the situation to identify their most important issues and concerns. The goal is to help clients form specific and concrete plans for how they will proceed. Issues to explore might include treatment options, financial concerns, euthanasia decisions, clients' short-term plans, and ways to connect clients with appropriate sources of support.

Because clients in crisis can behave irrationally or be angry, it is important to use *gentle confrontation* and *immediacy* when the need arises. Gentle confrontation is used to set limits on clients' behavior. Gentle confrontation can take many forms: it can be a question indicating that what a client has said is confusing; or a statement in which the client's belief system or interpretation of events is addressed.

The following is an example of gentle confrontation.

Mary: "You don't care at all about what happens to me or Biscuit!"
Veterinarian: "I can hear that you are very angry, Mary. However, we've been working very hard to help you and Biscuit. I'd like to know if you're upset about something specific we've said or done or if you're just angry about the whole situation."

Gentle confrontation may also be used to narrow the content of a client's conversation. During crisis, anxiety may cause some clients to ramble on about topics unrelated to their animals' care. They may also steer conversations off-track because they fear making difficult decisions or hearing what the veterinarian has to say. Gentle confrontation allows you to redirect rambling conversations (*e.g.*, "Mary, I'd like to hear more about your brother when we have more time, but we need to make some decisions about Biscuit's treatment now."). This strategy can help impose structure and set limits for clients who are feeling out of control.

The purpose of *immediacy* is to comment on the unspoken thoughts or feelings being shared *at the moment*. Immediacy can be used in a statement or question such as: "Mary, I get the feeling that you just now became angry with me for some reason, but I'm not sure why. Did I just say something to offend you?"

Unspoken thoughts and feelings may exist in crisis because clients want to avoid confrontations or protect their own feelings, or because intense emotions prevent them from identifying and speaking about what they are experiencing. Immediacy can be a powerful tool to deal with the more complex emotions presented by clients in crisis.

Once clients have expressed their emotions, concerns, and needs, you can move toward *decision-making*. The goal is to meet the client's needs with a specific plan of action. You should assist the client in assessing and prioritizing the situation and identifying the most important issues. Make sure to provide as many options and estimates as possible to help clients fully explore their resources before making any decisions. Ideally, the clients themselves should develop and implement their own plan (with your support and encouragement). Clients who find solutions on their own are much more invested in the outcome and are much less likely to blame you if the plan does not work out. When helping clients to identify alternatives and resources, you can act as the sounding board and calming presence needed to help clients think creatively for solutions.

FINANCIAL ISSUES

Financial issues are a significant factor in critical care. When a pet faces a life-threatening illness or injury, finances become an emotional issue for you and your clients. Never assume a client cannot afford treatment and always start the process by presenting the best treatment first. When appropriate, give clients permission to take finances into account (*e.g.*, "Mary, critical care can be expensive, and not all people can afford it. Even some of us who work here couldn't

Table 86-2. Veterinary Team Response to Clients in Crisis

To effectively intervene during crises, the entire veterinary team must act to meet both the medical needs of the animal and the emotional needs of the owner. Some strategies we suggest are:

- **Form a specific protocol for crisis situations.** Do not add to the chaos by being unprepared. Make sure all staff members know their "assigned duty" ahead of time.
- **Communicate.** Conference together as a team, sharing information among the staff as the crisis unfolds and providing updates as new information arises.
- **Work together with angry or manipulative clients.** Some clients in crisis may act out their frustrations by trying to "split" your staff or create conflict between you. To prevent this from happening, work with these clients as a team to communicate the same message.
- **Debrief.** Use regular staff meetings as a forum to discuss difficult cases and clients. Veterinary teams may find that debriefing provides an excellent way to end a difficult day, give positive and constructive feedback, and to provide mutual support.

Adapted from Durrance D, Butler C, Lagoni, L: Stat! Client in crisis! *Vet Tech* 20:8, 1999.

afford extensive medical treatment. I know that your financial limits say nothing about your love and commitment to Biscuit."). Each person and family has their financial priorities that do not necessarily reflect their level of compassion. The key is to uncouple finances from the perception of care and compassion on both sides.[6] Both you and your clients have financial constraints that you must live by—this does not mean that you both don't care deeply for animals. Depersonalize angry comments from your clients (their anger is usually about the situation, not you). With financial issues, it is helpful to write down options and details associated with the animal's treatment because clients in crisis often have difficulty remembering detailed information. It is also helpful to show clients the cost behind your fees. Explain the procedures you will perform and use pictures, models, handouts, and specimens to educate clients about your professional expenses. Explore other options while keeping financial responsibility on your clients. Your job is to give your best medical opinions, not to protect clients financially. The best that you can do is help clients understand the medical options (the pros and cons of each) and assist them in brainstorming financial alternatives such as credit cards, a short-term credit-agency loan, hospital payment plans, or paycheck advances.

Finally, when working with clients in crisis, it is essential that your entire veterinary team have predetermined policies in place. Supporting people in crisis can be emotionally and physically exhausting. It is important to lighten the load by working together with your colleagues in an organized manner so that no single individual has to manage a client alone (Table 86-2).

PATIENT EUTHANASIA AND DEATH

In CCUs, death comes in several forms. Death can occur from disease or injury or as a result of euthanasia. This section addresses the following key aspects:

euthanasia decision-making, client-present euthanasia protocols, sudden death, and resuscitation situations.

Euthanasia Decision-Making

For many clients, the decision to euthanize can be excruciating and they will often ask you for assistance. Typically, the primary issue with regard to euthanasia decision-making is quality of life, and you can encourage clients to define a bottom line for their animal. Quality is defined differently for each client and patient. For some clients, a quality life means their animal is able to urinate and defecate independently. For others, it might mean that the animal has a good appetite, is able to interact with the family, and can enjoy daily routines.

Perhaps the biggest issue influencing quality of life is pain. In response to a client's question, "Is my pet in pain?" you should be honest about the pet's condition. When clients ask, "Is there a chance?" it is important to not offer false hope, and to gently inform or remind clients of the animal's probability of regaining a quality life. In response to the almost-inevitable question, "What would you do?" it is essential to allow the client to make the decision, saying, for example, "There isn't a wrong decision. Biscuit will continue to have good and bad times, but there is nothing we can do to prevent his disease/injury from ending his life. You need to pick the time that feels right for you and for Biscuit." Allow clients who are struggling with this decision to spend time with their animal so that they can get a sense of their animal's needs.

When facilitating euthanasia decision-making for clients, it is often helpful to describe the euthanasia procedure. You should always ask clients if they have been present at euthanasia previously. Clients can then describe their experiences (positive or negative) and give you their perspective. Whether or not clients have had previous experience with euthanasia, you should walk all clients through the procedure step by step, so that you can help them to better grasp the reality of euthanasia and decide if it is timely and appropriate. This explanation generally takes a few minutes, and you can intersperse your description with gentle touches, pauses, or offering of tissues. This explanation used at Colorado State University's Veterinary Teaching Hospital is intended for adults, but can be easily simplified if children are present.[4]

> "Mary, have you ever been present at euthanasia before? *Continue with follow-up discussion.*
>
> "Mary, we will bring Biscuit to you in an exam room or outside if you prefer (when possible). We have some large mats that we can place on the floor or ground so that you and your family can be together with Biscuit. Biscuit will have already had an intravenous catheter in one of his rear (or fore) legs. The catheter[a] allows us to

[a] Using a previously-placed catheter during client-present euthanasia is strongly recommended because it creates the perception of a peaceful death. Without a catheter some clients perceive their animal to be "fighting" the euthanasia (when you take hold of the leg to give the injection, some animals will reflexively pull back, but this is often perceived by clients as "not wanting/ready to

administer the euthanasia solution more smoothly and do so without interfering with your desire to pet or hold Biscuit's head. Once Biscuit has been brought to you, you can spend some time alone with him if you desire.

Then, when it is time to proceed, we will begin the euthanasia process. The method we use involves three injections. The first injection is a saline flush to make sure the catheter is working. The second injection is an anesthetic, usually thiopental, which will place Biscuit in a plane of anesthesia, just as if he were undergoing surgery. At that point he will become relaxed and won't be aware of what is happening around him. The third injection is the euthanasia solution, usually pentobarbital sodium. This is the injection that will stop his brain, heart, and other bodily functions. All three injections are given within about 1 minute and once the final injection has been given, Biscuit's heart will stop beating within about 10 to 30 seconds. I will take a stethoscope and listen to Biscuit's heart so I can tell you when he has died.

Although death by euthanasia is peaceful and painless, Biscuit may urinate, defecate, twitch, or take a last breath or two as his body shuts down. In addition, his eyes will remain open in a sleepy sort of way. Do you have any questions about any of this?"

If the client expresses understanding, you can conclude with, "After Biscuit has died, you can stay with his body as long as possible." This explanation is intended for animals that are stable enough to be taken outside of the CCU for euthanasia, and would need to be modified for euthanasias occurring within the CCU.

Client-Present Euthanasia Guidelines

There are three key elements in facilitating sensitive client-present euthanasias: preparing the client for what to expect, empowering clients to create a meaningful goodbye, and creating a calm environment. Adults and children can be present at euthanasia if they know what to expect. The procedural description above contains many of the details that clients need to make an informed decision. Whatever the protocol, clients need to be informed about the number of injections, where they will be given, how quickly will they be given, and how long will it take for their pet to die. They also need to know how their animal will likely respond (vocalization, movement, eyes staying open) and what they as clients are allowed to do with their animal during the procedure (pet, hug, talk to, hold on lap). Clients need to be prepared for any medical equipment either present in the CCU or accompanying the animal to the euthanasia site, and any changes in their animal's physical condition (degree of consciousness, shaved areas, bruising, sutures, blood).

die"). Using a catheter prevents this potentially devastating last image and can help to prevent complicated grief reactions for your clients.

Clients need to be given permission to do what is important for them at the time of euthanasia, such as spending time alone with their pet (when possible), offering their pet a treat or a drink, saying a prayer, talking to their pet, or placing their pet on a special blanket or pillow. These simple rituals not only help to create a sense of ceremony, but also allow clients to combat feelings of helplessness, guilt, and being out of control. Clients can also be offered the opportunity to create a "linking object" either before or after the animal's death, such as clipping a tuft of fur or obtaining a clay impression of the animal's paw. As the name implies, items such as these help "link" the person to their pet long after the pet is gone.

If the animal must be euthanized in the CCU, a calm environment is more challenging to create. However, several measures can be taken. Minimize the number of people in the unit, and restrict access to the area as much a possible during the euthanasia. Radios or stereos should be turned off, and the critical care staff that must remain in the unit or are involved in the euthanasia should be encouraged to speak in low tones. Medical equipment can be minimized or covered up if appropriate. Regardless of where the euthanasia is performed, take care of consent forms, financial payments, and body care arrangements before the procedure whenever possible.

Following euthanasia, you can continue to facilitate a peaceful atmosphere. If the pet is euthanized in the CCU, offer the client a chance to spend time with their animal's body in a more private space. You can also ask clients to share special memories or stories. It is normal during such sharing for both you and your clients to feel emotion and respond accordingly. Clients typically see the tears of the veterinary team as validation of the uniqueness of their animal. Be aware that clients may express a broad range of thoughts and feelings and you may observe different reactions among family members. Remind clients that they did all that they could for their animal, but do not try to talk them out of feelings of guilt or remorse.

When clients leave, escort them out a back or side entrance if possible and when available, have a staff member remain with the pet's body until the client leaves. Clients almost always look back one last time, and when they see a friendly face petting their animal they are assured that their pet will be treated respectfully. If clients choose to stay until their pet's body is placed on a gurney or removed from the site, prepare clients that their animal's body will be limp when picked up, and take care to support the animal's head and move it gently. If a client is taking the animal's body, arrange the animal's body in a natural sleeping position, clean up bodily fluids, and tuck the tongue back into the mouth. You may even put tissue glue on the lower eyelids to keep the eyes shut. Clients generally prefer a cardboard box rather than a plastic bag if caskets are unavailable.

Sudden Death

Sudden death can occur soon after an animal arrives in the CCU or after a considerable stay. When there is no established rapport with clients and their animals die on arrival or within minutes after arriving, it can be particularly challenging for both you and your clients. It can be distressing for clients to have critically injured or ill animals taken from their arms and rushed away. You are likely to feel torn during these moments, wanting the owner to have time with the dying animal, but also feeling that the client's presence may pose a challenge to your job performance and the life of the animal. It is helpful to enlist the help of other staff to move clients to a private space and to give them as much information and decision-making power as possible.

When informing clients about the death of their animal, several steps can be taken. You should mentally prepare yourself for any response from the client, such as shock, anger, guilt, or hysteria. In a quiet place, give them a brief preparatory statement, such as, "Mr. and Mrs. Brown, I have some bad news that will be upsetting for you to hear." Then, give them the basic facts, telling them of the death up-front: "Biscuit has died. We performed CPR for 15 minutes and were unable to resuscitate him. I am so sorry." Do your best to absorb client's emotional responses without becoming defensive, hurried, or overly responsive. Instead, say things like, "I can imagine how hard this is," or "I know this is all overwhelming right now." You can offer more medical details then, or at a later time, and help clients mobilize their personal support system by suggesting that they call a supportive friend or family member.

When an animal has been in the unit for a day or more and then arrests or is found dead in the cage, owners often have to be called in the middle of the night or tracked down during the day. When delivering bad news over the telephone, it is important for you to be in a relatively quiet place. Do not leave notification of death on voicemail, or deliver the news to someone other than the owner(s) (*e.g.*, a secretary, coworker, or other relative). If you are calling a client at work, ask if it is an appropriate time. It can be helpful to give clients the option of hearing the news over the telephone or in person, saying, "Mrs. Brown, I have some news that will be upsetting to hear. Would you like me to tell you over the phone, or do you want to come into our clinic?" Most clients want to be told right then, but this gives them a choice and also a few seconds to prepare themselves for the news.

In either situation, once clients have been informed of their animal's death, they should be given the option of spending time with their animal's body in a private space. If possible, some clients may also want to see the CCU and the area in which their animal died. Again, it is important to arrange the body peacefully on blankets or pillows and to prepare owners for what to expect. Clients also appreciate you offering objects such as a clay imprint of the paw, the collar, or a clipping of fur.

Presence During Resuscitation

Research in the human medical arena suggests benefits from family presence during resuscitation.[7] Family members who were present during such efforts reported that, in addition to feeling that they have the right to be there, being present provided them with relief from wondering what was happening, allowed them to feel that their presence had provided comfort and protection to their loved one, and helped facilitate their grief process in later months. Family members participating in this study were prepared ahead of time for what to expect during a resuscitation situation or invasive procedure and had a nurse or chaplain with them during the procedure, explaining interventions, answering questions, and facilitating appropriate opportunities for family members to touch or speak to the patient. Family members who were combative, intensely emotional, or in an altered mental state were not offered the opportunity to be present. The majority of nurses and physicians supported family presence and although some were concerned about family disruptions during the procedure, no such incidents occurred.

Given that many companion animals are thought of as family members, you may decide to allow client presence during resuscitation in your veterinary hospital. If you do, make sure that you can devote one staff member exclusively for supporting and educating clients during resuscitation. This person will need to be prepared for any emotional responses from clients and should be given proper training to adequately educate and support clients. Your entire staff also must be thoroughly prepared ahead of time so that when clients are present during resuscitation, you work as a team in these challenging situations.

MAKING REFERRALS

When clients are in crisis, they often have needs that exceed your limits as a helper. Clients who confide intimate details of their lives may discuss mistakes about which they feel guilty, illnesses or disabilities with which they are coping, and even dangerous or illegal situations in which they are involved (*e.g.*, physical abuse,[b] alcohol or drug use). These instances go beyond the boundaries of your basic helping abilities and it is unwise, as well as unethical, for you to attempt to intervene in any way other than to connect clients with appropriate human service professionals and resources.

When you feel that a client may benefit from the support of an outside resource, it is essential to know how and where to make referrals. When selecting a referral source, use your community resources. These might include the telephone book, human hospitals, newspapers, online resources, and local religious organizations. National self-help organizations can also provide information on local services and chapters. Most national organizations offer hotline numbers on such topics as cancer, child abuse, suicide, and alcohol/substance abuse. When considering referrals for your clients, you should also use resources about which you have first- hand knowledge or have heard about from family or friends (Table 86-3). It is best to locate these resources ahead of time before you are in the midst of a crisis with your clients and feeling desperate for help yourself. You

[b] Currently, a veterinarian's duty to report child or animal abuse varies from state to state. The State Department of Professional Regulation for the Veterinary Medical Examining Board may have information pertaining to state statutes. Contact your state veterinary medical association and local veterinary societies for more information.[8]

Table 86-3. Building a Referral Network

When building a referral network for your clinic or hospital, research the most credible agencies and professionals. Then create a list of telephone numbers, e-mail addresses, and contact people for various types of resources, including the following:

Hotlines

- Crisis intervention
- Suicide prevention
- Substance abuse
- Domestic violence
- Child abuse
- Animal abuse

Mental Health Professionals

- Grief counselors
- Marriage/family therapists
- Substance abuse counselors

Community Resources

- Support groups
- Health services
- Clergy members
- Animal rescue/Adoption agencies
- Animal behaviorists
- Police/ambulance

Adapted from Durrance D, Butler C, Lagoni L: Stat! Client in crisis! *Vet Tech* 20:8, 1999.

want to refer your clients to the best resources in your community, not just the first available.

When making a referral, you want to be supportive and straightforward. The goal is to help clients feel empowered while simultaneously setting limits on your abilities as a helper. Over time, you will develop a repertoire of two or three ways in which you can smoothly and confidently let clients know about outside resources available to them. Some sample referral techniques are described in Table 86-4.

FOLLOWING UP

Some crisis situations require follow up after you have intervened (beyond writing a condolence letter/card or making a donation in the pet's memory). This may be a quick telephone call to a client, contact with the client's veterinarian, or other outside resources. The goal of following up is to determine if your clients have implemented the plans they developed at the time of crisis. Remember, your clients must ultimately choose solutions that are right for them. At this point, you want to encourage clients to find sources of ongoing emotional support so that you can step back and be free to support other clients coming in your door.

When you help clients successfully through intense emotions, it is not unusual for them to become strongly attached or overly reliant on you. They may believe that because you helped them through such a difficult time, you are the only one who truly understands them and they should look to you for future

Table 86-4. Referral Techniques

- **Self-Disclosure:** This skill normalizes, or gives credibility to others thoughts and feelings.

  "Mary, I can see how difficult Biscuit's death is for you. At the clinic, we work closely with someone who is skilled in assisting people like you who are experiencing grief over the death of their companion animal. I get feedback from many clients here that they there were helped by the services of this support person."

- **The Illusion of Choice:** This technique allows the client to feel empowered by the information, yet also able to make the decision for or against calling a professional.

  "Mary, since we initially covered the diagnosis, prognosis, and treatment options for Biscuit last week, I sense that you are still feeling overwhelmed by the information and confused as to what decision to make. I'd like to have you talk with someone that many of the clients here look to for support and guidance when faced with decisions regarding their pets' care. Let me give you the phone number."

- **The One-Down Approach:** This skill clearly establishes distinct boundaries, while still extending care beyond the illness or death of their companion animal.

  "Mary, I appreciate your trusting my professional judgment, yet I feel that what you are experiencing is beyond my expertise and professional training. I'd like to recommend someone who is trained and has extensive experience in working with people who are struggling with difficult decisions. Would you like me to give you their name and number?"

- **The Medical Analogy:** This technique facilitates clients who may be stagnant in their grief and unable to move beyond their emotions to active grieving. It can also assist those clients that need structure and direction in responding to the emotional situation.

  "Mary, if there was something physically wrong with you, I am confident you would seek medical attention. Like physical injuries, emotional stresses require attention from trained professionals. I know someone who may be able to help in your time of grief. With your approval, I would like to call them and let you set an appointment."

- **The Back-Door Approach:** This approach allows the client time to adjust to the idea that they as well as their family may need professional support.

  "Mary, I think it's beneficial for you to be thinking about your two children and their responses to Biscuit's death. I know a professional who is skilled in assisting both children and adults during emotional times. Before you leave, I will give you her name and you can call her at a later time."

Adapted from Lagoni L, Butler C, Hetts S: The Human-Animal Bond and Grief. Philadelphia: WB Saunders, 1994.

emotional support. Although you might want to make yourself available for a quick telephone call now and then, your goal should be helping your clients find long-term support. You must judge this on a client-by-client basis. When working with clients through crisis, you too, may develop your own personal feelings about them. The key is in knowing your own helping limits and deciding how much time you can personally and ethically give to your clients once the crisis has passed.

Helping clients through crisis takes commitment and practice. It also takes courage to confront sensitive issues rather than walking away from them. It is likely that you already use many of the skills discussed here in your practices. However, there are numerous educational programs that teach helping techniques and crisis intervention strategies. Some of these are offered within the field of veterinary medicine (Colorado State University provides such programs for veterinarians and veterinary professionals), and some are in the realm of human services. You may decide that you, and your staff, can use such programs to continue building your skills.

When you have the proper crisis intervention skills, you will have the confidence to remain calm, assured that no matter what happens, you will know how to handle a situation. You can also lower your own personal stress level and reduce your chances of professional burnout by knowing that you have supported your clients in a compassionate, professional manner. By responding appropriately to the medical needs of your patients and the "human" needs of your clients, you will enjoy a more fulfilling professional and personal life.

REFERENCES

1. Voith VL: Attachment of people to companion animals. *Vet Clin North Am Small Anim Pract* 15:289, 1985.
2. Lagoni L: The Argus Center Brochure, Colorado State University College of Veterinary Medicine and Biomedical Sciences, Fort Collins, CO, 1998.
3. Troutman C.M: The Veterinary Services Market for Companion Animals. Overland Park, Kansas, Charles Research Group and The American Veterinary Medical Association, Schaumburg, IL, 1988.
4. Lagoni L, Butler C, Hetts S: The Human-Animal Bond and Grief. Philadelphia: WB Saunders, 1994.
5. Durrance D, Butler C, Lagoni L: Stat! Client in crisis! *Vet Tech* 20: 8, 1999.
6. Durrance D, Lagoni L: I can't pay for treatment. *Vet Econ* June, 1999.
7. Meyers T, Eichhorn D, Guzzetta C, *et al.*: Family presence during invasive procedures and resuscitation. *Am J Nurs* 100:2, 2000.
8. Harvey A, Butler C, Lagoni L: Dealing with abuse: the role of veterinary professionals. *Vet Tech* 21:5, 2000.

87
Ethics in Veterinary Critical Care Medicine

Bernard E. Rollin

INTRODUCTION

In critical care medicine, as in veterinary medicine in general, the most problematic moral/conceptual dimension one confronts is the issue of whether veterinarians owe primary moral obligation to the animal and its interests or to the client. This question underlies virtually all of the pressing moral issues encountered in the field. Consider, for example, the problem of how long a clinician should keep a suffering animal alive, given our ever-increasing capacity to do so, and the client's lack of cognizance of, or lack of concern with, the degree to which the animal is suffering. Many clients want the animal kept alive at all costs for selfish reasons, and simply refuse to acknowledge the terrible price paid by the animal. In the same vein, in CCUs maintained in veterinary schools or other research institutions, the animal may be a research animal and the owner a zealous researcher interested primarily in milking every drop of data from that animal, again at considerable costs in pain and suffering to the animal. Another issue is the unowned animal brought to a CCU by a Good Samaritan who cares about the animal, but is not willing to assume financial responsibility. Additionally, there is the issue of a reasonable owner who wishes to have the animal treated not excessively, but enough to return the animal to relatively pain-free normalcy, but cannot afford the ever-burgeoning expenses of critical care. The issue of "cure" versus "care," with the latter often taking a back seat to the former in veterinary, as well as human, medicine is also central. Fixing the patient is given significant precedence over patient comfort. The measure of winning the battle against disease or injury is keeping the animal alive.

How one responds to these questions will almost certainly depend on how one answers what I have called "the fundamental question of veterinary ethics": to whom does a veterinarian owe primary obligation, owner or animal? If one adopts the *Pediatrician Model*, one serves the animal, with the client's interests shunted to the side if they are inimical to the animal's, as when the client will not spend money on a fixable animal, or, conversely, when a client spares no expense to keeping an animal in misery alive. On the other hand, if one adopts the *Garage Mechanic Model*, the veterinarian basically pursues the satisfaction of client interests or desires, with animal interests shunted to the side.

To understand the full significance of this pivotal question relative to the issues catalogued briefly early in our discussion, we must quickly address the nature of ethics. Three categories are relevant: social consensus ethics, personal ethics, and professional ethics

SOCIAL CONSENSUS ETHICS

Despite the unfortunate tendency on the part of what I have elsewhere called Scientific Ideology or the Common Sense of Science (for it is to scientific day-to-day practice what ordinary common sense is to ordinary life) to claim that ethics is simply a person's subjective opinions or predilections, that is patently false. Were ethics simply left to a person's subjective opinion, society would be chaotic, anarchy would prevail and life would be, as Thomas Hobbes put it "nasty, miserable, brutish, and short."

Thus all viable societies must possess what I have called a *social consensus ethic* that informs and is reinforced by all social laws and regulations. All of our laws, from municipal rules for zoning strip clubs and pornographic book stores away from elementary schools, to laws against discrimination, insider trading, and murder, are based on consensus insights about right and wrong, which enjoy social objectivity in the same way as do the rules of grammar or traffic.

It is no surprise that scientific ideology has put the scientific and medical communities at loggerheads with society in general.[1] This ideology is historically based in Newton's professed disdain for what could not be verified empirically. In the early 20th century, it was invoked to rid science of some mystical notions that had gradually entered various fields of science. Physics talked of absolute space and time that allegedly are independent of how they are measured. Biology invoked "life force" and "entelechy" to explain the essence of living matter. While successfully banishing these untestable concepts from science, it also threw out the baby with the bath water. Because ethical judgments could not be verified empirically—Wittgenstein once remarked that if one took inventory of all the facts in the universe, one would not find it a *fact* that killing is wrong—ethics too is banished from science and this banishment is trumpeted in the slogan that science is "value-free" and "ethics-free." Typical science textbooks throughout the 20th century proclaimed this notion in prefatory chapters and no less a figure in American science than the director of the National Institutes of Health once remarked that, although new technologies like genetic engineering are always controversial, "science should not be burdened by ethical considerations."

This ideology ramified in scientific and medical practice, leading to, among other things, cavalier treatment of human subjects in research, which treatment in turn led society to demand legislative and regulatory assurance that the research community is taking its ethical obligations seriously. Another component of scientific ideology further complicated the issue—the failure of veterinary and human medicine to focus on control of felt pain as a major component of practice.[2] Virtually no literature on animal analgesia, for example, could be found in veterinary medicine until after the federal laboratory animal laws of 1985 mandated that animals felt pain and that it needed to be controlled. In human medicine, the official definition of pain of the International Society for the Study of Pain makes the possession of language a precondition for feeling pain, and medical practice with neonates and infants has mirrored this highly questionable theory.[3] Although 90% of cancer pain in humans is controllable with today's analgesia modalities, 80% of such pain is in fact not controlled.[4] And until the late 1980s, open heart surgery on human neonates had been performed using paralytics, not anesthetics.

PERSONAL ETHICS

In addition to the social consensus ethic explained above, society leaves certain decisions of ethical import to an individual's personal ethic; such choices as what one eats, to whom one gives charity, and what one reads are left to one's (hopefully consistent and coherent) individual choice.

As society changes, decisions once the purview of the social ethic become relinquished to an individual's personal ethics, and vice versa. Sexual behavior among consenting adults provides an example of the former sort of change, whereas to whom one rents or sells one's property is an example of the latter. During the past 50 years, society has come to realize that private, uncoerced sexual activity is not its business, while also realizing that leaving renting and selling or hiring to individual choice led to unfair discrimination against minorities and women. In general, the social ethic appropriates behavior from personal ethics when leaving such behavior to individuals generates widespread injustice or unfairness.

PROFESSIONAL ETHICS

Finally, it is necessary to define *professional ethics*, which historically has erroneously been equated with intraprofessional etiquette in veterinary medicine and other professions. Professionals are people in society who perform highly significant tasks that require special skills and special privileges. Examples of such people are physicians and veterinarians, who are allowed to write prescriptions and perform surgery. Society by and large does not understand the details of such professions, and thus is unwilling to regulate them. Instead it essentially says to them: "You regulate yourselves the way we would regulate you given the social consensus ethic if we understood what you do, which we don't, but if you screw up we will know and will regulate you." Examples of what happens when professionals fail to follow this dictum are manifest. About 10 years ago, veterinary medicine almost lost extralabel drug use privileges to Congressional action when society became aware that some practitioners are endangering human health by indiscriminate use of antibiotics in animal feeds for growth promotion. Similarly, the biomedical research community was hammered with two pieces of federal legislation in 1985 when it became apparent that it was failing to provide proper care for laboratory animals.

In our ensuing discussion, we shall examine the five major ethical questions relevant to critical care medicine in terms of how we can illuminate the Fundamental Question of Veterinary Ethics by examining social ethics, personal ethics, and professional ethics.

If we look to the social consensus ethic historically for guidance on the question of the moral status of animals and thus on the Fundamental Question of Veterinary Ethics, we find a fairly unequivocal answer: Animals are property in the eyes of the law. This, in turn, seems to militate in favor of the Garage Mechanic View, pure and simple. Yet the situation is far more complex than that. In virtually all legal systems, going back to the Bible, the social ethic has constrained certain actions toward animals despite their property status. These actions traditionally are deliberate, willful, deviant, intentional, sadistic acts of cruelty toward animals or outrageous neglect.[5] These stipulations existed as much to protect society from sadists and psychopaths as to protect the animals, for it has long been known that such individuals may begin with abusing animals but graduate inexorably to abusing people.

During the past 30 years, it has become clear to society that the vast majority of animal suffering at human hands is not the result of what the anticruelty ethic constrains, but rather grows out of common, socially accepted practices with animals invisible to that ethic in areas such as agriculture, research on animals, toxicology, rodeo, hunting, trapping, circuses, indeed all "normal" uses of animals. A moment's reflection reveals that the amount of suffering in animals produced by such normal use vastly outnumbers what results from overt cruelty. (For example, the United States produces 8 billion broiler chickens per year, 80% of which go to market fractured or deeply bruised.) For reasons that I have detailed elsewhere, society began, for the first time in its history, to worry about the animal suffering that does not result from cruelty, wished to see it controlled, and needed other ethical notions beyond cruelty to articulate these concerns.[6]

But new ethics are not spun out of nothing. Ethical change comes out of recollection of implications of our prior ethical commitments. So it was inevitable that when society sought new ethical concepts to express its ethical concern for all varieties of pain and suffering occasioned by human use of animal, it would look to its ethical machinery for judging treatment of humans for a basis. And the relevant concepts to appropriate are obvious.

In brief essence, society is saying that if fair use of animals no longer occurs naturally and automatically as it did in husbandry, it needs to be artificially imposed by the legal and regulatory systems. Thus, in the past 20 years, the legal systems of all civilized countries have witnessed a vast proliferation of legislative proposals and laws designed to protect animals in all areas, with research and agriculture seeing the most dramatic laws (cf. the U.S. laboratory animal laws of 1985 and the Swedish law of 1988 abolishing confinement agriculture). In addition, we are seeing the concept of cruelty being modified to cover established and accepted practices where we now know that equal alternatives that do not cause as much suffering exist (cf. the U.S. Department of Agriculture being found guilty of cruelty for mandatory face branding of cattle during the dairy buyout of the 1980s).

This new state of affairs has major implications for social consensus morality regarding animal treatment. Although it is still true that animals are legally property, there are ever-increasing moral constraints entering the law on how they can be treated, even for human benefit. Indeed, a variety of philosophies and legal scholars are working toward a promissory change in the status of animals away from property.

What is quite real is the serious concern that society, and these new bills and laws, show for animal pain and suffering. (In fact, people are so concerned with animal suffering that it affects their economic choices. Disavowal of animal testing catapulted a cosmetic company called the Body Shop into a multimillion dollar business, and zoos as prisons are a thing of the past.) Consider the laboratory animal laws that have proliferated in the United States, Britain, and Europe during the past two decades, or the European food animal laws. Their concern is with ensuring that animals do not suffer or experience significant pain, distress, or suffering. In some countries, if an animal is experiencing unalleviable pain, the experiment must be terminated immediately. In all countries, early end points for experiments are designated to prevent suffering, and pain and distress must be controlled by proper use of anesthesia, analgesia, and sedation.

In all of these emerging laws, little attention is paid to preserving animal life per se; rather, the emphasis is on limiting pain and suffering. In fact, to my knowledge, nowhere do laws address the most senseless waste of animal life, the euthanasia of pet animals for convenience! The taking of animal lives for research, testing, or food is not addressed; the quality of that life is seriously addressed.

The most momentous of these new laws in the United States are the 1985 laws regulating the use of animals in research. At a conference on the legal mandate to control pain held in 1987, Hyram Kitchen pointed out that, being embodied in federal law, the mandate for control of pain in research animals sets the standard of practice that veterinarians must live up to or be (theoretically at least) legally actionable. This is directly relevant to a number of the issues we raised in critical care medicine. The first problem we raised is keeping a suffering animal alive: How long should one do this for an owner? For a researcher? How much suffering is justified by a cure? Are owner demands sacrosanct?

The issue is clear from the dictates of the social ethic with regard to a research animal in critical care: If euthanasia is the only way to control suffering, the animal should be euthanized. Intractable and prolonged suffering is not permitted under these laws. If the purpose of the experiment is realized, the animal must be terminated immediately, and no Animal Care Committee would ever permit a protocol requiring prolonged, uncontrolled pain.

The same logic, in my view, applies *mutatis mutandis* to an animal owned by a private individual. If society will not accept prolonged suffering in an animal for biomedical reasons (*i.e.*, reasons that benefit humanity in general), it will surely condemn the owner who keeps a suffering animal alive for egoistic (or egotistic) reasons, because he or she cannot bear to let go. Similarly, it would clearly be wrong to the consensus ethic to keep an animal alive heroically, and at considerable suffering cost, if the animal will never be capable of a decent (not perfect!) quality of life, for instance, if the animal will be unable to move or dramatically be wracked by pain.

Part of the emerging consensus social ethic is a respect for, and increasing demand for legal protection of, animal natures, what I call after Aristotle, the "pigness" of the pig, the "dogness" of the dog.[7] The fact is that the U.S. laboratory animal laws mandate "exercise for dogs" and "environments for primates that enhance their psychological well-being;" that the Swedish agricultural law of 1988 demands environments for animals that suit their psychological and biologic needs and natures, and that U.S. zoos now try to create *functionally* naturalistic environments for their charges, rather than aesthetically naturalistic environments that look good to us, all attest to the extent to which society worries about animal nature. In that light, a dog (or any other animal) suffering constant significant pain is no longer a dog—its normal life is subordinated to the pain, even as humans tell us that extreme pain leaves little else to focus on in life. Animals in pain may well suffer more than people in pain; at least we are capable of hope and anticipation of pain's end![8]

Thus I am arguing that whether the CCU client is a researcher or a pet owner, the emerging social ethic militates in the direction of the veterinarian acting as a pediatrician, not as a garage mechanic, at least as far as pain and suffering are concerned. In the case of a research animal, clinicians have explicit law on their side. In the case of a private owner, although the law is not explicit, it certainly sets the standard of practice on the side of stopping pain. Thus, a CCU clinician could say to a client, "We've gone far enough; keeping the animal alive at any cost involves too much suffering," and "going any further would not be allowed in research" and, "in addition, in my view violates my understanding of the Veterinary Oath," and he or she would have the moral force of federal law and society behind them.

Technically, though, the animal is still property, and a client could be intransigent. In this case, there are three options for the clinician:

1. Capitulate: You have done what you can.
2. Persuade: Use your Aesculapian authority (which is considerable and which we shall shortly discuss) to move the client to a different place, for example, by explaining the suffering, making the client watch, visit, and so forth.
3. Extract a commitment allowing you to keep the animal comfortable. Even if you truly believe that the animal should be euthanized, it is almost as reasonable to gain client support for keeping the animal unaware. In the first place, you forestall suffering. Second, there is a fine line between keeping an animal comfortable with increased analgesia and moving toward euthanasia. The former can well entail the latter.

Obviously some combination of (2) and (3) is probably optimal. Resorting to (1) on a regular basis would probably generate what I have elsewhere called "moral stress"—the tension between what one is doing and what one believes one *ought* to be doing—which ultimately erodes both personal health and job satisfaction.[9]

Thus, although the social ethic clearly determines the path a critical care veterinarian is obliged to take regarding a suffering research animal, it merely suggests, without compelling, the decision regarding a suffering companion animal. For even though federal law sets the standard of practice in theory, *de facto* there is no one to impose it on a private owner. At best it provides a powerful argument for the critical care clinician who must, in the end, appeal to his personal ethic in adjudicating such a situation. If the veterinarian holds strongly to the Pediatrician Model, he will strongly object to prolonging life at all costs. I believe that veterinarians, like physicians, enjoy a great deal of what Talcott Parsons called *Aesculapian authority*, the powerful, almost mystical authority that healers enjoy in all cultures. Deploying this authority by first of all convincing the client that you have the animal's best interest at heart and second by demonstrating your considerable experience with situations like the one in question, both go a long way toward securing client trust.

A special case, midway between research and private ownership, is the case of a client animal being used in an experimental research protocol for therapeutic purposes. In some ways, the use of animals with naturally occurring disease for research obviously represents a moral advance over creating the disease in experimental animals. But this sort of activity, for example in oncology, creates its own moral problems. In particular, the clinician-researcher usually has a vested interest in keeping the animal alive as long as possible for the understandable purpose of garnering data. The animal owner may be subtly (or not so subtly) swayed by the Aesculapian authority of the research-clinician to keep the animal alive for longer than she would be inclined to do. (Such researchers often build close emotional bonds with clients after many months or even years of therapy.) Thus the client may decide to take the animal home after a very dramatic invasive experimental therapy, say radical intestinal resection, amputation of the tongue, or removal of the mandible. The animal may have been stabilized in the research institution's CCU, but is by no means normal. While at home, the animal crashes, sometimes far away from the research institution, and the animal is brought to a local CCU. Because the local veterinarians may not be familiar with the intricacies of the protocol, they are faced with a suffering, failing animal about whose situation they may know very little. With the client-researcher complex strongly leaning toward keeping the animal alive, the CCU veterinarians are faced with controlling pain and suffering in an area in which they lack familiarity. Although end points for ordinary research animals are generally set by researchers in consultations with Institutional Animal Care and Use Committees, the euthanasia decision for client-owned research animals in the sort of situation we described is left to the client!

In my view, the CCU clinician should address this moral problem very directly and honestly. If the clinician believes that saving the animal or even keeping it comfortable requires specialized knowledge or facilities lacking in the practice, or believes that the animal cannot in fact be made comfortable, she should say so directly. She should explain to the client that, although perhaps

CCU clinicians at the research institution may have the specialized knowledge necessary to manage the suffering adequately, she is uncomfortable with the responsibility. In my view, by no means should this private clinician trade extra data for animal suffering, particularly if she embraces the Pediatrician Model. Once again, the spirit of current social ethics supports this decision.

Although typically a critical care clinician does not enjoy the long-term relationship with a client that allows you to put your arm around the client and say, "It's time to let go," the lack of such a relationship can also be a boon. Many oncologists who treat animals over a long period of time warn that directing clients toward euthanasia may well lead them to later blame the veterinarian for "killing my dog." The very fact that the critical care clinician steps into the picture only *in extremis*, for a relatively brief and dramatic moment, militates against long-term resentment and increases the power of your advice. If the client later resents you, it will not have the same effect on you professionally or emotionally as it does on a primary care clinician or oncologist. To put it crudely, you are able to focus more on the animal.

Our analysis is buttressed by looking at professional ethics. It is manifest that society expects veterinarians to champion animal welfare and lead in welfare reform.[10] This is clearly evidenced by the laboratory animal welfare laws in the United States and Britain designating veterinarians as responsible for ensuring research animal well-being. It is also something any veterinarian can confirm through ordinary experience. Though U.S. organized veterinarian medicine has been slow to shoulder this burden, society expects veterinarians to perform the same role with regard to all animals, including agricultural animals, race horses, zoo animals, wild animals, and companion animals. Once again, except for endangered species, the area of concern is animal suffering rather than animal life. We all know from personal experience that society unequivocally condemns people who will not euthanize a suffering animal (though we are split on suffering humans). It would therefore behoove organized veterinary medicine as a whole—and certainly the specialty of emergency/critical care veterinarians—to adopt as a principle of professional ethics that they are committed to not prolonging the life of an animal when suffering is uncontrollable, or when the prognosis is permanent suffering, pain, distress, or disability. The details of such a professional ethical position should of course be worked out by the professionals involved. This leaves room for professional judgment and flexibility, but some such principle would be of great social value both in setting out the ground rules regarding uncontrolled suffering, and pre-empting eventual loss of professional autonomy to legislation.

On the basis of the analysis we have hitherto developed, we can generate a response to the problem of pain control, the third ethical question we raised in our introductory paragraph; what we may call "care" versus "cure."

It is manifest that 20th century scientific medicine, human or animal, is captured by the ideology outlined above and, desirous of eschewing talk of unverifiable subjective states, has schematized the battle against disease, injury, or death as won or lost. If a disease is cured or life is prolonged, medicine wins; if not it loses. Little emphasis is placed on patient comfort—that is one reason the voluntary euthanasia issue has become so pronounced. Physicians routinely argue against morphine and marijuana for terminally ill patients. As one nursing dean said to me, "Physicians worry about *cure*, we worry about *care*." Patients whose situations are perceived as hopeless end up cared for by nurses, and it is all too revealing that the hospice movement, aimed at keeping patients comfortable and as pain free as possible, is almost totally a creation of, and staffed by, nurses, not doctors.

Veterinary medicine too, has been guilty of ignoring patient comfort.[11] For much of the 20th century, anesthesia has been confused with chemical restraint both in nomenclature and in practice. Surgical procedures such as spays, castrations, dehorning, wound repair, and others are performed with "bruticaine" on small and large animals, or with paralytic, curariform drugs, or visceral procedures have been performed with drugs like ketamine, which provide virtually no visceral analgesia but do immobilize. Killing of animals is often done with these paralyzing drugs via asphyxiation—a far cry from the "good death" embodied in the term "euthanasia." Early textbooks of veterinary anesthesia do not even mention pain control as a justification for anesthesia, and routine rationalization for not using anesthesia or analgesia have been rife: "The anesthetic bothers the animal more than the pain" or "The analgesia will allow the animal to reinjure itself," and so forth.

In today's society, enduring pain is not seen as a virtue or as building strength or character. Indeed, pain is a major biologic stressor that, if not alleviated, can retard healing and even promote morbidity and mortality. One can argue that one of the major causes of the movement in society toward scientifically unproven alternative medicine is that alternative practitioners openly address and sympathize with human and animal pain, suffering, and distress.

Our earlier discussions of the question of keeping animals alive are directly relevant to the issue of controlling pain and suffering. As detailed in our earlier reasoning, social ethics values control of animal suffering more than it values animal life, as do owners not blinded by selfish concerns. Thus the moral imperative for CCU veterinarians to keep animals as pain-free as possible seems to rule, and in some cases can be used to trump the selfish owner's willingness to keep the animal alive at all costs, because death can be a serendipitous sequel to controlling pain.

Obviously, not all pain can be controlled all the time. In some cases, like physical therapy, some pain must be accepted to return the animal to normalcy. There are no hard and fast rules for such situations; common sense and common decency should suffice. As a general moral principle, it is only reasonable not to control pain and suffering when controlling pain interferes with a clear and pressing health demand that leads directly to rapid return to normalcy (as in physical therapy).

When, however, one is tempted to withhold pain control one should bear in mind that, contrary to old Shibboleths, animals may actually suffer pain more intensely than humans. It used to be said that, lacking language and future concepts, animal pain is limited to the now, as opposed to human pain, which can be potentiated by fear and anxiety. (Thus part of the suffering of going to the dentist may be fear that he is Josef Mengele.) In response to that claim, I would argue that, lacking such concepts, animals have no *hope* of pain cessation, or anticipation of a future without pain, and thus they *are* their pain.

In the same vein, Ralph Kitchell has pointed out that the experience of pain has two elements, a sensory discriminative dimension and a motivational dimension.[12] Because animals lack the intellectual power humans have to reason out the source of pain and how to stop it, the motivational aspect may be stronger and thus animals may well suffer more than we do.

Thus keeping the animals comfortable should be a top moral priority for the CCU clinician. The social consensus ethic points in that direction, and the professional ethics of such clinicians should be developed to be in accord with that ethic. Control of animal pain, suffering, and distress should be a primary and articulated ethical imperative across all of veterinary medicine and should be made an unequivocal top priority in the Veterinarian's Oath.

The issue of clients who cannot afford to pay for CCU fees is one that leads to pervasive problems across veterinary medicine. Unlike human medicine, there is no social guarantee in veterinary medicine that a patient will get the requisite care. There is little animal health insurance in society, and what there is favors upper middle class animal owners. Unlike the situation for children, society does not yet see fit to guarantee medical care for animals, especially the costly sort of care entailed by CCU modalities. So euthanasia for animals belonging to poor people often presents itself as the only option.

In some cases, veterinary schools may run a clinic for indigent clients, both as a public service and as a way of educating veterinary students, but this sort of operation is relatively rare, and is not found in all (or even most) veterinary schools. Given that society is increasingly reluctant to allow veterinary students to practice surgery and other skills on unwanted companion animals slated for euthanasia, such clinics may well proliferate. But given that there are only some 30 veterinary colleges in the United States, even creating such clinics at every veterinary college would only deal with a very tiny percentage of such cases.

In large measure then, solutions to this problem will emerge from the personal ethics of veterinarians engaged in critical care. If a veterinarian strongly adheres to the Pediatrician Model, or strongly values the strength of the human-animal bond in at least some cases, for example, where the animal in question is all that gives meaning to the life of an elderly, lonely person, he may choose to do the requisite work at cost. But in many such instances, the owner in question can still not afford to pay. The veterinarian is then left with a dilemma—either euthanize the animal or do the work gratis. Although idealistic students are often inclined to working for free, they soon realize that they simply cannot afford to do this very often, particularly in critical care cases that are extremely consumptive of time and resources.

One solution that was quite prevalent in veterinary medicine in general during hard times earlier this century was barter. Often cash-poor clients may have a good deal to trade for veterinary services. I have heard of veterinarians trading their services for farm products such as eggs, milk, vegetables, or meat. I have also heard of barter for client labor, skilled or unskilled. Clients can trade house painting, fence building, lawn maintenance, snow removal, mechanical work, trash hauling, or general clean-up for care given to their animals. Alternatively, some veterinarians allow clients to pay a small amount each month, in effect extending long-term, low-interest credit to poor people.

In the end, however, there is only a limited amount that critical care veterinarians can do, as they will always encounter more hardship cases than can be managed by the approaches mentioned. State-of-the-art critical care is expensive and is likely to become even more expensive as new cutting-edge technology is incorporated.

A final related issue concerns the unowned animal requiring critical care, say a trauma victim brought in by a Good Samaritan or public servant such as a policeman, fireman, or animal control officer. The owner is unknown, and the animal rescuer is unwilling to assume financial responsibility. Obviously, as we saw earlier, even the most morally concerned veterinarian cannot do many such treatments without pay. What does one do?

Many of the considerations relevant to the indigent owner clearly apply here. But there are some new aspects worthy of note. Once again, the key to resolving the problem lies in the veterinarian's personal ethic. If one holds a Garage Mechanic view, the choice is simple—euthanize the animal. But if one leads toward the Pediatrician Model, the old difficulties arise.

One of my veterinarian colleagues has found a very solomonic solution to such cases. Unlike most veterinarians, he welcomes these situations. He first of all sees them as "continuing education from God," helpful in sharpening his clinical skills. Secondly, he has a unique agreement with the local newspaper. When such an animal is brought in, he photographically documents the animal's condition. He then proceeds to treat the animal to the full extent of his ability. When the animal returns to normalcy, he takes a new set of photographs. He then presents both sets of photos to the newspaper. The paper devotes a page to the "before" and "after" and offers the public the chance to adopt the animal if the owner does not claim the animal. In some cases, grateful new owners will pay my colleague. Even if this does not happen, my veterinarian friend argues that he has acquired, relatively cheaply, priceless publicity and advertising that he could not have bought for any amount of money!

Another option is for the local humane society to develop a fund covering unowned injured animals. Such funding drives are often quite successful, and in some areas come close to covering all the requisite expenses. Finally, some fortunate veterinarians have their own funding from rich clients precisely earmarked to cover such situations. In my view, it is not unethical, but rather, laudable for a veterinarian to solicit such funding and thereby perform a public service that furthers the social plausibility of the Pediatrician Model.

In sum, then, as long as society is in flux regarding the social ethic for animals, the ethical issues in critical care medicine will be solved by reference to reasonable implications from extant social ethics, collective professional ethical decisions, and the veterinarian's personal ethic. In the latter case, I would suggest that what we have called the Pediatrician Model can well serve as a practical moral beacon.

REFERENCES

1. Rollin BE: The Unheeded Cry: Animal Consciousness, Animal Pain and Science (expanded version). Ames, IA: Iowa State University Press, 1998.
2. Rollin BE: Pain and ideology in human and veterinary medicine. *Semin Vet Med Surg Small Anim* 12:55, 1997.
3. Rollin BE: Some conceptual and ethical concerns about current views of pain. *Pain Forum* 8:78, 1999.
4. Ferrell BR, Rhiner M: High-tech comfort: ethical issues in cancer pain management for the 1990's. *J Clin Ethics* 2:108, 1991.
5. Rollin BE: Animal Rights and Human Morality, 2nd ed. Buffalo, NY: Prometheus Books. 1992.
6. Rollin BE: Farm Animal Welfare. Ames, IA: Iowa State University Press, 1995.
7. Animal Rights and Human Morality.
8. Rollin BE: The ethics of pain control in companion animals. *In* Hellebrekers LS, ed.: Animal Pain. Utrecht: Van Der Wees, 2000, chap 2.
9. Rollin BE: Euthanasia and moral stress. *In* DeBellis R, ed.: Loss, Grief and Care. Binghamton, NY: Haworth Press, 1986, p 115.
10. Rollin BE: Veterinary Ethics: Theory and Cases. Ames, IA: Iowa State University Press, 2000.
11. McMillen F: Comfort as the primary goal in veterinary medicine. *J Am Vet Med Assoc* 212:1370, 1998.
12. Kitchell R, Guinan M: The nature of pain in animals. *In* Rollin B, Kesel M, eds.: The Experimental Animal in Biomedical Research, vol I. Boca Raton, FL: CRC Press, chap 12.

88
Advanced Directives and Do-Not-Resuscitate Orders

Charlotte A. Lacroix and Deidre Noling

INTRODUCTION

The sweat rolled down her forehead as she manually massaged "Jake's" heart. Dr. Criticare had not wanted to crack "Jake's" 15-year-old chest, but, felt she had no other choice since the hospital staff had been unsuccessful in contacting "Jake's" owner. This had been "Jake's" third run-in with an automobile since he had been a young dog. He just could not get enough of those tires. Despite "Jake's" grave prognosis and apparent pain, Dr. Criticare proceeded with her CPR efforts even though "Jake" was not likely to recover from this latest confrontation with a bumper.

Advanced directives and do-not-resuscitate (DNR) orders are two forms of directives that guide human health care providers as to the type and extent of medical care that should be provided to patients. Although rarely used in the veterinary clinical setting, such directives would allow pet owners to specify the type of medical care, if any, that should be provided to their pets in the event of an accident or life-threatening condition. Additionally, the use of directives would relieve some of the burdens experienced by veterinarians faced with making difficult decisions as how to proceed with the care of patients when there are no clear instructions from clients who are unavailable to make decisions.

Having owners consider the use of directives before the onset of an emergency allows more time to for them to think about the ethical, emotional, and financial ramifications associated with the consequences of their decisions. This is especially the case for owners who have a strong relationship with their pets, because they are likely to have the most difficulty grappling with these complex issues and making an informed decision as to what is the most appropriate course of medical treatment. Veterinarians who initiate discussions addressing the use of advanced directives can get owners to think about their pets' health, which ensures against impulsive and emotionally charged decisions that may not be in the best interests of the pets or owners.

The authors are not aware of any laws addressing the use of directives for veterinary practitioners, but, most states do have laws, known as right to die statutes, that set forth the scope and procedural requirements that apply to these directives in the human context. Although these laws do not regulate the veterinary community's use of advanced directives and DNRs, they could serve as guidelines for veterinarians who wish to use such directives and adopt hospital policies on their implementation.

The implementation of advanced directives and DNRs in the veterinary clinical setting is a daunting endeavor. Their use will require that veterinary practices adopt policies, draft forms, and train their veterinary and nonveterinary staff to discuss the numerous ethical issues associated with their use. Fortunately, the veterinary community does not need to "reinvent the wheel" but can look to the human medical field for guidance. Advanced directives and DNRs are commonly used in human hospitals, which have policies and forms that can be modified and tailored for use in veterinary hospitals.

WHAT IS AN ADVANCED DIRECTIVE?

Advanced directives used in the human medical field are instructions written by patients, usually long before they have become ill, that list the types of medical interventions that patients wish to receive in the event they lose their mental capacity to make decisions pertaining to their care. Individuals are usually prompted to consider these documents as part of their estate planning and the drafting of their wills. Laws about advanced directives vary from state to state, but, usually recognize two forms of advanced directives: the living will and the durable power of attorney for health care.

Advanced directives do not have the same implications in the veterinary setting, because it is the owners and not the pet patients that make decisions pertaining to the management of a pet's medical condition. However, they do have their place in assisting veterinarians in carrying out the wishes of their clients as it relates to the care of terminally ill pets. Owners who anticipate being unavailable to make medical decisions for their pets, either because of travel plans or their own illness, could use these directives to give themselves the peace of mind that their wishes will be carried out.

The Living Will

The advance directive known as a living will is a written document wherein patients specify in advance of a terminal illness or serious accident, the type of medical care they wish to receive should they lose their ability to make medically related decisions. Living wills allow physicians to manage their patients' medical conditions in accordance with their patients' wishes as opposed to leaving these very personal decisions to individual doctors, hospital ethics boards, or courts. Used by pet owners, living wills would provide veterinarians with guidance as to the appropriate medical interventions to pursue and, thus, eliminate the guessing games practitioners endure trying to "read" the minds of their clients. An example that can be tailored to a specific veterinary practice is set forth in Table 88-1.

Durable Power of Attorney for Health Care

A durable power of attorney for health care allows individuals to appoint others to make medical decisions on their behalf when they are unable to do

Table 88-1. Sample Living Will

LIVING WILL

ADVANCE INSTRUCTION FOR HEALTH CARE OF (Insert Pet's Name)

Pet's Name: __________; Species: __________; Sex: __________

EFFECTIVE DATE:

I, the undersigned owner of the pet identified above, certify that I am over 18 years of age, and make this statement as a directive to be followed if, for any reason, I become unable to participate in the decisions regarding the medical care of my pet.

I direct that if in the opinion of the attending veterinarian, my pet's medical condition becomes such that:

1. My pet's medical condition is terminal and hopeless, or death is imminent; or
2. My pet is in a state of permanent unconsciousness; or
3. My pet is suffering and it would be inhumane to keep my pet alive; or
4. There is no reasonable expectation that my pet will recover and regain a meaningful quality of life; or
5. My pet is in the terminal stage of an irreversible fatal illness, disease or condition; then, I direct that further treatment by life sustaining procedures, methods and devices involving further therapeutic or emergency care be withheld and withdrawn. I further direct that all treatments be limited to comfort and pain management measures only, even if they shorten my pet's life.

The life-sustaining procedures, methods and devices, and therapeutic or emergency care that shall be withheld and withdrawn, include, without limitation: surgery, antibiotics, cardiopulmonary resuscitation, respiratory support or life-sustaining treatment, and artificially administered feeding and fluids.

I hereby release any veterinarian or hospital from any legal liability for honoring this directive, and declare that any such veterinarian or hospital is acting in accordance with my directions.

Being of sound mind, I voluntarily execute this order, and I fully understand it.

____________________________ ______________

Owner's Signature Date

____

Owner's PRINTED name

so. Because these agents are appointed to substitute in their judgments for that of the patients, they usually are spouses, children, or close family members or friends who know the patients well and, therefore, are likely to arrive at the same medical decisions as the patients. This delegation to another is not directly relevant in the veterinary context, because it is not the pets but rather the owners who control the medical care delivered. Nonetheless, owners could delegate their rights to make such decisions to others whom they feel could make the appropriate decisions for their pets.

In the human context, if there is a dispute as to whether an agent's medical decision should be carried out, a court or governmental body may review the substituted decision to ensure that it is in fact in the best interests of the patient.

Such judicial or governmental scrutiny is unlikely to occur in the context of pets in the near future, because animals are still considered to be property and, as such, have no protectable rights. The only exception to this rule would be if the medical decision was considered to lead to cruel and inhumane treatment.

Table 88-2 presents an example of a medical power of attorney.

WHAT IS A DO-NOT-RESUSCITATE ORDER?

Do-not-resuscitate orders or DNRs instruct health care providers not to perform cardiopulmonary resuscitation or any other life-sustaining techniques to prolong a patient's life. Whereas advanced directives are written by patients, usually before they become ill, DNRs are directives issued by attending physicians after certain criteria have been met. Typically, before physicians will issue DNRs, patients must be terminally ill or afflicted with medical conditions for which resuscitation would be unsuccessful or harmful to the patient. Resuscitation ordinarily includes the full range of cardiopulmonary resuscitation techniques, including (1) establishing and maintaining an airway, (2) cardiac compression, (3) defibrillation, and (4) administrating cardiovascular medications. Unsuccessful resuscitations are those that are unlikely to be effective or, if effective, make it probable that the patient's medical condition will result in another cardiopulmonary failure shortly thereafter. In determining whether a resuscitation would be harmful, physicians, patients, and family members weigh the pain and suffering experienced by the patient with the likelihood that the resuscitation would be successful and lasting.

Before a DNR can be issued, attending clinicians must first have received consents not to resuscitate pets from their clients or clients' agents, and such consent must be noted in the medical record if no separate form is available. The consent must be informed, which means that the client has been apprised of (1) the reasons for the DNR and its consequences, (2) which treatments will be withheld, and (3) the availability of alternatives and their consequences. Additionally, clients should have had opportunities to ask questions and have been offered opportunities to seek second opinions.

As with advanced directives, the basis for using DNRs is to ensure that patients' wishes are honored and that their lives are not unnecessarily and painfully prolonged. Pet owners may wish to exercise similar prerogatives for their pets and those veterinary hospitals that provide clients with DNRs will not only provide clients with opportunities to become more involved in the critical health care decisions of their pets, but also, reduce the incidence of misunderstandings from mismatched expectations. More importantly, the use of DNRs will encourage owners to become actively involved and therefore assume responsibility for the difficult medical decisions they make on behalf of their pets.

A DNR is not lengthy nor complicated document, but it should contain at a minimum, the name of the pet, names and signatures of the veterinarian and client or client's agent, the words "Do Not Resuscitate" prominently displayed, and the effective date of the DNR (Table 88-3).

Table 88-2. Sample Medical Power of Attorney

MEDICAL POWER OF ATTORNEY

I, the undersigned owner, of *(Insert Pet's Name),* a *(Insert Age) (Insert Species and Breed),* certify that I am over 18 years of age, and appoint:

Name: ______________________________

Address: ______________________________

Phone: ______________________________

Fax: ______________________________

as my agent to make any and all health care decisions for my pet, except to the extent I state otherwise in this document. My agent shall follow my wishes as known to him or her either through this document or through other means. If my agent cannot determine the choice I would want for my pet, then my agent's decision shall be based on what he or she believes to be in my pet's best interest. This medical power of attorney takes effect if I become unable to make health care decisions for my pet and this fact is certified in writing.

The following sets forth limitations on the decision-making authority of my agent:

(Suggested limitations)

a. Agent's decisions must be made in accordance with the living will directive for my pet, executed on *(insert date).*

b. I agree to pay for all authorized services, as long as the costs for my pet's medical care does not exceed $

c. No limitations shall be imposed on my agent.

I understand that this power of attorney revokes any prior medical power of appointment and shall exist indefinitely from the date I execute this document unless I establish a shorter time or revoke the power of attorney. If I am unable to make health care decisions for my pet and this power of attorney expires, the authority I have granted to my agent shall continue to exist until the time I again am able to make health care decisions for pet.

(IF APPLICABLE) This power of attorney ends on the following date:

If the person designated as my agent is unable or unwilling to make health care decisions for my pet, I designate the following alternative person to serve as my agent to make health care decisions for my pet as authorized by this document.

Name: ______________________________

Address: ______________________________

Phone: ______________________________

I sign my name to this medical power of attorney on the ____ day of *(Insert month and yr)*

____

Owner's Signature

____

Owner's PRINTED name

Table 88-3. Sample Do-Not-Resuscitate Order

DO-NOT-RESUSCITATE ORDER

Pet's Name: ________; Species: ________; Sex: ________

EFFECTIVE DATE:

- I, the undersigned owner, or owner's agent, of the pet identified above, certify that I am over 18 years of age, and have been informed of the critical nature of my pet's medical condition.
- I hereby request that in the event my pet's heart and/or breathing should stop, **NO PERSON SHALL ATTEMPT TO RESUSCITATE MY PET.**
- This request is being given after *(Insert Name of Attending Veterinarian)* has discussed with me my pet's medical condition and the consequences of this order **NOT TO RESUSCITATE.**
- This order is effective on the date set forth above until it is revoked by me.

Being of sound mind, I voluntarily execute this order, and I fully understand it.

______________________________	______________
Owner's or Agent's Signature	Date
Owner's or Agents PRINTED name	
Veterinarian's Signature	Date
Veterinarian's PRINTED name	
Witness for Telephone Authorizations	Date
Witness' PRINTED name	

HOSPITAL POLICIES

Veterinarians who wish to use advanced directives and DNRs in their hospitals should concurrently adopt hospital policies that inform clients of their options to accept or refuse medical treatments for their pets and instruct hospital personnel on how to use such directives. An example of such a policy is displayed in Table 88-4.

ETHICAL CONSIDERATIONS IN THE USE OF DIRECTIVES

The use of advanced directives in the human medical field has evolved only after considerable discussion as to their ethical ramifications. The veterinary profession will be faced with different ethical issues than physicians, however, because animals are characterized as property under the law and there is neither recognition nor protection of their individual rights. The closest similarity in the human context is the medical management of critically ill patients who are mentally incompetent, which often includes minors, mentally handicapped

Table 88-4. Policy Guidelines

("Insert Hospital Name") Policy Pertaining to the Use of Advanced Directives and Do-Not-Resuscitate Orders (DNRs)

("Insert Hospital Name") has adopted the following policy pertaining to the use of advance directives and DNRs, to ensure that the medical decisions made on behalf of our clients' pets reflect owners' wishes, which have been clearly communicated to the hospital staff. Such directives shall be used only after clients have been fully informed of the medical condition of their pets and consequences of their decisions. These decisions should reflect a clear commitment to serve the needs and best interests of the patients and be made only after careful consideration by clients and attending veterinarians. The following guidelines have been developed to provide pet owners, veterinarians and hospital staff, with support and guidance in making decisions to withhold or withdraw life-sustaining treatments from our patients.

POLICY GUIDELINES

Definitions

- Advanced directives are documents by which clients provide instructions to their veterinarians as to the type and extent of health care that should be provided to their pets if they are not available to make decisions at the time such choices are medically required. There are two types of advanced directives, living wills and medical powers of attorney. Living wills guide veterinarians as to what types, if any, of life-sustaining treatments should be provided to terminally or critically ill pets. A medical power of attorney permits clients to appoint persons to make medical treatment decisions for their pets. If a living will has been completed for a pet, the appointee's decisions would be guided by that document.
- A DNR is provided by the veterinarian and requires the client's consent and signature. It serves to notify all attending medical personnel that no one is to use cardiopulmonary resuscitation to revive a patient, if the pet stops breathing or experiences cardiac arrest.

Procedure

- For pets that are admitted as critical care patients, terminally ill patients or are likely to require advanced directives and or DNRs, clients will be asked at each admission whether they have such documents. If so, copies of each will be placed in patients' medical records.
- For clients that have no directives for their pets, attending veterinarians and support staff may discuss the use of such directives if clients make a request or, if in the opinion of the veterinarians, such discussion is warranted based on the medical conditions of the patients.
- All discussions pertaining to directives and life-sustaining treatment must be recorded in the pets' medical records.
- If clients wish to sign a DNR, veterinarians and or support staff must indicate to the clients or agents, which medical treatments will be withheld and explain the rationale for such decisions. If a DNR is issued and signed, clients should be informed that even though certain treatments be withheld, other treatments will be provided to ensure their pets' comfort and relief from pain.
- If a pet suffers cardiac or respiratory arrest, cardiopulmonary resuscitation will be initiated unless a DNR order has been written and signed by a veterinarian and the client and put in the pet's medical record. Owners will be charged for resuscitation services in accordance with the hospital's fee schedule.
- Veterinarians and staff members who are unable to follow through with a client's directive must transfer the care of the patient to another veterinarian and or staff member, who will honor the client's wishes.

Table 88-4. Continued

Client Considerations
• Determining the specifics of advance directives for pets that are regarded as family members is difficult. Although owners cannot anticipate all the different medical decisions with which they may be faced, they should consider their treatment goals.
• Owners may wish to examine their attitudes toward the possible death of their pets and under what circumstances they would consent to a DNR.
• Some useful questions owners may wish to consider include, 1. Could you provide supportive care to a pet that was incontinent, partially or completely paralyzed, needed multiple medications per day, or had a condition that altered its behavior? 2. How active and healthy is your pet currently? How old is your pet? Has your pet lived most of its adult life? Would age and activity level play a role in your decision-making process? 3. Do religious beliefs or finances play a role in decisions about your pet's health care? 4. What role should other family members and your veterinarian play in your decisions? 5. How does your pet's quality of life effect your decision? What are your expectations? Some clients consider pets afflicted with blindness or that have an amputated leg, as unacceptable handicaps. At what point would you consider euthanasia or a DNR?

individuals, and elderly people who are no longer able make their own decisions. In such situations, many state courts recognize that family members, and not the doctors nor government officials, are best qualified to make substituted decisions for incompetent patients. Nonetheless, family members' decisions have been scrutinized by judges when the decisions were inconsistent with patients' interests or if there was evidence that they were contrary to the patients wishes.

Although no one can be sure of pets' wishes as it pertains to their care, a presumption that owners are best qualified to make such decisions is reasonable and, in fact, has been the standard followed by most veterinary practitioners. It becomes complicated, and the moral, ethical, and legal ramifications are not clear, when veterinarians and their staff substitute judgments that differ from those of their clients. One can speculate, however, that veterinarians who fail to honor directives that withhold medical treatment may subject themselves to lawsuits and risk being held accountable for damages. This would likely include the cost of all medical care that was provided subsequent to the veterinarian's decision to keep the pet alive.

CONCLUSION

The use of advanced directives and DNRs are not commonly used within the veterinary profession. Yet as the human-animal bond grows and the profession continues to improve its ability to extend the lives of its patients through advancements in technology, pharmacology, and medical and surgical techniques, there will be an increased need and demand for such directives. Directives from owners will encourage owners to consider the difficult decisions that arise in caring for critically or terminally ill pets and encourage them to consider their options when they are not under the stress and pressures of emotionally charged situations.

Additionally, the use of such directives will provide clearer guidance for veterinarians as to whether they should provide medical and or surgical support and, if so, to what extent. Because many of the issues that arise in drafting, interpreting, and carrying out directives are similar to those in the human medical professions, the forms and policies used in human hospitals can be useful starting points for veterinary hospitals. As to the moral, ethical, and legal issues that will surface from the use of such directives, only time will tell.

89
Disaster Preparedness, Response, and Triage

Wayne E. Wingfield and Lorna Lanman

"Chance favors only the prepared mind."
Louis Pasteur

INTRODUCTION

Throughout history disasters have exacted a heavy toll of death and suffering. In the past 20 years over 20 million humans have died worldwide and property damage easily exceeds $50 billion. To date, the United States has only experienced one truly massive disaster with thousands of deaths of humans; frequently, disasters in this country have easily affected millions of poultry, swine, and fish. When urban populations are struck by a disaster, many of the victims are animal owners because 56% of the households in the United States now have pets. In the past, the first priority of disaster relief was to protect and save human life. With the widespread emphasis on the human-animal bond, disaster agencies are now being called on to deal with more complicated animal-related issues.

Many factors point toward an increasing probability of mass casualty incidents. Among these factors are the increasing population in flood plains, seismic zones, ocean or lakeside housing developments, the transport of hazardous materials, the risks of chemical or nuclear facility mishaps, catastrophic fires and explosions, terrorism, and weapons of mass destruction, including animal disease agents as weapons.

The role of veterinarians in disaster preparedness is increasing and they are considered a first responder professional. Unfortunately, most veterinarians do not have minimal training, planning, or management skills related to disaster medicine. Veterinarians need to understand the components of disaster preparedness to integrate themselves with the official aspects of disaster management at the local, state, national, and even international levels. Our profession needs to assume a primary role in the veterinary medical aspects of disaster planning, management, triage, and patient care. This will only come with involvement and additional training. In the event of a true disaster, having only a few veterinarians and their hospitals trained are insufficient to provide assistance to a disaster preparedness program. A commitment of all the veterinarians in a community, state, region, and nation is absolutely necessary. The effects of any disaster can be minimized and or avoided by applying effective preventative strategies.

NATURE OF DISASTERS

There is no standard definition of "disaster." Traditionally, the term disaster is used to describe large-scale incidents that overwhelm the resources of the affected community. Because disaster medicine is multidisciplinary and depends on the integration of multiple levels of responders, the use of more concise definitions is essential. More frequently in the United States, the term "emergency" should be used to describe incidents that can be handled with existing community resources. It is certainly possible for an emergency to quickly overwhelm the local resources, especially in a small, rural community. This is less likely in larger metropolitan areas, provided an organized disaster plan is in place to guide the veterinary professionals responding to the incident. Thus, it seems it is more a functional impact on a specific area that is the key to determining whether an emergency exists or a true disaster occurs.

When disasters strike, destruction, injuries, and death occur. The impact varies widely according to the degree of warning given, the suddenness of onset, and animal density (*e.g.*, feed lots, confinement houses, etc.). The effects of any disaster can be minimized and or avoided by applying effective preventative strategies. The existence of county and community preparedness plans greatly increases the self-reliance and effectiveness of assistance, contributing to the decrease of disaster related mortality and morbidity.

The first order of business is to conduct vulnerability studies of each community or county, mapping specific locations of potential disasters and pinpointing potential associated risks; thus, each community or county knows the location of all animals potentially in harm's way. Inventorying existing resources to facilitate the rapid mobilization of all available resources during the emergency follows. Included is an up-to- date list of all trucks, trailers, and boats available to evacuate large animals; kennels, shelters, and fairgrounds for housing animals; and warehouses for storing food. Also, critical to any effective disaster response is the type of support expected from of ancillary agencies, such as police and fire departments, poison control, hazardous material responders, animal control, and search and rescue. The effects of man-made and natural disasters can be foreseen and contained; however, implementation of these appropriate preventative preparedness and mitigation measures are mandatory.

The next important portion of the disaster plan is putting the plan into action by training all parties involved. No recommendation will be effective without support of volunteer training and personnel management

Weapons of Mass Destruction (WMD)

No discussion on disaster medicine should exclude the topic of animal issues involved in WMD. Since the end of World War II, our nation has thought of WMD mainly as nuclear bombs, resulting in the establishment of the old Civil

Defense shelters, which included supplies for human field hospitals. In recent years, WMD that are a threat to our nation include biologic and chemical warfare in addition to nuclear radiation. All of these are potentially capable of creating a disaster involving humans and animals. As veterinarians, we must be educated in recognizing these diseases and conditions, and the appropriate treatment and decontamination of these potentially affected animals. More importantly, we must remember to protect our staff, the hospital, and ourselves when presented with these problems.

After the World Trade Center bombings in New York City in 1993 and 2001, our country realized that terrorism was no longer just a problem outside our borders, and we began to prepare for a myriad of forms of weapons of mass destruction causing mass casualties within our borders. Many terrorists are capable of obtaining nuclear warheads, but more likely they will resort to cheaper forms of WMD, such as biologic and chemical agents. We must plan for the inclusion of animals in these kinds of disasters and the following discussion will contain many of the WMD involving animals as well as humans.

Biologic Agents as WMD

Biologic warfare can be defined as the use of microorganisms or toxins derived from living organisms to induce death or disease in humans, animals, or plants. Animal disease agents have long been used as biologic warfare agents.[1] As far back as the 14th century, armies catapulted plague-infected corpses over their enemy's city walls.[2] Even as recently as 1984, members of a cult spread *Salmonella* over salad bars of four restaurants in Oregon causing illness in 700 people, all to influence an election. Most bacterial infections can be treated with antibiotics, assuming the offending organism is identified early enough and there are enough drugs on hand.

Animals may become sentinels in the event of a bioterrorism incident and veterinarians may be the first to diagnose. Economic targets such as livestock, crops, tourism, and transportation are likely to become terrorist choices. Even small outbreaks of exotic disease in livestock or crops could remove the United States from the large world market of agricultural products, which we have enjoyed for so long. Table 89-1 summarizes some of the agents likely to be involved in a biologic terrorist attack.

Chemical Agents as WMD

The attitude of many health care professionals has been that chemicals used as WMD have an outcome that is disastrous, defense is impossible, and that casualty and death rate will be high. In reality, chemical casualties can be saved and mortality can be minimized. The historical use of chemical warfare is well documented in the literature. These agents are usually grouped as nerve agents, vesicants, cyanide, pulmonary agents, riot control agents, and incapacitating agents (see Table 89-1). Nerve agents are the most toxic of the known chemical agents. They are hazards in their liquid and vapor states and can cause death within minutes after exposure. Most inhibit acetylcholinesterase in tissues and their effects are caused by the resulting excess acetylcholine.[3]

The effects of a vapor exposure maximize within 15 minutes, so by the time the animal is presented to your hospital, the symptoms will likely be at a peak or waning. With skin exposure, the effects may progress for hours after onset, or after decontamination, due to the absorption of the agent into the outer skin layers.

Most veterinarians are experienced in diagnosing and treating animals for organophosphate toxicity, and the clinical signs are similar: generalized fasciculations and twitching, miosis, and increased salivation. Medical management of the nerve agent intoxication consists, also, of a similar protocol: decontamination, ventilation, administration of the antidotes, and supportive therapy. The condition of the patient always dictates the need for each of these and the order in which they are given.

Vesicants, such as "mustard gas," have been used in wartime since World War I. Lewisite was also produced during World War I, although never used.[3] These products cause erythema (which looks like a sunburn), vesicles or blisters on the skin, and severe damage to the eyes, airways, gastrointestinal (GI) tract, and bone marrow stem cell suppression. Phosgene (CG) is also classified as a vesicant, but is a corrosive pulmonary agent. The nitrogen mustards (HN_1, HN_2, HN_3) are by far the most commonly available. Management of animals exposed to mustard is by immediate decontamination and symptomatic treatment of the lesions. This includes systemic analgesics for pain control, topical mydriatics and ophthalmic antibiotic ointments, soothing lotions and irrigation of the blistered areas, ventilation support, systemic fluids, antibiotics, bronchodilators, cough suppressants if needed, and antiemetics to control vomiting. Death usually results from pulmonary damage, pseudomembrane formation in the airways causing obstruction, and sepsis. The complicating issue with mustard, as opposed to lewisite and phosgene, is that it does not burn the skin and eyes initially, so decontamination is delayed, thus the effects are compounded the longer the substance stays on the skin and in the lungs.

Cyanide has been used in wartime, but due to its high volatility, it evaporates too quickly to kill large numbers of animals. With prolonged exposure, death results within minutes from seizures, respiratory, and cardiac arrest. The patient will elicit the odor of almonds. Because cyanide is attracted to methemoglobin, management is geared to neutralizing the cyanomethemoglobin molecules that are formed.[4]

Animals Exposed to Radiation[5]

Not only should we be aware of the effects of radiation from a terrorist attack, but also from accidents involving nuclear power plants, nuclear medicine equipment in hospitals, and accidents involving transportation of nuclear waste. Serious radiation events, in the last 10 years, involving human deaths have been rare; only five incidents have required disaster responses either by national and regional agencies and where outside medical resources were used in the response.

Table 89-1. Types of Agents Likely to be Used as Weapons of Mass Destruction

Type of Agent	Effects	Onset Time	Skin Decontamination	Immediate Care
Nerve GA (Tabun) GB (Sarin) GD (Soman) GF VX	VAPOR: Mild: small pupils, runny nose, muscle fasciculations, convulsions, apnea LIQUID: Fasciculation, sweating at site, GI effects, convulsions, apnea	VAPOR: seconds to minutes LIQUID: minutes to 18 h	0.5% bleach water	Atropine, pralidoxime, ventilation, diphenhydramine HCl, diazepam
Vesicants H (Sulfur mustard) HD (Sulfur mustard) L (Lewisite)	Erythema, blisters, irritation of the eyes, cough, respiratory distress	Hours, except immediate pain after contact with lewisite	0.5% bleach water	Immediate decontamination
Cyanide AC (Hydrocyanic acid or hydrogen cyanide) CK (Cyanogen chloride)	Loss of consciousness, convulsions, apnea	Seconds	None usually needed	Amyl nitrite, sodium nitrite, sodium thiosufite, ventilation
Pulmonary CG (Carbonyl chloride) PFIB (Perfluroisobutylene) HC (Smoke)	Respiratory distress, coughing	Hours	None usually needed	None, complete rest

Agent	Species	Symptoms	Treatment	Dosages
Anthrax (*Bacillus antracis*)	Humans	Nonproductive cough, acute gastroenteritis, small papule ulcers with black necrotic centers, edema	Ciprofloxacin	500 mg PO BID X 4 wk
			Doxicycline	100 mg PO BID X 4 wk
			Penicillin	2 million units IV q 2 h for penicillin-sensitive organisms
			Alternate drugs: Clindamycin, erythromycin, chloramphenicol	
	Dogs and cats	Lesions of face, mouth, and tongue, swelling of lips, head, and throat, severe gastroenteritis	Doxicycline	5 mg/kg IV followed by 5 mg/kg PO bid
			Ciprofloxacin	5–15 mg/kg bid
			Penicillin G	20,000 IU/kg IV, IM, or SQ q 4 h or 40,000 IU/kg PO q 6 h
	Horses	Colic, enteritis, respiratory distress, subcutaneous swelling on ventral neck, thorax, and abdomen, death in 2-4 days.	Penicillin G	25–50,000 IU/kg IV or IM q 6–12 h
	Cattle and sheep	Pyrexia, anorexia, bloody diarrhea, hematuria, stimulation and aggression followed by depression, tremors, respiratory distress, convulsions, edema of the ventral neck and thorax	Penicillin	40–60,000 IU/kg IM or SQ q 24 h

Table 89-1. Continued

Agent	Species	Symptoms	Treatment	Dosages
Plague (*Yersinia pestis*)	Humans	Bubonic: Flulike symptoms, cutaneous findings, buboes.	Streptomycin	30 mg/kg daily IM in divided dosages X 10 d
			Doxycycline	100 mg PO q12 h X 7 d
		Pneumonic: Rapidly fatal, bloody sputum, pyrexia lymphadenopathy	Chloramphenicol	1 g IV q 6 h
	Dogs and cats	Pyrexia, respiratory disease, suppuration of cervical lymph nodes	Doxycycline	5 mg/kg PO or IV followed by 5 mg/kg PO q 12 h
Tularemia (*Franciella tularensis*)	Humans	Pyrexia, chills, headache, non-productive cough, regional lymph nodes affected	Streptomycin	1 gm IM q 12 h X 10-14 d
			Gentamycin	3–5 mg/kg/d X 10-14 d
			Doxicycline	100 mg PO q 12 h X 14 d
			Alternative: Tetracycline	
	Dogs and cats	Pyrexia, depression, anorexia, icterus, pneumonitis, generalized lymphadenopathy, abscess formation in the liver or spleen	Doxicycline	5 mg/kg PO q 12 h
			Tetracycline	15 mg/kg PO q 8 h
			Gentamycin	2.2–4 mg/kg IV or IM q 8 h
	Horses	Acute septicemia with localization, especially in spleen and liver. Fever, anorexia, depression, cough, diarrhea, stiffness, and edema of limbs.	Gentamycin	1–4 mg/kg IM q 8–12 h
			Tetracycline	7.5 mg/kg IV q 12 h

	Sheep	Most commonly affected livestock species; acute septicemia, spleen and liver involvement, pyrexia, anorexia, depression, diarrhea, stiffness, edema of limbs, cough	Gentamycin	2.2 mg/kg IM q 12 h
Q Fever (*Coxiella burnetii*)	Humans	Tetracycline		500 mg PO q 6h X 5–7 d
		Doxicycline		100 mg PO q 12 h X 5–7 d
	Dogs and cats	Dogs: Encephalitis	Tetracycline	22 mg/kg PO q 8 h
		Cats: Subclinical fever, anorexia	Doxicycline	5 mg/kg PO q 12 h
	Sheep, goats, ruminants	Causes abortion, most infectious are asymptomatic		
VEE	Humans		Supportive therapy	Analgesics
				Anticonvulsants
	Horses	Prolonged fever, cerebral signs 4 d following infection, hyperesthesia, aggression, excitability, continuous chewing movements	Supportive therapy	Control seizures with phenobarbital sodium or diazepam

Transportation and radiation accidents are of great concern, but have historically had the one of the best safety records. Thus, we have become very complacent in our preparedness for these types of emergencies.

Understanding the type of radiation and their interactions will aid the veterinarian if presented with an animal exposed to radiation. There are three types of radiation exposure: external contamination, internal contamination, and irradiation. The form of radiation determines the type of exposure.[6] These forms of radiation include alpha particles, which are dense helium nuclei stripped of their electrons. They have no penetrating power past the keratinized layer of skin. Beta particles are high-energy electrons emitted from unstable nuclei and have a penetrating power of a few centimeters of tissue. Both of these forms of exposure pose a risk of secondary contamination to the attending veterinarian and staff; therefore, universal precautions and decontamination should be instituted as soon as possible. X-rays and gamma rays are high-energy photons that are greatly attenuated only after thicknesses of lead. Patients exposed to these forms will be irradiated and do not pose a secondary contamination risk.[6]

Alpha sources have a shorter range and do not penetrate the skin, but are more toxic in cases of internal contamination. Beta particles on the skin result in burns to skin. Because most symptoms produced from radioactive exposure are delayed, treatments for trauma and other medical problems should be initiated immediately. Never forget the protocol of the ABCs. When triaging an animal that has be exposed to radiation, one should remember that rapidly dividing cells, which are poorly differentiated and have a long mitotic period, are very radiosensitive. These include cells in the red marrow, epithelial cells of the GI system and lung, epithelium of the lens, germinative cells of the testis and ovary, and endothelial cells of blood vessels. The lymphocyte is considered the most radiosensitive cell type in the body and thus becomes the most reliable and most rapid means of assessing the amount of exposure and degree of radiation injury.[5] Clinical signs in animals include vomiting, diarrhea, anorexia, fever, and lethargy. Burns on the skin are prevalent signs when exposed to beta particles.

Treatment of radiation exposure begins with decontamination, if the radiation is of the alpha or beta type. Tincture of green soap has been touted as the soap of choice to remove these types of radiation from the skin. Because of the risk of contamination of the individual who is decontaminating the animal, universal precautions should be followed. These should include the use of a waterproof hospital gown, cap, face shield, waterproof booties, and double gloves where the inner glove layer is taped snuggly around the wrists of the caregiver. Treatment of GI disorders is with antiemetics and antidiarrheals, intravenous fluids, and antibiotics. If surgery is indicated for treatment of any trauma condition, it should be done within the first 24 hours, as the toxicity levels from anesthetics and analgesics increase starting about 24 hours after radiation exposure. Also, the complicating factors from pancytopenia arise around 36 hours after exposure. Radiation burns should be treated as any other burn.

Primary decontamination of exposed patients whether radiation or chemical is best done immediately at the site of the incident. Animals may not be given priority in an event involving humans and animals, so owners or helpful individuals may transport the exposed animals to your hospital. A contaminated hospital is an essentially closed hospital. Always protect yourself and staff.

Blast Overpressure Injuries

Bombings in Oklahoma City and The World Trade Center have reminded our nation that injuries from blast overpressure are no longer limited only to the military battlefield or an embassy in a foreign country. Unfortunately, critical care veterinarians of today and tomorrow may be presented with animals effected by blast injuries.

Blast overpressure is the sharp, instantaneous rise in ambient atmospheric pressure (Friedlander wave) following detonation of munitions or occupational accidents involving explosives.[7] Blast injuries may be classified as primary, secondary, or tertiary. Primary blast injury may cause severe internal damage without any visible external signs of injury, causing most injuries to gas-containing organs. Secondary blast injuries occur when flying debris cause penetrating wounds, and tertiary injuries are a result of the animal being impaled against a stationary wall or object.

Solid organs are much less affected by primary blast overpressure than are gas- or fluid-filled organs. The inner ear is the most sensitive organ to being damaged and becomes a good diagnostic parameter for assessing the severity of the blast. Retinal detachments may occur as well as intraocular hemorrhage. Damage to the lungs and GI tract may not be apparent initially; however, damage may be so severe as to cause sudden death. Air embolism is believed to be responsible for most of the sudden deaths that occurs within the first hour after blast exposure, especially if the animal gets up and moves around. Severity of pathology is significantly enhanced by exercise. The lung damage consists of ruptured alveoli resulting in air escaping into the vascular system, alveolar hemorrhage, interstitial edema, and pneumothorax.

If the intestines have ruptured, free gas is seen on abdominal radiographs. Rest and inactivity are critical in the initial management of blast injuries. Supportive care for the respiratory system with ventilation and chest tubes should be initiated immediately. Maintenance of circulation is necessary as hypotension from blood loss may be a factor; however, the risk of overhydration and resultant pulmonary edema must be addressed. If surgery is necessary, injectable anesthetics are preferred over positive pressure anesthesia so as not to worsen the pulmonary barotrauma or possibility of air embolism.

CASUALTY TRIAGE AND MANAGEMENT

Little is written regarding pets caught in disasters. Most frequently it is volunteers and rescuers who recover dogs and cats following a large scale disaster.[8] In a unique study following the fire storms in Oakland, California, that occurred in 1991, several observations associated with dogs and cats caught in a large-scale disaster are reported.[9] In this study, cats are apparently less likely to be evacuated than dogs. This is likely due to the solitary nature of the cat and the more family-oriented behavior of dogs. Pets are also abandoned during a disaster. This is likely

Table 89-2. Suggested Database Items to be Included in a Disaster Hotline for Animals

Date and time of the call
Is this a lost pet or a found animal?
Date the animal was lost?
Person initiating this call.
Address and telephone number of the caller.
Association of the caller with the pet (veterinarian, shelter volunteer, rescuer, other)
Were other locations searched for the pet? (shelters, neighbors, veterinary hospitals)
Pet's profile (species, age [<1 y, adult, >10 y]), breed, sex, color and markings, and photograph.
Tattoo or electronic chip ID
Known injuries to the pet.
Date and resolution (reunited with owner, returned to owner's address, adopted, euthanatized)

due to the lifestyle change of the family, loss of property or family members, and motivational priorities associated with the disaster. In North Carolina, following hurricane Floyd, hundreds of pets were abandoned, because many people had no home in which to return. The suddenness of the impending disaster leading to the evacuation of residents, plus the economic status of some of involved communities involved contributed to the demise of many dogs and cats. Many residents did not evacuate with their pets in this disaster. In one county, the number of rescued animals that were spayed or neutered was less than 10%, reinforcing the findings of the study done in the Oakland fire storms, that people who take their animals regularly to a veterinarian usually will evacuate with their pets, and those owners who do not may often leave their pets behind.

The large animal issue in North Carolina was most devastating, with nearly 30,000 hogs drowned along with 2.9 million chickens and turkeys, 680 cattle, and a dozen horses. With few evacuation resources available, most of these livestock producers were left to attempt evacuation of their animals. One farmer reported tearing his porch from his house and ferrying 40 hogs at a time out of the flooded barn and thus saving about 40% of his animals. Not only were these farmers devastated by the economic impact but also by emotional stress of watching their animals perish.

Numerous reports from individuals searching for their lost pet experience a trauma similar to other victims. Experiences in the Oakland firestorm and the North Carolina floods show the importance of a disaster "hotline" dedicated to lost or found animals. This hotline should be locally based and staffed, have adequate number of phone lines, and have an organized, computerized, database ready when called on to react.[9] Consistency in the database should be of paramount importance. Table 89-2 lists proposed information to be collected by the hotline. The longer an owner waits to search for a pet, the lower the chance of being reunited. Interestingly, animals wearing a collar with the owner's name and address have a 10-fold increased likelihood of being reunited.[9] Few pets are reunited with their owners 4 weeks after a disaster.[9] In North Carolina, a hotline was established, which also included collection of donations of money, small animal foods, large animal feeds, and volunteer opportunities. The North Carolina State College of Veterinary Medicine established and supported a large shelter/hospital for all the rescued and abandoned pets. Many of the animals rescued in other counties were transferred to this facility, leaving behind a Polaroid picture and detailed description of the animal and where the animal was found. All animals were examined by a veterinarian, vaccinated, wormed, treated for any injuries or ailments, and microchipped. Two additional Polaroid pictures were taken for that animal's record. A vast fostering system was established throughout the affected part of the state.

Individual veterinary patient medical care is an important, but only a very small part, of disaster relief. This relief has been roughly divided into three phases: (1) emergency, (2) rehabilitation, (3) and reconstruction. The response needs of each of these phases vary greatly by disaster type, severity, and duration. For sudden-onset disasters such as terrorism, earthquakes, and tornadoes, the emergency phase has been described as the "Golden 24-Hours." When this emergency phase commences, action is necessary to save lives, which includes search and rescue, triage, emergency medical attention, communication and transportation networking, and evacuation. Because of time constraints, the local population and volunteers deliver the vast majority of relief efforts during this phase from local resources and from adjacent lesser-affected communities. During the rehabilitation phase, essential services such as food and water distribution, and primary veterinary health care are re-established. Also during rehabilitation, search and rescue efforts generally turn to body recovery. Medical care focuses on definitive treatments and routine veterinary services. The rehabilitation phase may last days to months, depending on the severity of the disaster.

In North Carolina, how to dispose of the large number of carcasses created a monumental problem. Most of the chickens and turkeys were composted, but the thousands of hog carcasses all had to be incinerated. With only wet fuel available and only two operational incinerators, the task was a long drawn-out procedure with huge piles of dead hogs lying next to farmer's homes for many days. The reconstruction phase may take months to years and involve the overall structural and economic recovery of the area and restoration of all services. North Carolina's plight of having so many homes destroyed by the tremendous amount of water initiated the enormous challenge of housing all the displaced families in hundreds of travel trailers for many months. Most of those people had no means to take care of an animal, thus most never attempted to find their pets. The estimated number of pets reunited with their owners was less than 2%.

Hurricane Andrew hit Florida in 1992 and devastated not only homes, but approximately 25 veterinary hospitals.[10] Thousands of animals were killed, injured, separated from their owners, or left to fend for themselves, and the veterinary infrastructure was destroyed. The military was deployed to establish order to the many volunteer groups who arrived to establish their own emergency units. This coordinated the needed attention to emergency animal care, veterinary public health issues, and animal control. The lack of an Emergency Animal Relief Disaster Plan being in place before both of these devastating storms created an enormous delay in the response and the recovery phase.

Veterinary disaster medicine should concentrate their disaster expertise on building local emergency-response capacity through research, training, and preparedness. Cooperation and input should be provided to city and state disaster plans and drills. Communication with local emergency management agencies and established disaster organizations such as the American Red Cross is mandatory.

The U.S. Public Health System provides Disaster Medical Assistance Teams (DMAT) for humans and Veterinary Medical Assistance Teams (VMAT) to states, on request, in the event of a federally declared disaster. There are 25 level one DMAT teams and four VMAT teams in the United States and both of these types of teams are prepared to leave within a few hours notice and are equipped to set up field hospitals. The VMAT teams, which are sponsored by the AVMA, are also equipped to be mobile and to respond to field emergencies of both large and small animals. The main mission of the VMAT is to help support the local and state veterinary infrastructure and respond to matters of public health importance, in addition to primary patient care. Local organization of disaster response teams will serve the emergency phase best; however, when local and state resources are overwhelmed, the state can and should ask for federal assistance. With this in mind, this discussion will now focus on identification and triage of ill or injured animals.

THE VETERINARY DISASTER RESPONSE MODEL

Providing immediate veterinary care in disasters can be modeled after its human counterpart.[11] The operations plan of the medical (veterinary) disaster-response model organizes surviving veterinarians into teams capable of delivering immediate care after a disaster. The goal of these teams is to recognize the seriousness of injuries, stabilize the patient, and arrange for transport to intact shelters, kennels, or veterinary hospitals. The plan is divided into three phases according to the time elapsed since the initial disaster: hour 0 to 1, solo treatment areas; hours 1 to 12, disaster-veterinary medical aid centers; and hours 12 to 72, casualty collection points.

Phase 1: Solo Treatment Areas

Immediately after a disaster, the veterinarian would assess their surroundings. If animals in critical condition are present, solo treatment locations are developed where animals could be evacuated and their physical condition normalized with resources from a mobile "crash" module. The contents of such a module are listed in Table 89-3. Development and maintenance of these modules would likely be the responsibility of the veterinarian. Victims of the disaster

Table 89-3. Proposed Contents of a Mobile Crash Module

Maintenance of Circulation	Airway Management	Orthopedic Management	Miscellaneous
Atropine sulfate	Endotracheal tubes	Ketamine	Sodium bicarbonate
Epinephrine (1:1000)	Laryngoscope	Bupivacaine	Dextrose (50%)
Furosemide	Ambu bag and nose cones	Lidocaine	Diazepam
IV catheters	Thoracic drains	Emergency surgery pack (knife handle, blades, hemostats, needle holder, carmalt forceps, thumb forceps, sterile 4X4 gauze sponges, towel clamps)	Diphenydramine
Heparinized saline	Heimlich valves	Roll cotton	Foley catheters
Intraosseous needles	Dexamethasone SP	Kling gauze	Insulin (regular)
0.9% sodium chloride		1″ and 2″ adhesive tape	Methylprednisolone
Hetastarch		Vetwrap	Nasogastric tube
Oxyglobin			Normosol
IV needles			Orogastric (stomach) tube
Infusion sets			Mineral oil
Blood transfusion sets			Green soap
			Euthanasia solution
			Analgesics (fentanyl, morphine)

would be triaged as quickly as possible to a site with additional supplies—the disaster aid medical center. Whether this is a field tent or a designated veterinary hospital facility should be decided prior to the disaster. In humans, the goal is to spend no more than an hour in a solo treatment area unless debris or number of affected patients impedes travel. In that case, additional assistance is requested. Communication during this phase is either through runners, CB radios, or possibly cellular telephones.

Phase 2. Disaster-Veterinary Medical Aid Centers

There will be competition for these centers from human casualties. Prior planning by veterinarians designates hospitals scattered throughout the area as disaster-veterinary medical aid centers. This designation must be made prior to the disaster to publicize their locations, prepare for staffing, and for conducting mock disaster drills in preparation for the real event. It is not unrealistic to expect some of these centers to be victims of the disaster. Thus, contingency plans must include backup centers located at or near the original. Additional triage is performed at these centers.

"Triage" is a French word that means *to sort* (and was originally used to describe the sorting of wool!). Early in the management of disasters, rescue personnel often use a *s*imple *t*riage *a*nd *r*apid *t*reatment (START) technique (Fig.

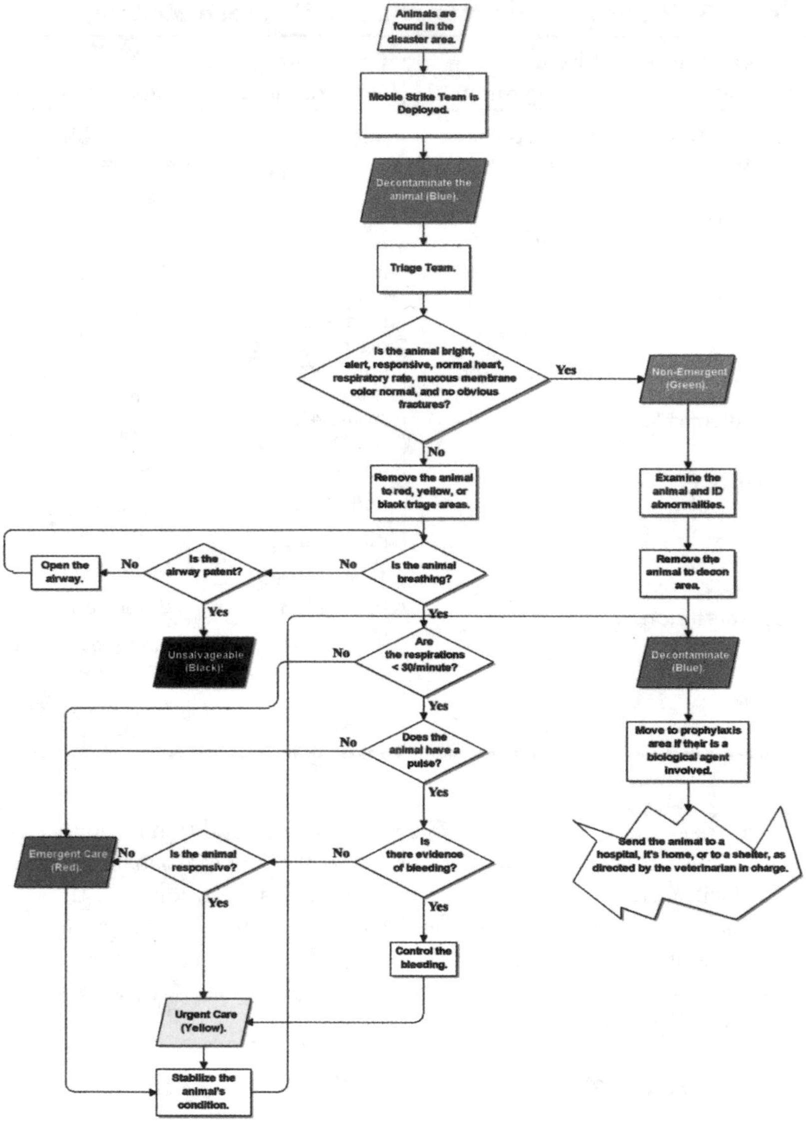

Figure 89-1
Simple triage and rapid transport (START). Animals that can walk are first identified and triaged to a "minor" category. The remaining animals are triaged using this algorithm.

89-1). In this approach one depends on a quick assessment of *r*espiration, *a*lertness, and *p*erfusion (RAP). If the animal can walk it is generally classified as a walking-wounded patient (priority III, nonurgent, "green" triage color) (Table 89-4 and Fig. 89-2). These animals are later reassessed after the more critical animals are triaged.

Table 89-4. Categories and Identification in Triage

Group	Color	Type of Injuries
Priority 1/Immediate	Red	Critical; may survive if simple lifesaving measures are applied.
Priority 2/Delayed	Yellow	Likely to survive if simple care is given within hours.
Priority 3/Nonurgent	Green	Minor injuries; care may be delayed while other patients receive treatment.
Priority 2 or 3*	Blue	Catastrophic: Patients unlikely to survive or those who need extensive care within minutes.
None (Dead or Dying)	**Black**	Dead or severely injured and not expected to survive.

* The blue category is often not used because it is difficult to triage accurately to this category. When used it is most likely for the benefit of the rescuer more than the animal. Many rescuers have difficulty placing live animals in the black category if they are still alive.

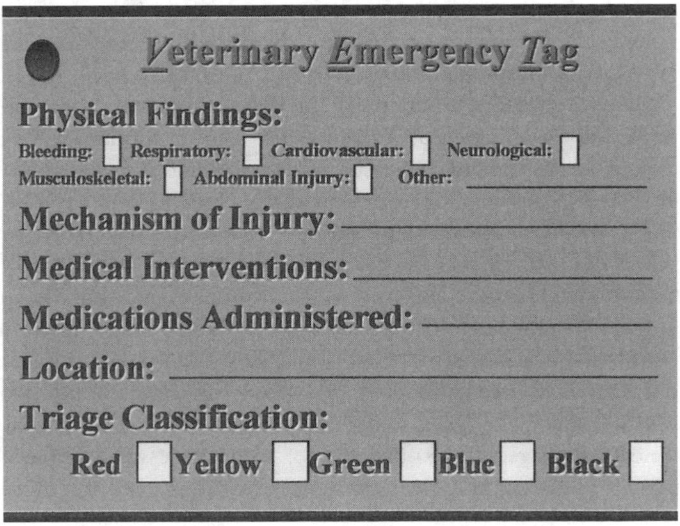

Veterinary Emergency Tag

Physical Findings:

Bleeding: ☐ Respiratory: ☐ Cardiovascular: ☐ Neurological: ☐
Musculoskeletal: ☐ Abdominal Injury: ☐ Other: ____________

Mechanism of Injury: ____________

Medical Interventions: ____________

Medications Administered: ____________

Location: ____________

Triage Classification:

Red ☐ Yellow ☐ Green ☐ Blue ☐ Black ☐

Figure 89-2
*V*eterinary *E*mergency *T*ag (VET) for color-coding triage victims.

Phase 3: Casualty Collection Points

In veterinary medicine, these sites likely would continue to be veterinary hospitals, kennels, or shelters. Uninjured, lost, less critical animals would ideally be moved to kennels and shelters after being entered into the uniform database and being tagged for identification (see below). As outsiders arrive at the disaster, they can be assigned to relieve veterinarians and volunteers in casualty collection facilities. Critical to these centers is the need for a mechanism for resupplying medical needs. This will be a difficult task if numerous human casualties exist.

TRIAGE DURING THE EMERGENCY PHASE

Figure 89-1 illustrates how a rescuer can move through a group of animals in a short period of time checking RAP. The animals are tagged into the triage categories (see Table 89-4). The only patient care interventions provided during early triage are the opening of the obstructed airway (extremely rare!) and direct pressure on obvious external hemorrhage. Hopefully the animal can then be transported with a color-coded triage tag, reassessed, and retriaged by the hospital staff at a disaster veterinary medical aid center and later at casualty collection points.

In veterinary disaster medicine, triage describes a medical decision-making process used to identify the most seriously affected body system in a sick or injured animal and then targets treatment to that body system. The goal of these aggressive medical efforts is to recognize, and then successfully treat, life-threatening emergencies.[12]

In disaster situations triage must be conducted with the purpose of doing the greatest good for the largest number of patients.[13] Rapid examination followed by classification of patients according to the urgency of their treatment needs is critical. Triage calls for an organized approach to multiple patients and ensures that the most critical animals are identified and normalized first. Triage in local disasters requires knowledge of available facilities and capacities immediately adjacent to the disaster as well as knowing this same information for facilities located just outside of the disaster area. Without doubt, conventional triage is only the first step in a dynamic decision-making process.

In human medicine, few articles address triage in disasters. In veterinary medicine, disaster medicine has concentrated on the many other facets of disaster preparedness and has also avoided a discussion of triage. Traditionally, in human medicine, triage systems have sorted victims into categories to determine their priority for treatment and transport. Varieties of colors, numbers, and symbols have been used to delineate triage categories based on degree of injury or illness (see Table 92-4 and Fig. 92-2). Triage is a learned skill. Placing patients in appropriate categories requires knowledge of injury assessment, anatomic and physiologic determinants, and clear awareness of the system, resources, equipment, and personnel available.

In veterinary medicine we are often faced with catastrophic casualty management (*e.g.*, poultry, swine, and fish) with large numbers of victims, severely limited medical resources, and poorly trained local rescue personnel. With these catastrophic casualties the animals remain at the scene for a protracted period of time and must be frequently reassessed. Triage is decentralized and often occurs at multiple sites in the disaster zone. To address these considerations, the *s*econdary *a*ssessment of *v*ictim *e*ndpoint (SAVE) system of triage is designed to identify animals most likely to benefit from the care available under austere conditions.

Care under the SAVE triage system is immediate and dynamic, rather than delayed and static. The methodology divides animals into three categories: (1)

those that will die regardless of how much care they receive; (2) those who survive whether or not they receive care; and (3) those who will benefit significantly from the austere interventions. Only those animals expected to improve receive more than basic care and comfort measures. In this way, resources can be focused appropriately. The decision to place an animal in a particular group is based largely on the experience of the triage team. This is because there is little to no information available regarding statistical probability of survival in veterinary patients. These are tough decisions but they must be made and adhered to. After the disaster resolves, the team can retrospectively examine decisions in hopes of improving performance at the next disaster.

TRIAGE SCENARIOS

Pre-existing Illness and Multiple Injuries. When a disaster affects a veterinary hospital and requires triage decisions, it must be remembered that an injury or illness to this hospitalized animal will confound the seriousness of the previous illness/injury. These multiple injuries should be considered synergistic and the prognosis is worse for an individual patient than the simple sum of the likelihood of survival for each injury. With pre-existing illness, multiple injuries, and advancing age, there is a worsening prognosis and these factors should thereby be taken into consideration when making triage decisions.

Newly Acquired Illnesses During Triage. Just because there is a disaster does not mean illness takes a few days off. There will be animals requiring renewal of prescriptions, having an exacerbation of an ongoing chronic illness (*e.g.*, acute on chronic renal failure), and even development of new illnesses (*e.g.*, diarrhea, salmonellosis). These animals will require treatment and should be seen by their regular veterinarian, if possible, or a veterinary colleague temporarily. For sure, these animals should not be included in the triage techniques.

Special Triage Resources. Occasionally an animal owner is recruited to assist with treatment of disaster victims. The poultry or swine producer, the owner/manager of a dog kennel or cattery, the animal attendants from the zoo, all know their species and are used to handling these animals. Moving these people to a treatment area and seeking their assistance can enhance outcomes. Undoubtedly, the addition of skilled hands to a disaster treatment team not only improves outcome but also increases effectiveness. Again, the guiding principle in disaster triage is to maximize the benefit to the most animals.

SYSTEMS TRIAGE IN DISASTERS

To quickly and efficiently triage and initiate lifesaving treatment on emergency patients, it is imperative to develop a "team approach." All veterinary clinical personnel should have a working knowledge of basic lifesaving procedures and equipment. Staff meetings should use a portion of their time for review and

Table 89-5. Essential Equipment in Triage

Oxygen
Crash cart with electrical defibrillator
IV catheter setup
IV fluids and Oxyglobin
Administration set and pressure infuser bag
Bandage materials
Electrocardiograph
Heat source for the patient
Thoracocentesis setup

updates on trauma priorities, basic cardiopulmonary resuscitation, emergency procedures, and individual duties and responsibilities. "Dry-runs" or practice drills can improve the team's speed and efficiency.[14-16]

If it is known that a disaster victim(s) is en route to the hospital, it is important to prepare for the patient's arrival by having certain equipment readily available and on a standby (Table 89-5). It is always best to be prepared for the worst possible scenario.

Initial Evaluation

On arrival of the disaster patient(s), an initial evaluation is done. Staff must stay calm, work quickly, and minimize patient stress, especially with cats.

A systematic, standardized approach to *every* emergency is essential (Table 89-6). Such an approach minimizes oversight during assessment of organ systems and anatomic areas. By having a standardized emergency response protocol, life-threatening problems can be identified, and immediate therapy initiated.

Adequate assessment and appraisal of the disaster patient consists of several components. Although these components are often discussed separately, in actual practice there is often no chronological separation of the entire appraisal and management scheme (Table 89-7). Several goals are accomplished simultaneously because diagnosis, treatment, and monitoring coincide. Some of the key issues in the triage of disaster patients are listed in Table 89-8.

Table 89-6. Systems Triage in Disasters[16]

1. Arterial bleeding
2. Respiratory system
3. Cardiovascular system
4. Transfusion and hemorrhage control
5. Neurologic system
6. Musculoskeletal system
7. Abdominal injuries

Table 89-7. The ABCDEs of the Primary Survey

• Airway	• Is the patient having difficulty breathing? Are there mandibular injuries that are interfering with the airway? Has a bite wound disrupted the larynx or trachea? Is subcutaneous emphysema present?
• Breathing	• Is the patient in respiratory distress? What is the color of the mucous membranes? Does the respiratory distress get worse with positional changes of the animal? Is there evidence of thoracic penetration or is there a flail chest? Are the peripheral veins distended?
• Circulation	• Is there evidence of hemorrhage? If there is an extremity fracture, how much swelling is present? Are the mucous membranes pale and tacky? Are the femoral pulses weak and rapid? Are the extremities cold? Is the pulse pressure weak?
• Disability	• Is there evidence of neurologic injury? What is the posture of the animal? Is the animal bright, alert, and responsive? Does the animal respond to painful stimuli? Are the pupils dilated, constricted, of equal size, and responsive to light? Is there an extremity fracture that might threaten a peripheral nerve?
• Examination	• Are there lacerations? Is there bruising and is this bruising getting worse? Are there multiple fractures? Is the abdomen painful? Is there evidence of debilitation or concurrent disease?

Table 89-8. Key Issues in the Management of Disaster Victims[16]

- Disasters frequently result in animals with trauma affecting multiple organ systems.
- An organized, systematic approach should be undertaken for *each patient.* This approach begins with an assessment of the respiratory, cardiovascular, and neurologic system and concludes with musculoskeletal management and the diagnosis of abdominal injuries.
- An aggressive diagnostic and therapeutic approach is taken toward each of the involved systems.
- Overtreatment of some complications can be just as hazardous as undertreatment. This is especially true of respiratory trauma and/or intra-abdominal hemorrhage.
- Constant monitoring and reassessment of the patient's status is mandatory.
- Each patient deserves frequent "hands on" special attention and lots of "tender loving care."

SUMMARY

Preparation and training will lead to confidence and improved emergency treatment of animals involved in any potentially chaotic event. Prior planning is mandatory and use of mock drills useful in preparing local veterinary hospitals to deal with preparedness, response, and triage.

REFERENCES

1. Stamp GL: Hurricane Andrew: the importance of coordinated response. *J Am Vet Med Assoc* 203:989, 1993.
2. Medical Management of Chemical Casualties Handbook, 2nd ed. Aberdeen Proving Ground, MD: U.S. Army Medical Research Institute of Chemical Defense, 1995.
3. Celantano J: Chemical agent overview. National Disaster Medical System Conference, 1998.
4. Celantano J: Biological agent overview. National Disaster Medical System Conference, 1998.
5. Anderson JH: Preparation for the consequences of terrorism. Proceedings of the Sixth International Veterinary Emergency and Critical Care Symposium, 1998.
6. Fong F, Schrader C: Radiation disasters and emergency department preparedness. *Emerg Med Clin North Am* 14:349, 1996.
7. Fong F: Radiation injuries. National Disaster Medical Systems Conference, 1998.
8. Huxsoll DL: The veterinarian's role in countering the consequences of bioterrorism. Proceedings of the Sixth International Veterinary Emergency and Critical Care Symposium, 1998.
9. Martin DG, Elsayed NM, Januszkiewicz AJ: Medical effects of blast overpressure. Sixth International Veterinary Emergency and Critical Care Symposium, 1998.
10. Heath SE, Dorn R, Linsbury LD, *et al.*: An overview of disaster preparedness for veterinarians. *J Am Vet Med Assoc* 210:345, 1997.
11. Heath SE, Kass P, Hart L, *et al.*: Epidemiologic study of cats and dogs affected by the 1991 Oakland fire. *J Am Vet Med Assoc* 212:504, 1998.
12. Schultz CH, DiLorenzo RA, Koenig KL, *et al.*: Disaster medical direction: a medical earthquake response curriculum [abstract]. *Ann Emerg Med* 20:470, 1991.
13. Kennedy K, Aghababian RV, Gans L, *et al.*: Triage: techniques and applications in decision-making. *Ann Emerg Med* 28:136, 1996.
14. Rodkey WG: Initial assessment, resuscitation and management of the critically traumatized small animal patient. *Vet Clin North Am Small Anim Pract* 10:561, 1980.
15. Faggella AM: First aid, transport, and triage. *Vet Clin North Am Small Anim Pract* 24:997, 1994.
16. Kovacic JP: Management of life-threatening trauma. *Vet Clin North Am Small Anim Pract* 24:1057, 1994.
17. Wingfield WE, Henik RA: Treatment priorities in multiple trauma. *Semin Vet Med Surg Small Anim* 3:193, 1988.

SECTION XIII
Appendices

Appendix 1
Units and Conversions

Temperature Conversion

°F	°C
212	100
111.2	44
109.4	43
107.6	42
105.8	41
104	40
102.2	39
100.4	38
98.6	37
96.8	36
95	35
93.2	34
91.4	33
89.6	32
87.8	31
86	30
32	0
°F = (9/5 °C) + 32	°C = 5/9 (°F − 32)

Tubing Sizes

French Size	Outside Diameter (mm)	Outside Diameter (inches)	Type of Device
1	0.3	0.01	Vascular Catheters Urinary Catheters
4	1.3	0.05	
8	2.6	0.10	
10	3.3	0.13	Urinary Catheters Feeding Tubes Endotracheal Tubes
12	4.0	0.16	
14	4.6	0.18	
16	5.3	0.21	
18	6.0	0.23	
20	6.6	0.26	Chest Drains Endotracheal Tubes
22	7.3	0.28	
24	8.0	0.31	
26	8.6	0.34	
28	9.3	0.36	
30	10.1	0.39	
32	10.6	0.41	
34	11.3	0.44	
36	12.0	0.47	
38	12.6	0.50	
40	13.2	0.53	
	1 F = ~3 mm		

Intravascular Catheter Sizes

Gauge	Outside Diameter (mm)	Outside Diameter (in)	Type of Catheter
26	0.45	0.018	Butterfly Needles
25	0.50	0.020	
24	0.56	0.022	
23	0.61	0.024	
22	0.71	0.028	Peripheral IV catheters
21	0.81	0.032	
20	0.91	0.036	
19	1.02	0.04	
18	1.22	0.048	Central IV catheters
16	1.62	0.064	
14	2.03	0.08	
12	2.64	0.104	Introducer Sheaths
10	3.25	0.128	

SI Units for Selected Clinical Laboratory Tests

Analyte	SI Units	Reference Range		Conversion Factor from Traditional to SI Units
		Dog	Cat	
Liver				
Alanine Aminotransferase	U/L	0–130	75–110	1.00
Albumin	g/L	22–35	25–39	10.0
Alkaline Phosphatase	U/L	0–200	0–90	1.00
Ammonia (resting)	μmol/L	20–80		0.5871
Aspartate Aminotrans-ferase	U/L	10–50	10–59	1.00
Total bilirubin	μmol/L	0–7	0–4	1.00
Conjugated bilirubin	μmol/L	0–3	0–1	—
Free bilirubin	μmol/L	0–7	0–4	—
Cholesterol	mmol/L	2.75–9.50	1.50–6.00	0.025
γ-GT	U/L	0–6	0–2	—
Glucose	mmol/L	3.3–8.7	3.5–9.0	0.55
Kidney-Electrolytes				
Urea Nitrogen	mmol/L	2.1–9.7	5–10	0.36
Creatinine	μmol/L	43–151	67–193	88.4
Calcium				
Total	mmol/L	2.24–2.95	2.23–2.90	0.25
Ionized	mmol/L	1.12–1.48	1.12–1.45	0.25
Chloride	mmol/L	105–122	112–129	1.00
Magnesium	mmol/L	0.8–1.2	0.8–1.2	0.41
Phosphorous	mmol/L	0.5–2.6	1.6–2.75	0.332
Potassium	mmol/L	3.6–5.8	3.7–5.8	1.0
Total carbon dioxide	mmol/L	18–30	14–26	1.00
Anion gap	mmol/L	15–25	15–25	—
Lactate	mmol/L	<2.0	<2.0	1.00
Pancreas				
Amylase	U/L	400–1800	700–2000	1.00
Lipase	U/L	50–1000	50–700	1.00
Muscle				
Creatine Kinase	U/L	0–460	0–580	—
Endocrine				
Thyroxine (T_4)	nmol/L	15–55	15–65	12.87
Cortisol	nmol/L	<30–300	<30–390	27.59
Coagulation				
Fibrinogen	g/L	1.5–3.5	1.5–3.5	0.01
Fibrin split products	mg/L	<10	<10	1

Table adapted from: Matthews KA: Veterinary Emergency and Critical Care Manual and Marino PL: The ICU Book

Appendix 2
Continuous Rate Infusions

A continuous rate infusion (CRI) is a precisely calculated amount of druug added to a specific volume and type of fluid. The mixture is then delivered as a continuous intravenous infusion. The efficacy of CRI drugs is increased through maintenance of steady-state concentrations of the drug.

Drugs Administered Via Continuous Rate Infusions

Drug	Formulation	CRI Dosage	Actions
Diazepam	5 mg/ml	0.1–0.04 mg/kg/hour	Anticonvulsant, ataractic
Diltiazem	5 mg/ml	0.2–0.5 mg/kg/hour	Calcium channel blocker
Dobutamine	12.5 mg/ml	2–20 μg/kg/minute	Synthetic catecholamine, positive inotrope
Dopamine	40 mg/ml	2–20 μg/kg/minute	Dopaminergic, B-agonist, norepinephrine precursor
Epinephrine	1:1000	1 μg/kg/minute	Alpha and beta agonist
Fentanyl	0.05 mg/ml	1–5 μg/kg/hour	Narcotic analgesic
Insulin (regular)	100 U/ml	1.1–2.2 U/kg/day	Hormone
Isoproterenol	0.2 mg/ml	0.04 μg/kg/hour	Beta-adrenergic agonist
Ketamine	100 mg/ml	1–3 μg/kg/minute	Neuroleptoanalgesia
Lidocaine	20 mg/ml (2%)	50–100 μg/kg/minute	Ventricular antiarrhythmic
Metoclopramide	5 mg/ml	1–2 mg/kg/day	Gastrointestinal stimulant, antiemetic
Nitroprusside	200 μg/ml	1–5 μg/kg/minute	Venous and arterial vasodilator
Procainamide	100 or 500 mg/ml	20–50 μg/kg/minute	Antiarrhythmic
Propofol	10 mg/ml	0.05–0.2 mg/kg/minute	Short-acting hypnotic

CALCULATIONS OF CONTINUOUS RATE INFUSIONS

The objective of CRI dosages is to determine how much drug must be added to a specific volume of intravenous fluid to achieve the required dosage. If the dosage is in μg/kg/minute, then the following equation will apply:

$$\mu g \times kg \times minute = \mu g \text{ required drug}$$

Since μg are given in the dosage orders, and kgs are given for the specific patient, only the number of minutes that a given volume of intravenous fluids will last must be calculated. Simply calculate the number of hours an infusion will last by dividing the volume in the bag by the fluid administration rate per hour. Then, multiply the number of hours by 60 minutes/hour to determine the number of minutes. Next, solve the following equation:

$$\mu g \times kg \times minutes = \mu g \text{ of required drug}$$

Then, divide the number of μg needed by 1000 to convert μgs to mgs.

Example: Give lidocaine CRI at 60 μg/kg/minute to a 15 kg dog. Add the lidocaine to 1000 ml of Normosol-R which is running at a rate of 41 mls/hour. How much lidocaine do you add to the 1000 mls of Normosol-R?

1. Calculate the number of minutes the 1000 mls of Normosol-R will last:
   - 1000 mls/41 mls/hour = 24 hours
   - 24 hours × 60 minutes/hour = 1440 minutes
2. Solve the equation:
   - 60 μg × 15 kg × 1440 minutes = 1,296,000 μg
3. Convert μg to mgs:
   - 1296000/1000 = 1296 mgs
4. Calculate the amount of drug needed per 1000 ml bag by dividing the amount of drug needed by the concentration of drug that you are using (2% lidocaine):
   - 1296 mgs/20 mg/ml = 64.8 mls of lidocaine
5. In order to be precise in your dosage, 64.8 mls of Normosol-R should be discarded and then the 64.8 mls of lidocaine added to the bag.

Sample Problems

1. "Goldie," a 30 kg golden retriever, is in oliguric renal failure. The doctor has ordered a dopamine CRI at 5 μg/kg/minute and a fluid rate of 121 mls per hour. How much dopamine will you add to 1000 ml of 0.9% Sodium Chloride solution?
2. "Maggie," a 25 kg Labrador retriever, was hit by a tractor (HBT). The electrocardiographic monitor is showing a continuous run of multiform ventricular tachycardia. The doctor orders a lidocaine CRI to be given at a rate of 80 μg/kg/minute. The fluid rate is set at 34 mls/hour. How much lidocaine will you add to 1000 mls of Normosol-R?
3. "Gretchen," a 7 kg miniature schnauzer, has pancreatitis and has been vom-

iting frequently. The doctor orders a metoclopramide CRI at 2 mg/kg/day. The fluid volume is set at 23 mls/hour. How much metoclopramide will you add to 1000 mls of Normosol-R?

4. "Sage," a 42 kg yellow Labrador retriever, is in recovery following an abdominal exploratory. The doctor orders a fentanyl CRI at 4 µg/kg/hour. The fluid volume is set at 55 mls/hour. How much fentanyl will you add to 1000 mls of 0.9% Sodium Chloride?

Answers

1. 1.86 mls of 40 mg/ml dopamine.
2. 1.76.5 mls of 20 mg/ml (2%) lidocaine.
3. 5.1 mls of 5 mg/ml metoclopramide.
4. 61 mls of 0.05 mg/ml fentanyl.

Appendix 3
Selected Reference Ranges

Hemodynamic Parameters

Parameter	Equation	Normal Range
Systemic Blood Pressure		
Systolic [SBP]	Direct measurement	90–140 mm Hg
Diastolic [DBP]	Direct measurement	60–90 mm Hg
Mean [MBP]	[SBP + (2 × DBP)]/3	70–105 mm Hg
Right Heart Pressure		
Central venous pressure [CVP]	Direct measurement	0–5 cm water
Right Atrial Pressure [RAP]	Direct measurement	2–6 mm Hg
Right Ventricular Pressure [RVP]	Direct measurement	15–25 mm Hg systolic 5–15 mm Hg diastolic
Pulmonary Artery Pressure		
Systolic [SPAP]	Direct measurement	15–30 mm Hg
Diastolic [DPAP]	Direct measurement	8–15 mm Hg
Mean [MPAP]	[SPAP + (2 × DPAP)]/3	10–20 mm Hg
Wedge [PAWP]	Direct measurement	4–9 mm Hg
Left Atrial Pressure [LAP]	Direct measurement	3–10 mm Hg
Cardiac Indices		
Cardiac Output [CO]	HR × SV/1000	100 mL/kg/min
Cardiac Index [CI]	CO/Body surface area	50–150 mL/kg/min/m^2
Stroke Volume [SV]	CO/HR × 1000	1–2 ml/kg/min
Stroke Volume Index [SVI]	SV/Body surface area	3–30 mL/kg/min/m^2
Systemic Vascular Resistance [SVR]	80 × (MAP-RAP)/CO	800–1700 dynes sec/cm^5
Pulmonary Vascular Resistance [PVR]	80 × (MPAP-PAWP)/CO	<250 dynes sec/cm^5
Left Ventricular Stroke Work [LVSW]	SV × (MAP-PAWP) × 0.0136	58–104 gm m/beat
Right Ventricular Stroke Work [RVSW]	SV × (MPAP-RAP) × 0.0136	5–10 gm m/beat
1.34 cm water = 1 mm Hg		

Oxygen Parameters

Parameter	Equation	Normal Range
Arterial		
Oxygen partial pressure [PaO_2]	Direct measurement	80–95 mm Hg
Carbon dioxide partial pressure [$PaCO_2$]	Direct measurement	33–38 mm Hg
Oxygen saturation [SaO_2]	Direct measurement	95–99%
Oxygen content [CaO_2]	$(0.0138 \times Hb \times SaO_2) + 0.031 \times PaO_2$	17–20 ml/dl
Venous		
Oxygen partial pressure [PvO_2]	Direct measurement	35–50 mm Hg
Carbon dioxide partial pressure [$PvCO_2$]	Direct measurement	35–43 mm Hg
Oxygen saturation [SvO_2]	Direct measurement	865–875%
Oxygen content [CvO_2]	$(0.0138 \times Hb \times SvO_2) + 0.031 \times PvO_2$	12–15 ml/dl
Oxygen Delivery Indices		
A-V Oxygen Content [Cao_2]	$Cao_2 - Cvo_2$	4–6 ml/dl
Oxygen Delivery [DO_2]	$Cao_2 \times CO \times 10$	950–1150 ml/dl
Oxygen Consumption [VO_2]	$C(a\text{-}v)o_2 \times CO \times 10$	200–250 ml/min
Oxygen Extraction Ratio [OER]	$[C(a\text{-}v)O_2/CaO_2] \times 100$	20–30%

Pulmonary Ventilation

Parameter	Equation	Units	Reference Range	
			Dog	Cat
Tidal volume [V_T]	7–10 ml/kg × BW (kg)	ml	—	—
Minute volume [V_E]	$V_T \times$ respiratory rate	ml/min	—	—
Dead space ventilation [V_D]	$V_E([PaCO_2 - P_ECO_2\})/PaCO_2$	ml/kg	—	—
Alveolar partial pressure of oxygen [P_AO_2]	$[P_{barometric} - P_{water}] \times FiO_2 - (PaCO_2) \times 0.8$	mm Hg	>100	>100
Arterial P/F ratio	PaO_2/FiO_2	—	>400	>400
Alveolar-arterial oxygen gradient [$A\text{-}aDO_2$]	$P_AO_2 - P_aO_2$	mm Hg	<10	<10
Intrapulmonary shunt fraction [Q_S/Q_T]	$Q_S/Q_T = \frac{(P_AO_2 - P_aO_2\}) \times 0.0031}{(P_AO_2 - P_aO_2\}) \times 0.0031 + (CaO_2 - CvO_2)}$	%	<5%	<5%

Acid-Base, Electrolyte, Renal Parameters

Parameter	Formula	Reference Range	
		Dog	Cat
Acid-Base			
Metabolic acidosis	$\Delta PaCO_2 \sim 1.2\ \Delta[HCO_3]$	—	—
Metabolic alkalosis	$\Delta PaCO_2 \sim 0.7\ \Delta[HCO_3]$	—	—
Respiratory acidosis			
Acute	$\Delta[HCO_3] \sim 0.1\ \Delta PaCO_2$	—	—
Chronic	$\Delta[HCO_3] \sim 0.3\ \Delta PaCO_2$	—	—
Respiratory alkalosis			
Acute	$\Delta[HCO_3] \sim 0.2\ \Delta PaCO_2$	—	—
Chronic	$\Delta[HCO_3] \sim 0.5\ \Delta PaCO_2$	—	—
Anion Gap	$[Na + K] - [HCO_3 + Cl]$	15–25	15–25
Bicarbonate deficit	0.6 × body wt (kg) × [22-measured bicarbonate]	0 ± 2	0 ± 2
Electrolyte			
Corrected sodium [hyper-glycemia]	$Na_{euglycemic} = [Na_{measured}] - 0.028\ (glucose - 100)$	Reference range	Reference range
Corrected sodium [hyper-lipidemia]	Decrease serum Na = plasma lipids [mg/dl] × 0.002	Reference range	Reference range
Corrected sodium [hyper-proteinemia]	Decrease serum Na = [Measured total protein] − 8 gm/dl × 0.25	Reference range	Reference range
Corrected chloride	$Cl\ corr = Cl \times \frac{Na\ (normal)}{Na\ (measured)}$	Reference range	Reference range
Corrected calcium	$Ca_{Corr} = Ca(mg/dl) - albumin\ (g/dl) + 3.5$	Reference range	Reference range
Renal			
Creatinine clearance	$Clearance_{creatinine} = \frac{[Creatinine_{urine}] \times Flow}{[Creatinine_{plasma}]}$	—	—
Fractional excretion of sodium [F_ENa]	$\frac{(Urine\ [Na] \times serum\ [Cr])}{(Serum\ [Na] \times urine\ [Cr])}$	<1	<1
Osmolality [mOsm]	2 × [Na] + glucose/18 + BUN/2.8	270–310	280–320
Water deficit [L]	0.6 [wt in kg] × [Na-140]/140	0	0
Colloid osmotic pressure [COP]	1.4 [globulin] + 5.5 [albumin]	24 ± 3	24 ± 3

Approximate Electrolyte Content [mEQ/L] of Gastrointestinal Fluids in the Dog

	Na	K	Cl	HCO_3	pH
Saliva	40–60	13–32	40–50	23	7.2–7.8
Stomach	40–80	10–20	100–140	0	1.4–7.0
Bile	171	5.1	66	61	6.6–7.4
Pancreas	149–162	4–5	71–106	135–148	7.1–8.2
Duodenum	138–156	5–9	103–139	5–20	6.5–7.6
Jejunum	126–152	4–10	141–155	5–27	6.3–7.3
Ileum	146–156	5–7	68–88	70–114	7.6–8.0
Colon	136–151	6–9	60–88	86–93	7.9–8.0

Source: DiBartola S: Fluid Therapy in Small Animal Practice, 1992, 2001

Index

Note that entries with *t* after them indicate tables; *f* indicates figures.